MW01268198

Tendon, Nerve and Other Disorders

Surgery of Disorders of the Hand and Upper Extremity Series

Tendon, Nerve and Other Disorders

Edited by

Raoul Tubiana MD FRCS(Ed)Hon
Associate Professor of Orthopedic Surgery
Institut de la Main
Paris, France

Alain Gilbert MD
Associate Professor of Orthopedic Surgery
Institut de la Main
Paris, France

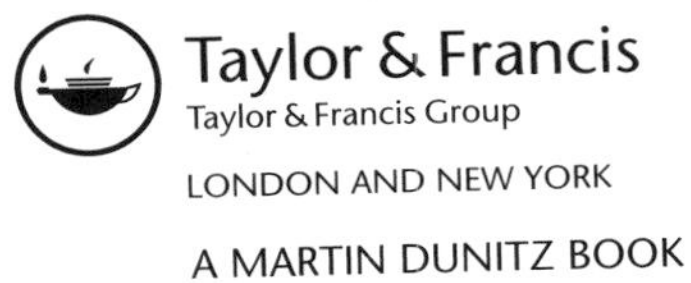

Taylor & Francis
Taylor & Francis Group
LONDON AND NEW YORK
A MARTIN DUNITZ BOOK

First published in the United Kingdom in 2005
by Taylor & Francis, an imprint of the Taylor & Francis Group,
2 Park Square, Milton Park, Abingdon, Oxfordshire, OX14 4RN

Tel.: +44 (0) 20 7017 6000
Fax.: +44 (0) 20 7017 6699
E-mail: info@dunitz.co.uk
Website: http://www.dunitz.co.uk

A CIP record for this book is available from the British Library.

Library of Congress Cataloging-in-Publication Data

Data available on application

ISBN 1-85317-494-7

Distributed in North and South America by

Taylor & Francis
2000 NW Corporate Blvd
Boca Raton, FL 33431, USA

Within Continental USA
Tel.: 800 272 7737; Fax.: 800 374 3401
Outside Continental USA
Tel.: 561 994 0555; Fax.: 561 361 6018
E-mail: orders@crcpress.com

Distributed in the rest of the world by
Thomson Publishing Services
Cheriton House
North Way
Andover, Hampshire SP10 5BE, UK
Tel.: +44 (0)1264 332424
E-mail: salesorder.tandf@thomsonpublishingservices.co.uk

Composition by Scribe Design, Ashford, Kent, UK

Printed and bound in Spain by Grafos SA.

Contents

Contributors

Christian Allende
Institut de la Main
Clinique Jouvenet
6 Square Jouvenet
75016 Paris
France

Yves Allieu
Department of Orthopaedic
Surgery II & Hand Surgery
Lapeyronie Hospital,
avenue du doyen Gaston Giraud
34295 Montpellier
France

Jean-Yves Alnot
Hand Surgery Service
Department of Hand Surgery
Hospital Bichat AP-HP
46, rue Henri-Huchard
75877 Paris
France

Peter C Amadio
Department of Orthopedics
Mayo Clinic E-14A
200 First Street SW
Rochester MN 55905
United States of America

Dimitri J Anastakis
Head of Surgical Programs, TWH
Associate Director Surgical
Services, UHN
399 Bathurst Street, FP4-142
Toronto, ON M5T 2S8
Canada

Rolfe Birch
Professor in Neurological
Orthopaedic Surgery
Royal National Orthopaedic
Hospital
Peripheral Nerve Injury Unit
Brockley Hill
Stanmore
Middlesex HA7 4LP
UK

Chantal Bonnard
Specialist in Plastic Surgery
FMH Clinique Longeraie
avenue de la Gare 9
1003 Lausanne
Switzerland

Jacques Borrelly
Department of Thoracic Surgery
Médipôle Saint Jacques
54320 Nancy-Maxeville
France

Giorgio A Brunelli
Professor of Orthopaedics
Brescia University Medical School
Via Campiani 77
25060 Cellatica (BS)
Italy

Dieter Buck-Gramcko
Am Heesen 14A
21033 Hamburg
Germany

Frank D Burke
Consultant Hand Surgeon
Pulvertaft Department of Hand
Surgery
Derbyshire Royal Infirmary
London Road
Derby DE1 2QY
UK

Michel Chammas
Department of Orthopaedic
Surgery II & Hand Surgery
Lapeyronie Hospital,
avenue du doyen Gaston Giraud
34295 Montpellier
France

Jean-Jacques Comtet
Professeur Emérite des Universités
Ancien Chirurgien des Hôpitaux
201 rue des Ecoles
01600 Miserieux
France

Lars B Dahlin
Department of Hand Surgery
Malmö University Hospital
SE-205 05 Malmö
Sweden

Zoe H Dailiana
Department of Orthopaedic
Surgery
University of Thessaly
22 Papakiriazi Street
41222 Larissa
Greece

Michael Davidsen
Arhus University Hospital
Arhus Kommunehospital
Department of Orthopaedics
Nørrebrogade 44
8000 Arhus C
Denmark

M Del Bene
Plastic and Hand Surgery
Department
Ospedale di Legnano
Via Candiani 2
20025 Legnano
Italy

Christian Dumontier
Institut de la Main, Paris
and Hôpital Saint Antoine
Orthopedic Department
184 rue du Faubourg St Antoine
75012 Paris
France

Alain Gilbert
Institut de la Main
Clinique Jouvenet
6 square Jouvenet
75016 Paris
France

Caroline Leclercq
Ancien Chef de Clinique-Assistant
des Hôpitaux de Paris
Institut de la Main
Clinique Jouvenet
6 Square Jouvenet
75016 Paris
France

Dominique Le Viet
Institut de la Main
Clinique Jouvenet
6 Square Jouvenet
75016 Paris
France

Göran Lundborg
Department of Hand Surgery
Malmö University Hospital
SE-205 05 Malmö
Sweden

Jean-Louis Mallet
Department of Orthopaedic
Surgery II & Hand Surgery
Lapeyronie Hospital,
avenue du doyen Gaston Giraud
34295 Montpellier
France

Michel Merle
Head of European Institute for
Hand Surgery
13, rue Blaise Pascal
54320 Nancy-Maxeville
France

Hanno Millesi
Professor Emeritus of Plastic
Surgery
University of Vienna Medical
School
Pelikanasse 15
A-1090 Vienna
Austria

François Moutet
Director of the Hand Unit
Hôpital A. Michalon
CHU de Grenoble BP 217 X
38043 Grenoble
France

Toshihiko Ogino
Department of Orthopaedic
Surgery
Yamagata University School of
Medicine
Iida-Nishi 2-2-2
Yamagata 990-9585
Japan

Luciano A Poitevin
Professor of Orthopaedics and
Anatomy
Buenos Aires University Hospital
and Buenos Aires Medical School
J.A. Pacheco de Melo 1999
Buenos Aires 1126
Argentina

Guy Raimbeau
Centre de la Main
2 rue Auguste Gautier
49100 Angers
France

Pier Luigi Raimondi
Plastic and Hand Surgeon
Casa di Cura Santa Maria
Viale Piemonte 70
21053 Castellanza (VA)
Italy

Michel Romain
Department of Functional
Rehabilitation B
Centre Hélio-Marin
30240 Le Grau du Roi
France

Jean-Claude Rouzaud
Department of Orthopaedic
Surgery II & Hand Surgery
Lapeyronie Hospital,
avenue du doyen Gaston Giraud
34295 Montpellier
France

Terri M Skirven
Director of Hand Therapy
The Philadelphia Hand Center
700 S. Henderson Road, #200
King of Prussia
Philadelphia, PA 19406
United States of America

Robert J Spinner
Assistant Professor of Neurologic Surgery and Orthopedics
Department of Neurologic Surgery
Mayo Clinic
200 First Street SW
Rochester MN 55905
United States of America

Raoul Tubiana
Associate Professor of Orthopedic Surgery
Institut de la Main
Clinique Jouvenet
6 Square Jouvenet
75016 Paris
France

Philippe Valenti
Institut de la Main
Clinique Jouvenet
6 Square Jouvenet
75016 Paris
France

William Williams
Consultant Orthopaedic Surgeon
Broomfield Hospital
Court Road
Chelmsford CM1 7ET
UK

Stuart W. Wilson
Department of Plastic & Reconstructive Surgery
South Manchester University Hospitals
Southmoor
Manchester M22 1PR
UK

Eduardo A Zancolli
Avenida Alvear 1535
Buenos Aires 1014
Argentina

Preface

Steadfast progress in our scientific knowledge and increased experience of hand surgeons have resulted in significant advances in hand surgery. We have already described this progress in most aspects of bone and skin disorders in the first volume in the series. This second volume focuses on three major topics: nerve, tendon and rheumatoid arthritis surgery.

Tendon and nerve injuries are frequent in the upper extremity, a limb whose main attribute is its mobility, and they are an important cause of functional incapacity. Understanding of their physiopathology has considerably increased in recent decades, and the routine use of microsurgical techniques has gradually transformed their treatment. Primary repair for both tendons and nerves has proved to be the best solution when local and general conditions are favourable. However, primary flexor tendon grafts are no longer performed, while autologous nerve grafts, introduced by Millesi, are the basis for reconstruction of segmental nerve defect.

Division of a tendon or of a nerve trunk leads to a local process at the site of injury with a distal loss of function, but the consequential effects are different for the nerve and for the tendon. Whereas a tendon division causes only a muscle contracture proximally, a nerve division involves both degeneration of the axon distally to the injury and structural and biochemical changes proximally in the nerve cell body. It can also lead to severe functional consequences in terms of reorganization at the cortical, subcortical and spinal levels, as described by Dahlin and Lundberg.

This volume includes not only repair of the peripheral nerves and of brachial plexus (brachial plexus lesions are mostly managed by hand surgeons), but also paralytic disorders of the upper limb.

Palliative surgery for peripheral nerves is quite standardized when there are possible motors for transfer. For associated peripheral or more proximal paralyses, the situation is more difficult, the motors are limited, sometimes only partially re-innervated and, as in obstetrical cases, with the problems of co-contractions.

Surgery is only one of the elements in the treatment of tendinous or nervous lesions: physiotherapy, for example, also plays a fundamental role. The more extensive the paralysis, the greater the role of associated non-surgical treatment.

Multidisciplinary work and working as part of a team are essential in order to keep abreast with increasingly sophisticated therapeutic techniques. This is also necessary for the management of some pathologic disorders of the upper extremity included in this book, and particularly for rheumatoid arthritis (RA).

Surgical treatment of RA has evolved with better understanding of the natural history of deformities, surgical experience of both early and late stages of the disorder, earlier diagnosis and progress in medical treatment. Development of new medical strategies aiming at a tight control of the inflammatory process and, if needed, biological agents such as anti-tumour necrosis factor (TNFα), are leading to a revision of surgical indications.

We would like to express our gratitude to all the authors who have contributed to this volume, and also to thank our publishers, Martin Dunitz, and editors Robert Peden and Giovanna Ceroni for their patient help.

Raoul Tubiana
Alain Gilbert

I Tendons

1 Acute traumatic injuries of the digital extensor mechanism

Yves Allieu, Michel Chammas, Jean-Louis Mallet, Michel Romain and Jean-Claude Rouzaud

Introduction

Extensor tendon lesions are wrongly considered as minor injuries, particularly on the dorsal part of the finger. Because of their subcutaneous position extensor tendons are particularly vulnerable in injuries of the dorsum of the hand. Failure to recognize these injuries, following a hasty clinical examination or an inappropriate treatment can lead to serious functional sequelae – compromising the function of the entire hand and necessitating difficult revisional surgery, long rehabilitation sessions and giving rise to important social and professional consequential effects.

Topographic zones

The anatomical and functional characteristics of the extensor mechanism vary in function with the topography at the level of the forearm, the wrist or the hand. In order to comply with the specificity of the lesions according to the level of injury of the extensor mechanism, an international classification (Kleinert and Verdan 1983) in eight zones is used (Figure 1.1). A ninth zone can be added to these eight zones, corresponding to the intramuscular part of the extrinsic tendons (Wehbé 1995, Doyle 1999), and a tenth zone representing the very proximal portion of the extensors (Wehbé 1995).

Vascularization and tendinous nutrition

The intratendinous vascularization adjacent to that of the flexor tendons at the level of zones VI, VII and VIII originates from an extratendinous source. The tendon nutrition is brought by the vessels at the level of zones VI, VII and VIII. In zone VII synovial diffusion is the major nutrient pathway, as for flexor tendons. At the digital level, vascularization of the extensor mechanism is supplied by the dorsal branches of the collateral arteries (Tubiana 1997). A fine vascular supply exists on the superficial and deep sides of the extensor mechanism.

Healing of the extensor mechanism

Healing of the extensor mechanism has not evoked as much interest as that of flexor tendons. At the digital

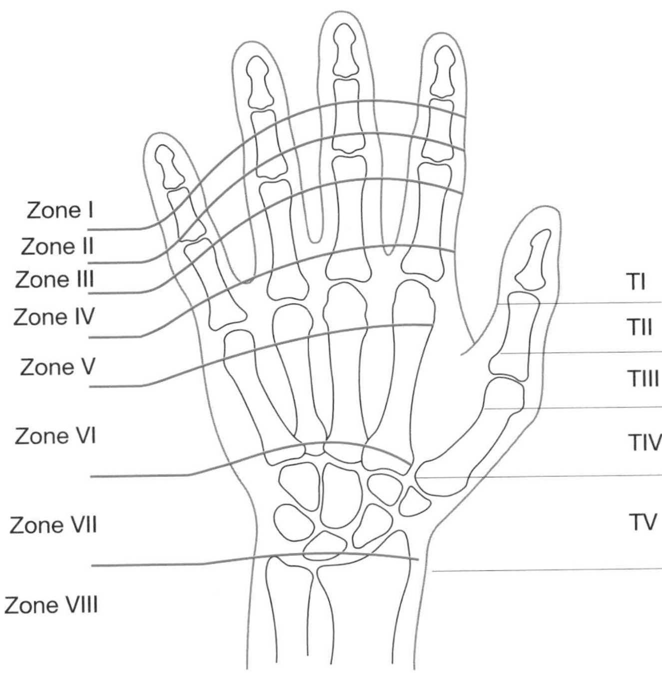

Figure 1.1

International classification of zones of extensor tendon injuries (according to Doyle 1999).

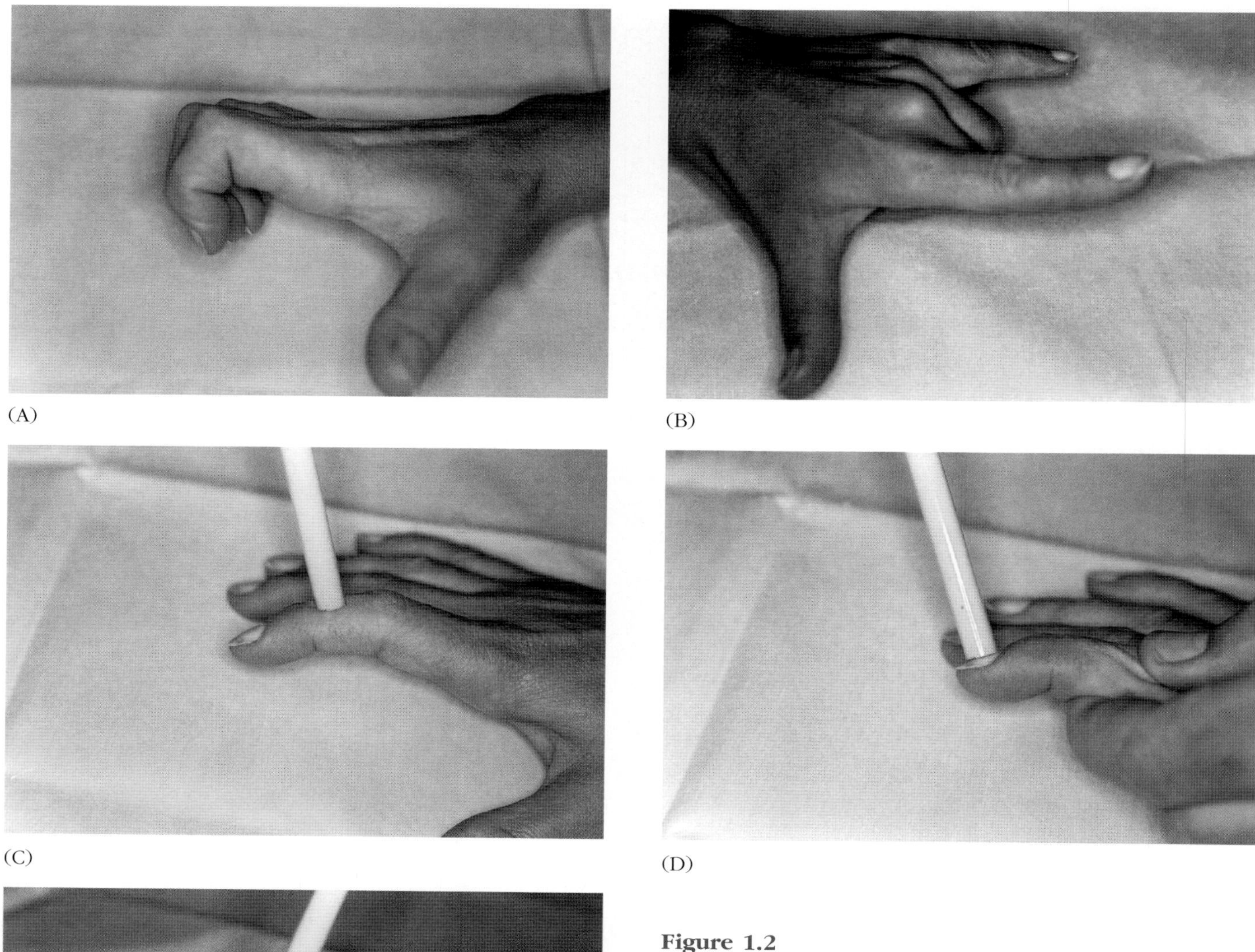

(A) (B) (C) (D) (E)

Figure 1.2

Examination of the extensor mechanism. (A) extensor digitorum communis, extensor indicis proprius and extensor digiti minimi; (B) extensor indicis proprius and extensor digiti minimi; (C) median band; (D) terminal band; (E) extensor palmaris longus.

level, and particularly in zone IV, the laminous tendinous aspect of the extensors, the absence of a sheath isolating the tendon from the cutaneous cover and from the bone and the fact that the major part of the tendon mechanism is extrasynovial can only favour the appearance of cutaneous and periosteal adhesions. This means that extrinsic healing by the paratendon has a clear advantage over intrinsic healing.

Clinical evaluation

Diagnosis of injuries of the extensor mechanism of the fingers can be wrongly interpreted if only a clinical examination is carried out. All wounds facing a tendinous pathway of the hand necessitate a surgical exploration at least under local anaesthesia. Beware of a hasty clinical examination carried out in an emergency situation.

This discussion of clinical evaluation will refer to the classification by zones established by the International Federation of Societies for Surgery of the Hand (Kleinert and Verdan 1983) (Figure 1.1). This classification serves as a reference, but also makes it possible to offer a therapeutic response for each topographic zone.

The examination of the extensor mechanism is analytical and carried out against resistance. A test against resistance that revives pain indicates a partial tendon injury. In this case, the possibility of an active extension without resistance can be totally maintained.

Metacarpophalangeal (MCP) extension of the long fingers allows testing of extensor digitorum communis (EDC), extensor indicis proprius (EIP) and extensor digiti minimi (EDM) (Figure 1.2A). The patient is asked to extend the index and small fingers (Figure 1.2B), in order to test the extensors belonging to the index and small finger independently. However, even in cases where the EIP is sectioned there is compensation by the EDC of zone II. The EDC must be analysed in a precise manner because of the possibility of compensation by the junctura in cases of tendon injury of the common extensor of the third and fourth fingers above these juncturae tendinosum.

The study of the proximal interphalangeal (PIP) extension mainly tests the central extensor tendon (Figure 1.2C). Beware of a possible compensation at the initial phase by the lateral bands.

Testing of distal interphalangeal (DIP) extension allows the study of lateral and terminal extensor tendons (Figure 1.2D). As far as possible it must be done in PIP extension and then in flexion in order to test the oblique retinacular ligaments.

At the thumb level the extensor palmaris longus (EPL) is tested with the hand placed flat on the table and the patient is asked to lift the thumb towards the ceiling (Figure 1.2E). Retropulsion of the thumb column is associated with an interphalangeal hyperextension; the EPL excursion is then evident. An interphalangeal extension without hyperextension is allowed in the case of a disruption of the long thumb extensor by the action of the intrinsic muscles of the thumb.

The EPB is tested by an active extension against resistance of the MCP joint.

Deformities of the long fingers are not constant at the first stage. It must be emphasized that the existence of a finger deformity at the initial phase of an injury of the extensor mechanism is not constant. Its absence does not by any means exclude a tendon lesion. The rapidity with which this deformity appears depends on the importance of the tendon lesion as well as on the hyperlaxity of the patient.

Boutonnière deformity

This deformity is related to a disruption of the median band behind the PIP joint. There is flexion of the PIP joint and hyperextension of the DIP joint, which is quite supple and reducible in the initial phase. This severe derangement is enhanced by the lateral and ventral displacement of the lateral bands. Hence, like a button in a buttonhole, the head of the first phalanx, penetrates into the tendinous detachment.

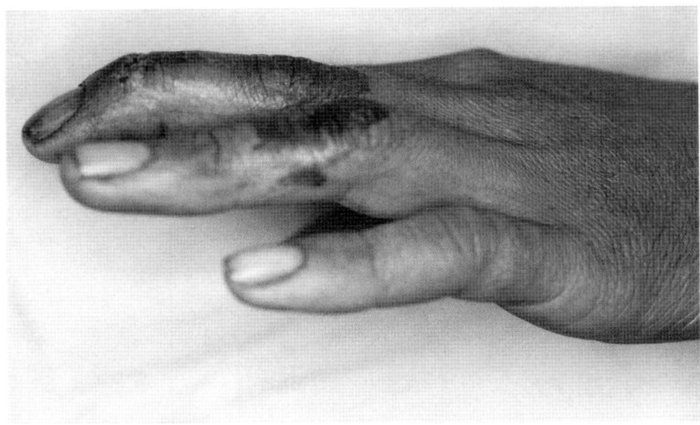

Figure 1.3

Mallet finger.

Mallet finger

This deformity is the result of a disruption of the two lateral bands or of the terminal band (Figure 1.3). The distal phalanx is flexed and cannot fully extend actively. This extension deficiency can be masked at the initial stage by the action of the oblique retinacular ligaments. However, if these are also injured the mallet finger is evident. The derangement of the extensor mechanism resulting from this is referred to as a swan-neck deformity where the interphalangeal flexion is accompanied by a PIP hyperextension position – which is an important functional handicap.

It is important to specify the nature of the trauma and the associated lesions, as described below.

Open injuries of the extensor mechanism

The peritendinous gliding structures are more or less seriously injured in these cases. The type of trauma – clean lacerations, crushing or tearing – as well as the importance of the concomitant lesions (joint opening, fracture, skin loss) constitute important elements for prognosis which influence the results of tendon repair. Foucher et al (1986) proposed a classification of loss of substance on the dorsal side of the proximal interphalangeal joint, a zone which is particularly exposed.

- Type I: loss of cutaneous substance
  Ia, intact paratendon
  Ib, injured paratendon
- Type II: loss of cutaneous and tendinous substance
  IIa, rupture of the tendon
  IIb, loss of tendon substance
- Type III: loss of cutaneous, tendinous and osteo-articular substance
  IIIa, joint opening
  IIIb, loss of substance of more than one-third of the joint surface
  IIIc, articular destruction.

Although in theory the lesions are often associated, this classification according to the magnitude and extent of the lesions is useful from the therapeutic point of view.

It must not be forgotten that all lesions of the extensor mechanism dorsal to a joint (zones I, III, V) are associated with articular lesions which must not be neglected in order to avoid septic risks. Septic injuries, particularly bites at the MCP level, associated tendon wounds and joint opening, run a major risk of septic arthritis which can delay the tendon repair in an emergency.

In the case of a phalangeal fracture associated with a lesion in zones II, IV or VI the gliding structures are seriously injured and the quality of the stabilization will be an important criterion for prognosis.

'Moulding machine'-type traumas frequently result in very severe and extensive multidigital complex lesions ranging from zones I to V. There is loss of multidigital cutaneous substance, phalangeal fractures and PIP and DIP destruction with extensive loss of substance of the extensor mechanism, without digital devascularization in most cases.

Trauma following traffic accidents involving the dorsal part of the hand mainly concerns zone VI and extends to zones V and VII. Interosseous muscle lesions are associated with metacarpal lesions.

Closed injuries by subcutaneous rupture

The peritendinous gliding structures are respected in these cases. The most common injury is known as the 'mallet finger' after rupture of the terminal band at the level of its insertion on the base of the distal phalanx with or without an osseous fragment (Figure 1.4). In rare cases, a rupture of the median band dorsal to the PIP joint can be observed, resulting in a boutonnière-type deformity.

Subcutaneous rupture of the long extensor of the thumb in zone V can be observed after a fracture of the distal radius, often with little or no displacement by tendinous ischaemia due to haematoma in the third compartment or extensor rupture due to the osteosynthesis pin.

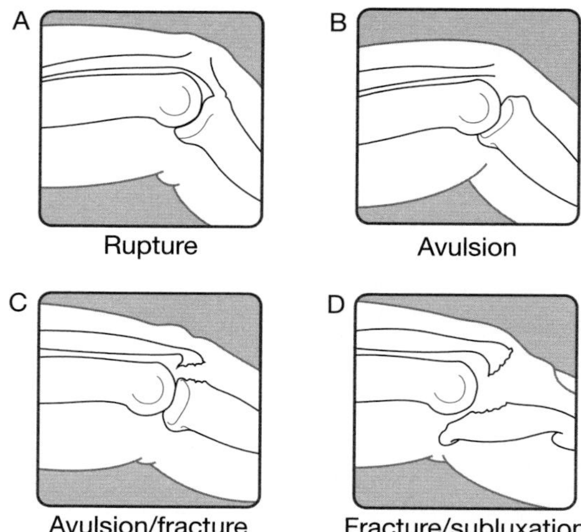

Figure 1.4
Different types of subcutaneous rupture of the extensor mechanism in zone I (according to Wilson and Fleming 1997): (A) rupture; (B) avulsion; (C) avulsion/fracture; (D) fracture/subluxation

After a direct shock (a punch) to the head of the third metacarpal (which is the most protruding), a rupture of the radial side of the sagittal band and of the transverse fibres of the intrinsics will bring about a dislocation of the extensor tendon on the ulnar side of the MCP joint.

Treatment

Lesions of the extensor mechanism must be treated as an emergency when the tendon lesion is facing a superficial joint (zones I, II, V) or if it is associated with an open fracture or is badly contaminated. In other cases an emergency treatment within 24 hours is acceptable if a local antiseptic has been applied. Treatment of closed injuries by subcutaneous rupture of the extensor mechanism must also be treated as early as possible, particularly if treatment by orthosis is preferred.

Therapeutic approaches

Joint immobilization

Treatment by orthosis

This splint allows a total extension of the joint at the seat of rupture of the extensor mechanism. The splint

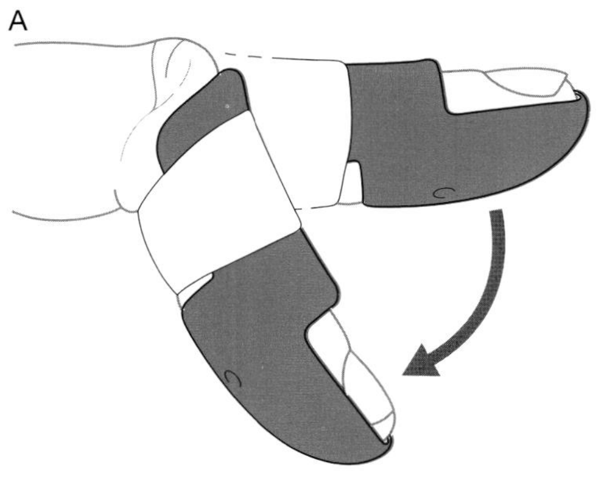

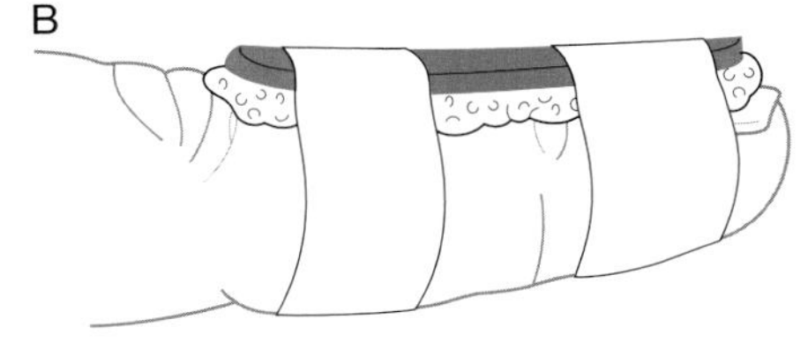

Figure 1.5
Splints which can be used in cases of mallet finger deformity (according to Doyle 1999). (A) Stack splint; (B) dorsal splint.

must be perfectly adapted and must not cause any cutaneous complications. In zone I, a Stack splint (which is available in several sizes) is very useful (Figure 1.5); however, the splint covers up the pulp and a dorsal splint moulded in slight hyperextension is preferable. In zone III a made-to-measure dorsal orthosis or a dorsal splint can be fitted by leaving the distal interphalangeal (DIP) and MCP joints free. A Capener splint allows a PIP active flexion and an elastic return in extension and is only used after a static splint.

Temporary joint pinning in extension

Percutaneous pinning can constitute the only treatment and is maintained for 3 weeks or more, after which it is replaced by a static orthosis for a total period of 6 weeks immobilization. This treatment is useful in uncooperative patients in case of a subcutaneous rupture of the extensor mechanism in zones I or III. The distal interphalangeal pinning needs to be axial or rather oblique, as in the PIP, in order to avoid pulp complications where the pin passes. This pinning can also be carried out in association with an open tendon repair and is maintained for 6 weeks or for only 3 weeks, after which it is replaced by a static extension orthosis which leads to less stiffening.

Immobilization and joint distraction

In cases of destruction with loss of joint substance, immobilization with joint distraction by external fixation or pins can prepare the way for a secondary reconstruction by arthroplasty or even by composite joint transfer.

Open tendon repair

Treatment of injuries of the extensor mechanism should under all circumstances include a tendon repair surgery procedure, followed by an appropriate, specific and controlled rehabilitation programme. This treatment must take into account all associated injuries and prime consideration must be given to cutaneous lesions.

Tendon sutures

The morphological differences between the zones situated distally and those situated proximally to the MCP joint are very important at the extensor level. The tendon shape varies from oval to a fibrous strip. The thickness varies too, for the long fingers the thickness is 1.5 mm in zones V and VI and 0.6 mm in zones I–IV (Doyle 1999).

Use of controlled mobilization techniques for the flexor tendons has influenced suture techniques as regards greater resistance of the wires and the type of stitches; the same developments have been noted for the treatment of extensor tendons. Controlled early postoperative mobilization techniques were progressively used for lesions in zones III and IV, which are the most difficult to treat. A greater suture strength should further improve the quality and rapidity of the results by facilitating early postoperative mobilization. Newport's experience – published in 1992 for zone VI (Newport and Williams 1992) and in 1995 for zone IV (Newport et al 1995) – confirms the superiority of the modified Kessler-type sutures (Figure 1.6) compared with simple or figure-of-eight techniques, and the possibility of controlled postoperative mobilization in a limited amplitude sector thanks to stronger sutures. These studies also pointed out the consequences of tendon shortening due to suture techniques, particularly in zone VI in terms of digital flexion loss (Newport and Williams 1992). Hence, this complication produced by a very tight suture must not be overlooked. In fact, MCP and PIP flexion deficiency progresses linearly when the shortening increases. The same rules apply to the strength necessary for finger flexion. For example, a shortening of 8 mm in zone VI results in a flexion deficiency of 23° at the MCP level and of 22° at the PIP level (Newport and Williams 1992). In zone III shortening must also be minimal in order to maintain flexion (Iselin 1997). Tendon plasty adjustments must be particularly precise.

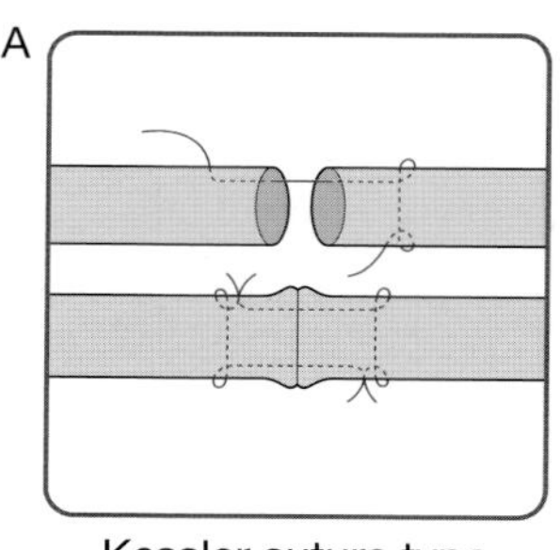

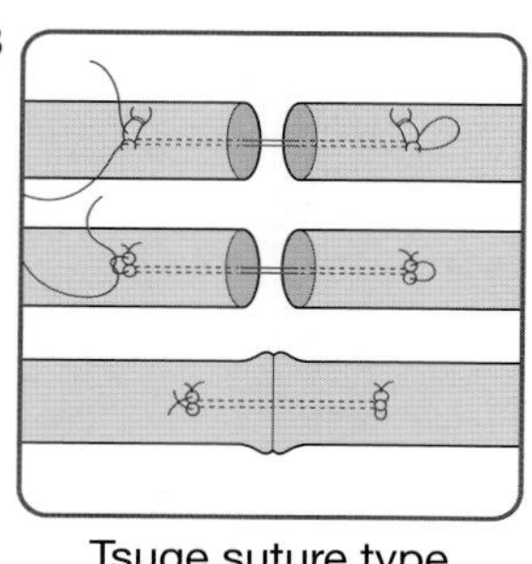

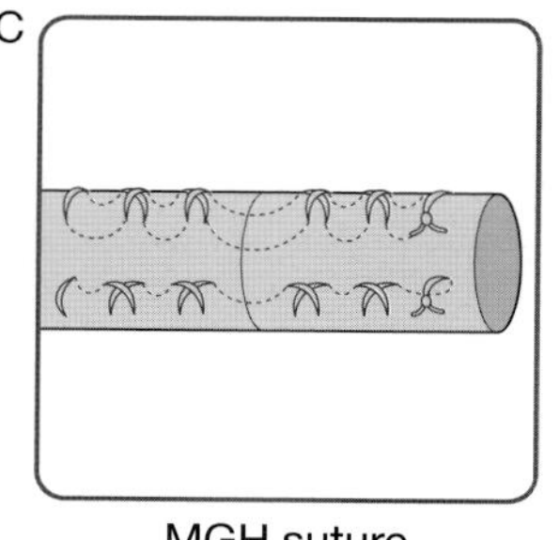

Figure 1.6

Types of intratendinous sutures of the extensor mechanism; (A) Kessler; (B) Tsuge; (C) MGH.

At present, suture techniques for extensor tendon injuries associate a modified Kessler-type suture (Doyle 1999) or a Tsuge suture with a non-absorbable or slow absorption PDS-type 3-0 or 4-0 thread with a 5-0 non-circumferential dorsal edge-to-edge suture at the level of the epitendon (Doyle 1999) (Figure 1.6). It is preferable not to make the suture knot or knots in the tendon extremities zone which could prevent healing, as in Tajima or Kessler Tajima-type sutures, because the thickness of the extensor mechanism is less important than that of the flexor mechanism. In zone VI, a four-thread suture called MGH (Figure 1.6) was recommended by Howard et al (1997) to allow active postoperative mobilization. As in the case of flexors, epitendinous edge-to-edge sutures increase the resistance of the sutures and maintain the extremities; a simple edge-to-edge suture or a Silfverskiold-type edge-to-edge suture can be used (Figure 1.7). This edge-to-edge suture cannot be used at the level of the lateral bands, where the Tsuge suture technique is preferable.

Tendon reinsertion

When the tendon injury is at the level of or very close to the distal tendon insertion, reinsertion must be carried out by one of the following approaches:

- through a transverse transosseous tunnel (allowing maintenance of the suture if there is a small tendon stump (Doyle 1999));
- a pull-out technique with a palmar button if the injury is in zone I;
- use of a Mitek mini anchor, on which is placed a 3-0 non-absorbable or absorbable thread (this is a very useful solution to avoid complications arising from the other methods); however, the price is a disadvantage;
- use of a Jenning's barb wire (Allieu 1977) which comes out mediolaterally in zone III (Foucher et al 1986) or at the nail extremity in zone I; it prevents digital mobilization and necessitates specific supervision with risks of cutaneous and septic complications, and as a result this system has disappeared.

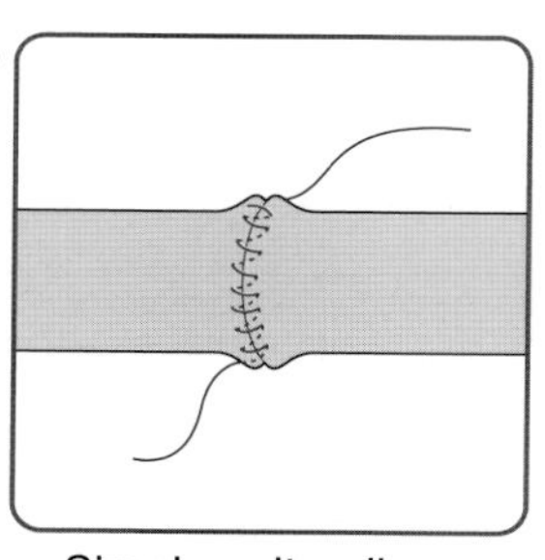

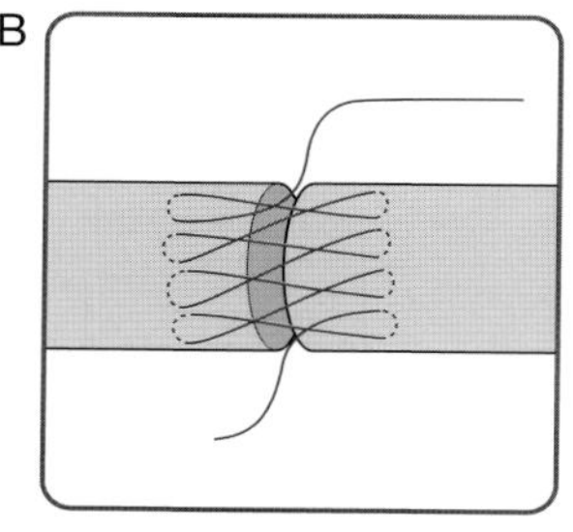

Figure 1.7

Types of epitendinous edge-to-edge sutures: (A) simple epitendinous edge-to-edge; (B) Silfverskiold epitendinous.

In cases of a torn bony fragment with tendon and displaced insertion, an osteosynthesis produced by pinning, cerclage or barb wire is possible.

Tendon plasty

These are specially indicated in cases of loss of tendon substance in zones II, III, IV and V. The following techniques are used:

- Snow-type plasty with a return distal flap (Snow 1973) for loss of substance in zone III, and 'banana split' plasty described by Foucher et al (1986) for loss of substance in zone III and/or IV and/or V. Snow's plasty consists of using a small median flap from the extensor mechanism in zone IV, then suturing it to the distal median band (Figure 1.8). For the 'banana split' plasty at the level of the index and small finger, in cases with clean extensors, the common extensor is sectioned proximally and turned over subcutaneously up to the PIP joint. At the level of the third and fourth fingers, half of the extensor tendon or a band is turned over. The tendon must be centralized at the dorsum of the MCP joint by a few lateral stitches.
- Plasty from Aiache-type lateral bands (Aiache et al 1970), used only in cases of limited injury to the median band (Figure 1.8).
- Joshi's cutano-tendon plasty (Joshi 1982), proposed in cases of cutano-tendinous loss of substance. One of the lateral bands is sectioned distally, then centralized by means of a proximal pedicled dorsolateral cutaneous flap and is finally placed at the level of the median band insertion at the base of P2.
- Short tendon grafting as a salvage procedure.

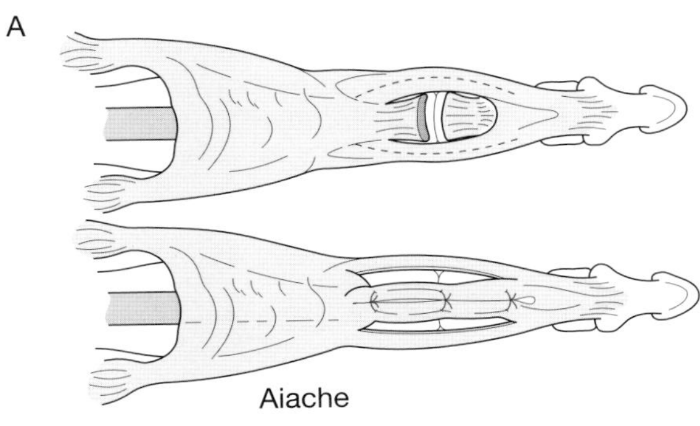

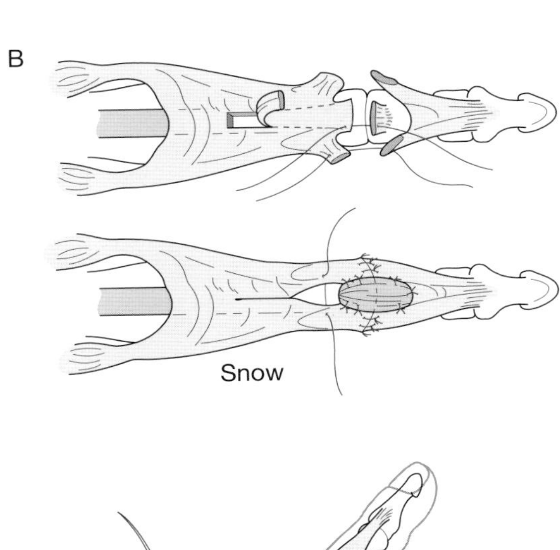

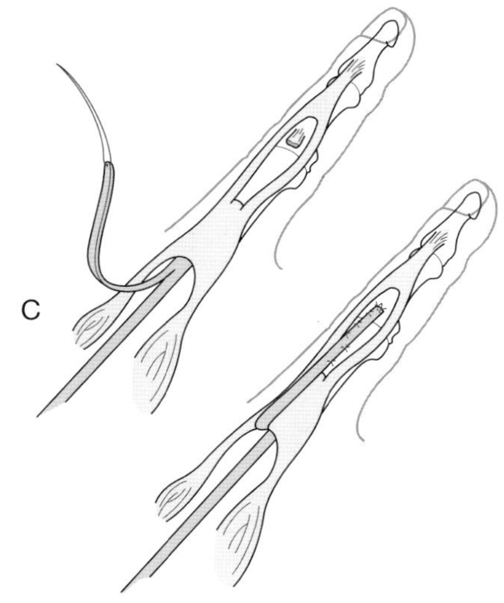

Figure 1.8
(A) Aiache, (B) Snow plasty (according to Doyle 1999) and (C) Foucher 'banana split'-type (according to Vaienti and Merle 1997) for median band reconstruction.

Tendon transfers

Tendon transfers are used in cases of loss of unitendinous substances or in cases of a small number of tendons mainly in zone VI.

Transfer of EIP on EPL is a classic approach (Schneider et al 1983, Saffer and Fakhoury 1987). This tendon can also be transferred in cases of loss of tendon substance on one or two ulnar digits.

The 'by-pass' technique described by Oberlin et al (1995) is proposed in case of complete unidigital loss of substance of the extensor mechanism extending to zone III. In this case, the EIP transfer is prolonged by a tendon graft up to the distal insertion of the median band.

In an emergency a tendon transfer can be carried out from an amputated finger (Foucher et al 1986). A terminolateral suture to the adjacent healthy tendon can also be carried out in case of loss of tendon substance, as in rheumatoid arthritis (Allieu et al 1997).

Interphalangeal arthrodesis

Proximal or distal interphalangeal arthrodesis can be the only therapeutic solution in an emergency when a tendon injury is associated with articular destruction. Proximal interphalangeal arthrodesis does not exclude the possible repair of the lateral bands in order to maintain an active DIP extension, because the oblique retinacular ligaments will no longer be active, the PIP joint being fixed in flexion. Distal interphalangeal arthrodesis can also be indicated in cases of loss of tendon substance in zone I and II without articular destruction.

Splinting and postoperative rehabilitation

Immobilization

Indications

For long fingers, postoperative immobilization is necessary for lesions in zones I and III. For zones V–VIII and more particularly for zones II and IV, postoperative controlled passive mobilization protocols are being used increasingly. Immobilization is preferable in cases of uncooperative patients, whether for psychological reasons or because of the patient's age, or in cases when suitable early rehabilitation is not possible.

Time period

The time period of immobilization for zones I–IV is 6 weeks; for zones V–IX, it is 3–6 weeks.

Type and position

For injuries in zones I and II, the MCP and PIP joints are left free, as well as the wrist. For injuries in zones III and IV, the MCP joint is flexed at 20–30° to relax the intrinsics, the wrist is immobilized at 40° extension (or 40° less than maximum extension) if the injury in zone IV extends to zone V. For zones V–VII, the MCP joint is in 0° extension and the wrist is in 40° extension. For zone IX, the orthosis includes the elbow flexed at 90°.

For the thumb, in distal zones TI and TII, the MCP joint can remain free. For more proximal injuries, splinting is performed, maintaining the thumb in extension and retropulsion and the wrist in extension.

Postoperative controlled passive mobilization

Assisted early passive mobilization using dynamic splinting to reduce adhesions was introduced in the treatment of extensor tendon lesions as early as 1972 by Allieu in order to protect the suture by Jenning's barb wire (Allieu 1977). In 1980 Laboureau and Renevey mentioned the application of the Kleinert method to the extensor mechanism. Later, protection by orthosis was considered sufficient to give up the barb wire technique and use only a fine atraumatic suture. Different teams published their results on assisted passive mobilization, either with a 'low profile' dynamic orthosis (Allieu et al 1984, Marin-Braun et al 1989, Le Nen et al 1993, Escobar et al 1998) (Figure 1.9), or with a Levame's apparatus (Frère et al 1984, Guinard et al 1993). To compensate for the stretching of the dynamic extension recall and to meet the specific constraints of each digit and of each patient, standardized spiral springs allowing a lengthening of 50 mm were proposed (Rouzand and Allieu 1987).

Long fingers: Zones V–VIII

Splinting

The orthosis for protection and assistance is placed 48 hours postoperatively. The wrist is placed in 30° extension (or 30° less than the maximum wrist extension), the sling is fitted under P1. This splinting is maintained in an uninterrupted manner for 4–5 weeks; it permits a rapid and early mobilization, under protection of the MCP joint and without risk of causing suture tension. This dynamic system can be transformed into a static splint at night for patients who are considered 'restless'.

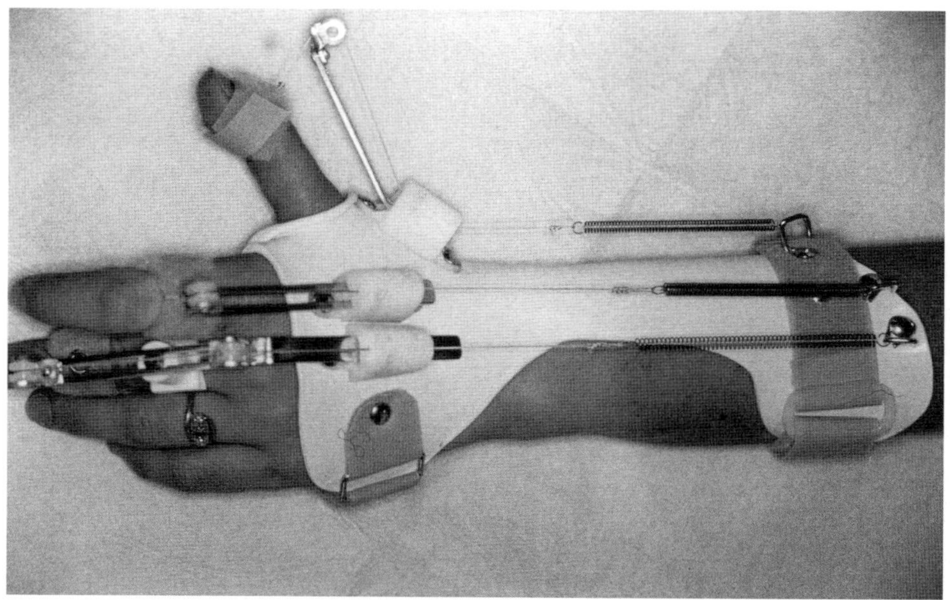

Figure 1.9

Orthosis for controlled passive mobilization.

Passive mobilization protocol

By the first week an active MCP flexion of 50–60° must be obtained with the orthosis. By the second week there must be 70° flexion in order to achieve 90° at the end of the third week. All these mobilizations are carried out with the wrist maintained in extension. The MCP joint can be mobilized by keeping the PIP joint in extension, or the PIP joint can be flexed by maintaining the MCP joint in extension. By the fourth week a combined MCP, PIP, DIP and wrist flexion can be carried out without force. At this stage complete flexion of the finger can be achieved.

Active mobilization protocol

Active mobilization in extension is forbidden before the third week, which is the time period necessary for soft tissue healing. However, it is possible to check the tendon excursion by the second week by an assisted active contraction at the end of the session. Simple active work is undertaken during the third week. For this the MCP joint will be in extension with the PIP and DIP joints in flexion. This type of work results in the best gliding at the level of the sagittal bands. Following this, the patient must be capable of performing a complete contraction at all amplitudes without resistance. Work against resistance can only be expected by the fourth week.

Special techniques according to the zones: Zone V

This can concern an isolated lesion of the sagittal band leading to a lateral tendon luxation. There is no tendon rupture in this case. It can be a lesion or slackening of the sagittal band. The two adjacent fingers must be placed in syndactyly and in extension of the MCP joint by means of a short orthosis. From 60° flexion onwards the tendons are luxated. The PIP and DIP joints are left free.

Special techniques: Zone VI

There are two possibilities for this zone (Frère et al 1984). In the case of a lesion distal to the juncturae, finger flexion leads to a relaxing of the injured digit. It is evident that a splint must not be applied to the adjacent fingers, this would cause stretching at the suture level. The fingers close to the injured digit must be kept free and must be maintained flexed during the mobilization of the injured digit in order to relax the suture.

In contrast to lesions situated distal to the juncturae, in the case of lesions proximal to the juncturae it is preferable to splint the adjacent fingers (Frère et al 1984) and maintain them in extension. Flexion of the adjacent fingers leads to a gap. The fingers must be maintained in extension so as not to provoke stretching at the suture level.

Special techniques: Zone VII

This zone passes under the dorsal retinacular ligament. It is the synovial sheath zone and it passes through each osteo-fibrous tunnel. There are potential adhesions in this zone. Mobilization must be carried out rapidly so as to provoke a gliding in the tunnel and pass the suture. The work proposed by Thomas et al (1986) – under protection of an orthosis with a dynamic extension system under the first phalanx – makes it possible to work separately on the wrist, on the metacarpophalangeal joint and on the interphalangeal joints.

Special techniques: Zones III and IV

Postoperative management is the same as that for extrinsic injuries, with a dynamic splint maintained for 5 weeks or more if a PIP extension deficiency appears. This splint leaves the wrist free and maintains the MP in flexion at 20°–30°, which relaxes the intrinsics, and the recall is done under P2. The PIP must be at 0° except during rehabilitation. An orthosis maintaining the wrist in 30° extension is used in zone IV lesions extending to zone V. Flexion progress is slow, progressing by levels up to 30° maximum flexion during the first 2 weeks and not exceeding 45° till the third week. Later on, active flexion amplitude is increased.

Thumb column

The same principles are applied to the thumb as for long fingers. The splint holds the wrist in 40° extension in order to relax the suture. The recall is done under P2, maintaining the thumb column in retropulsion for EPL lesions, more radially in abductor pollicis longus (APL) lesions, with thumb opening on the plane of the hand. The EPL splint is maintained for 5 weeks, bearing in mind the rupture risks related to precarious vascularization.

Contraindications for postoperative controlled mobilization

- Injuries in zones I, II and IX.
- Tendon graft repair.
- Patient not very cooperative due to age, psychological reasons or distance.
- Insufficient stabilization of the bone.

Tendon plasty is not a contraindication to post operative controlled mobilization (Foucher et al 1986, Oberlin et al 1995).

Early active mobilization protocol

This protocol introduced by Evans (1995) is based on different conclusions:

- Injuries in zones III and IV treated by prolonged immobilization are characterized by an insufficient excursion of the repaired tendon, a risk of slackening of the tendon suture by mobilization due to adhesions in zone IV (wide contact zone between the extensor mechanism and the first phalanx), and a frequent PIP flexion loss (Newport et al 1990, Doyle 1999).
- 30° of PIP flexion allows a tendon excursion of around 4 mm and causes a constraint of only 300 g at the tendon level, which can be borne by the suture (Evans 1995).

This protocol allows an active mobilization, progressively increasing in flexion and in extension of the PIP and DIP joints. This progression advances as long as active extension at 0° is possible. The orthoses are designed corresponding to the amplitude of the flexion desired. A PIP static orthosis is maintained by the patient except during rehabilitation sessions. The active extension/flexion amplitudes authorized are:

- First 2 weeks: PIP 0°/30° and DIP 0°/25°.
- Third week: PIP 0°/40° and DIP 0°/25°.
- Fourth week: PIP 0°/50°, then 0°/80°.

Indications

Long fingers

Zone I

For closed lesions, treatment by orthosis is indispensable up to the end of the second postoperative month. The PIP joint is left free for treatment of a mallet finger during the 6–8 week treatment period. After this, the DIP extension splint is maintained at night for 3 weeks and under circumstances when the finger is likely to receive a shock. In cases of disinsertion with loss of osseous fragment, treatment by orthosis is carried out if displacement reduction is obtained under orthosis. In the opposite cases and particularly in case of joint subluxation, an osteosynthesis is carried out with additional immobilization.

Open lesions require tendon repair and DIP pinning for 3 weeks followed by 3 weeks in an extension splint. In cases of loss of tendon substance without compensation by the oblique retinacular ligament and/or of DIP destruction, a DIP arthrodesis is justified.

Zone II

In cases of an open lesion of one of the bands, repair is not justified and early mobilization is carried out. If the two bands are injured, a tendon repair and DIP pinning for 3 weeks followed by a splint for 3 weeks will be necessary. In cases of loss of tendon substance without compensation by the oblique retinacular ligament, and/or of DIP joint destruction, a DIP athrodesis is justified.

Zones III and IV

For closed ruptures of the median band in zone III, treatment by orthosis is indispensable. The DIP joint is kept free in order to be mobilized in flexion in such a way as to pull the median band distally thanks to the lateral bands. On the other hand, the MCP joint is immobilized in 20–30° flexion during the first 4 weeks in order to relax the intrinsics. After that, an extension orthosis limited to the PIP joint for 2 weeks is sufficient. Following this, a static PIP extension orthosis is used during the night and a Capener-type dynamic PIP extension orthosis is used during the day with the possibility of active flexion. The time period will vary according to the quality and stability of extension obtained.

Open injuries require tendon repair and – depending on the associated lesions – either assisted early mobilization, or PIP pinning for 3 weeks, followed by a PIP extension splint for 3 weeks. In cases of PIP joint destruction, an arthrodesis or a temporary distraction before reconstruction is justified.

Zones V, VI, VII and VIII

This is a particular case of closed rupture of the radial sagittal band of the extensor mechanism at the dorsum of the metacarpophalangeal joint: if the rupture is initially recognized, treatment by a short metacarpal bracelet-type orthosis immobilizing the MCP joint in extension for 6 weeks is carried out (Inoue et al 1996; Doyle 1999). Beyond the second week, surgical treatment is possible and in cases where a simple suture is not possible, a reconstruction is performed if possible by passing a part of the extensor tendon around the radial collateral ligament of the MCP joint (Inoue et al 1996, Doyle 1999).

An isolated injury of an EIP extensor with compensation by the common extensor (or vice versa) can justify a decision not to repair the tendon, depending on the patient's needs for finger function. In other cases, tendon repair is permissible with assisted mobilization except when there are contraindications.

In the case of a 'banana split'-type reconstruction (Foucher et al 1986) for loss of substance in zone V, the extensor mechanism must be stabilized at the dorsum of the MCP joint by a tendon plasty at the palmaris longus (Vainti and Merle 1997).

In the case of loss of tendon substance extended to several areas at the level of zone VI with possible extension to zones V and VII, the cutaneous reconstruction will be a preliminary preparation for secondary tendon grafting unless the mechanized fibrosis compensates for the loss of extensor tendon substance. Implantation of Hunter stems in an emergency does not appear to be useful and carries a risk of sepsis.

In zone VII, the dorsal retinacular ligament can be partially opened if it obstructs the tendon excursion.

Zone IX

Muscular injuries can be associated with injury of the posterior interosseous nerve, thus justifying a combined repair if possible. In cases of serious muscular injuries and loss of nervous substance and according to the age of the patient, secondary tendon transfers can be indicated.

Thumb

Closed injuries

These injuries are rare in zone TI and justify an orthetic treatment such as that used for the mallet finger. In zones TV and TVI, a transfer of the EIP is possible for ruptures with loss of EPL substance.

Open injuries

Repair techniques are similar to those used for long fingers. Postoperatively, assisted passive mobilization is preferable for zone TIII and more proximal zones. For zones TI and TII, immobilization for 5 weeks in IP extension is allowed after repair, with MCP mobilization during this time period. In cases of loss of tendon substance of the EPL in zones TIV and TV, a transfer of the extensor indicis proprius is indicated.

Results

Methods of evaluation

Apart from the fact that sequelae of extensor tendon injuries arise from extension deficiency as well as from a digital flexion deficiency, some remarks concerning the methods of evaluation need to be made (Romain and Allieu 1998): a digital rolling deficiency will result in the same functional handicap whichever finger is injured. A PIP extension deficiency related to an injury in zones III or IV will be a greater handicap than the same deficiency spread over the three digital joints on account of a proximal lesion (zones V–VIII).

In long fingers, the total active motion (TAM) method is frequently used, either in an isolated way or integrated in a classification (Marin-Braun et al 1989, Guinard et al 1993, Escobar et al 1998):

- >220° = excellent
- 201°–220° = good
- 181°–200° = mediocre
- >181° = poor.

However, TAM, like all non-specific extensor classifications (such as those of Strickland, Kleinert, Buck-Gramcko or Miller), does not take into consideration the tenodesis effect of the wrist in extensor function. This is why we have set up the evaluation established by Romain and Allieu (1998) which specifically complies with the specifications of extensor function evaluation: by disassociating the measure of active extension and passive flexion, by eliminating the compensation by the MCP joint and by revealing the tenodesis effect of the wrist. This evaluation considers that the normal function of the fingers allows complete extension of the digital chain: wrist at 45° extension and a pulp to distal palmar crease contact, wrist in neutral position. Any deviation from these two positions is abnormal, particularly when the deviation is important. These two positions serve as a reference and we classify the results according to the importance of their respective deficiency and according to the lesional zone. Two measures are carried out:

1. Active extension measure, with the wrist placed at 45° extension: we measure the global angular deficiency of active extension of the digital chain (nail–metacarpal angle). This measure reveals a tendon slackening.
2. We measure the passive flexion of the fingers, with the wrist in neutral position and the MCP joint maintained at 90° flexion: pulp to distal palmar crease distance (PDPCD).

This measure shows an adhesion syndrome (stiffness in extension) or a tendon shortening. The PDPCD measure is standardized (Figure 1.10). A PIP extension deficit due

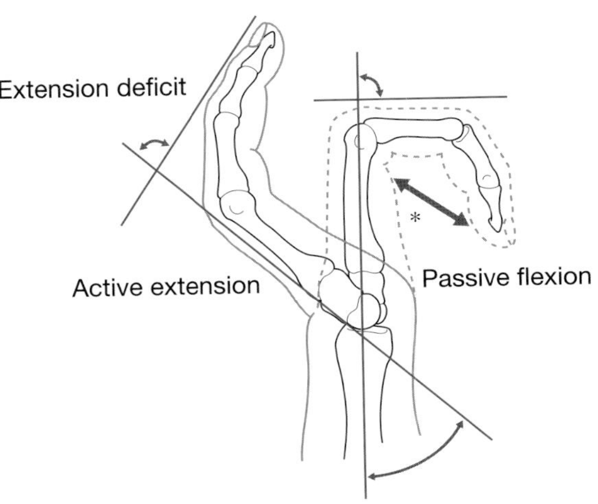

Figure 1.10
Principles of evaluation by Romain and Allieu (1998). *Indicates PDPCD.

Table 1.1 *Principles of evaluation by Romain and Allieu (1998)*

Parameter	*Excellent*	*Good*	*Mediocre*	*Poor*
PDPCD all zones	<1 cm	1–2 cm	2–3 cm	>3 cm
Extension deficit zones III and IV	<15º	15º–30º	30º–45º	>45º
Zones V–VIII	<30º	30º–60º	60º–90º	>90º

Table 1.2 *Classification of results after extensor pollicis longus repair according to Tubiana*

Parameter	*Excellent*	*Good*	*Mediocre*	*Bad*	*Poor*
Active flexion	>60º	>30º	<30º	<30º	>30º
Extension deficit	<15º	>30º	<15º	<30º	>30º

to an injury situated on the dorsal side of the finger in zones II or IV will be more harmful than the same angular deficit spread over the MCP, PIP and DIP joints, and appearing only when the wrist is in extension. This is why these same two extension deficits will be evaluated differently according to the lesional zone in our classification (Table 1.1).

It is also useful to measure the prehension strength (Guinard et al 1993), but the presence of associated lesions can interfere with the study of the tendon mechanism.

As regards the thumb, the evaluation of Tubiana (1997), like that of Allieu et al (1984), with the wrist in neutral position, analyses flexion and extension deficits separately (Table 1.2).

Clinical results

We have recently published the results of a 7-year retrospective study on emergency repair of 163 thumb and long finger injuries of extensor tendons in 115 patients. All the patients were treated in the department following the same protocol. Rehabilitation was carried out in a specific upper limb unit by the same physiotherapist. The evolution of functional progress as well as complications were registered as computer data. The results were analysed according to the evaluation by Romain and Allieu (1998). We thus registered 41% of adhesion syndromes (or tenodermodesis, in most cases without functional impact), 9% of ruptures of tendon sutures, 5% poor results, but 63% excellent results, 22.5% good results and 9.5% mediocre results.

Literature review

Controlled postoperative mobilization shortens the duration of treatment after tendon injury (Allieu et al 1984, Walsh et al 1994, Escobar et al 1998). Good and very good results have been observed in 76–98% of cases in long fingers and in 64–92% in the thumb following the evaluation method and the associated lesions (Allieu et al 1984, Marin-Braun et al 1989, Guinard et al 1993, Escobar et al 1998). Secondary rupture complication rates range from 0 to 2.5% (Allieu et al 1984, Marin-Braun et al 1989, Escobar et al 1998). Although the results differ in literature review (Chow et al 1989, Walsh et al 1994), the superiority of mobilization in comparison with postoperative immobilization, in terms of follow-up results, is evident only in zones III–V and in complex injuries (Allieu et al 1984, Chow et al 1989, Marin-Braun et al 1989, Escobar et al 1998) on condition that this mobilization is carried out from the second postoperative day onwards (Escobar et al 1998). A further delay will be harmful for the postoperative results (Walsh et al 1994, Escobar et al 1998). From zone VI onwards, for simple tendon injuries the results do not appear very different, except with regard to the duration of rehabilitation.

The main harmful factors which can influence the results after tendon repair are as follows (Allieu et al 1984, Frère et al 1984, Foucher et al 1986, Marin-Braun et al 1989, Newport et al 1990, Walsh et al 1994, Escobar et al 1998):

- associated fracture
- crushing or avulsion mechanism of injury
- work injuries
- important loss of cutaneous substance
- multidigital injuries.

References

Aiache A, Barsky AJ, Weiner DL (1970) Prevention of boutonniere deformity, *Plast Reconstr Surg* **46**: 164–7.

Allieu Y (1977) L'utilisation du barb wire de Jenning en chirurgie de la main. Note de catamnèse, *Ann Chir* **31**: 359–61.

Allieu Y, Chammas M (1997) Tendon transfers in rheumatoid arthritis. In: Hunter JM, Schneider LH, Mackin EJ, eds, *Tendon and Nerve Surgery in the Hand, a Third Decade* (Mosby: St Louis) 426–31.

Allieu Y, Asencio G, Gomis R et al (1984) Suture des tendons extenseurs de la main avec mobilisation assistée. A propos de 120 cas, *Rev Chir Orthop* **70**Suppl II: 68–71.

Chow JA, Dovelle S, Thomes LJ et al (1989) A comparison of results of extensor tendon repair followed by early controlled mobilisation versus static immobilisation, *J Hand Surg* **14B**: 18–20.

Doyle JR (1999) Extensor tendons – acute injuries. In Green DP, Hotchkiss RN, Pederson WC, eds, *Green's Operative Hand Surgery* (Churchill Livingstone: New York) 1950–87.

Escobar C, Le Nen D, Lefèvre C (1998) Mobilisation assistée de l'appareil extenseur des doigts après lésions traumatiques fraîches. A propos de 119 cas, *La Main* **3**: 33–41.

Evans R (1995) Immediate active short arc motion following extensor tendon repair, *Hand Clin* **11**: 483–512.

Foucher G, Debry R, Merle M, Dury M (1986) Le traitement des pertes de substances dorsales au niveau de l'articulation interphalangienne proximale des doigts, *Ann Chir Plast Esthet* **31**: 129–36.

Frère G, Moutet F, Sarorius C, Vila A (1984) Mobilisation contrôlée post-opératoire des sutures des tendons extenseurs des doigts longs, *Ann Chir Main* **3**: 139–44.

Guinard D, Lantuejoul JP, Gérard P, Moutet F (1993) Mobilisation précoce protégée par appareil de Levame après réparation primaire des tendons extenseurs de la main, *Ann Chir Main* **12**: 342–51.

Howard R, Ondrovic L, Greenwald D, Biomechanical analysis of four-strand extensor tendon repair techniques, *J Hand Surg* **22A**: 838–42.

Inoue G, Tamura Y (1996) Dislocation of the extensor tendons over the metacarpophalangeal joints, *J Hand Surg* **21A**: 464–9.

Iselin F (1997) Boutonnière deformity treatment. Immediate and delayed. In: Hunter JM, Schneider LH, Mackin EJ, eds, *Tendon and Nerve Surgery in the Hand, a Third Decade* (Mosby: St Louis) 580–1.

Joshi BB (1982) A salvage procedure in the treatment of the boutonnière deformity caused by a contact burn and friction injury, *Hand* **14**: 33–7.

Kleinert HE, Verdan C (1983) Report of the committee on tendon injuries, *J Hand Surg* **8A**: 794–8.

Laboureau JP, Renevey A (1980) Utilisation d'un appareil personnel de contention et de rééducation segmentaire élastique de la main type 'crabe', *Ann Chir* **25**: 165–9.

Le Nen D, Escobar C, Stindel E et al (1993) Mobilisation assistée après suture des tendons extenseurs à la main. A propos de 30 cas consécutifs, *Rev Chir Orthop* **79**: 194–9.

Marin-Braun F, Merle M, Sanz J et al (1989) Réparation primaire des tendons extenseurs de la main avec mobilisation post-opératoire assistée. Apropos d'une série de 48 cas, *Ann Chir Main* **8**: 7–21.

Newport M, Williams C (1992) Biomechanical characteristics of extensor tendon suture techniques, *J Hand Surg* **17A**: 1117–21.

Newport M, Blair W, Steyers C (1990) Long-term results of extensor tendon repair, *J Hand Surg* **15A**: 961–6.

Newport ML, Pollack GR, Williams CD (1995) Biomechanical characteristics of suture techniques in extensor zone IV, *J Hand Surg* **20A**: 650–6.

Oberlin C, Atchabayan A, Salon A et al (1995) The by-pass extensor tendon transfer. A salvage technique for loss of substance of the extensor apparatus in long fingers, *J Hand Surg* **20B**: 392–7.

Romain M, Allieu Y (1998) Bilan de la fonction des tendons fléchisseurs et extenseurs de la main, *Ann Chir Main* **17**: 259–65.

Rouzaud J, Allieu Y (1987) L'assistant dynamique chiffré par ressort spiralé étalonné dans l'orthèse de la main, *Rev Chir Orthop* **6**: 255–9.

Saffar P, Fakhoury B (1987) La réparation secondaire du long extenseur du pouce, *Ann Chir Main* **6**: 225–9.

Schneider L, Rosenstein RG (1983) Restoration of extensor pollicis longus function by tendon transfer, *Plast Reconstr Surg* **71**:533–7.

Snow JW (1973) Use of retrograde tendon flap in repairing a severed extensor tendon in the PIP joint area, *Plast Reconstr Surg* **51**:555–8.

Thomas D, Moutet F, Guinard D (1996) Postoperative management of extensor tendon repairs in zones V, VI, and VII, *J Hand Ther* **9**: 309–14.

Tubiana R (1997) Anatomy of the extensor system of the fingers. In: Hunter JM, Schneider LH, Mackin EJ, eds, *Tendon and Nerve Surgery in the Hand, a Third Decade* (Mosby: St Louis) 547–56.

Vaienti L, Merle M (1997) Lésions de l'appareil extenseur. In: Merle M, Dautel G, eds, *La Main Traumatique* (Masson: Paris) 233–50.

Walsh MT, Rinehimer W, Muntzer E et al (1994) Early controlled motion with dynamic splinting versus static splinting for zones II and IV extensor tendon lacerations, *J Hand Ther* **7**: 232–6.

Wehbé MA (1995) Anatomy of the extensor mechanism of the hand and wrist, *Hand Clin* **11**: 361–6.

Wilson RL, Fleming F (1997) Treatment of acute extensor tendon injuries. In: Hunter JM, Schneider LH, Mackin EJ, eds, *Tendon and Nerve Surgery in the Hand, a Third Decade* (Mosby: St Louis) 567–76.

2 Late reconstruction of the extensor tendons

Raoul Tubiana

This chapter describes different types of late extensor mechanism reconstruction, from forearm to fingertip. Late extensor tendon reconstruction proximal to the dorsal apparatus of the digits is in many ways similar to reconstruction for radial nerve palsy (see Chapter 10); the main difference is the risk of scarring and adhesion after injuries. In the fingers, the functional complexity of the extensor mechanism can result in late tendon imbalance, in many ways similar to rheumatoid deformities (see Chapter 36).

Late extrinsic extensor tendon reconstruction in the forearm and wrist

The musculotendinous junction of the extensor muscles is situated in the distal forearm. Tendons in the forearm can be injured by open or blunt trauma. At the wrist they can also be injured by attrition caused by osteophytes or bone displacement.

The most common rupture is of the EPL, following Colles fracture; the majority of such ruptures occur after undisplaced fractures (Helal et al 1982, Bonatz et al 1996), weeks to months after the original injury. The etiology of this delayed rupture is thought to be interruption of the tendon's vascularity as a result of hemorrhage and pressure.

Ruptures of the extensor tendons are quite common in rheumatoid patients; they may also result from arthritis of the distal radio-ulnar joint (Carr and Burge 1992). The extensor digiti minimi is usually the first to be ruptured. Further ruptures of the extensor digitorum communis may follow (see Chapter 34, Ruptures of the extensor tendons).

Tendon transfers are good procedures for restoring finger and wrist extension. Soft tissue coverage is required and may be performed with a free or local flap. When possible, tenolysis should be attempted first to restore motion.

Full passive joint mobility must be obtained before any reconstruction of the extensor mechanism is attempted. This can usually be obtained with a careful splinting and exercise program. If not, a two stage surgical program may be necessary; first a joint release followed by maintenance of full passive motion, then in a second stage, the extensor tendon reconstruction.

Intercalated tendon minigrafts have also been used to bridge a short tendon loss (Hamlin and Littler 1977). They are only effective if the muscle contractibility still has an adequate range of motion. However, tendon transfer is the most usual treatment for late extensor tendon ruptures.

The technique of tendon transfer for ruptures of the extensor tendons is described in Chapter 10.

Extensor tendon reconstruction in the dorsum of the hand

The most common severe injuries in this area are industrial, or motor vehicular. Often the skeleton has required stabilization. Skin coverage with an appropriate flap will allow staged extensor tendon reconstruction with silicone rods.

Delayed suturing remains feasible for a long time, especially in distal lesions, because the juncturae tendinum prevent retraction of the proximal end. However, delayed repair is not indicated in more proximal lesions because of the tension on the suture lines resulting from tendon retraction. It is preferable to suture the distal tendon to a neighbouring extensor, or use a tendon graft, or tendon transfer. Anastomosis to an adjacent tendon is the simplest solution, which of course necessitates the presence of a viable motor muscle. The anastomosis should lie in healthy (i.e. unscarred) tissue.

Finally, tendon transfers represent an excellent method of reactivating the digital extensors, an adjacent tendon of sufficient length being the first choice. When available, the extensor indicis proprius provides the ideal transfer because it can reactivate the extensor tendons of one or two fingers (Figure 2.1).

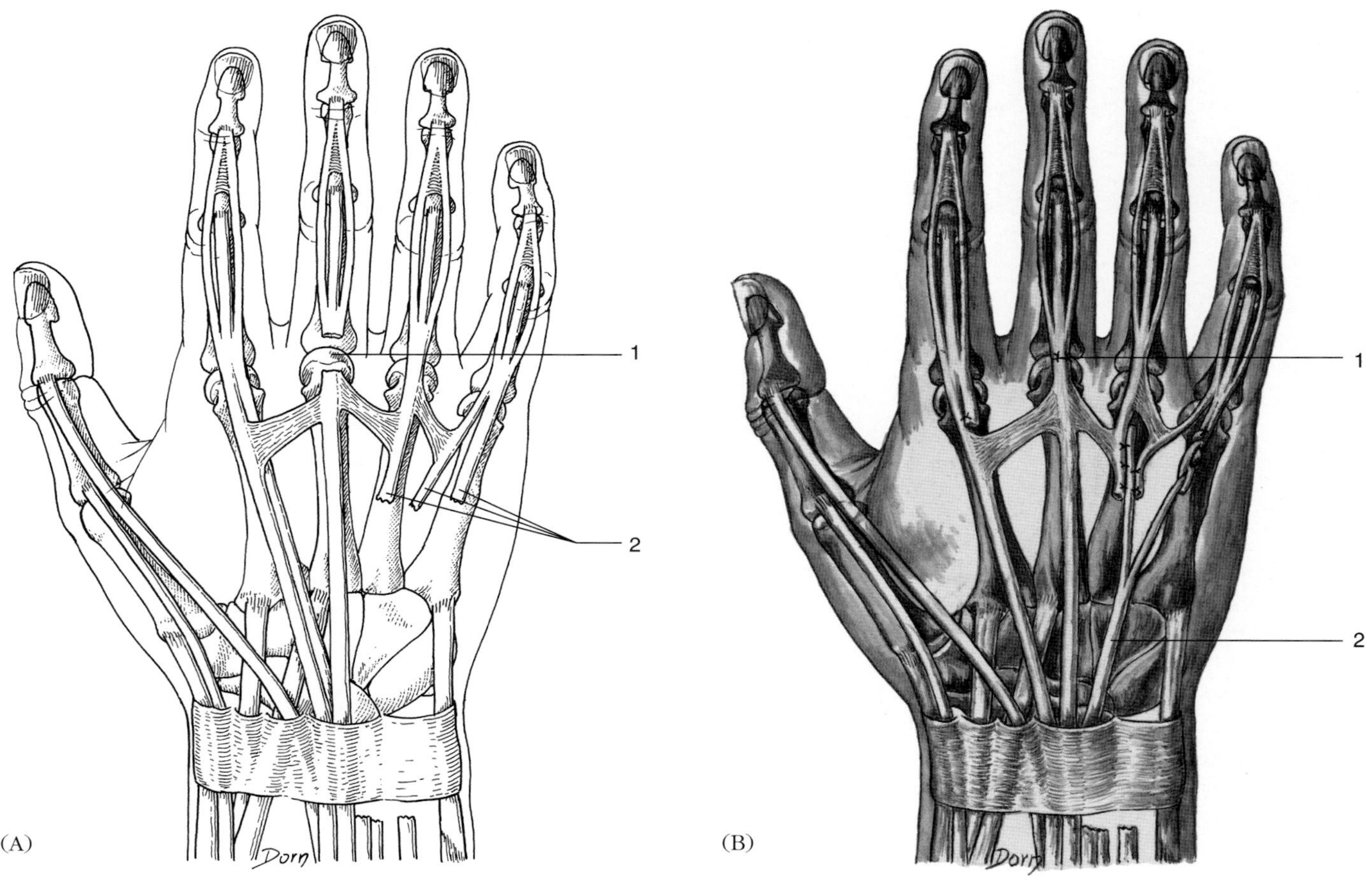

Figure 2.1

Extensor tendon reconstruction in the dorsum of the hand. (A) Extensor tendon lesions. (1) Distal laceration of the long finger EDC tendon – junctura tendinum prevents retraction of the proximal stump. (2) Severe retraction of EDC tendons IV, V and EDM in lesions proximal to the juncturae tendinum. (B) (1) Suture of the long finger EDC. (2) Transfer of the EIP to the EDC IV, V and EDM.

Complications

Among the secondary complications following late extensor tendon reconstruction in the dorsum of the hand are tendon adhesion and extensor tendon tightness. They may be responsible for the extensor plus syndrome (Kilgore and Graham 1977).

Extensor plus syndrome

This syndrome results from either shortening of the tendon or adherence of the tendon to the first part of the proximal phalanx at the extensor hood. It results in the inability to flex the proximal interphalangeal (PIP) and metacarpophalangeal (MP) joints simultaneously, although each joint can be flexed normally individually. The clinical test demonstrating this state is the opposite of the intrinsic plus test: flexion of the MP joint prevents flexion of the PIP joint, and conversely flexion of the PIP joint facilitates hyperextension of the MP joint. This test means that the extensor tendon, which passes dorsal to both the MP and PIP joints, before its insertion on the base of the middle phalanx, lacks the necessary range of motion to allow simultaneous flexion of the MP and PIP joints. Patients complain of the inability to flex the involved finger fully (Figure 2.2).

Extrinsic extensor tightness

Extrinsic extensor tightness is seen after extensor tendon repairs under excessive tension or when the muscle belly is contracted in the forearm. Tendon adhesion may follow any repair if there is important scarring to adjacent bone or fascia, particularly after metacarpal fractures or severe dorsal soft tissue injuries. The initial treatment consists of prolonged hand therapy. Surgical

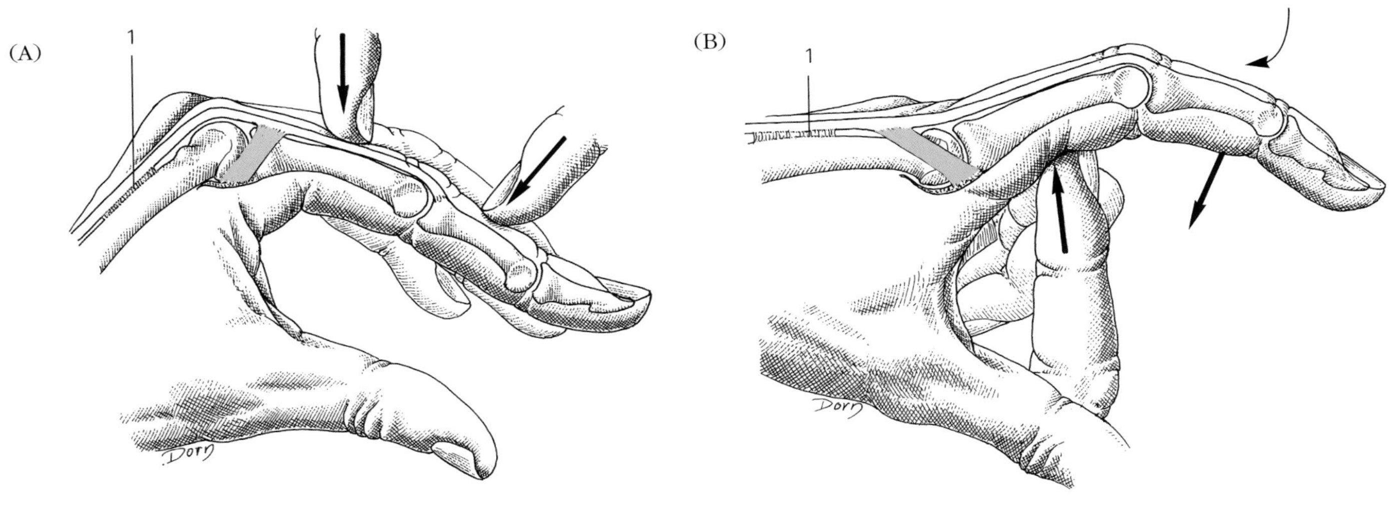

Figure 2.2
Extensor plus syndrome. 1. Tendon adhesion proximal to the MP joint. (A) Flexion of the MP joint prevents flexion of the PIP joint. (B) Flexion of the PIP joint facilitates hyperextension of the MP joint.

treatment cannot be considered before 6 months after tendon repair; it consists of extensor tendon tenolysis and/or extrinsic tendon release.

As regards extensor tendon release, Littler (1977) bases surgical correction of this problem on the concept of the double action of the extrinsic extensors and intrinsic muscles on extension of the distal phalanges. Because either group of muscles can act alone, in cases of extrinsic extensor tightness he proposes the resection of the central tendon and of the oblique fibers of the extensor hood over the proximal phalanx shaft. Of course, both the sagittal bands at the MP joint and the distal portion of the central tendon must be preserved, so as not to disturb the confluence of the central bands of the interosseous muscles. Burton (1993) suggests doing the operation under digital block (not a wrist block, which paralyses intrinsic muscles), permitting the patient to flex the digit so that the surgeon can monitor the extent of resection necessary. Physiotherapy is started immediately. The PIP joint is splinted in extension between the exercise periods (Figure 2.3).

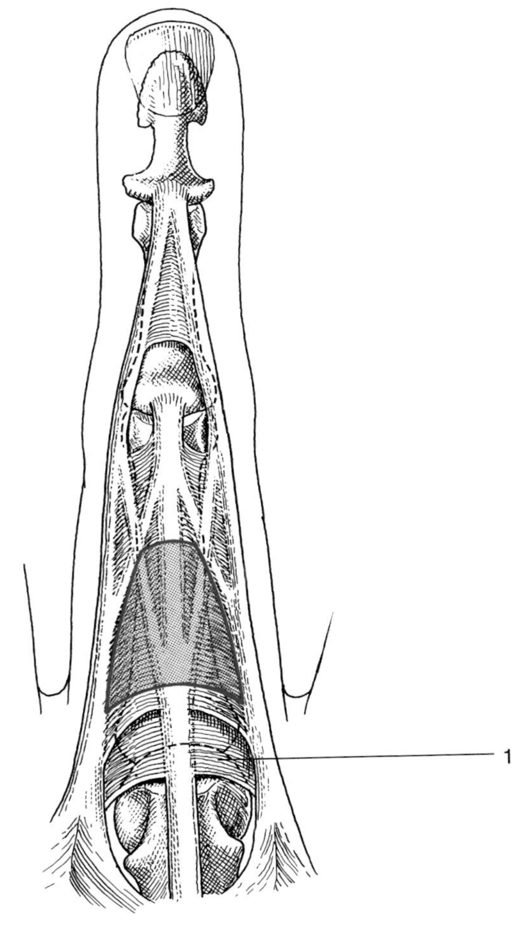

Figure 2.3
Extensor tendon release. Resection of the central extensor tendon and of the oblique fibres of the extensor hood (in red) (Littler 1977). 1. Sagittal bands.

Subluxation of the extensor tendons at the MP joint level

Each extrinsic extensor tendon crosses the dorsal aspect of the MP joint. It is held in the axis of the digit, particularly by the sagittal bands. These fibers arise from the extrinsic extensor, embrace the metacarpal head and insert into the volar plate. With MP joint motion, the sagittal (or shroud) fibres move back and forth in a sagittal plane (Figure 2.4 and 31.27).

(A)

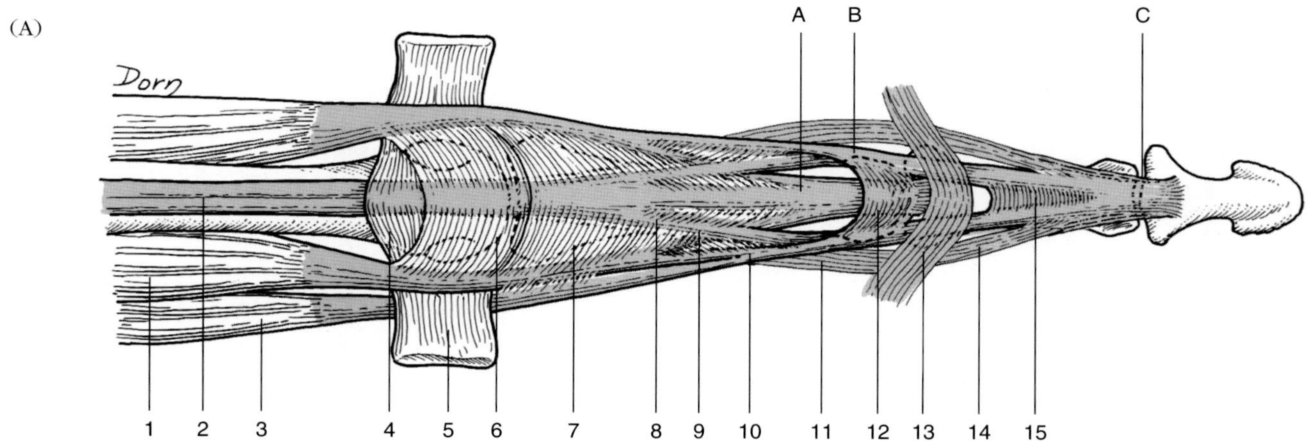

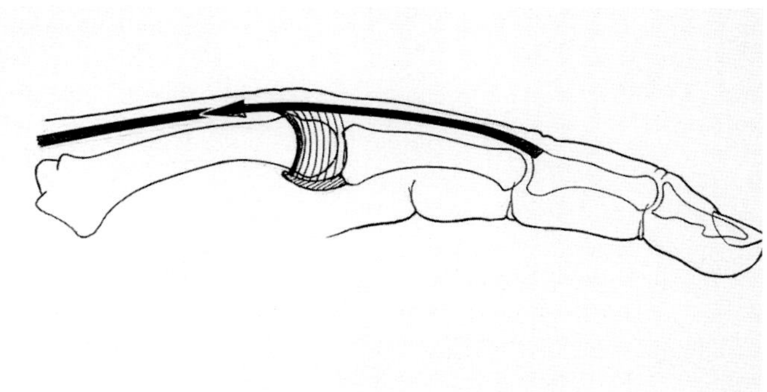

(B)

Figure 2.4

The extensor apparatus of the fingers. (A) Dorsal view. (1) Dorsal interosseous, (2) EDC tendon, (3) lumbrical, (5) sagittal band, (6) transverse intermetacarpal ligament, (7) transverse fibers of the extensor hood, (8) oblique fibers of the extensor hood, (9) lateral band of the extensor tendon, (10) interosseous central band, (11) interosseous lateral band, (12) spiral fibers, (13) oblique retinacular ligament, (14) transverse retinacular ligament, (15) triangular lamina. A, Central conjoint extensor tendon; B, lateral conjoint extensor tendon; C, terminal extensor tendon. (B) With MP joint motion, the sagittal bands inserted on the MP joint volar plate move back and forth. (See Figures 2.2 and 31.27)

When these structures are torn by trauma or stretched by arthritis, when the tendon is submitted to passive tension as in flexion, it tends to slide over the ulnar side of the joint. As the lesions become more severe, the tendon is displaced into the intermetacarpal valley and contributes to the maintenance of the flexion deformity and ulnar deviation of the MP joint. In addition, freed from its proximal attachment, the extensor tendon exerts an even stronger pull on the middle phalanx, forcing it into hyperextension. Such tendon displacement must be corrected, the difficulty being to maintain the tendon in its axis without impeding its gliding movement.

The most common cause of dislocation of the extensor tendon is rheumatoid arthritis; treatment of this condition is described in the sections on the treatment of rheumatoid finger deformities (Chapter 36). It often involves imbalances at the wrist level which should be corrected. Other possible etiologies are epileptic, congenital, degenerative and traumatic.

Delayed primary repair of the ruptured sagittal fibers is sometimes possible but technically difficult if the sagittal fibers have contracted; subluxation of the extensor tendon may be corrected by a dorsal tenodesis or a sling procedure.

Dorsal tenodesis

In dorsal tenodesis a distally based strip of extensor communis is raised from the tendon of the adjacent finger and passed through or around the extensor communis of the involved digit and sutured back onto itself. The procedure can be done under wrist block anesthesia to permit active motion when the tenodesis repair is being adjusted (Burton and Melchior 1997). Wheeldon (1954) used a portion of the junctura tendinum lapped over the extensor tendon and sutured the joint capsule on the radial side (Figure 2.5).

Sling procedures

In the sling procedure, the tendon strip is raised from the subluxating tendon itself and then sutured to the deep transverse metacarpal ligament (interglenoid ligament).

According to Helal (1974) a long strip is detached from the ulnar border of the subluxating EDC tendon, it is passed under the interglenoid ligament on the radial side

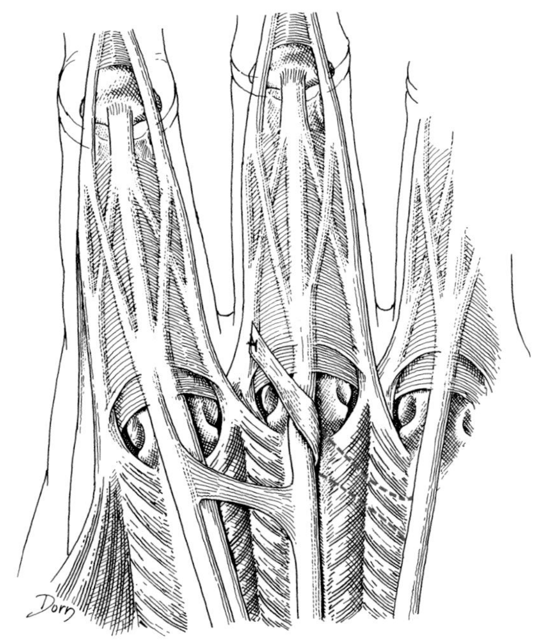

Figure 2.5

Subluxation of the long finger extensor tendon corrected by a portion of the junctura tendinum between the long and ring fingers, lapped over the subluxated tendon and sutured after correction to the MP joint capsule on the radial side (Wheeldon 1954).

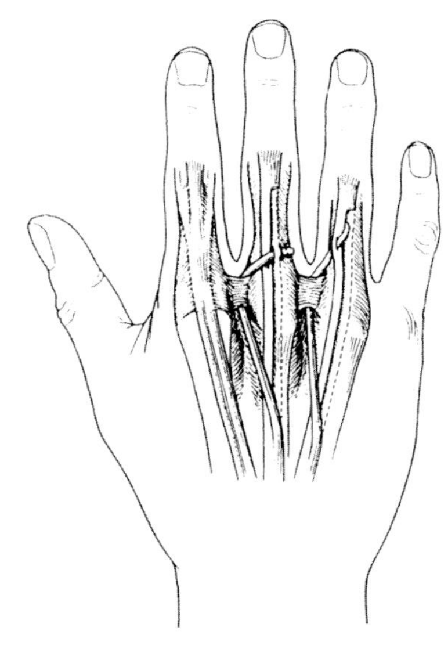

Figure 2.6

A long strip is detached from the ulnar border of the subluxated EDC tendons III and IV. It is passed under the transverse intermetacarpal (or interglenoid) ligament, which serves as a pulley, and after correction of the displaced tendon, is fixed to the extensor communis of the ring finger, or passed over the tendon and is fixed to the fibrous tissue on the ulnar side of the tendon (long finger) (Helal 1974).

of the involved finger, which serves as a pulley, and after correction is fixed to the fibrous tissue on the ulnar side of the tendon (Figure 2.6).

McCoy and Winsky (1969) used a proximally based slip from the radial side of the central extensor tendon, which was passed around the lumbrical tendon and sutured back to itself (lumbrical loop procedure) (Figure 2.7).

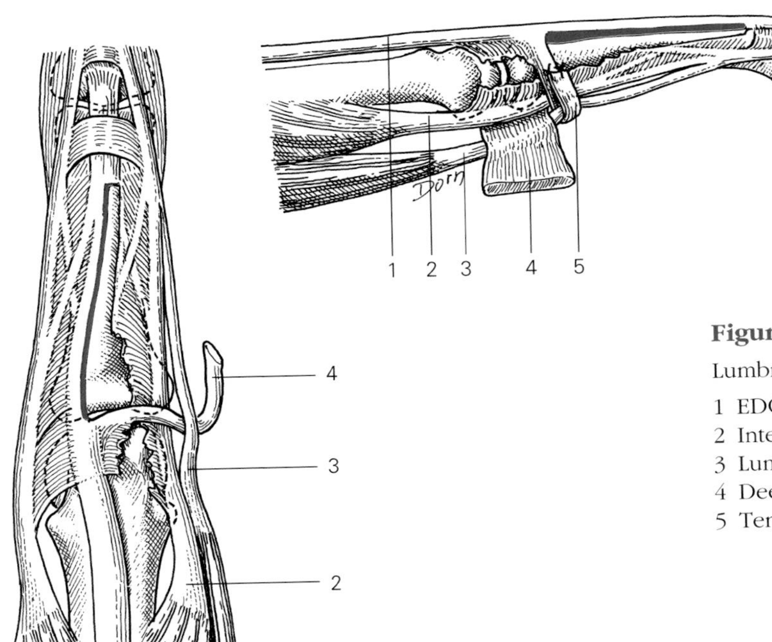

Figure 2.7

Lumbrical loop procedure (McCoy and Winsky 1969).

1 EDC tendon
2 Interosseous tendon
3 Lumbrical tendon
4 Deep transverse intermetacarpal ligament
5 Tendon slip from central extensor band

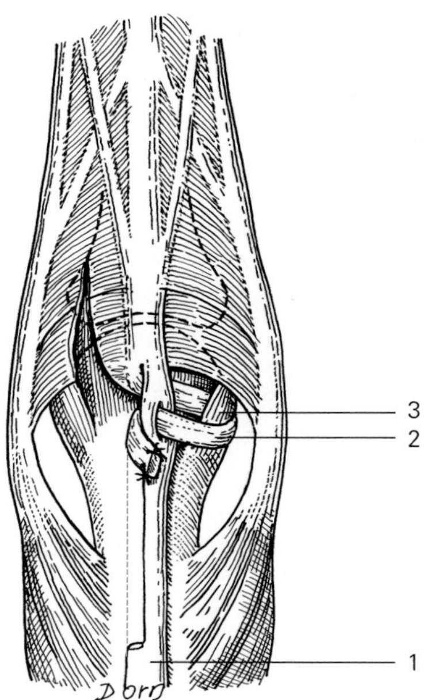

Figure 2.8
Carroll sling procedure (1987)
1 EDC tendon
2 Slip from the ulnar side of the EDC
3 Radial collateral ligament

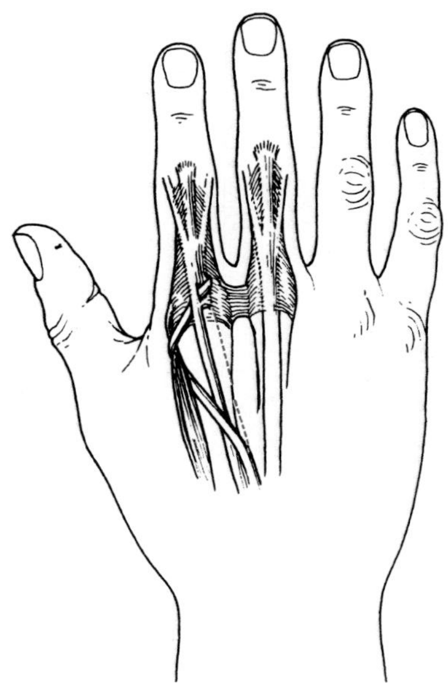

Figure 2.9
When the index finger is involved, the distal end of the EIP is detached and passed around the tendon of the first interosseous muscle.

Carroll et al (1987) use a distally based slip from the ulnar side of the EDC, wrapping it round the radial collateral ligament of the MP joint and then suturing it back to itself (Figure 2.8).

When the index finger is involved, the distal end of the extensor proprius is detached and passed around the tendon of the first dorsal interosseous muscle (Figure 2.9).

Non-operative treatment

Non-operative treatment of spontaneous and traumatic rupture of the extensor sagittal bands may be successful with plaster cast immobilization of the MP joint in full extension for 4 weeks, in early cases before contraction of the sagittal fibers (Ishizuki 1990).

Late reconstruction of the extensor mechanism of the thumb

Lesions of the extensor mechanism of the thumb require a careful physical examination because the IP and the MP joint of the thumb may be extended through the insertion of the intrinsic muscles of the thumb into the dorsal apparatus.

In the distal forearm and at the wrist level

The extensor tendons of the thumb form two groups which border the anatomical snuffbox. In each group, the ALP and EPB laterally, and the EPL medially, runs into a separate fibro-osseous compartment within its own synovial sheath (Figure 2.10). It is important not to use the same transfer for the EPL and for the APL and EPB, whose ranges of motion differ greatly (see Chapter 10).

Ruptures of the EPL are the most common lesions of the thumb extensor apparatus. The clinician should not be misled by the presence of extension movements at the distal thumb phalanx. The impossibility for the patient of moving the thumb ray into retroposition, with the thumb in abduction, is the sign of an EPL rupture. Exploration is effected through a curved longitudinal incision. The gap between the two tendon extremities is usually important. A tendon graft from the PL can be a solution; most authors use an EIP tendon transfer (Figure 2.11).

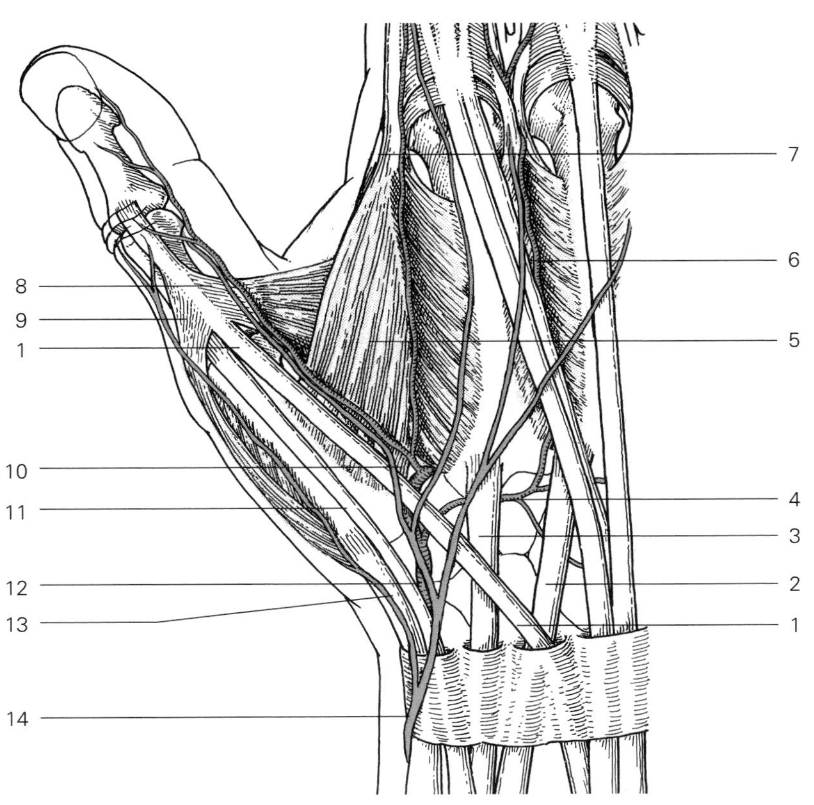

Figure 2.10

The extensor tendon of the thumb

1 EPL
2 ECRB
3 ECRL
4 Dorsal carpal artery
5 First dorsal interosseous
6 Second metacarpal artery
7 First lumbrical muscle
8 Adductor pollicis expansion to EPL tendon
9 APB expansion to EPL tendon
10 First dorsal metacarpal artery
11 EPB
12 Radial artery
13 APL
14 Sensory branch radial nerve

Figure 2.11

Rupture of the EPL tendon. EIP tendon transfer.

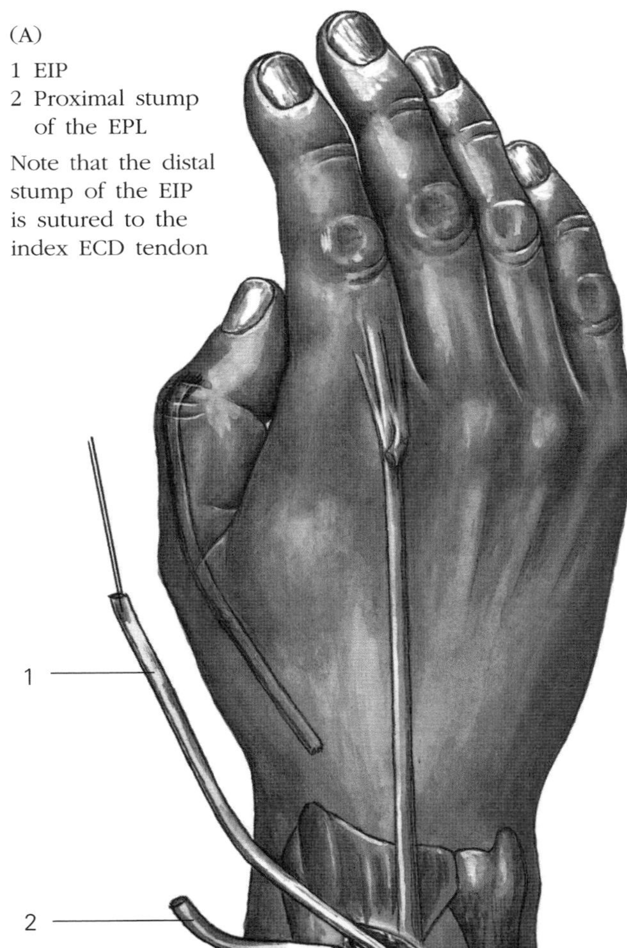

(A)

1 EIP
2 Proximal stump of the EPL

Note that the distal stump of the EIP is sutured to the index ECD tendon

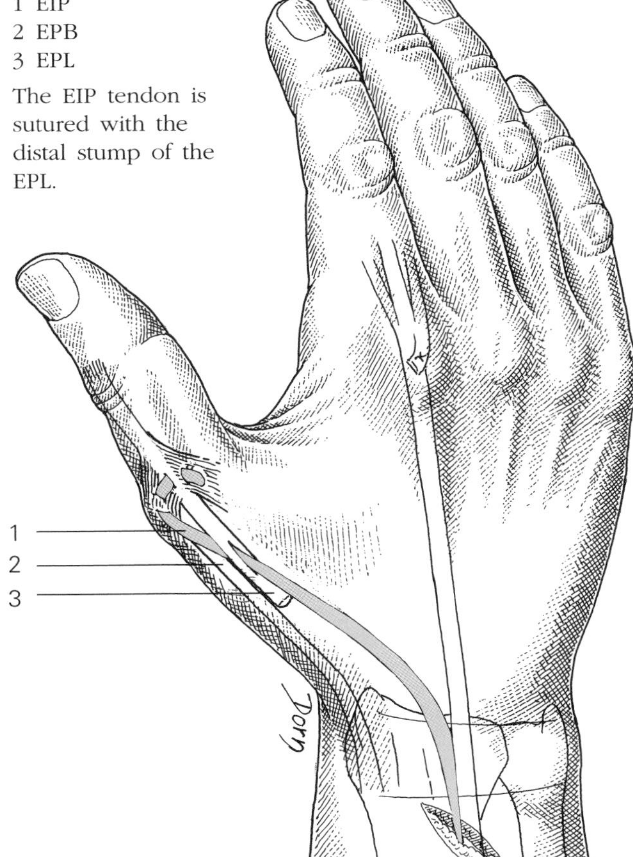

(B)

1 EIP
2 EPB
3 EPL

The EIP tendon is sutured with the distal stump of the EPL.

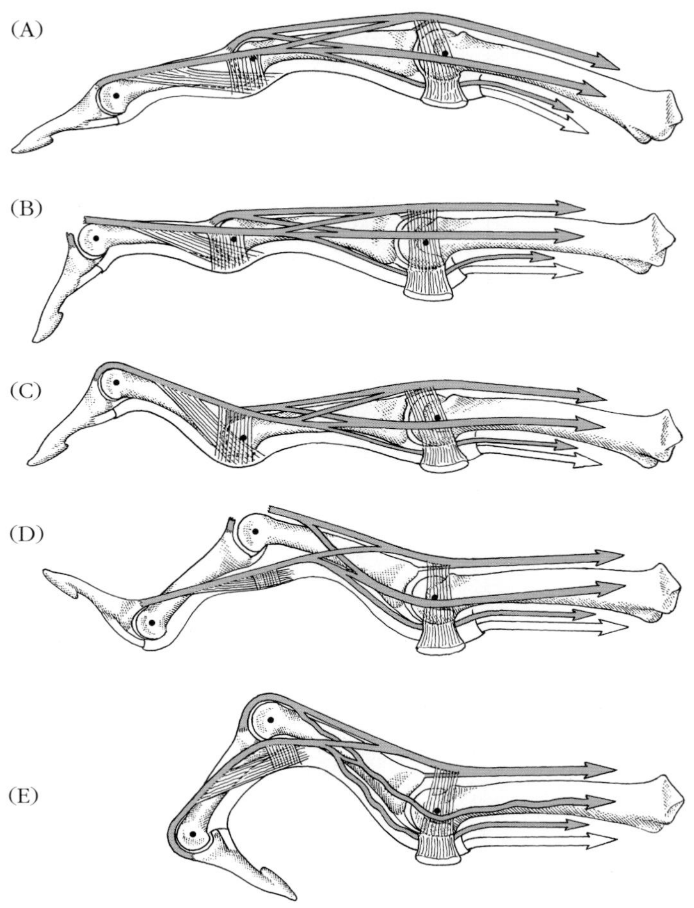

Figure 2.12

The extensor apparatus of the fingers. A lesion of the extensor mechanism at one level of the multiarticular chain may alter the balance of the three phalanges.

A Normal balance of the finger
B Mallet deformity
C Swan-neck deformity
D Boutonnière deformity
E Claw deformity

At the thumb level

A delayed tendon repair may be attempted if the distal joints have retained some mobility. If the joints have become fixed in too much flexion, arthrodesis may be indicated.

Chronic extensor mechanism imbalance in the fingers

The three finger joints, together with the three phalanges, constitute a multiarticular chain. A deformity at one level may alter the balance of the whole finger (Landsmeer 1958).

Deformities caused by chronic extensor mechanism imbalance can occur at each finger joint: MP, PIP or DIP (Figure 2.12). They are usually studied individually and authors use different classifications for each deformity. For a long time we have used different classifications for boutonnière and swan neck deformities (Tubiana 1988). Later (Tubiana 1999) we adopted a new classification in four stages that we use for all chronic finger deformities in association with a musculotendinous imbalance. This classification was inspired by Nalebuff's classification for rheumatoid swan neck (Nalebuff 1969). It differs because it takes into account the three finger joints and not just the PIP, and is general enough to be used for most finger deformities associated with a musculotendinous imbalance, whatever their type or etiology (Tubiana and Dubert 2000).

- Stage 1: Purely dynamic imbalance. There is no limitation of passive motion in any joint of the finger, whatever the position of the other two joints.
- Stage 2: Each finger joint has complete passive mobility; however, limitation of motion in one joint is influenced by the position of the joint in the multiarticular chain. The deformity may be caused by tenodesis, muscular contracture or tendinous adhesion.
- Stage 3: Fixed defomities without articular lesion. Limitation of joint mobility is not influenced by the position of the other joints. This limitation may be due to soft tissue contracture or adhesions. No articular surface alterations are seen on X-rays.
- Stage 4: Joint stiffness with bone and articular lesions.

This classification is easy to remember and avoids joint measurements in degrees. We believe that this assessment helps to clarify the therapeutic indications. It is particularly useful at the level of the PIP joint; however, it can be used at the DIP and MP levels.

Chronic mallet finger deformity

The term mallet finger denotes the persistent flexion of the distal phalanx resulting from a lesion of the terminal extensor tendon. Mallet finger deformities may result from several causes, the most frequent are traumatic but they are also common in rheumatoid patients with DIP joint synovitis (see the Chapter on rheumatoid arthritis).

Stage 1

In stage 1 the only deformity is the drop of the distal phalanx; there is no limitation of passive motion. There is some disagreement about when a mallet finger can be regarded as 'chronic' and when the non-surgical treatment applied to acute injuries becomes contraindicated.

Patel et al (1986) described good results with uninterrupted splint immobilization of the distal phalanx in

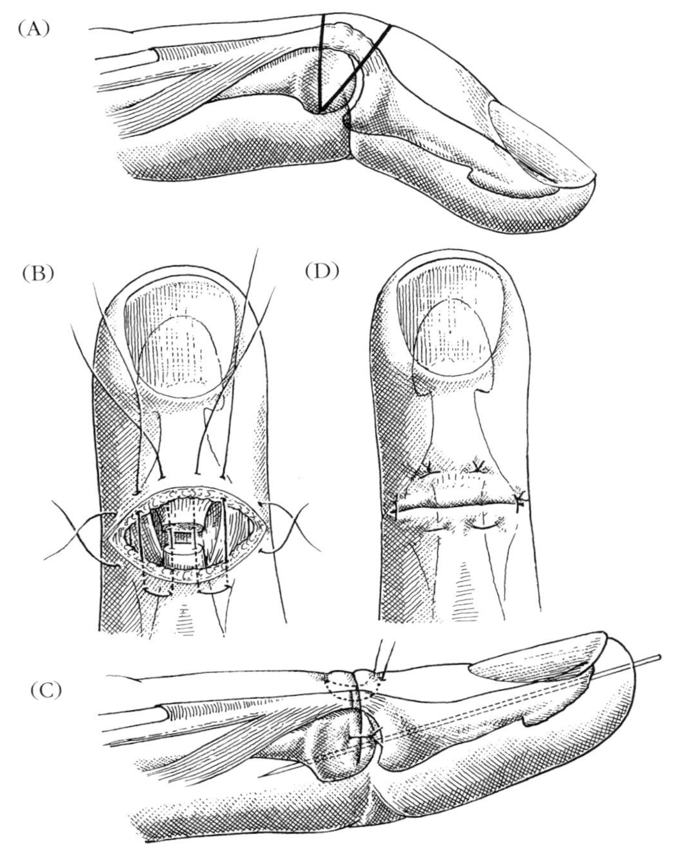

Figure 2.13

Correction of stage 1 chronic mallet finger. Mallet deformity.

A Excision of skin and tendon callus
B Mattress sutures are passed through the skin and tendon
C K-wire fixes the terminal phalanx in extension
D Sutures are tied

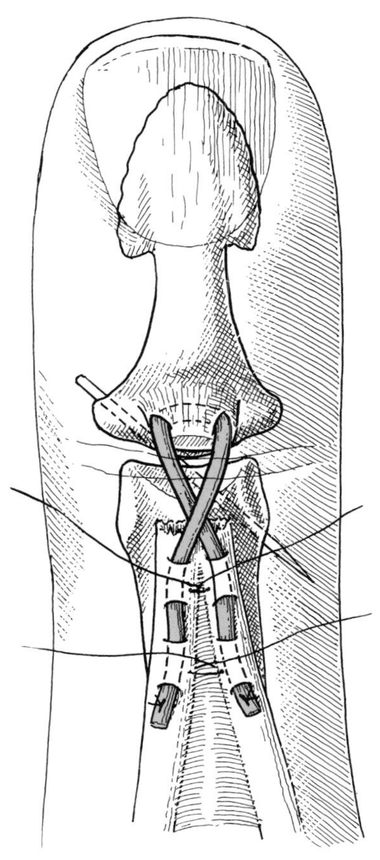

Figure 2.14

Tendon graft used to bridge a gap in the terminal extensor tendon.

extension for at least 8 weeks, beginning as late as 18 weeks. The history with respect to age of the lesion and type of injury is important. After 18 weeks, the percentage of failures after a non-operative treatment increases steadily with the age of the lesion.

Surgical treatment of stage 1 chronic mallet finger

Brooks (1976) and Iselin et al (1977) (Figure 2.13) have independently developed a technique that involves the following steps (Albertoni 1988).

- A transverse ellipse of skin, about 2–3 mm wide, is excised from the dorsal aspect of the DIP joint.
- The tendon callus at the same level is excised (about 2 mm wide), preferably without opening the capsule.
- Tenolysis of the proximal segment of the extensor aponeurosis is carried out over the middle phalanx.
- Three 4-0 monofilament nylon mattress sutures are passed en bloc through the skin, tendon and capsule on one side, and then on the other. The sutures are not tied immediately, but are crossed over to check that full extension of the joint can be obtained.
- Graner (1988) added a K-wire, which fixes the terminal phalanx in slight hyperextension.
- The sutures are then tied.
- The digit is externally splinted. The K-wire is left in place for 6 weeks.

Tendon grafts are used to correct a mallet finger after abrasion, with loss of tendon substance. The skin cover must be adequate, and the joint mobile. A thin tendon graft, 2 mm wide and 6 cm long, is taken from one of the wrist flexors. The middle part of the graft is anchored to the fibrous tissue at the base of the terminal phalanx. The two ends of the graft are then crossed over the midline and passed through the lateral extensor tendons. The distal phalanx is fixed in extension by a K-wire. The graft is adjusted by means of several stitches, whose knots are buried (Figure 2.14).

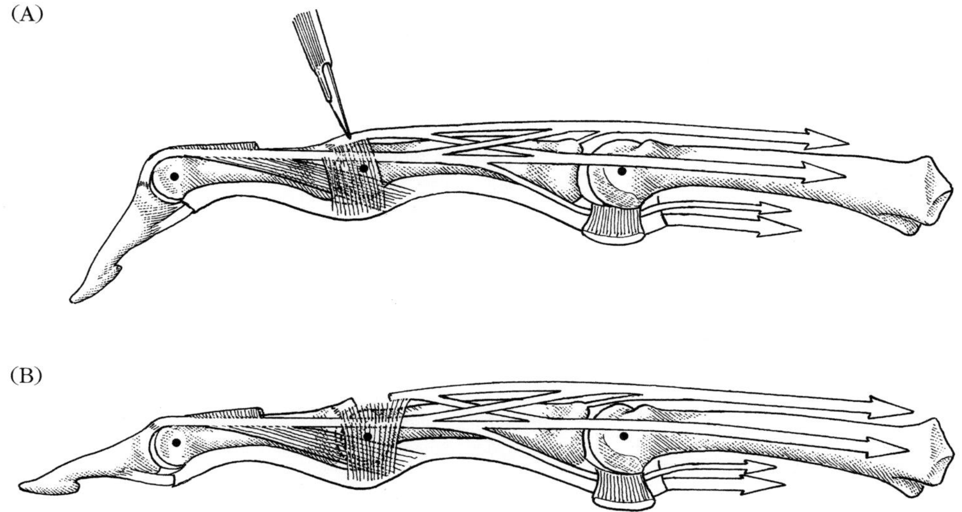

Figure 2.15

Tenotomy of the central extensor tendon.

A Division of the central extensor tendon (spiral fibres and other transverse structures at this level are spared)
B Proximal retraction of the extensor apparatus

Indications for surgical treatment
As results after surgical treatment are not always satisfactory – correction of the deformity may be incomplete and active flexion of the terminal phalanx may be reduced – stage 1 chronic mallet fingers should only be operated on if flexion deformity of the distal phalanx is important and interferes with manual function. However, the cosmetic aspect can also be of importance for some patients.

Stage 2

Stage 2 comprises chronic mallet finger with hyperextension of the PIP joint. PIP deformity is caused by excessive traction of the central extensor tendon inserted on the base of the middle phalanx, secondary to the rupture of the extensor terminal tendon at the level of the DIP. In stage 2, in spite of the deformity the two interphalangeal joints have a complete passive mobility.

The most physiologic treatment is a tenotomy of the central extensor tendon (Fowler 1949, Harris 1966, Bowers and Hurst 1978) (Figure 2.15). Dividing the central extensor tendon allows the terminal extensor tendon and the fibrous callus to retract proximally. There is little risk of a boutonnière deformity if the spiral fibers and other transverse structures that prevent the lateral extensor tendons from pulling apart are spared. The two interphalangeal joints are immobilized in extension for 3 weeks. Then, only the DIP is maintained in extension for 3 more weeks.

Littler's spiral tendon graft is another elegant and more sophisticated technique for correction of the deformities of the two interphalangeal joints, when both joints are mobile (see Figure 2.33).

Arthrodesis of the distal joint is the safest treatment if the swan neck deformity is increasing rapidly.

Stages 3 and 4

Fixed deformity is present in stages 3 and 4. Persistent flexion deformity of the distal phalanx, that is interfering with manual function, may benefit from fusion of the DIP joint in slight flexion (Stern and Kastrup 1998) (Figure 2.16).

Chronic boutonnière deformity

Division, avulsion or progressive elongation of the central conjoint extensor tendon over the PIP joint can cause a dynamic imbalance of the extensor linkage system. This central tendon lesion, whatever its etiology (traumatic, rheumatoid arthritis or osteoarthritis), involves alterations of the transverse retinacular fibers that lead to volar subluxation of the lateral extensor tendons and form a boutonnière (buttonhole) through which the fixed PIP joint protrudes. The proximal retraction of the central extensor tendon increases the traction on the distal joint, which becomes hyperextended.

Boutonnière deformity is a progressive condition. When left untreated, the dorsal central tendon and dorsal transverse retinacular fibers tighten and the lateral extensor tendons are restrained volar to the PIP joint axis. The oblique retinacular ligaments (ORL), which are inserted distally on the lateral tendons at the level of the middle phalanx and proximally on the fibrous flexor sheath and the periosteum of the proximal phalanx, also tighten, fixing the middle phalanx in flexion and the distal phalanx in extension. Haines (1951) and Zancolli (1968) have demonstrated this contracture by means of a clinical test.

In the absence of contracture of the oblique fibers, the distal phalanx can be passively flexed while the middle

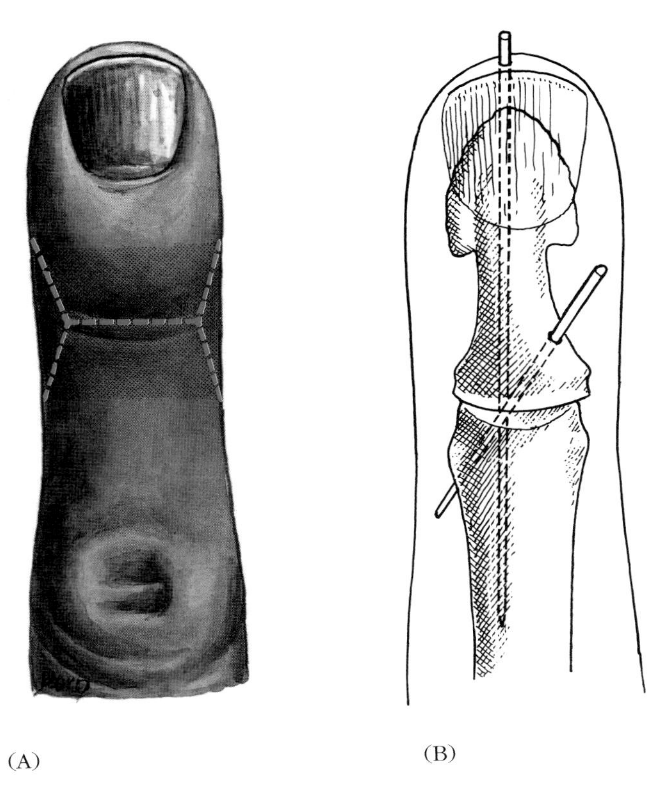

(A) (B)

Figure 2.16
Arthrodesis of the distal joint. (A) A four-flap exposure allows a large exposure of the joint. (B) An axial wire is placed through the DIP joint and a second oblique wire impedes rotation.

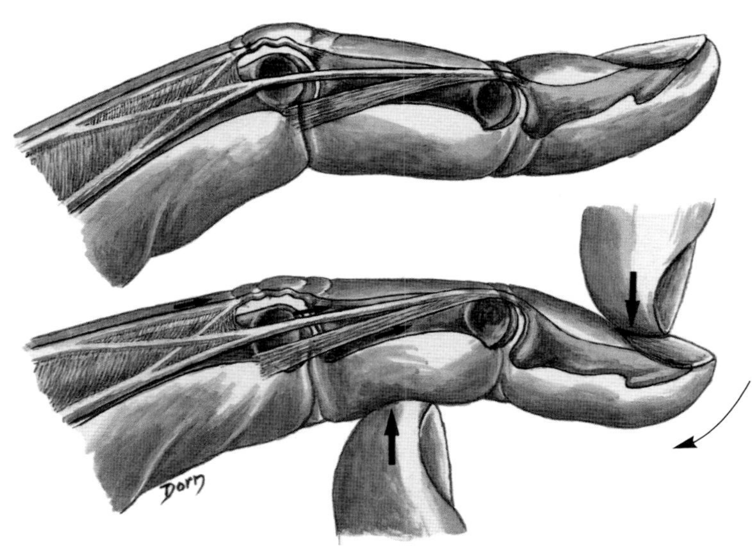

Figure 2.17
Boutonnière deformity stage 1. In the absence of contraction of the ORL, the distal phalanx can be passively flexed while the middle phalanx is maintained in extension. The Haines–Zancolli retinacular test is negative.

phalanx is maintained in extension, the retinacular test is then said to be negative (Figure 2.17). When these fibers shorten, passive extension of the middle phalanx prevents flexion of the distal phalanx and the retinacular test is termed positive (Figure 2.18). Secondary joint changes ensue.

Stage 1

There is no limitation of passive joint motion in any finger joint in stage 1. Splinting is indicated in extension at the PIP level, combined with active flexion exercises

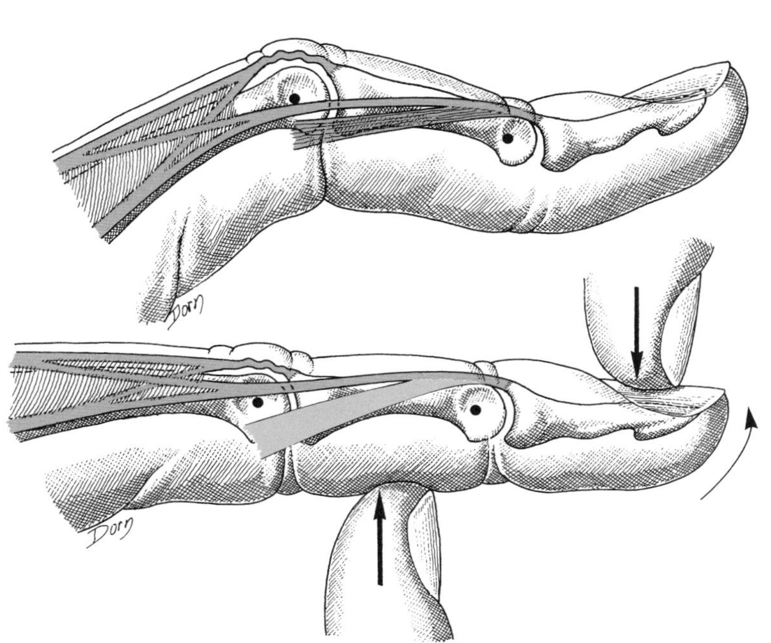

Figure 2.18
Boutonnière deformity stage 2. Each finger joint has complete passive mobility. However, when the middle phalanx is maintained in extension, flexion of the distal phalanx is not possible. The Haines–Zancolli test is positive because of the fixed contracture of the URL (in red).

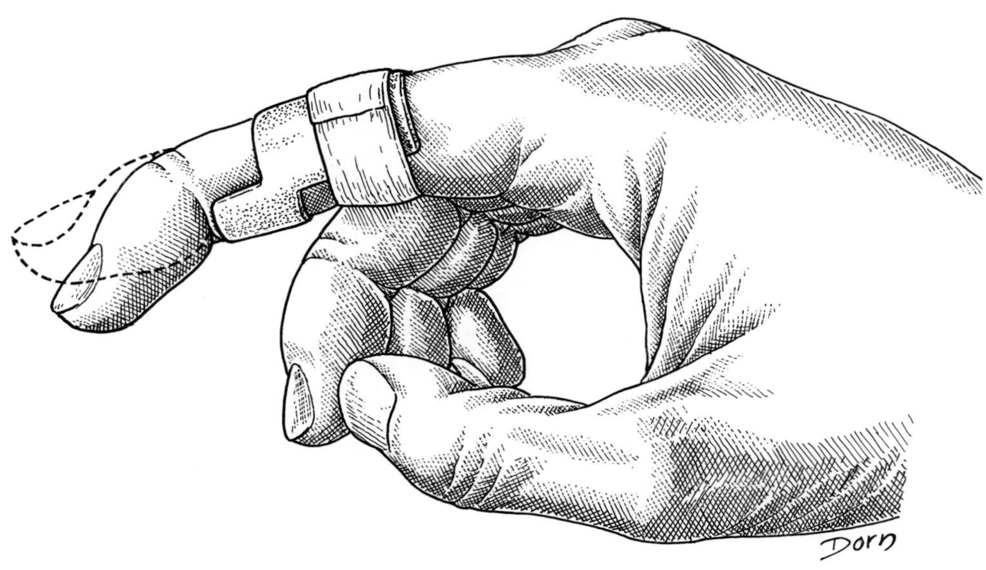

Figure 2.19

Stack's splint maintaining PIP joint in extension, leaving the DIP and MP joints free.

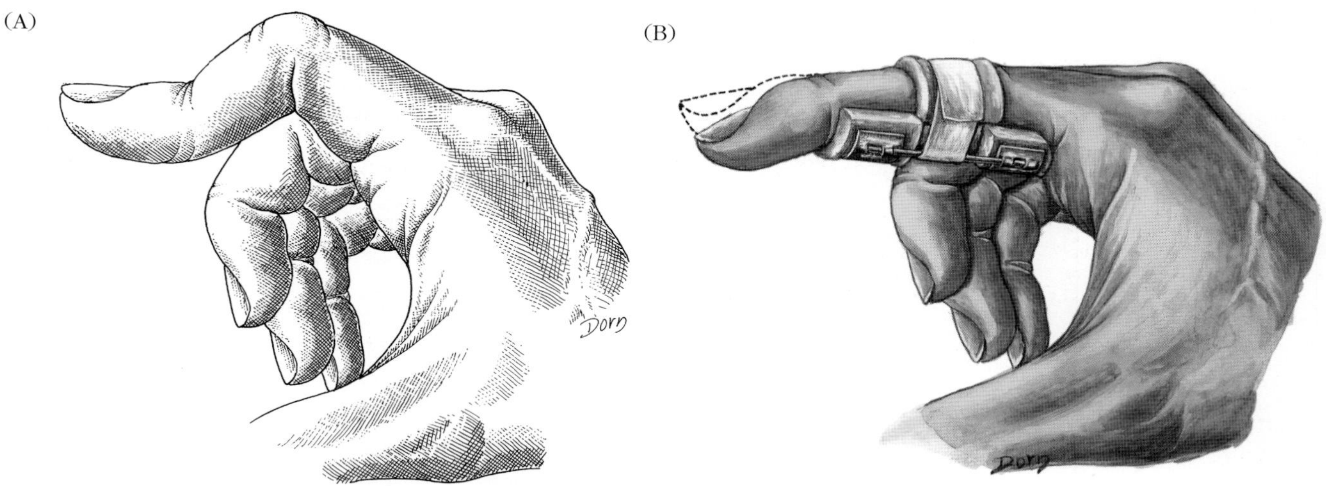

Figure 2.20

The Bunnell safety pin. As the correction of the PIP joint flexion contracture progresses, the strap on the splint is tightened on a daily basis.

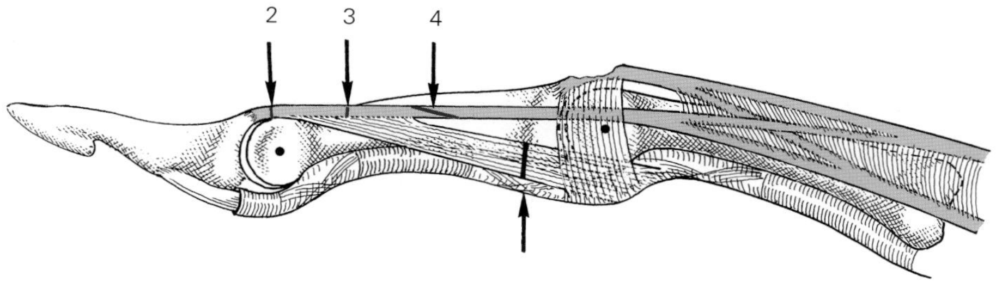

Figure 2.21

Different sites of tenotomy used in the treatment of boutonnière deformity.

1 Division of oblique retinacular ligament (ORL) (Zancolli 1968)
2 Tenotomy of terminal extensor tendon (Fowler 1949)
3 Tenotomy of terminal extensor tendon proximal to distal insertions of the ORL (Dolphin 1965)
4 Oblique tenotomy of lateral extensor tendons (our preferred procedure)

of the DIP. The PIP joint must be maintained in full extension, without allowing any flexion of that joint. A Stack-type splint for a dorsal Alumafoam splint (Figure 2.19) or a cast is equally acceptable. We do not use percutaneous pinning of the PIP joint.

Passive flexion exercises of the DIP prevent contracture and mobilize the lateral extensor tendons and ORL to their normal anatomic position. This splinting and exercise program must be maintained for 2–3 months to prevent recurrence. At the first sign of recurrent flexion, the splint is reapplied and worn continuously for an additional 2 weeks.

Stage 2

The tenodesis effect is seen in stage 2. When the middle phalanx is maintained in extension, flexion of the distal phalanx is not possible. The Haines-Zancolli retinacular test is positive. Fixed contracture of the ORL prevents passive flexion of the distal joint. However, passive correction of the flexor deformity at the PIP joint is still possible, as well as complete flexion of the three joints, and the complete closing of the finger is not disturbed. Corrective splinting with exercises is again indicated (Figure 2.20).

Surgical treatment may occasionally be considered, to correct the distal joint hyperextension, and will theoretically consist of a partial resection of the contracted oblique retinacular ligament (Zancolli 1968). Tenotomy of the terminal extensor tendon has been suggested by Fowler (1959) in an attempt to restore the balance of extensor forces. Division of the distal extensor tendon would correct hyperextension of the DIP joint and reduce the flexion of the PIP joint, when joints are supple and if there is no adhesion of the extensor apparatus (Figure 2.21).

A surgical shortening of the central extensor tendon has been advocated. Although it is technically possible, surgical correction is fraught with pitfalls, especially the risk of stiffness at the PIP level. Almost all fingers in stage 1 and many in stage 2 are best treated without surgery.

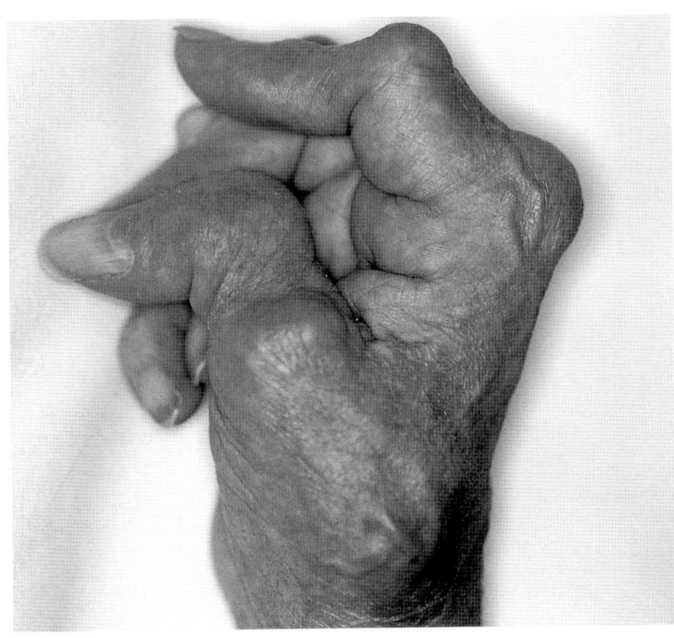

Figure 2.22

Boutonnière deformity – stage 2.

Stage 3

There is a fixed deformity with articular surfaces intact. Either the PIP or the DIP joint or both may present a limitation of motion that is not influenced by any position of the other finger joints (Figure 2.22). PIP flexion is still possible (Figure 2.23); however, complete closing of the finger is lost. Because flexion of the distal phalanx is responsible for the completion and strength of the grasp the evolution from stage 2 to stage 3 is of great functional importance. The progression of the contracture can be described as involving first the extensor apparatus, then volar plates and ligaments of the PIP and the DIP joints.

Conservative treatment with a combination of static and active splints over a period of at least 2 or 3 months should be attempted. As the correction of the PIP joint flexion contracture progresses the splint is altered. If the Bunnell safety pin is used, the strap on the splint is tightened on a daily basis (see Figure 2.20). This treatment is carried on for maximal recovery. If full passive extension of the PIP joint is achieved (this may require several weeks), the correction is maintained with a circular plaster cast permitting DIP flexion or with a dynamic splint for at least 4 more weeks. If, despite adequate conservative treatment, there is a persistent deformity, a useful range of PIP flexion may provide good function. In any event, splintage and physiotherapy constitute an essential step before any operation. Results from surgery are better when joint deformities are passively corrected preoperatively.

Surgical indications should take into account both the discomfort experienced by the patient and the possibilities of repair. It is difficult to evaluate how much the flexion deformity of the DIP joint bothers the patient, because this is measured not only by the degree of contracture but also by other factors – aetiology, profession, sex, esthetic considerations, and the finger involved (an extension deficit of the middle phalanx is less bothersome in the ulnar than the radial fingers).

The flexion deficit of the distal phalanx can be more disabling to the grip than the extension deficit in the PIP, especially in the ulnar fingers. On the other hand, recon-

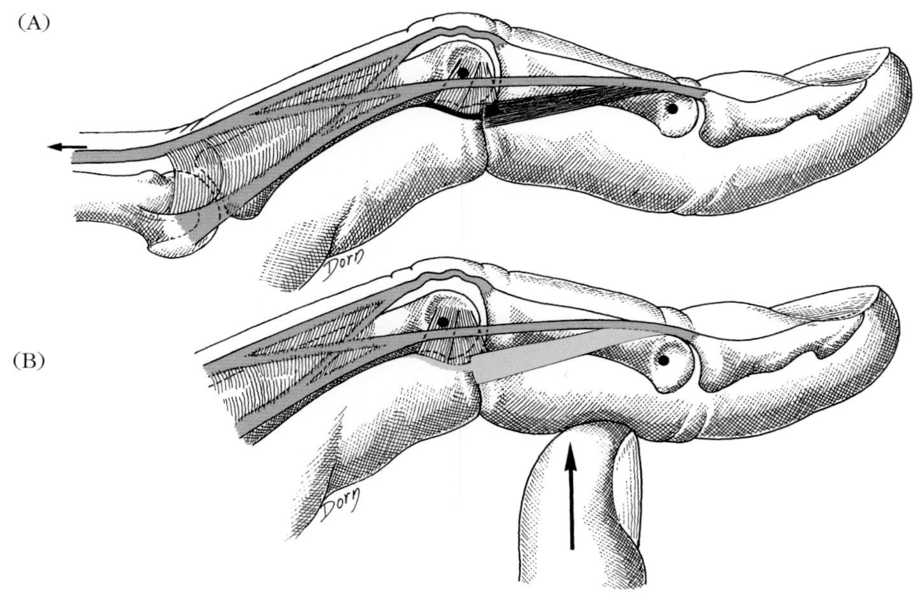

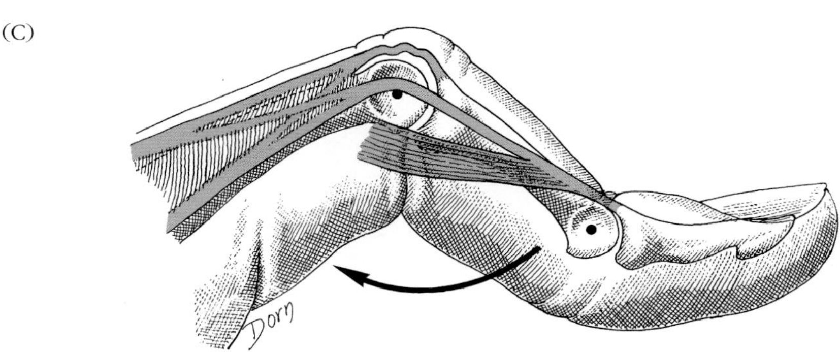

Figure 2.23

Boutonnière deformity stage 3. Limitation of PIP and DIP joint mobility caused by soft tissue contracture.

A Proximal retraction of extensor apparatus causing MP joint hyperextension
B Contracture of ORL limiting flexion of distal phalanx. Contracture of PIP joint volar plate and accessory collateral ligaments limiting extension of PIP joint
C However, PIP joint flexion is still possible

The flexion deficit of the distal phalanx can be more disabling to the grip than the extension deficit in the PIP joint, especially in the ulnar fingers.

struction of the extensor apparatus at the PIP joint is difficult, scarring is much more important in a traumatic boutonnière than in a rheumatoid boutonnière deformity, and surgery must not jeopardize flexor function in an attempt to gain extension. Therefore, indications for surgery should be cautiously defined, and the candidate should be selected carefully (Steichen et al 1982).

Many surgical procedures have been proposed for fixed boutonnière deformity. They include two distinct steps: the surgical correction of the deformities and the repair of the extensor apparatus. The surgical correction of a boutonnière deformity requires a rebalancing of the extensor system, deviating the excess of tone at the distal joint to the proximal joint (Littler and Eaton 1967). Both the extension deficit of the PIP joint and the flexion deficit of the distal joint must be corrected. Correction of the flexion contracture at the PIP joint is usually achieved by liberation of the posterior structures.

Structures are usually not clear in a chronic, boutonnière deformity, especially of traumatic origin, where the different elements of the extensor apparatus meet in a sheet of fibrous tissue that covers the joint (Figure 2.24). The central extensor tendon and the two lateral extensor tendons are located. Repair of the extensor apparatus includes shortening of the central extensor tendon and correction of the volar subluxation of the lateral extensor tendons.

Reconstruction of the central extensor tendon is the simplest way to restore the anatomical situation, but it is only possible when the tissue loss is limited. The fibrous callus on the central tendon is resected for about 3 mm (Figure 2.25). The shortened central tendon is sutured (Figure 2.26). The volar subluxation of the lateral extensor tendons is corrected; these are sutured one to the other at their distal end (Figure 2.27). The distal phalanx is flexed (Figure 2.28). If this is not possible, an oblique tenotomy of the lateral extensor tendons is performed (Figure 2.29).

Several possibilities then exist:

1. The two interphalangeal joints can be placed passively in extension or in flexion.
2. Passive extension of the PIP joint is obtained but it is not possible to flex the distal joint completely, regardless of the position of the PIP joint. This may be caused by either adhesion of the distal part of the extensor apparatus or stiffness of the DIP joint.

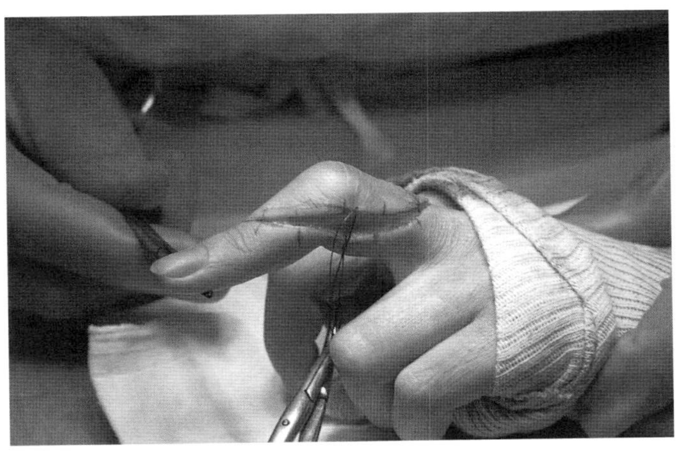

(A)

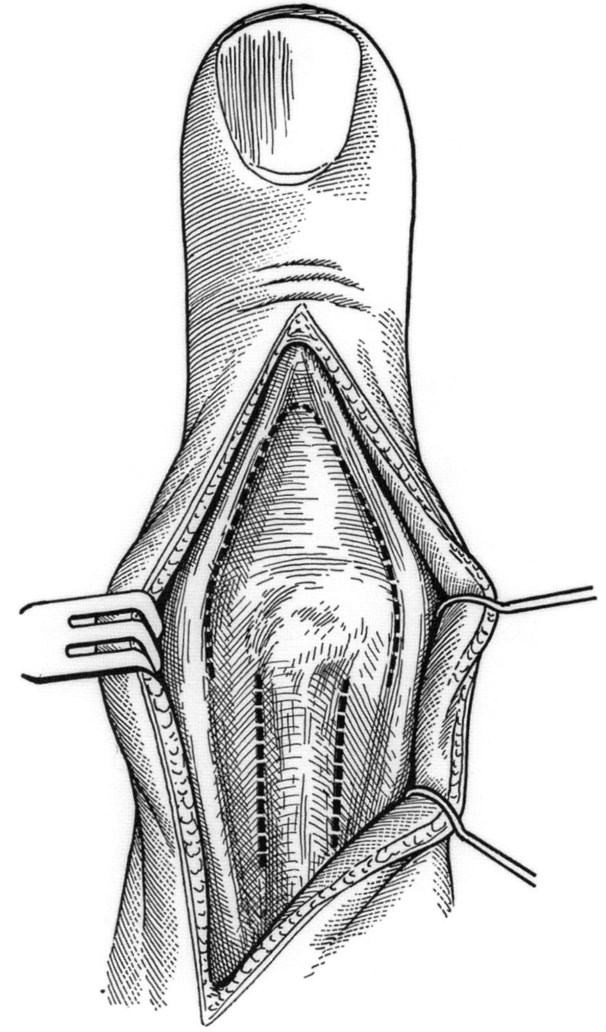

(B)

Figure 2.24

(A) A dorsal longitudinal curved incision is made over the PIP joint. The approach should be large in order to permit wide access to the extensor apparatus. (B) The central and the two lateral extensor tendons are located.

2. Passive extension of the PIP joint is not obtained by liberation of the posterior structures.

A liberation of the anterior structures is considered. The fibrous flexor tendon sheath is opened at the level of the pulley C1. Any tenosynovitis of the flexor tendons should be removed and the freedom of the tendons should be tested. If necessary, the proximal 'check reins' of the volar plate are divided. Care must be exercised when freeing the joint, so that excessive surgery does not lead to hyperextension of the PIP joint resulting in a swan neck deformity. (See also 'The rheumatoid boutonnière deformity' in Chapter 36.)

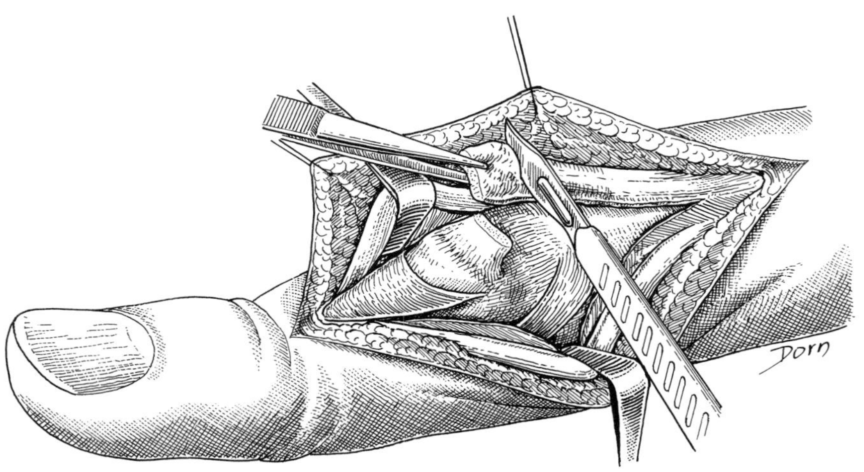

Figure 2.25

Shortening of the central extensor tendon for about 3 mm. The distal insertion of the tendon is preserved.

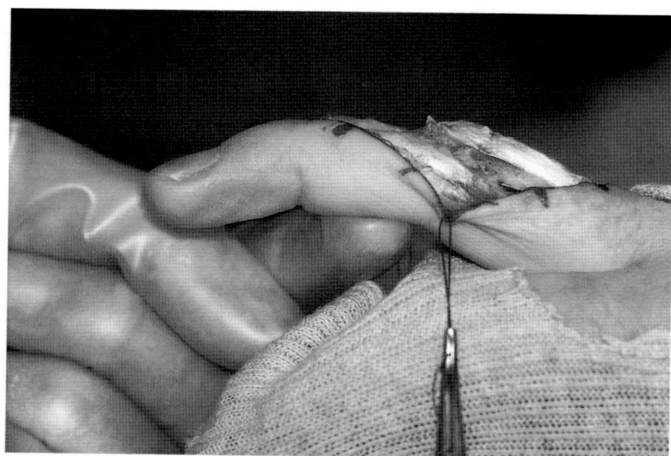

Figure 2.26
The central tendon is sutured to itself.

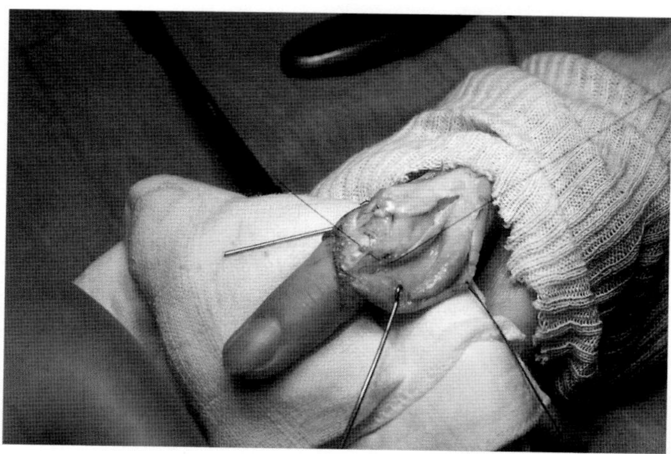

Figure 2.27
The volar subluxation of the lateral extensor tendon is corrected.

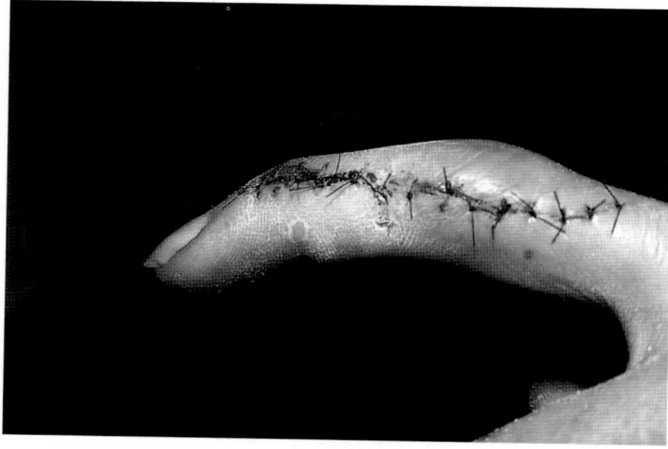

Figure 2.28
The distal phalanx is flexed. Skin sutured.

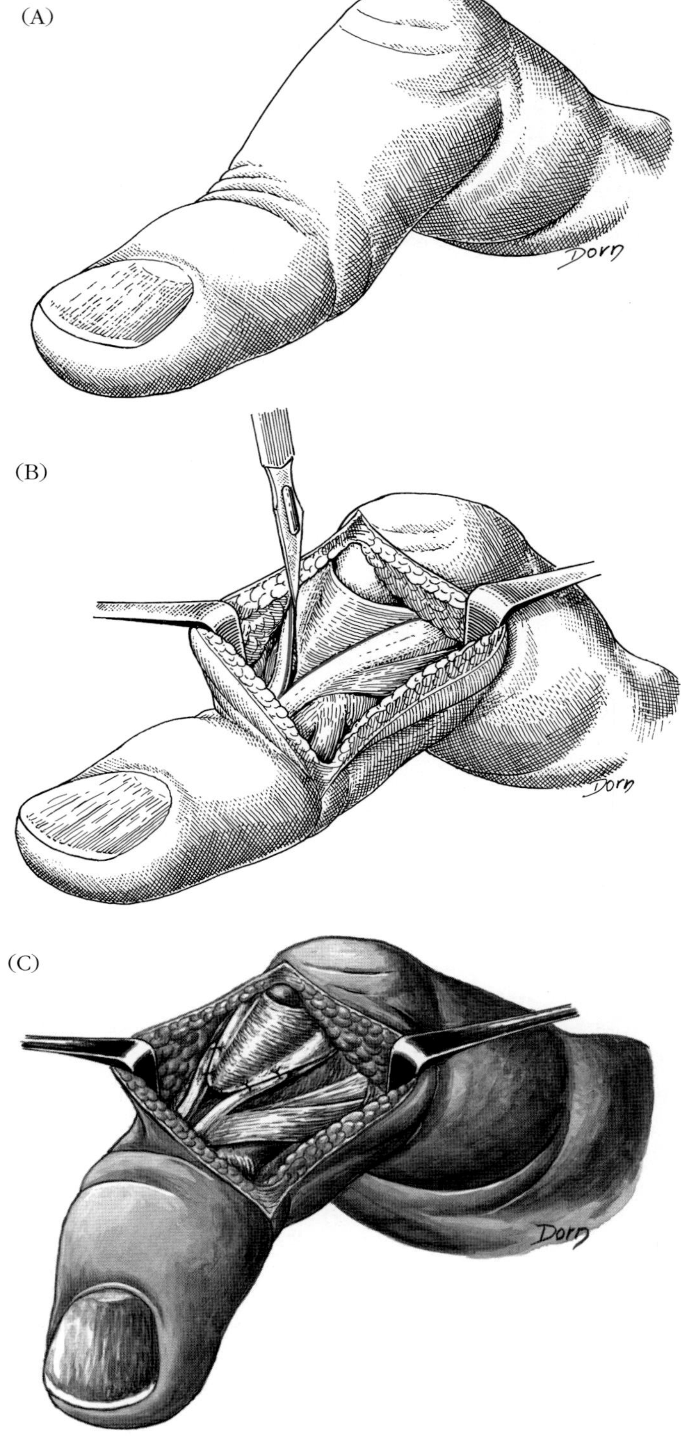

Figure 2.29
Oblique tenotomy of the lateral extensor tendons.

A Incision on the dorsum of the middle phalanx
B The extensor apparatus at the level of the idle phalanx is freed with a blunt spatula passed under the lateral tendons. Then the two lateral tendons are divided obliquely
C The distal phalanx is flexed. The obliqueness of the division allows lengthening of the distal extensor apparatus without loss of control between the ends of the divided tndons

Stage 4

Radiography shows significant articular lesions at the PIP level. In cases of severe fixed flexion deformity of the PIP joint, arthrodesis of the PIP joint is a reliable procedure. It can be combined with an oblique tenotomy of the two lateral extensor tendons to obtain flexion of the distal phalanx.

Arthroplasty of the PIP joint provides another alternative when the extensor system is salvageable.

Tenotomy of the lateral extensor tendons can also be done alone if the lack of distal joint flexion is more disabling than the lack of PIP joint extension (Figure 2.29).

In cases of stiffness of the distal joint, it may be useful to free the volar plate and hold the joint in 30° of flexion with a temporary K-wire.

Chronic swan neck deformity

Swan neck deformity is a posture of the finger in which the PIP joint is hyperextended and the DIP joint is flexed. Swan neck is the reciprocal of the boutonnière. Swan neck deformity is not the result of a direct injury of the extensor apparatus of the finger. This deformity is a dynamic finger imbalance caused by excessive traction of the central extensor tendon inserted on the base of the middle phalanx. Hyperextension of the PIP joint causes dorsal displacement of the lateral extensor tendons toward the midline. Their line of action being thus shortened, their extensor effect on the distal phalanx consequently diminishes and at the same time the FDP tendon, stretched by the PIP joint hyperextension, has its action reinforced. The result is a deformity that combines PIP hyperextension with DIP flexion (Figure 2.12C). It is important to realize that the DIP posture is dependent on the PIP posture. Any factor at any level of the osteoarticular chain that reinforces traction of the extensor tendon on the base of the middle phalanx may give rise to a swan neck deformity. These lesions have a variety of etiologies: traumatic (fractures, dislocations with deviation of the tendons, volar plate injury at the PIP joint, or mallet deformity), spastic conditions, rheumatoid arthritis, generalized systemic ligamentous laxity, etc. The multiplicity of causes explains the number of procedures proposed for the correction of this deformity. Treatment must be directed at the etiology whenever possible, and correct the deformity. Any skeletal deviation that accompanies swan neck deformity should be corrected, since re-establishing the alignment of the skeleton will rebalance the extensor mechanism. The PIP joint volar plate laxity must also be corrected, to prevent recurrence of the deformity. As this dynamic imbalance can progress to a fixed deformity of the PIP joint in extension, it is important to treat swan neck deformity at an early stage, when it is still correctable.

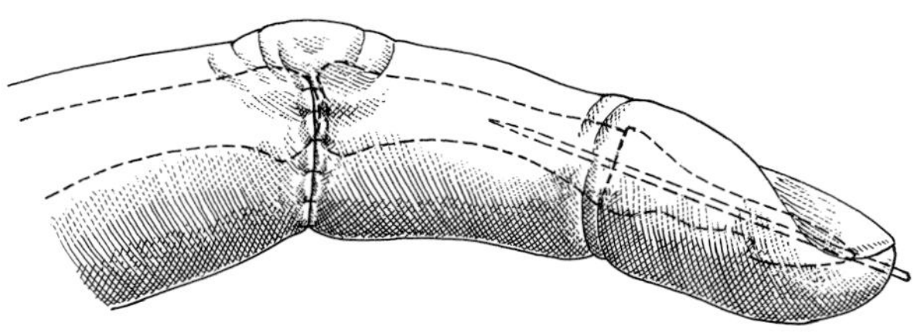

Figure 2.30
Dermadesis associated with DIP joint fusion.

Stage 1

There is no limitation of passive motion in any finger joint at this stage.

Tenotomy of the central extensor tendon (Fowler 1949) is theoretically the most physiological treatment for correction of the dynamic finger imbalance. This technique has already been described (see Chronic mallet finger, stage 2). However, because of the risk of creating a boutonnière deformity, most authors use other methods to prevent PIP joint hyperextension, such as dermadesis (Figure 2.30), sometimes associated with PIP fusion or a flexor superficialis tenodesis.

Flexor superficialis tenodesis is the simplest passive method of correction. One slip of the FDS is divided 2 cm proximal to the PIP joint, but is left attached distally. It is used to prevent hyperextension of the PIP joint. The slip is fixed to the flexor tendon sheath, proximally to the PIP joint (Figure 2.31) and preferably on the opposite side in order to have a double effect; it will act as a check rein against extension of the PIP joint and as a pulley for the flexor. However, it does not directly correct the distal joint flexion. The PIP joint is then temporarily fixed in 20° flexion with a K-wire.

An attachment into the distal extremity of the proximal phalanx is indicated for the spastic hand, where a strong tenodesis is necessary (Figure 2.32).

Stage 2

The three finger joints have a complete passive mobility; however, one joint has a limitation of motion influenced by the position of another joint. Two mechanisms are responsible for the deformity.

1. The oblique retinacular ligament (ORL) has lost its tenodesis action on the PIP joint preventing its hyperextension; the ORL should be reconstructed.
2. IPP flexion is limited by a tenodesis effect of MP joint extension on the intrinsic muscles.

Oblique retinacular reconstruction

Littler and Eaton (1967) have given the principle of the method for ORL reconstruction and have successively

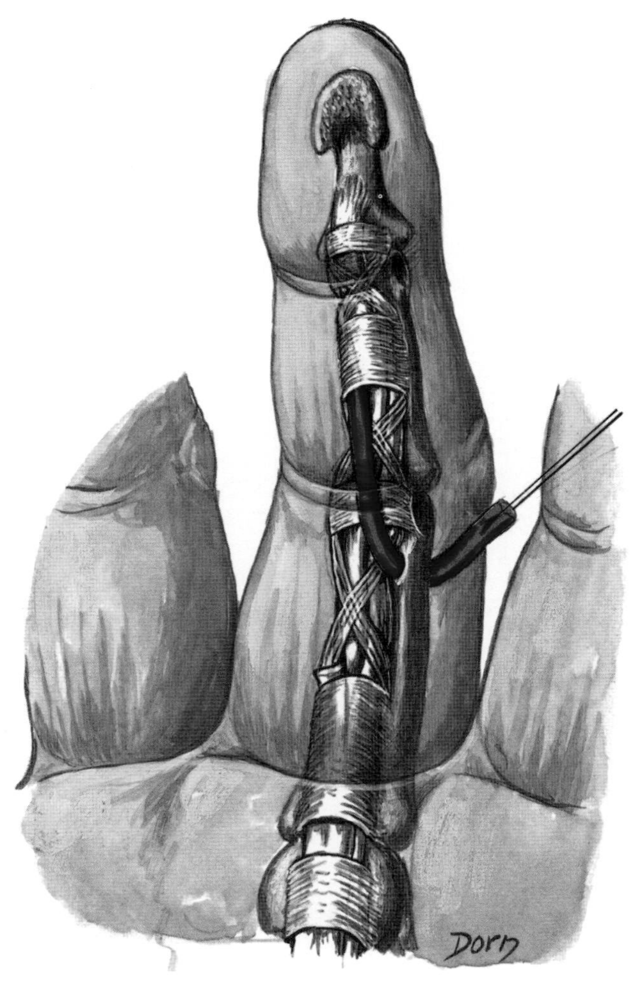

Figure 2.31

Flexor superficialis tenodesis. The FDS slip is usually fixed to the flexor tendon sheath. In some patients, particularly on spastics, a stronger attachment into the bone is preferable.

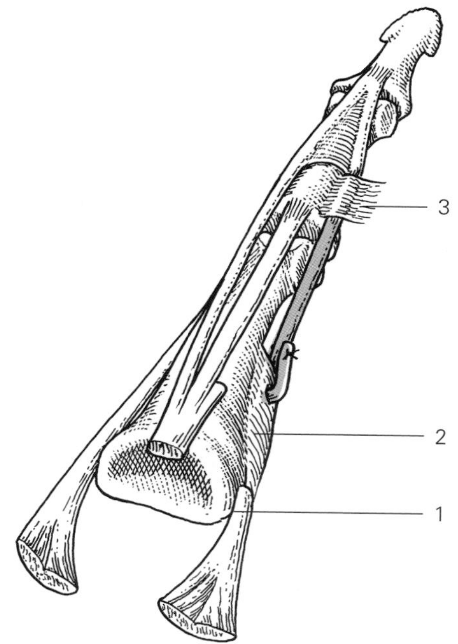

Figure 2.32

Oblique retinacular reconstruction.

1 Interosseous muscle
2 Flexor tendon sheath
3 Cleland's ligament

described several techniques. They suggested reconstruction of an ORL, held volar to the PIP joint axis, thus serving as a check rein to prevent PIP hyperextension. This ligament also serves as passive tenodesis of the DIP joint into extension as the PIP actively extends. The lateral band technique was the original procedure. Exposure was through a long lateral incision on the ulnar aspect of the finger. The ulnar lateral extensor tendon was divided at the musculotendinous junction at the base of the proximal phalanx. This band is freed down to its distal dorsal insertion, which is left intact, and rerouted volar to Cleland's ligament, volar to the PIP joint. The original proximal attachment was through a window in the proximal flexor tendon sheath at the A2 level (see Figure 2.31).

For a more secure repair, a lateral extensor band may be rerouted volarly across the digit and then through the bone of the proximal phalanx (Burton 1993) (Figure 2.33A). Use of a lateral extensor band is indicated if intrinsic tendon tightness is present, as it releases the interosseous muscles on one side of the finger. A modification of this technique uses a tendon graft (the PL if available): it is the spiral ORL (Thompson et al 1978). This technique is preferred if the quality of the extensor tendon is poor (Figure 2.33B, C and D).

Zancolli uses another technique: the lateral extensor tendon translocation (E. Zancolli, personal communication, 1986). The lateral extensor tendon on the radial side is freed at the level of the PIP joint. It is subluxated volarly in front of the volar plate and maintained in this position by suture of the volar plate to the FDS tendon. An ORL is created (Figure 2.34).

Intrinsic muscle contracture

The Bunnell–Finochietto test indicates an intrinsic muscle contracture: when the MP joint is in extension, the intrinsic muscles are tightened and PIP joint flexion is limited. If the MP joint is allowed to flex, PIP joint flexion is increased (Figure 2.35). Post-traumatic interosseous contracture is usually caused by edema, prolonged immobilization, and muscle ischemia.

In patients with swan neck and intrinsic muscle contracture, without any MP joint disorder, a distal intrinsic release (Littler 1954) is indicated. A triangular

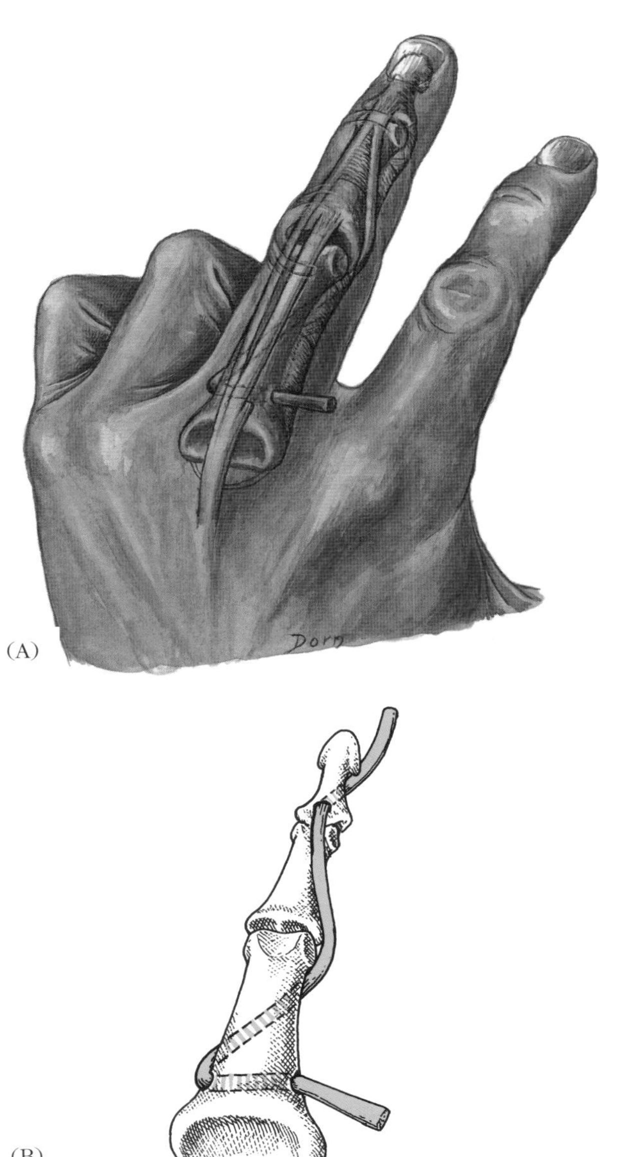

(A)

(B)

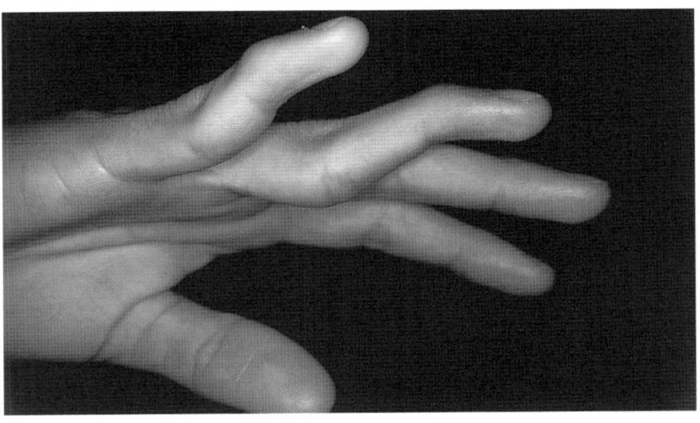

(C)

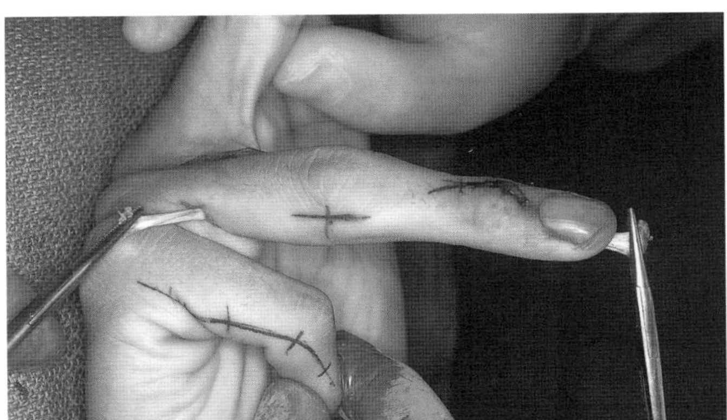

(D)

Figure 2.33

(A) The lateral band spiral ORL procedure (Burton). (B) The tendon graft spiral ORL procedure (Thomson, Littler, Upton). (C) Supple swan neck deformity. (D) Traction on the two extremities of the spiral ORL tendon graft corrects the deformity. Tension is adjusted so that the PIP joint is in 20° flexion and the DIP joint at 0°.

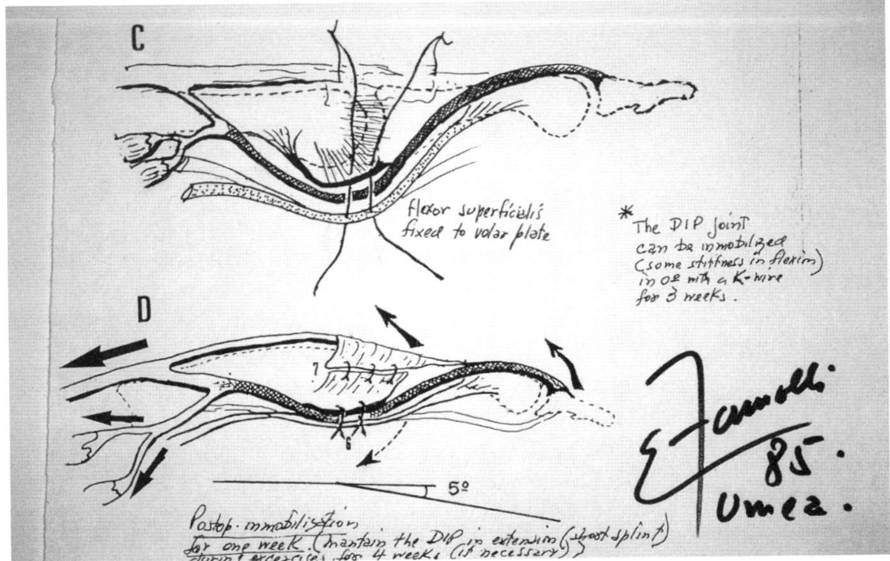

Figure 2.34

Lateral extensor tendon translocation (Zancolli). (See also Figure 36.13 in the section on Rheumatoid swan-neck.)

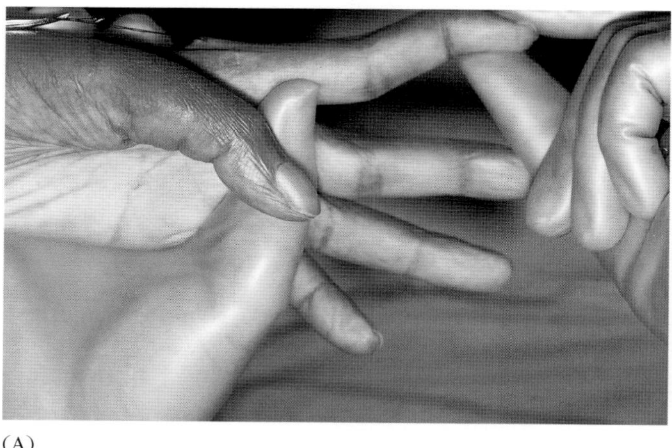

(A)

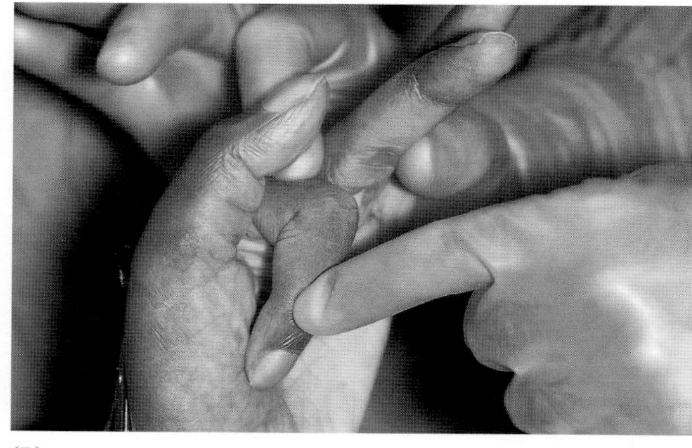

(B)

Figure 2.35

The Bunnell–Finochietto test. (A) When the proximal phalanx is maintained in extension, the distal phalanges cannot be flexed. (b) Flexion of the proximal phalanx allows flexion of the distal phalanges.

(A)

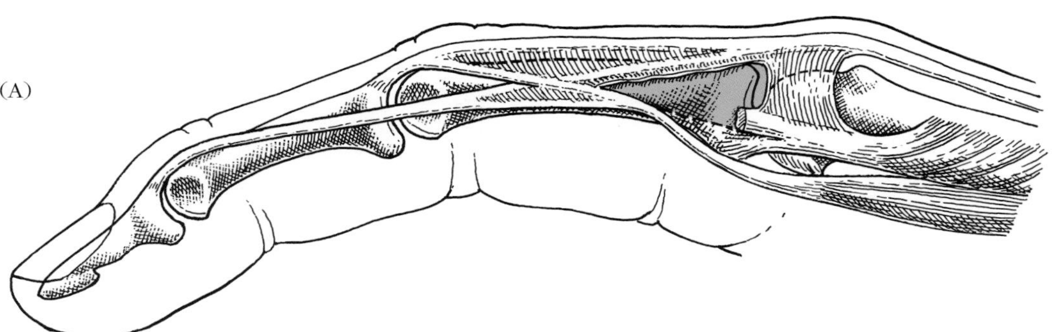

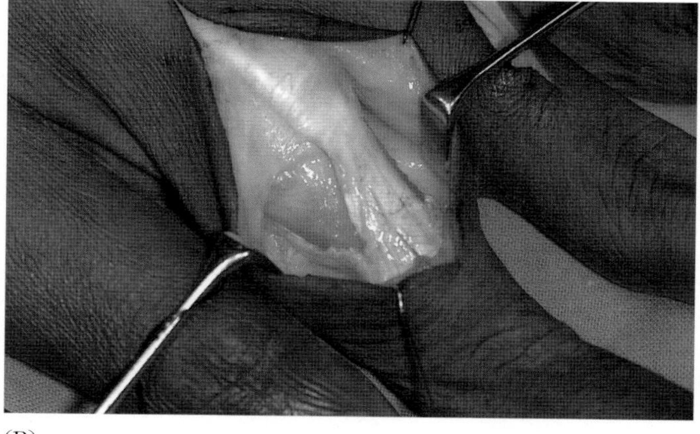

(B)

Figure 2.36

Distal intrinsic release (Littler). (A) Triangular reaction of the oblique fibres of the interosseous hood and of the central band of the interosseous tendon. (B) In rheumatoid patients with ulnar drift, the ulnar intrinsics become tighter than the radial intrinsics. The release on the ulnar side of the finger is usually sufficient.

resection of the oblique fibers of the interosseous hood and of the central band of the interosseous tendon is performed (Figure 2.36). The central tendon, the lateral bands of the extensor, and the transverse fibers of the intrinsic aponeurosis are preserved.

In post-traumatic interosseous contracture involving both the MP and the PIP joint, extensive release of the dorsal aponeurosis over the tight muscles is performed. If the muscles are necrotic, contracture may be relieved by transecting the interosseous tendons proximal to the MP joint (Figure 2.37). Lumbrical function may be preserved. If the interossei retain their contractility and some function remains, the muscles may be relaxed by an interosseous muscle slide (Figure 2.38).

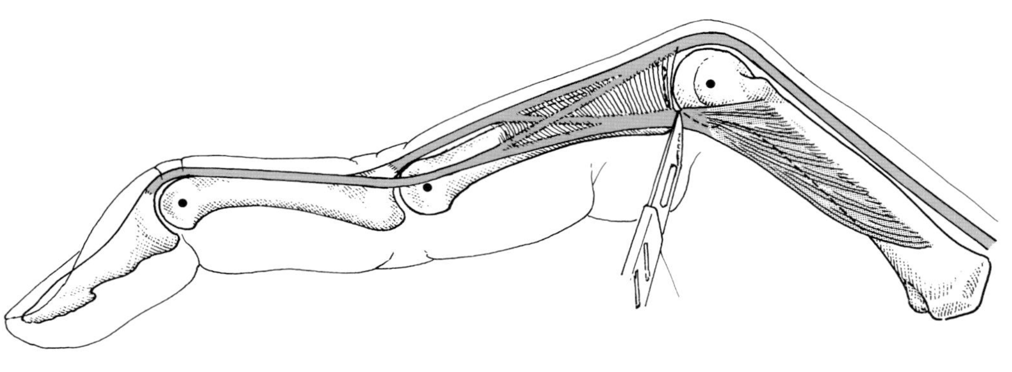

Figure 2.37
Interosseous contracture. Division of interosseous tendon proximal to MP joint.

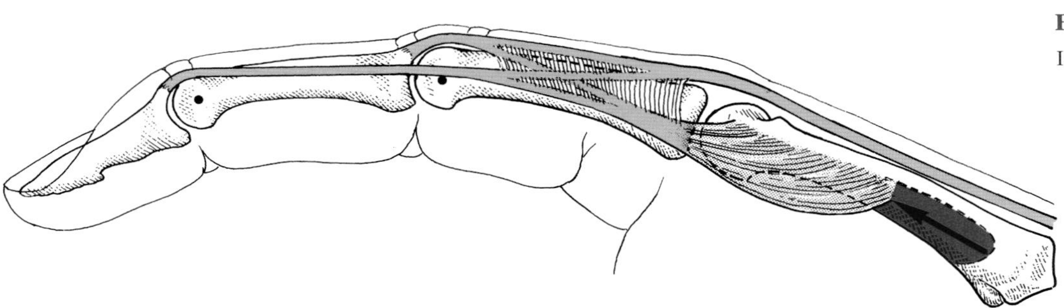

Figure 2.38
Interosseous muscle slide.

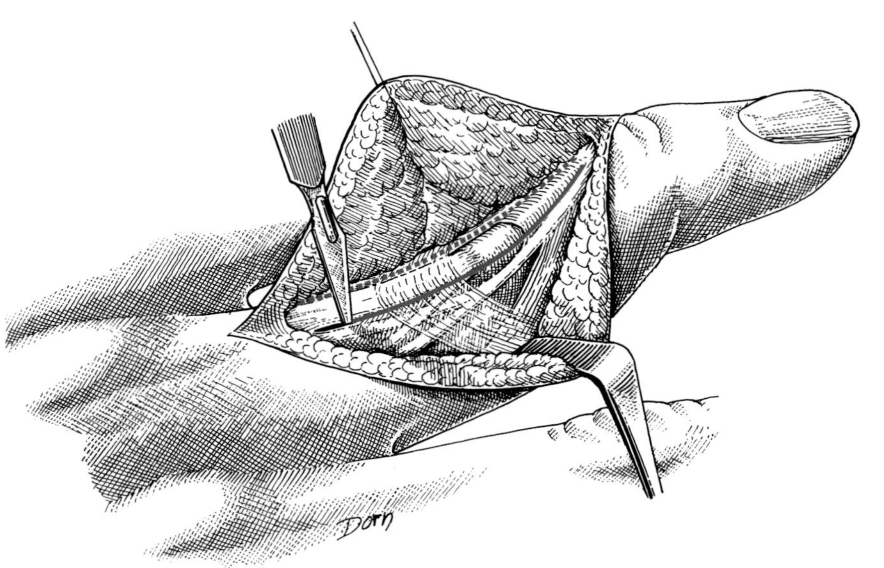

Figure 2.39
Soft tissue release (Nalebuff 1999). Longitudinal incisions along the central extensor tendon. The two extensor lateral tendons are tenolysed and mobilized to recover thir normal volar shift.

In patients with swan neck and associated MP joint deformity, often seen in rheumatoid patients, a metacarpal joint arthroplasty with resection of the metacarpal head, sometimes associated with an ulnar intrinsic muscle release, will reduce the risk of tightness recurrence (see the section on rheumatoid swan-neck).

Stage 3

There is fixed deformity with articular surfaces intact; limitation of joint motion is not influenced by the position of other finger joints. Contracture of the extensor apparatus, of the skin, and later of para-articular structures fixes the deformity. Limitation of PIP joint flexion has serious consequential functional effects for the completion of the grasp. In rheumatoid patients, gentle manipulation into flexion, associated with splinting and an exercise program, may progressively correct the deformity. If not, the clinician should proceed to a dorsal soft tissue release (Figure 2.39; see technique of soft tissue release in the chapter on 'Treatment of rheumatoid finger deformities') followed by a PIP joint

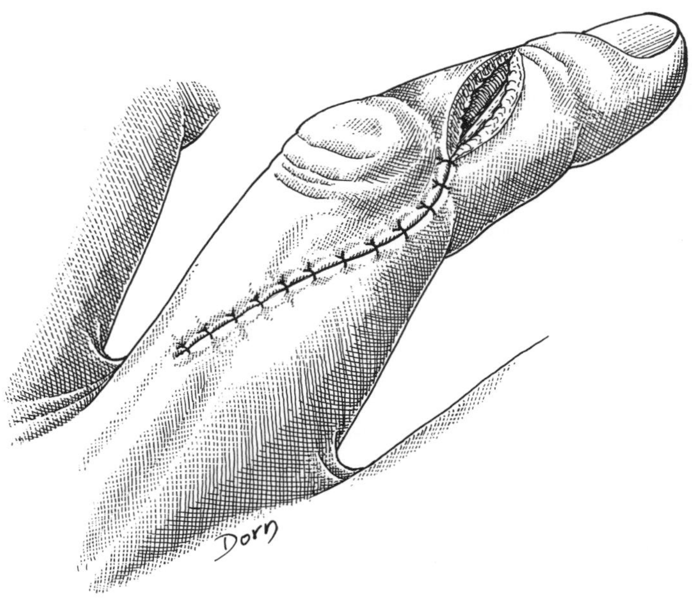

Figure 2.40
The incision is closed proximally so that the extensor apparatus is covered at the PIP joint level. The distal third of the incision over the middle phalanx is left open.

tenodesis to prevent recurrence of the deformity. An exploration and assessment of the flexor tendons may be made through a palmar incision to be sure that their excursion is normal. It is rarely necessary to release the PIP joint collateral ligament or to lengthen the central tendon. Often, because of the skin contracture the distal third of the incision over the middle phalanx should be left open (Nalebuff and Ferrano 1999) (Figure 2.40). In rheumatoid patients, this soft tissue release may be associated with MP joint arthroplasty (see the Chapter on Rheumatoid arthritis).

Stage 4

Joint stiffness with PIP articular surface lesions. The only two surgical alternatives are arthroplasty or fusion of the PIP joint; the choice depends mostly on the condition of the two other joints of the finger. A PIP joint fusion is preferably used for the index finger and a PIP joint arthroplasty for the ulnar fingers.

Chronic extensor mechanism imbalance at the MP joint level

The same classification can be used for chronic musculotendinous imbalance at the MP joint level: MP lateral deviation, MP joint flexion deformity, and MP joint hyperextension deformity.

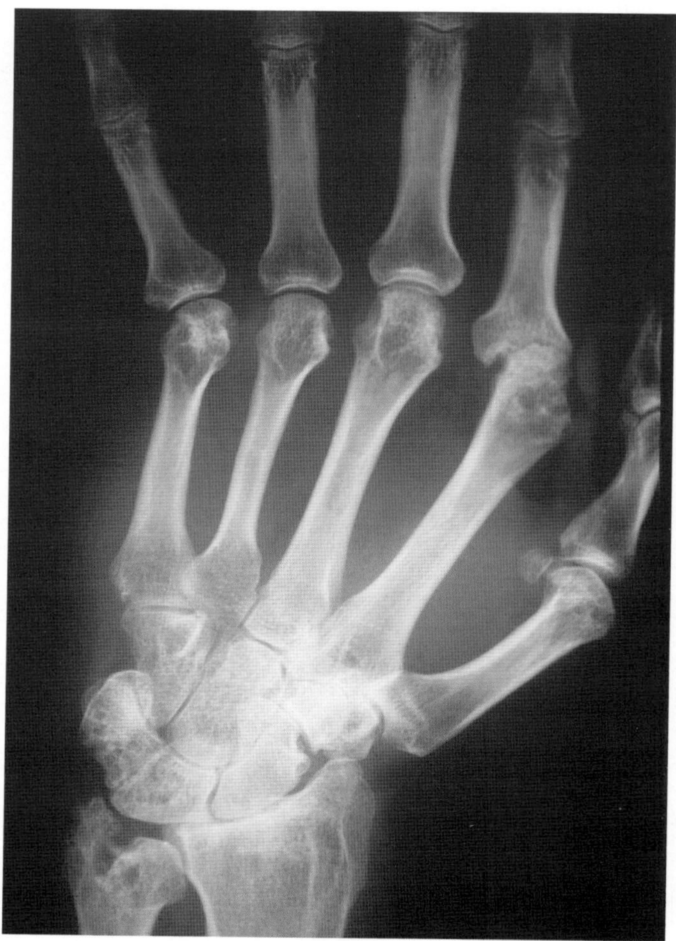

Figure 2.41
MP joint ulnar deviation associated with a radial deviation of the wrist.

MP joint lateral deviation

Lateral deviations of the fingers are mostly ulnar and are often associated with a radial deviation of the wrist (Figure 2.41). However, radial deviations of the fingers are possible, particularly in juvenile arthritis, often associated with an ulnar deviation of the wrist (Figure 2.42). Wrist deviation should be corrected before finger lateral deviation.

Stage 1

The deviation is passively reducible, each finger joint has a complete passive mobility, there is no deformity of the PIP joint. The extensor tendon is usually subluxated on the ulnar side of the MP joint. Surgery on the finger is rarely indicated at this stage. In rheumatoid patients MP joint surgical synovectomies are rarely performed because of the high incidence of recurrence. A non-surgical treatment is usually preferred at this stage.

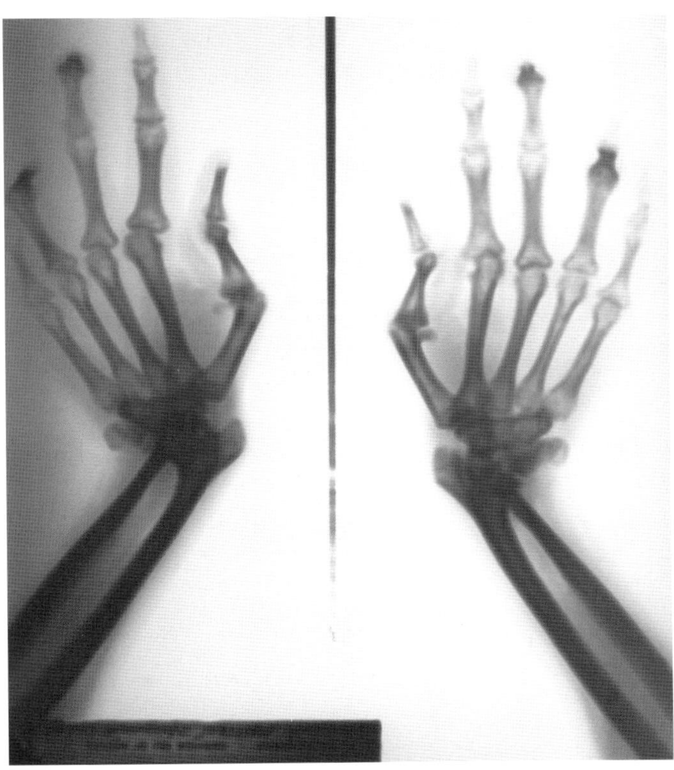

Figure 2.42
Radial deviation of the fingers associated with an ulnar deviation of the wrist, particularly in juvenile arthritis.

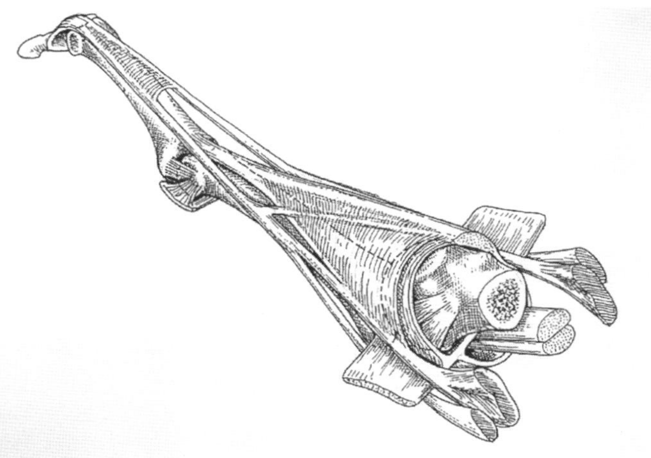

Figure 2.43
Finger deviation associated with extensor tendon subluxation may increase the extensor tendon traction on the base of the middle phalanx and produce a swan neck deformity.

Stage 2

The deviation is still passively reducible and each finger joint has a complete passive mobility. However, subluxation of the extensor tendon associated with the finger deviation may increase the extensor tendon traction on the base of the middle phalanx and may produce a swan neck deformity (Figure 2.43).

The situation is similar to a stage 2 swan neck deformity caused by a tenodesis effect. Surgical correction is indicated before the deformity becomes fixed. An intrinsic release is performed; the extensor apparatus should be realigned over the middle of the MP joint and the PIP joint hyperextension must be corrected to prevent recurrence of the deformity. A cross intrinsic transfer should be avoided as it may accentuate the swan neck deformity.

Stage 3

There are fixed deformities; finger deviation is not reducible. Articular surfaces are intact but often the MP joint is subluxated in rheumatoid patients. A soft tissue release is performed, usually in conjunction with an MP joint arthroplasty. The resection of the metacarpal head will reduce intrinsic muscle tightness. In the little finger, the ADM tendon is divided but the FDM tendon is preserved.

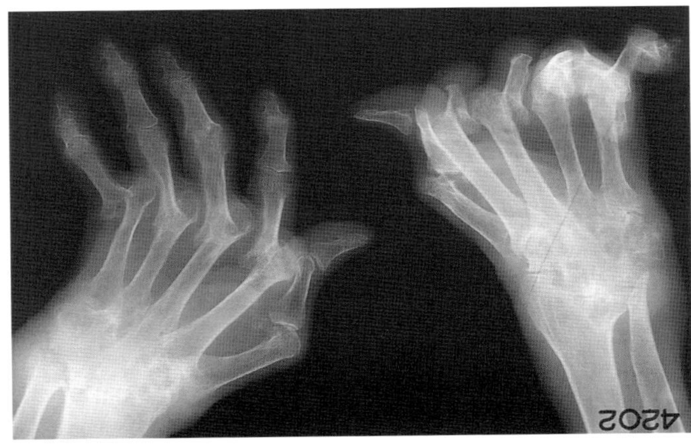

Figure 2.44
Ulnar deviation of the finger with destruction of the MP joints. Stabilization of the wrist in good position should precede MP joint arthroplasties.

Stage 4

Lesion of the articular surface (Figure 2.44). MP joint arthroplasty is associated with a soft tissue release and a realignment of the extensor apparatus.

MP joint flexion deformity

MP join flexion deformity may be caused by intrinsic muscle contracture or MP joint lesions.

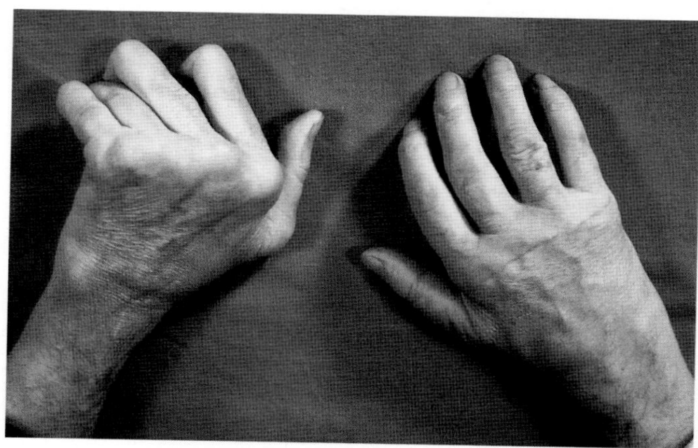

Figure 2.45

MP joint flexion deformities stage 4, corrected by MP joint arthroplasties.

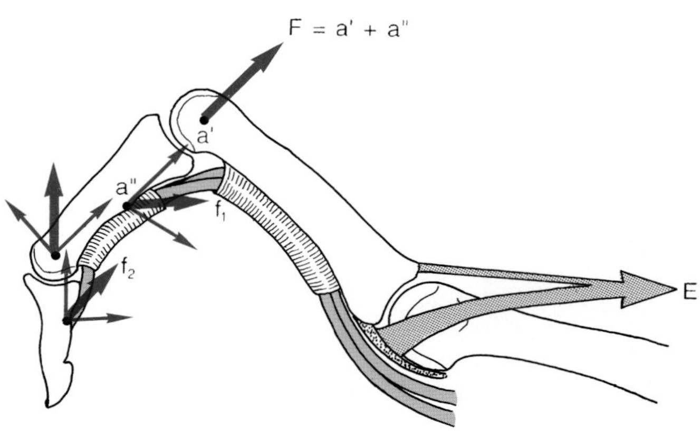

Figure 2.46

The claw hand consists of hypertension of the proximal phalanx caused by intrinsic muscle paralysis. The EDC (E), which exhausts its action at the level of the proximal insertion on the MP joint volar plate, has no effect on the distal phalanges (see Figure 12.5).

Stage 1

No limitation of passive motion in MP and IP joints. Splintage is indicated, sometimes associated with an MP joint synovectomy in rheumatoid patients.

Stage 2

Tenodesis effect: the Bunnell–Finochietto test indicates an intrinsic muscle contracture (see Figure 2.35).

In patients without MP joint disorder, a distal intrinsic release as described by Littler (1964), (see Swan neck deformity, stage 2) restores flexion of the distal phalanges when the proximal phalanx is held in extension.

Stage 3

Fixed flexion deformity; passive mobility of the MP joint is limited. Articular surfaces are intact. A soft tissue release is indicated. The intrinsic muscle tendons are divided at the myotendinous junction. An MP joint arthroplasty with resection of the metacarpal head may contribute to releasing the tension of the soft tissue contracture, especially when MP limitation of extension is associated with a swan neck deformity.

Stage 4

Articualr lesions. MP flexion deformity, associated with MP joint subluxation and intrinsic muscle tightness is an excellent indication for an MP joint arthroplasty (Figure 2.45).

MP joint hyperextension deformity

This deformity has two main causes: intrinsic muscle paralysis and extensor mechanism imbalance as seen in chronic boutonnière deformity.

The intrinsic muscles of the fingers flex the proximal phalanx and extend the distal phalanges. Their paralysis produces a claw hand deformity which consists of hyperextension of the proximal phalanx while the two distal phalanges are in flexion (Figure 2.46).

Stage 1

There is no limitation of passive motion in any joint of the finger. The claw deformity is correctable by stabilization of MP joint. The Bouvier test (1851) maintaining the MP joint in slight flexion allows extension of the distal phalanges (Figure 2.47). The claw is actively corrected by tension of the long extrinsic extensor muscles. In these cases, MP hyperextension can be prevented passively by capsulodesis or tenodesis, or by the dynamic action of a tendon transfer (Figure 2.48). The cause of the claw should also be treated by ulnar nerve repair or extensor mechanism repair.

Stage 2

The claw is not actively correctable. There is a deficit of the extension of the distal phalanges despite the maintenance of the MP joint in flexion. In most cases, when

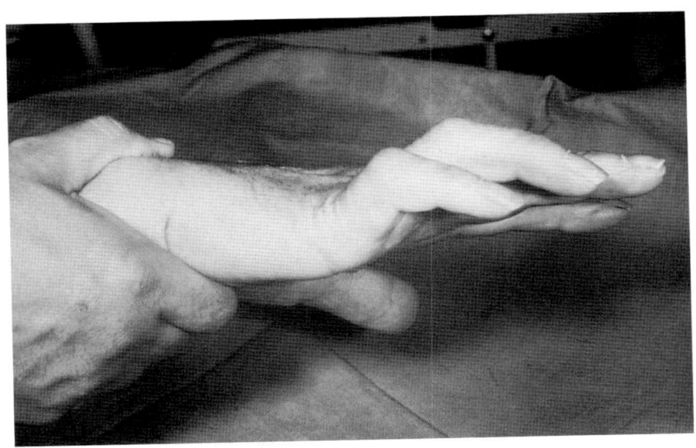

(A)

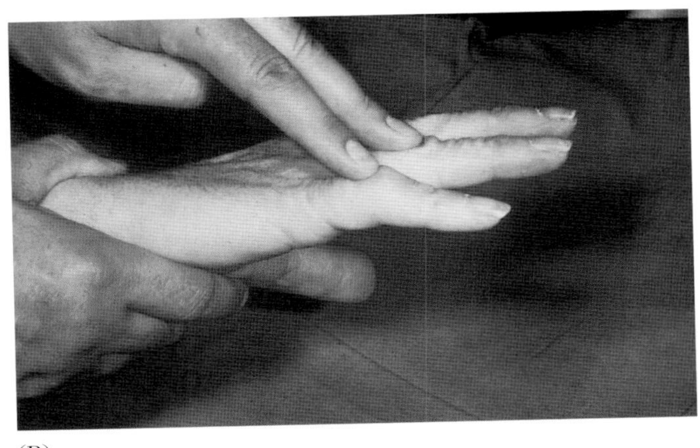

(B)

Figure 2.47

(A) Claw hand. (B) Prevention of hypertension of MP joints allows extension of distal phalanges (Bouvier's test).

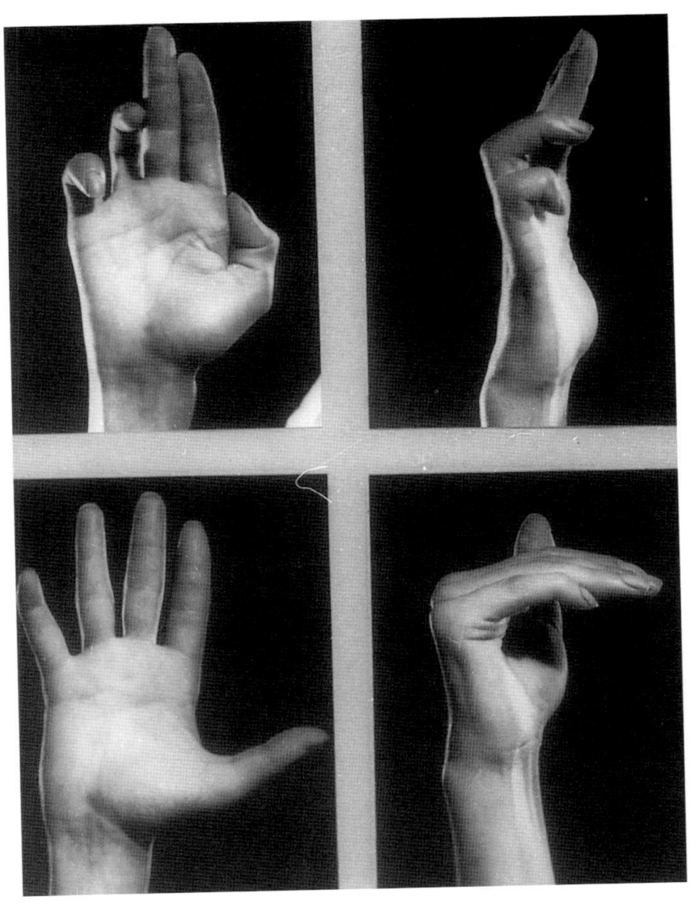

Figure 2.48

Ulnar nerve paralysis. Claw deformity of the two ulnar fingers. Deformity is corrected by a tendon transfer.

the joints are supple, this indicates a lesion of the extensor apparatus: adhesion of the extensor tendon proximal to the MP joint or lesion of the extensor mechanism at the PIP joint level (Figure 2.49).

Adhesion or synovitis of flexor tendons is another cause of limitation of the extension of the PIP joint. If extension of the PIP joint is greater when the MP joint is more flexed, the tenodesis effect is volar and corresponds to adhesions of the flexor tendons proximal to the MP joint.

Stage 3

Fixed deformities. Limitation of passive mobility at the MP or PIP level is not influenced by the position of another finger joint. Articular surfaces are intact.

Corrective splinting with exercises is necessary before any surgical repair. A tendon transfer may be possible, if the joints gain sufficient passive motion (Figure 2.50).

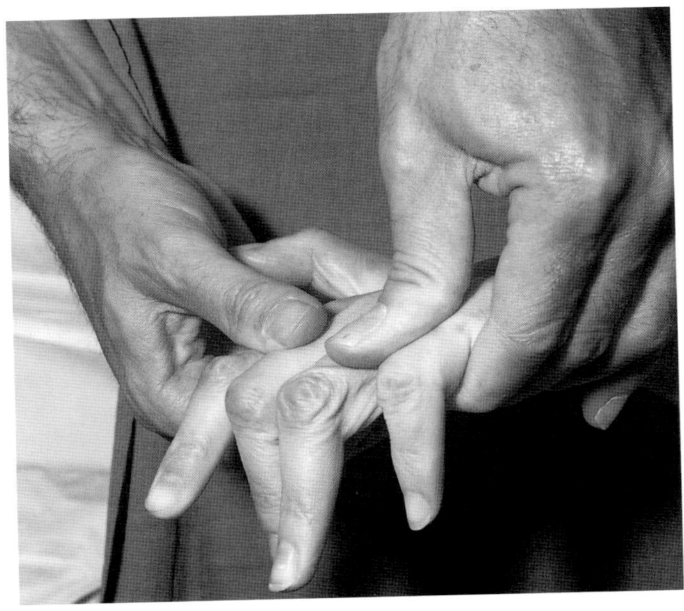

Figure 2.49

The claw is not actively correctable.

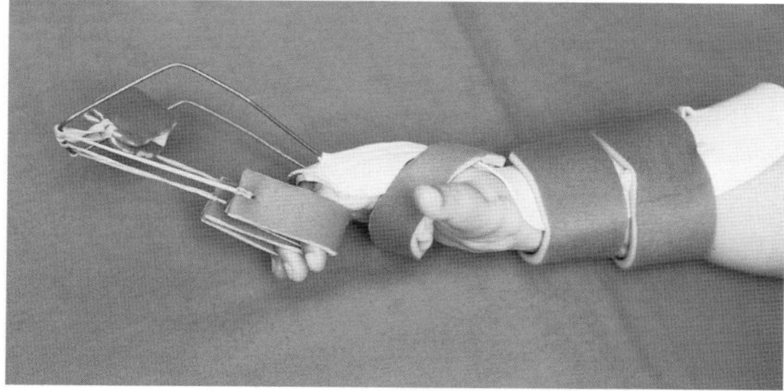

Figure 2.50

Corrective splinting associated with exercises may gain sufficient passive motion to allow a tendon transfer (see Chapter 12).

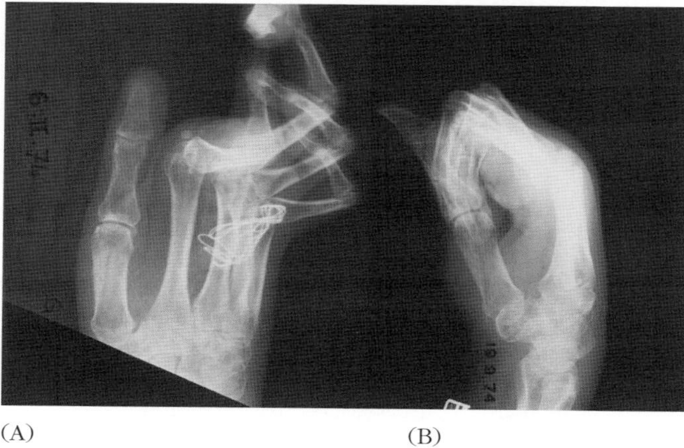

(A) (B)

Figure 2.51

Paralysis of the intrinsic muscles. (A) Fixed deformity in hyperextension of the MP joints (B) treated by MP joint arthroplasty.

Stage 4

Fixed deformities with articular lesion. At the PIP level a fusion may be indicated in a functional position. At the MP joint level an MP joint arthroplasty is sometimes possible in assiciation with a tendon transfer (Figure 2.51).

References

Albertoni WM (1988) The Brooks–Graner procedure for correction of the mallet finger. In: Tubiana R, ed, *The Hand*, vol 3 (WB Saunders: Philadelphia) 97–100.

Bonatz E, Kramer TD, Masear VR (1996) Rupture of the extensor pollicus tendon, *Am J Orthop* **25**: 118–22.

Bouvier (1851) Note sur un cas de paralysie de la main, *Bull Acad Med* **27**: 125.

Bowers WH, Hurst LC (1978) Chronic mallet finger. The use of Fowler's central slip release, *J Hand Surg* **3**: 373–6.

Brooks D (1976) Personal communication cited by Albertoni WM (1988) The Brooks–Graner procedure for correction of the mallet finger. In: Tubiana R, ed, *The Hand*, vol 3 (WB Saunders: Philadelphia) 97–100.

Burton RI (1993) Extensor tendons. Late reconstruction. In: Green DP, ed, *Operative Hand Surgery*, 3rd edn (Churchill Livingstone: Edinburgh) 1955–88.

Burton RI, Melchior JA (1997) Extensor tendons. Late reconstruction. In: Green DP, ed, *Operative Hand Surgery*, 4th edn (Churchill Livingstone: Philadelphia) 1988–2001.

Caar AJ, Burge PD (1992) Rupture of extensor tendons due to osteoarthritis of the distal radio-ulnar joint, *J Hand Surg* **17B**: 594–696.

Carroll CIV, Moore JR, Weiland AJ (1987) Post-traumatic ulnar subluxation of the extensor tendons: a reconstructive technique, *J Hand Surg [Am]* **12**: 227–31.

Dolphin JA (1965) The extensor tenotomy for chronic boutonnière deformity of the finger, *J Bone Joint Surg [Am]* **47**: 161–4.

Duchenne GBA (1867) Physiologie des mouvements (English edition translated by EB Kaplan, Physiology of motion; Philadelphia: Lippincott, 1949).

Finochietto R (1920) Retraction de Volkman de los musculos intrinsecos de la manos. Societad de Cirurgia de Buenos Aires. Tomo IV.

Fowler SB (1949) Extensor apparatus of the digits, *J Bone Joint Surg [Br]* **31**: 477.

Fowler SB (1959) The management of tendon injuries, *J Bone Joint Surg [Am]* **41**: 579–80.

Graner O, cited by Albertoni WM (1988) The Brooks–Graner procedure for correction of the mallet finger. In: Tubiana R, ed, *The Hand*, vol 3 (WB Saunders: Philadelphia) 97–100.

Haines RW (1951) The extensor apparatus of the finger, *J Anat* **85**: 251–9.

Hamlin C, Littler JW (1977) Restoration of the extensor pollicis longus tendon by an intercalated graft, *J Bone Joint Surg* **59A**: 412.

Harris C (1966) The Fowler operation for mallet finger, *J Bone Joint Surg* **48A**: 612.

Helal B (1974) The reconstruction of rheumatoid deformities of the hand, *Br J Hosp Med* **617**: 226.

Helal B, Chen SC, Iwegbu G (1982) Rupture of the extensor pollicis longus tendon in undisplaced Colles' type of fracture, *Hand* **14**: 41.

Iselin F, Levame J, Godoy J (1977) A simplified technique for treating mallet fingers: tenodermodesis, *J Hand Surg* **2**: 118–21.

Ishizuki M (1990) Traumatic and spontaneous dislocation of extensor tendon of the long finger, *J Hand Surg* **15A**: 967.

Kilgore ES, Graham WP (1977) The extensor plus finger. In: Neumeyer WL, Brown LG, eds, *The Hand, Surgical and Nonsurgical Management* (Lea & Febiger: Philadelphia) 159–67.

Landsmeer JMF (1958) A report on the coordination of the interphalangeal joints of the human finger and its disturbance, *Acta Morphologic Nederlando-Scandinavica* **2**: 59–84.

Littler JW (1954) Quoted by Harris C and Riondan DC. In: Intrinsic contracture of the hand and its surgical treatment, *J Bone Joint Surg* **36A**: 10–20.

Littler JW (1977) Principles of reconstructive surgery of the hand. In: Converse JM, ed, *Reconstructive Plastic Surgery*, 2nd edn, vol 6 (WB Saunders: Philadelphia).

Littler JW, Eaton RG (1967) Redistribution of forces in correction of boutonnière deformity, *J Bone Joint Surg [Am]* **49**: 1267–74.

McCoy FJ, Winsky AJ (1969) Lumbrical loop operation for luxation of the extensor tendons of the hand, *Plast Reconstr Surg* **44**: 142–6.

Nalebuff EA (1969) Surgical treatment of finger deformities in the rheumatoid hand, *Surg Clin North Am* **49**: 833–46.

Nalebuff EA, Terrono A (1999) Surgical treatment of the swan neck deformity in rheumatoid arthritis. In: Tubiana R, ed, *The Hand*, vol V (WB Saunders: Philadelphia) 258–68.

Patel MR, Shekhr SD, Bassini-Lipson L (1986) Conservative management of chronic mallet finger, *J Hand Surg* **IIA**: 570.

Stack HG (1971) Buttonhole deformity, *Hand* **3**: 152–4.

Steichen JB, Strickland JW, Call WH, Powell SG (1982) Results of surgical treatment of chronic boutonnière deformity: an analysis of prognostic factors. In: Strickland JW, Steichen JB, eds, *Difficult Problems in Hand Surgery* (CV Mosby: St Louis) 62–9.

Stern PJ, Kastrup JJ (1998) Complications and prognosis of treatment of mallet finger, *J Hand Surg* **13A**: 329.

Thompson JS, Littler JW, Upton J (1978) The spiral oblique retinacular ligament (SORL), *J Hand Surg* **3**: 482–7.

Tubiana R (1968) Surgical repair of the extensor apparatus of the fingers, *Surg Clin North Am* **48**: 1015–31.

Tubiana R (1988) *The Hand. The Boutonnière Deformity*, vol 3 (WB Saunders: Philadelphia) 106–24.

Tubiana R (1999) Extensor tendons: In: Tubiana R, Gilbert A, Masquelet A, eds, *An Atlas of Surgical Techniques of the Hand and Wrist* (Martin Dunitz: London).

Tubiana R, Valentin P (1964) Anatomy of the extensor apparatus and the physiology of the finger extension, *Surg Clin North Am* **44**: 897–918.

Tubiana R, Dubert T (2000) Classification des déformations des doigts longs liées à un déséquilibre musculo-tendineux, *Chir Main* **1**: 7–14.

Wheeldon FT (1954) Recurrent dislocation of extensor tendons, *J Bone Joint Surg [Br]* **36**: 612–17.

Zancolli E (1968) *Structural and Dynamic Bases of Hand Surgery* (JB Lippincott: Philadelphia) 105–6.

3 Primary repair in flexor tendon lesions

Ph Valenti

Introduction

Recent progress in understanding the function of the digital sheath, the pulley system, the vascularization of flexor tendons and tendon healing is very useful for the adaptation of surgical techniques to repair acute injuries of flexor tendons and for the proposal of an 'ideal' program of postoperative rehabilitation. Associated lesions (artery, nerve, bone, skin) should be repaired at the same time. Use of the strongest sutures and controlled passive motion followed by controlled active motion prevent the majority of complications such as rupture, tendon adhesion and proximal interphalangeal (PIP) joint contracture.

Anatomy and physiology of the flexor tendon

Topographic regions

Anatomy, physiology, surgical repair and expected results vary with the location of the flexor tendon injury. We use the classification in five zones established by the international Federation of Societies for Surgery of the Hand (Kleinert and Verdan 1983). From distal to proximal, the zones for the finger can be described as follows:

- Zone I. Distal to the insertion of the flexor superficialis.
- Zone II. Digital canal which is common to the profundus and the superficialis at the level of the chiasma; beginning at the distal palmar line and ending at the middle part of the second phalanx; this is Bunnel's 'no man's land'.
- Zone III. Between the distal part of the anterior retinacular ligament and the distal palmar line.
- Zone IV. Carpal tunnel.
- Zone V. The wrist.

Three zones are described for the thumb:

- Zone TI. A2 pulley and the insertion of the flexor pollicis longus (FPL).
- Zone TII. This is limited by the proximal part of the A1 pulley and the distal part of the oblique pulley.
- Zone TIII. Thenar eminence.

Nutrition of flexor tendon

The nutritive mechanism of the flexor tendon in the digital canal depends on the blood supply from the vincular system, the longitudinal intrinsic vessels and the synovial fluid. Good gliding of the repaired tendon in the narrow digital canal, particularly in the 'no man's land' area, depends on an atraumatic repair and a good knowledge of the detailed anatomy of these complicated systems.

Four transverse communicating branches of the digital arteries enter the digital canal and seem to play an important role in the blood supply to the vincular system of the flexor tendons (Lundborg et al 1977, Ochiai et al 1979). Schematically, there are two kinds of vincula; the short and long vincula. The vincula brevia are situated close to the insertion of the deep and superficial flexor tendons. The vinculum brevis (VBS), which supplies the flexor digitorum superficialis (FDS) originates at the level of the neck of the proximal phalanx. This VBS approaches the dorsal aspect of the superficialis flexor tendon at the level of Camper's chiasma. Volar to the chiasma, a vinculum longus (VLP) continues the vinculum brevis and approaches the dorsal aspect of the flexor digitorum profundus (FDP). There is also a VBP distally, close to the insertion of the FDP and a vinculum longus (VLS) proximally at the level of the base of the proximal phalanx.

The superficialis and profundus flexor tendons are covered by a synovial sheath which is reflected at the level of the distal palmar line for the index, long and ring fingers but at the level of the wrist for the little finger and the thumb (Strauch and De Moura 1985). The proximal reflection of the sheath has many synovial folds, which allow longitudinal movement. Moreover, the vascular network inside the sheath, close to the reflected point, is well developed; distally it ends abruptly with numerous terminal microvascular loops. The distally volar zone is less vascularized but the intrinsic longitudinal vessel perforates into the deep layers of the tendon. The synovial fluid allows good gliding of the tendon and also allows good nutrition (Weber 1986). These flexion and extension movements of the finger create a 'pump effect' which allows nutrition of the tendon, particularly on the avascular volar area of the tendon. Amadio et al (1985) reported that the synovial fluid was not sufficient to nourish the flexor tendon if the vincular system was avulsed.

Intrinsic longitudinal vessels distal to the bone insertion and proximal to the continuity of the muscle supply the tendon for a few centimetres on each extremity. Outside the digital canal the vascularization of the flexor tendons depends on a well developed vascular network on their surface and in their interior.

To summarize the vascular supply of the flexor tendons in the digital canal, the following points can be noted for the FDS:

- VBS at the neck level of the proximal phalanx.
- VLS at the base level of the proximal phalanx.
- Synovial fluid in the proximal reflection of the synovial sheath.
- Intrinsic longitudinal vessels from the palm region.
- Intrinsic longitudinal vessels from the insertion of the middle phalanx.

and for the FDP:

- VBP distally, at the neck level of the middle phalanx.
- VLP through the chiasma, continuity of the VBS.
- Synovial fluid in the proximal reflection of the synovial sheath.
- Intrinsic longitudinal vessels from the palm region.
- Intrinsic longitudinal vessels from the insertion of the distal phalanx.

The vincular system and proximal inflow from the proximal synovial reflection and intrinsic vessels are separate. Between these systems, there is an avascular zone on the volar aspect of the flexor tendon about 1 mm thick; at the PIP joint level for the FDP and proximal to the chiasma for the FDS.

Pulley system

The synovial sheath is reinforced by a fibrous pulley system delimiting the digital canal. This system is composed of five annular pulleys and three cruciform pulleys (Doyle 1988, 1990, Lin et al 1989). The first, third and fifth annular pulleys arise from the volar plate of the metacarpophalangeal (MP) joint, PIP joint and distal interphalangeal (DIP) joint, respectively. The second and the fourth annular pulleys arise from the proximal and middle phalanx, respectively, and are thicker and broader than the others. The first cruciform pulley is located between the second and third annular pulleys; the second cruciform between the third and fourth annular pulleys and the third cruciform just proximal to the DIP joint. The cruciform pulleys participate in the production of synovial fluid. The distal part of the transverse fibres of the palmar aponeurosis, close to the beginning of the membranous synovial sheath, called the palmar aponeurosis pulley, must be considered part of the finger pulley system; vertical fibres anchor on each side of the synovial sheath and are attached to the deep transverse metacarpal ligament. The main function of this digital fibrous pulley system is to maintain the flexor tendon close to the bone to allow complete flexion of the finger. The palmar aponeurosis pulley is especially useful if either one or two annular pulleys are absent. Moreover, the average breaking strength (16.5 kg) of the palmar aponeurosis is superior to the A2 pulley (14 kg) (Manske and Lesker 1983). The loss of flexion increases if the A2 and A4 pulleys are absent.

Tendon healing process

The process of tendon healing is not yet completely understood. Two processes seem to cooperate in the healing of tendon injuries: extrinsic healing (which for many years has been described as the main factor) involving the surrounding tissues, and intrinsic healing of the tendon, which involves the tendon itself and the synovial sheath.

Extrinsic healing is enhanced by vascular and cellular ingrowths from the surrounding tissues. The callus which is formed allows the cicatrization of the tendon but also restricts its mobility, particularly in zone II. To prevent ingrowth adhesion, biomechanical agents such as anti-inflammatory agents, steroids, antihistamine and hyaluronic acid have been proposed (Amiel et al 1989, Hagberg 1992). However, microsurgical techniques and new sutures combined with an atraumatic approach are helpful in decreasing this risk of adhesion formation. Nevertheless, many factors, such as the nature of the trauma (avulsion, blunt injury, crush injuries) and the associated lesions (vascular, nerve, skin loss, fracture) increase the risk of adhesion. Gelberman and colleagues (1990) reported the benefits of protected passive mobilization on the tensile strength and gliding function compared with complete immobilization of repaired tendons.

Some in vitro studies have shown that the tendon cells themselves possess a potential for repair. Lundborg et al (1980) proved that a flexor tendon that is cut and isolated in a synovial fluid environment, without a vascular supply, is able to heal without any adhesion formation. So, during our atraumatic approach and repair, it is assumed that the synovial sheath should be preserved as much as possible (Lundborg et al 1980, Lister 1983, Saldana et al 1987, Peterson et al 1990).

Surgical technique in primary flexor tendon repair

General considerations

In general, repair of the flexor tendon is currently performed in an emergency situation. In cases such as crush injuries or dirty trauma, the surgeon should convert a contaminated wound to a cleaner wound by debridement. All the lesions (fracture, neurovascular bundles, skin loss) are repaired during the same operating procedure as the flexor tendon. However, if the surgeon does not possess the knowledge to treat this kind of lesion it would be better to delay this repair until a more appropriate time (Schneider et al 1977).

All flexor tendons must be repaired in an operating room with proper instrumentation and under magnification so as to allow an atraumatic repair. Before the operation, the wound should be cleaned carefully and sometimes the administration of intravenous antibiotics just before, during and 6 hours after surgery is indicated. The repair is made under axillary block anaesthesia with a pneumatic tourniquet at the level of the arm. Just before wound closure, the tourniquet is released to obtain good homeostasis and to prevent haematoma, infection, fibrosis and potential adhesion.

Exposure incision

The skin wound should be debrided and enlarged to provide good visibility of the tendon and to allow an atraumatic anatomical repair to be carried out. Modalities of the extension of the wound depend on the shape of the initial lesion and the position of the finger; an oblique skin laceration can be extended with a palmar zigzag approach (Bruner's incision) (Figure 3.1); a transverse skin laceration can be extended via a midlateral approach. A palmar zigzag approach affords an excellent exposure but can create adhesions and scar tissue over the flexor tendon. The midlateral approach allows a direct repair of the flexor tendon and leaves back the neurovascular bundle with vascular transverse branches. Straight and midpalmar incisions which cross flexor creases should be avoided, as the sharp angle in the skin flap could lead to tip necrosis. The wound should be enlarged distally when the tendon section has occurred in flexion or proximally in finger extension trauma.

Sometimes the proximal end of the tendon is retracted into the palm and a transverse incision at the level of the palmar crease will be necessary if massage of the flexor tendon in the area of the MP and wrist flexion has failed. Then we use a silicone tube which is passed retrograde into the palm, through the superficialis chiasma until the proximal stump. This proximal tendon is attached to the tube and pulled distally, bringing the tendon to the wound. This procedure avoids traumatic lesion of the digital sheath and potential adhesion formation (Figure 3.2) (Sourmelis and McGrouther 1987).

The digital flexor tendon sheath is opened between the annular pulley with an L-shaped incision (Lister's technique) (Lister 1983). Annular pulleys (particularly A2 and A4) should be spared or repaired to prevent bowstringing. When possible, the sheath should be closed with a fine suture material after flexor tendon repair. Sometimes, if the damage to the sheath has been severe, it is necessary to excise the portion of the sheath

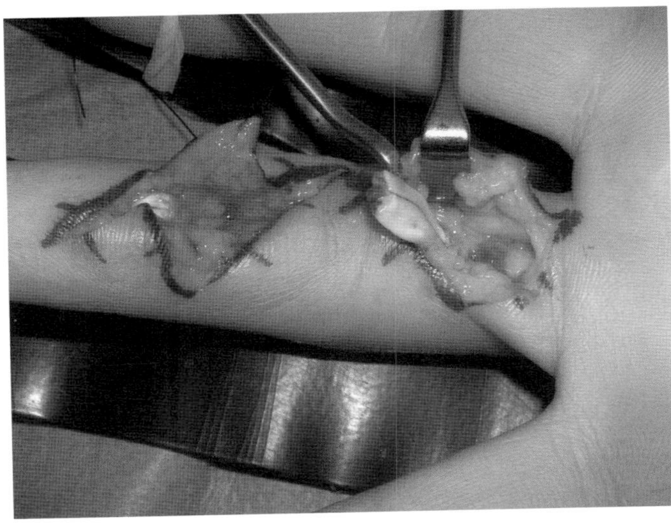

Figure 3.1
Isolated section of the FDP; Bruner's incision to retrieve and to expose the tendon stumps.

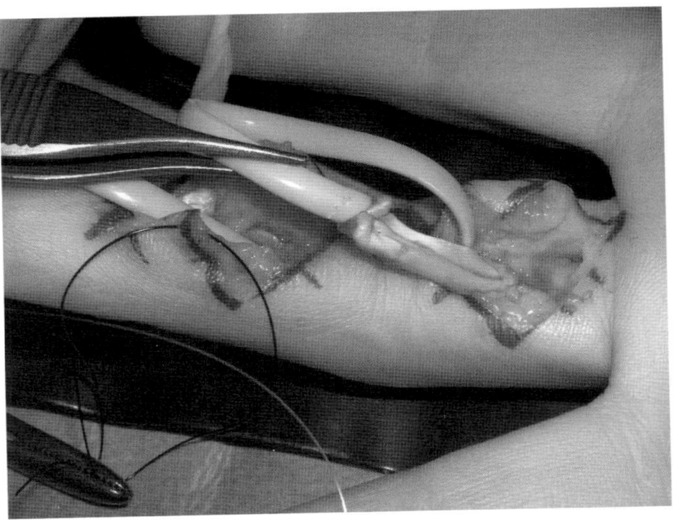

Figure 3.2
A silicone tube to bring the proximal tendon stump to the desired level to avoid potential formation of adhesions.

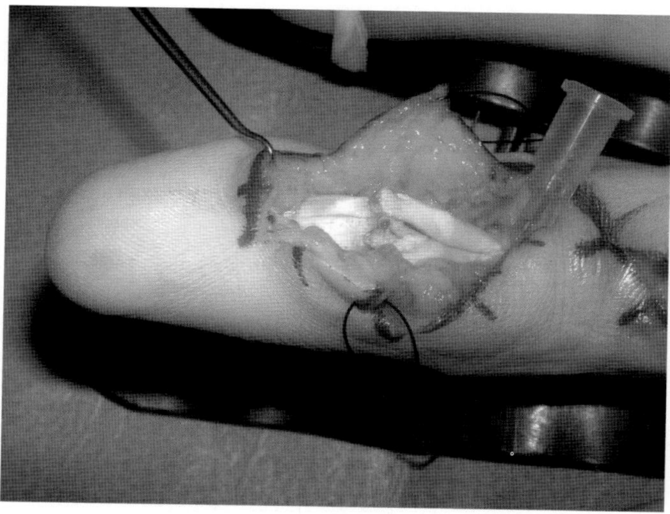

Figure 3.3
Temporary fixation of the proximal tendon stump with a needle to facilitate repair.

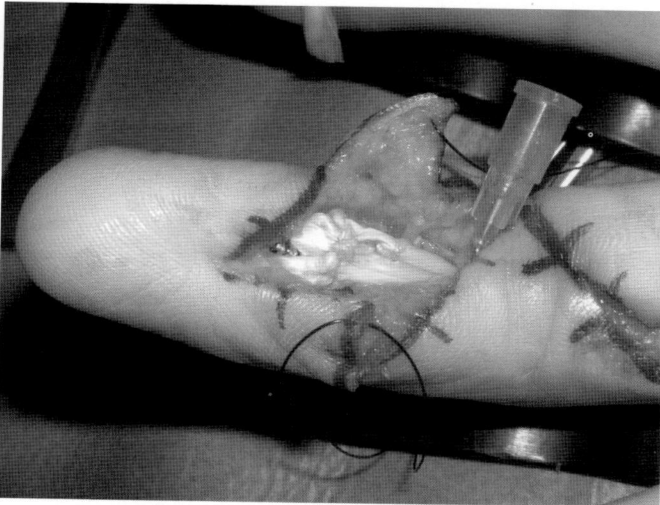

Figure 3.4
Tenofix fixation: new material.

around the repaired tendon to avoid an impingement or a trigger finger. When the lesion is not a clean cut, refreshing of the flexor tendon becomes necessary and we use a sharp blade or a nerve cutting instrument. The debridement should always be minimal to avoid tension over the suture. An approximation of the tendon's stumps is facilitated by a needle which blocks the stump proximally and makes it possible to perform the suture technique without tension and with less difficulties (Figure 3.3).

Suture technique

Several suture techniques have been reported but none have been universally accepted. Furthermore, the modified Kessler suture with two sutures (Tajima 1984) and a 'grasping' suture (Strickland 1985, 1989) with the knots inside the cross-section have been accepted by the majority of authors. A running epitendinous suture increases the tensile strength and allows good gliding of the tendon repaired in the digital sheath. However, this kind of suture does not allow immediate active rehabilitation. Therefore, experimental studies have been done to improve the suture material and the suture technique itself.

The 'ideal' material should be non-reactive, small calibre, but strong and pliable. Nylon 3/0 is recommended for the central suture and nylon 5 or 6/0 for the epitendinous running suture (Taras et al 2001).

The 'ideal' suture would be a 'locking' or a 'grasping' suture (Barrie et al 2001, Wada et al 2001) with four or six strand sutures (Savage and Risitano 1989, Dinopoulos et al 2000) added to a running epitendinous locking suture (Wade et al 1989). The initial resistance of this kind of suture is twice that of a traditional suture and allows an immediate active rehabilitation programme. Tsuge's suture (Tsuge 1975) makes it possible to perform a 'locking' suture easily, but with a knot left over the tendon, which can create a conflict with the sheath or the pulley system. This new suture increases the strength of repair, facilitates early active motion and decreases the risk of gap formation or early rupture of the tendon.

A new material characterized by its high traction resistance just been reported: it comprises two intratendinous, stainless steel anchors, which are joined by a multifilament stainless steel suture. This permanent implant is designed to hold the severed tendons in approximation until the tendon has healed (Figure 3.4).

A longer follow-up is required before these advancements can be universally accepted; protected passive mobilization of the flexor tendon is still widely used.

Postoperative management

A dorsal plaster splint is applied, postoperatively, from the proximal forearm to the fingertips in 'intrinsic position': the wrist is held with 20° of palmar flexion, the MP joints in 60° of flexion and the PIP and DIP joints in full extension to avoid flexion contracture. Two options are possible: immobilization for 4 weeks or early mobilization following specific protocols.

Immobilization is still indicated in children or in patients who are not cooperative. The mobilization will begin in the fifth week, combining active and passive motion under a protected dorsal plaster splint; mobilization

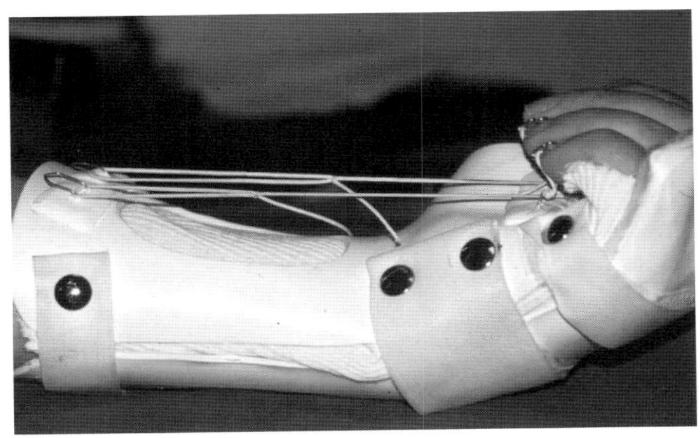

Figure 3.5
Kleinert's technique with a palmar pulley system at the level of the distal palmar crease; passive flexion.

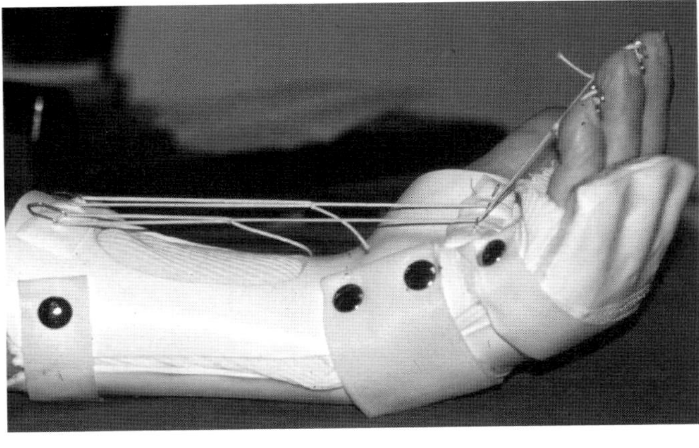

Figure 3.6
Kleinert's technique: active extension against a dorsal splint.

against resistance is begun in the seventh week. The rate of complications (e.g. rupture, gap) is very low, but adhesion formation occurred in the majority of repairs, which requires a tenolysis and is sometimes difficult. Strickland and Glogovac (1980) and Lister et al (1977) proved the benefit of early mobilization for tendon healing and final end result in a series of flexor tendon repairs in zone II. Controlled passive mobilization allowed patients to obtain 36% excellent results, 24% poor results and 4% had ruptures; immobilization produced no excellent results, 44% poor results and 16% had ruptures.

Gelberman et al (1990, 1991a, 1991b) reported the superiority of early mobilization and the major advantages: improvement of tendon gliding (low rate of production of soft tissue adherences), of intrinsic tendon healing with a remodelling of the suture, of tensile strength decreasing the risk of gap formation with an incomplete finger flexion. The high risk period for rupture is between days 5 and 10 postoperatively and the hand therapist should be very cautious during active motion.

Kleinert et al (1967) proposed passive and active mobilization under a protected dorsal plaster splint with the wrist in 20° of flexion, MP joint in 70° of flexion and the finger able to extend completely. An elastic band traction attached to a nylon loop, which was fixed through the nail, held the finger in flexion but allowed it to be actively extended against the dorsal splint. During the first 4 weeks, the patients performed active extension of the finger for several half-hour periods daily.

The rubber band traction is detached for the rest of the day and during the night to prevent flexion contracture of the interphalangeal joint. The movement should be controlled at the beginning by the hand therapist with the elbow flexed and pronated to relax the flexor muscles. During the fifth and sixth weeks, active flexion is begun under the protection of a dorsal splint. This method is an excellent technique but highly demanding for the surgeon, therapist and patient, and a control each week is necessary to prevent a gap or a rupture at the site of the repair.

A palmar pulley at the level of the distal palmar crease improves the range of flexion of the fingers and better results have been reported. After repairing the FPL, MP and IP joints of the thumb are held in 20° of flexion and the palmar pulley is located on the ulnar side of the hand (Figures 3.5 and 3.6).

Duran and Hauser (1975) proposed controlled passive motion for the flexor tendon lesion in zone II. The wrist is placed in 20–30° of flexion, the MP joint in 60° of flexion and the PIP and DIP joints in extension. Controlled passive motion is used for 4 weeks, by the hand therapist each day and by the patient twice a day with six to eight motions for each tendon per session. This method allows 3–5 minute movements at the repair site to prevent firm adhesion formation. A rubber band traction is attached to the wrist for a week and active exercises for 2 weeks are done with the protection of a dorsal splint.

Strickland (1985) modified Duran's technique. He increased the frequency and duration of the passive exercises each day. The PIP and DIP joints are mobilized separately through several repetitions of full passive flexion and extension. A specially trained therapist worked closely with the hand surgeon and many controls are essential during the first 5 weeks. To improve active flexion after 5 weeks, the Bunnel block technique (Bunnel 1956) can be used: the MP joint is blocked in extension and the PIP joint is actively flexed; the PIP joint is blocked in extension and the DIP joint is actively flexed. If there is a limited extension of the finger beyond 6 weeks, dynamic splinting may be necessary. Six months are necessary to obtain complete motion (particularly in children) and this is the minimal period before considering tenolysis.

Chow et al (1988) reported excellent results in a multicentre study of flexor tendon lacerations in zone II. They used rubber band traction incorporating a palmar pulley (distal palmar crease) which increased passive flexion at the PIP and MP joints. This modification increases the tendon excursion in the sheath and the differential gliding between superficialis and profundis tendon. For the first 4 weeks, full passive extension and flexion were performed under the control of a hand therapist, added to the active extension programme against the rubber band traction. For the fifth and sixth weeks, the rubber band traction is removed and active and passive full flexion and extension are performed. The supervision of a hand surgeon and a hand therapist is essential to prevent contracture at the interphalangeal joints.

Early active flexion exercises following flexor tendon repair in zone II have been reported by many authors (Becker et al 1979, Savage and Risitano 1989, Small et al 1989, Bellemère et al 1998). Improvements in the quality and resistance of the suture are essential to perform this rehabilitation programme, to avoid a gap or rupture of the tendon at the repair site. Indications are limited to cleanly cut tendons, motivated and intelligent patients with a specialized therapist and close supervision by a hand surgeon.

Currently, magnetic resonance imaging is very helpful for diagnosing this kind of complication and for differentiating gap or adhesion formation, particularly in zone II after repair of superficialis and profundus tendon injuries.

Features of primary repair in each specific zone

Zone I

Traumatic lesion involves only the FDP. The proximal stump is easy to find because the intact vincular system limits the retraction of the tendon. The tendon can be repaired directly if the distal stump is more than 1 cm proximal to the insertion. If the distal stump is less than 1 cm from the insertion, reinsertion of the proximal tendon into the distal phalanx is recommended. The attachment is double: at the palmar aspect of the base of the distal phalanx to a subperiostal flap; distally at the midlevel nail plate after passing through the distal phalanx (Foucher et al 1986). The A5 pulley is frequently partially opened but the A4 pulley should be preserved to prevent bowstringing.

Avulsion of the FDP is a relatively common injury in athletes but the diagnosis is often made late. This injury occurs mostly in the ring finger but any finger can be involved. The diagnosis, unavailable in an emergency situation, is made when the athlete is not able to flex the distal phalanx actively. A lateral radiograph should be routinely carried out, to look for a small bone at the level of the DIP or PIP joint providing from the distal phalanx. The prognosis of this lesion depends on three main factors:

1. The degree of retraction of the tendon and then the remaining nutritional supply of the avulsed tendon.
2. The delay in making a diagnosis.
3. The presence of a large bony fragment.

Leddy and Parker (1977) classified this lesion into three types:

- Type I: FDP is retracted into the palm with destruction of the vincular system. In an emergency, it is reasonable to try a reinsertion of the FDP, but there is a high potential for adherence formation and a dysfunction of the FDS. Secondarily, it is preferable to do nothing or an excision of the FDP with a fusion or a tenodesis of the DIP joint.
- Type II: FDP is retracted at the level of the PIP joint and the vincular system is preserved. This is the most common type. A small bone fragment can be found on the lateral radiograph blocked into the A3 or A2 pulley. Reinsertion should be performed early or at a later point (but within 3 months) if the vascular supply of the tendon is preserved and can produce a satisfactory result (Figures 3.7 and 3.8).
- Type III: There is a large bony fragment from the distal phalanx, caught in the A5 or A4 pulley. Retraction is limited and vascularization of the tendon is spared. The prognosis is excellent after an anatomic reinsertion, as soon as possible, into the distal phalanx. An active rehabilitation programme should be started immediately under a protective dorsal splint.

Robins and Dobyns (1975) reported a type IIIA lesion: a fracture of the distal phalanx resulted in a large detached bony fragment at the level of the DIP joint associated with an avulsion of the FDP retracted at the level of the PIP joint (sometimes a small fragment is diagnosed on the lateral radiographs at the level of the PIP joint). Treatment is difficult and should comprise a reduction and an internal fixation of the distal phalanx associated with reinsertion of the avulsed tendon.

When the avulsion is misdiagnosed in an emergency situation, the late treatment depends on the presence of symptoms (swelling, tenderness, tumefaction, pain) and the degree of motivation of the patient. If the patient reports problems at the base of the finger, the FDP should be excised. Fusion or tenodesis of the DIP joint can be indicated if the distal phalanx is unstable with an excessive dorsal extension with weakness of pinch. Reconstruction of the FDP with two-stage flexor tendon grafting is indicated in carefully selected patients; musicians and skilled technicians, if motivated, may require this sophisticated operation. Complications such as adherences, contracture of the PIP joint or worse

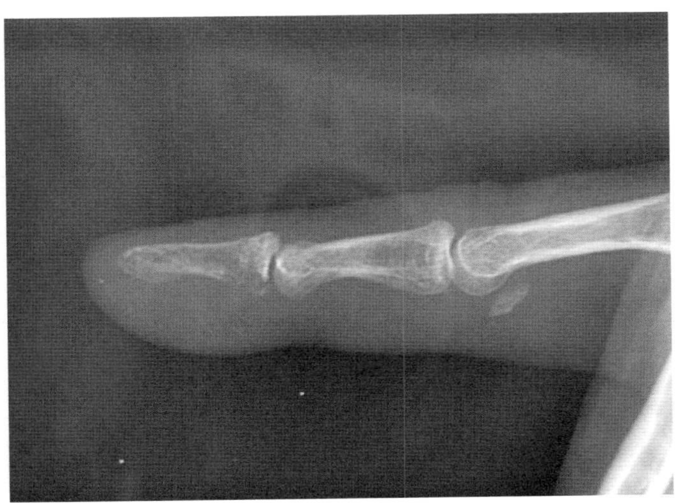

Figure 3.7

Avulsion of the FDP. Type II: small bone fragment blocked into the A3 pulley.

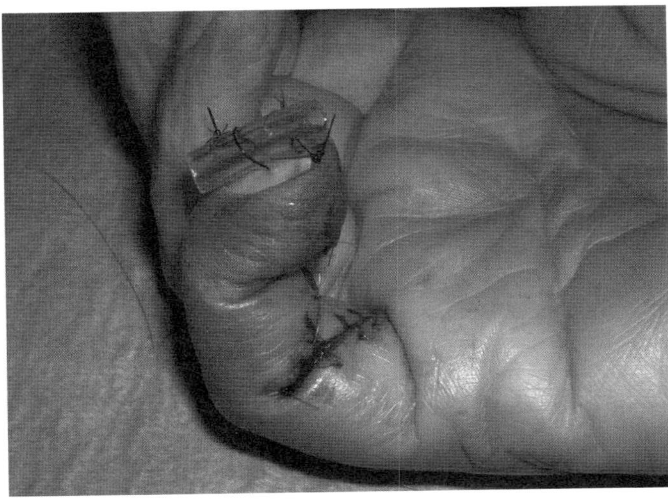

Figure 3.8

Reinsertion of the avulsed tendon through the distal phalanx and fixed on the nail plate.

Zone II (Figures 3.9, 3.10 and 3.11)

Traumatic lesion of the finger involves the FDP and FDS, which are frequently retracted into the palm. We recommend repairing both: repair of the FDS preserves the vinculum system which supplies the FDP and retains a smooth bed for the gliding of the FDP. If the FDS is excised, the vinculum system is removed at the same time and if there is a rupture of one tendon, the other can continue to flex the finger. However, frequently adherences between the two tendons occur at the repair site and tenolysis becomes necessary after 6 months to prevent a secondary rupture. We recommend atraumatic retrieval and repair of the two tendons.

In the thumb the FPL slips into the palm, making retrieval difficult. A small transverse incision at the wrist level allows the proximal stump to be located easily. This function of the FDS should be carefully explained to the patient.

In the thumb, when direct repair is not possible, tendinous lengthening procedures can advance the proximal stump by 1–3 cm. At the wrist level, a Z lengthening (Urbaniak 1985) can produce an advancement of about 2 or 3 cm and more proximally a fractional lengthening at the musculotendinous junction (Leviet 1986) allows an advancement limited to 1 cm. The A1 pulley should be preserved, but the A2 pulley can be partially excised without functional loss.

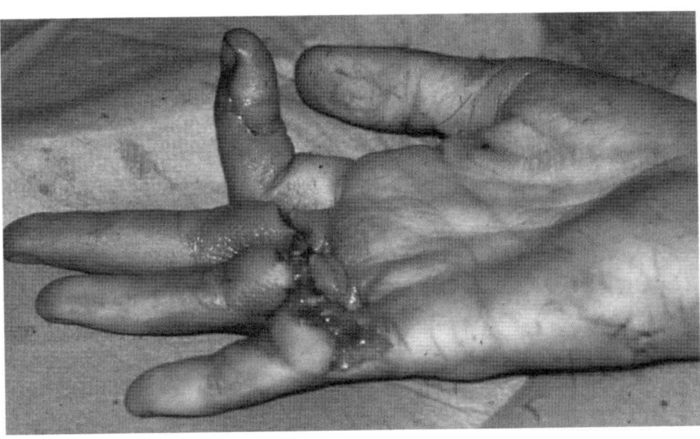

Figure 3.9

Flexor tendon injuries in zone II, Bunnell's "no man's land".

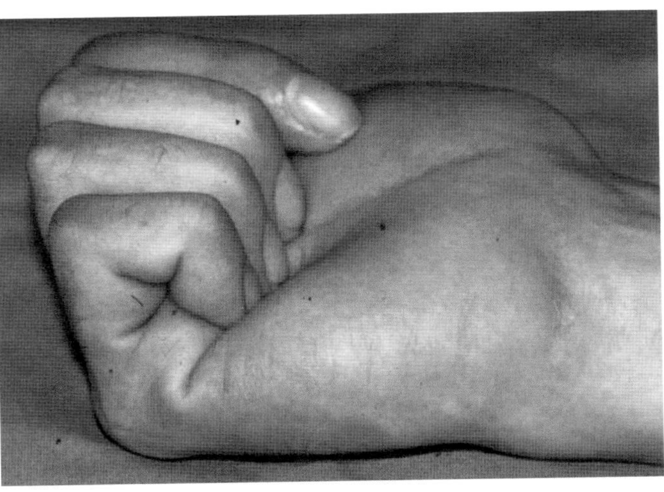

Figure 3.10

Result in flexion after modified Kessler suture and Kleinert's rehabilitation.

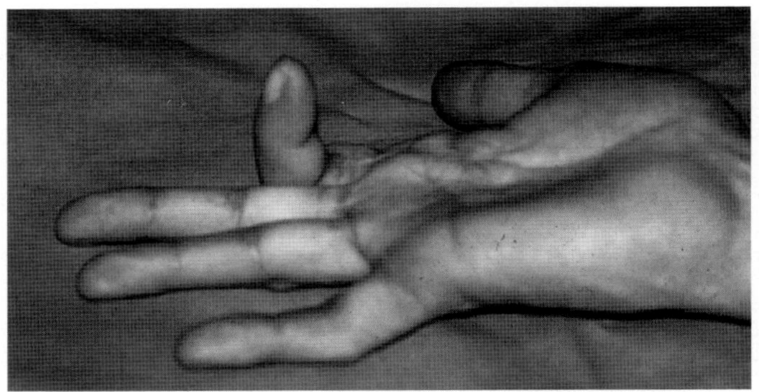

Figure 3.11
Result in extension after 6 months of follow-up.

simple approach avoids damage of the thenar eminence, the cutaneous branch of the median nerve and opening of the carpal tunnel. A silicone tube with the same technique as that used for the finger can bring the tendon atraumatically to the initial wound for direct suture or transosseous fixation. The A1 or oblique pulley should be preserved or reconstructed with aponeurosis of the abductor pollicis brevis (Leviet 1986) to prevent limited motion and bowstringing.

Zone III

Traumatic tendon injuries are associated with damage of the neurovascular bundles and must be repaired. The FDP and FDS should be repaired and the A0 pulley should be preserved.

Zone IV

Tendon injuries are rare here, because the annular anterior ligament, which is thick, protects this area. So, in a crush lesion, multiple tendons can be involved, associated with the median nerve (motor and sensory branches), palmar arch or motor ulnar nerve. Complete opening of the carpal tunnel is recommended to repair all the lesions.

Zone V

The main structures are superficial and tendon lesions are multiple and associated with the radial or ulnar arteries and median and ulnar nerves. The prognosis in zone III, IV and V is good and return of complete motion is the rule (Rogers et al 1990) after 6 months. Rupture or adherences with secondary bridge graft or tenolysis are rare compared with lesions in zone II.

Difficult indications in primary repair

In major trauma, flexor tendon injury is associated with skin loss, neurovascular lesions, phalanx fracture and tendon loss. Classical direct suture without traction cannot be performed. If advancement procedures are not sufficient, two options can be used. In zone III, IV or V a bridge graft can restore tendon continuity. A local or regional flap covers the repair and decreases potential adhesion formation. In zone II, the flexor tendon sheath and pulley are frequently damaged and a transitory silicone tube is necessary to create a digital sheath with good gliding potential. Reconstruction of the pulleys and repair of the neurovascular bundle and skin are done during the first operation. A secondary graft into the new digital sheath will allow the physician to restore capacity of finger flexion (Hunter procedure).

Is it necessary or dangerous to repair an isolated lesion in zone II of the FDP? If the proximal stump is not retracted into the palm and the contusion of surrounding soft tissue is limited, a direct atraumatic suture is recommended. But if the vinculum system is avulsed with a high potential for local fibrosis, it is less dangerous for the function of the FDS and the capacity of finger flexion to propose a DIP tenodesis or fusion.

In partial flexor tendon laceration, the surgical technique depends on the percentage of cross-sectional area of tendon involved: if it is less than 20% of the diameter of the tendon, the tendon should be rounded off by resection of the flap; a partial resection of the pulley could help to avoid a trigger finger (Frewin and Scheker 1989); if it is between 20 and 50%, a simple peripheral running suture should be sufficient; if it is more than 50%, a core through the injured part of the tendon and a peripheral suture should be preferred.

Evaluation of results of primary repair in flexor tendon lesions

Many methods have been reported for evaluating the results after tendon repair. In 1976 the American Society of Hand Surgery proposed a method which measured the active flexion of MP, PIP and DIP joints and decreases in loss of extension for each joint. This value was compared to the healthy contralateral finger.

Buck-Gramcko (1976) measured the distance pulp–palmar, active extension loss and total active motion (TAM) of the finger. A little sophisticated, this method is lengthy and difficult to reproduce for each patient in consultation.

Tubiana (1986) proposed a method of evaluation based on the PIP joint. This method evaluated the position of the second phalanx compared to the position of the metacarpal; then the loss of active extension and active flexion of the finger can be measured precisely. This method allows evaluation of global function of the finger but not the arc of mobility.

Strickland (1989) reported a simple and useful method which counted the TAM of PIP and DIP joints. This method ignores the MP joint, which is not under the

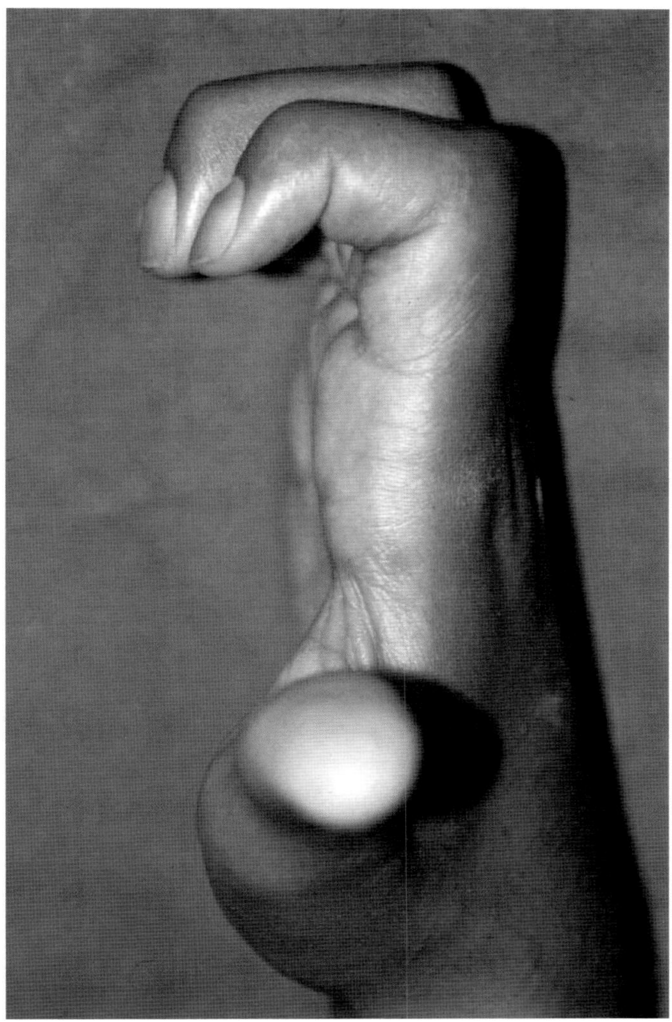

Figure 3.12
Strickland's evaluation of the flexor tendon repair: this method ignores the MP joint.

control of the flexor tendon, and compares TAM to the contralateral finger to obtain a percentage (Figure 3.12).

Conclusion

Many advances have been made in the understanding of tendinous healing – e.g. suture technique, rehabilitation programmes – but some factors have an important influence on outcome: the kind of initial injury (clean cut, contusion, avulsion), associated lesions (bone, neurovascular bundle, skin) and local lesions (irreparable sheath, damaged pulley), particularly in zone II. However, some factors are essential for achieving a good result: an atraumatic (microscope) and anatomic suture with a high potential of resistance to permit immediate active motion and a motivated patient who is able to understand and to follow postoperative physiotherapy under the control of a hand therapist and a hand surgeon.

References

Amadio PC, Hunter JM, Jaeger SH, Wehebe MA, Schneider LH (1985) The effect of vincular injury on the results of flexor tendon surgery in zone 2, *J Hand Surg* **10A**: 629–32.

Amiel D, Ishizue K, Billings E et al (1989) Hyaluronan in flexor tendon repair, *J Hand Surg* **14A**: 837–43.

Barrie KA, Tomak SL, Cholewicki J, Merrell GA, Wolfe SW (2001) Effect of suture locking and suture caliber on fatigue strength of flexor tendon repair, *J Hand Surg* **26A**: 340–6.

Becker H, Orak F, Duponselle E (1979) Early active motion following a bevelled technique of flexor tendon repair: repair of fifty cases, *J Hand Surg* **4**: 454–60.

Bellemère Ph, Chaise F, Friol JP, Gaisne E, Le Lardic C (1998) Résultats de la mobilisation active précoce après réparation primaire des tendons fléchisseurs, *La Main* **3**: 221–33.

Buck-Gramko D (1976) A new method for evaluation of results in flexor tendon repair, *Handchirurgie* **8**: 65–9.

Bunnell S (1956) *Surgery of the Hand*, 3rd edn (JB Lippincott: Philadelphia).

Chow A, Thomes LJ, Dovelle SW, Milnor WH, Jackson JP (1988) Controlled motion rehabilitation after flexor tendon repair and grafting. A multi-centre study, *J Bone Joint Surg* **70B**: 591–5.

Dinopoulos H, Boyer MI, Burns ME, Gelberman RH, Silva MJ (2000) The resistance of four and eight strand suture technique to gap formation during tensile testing: an experimental study of repair of canine flexor tendons after 10 days of in vivo healing, *J Hand Surg* **25A**: 489–98.

Doyle JR (1988) Anatomy of the finger flexor tendon sheath and pulley system, *J Hand Surg* **13A**: 473–84.

Doyle JR (1990) Anatomy and function of the palmar aponeurosis pulley, *J Hand Surg* **15A**: 78–82.

Duran RJ, Hauser RG (1975) Controlled passive motions following flexor tendon repair in zones two and three. In: *AAOS Symposium on Tendon Surgery in the Hand* (Mosby: St Louis) 105–11.

Foucher G, Merle M, Hoang Ph (1986) Suture du tendon fléchisseur profond au niveau de la partie distale du "No Man's land", *Rev Chir Orthop* **72**: 227–9.

Frewin PR, Scheker LR (1989) Triggering secondary to an untreated partially cut flexor tendon, *J Hand Surg* **14B**: 419–21.

Gelberman RH, Vandeberg JS, Manske PR, Akeson WH (1985) The early stages of flexor tendon healing: a morphologic study of the first fourteen days, *J Hand Surg* **10A**: 776–84.

Gelberman RH, Woo SLY, Amiel D, Horibe SH, Lee D (1990) Influences of flexor sheath continuity and early motion on tendon healing in dogs, *J Hand Surg* **15A**: 69–77.

Gelberman RH, Siegle DB, Savio LY et al (1991a) Healing of digital flexor tendons: importance of the interval from injury to repair, *J Bone Joint Surg* **73A**: 66–75.

Gelberman RH, Steinberg D, Amiel D, Akeson W (1991b) Fibroblast chemotaxis after tendon repair, *J Hand Surg* **16A**: 688–93.

Hagberg L (1992) Exogenous hyaluronate as an adjunct in the prevention of adhesions after flexor tendon surgery. A controlled clinical trial, *J Hand Surg* **17A**: 132–6.

Kleinert HE, Verdan C (1983) Report of the committee on tendon injuries, *J Hand Surg* **8**: 158–62.

Kleinert HE, Kutz JE, Ashbell TS, Martinez E (1967) Primary repair of lacerated flexor tendons in "No man's land", *J Bone Joint Surg* **49A**: 577.

Leddy JP, Parker JW (1977) Avulsion of the profundus tendon insertion in athletes *J Hand Surg* **2**: 66.

Leviet D (1986) Flexor tendon lengthening by tenotomy at the musculotendinous junction, *Ann Plast Surg* **17**: 239–46.

Lin GT, Amadio PC, Cooney WP (1989) Functional anatomy of the human digital flexor pulley system, *J Hand Surg* **14A**: 949–56.

Lister G (1983) Incision and closure of the flexor sheath during primary tendon repair, *Hand* **15**: 123–35.

Lister GD, Kleinert HE, Kutz JE, Atasoy E (1977) Primary flexor tendon repair followed by immediate controlled mobilization, *J Hand Surg* **2**: 441–52.

Lundborg G, Myrhage R, Rydevick B (1977) The vascularization of human flexor tendons within the digital synovial sheath region. Structural and functional aspects, *J Hand Surg* **2**: 417–28.

Lundborg G, Hansson HA, Rank F, Rydevick B (1980) Superficial repair of severed flexor tendons in synovial environment: an experimental, ultrastructural study on cellular mechanisms, *J Hand Surg* **5**: 451–61.

Manske PR, Lesker PA (1983) Palmar aponeurosis pulley, *J Hand Surg* **8**: 259–63.

Ochiai N, Maatsui T, Miyaji N, Merklim RJ, Hunter JM (1979) Vascular anatomy of flexor tendons. 1 – Vincular system and blood supply of the profundus tendon in the digital sheath, *J Hand Surg* **4**: 321–30.

Percival NJ, Sykes PJ (1989) Flexor pollicis longus tendon repair: a comparison between dynamic and static splintage, *J Hand Surg* **14B**: 412–15.

Peterson WW, Manske PR, Dunlap J, Horwitz DS, Kahn B (1990) Effects of various methods of restoring flexor sheath integrity on the formation of adhesions after tendon injury, *J Hand Surg* **15A**: 48–56.

Robins PR, Dobyns JH (1975) Avulsion of the insertion of the flexor digitorum profundus tendon associated with fracture of the distal phalanx. A brief review. In: *AAOS Symposium on Tendon Injury in the Hand* (CV Mosby: St Louis) 151–6.

Rogers GD, Henshall AL, Sach RP, Wallis KA (1990) Simultaneous laceration of the median and ulnar nerves with flexor tendons at the wrist, *J Hand Surg* **15A**: 990–5.

Saldana MJ, Ho PK, Lichtman DM, Chow JA, Dovelle S, Thomes LJ (1987) Flexor tendon repair and rehabilitation in zone II: open sheath technique versus closed sheath technique, *J Hand Surg* **12A**: 1110–14.

Savage R, Risitano G (1989) Flexor tendon repair using a "six strand" method of repair and early active mobilisation, *J Hand Surg* **14B**: 396–9.

Schneider LH, Hunter JM, Norris TR, Nadeau PO (1977) Delayed flexor tendon repair in no man's land, *J Hand Surg* **2**: 452–5.

Small JO, Brennen MD, Colville J (1989) Early active mobilization following flexor tendon repair in zone 2, *J Hand Surg* **14B**: 383–9.

Sourmelis SG, McGrouther D (1987) Retrieval of the retracted flexor tendon, *J Hand Surg* **12B**: 109–11.

Strickland JW (1985) Results of flexor tendon surgery in zone II in flexor tendon surgery, *Hand Clin* **1**: 167–9.

Strickland JW (1989) Flexor tendon surgery. Part I: Primary flexor tendon repair, *J Hand Surg* **14R**: 261–72.

Strickland JW, Glogovac SV (1980) Digital function following flexor tendon repair in zone II: a comparison of immobilization and controlled passive motion techniques, *J Hand Surg* **6**: 537–50.

Tajima T (1984) History, current status, and aspects of hand surgery in Japan, *Clin Orthop* **184**: 41–9.

Taras JS, Raphael JS, Marczyk SC, Bauerle WB (2001) Evaluation of suture caliber in flexor tendon repair, *J Hand Surg* **26**: 1100–4.

Tsuge K, Ikuta Y, Matsuhi Y (1975) Intratendinous tendon suture in the hand; a new technique, *J Hand Surg* **7**: 250–5.

Tubiana R, Gordon S, Grossman J, McMeniman P (1986) Evaluation des résultats après réparation des tendons fléchisseurs des doigts. In: Tubiana R, ed, *Traité de Chirurgie de la Main*, Vol 3 (Masson: Paris) 281–6.

Urbaniak J (1985) Repair of flexor pollicis longus, *Hand Clin* **1**: 69–76.

Wada A, Kubota H, Miyanishi K et al (2001) The mechanical properties of locking and grasping suture loop configurations in four strand core sutures technique, *J Hand Surg* **25B**: 548–51.

Wade PJF, Wetherell RG, Amis AA (1989) Flexor tendon repair: significant gain in strength from the halsted peripheral suture technique, *J Hand Surg* **14B**: 232–5.

Weber ER (1986) La réparation des tendons fléchisseurs dans le canal digital. Rôle nutritionnel du liquide synovial. In: Tubiana R, ed, *Traité de Chirurgie de la Main*, Vol 3 (Masson: Paris) 209–14.

4 Flexor tendon grafts

Raoul Tubiana

History of tendon grafting

The first attempt at tendon grafting was at the end of the nineteenth century. The exact dating has been made more difficult by the confusion surrounding the term tendon transplant, which should be used only to describe a tendon graft, although it was used inaccurately to signify a tendon transfer. In 1881 Heuck, a German surgeon, repaired an extensor pollicis longus using a tendon graft. In 1886, at the Surgical Society of Paris, Peyrot reported a case of 'transplantation in man of the tendon of a dog' to replace the flexor tendons of a middle finger. One year later (1887) at a meeting of the same society Monod reported a case in which a 5-cm tendon graft taken from the Achilles tendon of a rabbit was used to repair the extensor pollicis longus. Robson (1889) took a tendon from an injured digit to fashion an extensor graft on the same hand.

The beginning of the twentieth century saw extensive clinical and experimental work being done, especially in Germany, by Lange (1900), Kirschner (1909), Rehn (1910), and more particularly by Biesalski (1910) from Berlin. The latter reconsidered the problem of adhesion and the action of tension on sutures, and his work had a profound influence on his contemporaries. In 1912, Lexer from Iena published the results of the first series of 10 autografts of flexor tendons. In the USA, Lewis and Davis, in 1911, made an experimental study of direct tendon and fascial transplant. Leo Mayer, who had worked in Lange's Department in Munich, published three articles (1916a,b,c) on 'The physiological method of tendon transplantations'. In these he described the anatomy and physiology of the peritendinous structures and mentioned the necessity for a precise surgical technique which he called the 'physiological method'. He also stressed the importance of ensuring the correct tension of the transfer and the necessity for preserving the gliding planes.

While the clinical applications of Mayer's work were directed more toward the foot and the ankle joint, Bunnell in San Francisco turned his interest increasingly toward surgery of the hand. Between the time of his first article on tendon repair in the fingers, published in 1918, and his masterly book, *Surgery of the Hand*, whose first edition was published in 1944, he formulated the principles that now form the basis of tendon surgery.

At that time, primary suturing of flexor tendons was almost always doomed to failure in the digital canal. Although the tendon healing was usually satisfactory, adhesions were so extensive that tendon mobility was nil. In the face of these consistently poor results following primary suturing in what he called the 'no man's land', Bunnell in 1922 gave this advice: 'Close the skin, wait for the wound heal, then perform a secondary repair as follows: excise the two flexors and graft the profundus tendon alone from the lumbrical to the digital extremity'.

This teaching was held as a dogma by generations of surgeons for the treatment of lesions within the 'no man's land' (Littler 1947, Pulvertaft 1948, Boyes 1950, 1971). Progress in the technique of primary tendon suture (Verdan 1952, Kleinert et al 1973) has considerably reduced the indications for primary tendon grafting..

Now, tendon grafting is mostly used as a secondary reconstruction of tendon injuries. Non-vascularized tendon grafts require peripheral adhesions in order to survive; however, adhesions have a detrimental effect on sliding. Numerous techniques have been described that aim to decrease adhesion.

Allografts (homologous) and xenografts (heterologous)

In practice, most grafts are autogenous. However, the possibility of using preserved grafting material has been considered. This would allow the creation of tendon banks and obviate the need for autogenous grafts.

For many years, Iselin (1975) has advocated the use of cellular grafts preserved in a mercurial solution of Cialit, 1 in 5000 (1 g of Cialit powder in 5 liters of sterile water). These grafts are easy to handle and are immunologically more inert than fresh grafts containing live cells. Seiffert and Schmidt (1971) have followed the life cycle of these grafts by radioactive labeling techniques (^{14}C-proline) and have shown that the collagen is gradually replaced and the allograft is repopulated in 6 or 8 weeks.

In a series of experiments in dogs in which homologous freeze-dried grafts were transplanted into the digital sheaths, Potenza (1964) showed that the graft is well tolerated. As Potenza has pointed out, the term 'dead graft' is too often applied to allografts and heterografts, for although the cells themselves disappear, extracellular collagen remains.

Composite tissue tendon allografts

Peacock (1959) carried out a series of fascinating experiments on homologous transplantation of the whole flexor tendinous apparatus of the digits with a view to applying his methods to the human hand. His basic premise is that adult tendons and their sheaths are devoid of cells capable of synthesizing collagen. If the tendon sheath could be taken intact with its contents, the scarring would proceed between the recipient's bed and the outside of the sheath. Animal experiments confirm this view.

This method has been used successfully in man by several surgeons (Peacock 1960, Hueston et al 1967); Chacha (1974) has used composite autogenous grafts taken from the flexor apparatus of the toes (second toe), first in the monkey and then in man, with interesting functional results.

Reconstructing the fibrous tendon sheath

The attitude toward the flexor sheaths has changed considerably over the years. For a long time, the tendency was to resect as much of the sheaths as possible and to preserve only narrow pulleys. The reasoning was that the sheaths formed a barrier against vascularization of the graft and that there was a risk of the grafts becoming adherent to a fixed structure. Since the studies of Peacock (1965), Potenza (1964), Lundborg (1977), Matthews and Richards (1974), Doyle and Blythe (1975), Manske et al (1978) and many others, the mechanical and nutritional actions of the digital flexor sheath are better understood. The most important pulleys must be reconstructed around the graft. In some cases, it seems preferable to reconstruct the tendon sheath around a tendon implant, to prevent adhesions.

Reconstruction of a pseudo-tendon sheath

In 1963 Carroll and Basset used silicone rods to induce pseudo-sheath formation. Hunter (1965) progressively developed a two-stage procedure using a silicone rod for preliminary preparation of a pseudo-sheath. The basic concept of this technique is that when a pseudosynovial sheath is formed in response to a biologically inert implant, the cells adapt so that they can effectively accept the tendon graft. Hunter's technique is now widely used and will be discussed later.

Although the reconstruction of a fibrous tendon sheath represents progress, the non-vascularized tendon graft is placed in a more or less sclerotic receiver site with the difficult antagonistic purposes of realigning and sliding at the same time.

Pedicle tendon graft

In 1965 and 1969, Paneva-Holevich from Sofia reported a new technique for secondary reconstruction of flexor tendon injuries in zone II. The operation involves use of the superficial flexor of the same finger as a pedicled graft after suturing it at an earlier operation to the flexor profundus at the lumbrical muscle level. Later, this procedure was combined with the Hunter two-stage technique (two-stage tendon plasty) (Kessler 1972).

For Guimberteau (2001) a tendon graft can only be conceived of as an element in association with its surrounding sheaths to form a sliding unit. In 1989 Guimberteau et al described a salvage procedure in secondary flexor tendon repairs, using a vascularized sliding unit composed of a flexor tendon (usually the flexor superficialis of the annular digit) and its surrounding sheath, islanded on a branch of the ulnar artery.

Summary

In conclusion, during the last century tendon grafting has been the subject of numerous studies which have given rise to a variety of different techniques. This ingenious method is still evolving and seems to be mostly indicated for secondary tendon repairs. Inadequate skin cover, inadequate pulley system, joint contracture, and extensive damage to the tendon bed, are considered as contraindications for a primary tendon repair. This means that one-stage tendon graft is now only indicated if the soft tissues are supple, passive mobility is complete, and at least pulleys A2 and A4 are present.

Single-stage tendon graft

Exposure

The volar zig-zag incision (Bruner 1967) (Figure 4.1) or a 'hemi-Bruner' for the finger (Figure 4.2) are generally

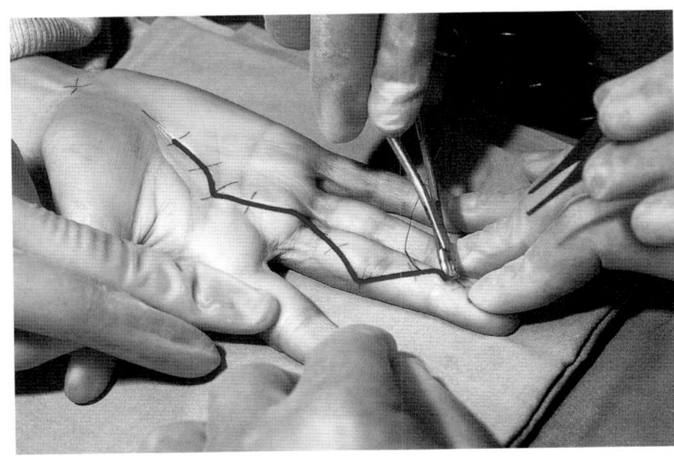

Figure 4.1
Volar zig-zag incision (Bruner).

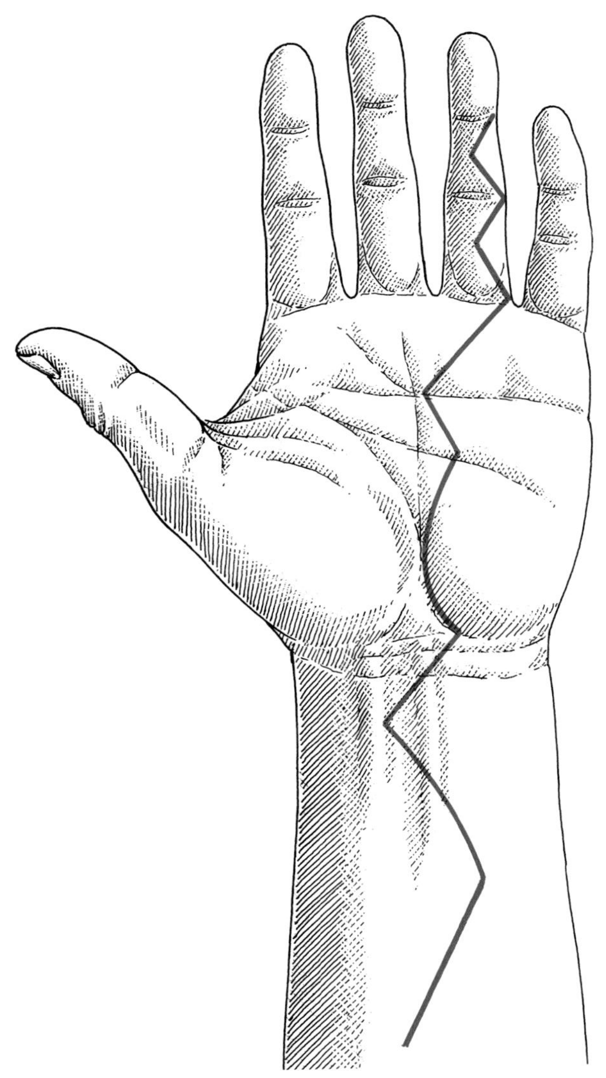

Figure 4.2
'Hemi Bruner' zig-zag incision for flexor tendon graft.

used for flexor tendon surgery. Previous incisions can be incorporated into a modified zig-zag Bruner incision. Complete exposure of the flexor tendon from the proximal part of the palm to the distal phalanx is required. At the digital extremity, the incision is placed on the side of the finger not used for tactile function. In the palm, the proximal repair site should not be directly beneath a suture line.

Graft bed preparation

Starting at the site of injury, the membranous portion of the sheath is incised, until the retracted tendon ends are located. As much as possible of the annular pulleys is preserved. Careful dissection of the adherent tendons should also leave the periosteum and the volar plates intact.

A 1-cm stump of distal profundus tendon is preserved. The distal stump of the superficialis, over the proximal interphalangeal (PIP) joint, is also preserved if the tendon remnant does not contribute to a flexion deformity; it provides a good bed for the graft and prevents PIP joint hyperextension. In cases of fibrous sheath shrinkage, the clinician can try to distend the sheath by gentle stretching, using a curved hemostat. In the palm, excision of all rigid fascia is indicated. If the remaining portion of the fibrous sheath is inadequate to allow a satisfactory function of the graft, a reconstruction of the pulley system is necessary. Most authors now believe that it is safer not to perform this reconstruction at the same time as the tendon graft.

Choice of the motor muscle

At the palm level the superficialis and profundus tendon are carefully separated. The profundus is transected at the lumbrical level. A longitudinal distraction is applied on each tendon to test its excursion. This distraction is gradually increased after about 2 minutes. The tendon with the longest excursion is chosen as the motor muscle, this is usually the profundus.

Selection of the tendon graft

Several factors must be considered when making the choice between the many potential tendon grafts: length, diameter, viability, possible sequelae at the donor site, and ease of suturing. Our choice in order of preference is as follows:

- *The palmaris longus tendon*, which is accessible in the same operative field and gives a thin graft, long

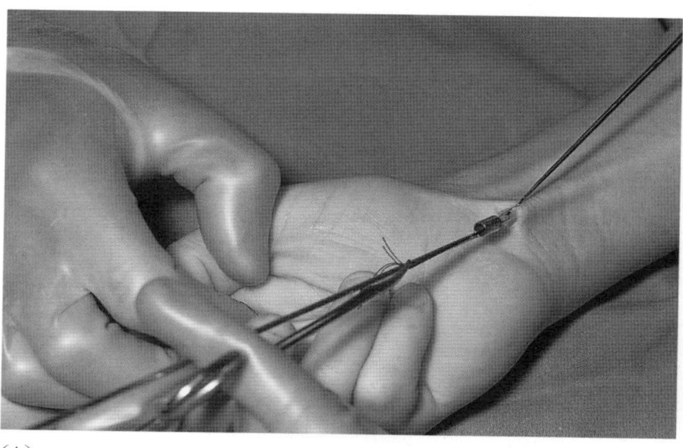

(A)

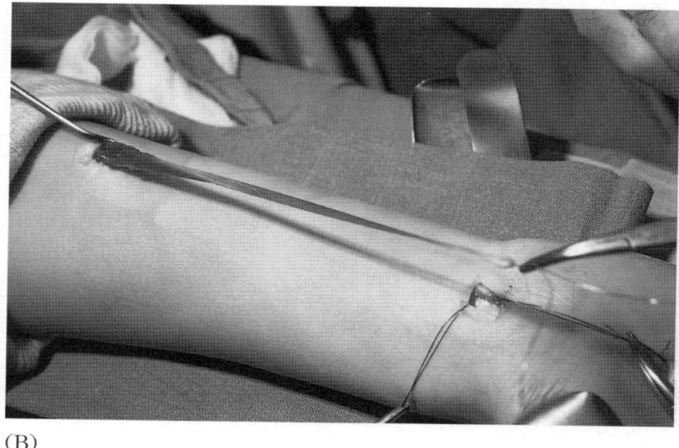

(B)

Figure 4.3
(A and B) Taking a palmaris longus tendon graft via two short incisions at the wrist and on the forearm, using a blunt stripper.

enough to run from the tip of the finger to the proximal part of the palm. It is taken through two small incisions, at the wrist and on the forearm, or by using a blunt stripper (Figure 4.3A and B). The presence of the palmaris is easy to determine preoperatively, it may be absent in about 15% of patients.

- *The plantaris* is useful for a long graft (fingertip to wrist) or for providing two finger grafts. However, unlike the palmaris longus, its presence cannot be ascertained preoperatively. The graft is usually taken on the lateral lower limb. The medial border of the Achilles tendon is exposed. If the plantaris is present, it is taken with a Brand's blunt stripper, or through a second 6-cm long incision at the superomedial of the calf, two finger-breadths behind the medial aspect of the tibia (Figure 4.4).
- *Extensor digitorum longus of second, third and fourth toes* are, after the plantaris, the tendon of choice for staged reconstruction with implant, and also when three or four grafts are necessary (Figure 4.5). They are removed using a tendon stripper through multiple transverse incisions.
- *The flexor superficialis tendon of the same digit* (except the little finger), if the retinacular system is large enough to accept this voluminous graft. If the superficialis is intact, it should never be utilized as a graft.
- Other alternative tendon donor sites include the extensor digiti minimi, the index finger common extensor tendon, or the extensor indicis proprius.

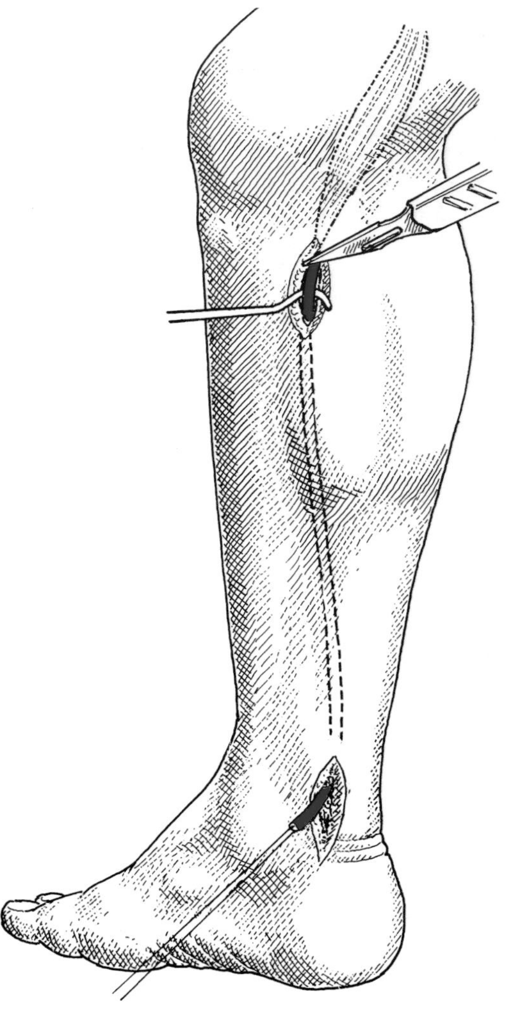

Figure 4.4
Taking a long graft of plantaris via two medial incisions on the leg.

Fixation of the graft

The tendon graft is left in place until its new bed is completely ready. The graft is then placed in its bed,

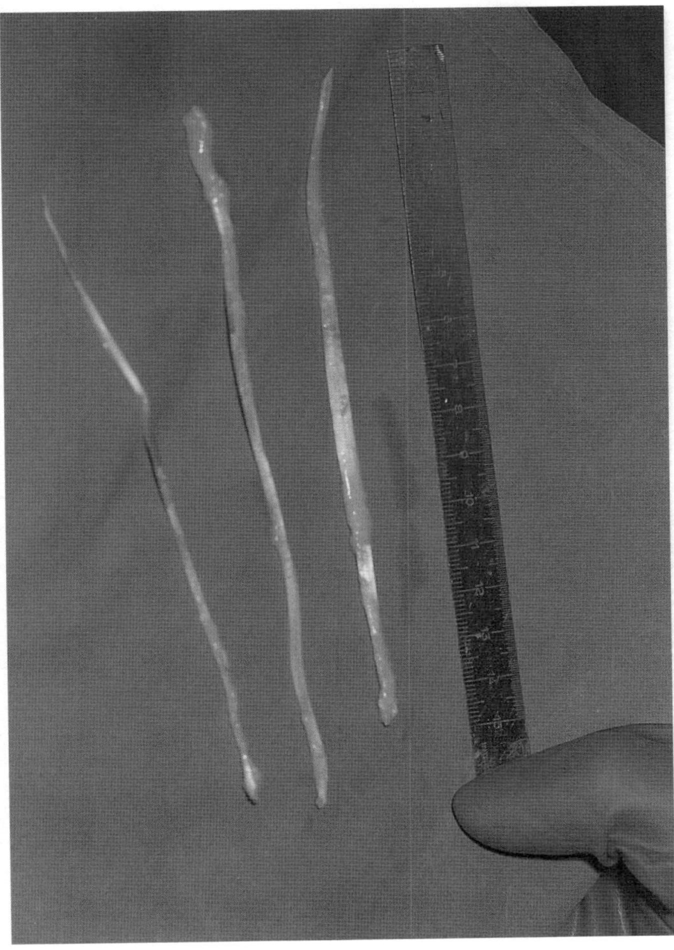

Figure 4.5

Extensor digitorum longus of second, third, and fourth toes used for grafting three flexor profundus tendons in the same hand.

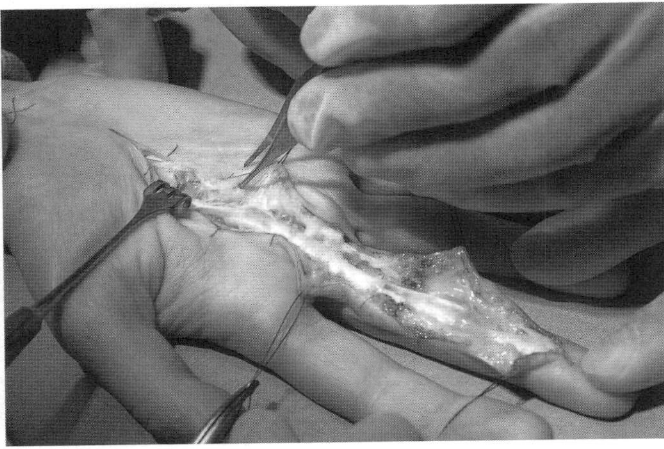

(A)

(B)

Figure 4.6

Flexor tendon graft. (A) The proximal fixation of the graft should lie in a zone where the tissues are mobile, away from fixed fibrosis structures. There are two favorable sites: the proximal part of the palm and the distal forearm. (B) The graft is passed under the remaining pulleys.

under the remaining pulleys (Figure 4.6A and B). Some surgeons prefer to fix the proximal end of the graft first and find it easier to adjust its tension distally. For similar reasons, other surgeons prefer to tether the distal end first on a fixed bony joint. Whatever the choice of the first fixation, the tension of the graft will be determined at the other extremity. The skin of the finger must be closed, by placing temporary bands of tape around the finger, because it constitutes an important element in the regulation of tension.

The distal end of the graft is attached to the distal phalanx and either a pull-out (Figure 4.7) or a pull-through suture (Figure 4.8) is used to secure the tendon into the bony cavity.

The technique at the proximal junction is determined by the diameter of the graft. When there is a discrepancy between the motor tendon and a thin graft, the fish-mouth Pulvertaft procedure is used (Figure 4.9). If both tendons are of equivalent caliber, an end-to-end type of suture is preferable. However, regardless of whether the proximal or distal end is sutured first, the important point is to ensure the correct adjustment of tension in the graft.

First the excursion of the motor muscle is tested by pulling its tendon with the aid of a traction suture. The motor tendon is then immobilized halfway through its course by a needle transfixing the skin and the tendon transversally. The length of the graft is such that with the wrist held in neutral position, the grafted finger is flexed 15° more than the adjacent digits; in normal position of function, the fingers on the ulnar side are more markedly flexed than those on the radial side (Figure 4.10).

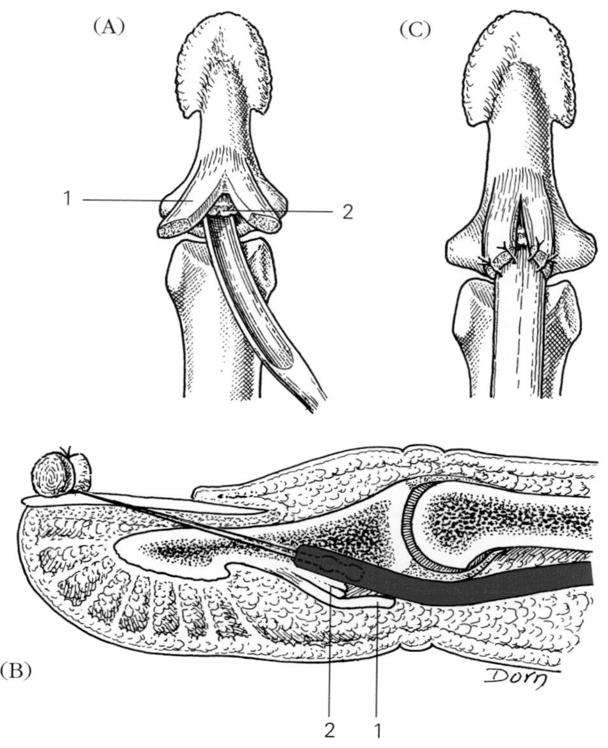

Figure 4.7

Distal pull-out fixation of the graft (Bunnell 1956).

1 Distal extremity of the FDP tendon
2 Osteoperiostal flap
(A) The distal extremity of the FDP tendon is divided in the midline. A small gouge raises an osteoperiostal flap beneath the tendon. The bone underneath and the nail are perforated obliquely with an awl or a drill. A straight needle is passed in a retrograde direction through the nail (distal to the lunula) and the bony tunnel (since it is easier to insert the blunt end first through the ungual orifice). Both ends of the core suture inserted in the graft extremity are threaded through the needle hole
(B) The tip of the graft is driven into a small bone niche. A transosseous anchoring suture is attached over a small pad or a button. The small bone flap raised by the gouge is reapplied over the graft.
(C) The extremities of the FDP tendon are sutured to the graft to hold it in its niche

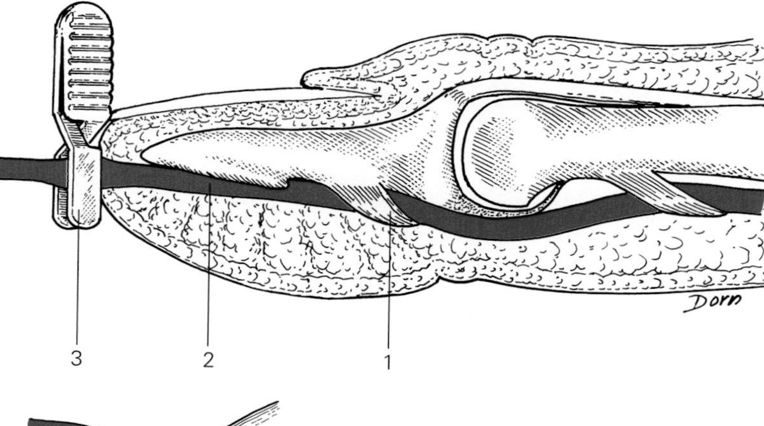

Figure 4.8

Distal pull-through fixation of the graft (Pulvertaft)

1 FDP tendon distal end
2 Tendon graft
3 Arterial clip

The graft is passed through the FDP extremity, then is drawn through the finger pulp with a Reverdin needle. The protruding part is clasped by an arterial clip. The tension is adjusted by allowing the graft to slip back or by withdrawing it.

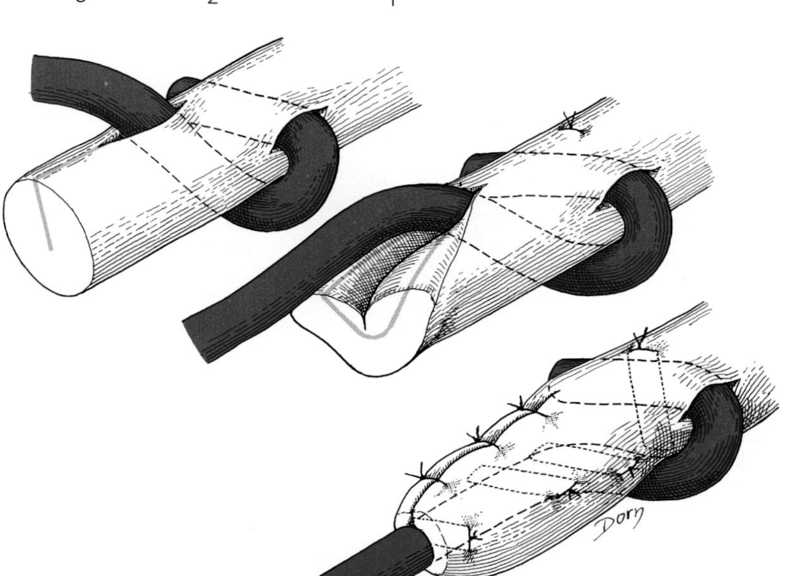

Figure 4.9

Pulvertaft 'fish-mouth' procedure used to join two tendons of different calibre, each passage of the thin tendon being at 90° angles to the previous channel. The extremity of the broader tendon is moulded around the thinner one. At each transfixation a U suture is passed through both.

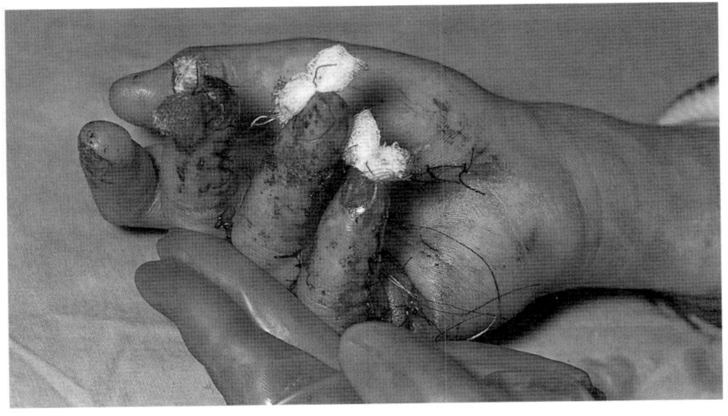

Figure 4.10
The grafted fingers are flexed 15° more than the normal position of function.

A first estimation of tension is made and a landmark stitch is used (or an arterial clip at the extremity of the finger). Next the wrist is flexed and extended. With the wrist in about 40° of flexion, it should be possible to extend the grafted finger; full wrist extension should carry the pulp of the flexed finger to within 3 or 4 cm of the palm. If tension is incorrect, adjustment is made.

Hemostasis and closure

The tourniquet is released and meticulous hemostasis is achieved. The wrist and fingers are maintained in a relaxed position by a dorsal plaster splint, the wrist in 30° of flexion, the MP joints in about 70° of flexion and the IP joints are held in extension.

Postoperative care

The splintage is identical to that described for primary flexor tendon repair. An early protected mobilization program is started in the dorsal blocking cast. At 4 weeks, the pull-out suture is removed, along with the dorsal splint, but because of the avascular nature of the graft, the strengthening exercises are delayed until 9–10 weeks after the graft (Figure 4.11).

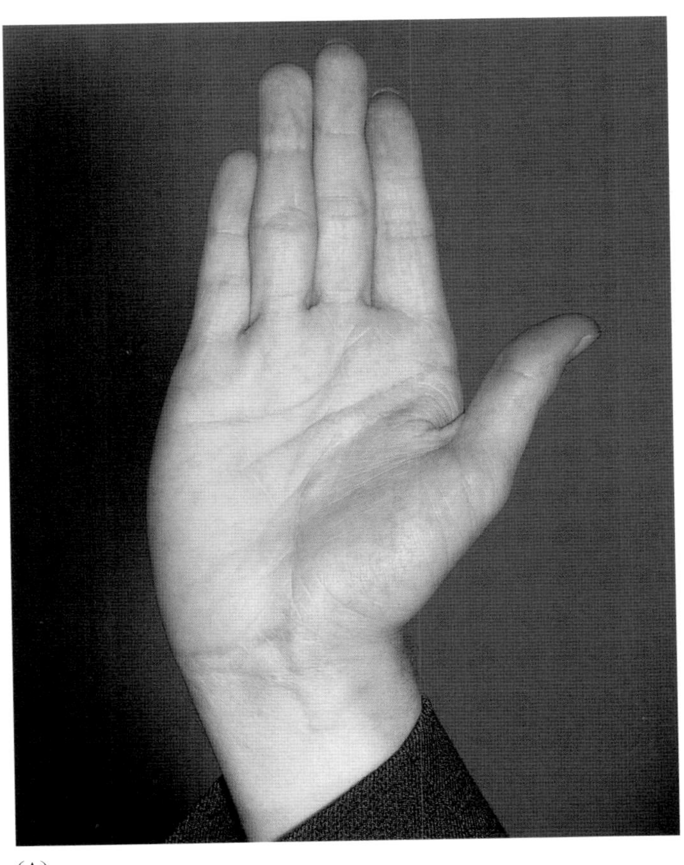

(A)

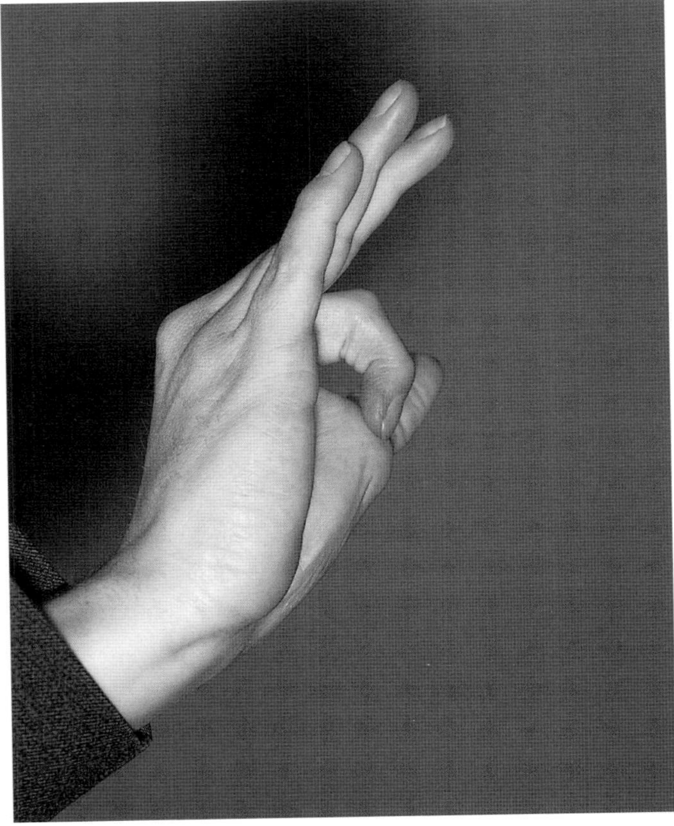

(B)

Figure 4.11
(A and B) Result of a flexor tendon graft on the index finger.

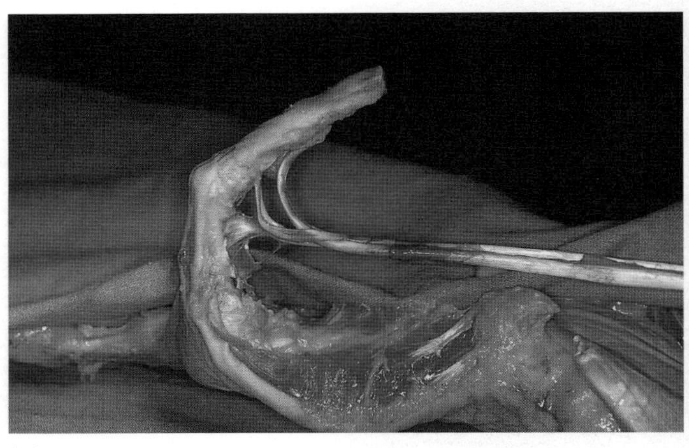
(A)

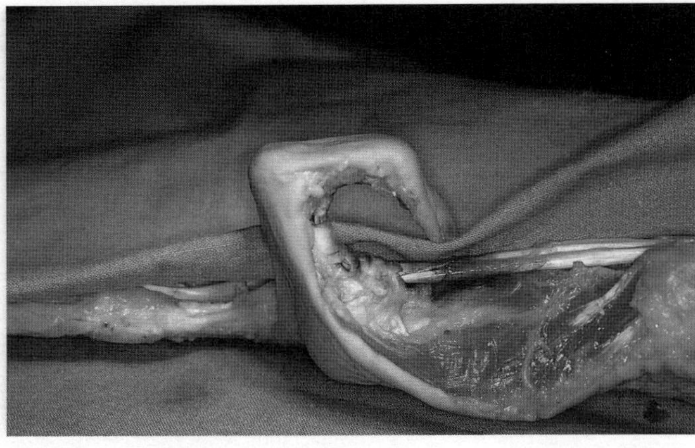
(B)

Figure 4.12
Role of the pulleys: (A) flexion of a finger without the pulley system; (B) flexion of the same finger after reconstruction of the pulleys.

Staged flexor tendon reconstruction using tendon implant

The staged reconstruction with silicone rod described by Hunter and associates (1971) is used to convert an unfavorable tendon bed into one that is much less prone to adhesions after tendon grafting.

During the first stage, the scarred tendon is resected and replaced with a 'tendon implant'. In addition, incompetent pulley systems are reconstructed and any capsular contractors are released.

At a later time, the implant is removed and tendon grafting is performed when normal gliding biomechanics and a fluid nutrition system have been re-established, so that predictable adhesion-free function of the graft can be achieved.

Indications

Flexor tendon reconstruction using a tendon implant is indicated when the tendon bed is scarred and a one-stage tendon graft will probably fail because of extensive scarring, limitation of passive mobility, or the requirement for pulley reconstruction.

In acute trauma, the tendon implant may be used if the wounds have been adequately debrided; when the injury requires simultaneous fracture fixation with flexor tendon repair, use of a tendon implant in the flexor system should be considered.

This procedure may also be indicated for grafting a profundus tendon through an intact superficialis when the profundus tendon is scarred.

In replantation surgery, the use of an implant in the flexor system when flexor tendons are damaged through a wide zone can keep the digital canal open. The implant enables passive flexion and active extension.

Acute infection is an absolute contraindication to this procedure.

Surgical techniques

Passive tendon implants

The most popular implant design is the passive implant. In passive gliding, the distal end of the implant is securely fixed to bone or tendon while the proximal end glides freely in the proximal palm or forearm. Movement of the implant is provided by active extension and passive flexion of the digit. A new biologic sheath begins to form around the implant during the period of gliding that follows stage 1 surgery. The new sheath develops a fluid system that supports gliding and nutrition for the tendon graft after stage 2. The implant usually can be replaced by a tendon graft after 3 months.

Stage I

Exposure of the flexor tendons and their excision is the same as for a one-stage tendon graft. All pulley material is preserved. The excised tendon is set aside for possible use in pulley reconstruction.

If joint flexion deformities are not relieved by tendon and scar excision, volar plate and accessory collateral ligament releases are carried out. Scarred or shortened

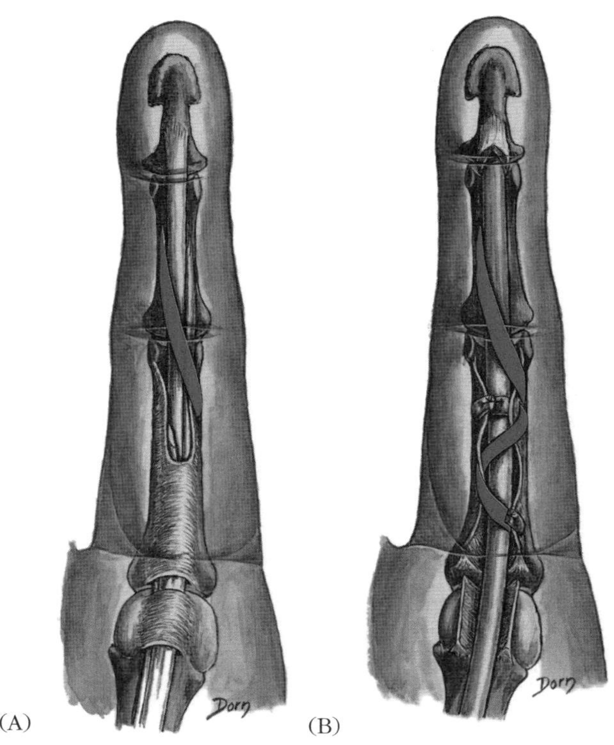

Figure 4.13

Pulley reconstruction using (A) insertion band of the FDS at the level of the middle phalanx to reconstruct A4 and (B) a PL tendon graft for A2 reconstruction. The extremity of the tendon graft may be fixed to the bone.

lumbrical muscle is resected to prevent the problem of a 'lumbrical plus' finger.

An incision is made above the wrist in the ulnar half of the forearm. A silicone implant of an appropriate size is selected, usually 4-mm for an adult male. It is sutured to the superficialis in the palm and brought proximally to the forearm through the carpal tunnel. The trial implant is then threaded distally into the pulley system. It should glide passively without resistance.

The implant is solidly sutured to the distal profundus stump with a 4-0 non-absorbable suture woven throughout its distal end (Figure 4.12); care is taken to place the suture through the central Dacron core.

Pulley reconstruction

When the pulley system is inadequate, it must be reconstructed (Figure 4.13A and B). The tail of the superficialis can be used for A4 reconstruction (Figure 4.14).

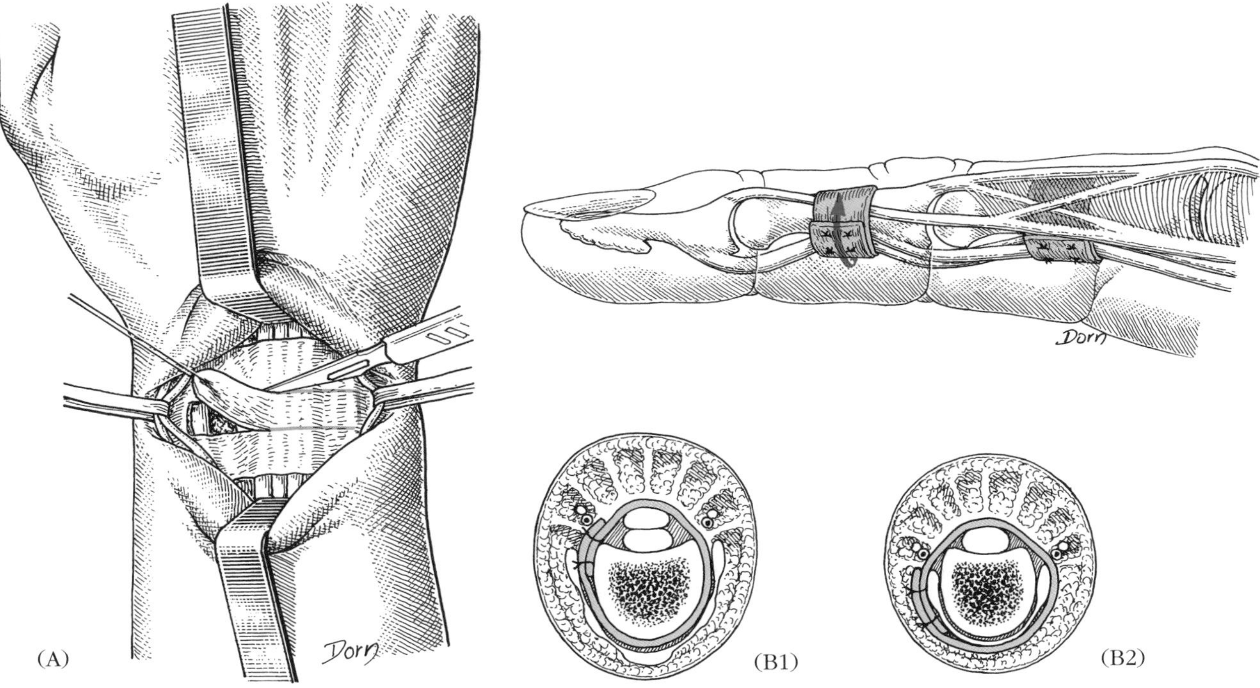

Figure 4.14

Pulley reconstruction (from Lister 1979)

A A strip 8 cm long and 1 cm broad may be taken from the extensor retinaculum. Retinacular or pulley tissue may also be taken on the dorsal aspect of the foot. Retinacular tissue is similar to flexor tendon sheath and seems preferable mto a tendon graft for pulley reconstruction

B The strip from the extensor retinaculum is passed around the phalanx and the tendon, deep to the extensor tendon over the proximal phalanx (1) and superficial to it over the middle (2)

The overlapped repair is rotated around to the side of the digit

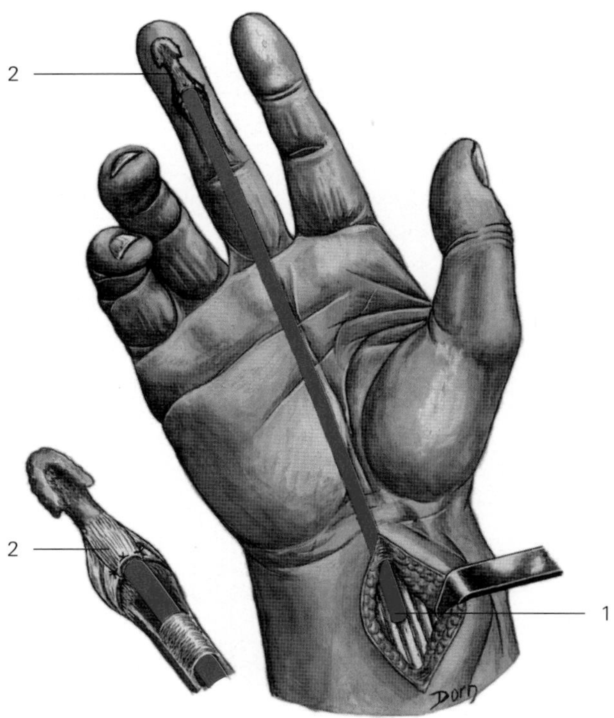

Figure 4.15

Hunter staged tendon reconstruction, stage 1

1 Proximal free extremity of the silicone implant (in red)
2 The distal extremity is solidly sutured to the distal FDP stump

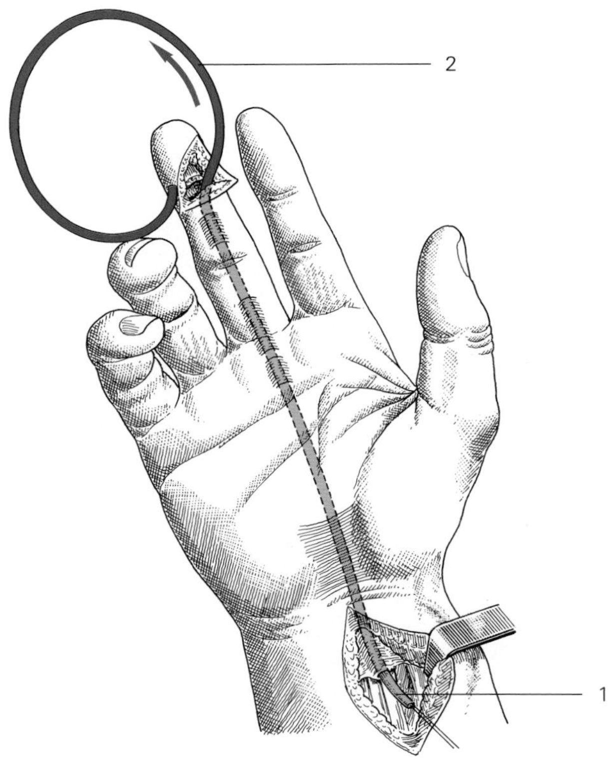

Figure 4.16

Hunter staged tendon reconstruction, stage 2

Three months later, a long tendon graft (1) is sutured to the proximal end of the implant (2) and is pulled through the carpal tunnel, the palm, and the digital canal

Various techniques using tendon grafts wrapped several times around the implant or a band taken from the dorsal retinaculum of the wrist (Lister 1979) have been described (Figure 4.15). At least A2 and A4 are necessary but better mechanics would be restored if more pulley support were supplied (Hunter and Cook 1980). The pulleys must not be bulky or too close to the joint or they may act as a mechanical block to flexion by abutting on one another.

The pulley should be located just beyond the widest part of the condyle at the metaphyseal–diaphyseal junction. This location offers the dual benefit of limiting pulley tension and maintaining good finger function by restricting bowstringing. In this way, tendon excursion for joint motion is kept within physiologic range (Hunter and Salisbury 1971).

The implant is trimmed to the appropriate length so that the proximal end can be seen 1–2 inches proximal to the wrist crease on full extension of the finger.

Buckling of the implant may occur distal to a tight pulley. If buckling does occur, it must be corrected by pulley reconstruction before closure, otherwise synovitis may develop.

Digital nerve repairs are completed if needed. The wrist and fingers are maintained in a relaxed position by a dorsal plaster splint. Passive motion exercises are started early, on the fifth day, except in cases of nerve suture. During the interval between stage 1 and stage 2, the joints are mobilized and should regain full passive motion.

Reconstructed pulleys must be protected with a pulley ring. After 3 months, the hand is usually soft, ready for grafting.

Stage 2

The distal portion of the finger incision is opened and the proximal incision is reopened in the distal forearm. The fascia is excised and the implant is located within its new sheath. The motor tendon is selected. Usually the common profundus muscle its used to motor the long, ring, and little fingers. For the index finger, the profundus of the index or sometimes the superficialis is used. A long tendon graft is necessary – the plantaris or, if it is absent, one of the long extensors of the three central toes.

The graft is sutured to the proximal end of the implant and pulled through the carpal tunnel, the palm, and the digital canal (Figure 4.16). The implant is discarded. The distal and the proximal junctures are secured in the same manner as is utilized for a one-stage graft. It is preferable that the operated finger be placed in slightly greater flexion than that of the uninjured digits. An early protected motion program is initiated 5 days after surgery.

Active tendon implants

Active tendon implants (Hunter et al 1988) are intended to be a temporary tendon replacement. They can be used in workers who are permitted to return to their occupations for extended periods of time while a new sheath is forming in the finger, palm, and forearm.

The placement of active tendon implants uses the same incision and follows the same general guidelines for insertion as those described for passive tendon implants.

Distal fixation

The distal fixation must be secured to bone in a way that will provide a strong, durable junction. A metal plate which is fixed directly to the bone can be used (Holter, Hausner design). A porous polyester cord technique is preferable for small fingers, the cords pass through the pulleys more easily than the metal plate. The porous cords are passed through drill holes in the bone. The length of the tendon is estimated.

If the patient can be aroused from anesthesia, an accurate assessment of the muscle amplitude is possible. Otherwise, the operated finger should lie in extension during wrist flexion and show a position of balance with the adjacent fingers on wrist extension.

The proximal junction

Active tendon implants have two types of proximal junctions. The preformed silicone loop allows the motor tendon to be passed through it so that the patient's own tendon can be secured to itself. The implants without a loop terminate with two free porous cords. Each of the cords is woven through the proximal tendon in criss-cross fashion. A protective postoperative splint is removed after 3 weeks.

Therapy is initiated on the first postoperative day, it begins with passive hold exercise. A contracture control program is initiated during the second postoperative week.

A minimum of 4–6 months is required between stage 1 and stage 2 to facilitate hand reconditioning.

Stage 2

Stage 2 surgery consists of removal of the active tendon graft, insertion of a tendon graft through the pseudo-sheath, and initiation of postoperative therapy to facilitate gliding of the graft.

Pedicle tendon graft

Paneva-Holevich (1965) described a technique involving, in unfavorable cases, the use of the flexor superficialis as a pedicle graft after suturing it at an earlier operation to the flexor profundus tendon of the same finger.

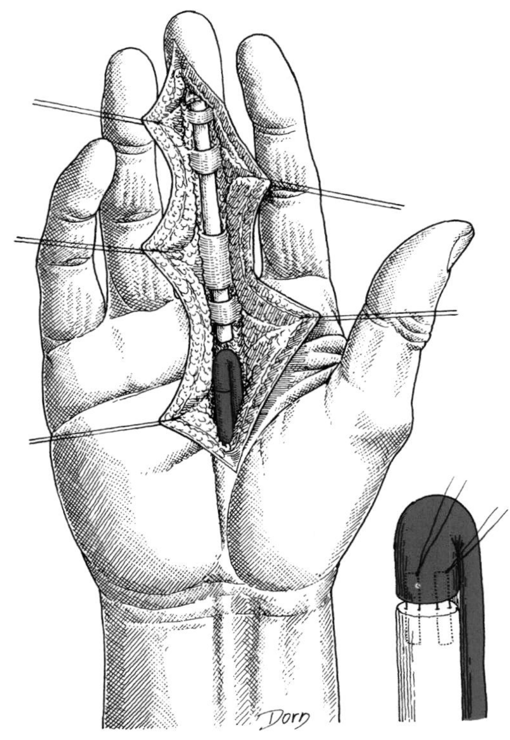

Figure 4.17
Pedicle tendon graft (Paneva-Holevich 1988). Stage 1: suturing of the proximal stumps of the FDS and FDP (in red) in the palm, implantation of a silicon rod in the digital canal.

First stage

The flexor profundus tendon is divided in the palm at the lumbrical muscle level. The flexor superficialis is cut 3 cm more distally and the cut ends of the two tendons are sutured end-to-end (Figure 4.17).

Since 1977, the author has added at this stage the excision of the digital portion of the flexor tendons and the preparation of the pseudo-sheath by the introduction of a silicone rod in the digital canal, which is fixed distally to the stump of the profundus. Annular pulleys are preserved or reconstructed as in Hunter's technique.

Second stage

Two to three months after the first stage, a long zig-zag incision is performed between the palm and the distal third of the forearm. The carpal retinaculum is opened

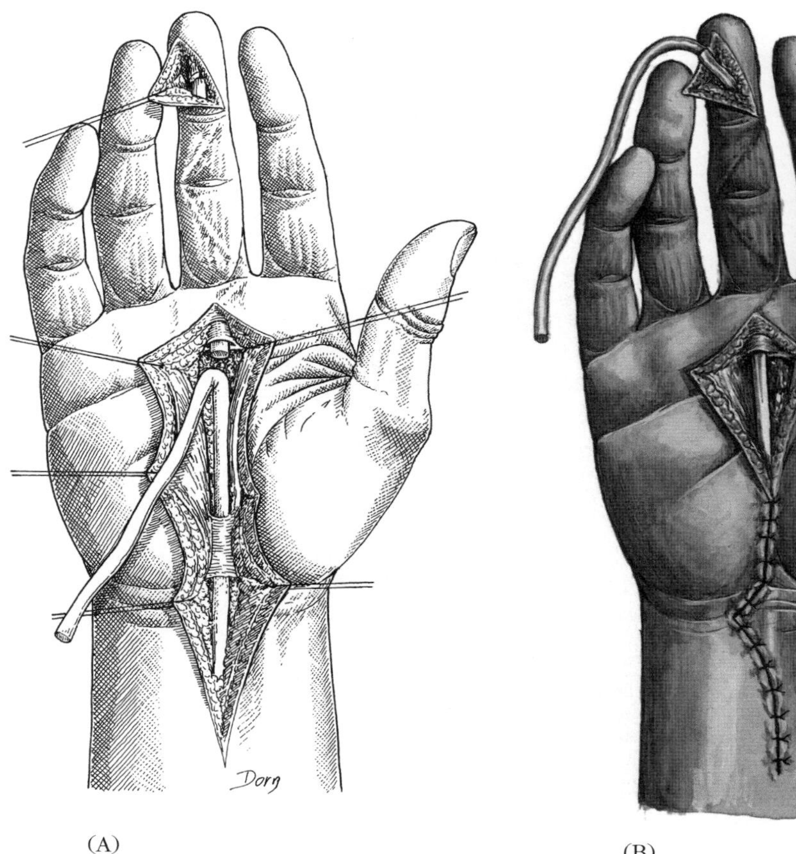

Figure 4.18

Pedicle tendon graft, stage 2

(A) The pedicle graft (from the FDS) is divided at its musculotendinous junction and rotated distally

(B) The graft is sutured to the proximal end of the silicone implant and pulled through the digital canal

in a zig-zag fashion. The involved flexor superficialis tendon is identified, and is divided at its musculotendinous junction. The pedicle graft is rotated distally. Adhesions are excised.

By flexing the digit, the proximal end of the silicone implant is exposed, in a blind synovial cul-de-sac, which is opened. The end of the pedicle graft is temporarily sutured to the implant (Figure 4.18). An incision is made at the level of the distal phalanx. The implant is pulled out until the end of the pedicle graft emerges in the wound. The end of the graft is fixed to the distal phalanx under physiological tension.

An early motion program is initiated on the fifth day, with the protection of a dorsal blocking cast.

The superficialis finger

The concept of the superficialis finger, initially described by Osborne (1968), has been suggested as a means of salvage for the finger affected by severe adhesions or failed tendon graft procedures associated with bone and neurovascular injury. In these situations, a more limited goal of a one-tendon, two-joint flexor system is justified to restore functional motion to the metacarpophalangeal (MP) and PIP joints, with arthrodesis of the DIP joint.

The indications for the superficialis finger operation are: inadequate DIP joint caused by arthrosis or extensor insufficiency, distal junction rupture of a tendon graft, multiple digit injuries, and multiple prior failed procedures on the flexor tendon system.

A staged superficialis tendon reconstruction with silicone implant and secondary tendon grafting is performed.

Arthrodesis of the DIP joint is performed before establishing the tendon junction, to avoid excessive manipulation of the tendon to bone attachment.

After surgery, a splint is applied with the wrist in 30° of flexion, with the MP joints in extension. Postoperative management is the same as that for a flexor tendon graft; however, the DIP joint must be protected with a thermoplastic splint.

Grafting the flexor profundus tendon in the presence of a flexor superficialis

In cases of a division of the flexor profundus tendon or an avulsion of its distal extremity, without damage of the superficialis, the clinician may elect to perform a tendon graft. The graft should be thin (the plantaris) and should

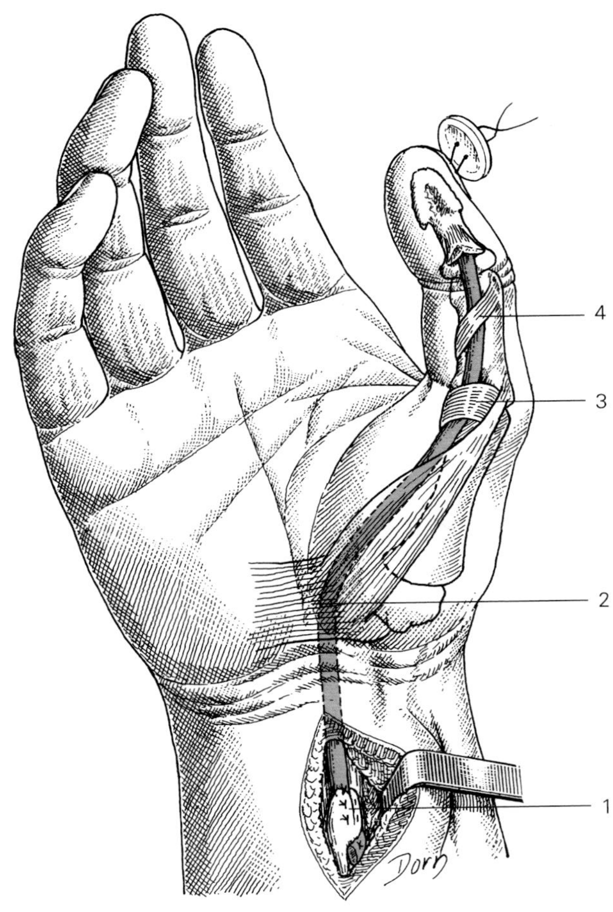

Figure 4.19
Flexor tendon graft in the thumb
1 Proximal fixation in the distal forearm
2 Flexor retinaculum
3 A1 pulley
4 Oblique pulley

be placed within the fibrous sheath, alongside the flexor superficialis tendon and not through it (because it might then injure the meso tendon).

The proximal and distal extremities of the graft are fixed with the wrist, MP and PIP joints straight and the DIP joint in 40° of flexion.

A dorsal splint is then used, maintaining the wrist flexed at 30° and the MP joint at 70°. The two interphalangeal joints are placed in slight flexion. After one week, active flexion of the wrist, MP, and PIP joints is started, while the DIP joint is maintained in extension. After 3 weeks active flexion of the DIP joint is allowed while the other joints remain flexed. At the fifth week, the distal phalanx is actively flexed, with the PIP joint maintained in extension. Some authors advocate a two-step procedure (Versaci 1970, Wilson 1980), the flexor profundus graft being preceded by the placement of a silicone implant. Such an approach is not always required, as shown by the satisfactory results of one-stage grafts (Pulvertaft 1960, Stark 1977). It would be a useful approach if a pulley reconstruction or a liberation of a stiff joint was required.

Flexor tendon grafting in the thumb

The technique is similar to that described for flexor grafts in the fingers. The graft is passed along the original course of the FPL into the thumb. At least one strong pulley opposite the proximal phalanx is essential. The proximal fixation of the graft may be done in the palm, but is usually performed at the wrist level, at a safe distance from the carpal tunnel (Figure 4.19). The palmaris longus usually provides a suitable graft.

The tension of the graft is adjusted, with the wrist in neutral position and the thumb in anteposition and moderate flexion of all joints, so that the tip of the thumb is in contact with the index finger pulp. A trial is conducted with only one suture. Full passive extension of the wrist produces complete thumb flexion, whereas full passive wrist flexion allows thumb extension. When the tension is correct, the junctions are completed.

A two-stage tendon graft with implant is required if there is severe scarring and joint contractures. The proximal end of the silicone implant is positioned deep in the wrist, adjacent to the FPL proximal tendon stump.

References

Biesalski K (1910) Über Sehnenscheidenauswechslung, *Deutsche Med Wochnschr* **36**: 1615–18.

Boyes JH (1950) Flexor tendon grafts in the fingers and thumb. An evaluation of end results, *J Bone Joint Surg* **32A**: 489.

Boyes JH, Stark HH (1971) Flexor tendon grafts in the finger and thumb. A study of factors influencing results in 1,000 cases, *J Bone Joint Surg* **53A**:1332.

Bruner JM (1967) The zig-zag volar digital incision for flexor tendon surgery, *Plast Reconstr Surg* **40**: 571–4.

Bunnell S (1918) Repair of tendons in the fingers and description of two new instruments, *Surg Gynecol Obstet* **26**:103.

Bunnell S (1922) Repair of tendons in the fingers, *Surg Gynecol Obstet* **35**: 88–97.

Bunnell S (1944) *Surgery of the Hand* (Lippincott: Philadelphia).

Caroll RE, Bassett AL (1963) Formation of tendon sheath by silicone rod implants, *J Bone Joint Surg* **45A**: 884–4.

Chacha P (1974) Free autologous composite tendon grafts for division of both flexor tendons within the digital theca of the hand, *J Bone Joint Surg* **56A**: 960–78.

Doyle JR, Blythe WF (1975) The finger flexor tendon sheath and pulleys: anatomy and reconstruction. In: *AAOS Symposium on Tendon Surgery in the Hand* (CV Mosby: St Louis).

Graham WC (1947) Flexor tendon grafts to the finger and thumb, *J Bone Joint Surg* **29**: 593–9.

Guimberteau JC, Goin JL, Panconi B, Schumacher B (1989) Tendon ulnar artery island flap in hand surgery: technique, indications, *Eur J Plast Surg* **12**: 12.

Guimberteau JC (2001) *New Ideas in Hand Flexor Tendon Surgery. The Sliding System. Vascularized Flexor Tendon Transfers* (Institut Aquitain de la Main: Aquitaine Domaine Forestier).

Heuck G (1881) Ein Beitrag zur Sehnenplastik, *Zentralbl Chir* **9**: 289–92.

Hueston JT, Hubble B, Rigg BR (1967) Homografts of the digital flexor tendon system, *Aust NZ J Surg* **36**: 269.

Hunter JM (1965) Artificial tendons. Early development and application, *Am J Surg* **109**: 324.

Hunter JM (1983) Staged flexor tendon reconstruction, *J Hand Surg* **8**: 789.

Hunter JM (1984) Active tendon prosthesis – techniques and clinical experience. In: Hunter JM, Schneider LH, Mackin EJ, eds, *Tendon Surgery in the Hand* (CV Mosby: St Louis).

Hunter JM, Salisbury RE (1971) Flexor tendon reconstruction in severely damaged hands. A two stage procedure using a silicone dracon reinforced gliding prosthesis prior to tendon grafting, *J Bone Joint Surg* **53A**: 829–58.

Hunter JM, Schneider LH, Fiette VG (1979) Reconstruction of the sublimis finger, *Orthop Trans* **3**: 321.

Hunter JM, Cook JF, Konikoff JJ, Merklin RJ, MacKin GA (1980) The pulley system, *Orthop Trans* **4**: 4.

Hunter JM, Singer DI, Jaeger SH, MacKin EJ (1988) Active tendon implants in flexor tendon reconstruction, *J Hand Surg* **13A**: 849–59.

Iselin F (1975) Preliminary observations on the use of chemically stored tendinous allografts in hand surgery. In: *AAOS Symposium on Tendon Surgery in the Hand* (CV Mosby: St Louis) 66.

Kessler F (1972) Use of pedicled tendon transfer with silicone rod in complicated secondary flexor tendon repairs, *Plast Reconstr Surg* **49**: 439–43.

Kirkpatrick WH, Kobus RJ (1992) The superficialis finger procedure, *Oper Tech Orthop* **3**: 303.

Kirschner M (1909) Über freie Sehnen und Fascientransplantation, *Beitr Klin Chir* **65**: 472–503.

Kleinert HE, Kutz JE, Atasoy E et al (1973) Primary repair of flexor tendons, *Orthop Clin North Am* **4**: 864.

Lange F (1900) Über periostale Sehnenverpflanzungen bei Lahmungen, *Munch Med Wochenschr* **47**: 486–90.

Lewis D, Davis CB (1911) Experimental direct transplantation of tendon and fascia, *JAMA* **57**: 540–6.

Lexer E (1912) Die Verwertung der freien sehnentransplantation. *Langenbecks Arch Klin Chir* **98**: 818–52.

Lister GD (1979) Reconstruction of pulleys employing extensor retinaculum, *J Hand Surg* **4**: 461–4.

Littler JW (1947) Free tendon grafts in secondary flexor tendon repair, *Am J Surg* **74**: 314.

Lundborg G, Myrhage PD, Rydevik B (1977) The vascularization of human flexor tendons within the digital synovial sheath region, structural and functional aspects, *J Hand Surg* **2**: 417–27.

Manske PR, Whiteside LA, Lesker PA (1978) Nutrient pathways to flexor tendons using hydrogen washout technique, *J Hand Surg* **3**: 32–6.

Matthews P, Richards H (1974) The repair potential of digital flexor tendons, *J Bone Joint Surg* **56B**: 618.

Mayer L (1916a) The physiological method of tendon transplantations. I. Historical: anatomy and physiology of tendons, *Surg Gynecol Obstet* **22**: 182.

Mayer L (1916b) The physiological method of tendon transplantations. II. Operative technique, *Surg Gynecol Obstet* **22**: 198.

Mayer L (1916c) The physiological method of tendon transplantations. III. Experimental and clinical experiences, *Surg Gynecol Obstet* **22**: 472.

Mayer L (1936) Reconstruction of digital tendon sheaths, *J Bone Joint Surg* **18**: 607–16.

Monod (1887) Plaies des tendons: greffe tendineuse, *Bull Mem Soc Chir Paris* **13**: 297–9.

Osborne GV (1968) The sublimis tendon replacement technique in tendon injuries, *J Bone Joint Surg* **42B**: 647.

Paneva-Holevich E (1965) Two stage plasty in flexor tendon injuries of the finger within the digital synovial sheath, *Acta Chir Plast* **7**: 112–14.

Paneva-Holevich E (1969) Two stage tenoplasty in injury of the flexor tendon of the hand, *J Bone Joint Surg* **5A**: 21–32.

Paneva-Holevich E (1988) Late repair in zone II flexor tendons in unfavourable cases (pedicle tendon graft). In: Tubiana R, ed. *The Hand* vol. 3: 280–96, Philadelphia, WB Saunders.

Peacock EE (1959) A study of the circulation in normal tendons and healing grafts, *Ann Surg* **149**: 414.

Peacock EE (1960) Homologous composite tissue grafts of the digital flexor mechanism in human beings, *Plast Reconstr Surg* **25**: 418–21.

Peyrot (1886) Transplantation chez l'homme d'un tendon emprunté à un chien. Guérison avec rétablissement partiel de la fonction, *Bull Mem Soc Chir Paris* **12**: 356–61.

Potenza AD (1964) The healing of autogenous tendon grafts within the flexor digital sheath in dogs, *J Bone Joint Surg* **46A**: 1462–84.

Pulvertaft RG (1948) Repair of tendon injuries in the hand, *Ann R Coll Surg Engl* **3**: 3.

Pulvertaft RG (1956) Tendon grafts for flexor tendon injury in the fingers and thumb, *J Bone Joint Surg* **38B**: 174.

Pulvertaft RG (1960) The treatment of profundus division by the free tendon graft, *J Bone Joint Surg* **42A**: 1363–71.

Rehn E (1910) Die homoplastiche Sehnentransplantation in Tierexperiment, *Beitr Klin Chir* **68**: 417–47.

Robson AWH (1889) A case of tendon grafting, *Trans Clin Soc London* **22**: 289.

Schneider LH (1999) Flexor tendons – late reconstruction. In: Green DP, ed. *Operative Hand Surgery* (Churchill Livingstone: New York) 1898–949.

Seiffert K, Schmidt KP (1971) *Preserved Tendon Grafts in Hand Surgery*, Trans Fifth Int Congr Plast Surg (Butterworths: London).

Stark HH, Zemel NP, Boyes JH, Ashworth CR (1977) Flexor tendon graft through intact superficialis tendon, *J Hand Surg* **2**: 456–61.

Tubiana R (1960) Greffes des tendons fléchisseurs des doigts et du pouce. Technique et résultats, *Rev Chir Orthop* **46**: 191–214.

Tubiana R (1965) Incisions and techniques in tendon grafting, *Am J Surg* **109**: 339–44.

Tubiana R (1988) Flexor tendon grafts in the hand. In: Tubiana R, ed, *The Hand*, vol 3 (WB Saunders: Philadelphia) 217–43.

Urbaniak J (1974) Vascularization and the gliding mechanism of free flexor-tendon grafts inserted by the silicone-rod method, *J Bone Joint Surg* **56A**: 473.

Verdan C (1952) *Chirurgie réparatrice et fonctionelle des tendons de la main*, Paris, Expansion Scientifique Française.

Verdan C (1960) Primary repair of flexor tendons, *J Bone Joint Surg* **42A**: 647–57.

Verdan C (1972) Half a century of flexor tendon surgery, *J Bone Joint Surg* **54A**: 472.

Versaci AD (1970) Secondary tendon grafting for isolated flexor digitorum profundus injury, *Plast Reconstr Surg* **46**: 57–60.

Weecks PM, Vray RC (1976) Rate and extent of functional recovery after flexor tendon grafting with and without silicone rod preparation, *J Hand Surg* **1**: 174.

Wilson RL, Carter MS, Holdeman VA, Lovett WL (1980) Flexor profundus injuries treated with delayed two-staged tendon grafting, *J Hand Surg* **5**: 74–8.

5 Rehabilitation after tendon injuries

Terri M Skirven

Introduction

Tendon rehabilitation has evolved over the last several decades and has been based on the evolving understanding of tendon nutrition and healing and the factors that influence it as well as on the development of surgical technique. This evolution is reflected in the progression in clinical practice from initial immobilization of repaired tendons to early controlled passive motion to most recently immediate active motion.

Historical perspective

Mason and Allen's experiments published in 1941 supported the practice of initial immobilization of repaired tendons. They studied the rate at which a repaired tendon regains its tensile strength in a canine model. Mason and Allen reported two significant findings. First there was a profound decrease in tensile strength with softening of the tendon ends with the lowest values measured 4–5 days after repair. The softened tendon stumps had little holding power, and the suture pulled out of the tendon when stress was applied. Although strength gradually increased for up to 16 days, the repair was considered incapable of responding favorably to externally applied stress during this time. The second finding was that after 19 days the strength of the repair increased directly with the stresses applied to it. These findings influenced clinicians to immobilize tendons for 3 weeks before allowing active tendon gliding.

Potenza's research reported in 1963 also supported the practice of initial immobilization of tendon repairs. In a canine model, he studied the healing response of repaired tendons that were encased in a synthetic tube that was intended to block the ingrowth of adhesions. He found aseptic necrosis of the tendon at 32 days following repair, with no intrinsic healing activity observed in the tendon itself. He believed that the degeneration of the tendon within the tube represented an anutritional and avascular phenomenon. Potenza concluded that no intrinsic fibroblastic response from the injured tissue occurred and that healing depends on extrinsic cellular ingrowth. Rather than prevent adhesions, he concluded that they were necessary and should be allowed to form without disruption, thus supporting the concept of immobilization during the early stages following flexor tendon repair.

Peacock (1965) subsequently proposed the 'one wound' concept, which supported the extrinsic healing theory. The 'one wound' concept refers to the fact that the early process of wound healing is the same in all tissues involved in the injury. During the first stage of healing, the inflammatory stage, the tendon wound site is filled uniformly with leucocytes, macrophages, fluids and other inflammatory elements, which leave the vascular system. During the second stage of proliferation or fibroplasia, fibroblasts synthesize and extrude collagen. Peacock stated that the fibroblasts migrated from adjacent areas and that the tendon itself did not contain many cells capable of synthesizing collagen. Initially the collagen is in a random network that links all parts of the wound. It is during the next phase of remodeling that differentiation of the scar between different parts of the wound occurs. With a successful repair the collagen between the tendon ends becomes reoriented into polarized parallel bundles that have great strength similar to normal tendon, while the collagen between the tendon and adjacent tissues remains highly elastic and mobile and randomly oriented (Beasley 1981)

What factors influence this remodeling and differentiation? Peacock found that the amount of trauma and subsequent tissue damage was related to the extent of remodeling. The lesser the trauma the more successful and complete the remodeling. Also, he believed that newly synthesized scar remodels in response to inductive influences of the tissue with which it is in intimate contact. Other factors relevant to postoperative management are motion and stress. Longitudinal stress and shearing force transmitted by muscle pull along a repaired tendon provokes polarization of the collagen fibers and hence promotes developing strength (Beasley 1981). The reality, however, is that scar remodeling following initial immobilization is not a predictable process and that tendon adherence with some limitation of motion invariably results. The desire to improve the functional outcome of flexor tendon repairs led to the investigation of alternative mechanisms of healing.

Because the response of the tendon to injury is dependent upon its nutrition, many investigators focused on defining more precisely the nutrient pathway to the flexor tendon within the sheath. The tendon passes freely through the sheath with attachment solely by two narrow bands of tissue known as vincula. Early investigators thought that these provided a mechanical supporting function, but ultimately recognized the vincula as the vascular line to the tendon. Vascular injection studies revealed an intricate intratendinous network derived from three sources: the vinculum longum, vinculum brevi, and longitudinal palmar vessels (Matsui and Hunter 1997). These studies showed that the intratendinous vessels are located on the dorsum of the tendon and that there are significant areas of avascularity on the volar surface of the tendon and in the zones of the pulleys. These studies led some to conclude that a cooperative system of nutrition, including the intrinsic vasculature and the synovial fluid, was involved in nourishing the tendon.

Manske et al in the late 1970s did a series of experiments to determine the relative importance of synovial fluid diffusion compared to vascular perfusion in the nutrition of flexor tendons. He found that the process of diffusion functioned more quickly and completely than did perfusion and was a relatively more important pathway for tendon nutrition.

About the same time, Lundborg and Rank (1978) studied the healing of rabbit tendons in a synovial environment without vascular supply and found that healing occurred without adhesions. They concluded that an intrinsic healing potential existed with nutrition supplied by synovial fluid. Studies by Manske et al (1978a, 1978b) and Gelberman et al (1986) further supported the concept of the intrinsic healing potential of tendons.

With the existence of an intrinsic healing potential fueled by a synovial fluid nutrient pathway established, investigators began to study those factors believed to influence or promote this mechanism of healing over extrinsic healing with adhesion formation. Clearly intrinsic healing without adhesion formation is desirable from the standpoint of preserving function and tendon gliding. Since immobilization supports adhesion formation, investigators began to study the effects of early motion following tendon repairs. Gelberman et al (1980a, 1980b, 1981, 1982) and Woo et al (1981) studied the effects of motion on the healing of canine flexor tendons compared with immobilization. Their results were striking. The tendons treated with early motion showed higher tensile strength and improved gliding function over the immobilized group at each postoperative interval assessed. Early motion stimulated a reorientation of blood vessels to a more normal pattern, whereas immobilization beyond 3 weeks resulted in a random vascular pattern. DNA content was assessed as an index of tissue cellularity and repair activity. The tendons that were treated with motion showed a significant increase in DNA, whereas the immobilized tendons were not altered. Gelberman et al also found an absence of adhesion formation and restoration of a gliding surface with the early motion group compared with the dense adhesions seen with the immobilized tendons, which obliterated the space between the tendon and the sheath. They concluded that early motion was the trigger for stimulating an intrinsic repair response.

What is the biologic basis for this conclusion? Gelberman et al proposed three possible explanations (Gelberman et al 1987, Gelberman and Woo 1989). (1) The repeated tendon excursions interrupt connections between the repair site and the periphery by mechanical disruption. (2) The rapid reinstitution of the function of the tendon induces the intrinsic healing response. (3) Ingrowth of cells from the tendon sheath during the initial phase of healing may overwhelm the repair process of the epitenon. Early motion may block an inhibitory response by denying access of the inflammatory tissue to the repair site.

Another study of interest and supportive of Gelberman's findings was reported by Hitchcock et al (1987), who found that tendons subjected to early motion following repair showed a progressive increase in tensile strength from day one and that the initial loss of strength as reported by Mason and Allen (1941) was not inevitable.

The concept of early motion was not a new one. In the 1960s, Kleinert and Duran advocated early controlled motion as a means of producing less restrictive adhesions and thus resulting in better tendon glide (Duran and Houser 1975, Lester et al 1977, Slattery and McGrouther 1984, Duran et al 1990). Both techniques involved passive flexion with blocked extension, with Kleinert advocating active extension and Duran et al describing passive extension. Later investigators described passive programs that incorporated elements of both approaches with modifications in keeping with new insights regarding tendon excursion and differential tendon glide (Strickland and Glogovac 1980, Chow et al 1987, Strickland 1989). Kleinert and Duran's protocols and modifications will be discussed in more detail later in this chapter.

Clinical studies (Strickland and Glogovac 1980) comparing early passive motion with immobilization found that tendons treated with early motion had a greater average total active motion and a greater percentage of excellent results when compared with tendons treated with immobilization. However, the technique of early controlled motion was not without complications and results were not consistently good. Seradge reported in 1983 that the incidence of failure and tenolysis following flexor tendon repair and treatment with early motion was directly related to elongation at the repair site. Pruitt et al (1991) described a method of cyclic stress analysis of flexor tendon repairs using tendons from human cadavers. They found that light repetitive stress applied to a flexor tendon repair, even when less than required to produce gapping in load to failure tests, can result in large gap formation at the repair site. They found that the epitenon suture reduced gap formation.

Kessler (Kessler and Nissim 1969) and others questioned whether passive motion produced any significant tendon motion at all. The suture site may not glide proximally during passive flexion; rather the segment of the tendon distal to the repair site may kink or buckle during passive flexion and then be stretched during limited active extension. Kessler pointed out that gliding of the suture site takes place only by active flexion of the operated digit.

The search has continued for a method of management to consistently control adhesion formation and improve functional outcomes following tendon repair. Most recently, investigators have focused on the development of suture techniques capable of withstanding the forces imparted to the tendon with active motion, combined with the development of splinting and controlled active motion programs. An important consideration with these programs is the breaking strength of the suture and the tensile demands on the normal tendon, which occur with active, passive, and resisted motion. Strickland (Strickland and Cannon 1993) as well as other investigators have based their programs on the findings of Urbaniak (1974) who studied the tensile demands on the digital flexors of human subjects with motion. He found that passive finger flexion generated a force of 200–300 grams; active flexion against mild resistance did not exceed 900 grams; active flexion against moderate resistance did not exceed 1500 grams, and strong digital flexion produced more than 5000 grams of stress on the tendon.

Strickland's early active motion protocol for primary flexor tendon repairs requires a four-strand repair using 3-0 or 4-0 braided synthetic suture with a running lock peripheral epitendinous suture, the lowest breaking strength of which at 1 week is 2150 grams (Strickland and Cannon 1993). Strickland concluded that a light active muscle contraction which generates 800–1500 grams of force is within the margins of safety for this type of repair. Strickland's protocol as well as protocols developed by Silfverskiold and May (1994) and Evans and Thompson (1997) are representative of detailed programs of early active motion. These programs are based on careful consideration of the tensile strength of the particular repair technique, and the tensile demands imparted to the repaired tendon during active motion with the wrist and digits in controlled positions. These programs will be discussed in detail in the following sections.

Phases of rehabilitation

Postoperative management for tendon repairs is based upon stages of wound healing and can be conceptualized in phases. Phase one is the protective phase from 0 to 4 weeks, when the strength of the repair is basically that of the suture and any motion program must observe the tensile limits of the repair. Any scar tissue that has formed is weak and easily disrupted by force. The transitional phase is from 4 to 6 weeks when repair strength increases due to the beginning of scar tissue maturation and the tensile demands on the repair are increased, but caution still must be observed not to overcome the capability of the repair. The extent of scar formation is assessed at this point by the amount of initial tendon excursion. The better the excursion at this phase the more the tendon is protected from excessive forces, because it is assumed that adhesion formation is minimal and the tendon is at greater risk of rupture. The third phase is full mobilization, which generally begins at 6 weeks and is gradually increased over time as the scar tissue increases in tensile strength.

Flexor tendon management

Flexor tendon zones

The level of the tendon injury in relation to the surrounding tissue is important in predicting the outcome following repair and rehabilitation.

Zone I extends from the mid-portion of the middle phalanx to the base of the distal phalanx. This is the area of the insertion of the flexor digitorum profundus (FDP) and is distal to the insertion of the flexor digitorum superficialis (FDS). Injury here will involve only the FDP and loss of distal interphalangeal (DIP) joint flexion will result.

Zone II extends from the level of the distal palmar crease to the mid-middle phalanx level. This is the area of the flexor sheath, a synovial lined fibro-osseous tunnel that houses both flexor tendons in this zone. This zone has been referred to as 'no man's land' because of the potential for poor results following injury and repair here. Adhesions that form in this zone tend to be very restrictive because the flexor tendon sheath is a fixed structure. The adhesions that form tether the tendon to the sheath and are difficult to remodel sufficiently to permit tendon glide. With the use of early motion programs the prognosis for injury and repairs in this zone has greatly improved. Lacerations in this zone may involve one or both tendons. Also, the position of the hand at the time of the laceration is an important consideration. If the hand is flexed when the tendon is lacerated, the level of the tendon laceration will actually be distal to the level of the skin laceration. If the digit is extended at the time of the laceration, then the tendon injury site and the skin injury site are at the same level.

Zone III refers to the mid-palm area from the metacarpal neck to the distal edge of the transverse carpal ligament. Prognosis is better in this zone compared with zone II, because adhesions that form here are less restrictive as there are no fixed structures on which the tendon can become adherent.

Zone IV is the carpal canal area. This zone underlies the transverse carpal ligament. Both tendons and the FDS alone may be injured here. The median and ulnar nerves are vulnerable with injuries in this zone. Intertendinous adhesions frequently will form in this zone due to the proximity of the tendons to one another. Adhesions between the tendons and the overlying transverse carpal ligament may also form and tend to be more restrictive because of the unyielding nature of the transverse carpal ligament.

Zone V extends from the musculotendinous juncture to the proximal edge of the transverse carpal ligament. Adhesions that form here are more easily remodeled to permit tendon glide because there are no fixed structures for the tendon to become adherent to. Injury here is frequently accompanied by major nerve trauma.

Zones of the thumb

Zone I covers the area distal to the metacarpophalangeal (MCP) joint of the thumb. Zone II involves the pulley area at the level of the MCP joint. Zones III, IV and V correspond to the zones described for the other digits.

Flexor tendon excursion

The goal of postoperative flexor tendon rehabilitation is to achieve maximum tendon excursion while protecting the tendon from rupture. Tendon excursion studies have helped to shape and define postoperative therapy protocols. Verdan (1960) reported that the normal excursion of the FDP and the FDS at the mid-palm level, which is required to produce full MCP, proximal interphalangeal (PIP) and DIP joint flexion, was about 2.5 cm. Full PIP and DIP flexion required 16 and 17 mm of FDS and FDP movement respectively at the proximal phalanx level. The excursion of the FDP over the middle phalanx to produce full DIP flexion was only 5 mm (Urbaniak 1979).

McGrouther and Ahmed (1981) related tendon excursion to joint motion. They found that passive MCP joint motion produces no related flexor tendon motion. DIP motion produces excursion of the FDP on the FDS of 1 mm per 10° of DIP joint motion. PIP joint motion produces FDP and FDS excursion together, relative to the sheath, of 1.3 mm per 10° of PIP motion.

Horibe et al (1990) studied tendon excursions relative to the tendon sheath. They found that the amount of tendon excursion was very small in regions distal to the joint in motion. They concluded that in order to achieve glide of a repair, the joints distal to the repair must be moved. Tendon excursion relative to the tendon sheath was the highest during PIP joint motion: 1.7 mm per 10° of joint motion. Results suggest that PIP motion is critical in minimizing adhesions between the tendons and the sheath following tendon repair in zone II.

McGrouther and Ahmed (1981) reported that complete excursion of the FDP and differential excursion between the FDP and the FDS could be accomplished only through motion of the DIP joint. This finding led to the use of a palmar pulley on the splint used with the Kleinert protocol. The dynamic traction of the involved digit was directed through the palmar pulley, resulting in greater DIP joint flexion (Chou et al 1988).

The effect of postoperative swelling and scar certainly influences excursion. Silfverskiold et al (1992) studied tendon excursion and gap formation following FDP repair in zone II. They placed metal markers in the FDP on each side of the repair during the operation. Postoperative gapping and tendon excursion were measured on X-ray film. They found that with early passive flexion of the PIP, mean tendon excursion along the proximal phalanx per 10° of flexion varied between 76% and 90% of that was subsequently obtained with normal active flexion in the same digit and joint. Passive flexion of the DIP was less efficient with excursions along the mid phalanx per 10° of joint motion of only 39% and 63% of the corresponding excursion recorded during active flexion. Silfverskiold et al concluded that overall clinical results could be expected to improve if tendon excursions could be increased during the early controlled motion phase, especially those excursions related to DIP joint motion. This led to the development of their early active motion program.

Duran's protocol (Duran and Houser 1975, Duran et al 1990) emphasized the importance of interphalangeal joint motion to produce excursion of the FDP relative to the FDS and its important in preventing cross-union between the FDS and the FDP in zone II. Duran asserted that 3–5 mm of glide of the repaired tendon was necessary to minimize restrictive adhesions. More recently, emphasis has been placed on producing as large a controlled range of motion as possible based on the assumption that the ultimate active tendon excursion would increase in a similar fashion and that clinical results correlate to the magnitude of excursion obtained during the healing phase. Studies by Silfverskiold et al (1992) support this practice. Their excursion studies showed a positive correlation between the magnitude of tendon excursion obtained during the early motion period and subsequent clinical results in terms of active interphalangeal joint range of motion.

Clinical evaluation

Following tendon repair and rehabilitation, total active motion (TAM) and total passive motion (TPM) measurements are used to assess outcome. Total active motion is calculated by adding the measurement of MCP, PIP, and DIP joint flexion in a fisted position and subtracting the sum of any extension deficits at these joints. Strickland (1989) advocates a formula, which omits the measurements at the MCP joint. TAM is calculated using only the measurements at the PIP and DIP joints and is divided by 175 multiplied by 100 to give the percentage of normal PIP and DIP motion. A score of 175 represents the normal TAM of these joints in most individuals. Strickland grades flexor tendon repairs from poor to excellent based on the return of normal motion. Excellent means 75–100% of return; good means 50–74% of return; fair equals 25–49% of return; and poor is 0–24% of return.

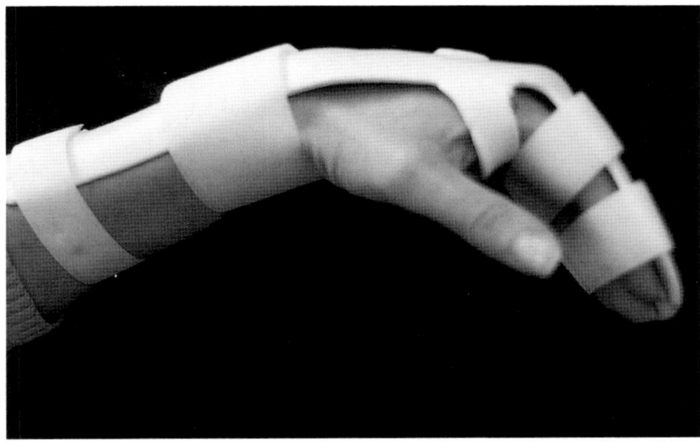

Figure 5.1
Dorsal block splint used following flexor tendon repair. Wrist and MCP joints are flexed with the IP joints in neutral extension.

Approaches to therapy

There are three basic approaches to the postoperative management of flexor tendon repairs: initial immobilization, early passive motion, and immediate active motion. Initial immobilization during the first 3 weeks of healing is the traditional and conservative method of management. This approach may be used for children and those patients who are judged by the surgeon to be unreliable or incapable of following the early motion programs and who are at risk for rupture due to poor compliance or comprehension. Another indication for initial immobilization is for cases when other structures are injured and require immobilization to prevent disruption.

Early passive motion is used for patients who are capable of following the home program instructions and observing the precautions involved in the early motion program. Early active motion is used in cases where the surgeon has selected a suture and suture technique which has the tensile capability of withstanding the forces involved with a light active muscle contraction during the early weeks of healing. This method of management requires the greatest level of patient comprehension and compliance. All techniques require a knowledgeable and experienced hand therapist.

Immobilization

Patients who are treated with initial immobilization following a flexor tendon repair are typically placed in a plaster cast or splint with the wrist and the MCP joints positioned in flexion and the IP joints allowed neutral extension. The cast is generally held in place for 3 weeks. After 3 weeks, the cast is removed and a dorsal thermoplastic splint is made positioning the wrist and the MCP joints as in the cast unless otherwise specified by the surgeon (Figure 5.1). Following 3 weeks of immobilization there is invariably stiffness of the digital joints and restricted tendon excursion. Typically, the patient begins active digital flexion within the confines

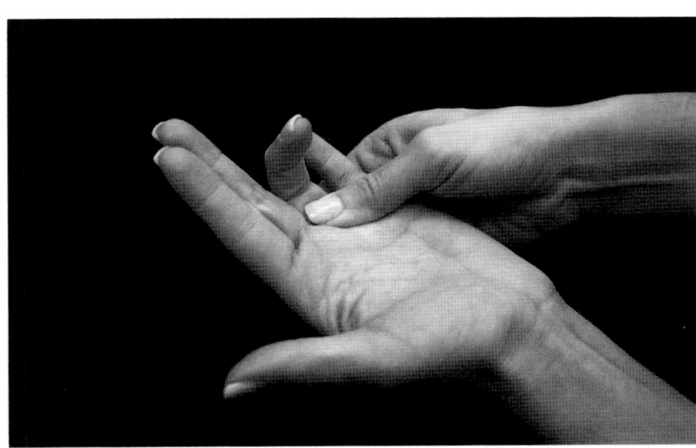

(A)

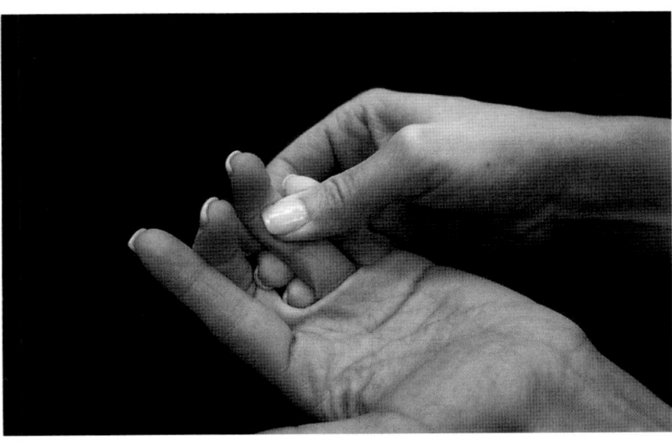

(B)

Figure 5.2
Blocking exercises are performed to increase tendon glide. (A) PIP flexion performed with the MCP joint supported in neutral extension. (B) DIP joint flexion performed with the PIP joint supported in extension.

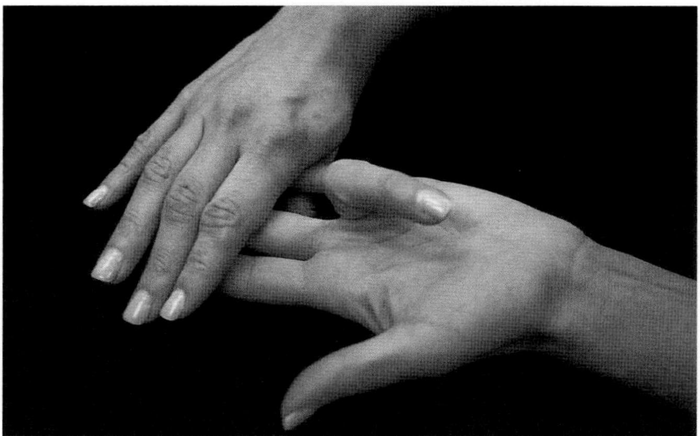

Figure 5.3
Flexor digitorum superficialis tendon glide is isolated from flexor profundus glide by holding the adjacent digits in extension during active flexion of the PIP joint.

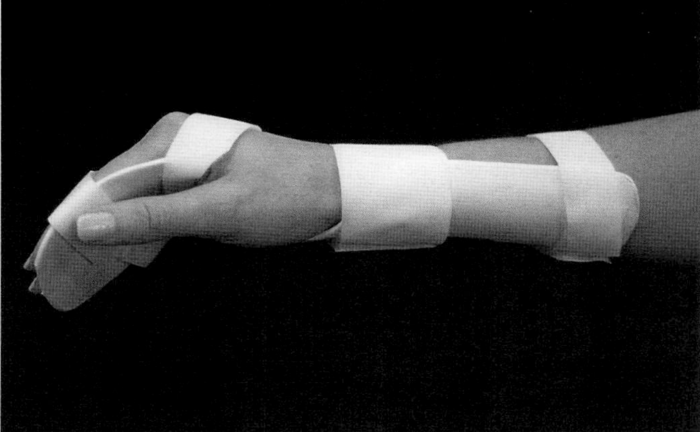

(A)

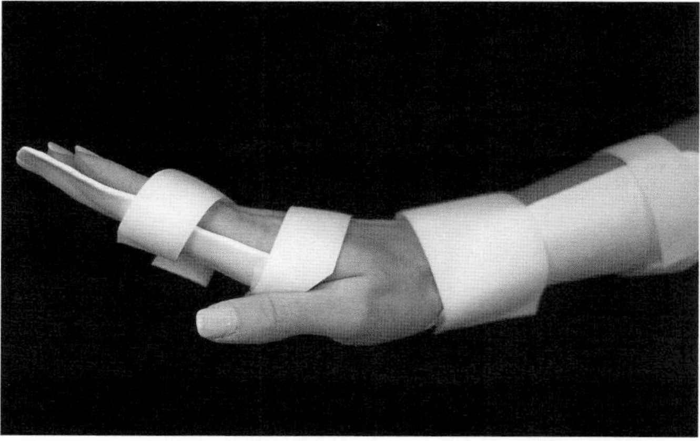

(B)

Figure 5.4
Thermoplastic splint used to overcome flexor tendon tightness and adherence with loss of extension. (A) Wrist and digits are positioned so that the flexor muscle tendon unit is held at full length without stress. (B) Over subsequent weeks, the splint is serially adjusted, positioning the wrist and digits in greater extension.

of the splint. Passive flexion is allowed but no passive extension, no extension outside of the splint, and no blocking exercises for flexion are allowed. From the fourth to sixth weeks, the dorsal block splint is adjusted each week to permit greater wrist extension toward neutral and exercises continue. At 6 weeks, the dorsal block splint is usually discontinued, although the patient may be advised to use the splint for protection in selected situations. At this time active wrist and finger extension begins, avoiding simultaneous wrist and finger extension to prevent overstress of the repair. The fisting exercises continue and blocking exercises can begin. Blocking refers to the technique of stabilizing the proximal joint in neutral extension during active flexion exercises. For example, for PIP flexion exercises, the MCP joint is held in neutral extension while the patient attempts active PIP flexion exercises. For DIP joint flexion, the PIP joint is held in extension as the patient attempts to flex the DIP joint (Figure 5.2A and B). To isolate the FDS gliding from the FDP, adjacent digits are held in extension while the patient attempts to flex the PIP joint of the involved digit (Figure 5.3).

Finger extension may be limited secondary to tightness or adhesions of the flexor musculotendinous unit. Serial splinting is an effective way to deal with this problem. A volar wrist splint with an extension to include the involved digits is molded with the wrist and digits positioned so that the flexor muscle tendon unit is held at full length without stress. Over subsequent weeks, the splint is serially adjusted, positioning the wrist and digits in greater extension (Figure 5.4A and B).

PIP flexion contractures are not uncommon, particularly after zone II injuries/repairs. Contracture correction splints may be used at 8 weeks. Contractures of ≤30° generally respond to a three-point extension-style splint. PIP joint contractures >30° respond best to dynamic splinting which is constructed to stabilize the proximal MCP joint and to provide a 90° angle of dynamic pull from the middle phalanx to the outrigger of the splint (Figure 5.5). The dynamic traction is applied with a low intensity level of stress to the involved joint. Low load prolonged stress to the contracted joint is recommended over brief, high intensity stress.

At 8 weeks, an increase in the stress applied to the flexor tendon is added to the program in the form of resistive exercises. The muscle contraction prompted by the addition of resistance is stronger and increases the demand on the tendon to glide proximally. Putty in graduated levels of resistance is a convenient method of resistive exercise and can be used for a home program.

Physical agent modalities such as hot packs, paraffin wax, and continuous mode ultrasound are helpful for

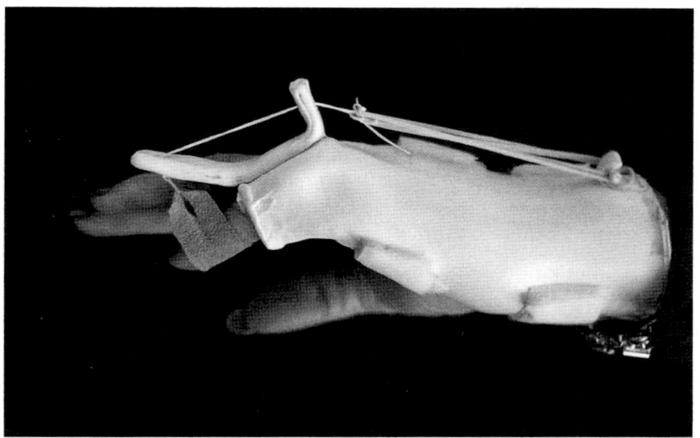

Figure 5.5
Dynamic splint used to correct a PIP joint flexion contracture. The MCP joint is stabilized with dynamic traction applied to the PIP joint in the direction of extension. The angle of pull of the dynamic traction must be at a 90° angle to the middle phalanx.

their effect of increasing the extensibility of the soft tissue and scar. Used prior to exercises, stiffness is diminished and the patient's efforts are facilitated. Electrical stimulation and biofeedback may be used to enhance the patient's efforts and to inhibit cocontraction during flexor tendon gliding exercises. Full resistance and work hardening generally begins at 10–12 weeks.

Cifaldi-Collins and Schwarze (1991) evaluated the results of flexor tendons treated with initial immobilization and an early progressive resistance program. The repaired tendons were immobilized for an average of 3.5 weeks. Patients were instructed in a program of differential tendon gliding exercises performed within a dorsal protective splint. After 2–3 days TAM was evaluated and compared with TPM. If the TAM was 50% less than the TPM, then extensive adhesion formation was presumed to be present and blocking exercises were initiated for tendon gliding. Gentle putty exercises began at 4 weeks for these cases and dynamic splinting for contracture correction. They found that the immobilized tendons treated with early progressive resistance compared favorably with tendons treated with early motion and there were no ruptures.

Early passive motion

In the early 1970s two protocols for early controlled passive motion were introduced. These protocols developed by Kleinert and colleagues (Lester et al 1977) and Duran and Houser (1975) form the basis for the early passive motion protocols used with some variations. These protocols were developed to minimize restrictive adhesion formation and in the Duran approach, to minimize cross-union between the FDP and the FDS in zone II. The later work of Gelberman and others as previously discussed confirmed the existence of intrinsic healing which was facilitated by early motion and which also minimized and modified adhesion formation to preserve tendon gliding function.

These programs are based on the understanding that the ultimate recovery of active flexor tendon excursion depends upon the passive tendon excursion obtained during the first phase of the early controlled passive motion programs.

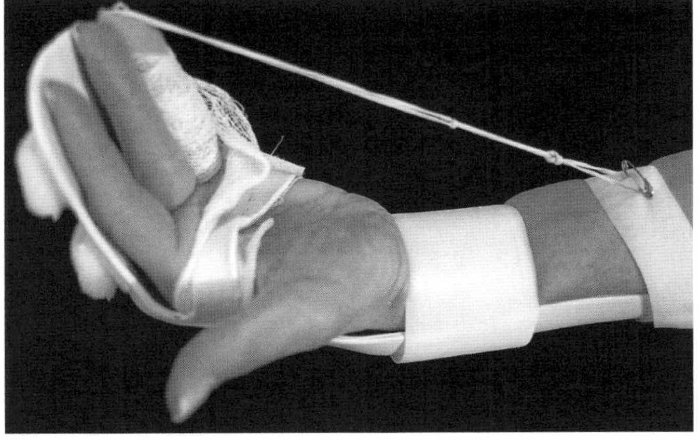

(A)

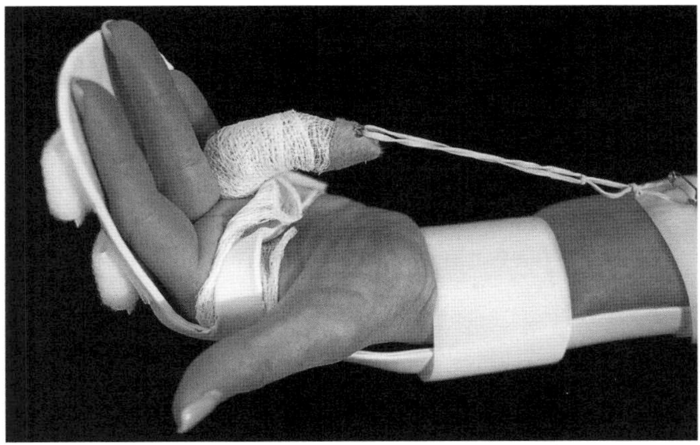

(B)

Figure 5.6
Kleinert method of controlled passive motion. (A) The involved digit extends actively to the limits of the dorsal protective splint against the resistance of the elastic traction. (B) The digit is pulled back to the flexed posture by the action of the dynamic traction.

Kleinert technique

The Kleinert protocol calls for the initiation of controlled passive motion within 24 hours post surgery. A dorsal splint is applied with the wrist and the MCP joints in a flexed posture with the IP joints in neutral extension. The splint is typically custom-made by the hand therapist and is made from a low temperature thermoplastic. Elastic traction is applied to the nail of the involved digit as well as to the adjacent digits. The elastic traction is attached to a volar and proximal attachment point, usually on the volar Velcro® strap of the splint. The tension of the traction should be enough to hold the fingers toward the palm, but light enough to permit the fingers to extend to the limit of the dorsal splint. The patient is instructed to extend to the limit of the splint against the resistance of the elastic and then to relax and allow the rubber band to pull the fingers back to a flexed posture (Figure 5.6A and B). This exercise is performed 10 times each hour. Kleinert et al based this program on the finding that resistance to the action of one group of muscles results in synergistic relaxation of its antagonist. Kleinert used EMG to confirm that the flexor muscle tendon unit was relaxed during active extension against the resistance of the rubber band and therefore would not be at risk for rupture. Of interest is Tajima's finding that when resistance to interphalangeal extension is strong either from elastic traction or from edema, the FDP often contracts simultaneously with active contraction of the lumbricals during the extension phase of Kleinert's protocol (Tajima 1997). He determined this through EMG and theorized that this takes place because the power of interphalangeal extension will be stronger if the FDP contracts and prevents distal shifting of the lumbrical origin during lumbrical contraction.

At 4–6 weeks, the dorsal splint is discontinued and the repaired tendon is protected with wrist cuff and elastic traction holding the digit in flexion (Figure 5.7). Usually, a protective night splint is used to prevent a flexion contracture at the PIP joint, which could develop due to the positioning of the digit in flexion with the wrist cuff and nail traction. The night splint is positioned with the wrist at neutral and the MCP joints flexed and the IP joints positioned in neutral extension. At this time, active flexion and extension exercises are begun with no blocking or resistance permitted and no passive extension or simultaneous wrist and finger extension. Active motion exercises are delayed in cases where the initial tendon motion is good, indicating minimal adhesion formation and greater risk for rupture. At 6 weeks, the wrist cuff is discontinued, and a splint is worn only to position the PIP joint to prevent flexion contractures and in selected situations for protection. Active exercises continue and blocking exercises may begin.

Modifications to the Kleinert program include the addition of a palmar pulley (Figure 5.8) to direct the flexion traction to the palm and result in greater DIP joint flexion. McGrouther and Ahmed's studies found that complete FDP excursion and differential excursion between the FDS and the FDP could only be accomplished with full DIP joint flexion (McGrouther and Ahmed 1981). A palmar pulley can be added by attaching a safety pin to the palmar strap at the level of the distal palmar crease as in the Brook Army Hospital splint designed by Thomes (Chow et al 1987). Alternatively, a small pulley can be fashioned from a paperclip and fixed to the plastic palmar piece of the splint. The Kleinert Post-op Flexor Tendon Traction Brace (PFT) was developed to control resistance to finger extension during the active extension exercises using a spring-loaded roller

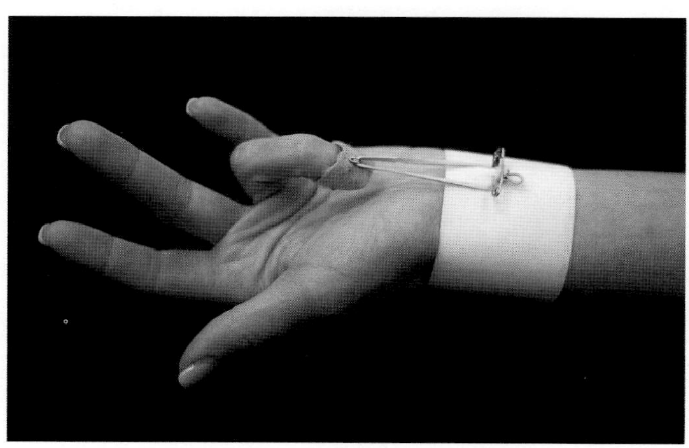

Figure 5.7

Wrist cuff with dynamic traction positioning the involved digit in flexion, used as a transitional method of protecting the repaired flexor tendon.

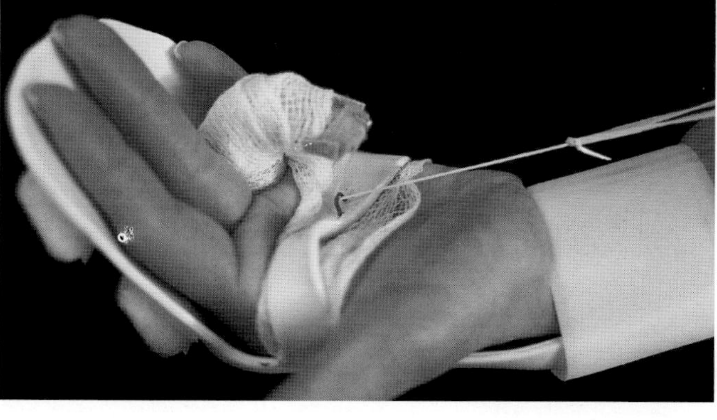

Figure 5.8

Kleinert method modified with the use of a palmar pulley, achieving greater DIP joint flexion. McGrouther and Ahmed's studies found that complete FDP excursion and differential excursion between the FDP and FDS could only be accomplished with full passive DIP joint flexion (McGrouther and Ahmed 1981).

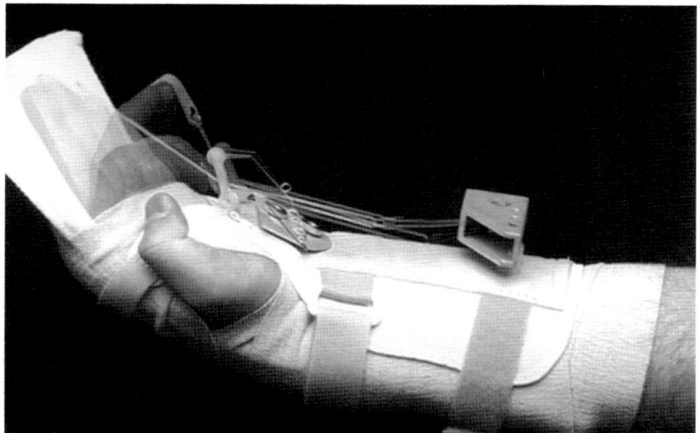

Figure 5.9
The Kleinert postoperative flexor tendon traction brace was developed to control resistance to finger extension during the active extension phase of the Kleinert method using a spring-loaded roller bar.

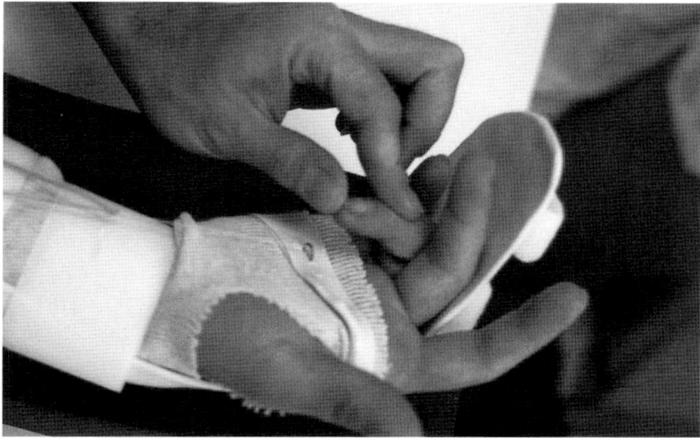

(A)

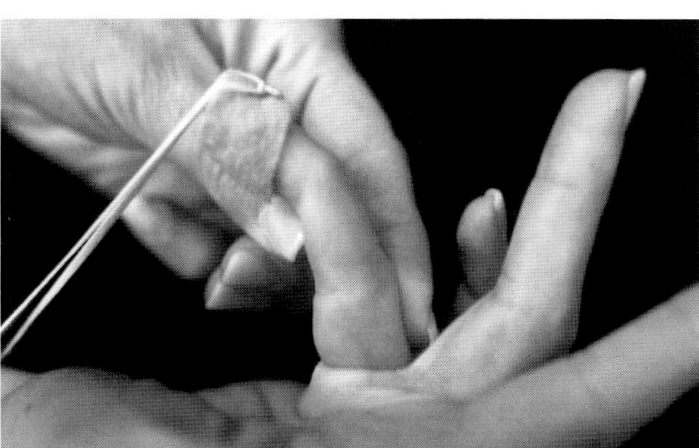

(B)

Figure 5.10
Duran technique. (A) Passive DIP joint extension with the MCP, PIP, and wrist flexed glides the FDP suture site away from the FDS suture site. (B) Passive PIP extension with the wrist, MCP, and DIP flexed glides both suture sites away from the site of the injury.

bar (Figure 5.9). This was intended to insure that the patient could achieve full finger extension within the splint and to prevent a flexion contracture from developing.

Another modification is to detach the traction at night when sleeping and secure the digits to the dorsal splint with Velcro straps. This will maintain the PIP joints in a neutral position and help to prevent the development of a flexion contracture, which is a risk with the continuous positioning of the digit in flexion, particularly overnight when no active extension exercises are being performed. Some clinicians fear that patients may inadvertently grip or flex their digits when sleeping, overcoming the Velcro straps. To minimize this risk, a detachable foam-lined volar splint, supporting the digits to the dorsal portion of the splint, can be used in place of the straps.

Duran technique

Duran and Houser (1975) designed their program specifically for tendon repairs in zone II to prevent cross-union between the FDS and the FDP. Through intra-operative measurement Duran and Houser observed that 3–5 mm of tendon glide was sufficient to prevent restrictive adhesion formation. They determined that passive DIP extension with the PIP and the MCP joints flexed glides the FDP suture site away from the FDS suture site. Passive PIP extension with the MCP and the DIP flexed glides both suture sites away from the injury site (Figure 5.10A–D). The dorsal splint in the Duran protocol positions the wrist in 20° of flexion and extends to the PIP joints with the MCP joints in a relaxed position of flexion. The Duran splint also includes rubber band traction to pull the digits into flexion when not exercising for the purpose of protecting the repair from stress.

Exercises are performed within the splint and include passive DIP extension with the PIP and MCP joints flexed and passive extension of the PIP with the DIP and MCP joints flexed. These are performed twice daily for 6–8 repetitions. Although Duran's original protocol calls for this limited frequency of exercise, the more common practice is hourly exercise.

At 4.5 weeks, the dorsal splint is discontinued and nail traction to a wrist cuff is used. Active extension is allowed with passive flexion by the elastic traction. At 5.5 weeks the wrist cuff is discontinued and active flexion begins. The following exercises are begun: DIP joint blocking to isolate FDP tendon glide; isolated FDS exercises are performed by holding the adjacent digits in extension and flexing the PIP of the involved digit; fisting exercises; and passive PIP and DIP extension with the tendon on slack accomplished by flexing the wrist and the MCP joints. At 7.5 weeks dynamic splinting can begin to correct flexion contractures, and resistance can begin with putty. At 10–12 weeks, splinting for contracture correction is continued and power gripping is allowed.

Modified programs

In practice the Duran and Kleinert programs are frequently modified and combined. For example, a combined Kleinert–Duran program includes a dorsal splint with elastic traction from the nail to a volar attachment point pulling the involved digit into a flexed position toward the palm. Hourly exercises are performed and include the following: active extension of the digit to the splint against the resistance of the elastic traction; passive return of the digit to a flexed position through the action of the elastic traction; further manual passive flexion of the digit to the distal palmar crease; passive DIP joint extension with the PIP and MCP joints flexed; and PIP joint extension with the MCP and DIP joints flexed. These exercises are typically performed 10 times hourly. The nail traction is usually detached at night and the digit is held to the dorsal block splint with Velcro straps when the patient is sleeping.

Related approaches and programs

Gelberman et al (1987) has described continuous passive motion (CPM) for the postoperative management of primary flexor tendons (Figure 5.11). These investigators conducted a multicenter study comparing the results of CPM with early controlled passive motion. CPM was applied within 24 hours postoperatively, and was held for 6 weeks at 8 hours per day. Active motion was begun at 4 weeks. At all other times when the CPM was not in use, a standard dorsal block splint was used and a controlled motion program was followed. The results of this study showed that the patients treated with CPM achieved a greater TAM compared with controls treated with a standard early motion approach. The authors' conclusion was that the duration of the controlled motion interval is significant in the postoperative management of flexor tendon repairs, i.e. a greater number of cycles or repetitions yield a better result. The pitfall of CPM for this application is the risk of tendon rupture that exists due to machine malfunction or with patient error in the application of the CPM machine and the change of the CPM to the standard dorsal block splint. A high degree of comprehension and compliance is a requirement for the use of CPM for flexor tendon repairs.

Evans zone I protocol

Prompted by the frequently suboptimal results of flexor tendon repairs in zone I even with early passive motion, Evans (1990) developed a protocol specifically for repairs of the FDP in this zone. Evans cited gap formation, elongation at the repair site, and adhesions between the tendon and surrounding injured tissues as the reasons for the poor results often seen. She proposed a protocol of splinting and controlled passive motion designed to address these problems. The dorsal splint in this protocol places the wrist in 30–40° of flexion and the MCP joints at 30° of flexion. A small separate dorsal splint is made and worn within the dorsal block splint to block the DIP joint at 45° (Figure 5.12). The purpose

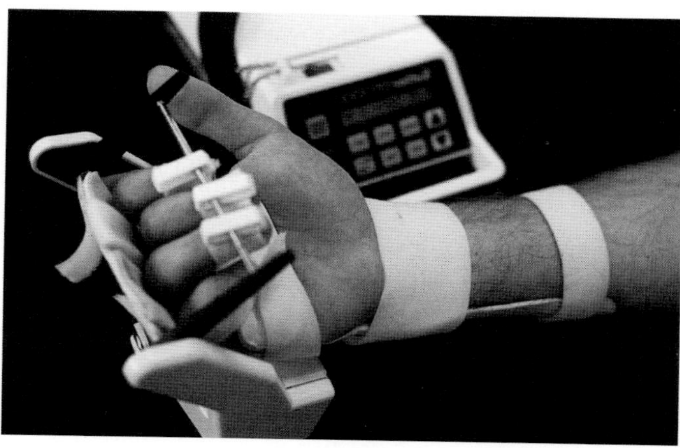

Figure 5.11

Continuous passive motion used following primary flexor tendon repairs. Gelberman's multicenter study led to their conclusion that the duration of the controlled motion interval is significant, i.e. a greater number of cycles or repetitions yield a better result (Gelberman et al 1987).

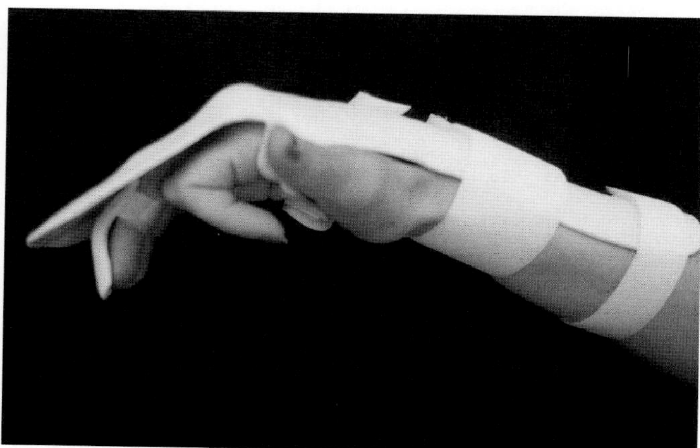

Figure 5.12

Splint used for Evans zone I flexor tendon protocol. A small separate dorsal DIP joint splint is worn within the dorsal block splint to block the DIP joint at 45°. The purpose is to place the suture site proximal to the injury site to decrease the chance of adherence of the tendon at the injury site.

is to position the tendon suture site proximal to the injury site to decrease the chance of adhesions at the injury site. The splint is applied at 24–48 hours post surgery. Exercises described include the following: passive motion of the DIP joint within the splints to 75°; passive composite flexion of the involved digit to the distal palmar crease; a modified passive hook fist in the splint (MCP joints are at 30° of flexion versus neutral); passive PIP extension with the MCP joints flexed; and position and hold exercise for the FDS. This is performed by holding the adjacent digits in extension within the limits of the splint and positioning the PIP joint of the involved finger in flexion and asking the patient to attempt to lightly hold it there actively. This last exercise is done to avoid adhesions between the FDS and the FDP and to insure that the function of the intact FDS is not compromised by the injured FDP.

The therapist performs two exercises with the splint removed. The first is extension of the wrist to 10° with the digits passively flexed. The second is a passive hook fist with the MCP joints at neutral and the wrist in maximal flexion. At 21 days, the DIP joint splint is discontinued and full place and hold fist exercises are begun. At 28 days, wrist tenodesis exercise is introduced, e.g. active wrist extension with fingers flexed and wrist flexion with the fingers extended. Hook fisting and gentle isolated FDS exercises are begun at this time. At 32 days, attempts can be made to recover full DIP joint extension.

Clinical problem solving

The protocols described must be modified based on individual patient characteristics. Most often what is modified is the timing of introduction of increasing levels of stress to the repaired tendon. Stress is applied in the form of active, assisted or resisted motion, and extension. The timing of the initiation of active motion is critical. If applied too early before the tendon has developed sufficient tensile strength, rupture can result. If applied too late, restrictive adhesion formation can seriously limit tendon function. Generally at about 3–3.5 weeks, the hand surgeon tests the tendon for active glide. If the tendon appears to be actively gliding well (> 50% of full motion) then active exercises may be delayed until 6 weeks postoperatively. The tendon that is moving well early on is presumed to have minimal scar formation and may be at greater risk for rupture. Therefore protection is maintained for a longer period of time. Conversely, if the tendon at 4 weeks shows poor active excursion, then active exercises and sometimes even blocking exercises may begin.

When beginning active flexion, the least stressful to the tendon is place and hold fisting. The digits are passively placed in a fist and the patient is asked to hold the fist with a light muscle contraction. Next, differential tendon gliding exercises can be introduced as described by Wehbe and Hunter (1985). The sequence begins with full extension of the digits. Then a hook fist is performed, where the greatest differential excursion occurs between the FDS and the FDP. The full fist is next with the fingers touching the distal palmar crease. The FDP has the greatest excursion with the full fist. The last position is the straight fist, which involves the greatest excursion of the FDS (Figure 5.13A–D). Next in terms of stress to the tendon are blocking exercises where the MCP joint is supported in neutral and the patient flexes

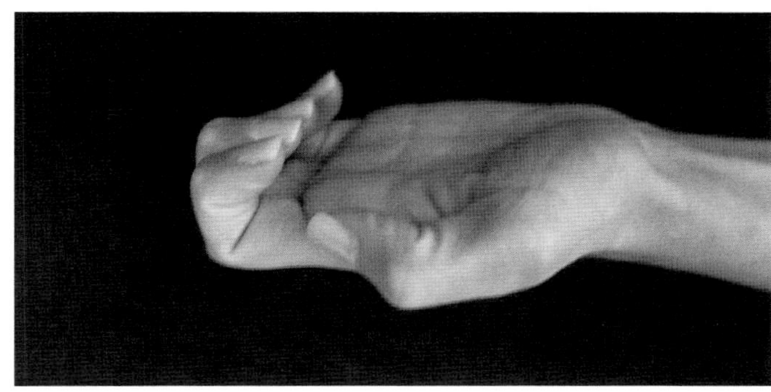

(A)

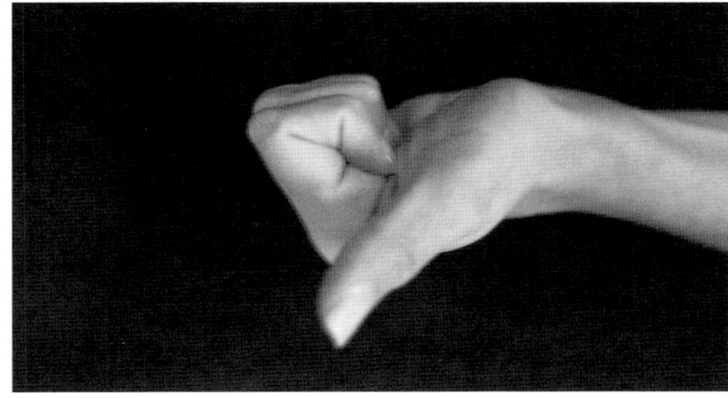

(B)

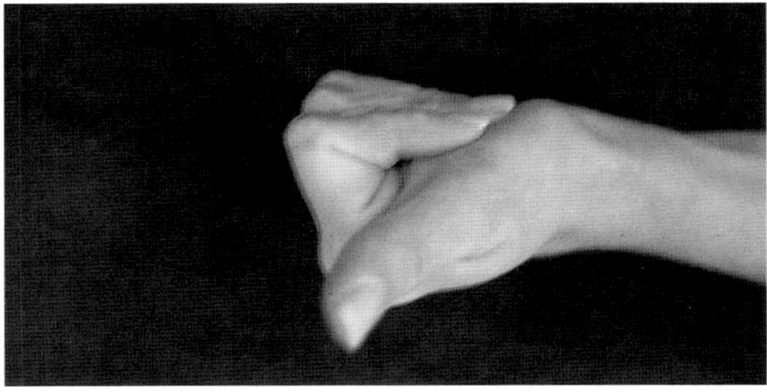

(C)

Figure 5.13

Tendon gliding exercises. (A) A hook fist requires the greatest differential excursion between the FDS and the FDP. (B) The full fist requires the greatest excursion of the FDP. (C) The straight fist involves the greatest excursion of the FDS.

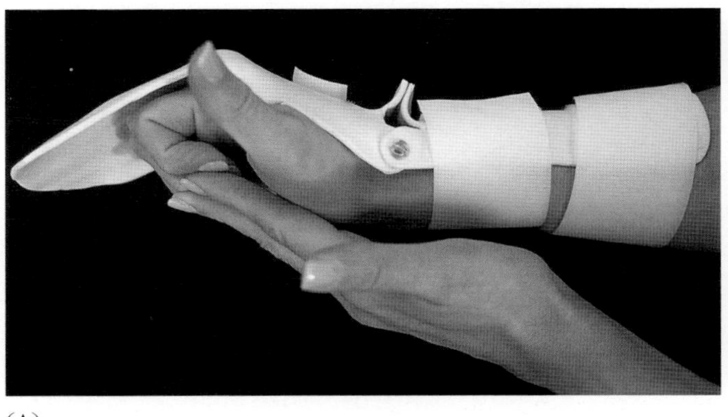

(A)

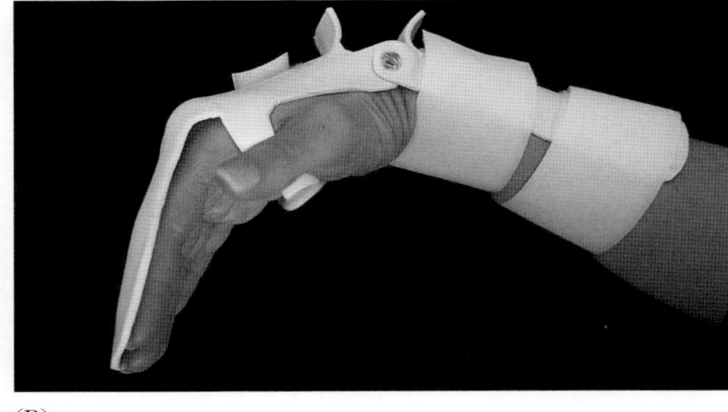

(B)

Figure 5.14

Indiana method tenodesis splint. (A) In the splint the patient passively flexes the digits and actively extends the wrist to the 30° allowed by the splint, then lightly contacts and holds the digits in the flexed posture for 5 seconds. (B) Then, the patient relaxes and allows the wrist to fall into flexion with the digits extending to the limits of the splint through tenodesis effect.

at the PIP joint. Then the PIP joint is supported in neutral and the patient attempts to flex the DIP joint. The stress to the tendon with blocking exercises can be increased by positioning the wrist in extension while performing the blocking exercises. Putty exercises are the next level of stress, where the patient attempts to flex the digit against the resistance of the putty, graded from light to heavy resistance. This requires a more forceful muscle contraction than the previous exercise and greater stress is imparted to the tendon. Full strengthening including power gripping, and lifting is the final phase of stress. Usually this is not initiated earlier than 12 weeks postoperatively and in some cases may be delayed longer.

Another clinical problem is limitation in extension that results following the initial protection in the flexed posture. Caution must be observed when attempting to restore extension. Again, if the tendon is stressed too soon before sufficient tensile strength has developed, attenuation at the repair site could occur. This would result in improved extension, but a loss in active flexion. Generally, active extension outside the limits of the dorsal block splint begins at 6 weeks and passive extension at 8 weeks. After the dorsal block splint is discontinued, a static splint may be worn at night and intermittently during the day to position the flexor muscle tendon unit at length with the PIP joint as close to neutral as possible. When treating the extension deficit a distinction must be made between a joint contracture or tendon–muscle unit length deficit. To determine the difference, PIP and DIP joint extension is evaluated with the MCP and wrist joints in extension and compared to PIP and DIP joint extension with the wrist and the MCP joints flexed, which puts the flexor tendon on slack. If PIP and DIP joint extension is limited when the MCP and wrist joints are extended, but they have full extension when the wrist and MCP joints are flexed, the limitation is caused by a muscle–tendon adherence or length problem. If PIP joint extension is limited regardless of the proximal joint position, this indicates a joint limitation. Joint restrictions are generally treated best with dynamic splinting or serial casting; and muscle–tendon unit length problems are usually treated with serial static splinting incorporating the wrist as well as the involved digits.

Early active motion

The most recent development in the postoperative management of flexor tendon repairs is the use of active motion exercises within the first 24 hours post repair. The protocols described are based on the use of specific suture techniques and suture materials that are capable of withstanding the stresses involved with active motion. The parameters for the therapy protocols are based on an understanding of the tensile demands on the tendon with active motion in various positions of the wrist and MCP joints. One of the most detailed protocols has been described by Strickland and Cannon of the Indiana Hand Center (Strickland and Cannon 1993). Their program utilizes a four-strand Tajima and horizontal mattress repair with running lock peripheral epitendinous suture. The repair strength of this suture remains above 1800 grams at 3 weeks, which is capable of handling the demands of a light muscle contraction, which should not exceed much more than 800 grams. The protocol is based on the fact that the least tensile demand during active flexion occurs with the wrist in 45° of extension and the MCP joints at 90° flexion. Additional requirements for this protocol are a motivated and intelligent patient, minimal to moderate edema, and minimal wound complications.

Two splints are used during the first 4 weeks of this protocol: a dorsal block splint with the wrist in 20° of flexion and the MCP joints at 50° of flexion; a tenodesis splint is also made at this point which allows the wrist to extend to 30° and full volar wrist flexion (Figure 5.14A and B). The digits are blocked dorsally in the splint at the MCP joints at 60° flexion. From 0 to 4 weeks the patient wears the dorsal block splint and every hour performs the Duran method of early passive motion. Also every hour, the dorsal block splint is removed and the tenodesis splint is applied. In the tenodesis splint, the patient passively flexes the digits and extends the wrist to the 30° limit allowed by the splint, then lightly contracts and holds the digits in the flexed posture for 5 seconds. Then, the patient relaxes and allows the wrist to fall into flexion. This routine is performed 25 times each hour. The tenodesis splint is removed and the dorsal block splint is reapplied until the next hour. Obviously, this protocol requires a high level of comprehension and compliance on the patient's part.

At 4 weeks, the dorsal block splint is continued for protection but can be removed during exercises. The exercises are performed 25 times every 2 hours. The tenodesis exercises continue with the digits passively flexed while simultaneously extending the wrist. The patient actively holds a light muscle contraction then drops the wrist into flexion, which through tenodesis allows the digits to extend. Active flexion and extension of the digits and wrist are performed with a light muscle contraction. The patient is instructed to avoid simultaneous wrist and finger extension to prevent elongation at the repair site. At 5 weeks, active flexion of the interphalangeal joints with the MCP joints extended followed by full digit extension is permitted. Blocking can begin at 6 weeks only if active flexion to the distal palmar crease is > 3 cm. Passive extension can begin at 7 weeks, strengthening at 8 weeks, and unrestricted use at 14 weeks.

Silfverskiold and May (1994) have described a protocol involving active extension and active/passive flexion. Their protocol is used for flexor tendons repaired with a modified Kessler and epitendinous circumferential cross-stitch. At 1–3 days post surgery a dorsal block splint is applied with the wrist neutral, the MCP joints at 50–70° of flexion, and the interphalangeal joints extended. Elastic traction is applied to all fingertips, pulled through a palmar pulley and attached to a proximal attachment point. All four fingers are included regardless of how many tendons are repaired, in order to avoid inadvertent stress to the repaired tendon that might occur with uncontrolled active motion of the adjacent uninvolved digits. Hourly exercises are performed with 10 repetitions and include active extension to the splint, passive flexion by the elastic traction, and further manual passive flexion to the distal palmar crease. During the passive flexion the patient is permitted to perform an active muscle contraction for 2–3 seconds. No unassisted active flexion is allowed without supervision by the therapist or the surgeon. To check the strength and effect of these active contractions and under the supervision of the surgeon or therapist, unassisted active motion is performed to produce at least 80° at the PIP joint and at least 40–45° of flexion at the DIP joint. These checks of unassisted active motion are performed once weekly. To ensure full active extension within the splint, the patient is taught to unload the rubber bands during the active extension phase of their exercise routine. At night the elastic traction is detached and the fingers are splinted in extension within the dorsal block splint. At 4 weeks, the splint is removed and unassisted active finger flexion and extension exercises are begun. At 6 weeks, gentle resisted flexion is allowed. At 8 weeks, progressive resistive exercise is started, and at 3 months power gripping is allowed.

Evans and Thompson (1992) studied the internal and external forces acting on the repaired tendon during active flexion, and did an extensive literature review of studies reporting the tensile strengths of various tendon repair techniques. Based on their findings, Evans developed an active motion program for the flexor tendon repaired with a standard repair (modified Kessler with epitendinous suture). Evans combines a standard program with a component of immediate active motion. The standard program, which is performed under the supervision of the therapist as well as by the patient on a home program basis, includes a dorsal block splint with the wrist at 30–40° flexion, MCP joints at 45° flexion, and the PIP and DIP joints at neutral. Four-finger traction is directed through a palmar pulley and allows resisted active extension to the splint with passive return of the digits to the flexed position. The program is supplemented with manual passive flexion of the digits to the distal palmer crease and active PIP and DIP joint extension with the MCP joints held in full flexion passively by the uninvolved hand. At night the traction is discontinued and the fingers are held to the dorsal block splint with Velcro straps.

The immediate active short arc motion program supplements this standard program and is performed only under the therapist's supervision. The active hold component is preceded by slow passive motions from the relaxed position to the composite fist position performed by the therapist to reduce visco-elastic resistance and displace fluids of edema. The active hold component is then performed with the wrist in 20–30° of extension, the MCP joints at 80° of flexion, 75° of PIP flexion and 30–40° of DIP flexion. The therapist places the hand in this position and instructs the patient to gently hold this position. The effort exerted by the patient is monitored with a Haldex strain gauge to insure that force does not exceed 15–20 grams. Evans and Thompson determined that internal tendon forces will be the least in the middle ranges of wrist and digital joint motion. They determined that active motion in this position is compatible with a standard modified Kessler repair with an epitendinous suture, and that the position of full flexion is not, since the forces in this position exceed the tensile strength of the conventional repair.

The short arc motion exercises are followed by wrist tenodesis exercises. The therapist actively holds the fingers of the injured hand into the palm and extends the wrist to 30–40° followed by passive wrist flexion to 60°, while the fingers are allowed to position in extension through natural tenodesis action. At 21 days, the patient is permitted to perform the active hold exercises without supervision and the therapy program proceeds according to the standard passive motion program.

The early active motion programs for repaired flexor tendons, while promising improved results, are not without risk. These programs require an experienced therapist who is very familiar with the guidelines for active motion in terms of the suture techniques capable of holding up to active motion as well as familiarity with the other factors affecting tendon response to movement. Close communication is essential between the surgeon and therapist. The decision to use an active motion approach is generally made by the surgeon and is based on judgement regarding the strength of the repair technique used and anticipated patient compliance.

Extensor tendon injuries

General considerations

Because of their complexity, injuries to the extensor tendon system can lead to significant deformity and dysfunction. This is particularly true with injuries undergoing delayed treatment. Initially, the extent of injury may not be apparent. With time, the injury can progress to a fixed deformity with adaptive shortening or attenuation and displacement of the involved structures. When treatment is delayed, the prognosis for a satisfactory outcome is not as favorable as it would be with early treatment. Reconstruction is often needed when extensor tendon injuries are treated late.

Typical problems seen following extensor tendon laceration and repair include adhesions, which limit extensor tendon excursion. There will be a limitation in active extension of the involved digit and full digital flexion may be restricted due to tendon tightness and/or adherence.

There are some important differences between the flexor and extensor tendons. For example, fibro-osseous tunnels are less prevalent along the extensor system and therefore are less commonly a factor in generating restrictive adhesion formation. In general, the adhesions that do form cause less restriction since the dorsal skin is not tethered as the volar skin is, and moves with the tendon to which it is adherent. Incomplete injuries to the extensor mechanism may initially be masked by the unaffected components. There are many interconnections and links to the extensor mechanism. Eventually, however, the untreated injury leads to attenuation, slippage, and displacement of the involved structures and ultimately fixed deformity if not treated.

Tendon length is just as critical with extensor repairs as with flexors. A millimeter or two of extra length can result in an extensor lag and if too tight can limit flexion. This fact emphasizes the need for careful postoperative positioning.

Extensor muscle force is greatly exceeded by that of the flexor muscles. The importance of this fact is that the repaired extensor needs protection from too great a pull by the flexors.

Guidelines and goals for therapy

In treating the extensor tendon injury, it is important to consider the following: the level of injury, the specific anatomic structures involved, and the anatomic features which influence healing at this level, the surgical procedure performed, and the usual postoperative protocol. The goals of therapy are to restore the tensile strength of the repaired tendon, to restore tendon gliding and extensibility, and to maintain or restore joint mobility.

Management by zone of injury

The extensor tendons are classified according to zones and injuries are managed accordingly.

Zones I and II

Zone I is the area over the dorsal DIP joint and zone II is the area over the dorsal surface of the middle phalanx. In these zones, the conjoined lateral bands converge over the dorsum of the middle phalanx to form the terminal tendon inserting at the base of the distal phalanx. The triangular ligament is a sheet of transversely oriented fibers located over the middle phalanx between the insertion of the central slip and the terminal tendon. This ligament holds the lateral bands dorsally preventing displacement volarly. The oblique retinacular ligament inserts distally on the base of the distal phalanx adjacent to the terminal tendon on either side. Proximally and volarly, it inserts into the flexor sheath at the PIP joint level. This ligament links the motion of the PIP and DIP joints. Injury at this level involves disruption of the terminal tendon at its insertion, resulting in loss of DIP joint extension. This is referred to as a mallet finger. With attempts at extension, tension is transmitted to the central slip and lateral bands, and sometimes this results in PIP joint hyperextension – especially if the PIP volar plate is lax – resulting in a swan-neck deformity. Injury is usually caused by forcible flexion of the DIP joint.

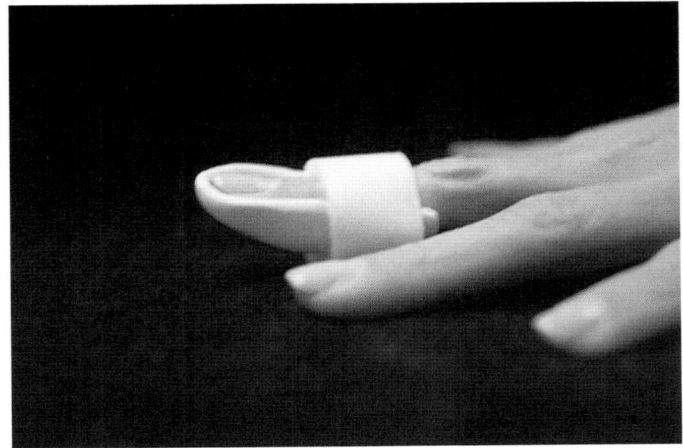

(A)

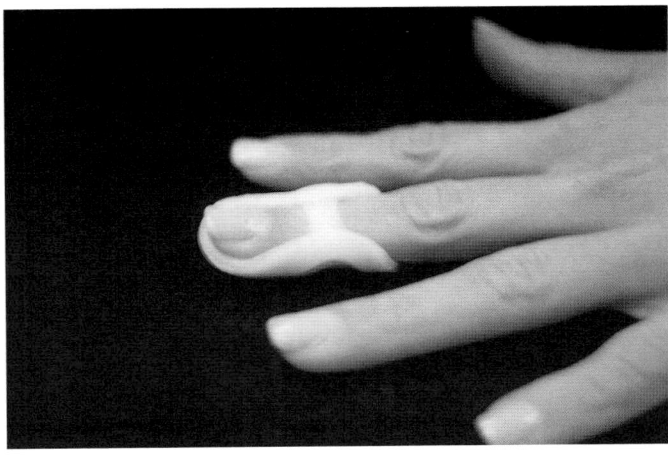

(B)

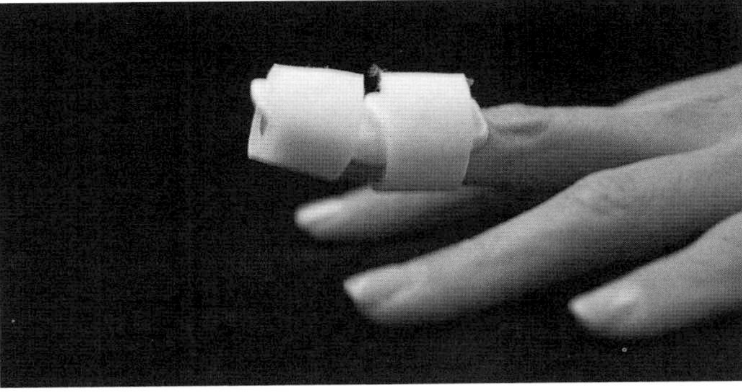

(C)

Figure 5.15
Mallet finger splints. (A) Volar gutter splint. (B) Figure 8 splint. (C) Dorsally based splint. The mallet splint must hold the DIP joint continuously in extension for 6 weeks.

Injury can also result from a crush injury, dorsal DIP joint dislocation, or laceration over the dorsum of the DIP joint and middle phalanx.

Injury can involve the tendon alone, the tendon with a chip of bone, or fracture of the dorsal cortex of the distal phalanx with the tendon attached to a large fragment. Injuries may be open or closed. There may be only a mild stretch or tendon attenuation resulting in a lag of 15–20°. With a rupture of the tendon with a bony chip a greater extension lag will result in the range of 40–45°. If the oblique retinacular ligament is intact, then weak extension will be possible at the DIP joint. If there is a laceration down to the capsule, a 90° lag will be present.

For closed injuries involving the tendon or a small chip of bone, treatment is usually conservative. The DIP joint is splinted in extension for a period of 6 weeks. The splint used must support the DIP joint without slipping and it should not limit PIP joint motion. A custom-fabricated thermoplastic splint may be made which holds the DIP joint in extension (Figure 5.15A–C). Prefabricated splints for DIP joint extension may also be used, but it is important to insure that the splint fits properly and maintains the DIP joint in extension for 6 weeks. Important to the successful management of mallet fingers is patient education and monitoring of the splint over the course of the 6 weeks. The patient is instructed not to remove the splint and to check the fit of the splint to insure that it does not slip or change position. The patient is also instructed to perform PIP joint range of motion exercises to maintain the motion of this joint. Skin care is important with mallet finger splints. The splint usually involves a strap or plastic over the dorsum of the DIP joint and skin breakdown is a risk. The patient is instructed to carefully check their skin without interrupting the extended finger position. At night the patient can be advised to tape the splint in place so that the splint does not slip off while the patient is sleeping. During this time, the surgeon or therapist should see the patient to monitor both splint fit and skin condition. At 6–8 weeks, the patient is allowed to remove the splint and use it at night only for the next 2 weeks. Active fisting can begin to restore DIP joint flexion and to strengthen DIP extension. Overzealous efforts to restore DIP joint flexion should be avoided to prevent attenuation of tendon scar and reoccurrence of extensor lag. At 8–10 weeks, if the DIP joint lacks full flexion, light DIP blocking can be performed. The splint is continued during the night if an extensor lag is present. If there is no lag, the splint may be discontinued at this time. Putty

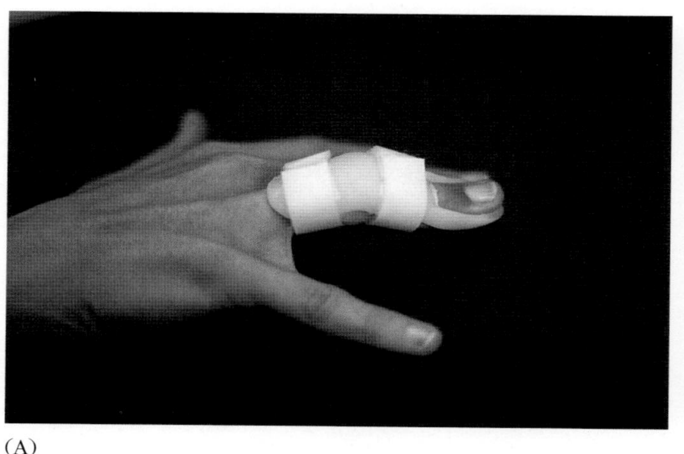

(A)

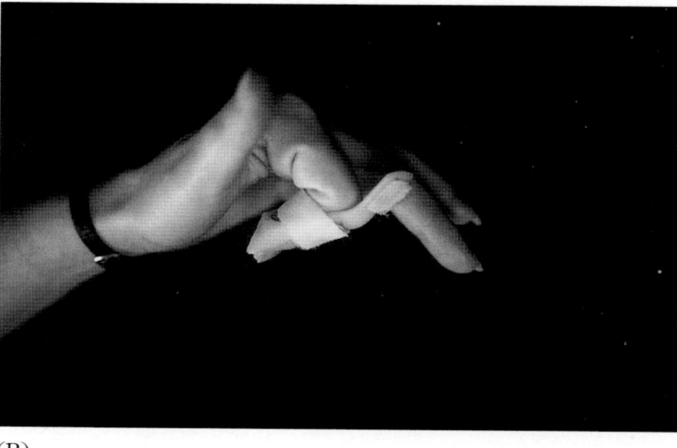

(B)

Figure 5.16

Splint used for a mallet injury with PIP hyperextension. (A) Splint supports the DIP joint in extension and blocks the PIP joint from full extension. (B) Splint allows PIP flexion while maintaining the DIP joint in the extended position.

exercises can begin at this time to restore grip strength as needed.

If a swan-neck deformity is present as a result of injury at this level, a splint can be made which blocks PIP extension and allows PIP flexion and supports the DIP joint in extension (Figure 5.16A and B). This splint is used for 3 weeks and then changed to a DIP extension splint for an additional 3 weeks.

When surgical repair is performed with tendon suture or reduction and pin fixation of a bony fragment, a splint is made protecting the DIP joint and the pin. Pin site care is incorporated, as well as PIP joint range of motion. The phase of mobilization begins at 6 weeks and progresses in the same manner as for conservative management. When the injury involves a large bony fragment and pin fixation is required, it is often difficult to regain DIP joint mobility and more intensive therapy may be required. For a persistent limitation in DIP joint flexion, elastic flexion straps can be used or dynamic flexion splints. If this injury is treated late, that is up to 2–3 months after the injury, splinting may still be tried but a longer duration may be needed (such as 8 weeks) and there may be a residual extensor lag.

Zones III and IV

Zone III refers to the dorsal PIP joint and zone IV refers to the dorsum of the proximal phalanx. In the region of the mid-shaft of the proximal phalanx, the extensor tendon splits into a central slip and two lateral slips. The central slip goes on distally to insert into the base of the middle phalanx. The lateral slips diverge laterally to join with the tendons of the interossei and lumbricals to form the conjoined lateral bands. At the dorsum of the proximal phalanx just distal to the MCP joint, the lateral tendons of the interossei give off transverse fibers, which run dorsally over the extensor tendon. These are located over the mid-shaft of the proximal phalanx and allow the intrinsics to flex the MCP joint. At the distal third of the proximal phalanx, oblique fibers are given off from the interossei tendons and insert into the base of the PIP joint with the central slip. These are called oblique fibers and aid in PIP extension.

The transverse retinacular ligament extends from the edges of the lateral bands and goes to the volar side of the PIP joint. They serve to prevent dorsal migration of the lateral bands. With flexion, the lateral bands shift volarly, and with extension, slip dorsally.

Injury may occur as a result of forced flexion of the PIP joint, closed trauma to the PIP joint, knife or glass laceration, or anterior dislocation of the PIP joint. With injury in this zone the central slip is disrupted. If the triangular ligament is torn, volar migration of the lateral bands can occur, resulting in loss of PIP joint extension. With attempts at extension, the pull is concentrated at the DIP joint level, resulting in DIP joint hyperextension. With time the lateral bands shorten, and contracture of the transverse retinacular ligament and the oblique retinacular ligament occurs, resulting in loss of DIP joint flexion and a PIP flexion contracture. This is termed a boutonnière deformity, where the finger will rest with the PIP joint in flexion and the DIP joint in hyperextension.

With acute closed injuries, management is usually conservative. Surgery is required for open injuries or for injuries treated late where established deformity is present and surgical correction is needed. The conservative method of management for acute closed zone III and IV injuries involves splinting of the PIP joint in extension with the DIP joint free for 6 weeks. The splint

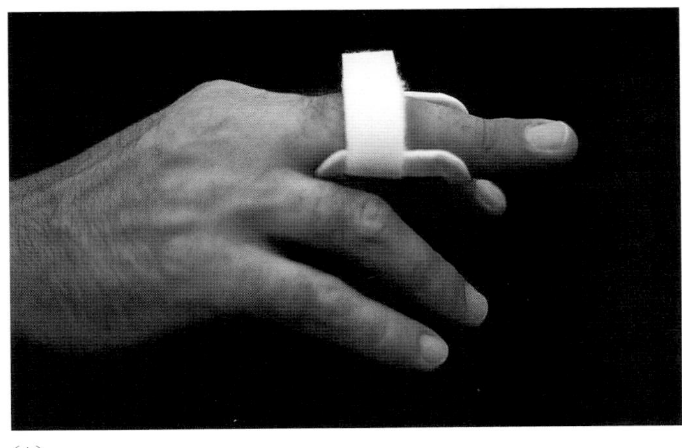

(A)

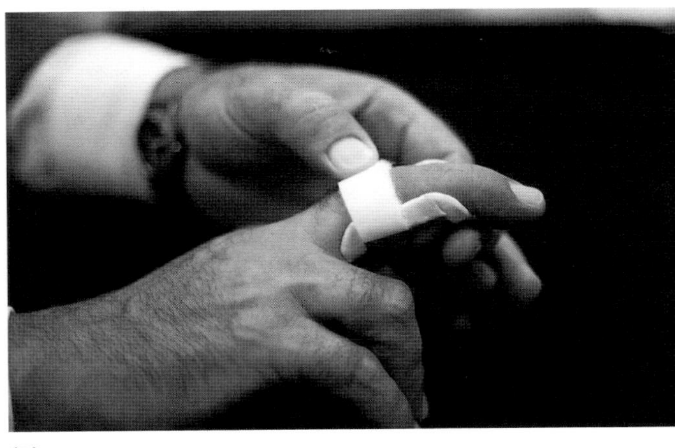

(B)

Figure 5.17

(A) Splint used for zone III–IV extensor tendon injuries positions the PIP joint in full extension. (B) The DIP joint must be left unrestricted to allow flexion.

used can be a thermoplastic gutter splint or a plaster cylinder cast. The important features of the splint include positioning of the PIP in full extension with no restriction of DIP joint range of motion (Figure 5.17A and B). The patient is instructed to keep the splint on at all times and to perform DIP joint flexion exercises. DIP joint flexion exercises are emphasized to prevent shortening of the oblique retinacular ligament, promote lateral band gliding, and preserve DIP joint motion. At 6 weeks, active motion of the PIP joint can begin. The PIP extension splint is continued at night and intermittently during the day depending upon the presence and extent of extensor lag. At 8 weeks, passive PIP flexion exercises can be done to restore PIP flexion if this is a problem. Putty exercises can begin, providing resistance to flexion as well as resistance to the extensor tendon to increase excursion in the zone III–IV area. A common problem with this injury is the difficulty in balancing flexion and extension exercises. As flexion is restored at the PIP joint, extension can be weakened – possibly due to immaturity and attenuation of the tendon scar. A reasonable strategy is to allow gradual recovery of flexion while monitoring and gently stressing extensor function. The balance of exercises and splinting is adjusted according to the extent of the extension deficit.

Injuries in zones III–IV treated late often have a fixed flexion contracture at the PIP joint and a hyperextension deformity at the DIP joint. Conservative management first addresses correction of the flexion contracture through serial cylinder plaster casts or dynamic splinting of the PIP joint (Figure 5.18A and B). Often DIP flexion splinting can be incorporated with the PIP extension splint. Once the contracture is corrected, the PIP joint is maintained in extension for a total of 6–8 weeks of splinting. At 8 weeks, the PIP joint can be mobilized

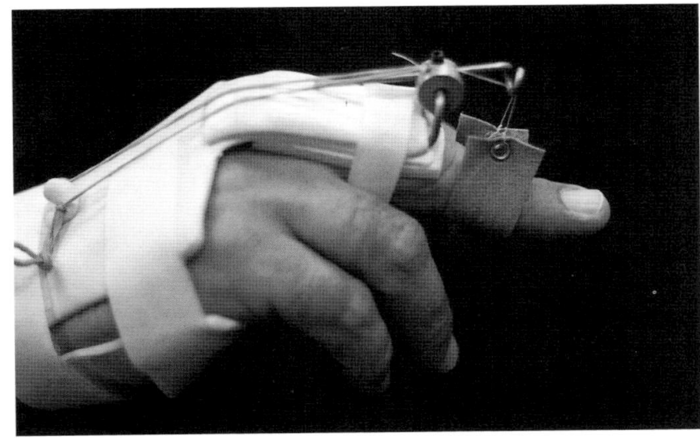

(A)

(B)

Figure 5.18

Correction of a fixed PIP flexion contracture through the use of (A) dynamic PIP extension splint; (B) serial cylinder plaster casts.

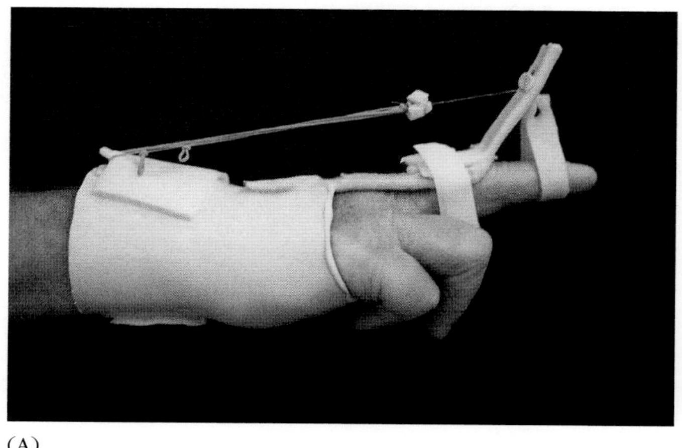

(A)

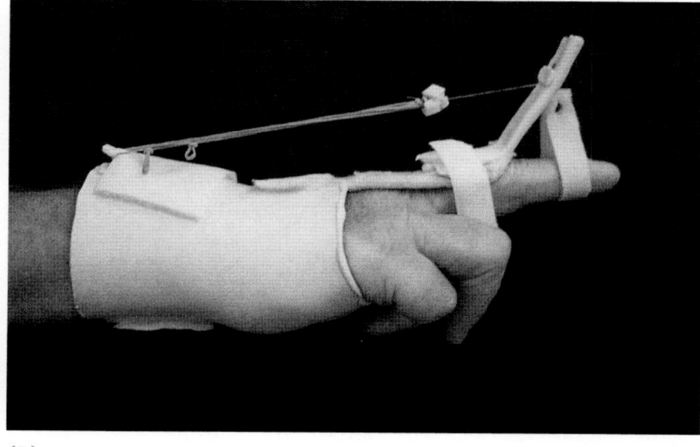

(B)

Figure 5.19

Dynamic extension splint described for repaired extensor tendons in zone III. (A) Splint holds the PIP joint in extension at rest with the MCP joint supported by the splint base. (B) Active flexion of the PIP joint in the splint stopped at 30° by a stop on the splint outrigger.

actively and the splint is continued at night and intermittently during the day. The frequency of daytime splinting is based upon the degree of limitation of PIP extension versus the flexion deficit, and efforts are balanced in favor of the greater deficit. If there is difficulty in recovering flexion of the digit, flexion straps, loops, or dynamic splints can be used.

Traditional management following surgical repair of the central slip and lateral bands generally involves splinting of the wrist and the involved and adjacent digits in extension for 2 weeks. At 2 weeks, the splint is changed to a finger-based splint supporting the PIP joint in extension. The DIP joint is also supported for another 2 weeks if the lateral bands were repaired. DIP joint range of motion (ROM) exercises are then performed in the splint. At 6 weeks, active PIP joint range of motion can begin and also fisting. The splint is continued and worn between exercises and at night. Massage of incision scars can be done and modalities can be used to increase scar extensibility and facilitate exercises. At 8 weeks, the splint is used at night only and light passive ROM exercises can be done if needed to recover flexion; light putty exercise for strengthening of grip; and light resistance for extension. If there is no extensor lag, and a limitation in flexion is present, splinting to restore digital flexion can begin at this time.

The use of early controlled motion following surgical repairs of extensor tendons in zones III–IV is an option advocated by some investigators. Walsh et al (1994) evaluated the results of patients with repairs of the extensor tendon in zones III–IV treated with early controlled motion compared to immobilization. The splint used for early controlled motion was a hand-based splint with the MCP joint supported in a neutral position and the PIP joint supported dynamically in extension. PIP joint flexion is allowed but is limited to 30° by a built-in stop on the splint (Figure 5.19A and B). The dynamic splint and early controlled motion was begun at 2–7 days following surgery. In the splint the patient was instructed to actively flex at the PIP and was limited by a stop on the dynamic traction to 30° of flexion. Exercises were performed as 10 repetitions every 2 hours, allowing the dynamic extension to extend the PIP joint. Patients were also instructed to flex the MCP joint to 30° with the PIP joint in extension. The splint was discontinued at 4 weeks and full active motion was begun. Passive and resisted flexion were begun at 6 weeks postoperatively. The static group was held in a static splint with the PIP in extension and the MCP joint in from 0° to 70° of flexion according to the physician's preference. The authors found no statistical difference between the static and dynamic groups. Good and excellent results were obtained with both methods of management. However, they found that fewer therapy visits were required and the visits were of shorter duration with the tendons treated with early motion. Their conclusion was that early controlled motion of extensor tendon repairs in zones III and IV appears to be safe and yields comparable results to those treated with immobilization but in a shorter time period and with fewer visits.

Evans has described a protocol for early active short arc motion of the repaired central slip, basing this on an analysis of tensile strengths of various tendon repairs and consideration of force application in terms of anatomic position (Evans and Thompson 1992). Evans determined that the repaired central slip would glide the recommended 3–5 mm with 30° of active PIP flexion and extension. Force application to the central slip with

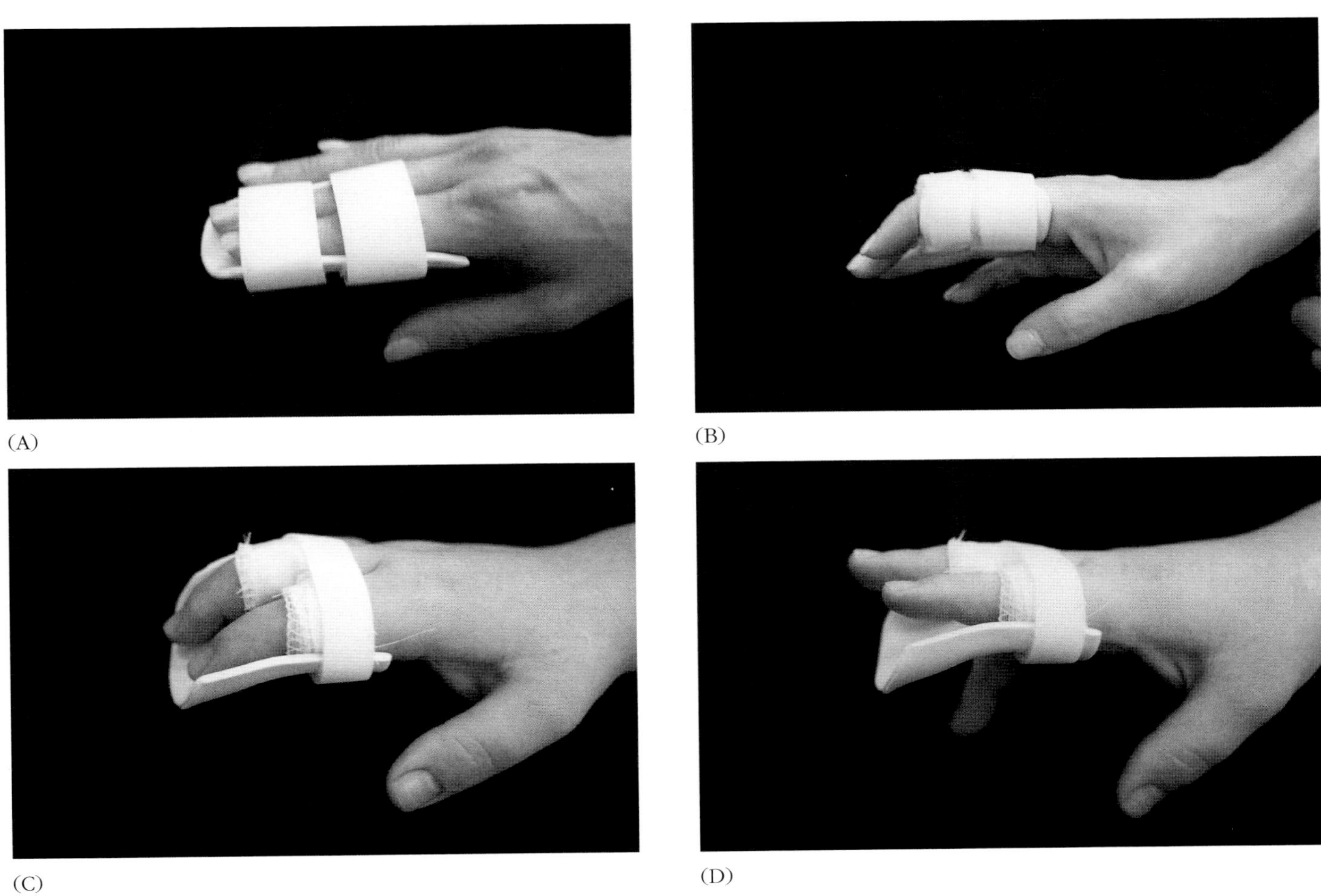

Figure 5.20
Evans short arc motion splints for the repaired central slip. (A) Volar gutter splint supporting the PIP and DIP joints in extension used all the time except at rest. (B) PIP extension splint with the DIP joint free to allow DIP joint exercises. (C) Exercise template splint allowing 30° of PIP extension and 20–25° of DIP joint flexion with extension to neutral.

active extension is estimated at 290 grams. The lowest tensile strength with extensor tendon repairs studied reported a 2 mm gap for the mattress suture when force application reached 488 grams. The conclusion is that the early short arc motion for repaired extensor tendons was safe and physiologically desirable.

Evan's early active short arc motion program begins 24–48 hours postoperatively. A volar gutter splint is worn supporting the PIP and DIP joints in extension all the time except for during exercises. Two exercise splints are made. The first is a PIP extension splint with the DIP free to allow DIP flexion and extension exercises. The second is an exercise template splint allowing 30° of PIP flexion and 20–25° of DIP flexion with active extension allowed of both PIP and DIP joints to neutral (Figure 5.20A–C). Every hour, 10–20 repeats of PIP and DIP joint exercises are performed using the two splints. The PIP extension is performed with the wrist flexed and the MCP at neutral. The patient is instructed in a technique which Evans calls 'minimal active tension', i.e. the minimal force required to overcome the elastic resistance of the antagonistic muscle–tendon unit. After 2 weeks, during the third postoperative week, if no lag develops, 40° of PIP motion is permitted. The template splint is remolded to allow the 40° of motion. At the fourth postoperative week, 50° is allowed. Hereafter PIP motion is gradually increased with continuous monitoring and adjustments for PIP extensor lags. Evans and Thompson (1992, 1997) reported the results of 64 digits with open injury and repair of zone III extensor tendons in 55 patients comparing conservative treatment of immobilization for 3–6 weeks post surgery with those treated with the early short arc motion protocol. This study showed that patients treated with the short arc motion protocol demonstrated significantly better results than those treated with immobilization. No patient in the short arc motion group developed an extensor lag or a boutonnière deformity.

Zones V–VI

Zone V refers to the area over the MCP joint and zone VI is the area over the dorsum of the hand. Six extensor tendons travel over the dorsum of the hand surrounded by fascia. The juncturae tendinum are intertendinous bands that diverge distally from the ring extensor tendon to join the extensors of the small and long fingers at the level of the metacarpal neck. This structure limits independent extension of these three joints. When the little and long fingers are flexed, the juncturae pull the ring extensors distally rendering it slack and limiting extension. MCP joint flexion of the ring finger has little effect on the long and small fingers since the fibers proceed distally. If the small and long fingers are lacerated proximal to the juncturae, they can still extend weakly by virtue of the ring finger and the intact connection to the lacerated tendons by the juncturae. The sagittal bands (also termed the dorsal hood or transverse lamina) are sagittally directed fibers, which surround the MCP joint and attach firmly to it. They attach volarly into the MCP joint volar plate. With flexion, the sagittal bands are pulled distally and with extension they are pulled proximally. Their function is to prevent bowstringing of the extensor tendon, to maintain it in the midline of the joint, and to allow extension of the MCP joint. The power of the extensor tendon can be transmitted distally with a block to MCP joint hyperextension since there is no tethering of the tendon to the proximal phalanx. The extensor indicis proprius and the extensor digit minimi allow independent extension of the index and small fingers.

Injuries in these zones may be caused by lacerations, metacarpal fractures, fist impact injuries, and bite wounds. If the sagittal bands are injured, the stability of the extensor tendon over the MCP joint will be disrupted. During flexion the extensor tendons will displace relative to the MCP joint. Injury to the tendon in zone VI will result in an extensor lag of a degree that depends on the relative level of the laceration to the junctura tendinae. Following repair the extensor tendon may become adherent to the surrounding tissue and limit full composite flexion and full active extension. Extensor tendon repairs can be treated with either initial immobilization or early controlled motion. If treated with immobilization, the wrist and digits are splinted for 2–4 weeks with the wrist in 20° of extension and the MCP joints in 15° of flexion, and the interphalangeal joints extended. After 2–4 weeks, the splint may be adjusted to free the IP joints and allow IP joint range of motion in the splint. If the injury to the tendon is distal to the juncturae tendinae, the adjacent digits can be splinted in slight flexion and the involved digit in extension (Figure 5.21). This permits distal advancement of the proximal stump of the severed tendon and takes pressure off the anastomosis. If the laceration is proximal to the juncturae, then all MCP joints are splinted in extension. At 4–5 weeks, guarded motion can begin. Extensor tendon gliding exercises are performed by extending at the MCP joints with the IP joints flexed. The patient can also flex at the MCP joints with the IP joints extended to avoid tension at the tendon repair site. Wrist flexion is allowed with the digits extended. Scar massage may be done to mobilize adherent incision scars. The splint is continued at this time between exercise sessions and at night. At 6 weeks, full fisting is allowed and the splint is worn at night and for protection during the day. At 8 weeks, passive flexion exercises can be done if needed and light resistance may begin with light putty. The static splint can be discontinued at this time unless an extensor lag is present. Common problems that can occur at this level include extensor lags secondary to adhesion formation, limiting the full excursion of the extensor tendon. Extensor gliding exercises are emphasized and flexion exercises are limited to prevent overwhelming the extensor tendon. Light resistance can be applied to the extensor tendon using light putty and a dynamic extension assist splint may be helpful to assist the extensor tendon and prevent overpull by the flexors. Another problem that is common is tendon adherence and tightness that limits composite finger flexion. It is important to distinguish between a joint contracture and tendon tightness. First evaluate PIP joint flexion with the MCP joint in extension. Then evaluate PIP joint flexion with the MCP joint flexed. If the PIP joint flexes further with the MCP joint in extension, this indicates that the extensor tendon is tight or adherent and cannot lengthen to allow full digital flexion. The splint that is used to restore flexion must incorporate all joints in a composite fist position.

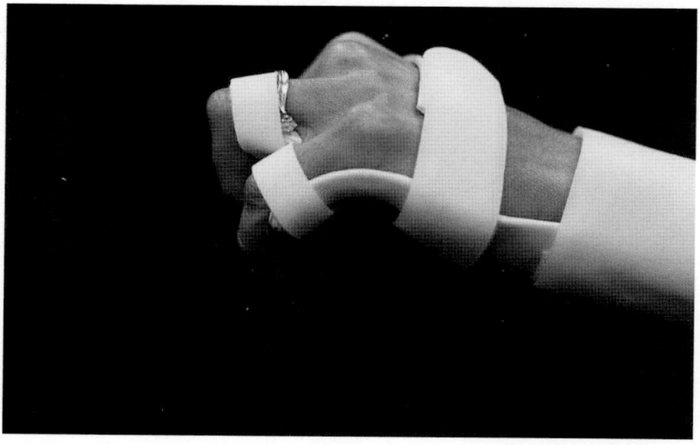

Figure 5.21

Splint used when the injury is distal to the juncturae tendinae. The involved digit is splinted in extension while the adjacent digits are splinted in slight flexion. This permits distal advancement of the proximal stump of the severed tendon and reduces tension at the tendon repair site.

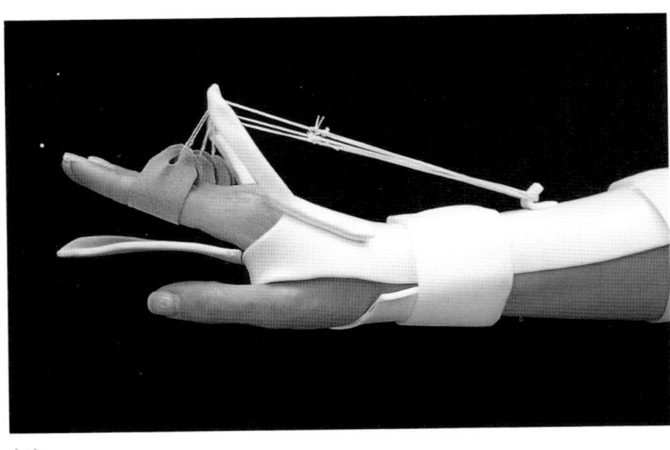

(A)

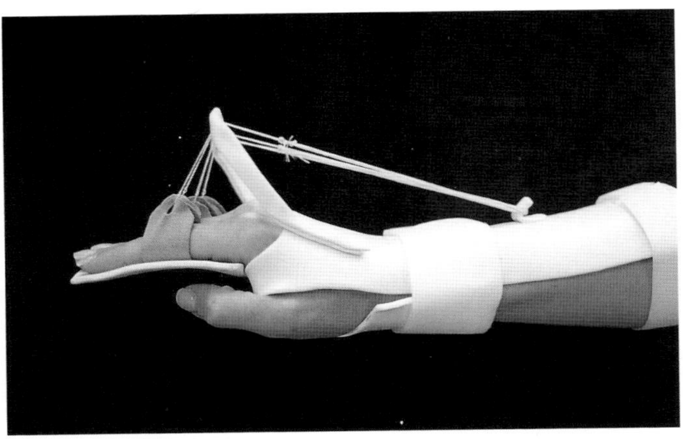

(B)

Figure 5.22

Evans splint used for early motion for extensor tendon repairs in zones V, VI, and VII. (A) A dynamic extension outrigger splint holds the digits in neutral extension. (B) Active flexion is permitted, blocked by a volar splint at 30° of flexion at the MCP joints with the PIP and DIP joints extended.

Early passive motion is applicable for injuries in zones V, VI and VII because of the propensity for restrictive adhesion formation in these zones. The extensors in zones V and VI are encased in paratenon and generally respond to injury with restrictive scar. The tendons in zone VII are similar to the flexors in zone II in that they are enclosed in synovial sheaths at this level. Evans (1989) has described an extensive protocol for early motion in zone V, VI, and VII injuries. The rationale for the parameters are based in part on the work of Kleinert, Duran and Gelberman. As discussed previously, these investigators found that superior tendon healing resulted when the tendon was subjected to early protected motion. The concept of reciprocal relaxation of the muscle tendon unit is cited. That is, with active contraction of one muscle against resistance, the antagonist will reciprocally relax, thereby protecting it from stress. Also, Duran's assertion that 3–5 mm of glide is needed to minimize restrictive adhesion formation is also cited. Evans and Burkhalter (1986) calculated how much range of motion was required to produce 5 mm of tendon glide. They determined that 16 mm of excursion takes place at the MCP joint with full flexion; therefore to produce 5 mm of glide, 30° of range of motion is required. For the thumb, 60° of interphalangeal flexion is required to produce 5 mm of glide.

At 3–5 days postoperatively, a splint is applied which is dorsally based and positions the wrist at 40° of extension. A dynamic extension outrigger is attached and adjusted to hold the MCP joints and interphalangeal joints in neutral or full extension. A volar splint is applied which serves to block flexion of the digits at 30° of flexion at the MCP joints with the interphalangeal joints straight (Figure 5.22A and B). The patient is instructed to perform active MCP joint flexion in the splint with passive pull back to the extended position by the dynamic traction and this is performed five times every 2 hours. Passive interphalangeal joint range of motion is performed with the MCP joints in extension. At night a static wrist and hand splint is used to maintain the position of the wrist and digits. At 3–4 weeks, the standard therapy protocol can begin with active extensor tendon gliding exercises. The dynamic splint is continued during the day and the static splint at night for another 3 weeks.

More recently, Evans and Thompson (1997) described an active component to supplement the passive protocol. The short arc motion is preceded by slow repetitious passive motions to reduce resistance secondary to edema and tight joints. The IP joints are moved through at least 70–80° of passive motion while the wrist and the MCP joints are held by the therapist in extension. With the wrist and IP joints held in extension, the MCP joints are passively moved to 30° for the index and long and to 40° for the ring and small fingers. With all the digital joints held at 0°, the wrist is passively moved to 20° of flexion with the repair level in zones V, VI, and to 10° of extension with repair in zone VII. The active extension component of the early motion program involves positioning the wrist in 20° of flexion with the digits extended fully and the patient is asked to hold this position with minimal tension. This active hold is repeated 20 times with the MCP joints brought to 30° of flexion and back to the 0° extension position for each repetition of active holding. At 4 weeks, the standard program begins. Evans (1989) reported clinical results which demonstrate significantly improved gliding of tendons treated with early passive and short arc motion compared with tendons treated with immobilization.

Zones VII and VIII

Zone VII is located over the dorsum of the wrist and zone VIII is located over the distal end of the forearm. The extensor digitorum communis muscle is the most superficial muscle on the dorsum of the forearm. In the lower third of the forearm, it divides into four tendons, which pass under the dorsal carpal ligament where they are surrounded by a synovial sheath. The extensor digiti minimi passes in a separate ulnar compartment and the extensor indicis proprius travels with the extensor digitorum communis. The synovial sheath and dorsal retinaculum act as pulleys to maintain the relationship of tendon to bone to allow for changes in movement direction. The mechanism of injury is usually the result of a laceration or rupture due to weakening of the tendons secondary to rheumatoid arthritis. The response of the tendon to injury is characterized by rapid contracture of the proximal end of the tendon, emphasizing the importance of early repair. Adherence at the dorsal retinaculum is often a problem, limiting full extensor excursion and limiting flexion by passive restraint. Repairs of tendons in these zones are usually immobilized for 4.5–6 weeks. The wrist and MCP joints are positioned in extension and the specific position is that which relieves any tension at the repair site. If only the wrist extensors are involved, the wrist is positioned in extension and the MCP joints can be left free. At 4.5 weeks, active wrist extension is permitted for wrist extensor tendon repairs. At 5–6 weeks, wrist flexion is allowed actively. The splint is continued for protection at all times. At 6–7 weeks, the splint is worn at night only and as needed for protection during the day. Gentle passive wrist flexion can begin and dynamic splinting as needed to gain wrist flexion. At 8 weeks, light resistive exercise can begin.

For finger extensor tendon repairs at this level, it is important to isolate finger extensor and wrist extensor tendon activity to prevent cross-union. Scar massage is needed to mobilize adherent incision scars and modalities to increase scar and soft tissue extensibility and to facilitate exercise. Protective splinting is usually maintained up until 8 weeks following surgery and resistance can begin at 8 weeks. Common problems include extensor tendon adherence limiting active extensor tendon excursion and passively restricting wrist and finger flexion. Dynamic splinting can be used to overcome limitations in flexion.

Thumb extensor tendon injuries.

The extensor pollicis longus (EPL) functions to hyperextend the thumb; the extensor pollicis brevis (EPB) is the prime MCP joint extensor. Thumb extensor tendon injuries are also classified by zones. Zone I is the area over the thumb interphalangeal joint and is the area of the insertion of the EPL, at the base of the distal phalanx of the thumb. Zone II is the area over the proximal phalanx and injury here involves the EPL tendon and the tendons of insertion of the intrinsic muscles of the thumb. Zone III is the area over the MCP joint of the thumb where the extensor pollicis brevis inserts at the base of the proximal phalanx. With injury to the EPB, there will be loss of MCP joint extension, and a boutonnière deformity of the thumb results with IP joint hyperextension and MCP joint flexion. Zone IV is the area over the thumb metacarpal and injuries here can involve both the EPB and the EPL. Zone V is at the level of the wrist. The EPL and the EPB along with the abductor pollicis longus lie in synovial lined compartments. Injury at this level frequently results in adherence under the retinaculum. Postoperative management at all levels generally involves 4 weeks of immobilization with the wrist and thumb supported in extension. The wrist is in 15° of extension and the thumb is extended at the CMC, MCP, and IP joints. At 4 weeks, active motion can begin with extensor tendon gliding. The thumb splint is worn at night and between exercise sessions. At 6 weeks, passive range of motion can begin and the splint is gradually discontinued. At 8 weeks, flexion splinting can begin if there is a limitation in flexion and resisted flexion and extension is allowed.

Early controlled motion can be used with parameters as discussed for the digital extensors.

Summary

Rehabilitation of the patient with a tendon injury is a challenging process. The repaired tendon must be simultaneously protected from disruption and moved in a controlled fashion. While measures are necessary to protect the repaired structures, early controlled motion is required to enhance healing and function. Appropriate intervention at the correct phase of healing is based on an understanding of tendon and soft tissue healing and the factors that influence repair and function. Coordination between the surgeon and the therapist is essential. Tendon injuries can profoundly affect hand function and appropriate therapy and rehabilitation are essential to preserve function to the fullest extent possible.

References

Beasley RW (1981) *Hand Injuries*, WB Saunders: Philadelphia, 242–52.

Cifaldi-Collins D, Schwarze L (1991) Early progressive resistance following immobilization of flexor tendon repairs, *J Hand Ther* **4**: 111–16.

Chow J, Thomes L, Dovelle S et al (1987) A combined regimen of controlled motion following flexor tendon repair in 'no man's land', *Plast Reconstr Surg* **79**: 447–53.

Chow JA, Thomes LJ, Dovelle S et al (1988) Controlled motion rehabilitation after flexor tendon repair and grafting, *J Bone Joint Surg (Br)* **70–B**: 591–5.

Duran RJ, Houser RG (1975) Controlled passive motion following flexor tendon repairs in zones 2 and 3. In: American Academy of Orthopedic Surgeons: Symposium on Tendon Surgery in the Hand. (CV Mosby: St Louis).

Duran RJ, Coleman CR, Nappi JF, Klerekoper LA (1990) Management of flexor tendon lacerations in zone 2 using controlled passive motion postoperatively. In: Hunter JM, Schneider LH, Mackin EJ, Callahan AD, eds, *Rehabilitation of the Hand* CV Mosby: St Louis, 410–16.

Evans R (1989) Clinical application of controlled stress to the healing extensor tendon: a review of 112 cases, *Phys Ther* **68**: 1041–9.

Evans R (1990) A study of the zone 1 flexor tendon injury and implications for treatment, *J Hand Ther* **3**: 133–45.

Evans RB, Burkhalter WE (1986) A study of the dynamic anatomy of extensor tendons and implications for treatment, *J Hand Surg* **11A**: 774–9.

Evans RB, Thompson DE (1992) An analysis of factors that support early short arc motion of the repaired central slip, *J Hand Ther* **5**: 187–201.

Evans RB, Thompson DE (1997) Immediate active short arc range of motion following tendon repair. In: Hunter JM, Schneider LH, Mackin, eds, *Tendon and Nerve Surgery in the Hand: a Third Decade* CV Mosby; St Louis, 362–93.

Gelberman RH, Woo SL-Y (1989) The physiological basis for the application of controlled stress in the rehabilitation of flexor tendon injuries, *J Hand Ther* **2**: 66–70.

Gelberman RH, Menon J, Gonsalves M, Akeson WH (1980a) The effects of mobilization on the vascularization of healing flexor tendons in dogs, *Clin Orthop* **153**: 283–9.

Gelberman RH, Vand Berg JS, Lundberg GN, Akeson WH (1980b) Flexor tendon healing and restoration of the gliding surface: an ultrastructural study in dogs, *J Bone Joint Surg* **65A**: 583–95.

Gelberman RH, Amiel D, Gonsalves M et al (1981) The influence of protected passive mobilization on the healing of flexor tendons: a biomechanical and microangiographic study, *Hand* **13**: 120–5.

Gelberman RH, Woo SL-Y, Lothringer K et al (1982) Effects of early intermittent passive mobilization on healing canine flexor tendons, *J Hand Surg* **7**: 170–5.

Gelberman RH, Manske PR, Akeson WH et al (1986) Flexor tendon repair, *J Orthop Res* **4**: 119–25.

Gelberman RH, Nunley JA, Osterman AL et al (1987) Influences of the protected passive motion interval on flexor tendon healing: a prospective randomized clinical study, *Clin Orthop* **264**: 189–96.

Hitchcock TF, Light TR, Bunch WH et al (1987) The effect of immediate constrained digital motion on the strength of flexor tendon repairs in chickens, *J Hand Surg* **12A**: 590–5.

Horibe S, Woo S, Spiegelman J et al (1990) Excursion of the flexor digitorum profundus tendon: a kinematic study of the human and canine digits, *J Orthop Res* **8**: 167.

Kessler I, Nissim F (1969) Primary repair without immobilization of flexor tendon division within the digital flexor sheath, *Acta Orthop Scand* **40**: 587–601.

Lester GD, Kleinert HE, Kutz JE et al (1977) Primary flexor tendon repair followed by immediate controlled mobilization, *J Hand Surg* **2A**: 441–51.

Lundborg G, Rank F (1978) Experimental intrinsic healing of flexor tendons based upon synovial fluid nutrtion, *J Hand Surg* **3**: 21–31.

McGrouther DA, Ahmed MR (1981) Flexor tendon excursions in 'no man's land', *The Hand* **13**: 129–41.

Manske PR, Bridwell K, Lesker PA (1978a) Nutrient pathways to flexor tendons to chickens using tritiated proline, *J Hand Surg* **3**: 352–7.

Manske PR, Whiteside LA, Lesker PA (1978b) Nutrient pathways to flexor tendons using hydrogen washout techniques, *J Hand Surg* **3**: 32–6.

Mason JL, Allen HS (1941) The rate of healing tendons: an experimental study of tensile strength, *Ann Surg* **113**: 424.

Matsui T, Hunter JM (1997) Injury to the vascular system and its effect on tendon injury in no man's land. In: *Tendon and Nerve Surgery in the Hand: a Third Decade* CV Mosby: St Louis.

Peacock EE (1965) Biological principles in the healing of long tendons, *Surg Clin North Am* **45**: 461–76.

Potenza AD (1963) Critical evaluation of flexor tendon healing and adhesion formation within artificial digital sheaths: an experimental study, *J Bone Joint Surg* **45A**: 1217–33.

Pruitt DL, Manske PR, Fink B (1991) Cyclic stress analysis of flexor tendon repair, *J Hand Surg* **16A**: 701–7.

Seradge H (1983) Elongation of the repair configuration following flexor tendon repair, *J Hand Surg* **8**: 182–5.

Silfverskiold KL, May EJ (1994) Flexor tendon repair in Zone 2 with a new suture technique and an early mobilization program combining passive and active motion, *J Hand Surg* **19A**: 53–60.

Silfverskiold KL, May E, Tornvall A (1992) Gap formation during controlled motion after flexor tendon repair in zone 2: a prospective clinical study, *J Hand Surg* **17A**: 539.

Slattery P, McGrouther D (1984) A modified Kleinert controlled mobilization splint following flexor tendon repair, *J Hand Surg* **9**: 34.

Strickland JW (1989) Biologic rationale, clinical application and results of early motion following flexor tendon repair, *J Hand Ther* **2**: 71–83.

Strickland JW, Cannon NM (1993) Flexor tendon repair – Indiana method, *Indiana Hand Center Newsletter* **1**: 1–19.

Strickland JW, Glogovac SV (1980) Digital function following flexor tendon repair in zone 2: a comparison of immobilization and controlled passive motion techniques, *J Hand Surg* **5**: 537.

Tajima T (1997) Indication and technique for early postoperative motion after repair of digital flexor tendon particularly in Zone 2. In: Hunter JM, Schneider LH, Mackin EJ, eds, *Tendon and Nerve Surgery in the Hand: a Third Decade* CV Mosby: St Louis, 324–31.

Urbaniak JR (1974) Tendon suturing methods: analysis of tensile strength. In: American Academy of Orthopedic Surgeons: Symposium on Tendon Surgery in the Hand. AAOS: Park Ridge, Il. 307.

Verdan C (1960) Primary repair of flexor tendons, *J Bone Joint Surg* **42A**: 647–57.

Walsh MT, Rinehimer W, Muntzer E et al (1994) Early controlled motion with dynamic splinting versus static splinting for zones III and IV extensor tendon lacerations: a preliminary report, *J Hand Ther* **7**: 232–6.

Wehbe M, Hunter JM (1985) Flexor tendon gliding in the hand. I: in vivo excursions. II: Differential gliding, *J Hand Surg* **10**: 570.

Woo SL-Y, Gelberman RH, Cobb NG et al (1981) The importance of controlled passive motion on flexor tendon healing: a biomechanical study, *Acta Orthop Scand* **52**: 615–22.

II Nerve and paralysis

6 Nerve repair: experimental and clinical update

Lars B Dahlin and Göran Lundborg

Nerve injury and repair – the problem

Injuries to the upper extremity and hand are a common problem, and two-thirds of these patients, mainly men, are below the age of 30 years (Angermann and Lohmann 1993, Beaton et al 1994). Many of the injuries involve the peripheral nerve trunks in the upper extremity and they may even include the brachial plexus. A far lower number of nerve injuries affect the nerve trunks in the lower extremity and they may require nerve grafting (Trumble and Vanderhooft 1994, Trumble et al 1995, Kline et al 1998, Allan 2000). The peripheral nerve lesion leads to severe and in many cases permanent impairment of the function of the limb. This is particularly evident in the hand, which performs fine manipulative tasks. Understanding of the pathophysiology of nerve injuries has increased during the last 20–30 years (Lundborg 2000a), but the methods available to repair such nerve injuries are still limited. Even though microsurgical techniques to approximate the two nerve ends of a transected nerve trunk have been introduced, the results are still far from ideal (Birch and Raji 1991). At present clinicians can only adapt the epineurial and perineurial sheaths of the transected nerve trunks, but they cannot, for example, influence the orientation of the outgrowing axons.

The principles of the regeneration process after a nerve injury and repair of a nerve trunk were outlined at the beginning of the twentieth century by Ramon y Cajal (Cajal 1928). New biological techniques have been introduced to examine what happens at the molecular and cellular level, but the clinical setting still lacks the means to improve the results. The nervous system is a unique system as regards the repair process. Injury and reconstruction involve not only a local process at the site of injury, but processes also occur at the spinal cord, in the dorsal root ganglia (DRG) and in the brain. Transection of the nerve trunk leads to a local injury at the site of injury. However, degeneration of the axon takes place distally to the injury, and structural and biochemical changes occur proximally in the nerve cell body located in the spinal cord or in the DRG (Eriksson 1997). Furthermore, the injury also leads to severe functional consequences in terms of reorganization at the cortical, subcortical and spinal levels (Merzenich et al 1983, Wall and Kaas 1986, Wall et al 1986, Merzenich and Sameshima 1993, Lundborg 2000b). It is disappointing to see the non-optimal results after a nerve injury and repair, but this reflects the complexity of the lesion, where the events at several levels – at the target level (muscle and sensory receptors), distal nerve segment, site of injury, proximal nerve segments, the nerve cell body in the spinal cord and DRG and the cortical and subcortical levels in the brain – contribute to outcome. The purpose this chapter is to review the injury and regeneration process of a peripheral injury from the basic as well as from the clinical point of view.

The site of injury

Following transection of the nerve trunk there is a biological battlefield, with general inflammation occurring at the site of injury (Figure 6.1). The blood–nerve barrier at the site of injury and also distal to the injury is broken down (Olsson 1966). Inflammatory cells invade the area of the injury concomitant with the bleeding at the site of injury and the formation of an oedema. The events that occur between the transected nerve segment have been extensively studied using the silicone tube model, and it is known that inflammatory cells and mediators accumulate very early in the process (Danielson et al 1993, Dahlin et al 1995). The presence of macrophages has been of interest, as these cells can stimulate non-neuronal cells like Schwann cells and fibroblasts to proliferate and produce neurotrophic factors (Brown et al 1991, Monaco et al 1992, Gehrmann and Kreutzberg 1993, Dahlin 1995, Miyauchi et al 1997).

In the gap between the nerve segments, where fluid accumulates, a fibrin matrix containing macrophages is formed at an early stage (Dahlin 1995). If the matrix is stable Schwann cells migrate into the matrix from both the proximal and the distal nerve segments (Torigoe et al 1996). The migration of Schwann cells from the proximal nerve segment is slightly more extensive, as they are

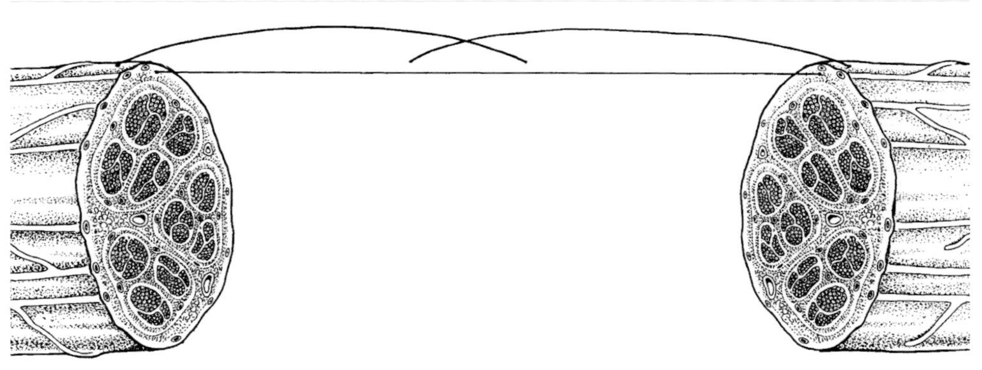

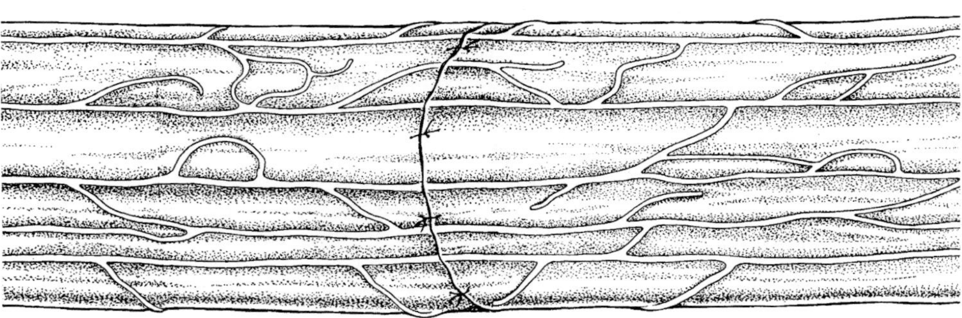

(A)

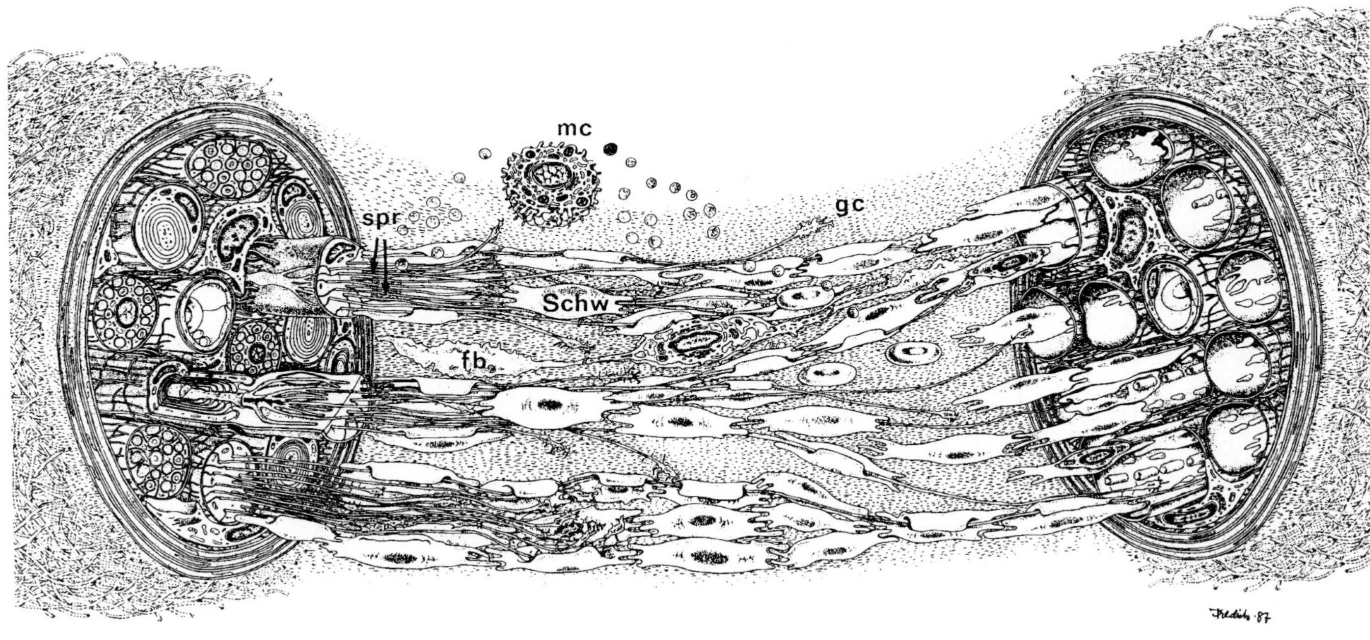

(B)

Figure 6.1

Two diagrams showing the problem from different views. (A) The surgeon can only adapt the epineurial sheath, but at the microscopic level (B) there is a biological battle field: spr, sprouts; Schw, Schwann cell; fb, fibroblast; mc, macrophage; gc, growth cone. Reproduced with permission from Lundborg G, ed. *Nerve Injury and Repair*. Churchill Livingstone: London, 1988.

followed and probably stimulated by the outgrowing axons (Torigoe et al 1996, Brandt et al 1999a), i.e. the axon and the Schwann cells exist in symbiosis. The distal part of the axon in the proximal segment forms after the transection sprouts with growth cones (Letourneau et al 1991). From each growth cone philopodia develop, which palpate the surroundings and try to reach the distal nerve segment and the formed bands of Büngner (see below). Cajal demonstrated the phenomenon of neurotropism (chemotropism) early in the twentieth century (Cajal 1928), which is a preferential growth of the outgrowing axons towards a distal nerve segment rather than towards other types of tissue such as tendons, muscle, etc. The phenomenon has been verified by many authors (Nachemson 1988, Dobretsov et al 1994, Kuffler 1994, Kuffler and Magwinoff 1994, Lundborg et al 1994a).

The distal nerve segment

Following transection of the nerve trunk, the proximal and distal parts of the axon retract from each other and swell. The swelling is due to a continuous accumulation of axoplasmic material transported by axonal transport, which occurs in the distal part of the axon for a short time period and occurs continuously in the axon proximal to the injury. The distal parts of the axon degenerate along with their myelin sheath (Wallerian degeneration) due to activation of calcium-dependent proteases. The blood–nerve barrier is broken down and oedema is formed in the distal nerve segment, particularly where macrophages invade that segment. Macrophages are usually found in very limited numbers in an intact nerve. The role of the macrophages is phygocytosis of myelin and axonal debris, together with the Schwann cells (Williams and Hall 1971, Gibson 1979, Beuche and Friede 1984, Stoll et al 1989). The Schwann cells seem to internalize and degrade the myelin sheath into myelin balls which are subsequently transferred to and phagocytosed by the macrophages (Williams and Hall 1971, Stoll et al 1989). Simultaneously, the non-neuronal cells in the distal nerve segments start to proliferate within the basal lamina. The cells consist of ≥70% Schwann cells (Siironen et al 1994) and the bands of Büngner are formed (Schwann cell columns). The basal lamina remains intact during Wallerian degeneration. However, the Schwann cells can probably modify the basal lamina with respect to composition and orientation of neurite-promoting molecules, e.g. laminin-2 (merosin) (Agius and Cochard 1998), thereby promoting the elongation of axons. The macrophages release a broad spectrum of substances and it has been suggested that the release of interleukin-1β may induce nerve growth factor (NGF) synthesis in Schwann cells and fibroblasts (Lindholm et al 1987). NGF, which in uninjured nerves is present at a low concentration, is upregulated in a bimodal way in the distal nerve segment following nerve injury (Heumann et al 1987, Thoenen et al 1988).

The Schwann cells, fibroblasts and the outgrowing axons all express NGF receptors (Taniuchi et al 1986, 1988, Raivich et al 1991). There are specific high affinity receptor tyrosine kinases including the NGF-receptor trkA (tyrosine receptor kinase A; p140) and low affinity NGF receptor called p75 (Canossa et al 1996). NGF is only one neurotrophic factor that contributes to the complex biochemical changes that occur at the site of injury, in the distal nerve segment and around the nerve cell bodies. This is a prerequisite for the regeneration process. NGF belongs to the neurotrophin family and other important members of this family are brain-derived neurotrophic factor (BDNF), neurotrophin-3 (NT3), neurotrophin-4/5 (NT4-5) and neurotrophin-6 (NT6), which all bind to specific receptors necessary to activate intracellular signalling. The activation processes, including autophosphorylation of specific tyrosine residues in the cytoplasm with its subsequent biological function in the cell, are important steps for initiating the regeneration process (Wiklund 1999). Other families of neurotrophic factors are the neuropoetic cytokines CNTF (ciliary neurotrophic factor) and interleukin-6 and fibroblast growth factors (FGFs) (Friedman and Greener 1999, Terenghi 1999, Weisenhorn et al 1999). In addition, further groups include insulin-like growth factors (IGF), leukaemia inhibitory factor (LIF) and glia-derived neurotrophic factor (GDNF). NGF only affects sensory nerves, motor neurons are not affected as they lack trkA receptors. However, motor neurons do respond to BDNF, which is mediated by high affinity receptors trkB and trkC (Barbacid 1995, Novikov 1999). The upregulation of BDNF in the distal nerve segment also has a different temporal pattern compared with NGF (Meyer et al 1992).

In the distal segment there are also neurite-promoting factors which support the outgrowing axons. The glycoproteins laminin and fibronectin (Manthorpe et al 1983, Davis et al 1987) and the adhesion molecules such as N-CAM, L1, myelin-associated glycoprotein (MAG) and TAG-1 are examples of supportive factors (Martini and Schachner 1988, Walsh and Doherty 1996). It has been suggested that repulsive factors for growth control are also involved in the process (Keynes and Cook 1990) – such as semaphorins (Tanelian et al 1997, Chen et al 1998).

The reaction of the nerve cell body

The nerve cell body, located in DRG (sensory neurons) and in the spinal cord (motor neurons), goes through profound structural and biochemical changes following transection of its peripheral axon. However, transection of the central process of the neuron in DRG has very little influence on the biochemistry and regeneration capacity of that part of the neuron (Reimer and Kanje 1999). For example, transection of the central part of DRG neuron has little or even no effect on the expression of GAP-43 (Schreyer and Skene 1991, 1993), β–tubulin (Oblinger and Lasek 1988), substance P (Henken et al 1990) and other neuropeptides (Reimer and Kanje 1999). Therefore, the outgrowth of the central process is poor and slow and reinnervation of the central targets usually does not occur. In contrast, the peripheral axons can – compared with the central process – more or less successfully reinnervate their peripheral target following an injury. After a transection, a crush and even a compression injury of the peripheral nerve trunk, the nerve cell body of sensory neurons undergoes profound changes in structure (Lieberman 1971, Dahlin et al 1987) and alteration in expression of a variety of proteins, e.g. β–tubulin (Oblinger and Lasek 1988) and GAP-43 (Schreyer and Skene 1991, 1993). Structural proteins such as neurofilament proteins are downregulated (Oblinger and Lasek 1988). Several neuropeptides in DRG neurons are affected after injury where the synthesis of galanin, NPY, VIP and PACAP is increased, but with a different time course (Hökfelt et al 1987, 1994, Wakisaka et al 1991, Noguchi et al 1993, Sundler et al 1996, Jongsma et al 2000), while the synthesis of substance P is decreased (Bisby and Keen 1986). The alteration of protein synthesis is preceded by upregulation of immediate-early genes such as *c-jun* and *c-fos*, which are induced very early after the injury (Koistinaho et al 1993).

The growth cone – which is the outgrowing axon's navigation unit – is influenced by the local phenomenon of cell proliferation and the growth factors (Letourneau et al 1991). However, to obtain an optimal regeneration process there has to be a continuous adjustment of the neuronal protein synthesis and therefore signals are involved in the communication between the growth cone and the nerve cell body. Such signals are probably transferred by retrograde axonal transport, although detailed information about the signals in this communication is not available. The signal transduction, which takes place both in the nerve cell body and at the growth cone level, comprises biochemical events between the binding of a factor to a cell surface and the physiological outcome of such a process. The transduction process involves protein phosphorylation performed by protein kinases which are probably of utmost importance as a signal pathway to control cellular proliferation and differentiation (Wiklund 1999). The signals that are transferred in a retrograde fashion may regulate the cell body machinery either by stimulation or repression of the transcription of certain genes. These signals may be target-derived, but may also be produced locally at the site of lesion ('injury factor'). LIF has been suggested to be an 'injury factor' regulating transcription of galanin in the neuron (Sun and Zigmond 1996). Furthermore, the neuron may also use substances normally transported in the axon to change the production machinery. Such substances may be modified by phosphorylation at the tip of the transected axon and thereby convey new information on the return to the cell body.

Following transection of a nerve trunk some neurons in the DRG and spinal cord may not survive and therefore a cell loss has been observed (Purves and Njå 1978). Even after an immediate microsurgical repair of the nerve there may be a 20–40% loss of neurons in the DRG (Himes and Tessler 1989, Liss et al 1994) and if the reinnervation is prevented the loss can be even greater (Liss et al 1994). The cell loss not only includes the sensory neurons, but also motor neurons (Li et al 1994, 1998, Novikova et al 1994, Martin et al 1999). The cell loss is probably due to apoptosis and necrosis (Hou et al 1998, Sastry and Rao 2000) and may be induced by oxidative or nitrosative stress (Martin et al 1999). The cell loss also includes the satellite cells (Hou et al 1998). It is interesting to note that macrophages migrate into the DRG after a peripheral nerve injury (Lu and Richardson 1991).

The neuronal cell loss in the DRG has been reported to depend on the proximity of the injury to the perikaryon and of course it is affected by the point in time after the injury at which the analysis is performed (Ygge 1989). It has also been reported that the neuronal loss caused by a crush injury is not different from that observed by a permanent axotomy, which would indicate that the survival of the neuron is not dependent on the possibility of axonal growth after axotomy (Degn et al 1999). However, if neurotrophic factors such as NGF (to sensory neurons) and BDNF or GDNF (to motor neurons) are administered the cell loss is markedly diminished (Li et al 1994, 1995, Novikov et al 1995, 1996, 1997, Ljungberg et al 1999, Wiberg et al 1999). For the motor neurons the mechanism for BDNF to act as a promotor for neuronal survival may be through blockage of nitric oxide synthesis (Novikov et al 1995). It should be noted that the population of DRG neurons could be roughly divided into large (positive for trkC), median (positive for trkA, trkB and trkC) and small (positive for SP, CGRP and trkA) cell bodies (Averill et al 1995, Kvist Reimer 2000, Mu et al 1993). NGF seems to mainly affect CGRP-positive neurons, while limited effects on SP-positive neurons are observed (Wiberg et al 1999). It has also been reported that NGF can upregulate expression of PACAP in small to medium sized neurons in both intact and injured DRGs, while NT3 decreases the PACAP expression observed with axotomy in many medium to large sized neurons (Jongsma et al 1999). In the future increased knowledge about the dynamics of neuropeptide alterations after nerve injuries may help clinicians to treat and prevent the pain that may occur after such injuries, since neuropeptides probably have a crucial role for pain modulation. In this context other substances such as tumour necrosis factor-alpha (TNF-α) should also be considered (Müller and Stoll 1998).

Factors influencing the growth direction of regenerating axons

There are many factors that could affect the outgrowing axons and influence the growth direction. These factors may influence the growth cones locally, as discussed above. Cell surfaces and polarized structures and interfaces between various tissue layers can guide the outgrowing axons by contact guidance. An example of such guidance is the fibrin matrix that is formed between the two segments of a transected nerve. The diameter of such a fibrin matrix is influenced by the diameter of the nerve segment and affects the number of outgrowing axons (Zhao et al 1993). Cajal introduced the term neurotropism (or chemotaxis) where axons from the proximal nerve preferentially grow towards a nerve graft or a distal nerve segment regardless of the alignment of this segment (Cajal 1928). Such a phenomenon may be explained by diffusion of substances from the distal target (Kuffler and Magwinoff 1994, Kuffler 1996, Zheng and Kuffler 2000). On the motor side the pruning concept has been introduced by Brushart, who concludes that the motor Schwann cell tubes maintain a specific identity that could be recognized by regenerating axons (Brushart and Seiler 1987, Martini et al 1992, Brashart 1998). Maki's group has emphasized that there is a selective mechanism in sensory regeneration but not in motor regeneration (Maki et al 1996a, 1996b, Iwabuchi et al 1999). The issue of specificity is complex and several types have been suggested: tissue specificity, fascicular or nerve trunk specificity, sensory versus motor specificity, topographic specificity and end-organ specificity (Brushart 1998, Lundborg 2000a).

Stimulation of nerve regeneration

Experimentally, various procedures have been used to stimulate and improve the regeneration process. A number of substances, such as various neurotrophic factors and hormones, have been administered systemically or locally via different conduits or via osmotic pumps (Lundborg 2000a). Many of these substances have been reported to improve the regeneration process by, for example, increasing the rate and number of myelinated axons and even the degree of functional recovery. However, no substance has ever been used and reported clinically to improve nerve regeneration. It is still not known which factor or factors should be administered, how they should be applied, in what combination, at what dose or at what time point in the process they should be used. In reconstructive procedures where various conduits are applied between the severed nerve trunks, cultured Schwann cells have been used (Guénard et al 1992, Gulati et al 1995, Ansselin et al 1997, Levi et al 1997, Nishiura et al 2001, Rodriguez et al 2000, Verdu et al 2000). The advantage of using living cells as a source would be that they could adjust the production of substances in a more meticulous way than a synthetic slow-release conduit. In the future the use of genetically modified cells may create a more efficient Schwann cell that can operate in close connection with the regenerating axon (Menei et al 1998, Sorensen et al 1998).

Other substances have been successfully used experimentally such as thyroid hormones (Danielsen et al 1986, Voinesco et al 1998, Barakat-Walter 1999), growth hormones (Kanje et al 1988) and immunosuppressants (FK-506) (Gold et al 1995). Of those, FK-506 is used clinically in connection with hand transplantation. some reported results give an impression of a high rate of axonal outgrowth (Dubernard et al 1999, Jones et al 2000).

Non-invasive techniques can be used to stimulate axonal outgrowth. Application of electromagnetic fields and hyperbaric oxygen treatment have been used experimentally and can enhance nerve regeneration (Sisken et al 1989, Haapaniemi et al 1998). However, hyperbaric oxygen treatment of peripheral nerve injuries has not been used clinically in Western countries. Again, factors such as duration of treatment and level of pressure are unknown and the possible neurotoxic effects of the use of high pressure should also be considered.

The conditioning lesion – timing of surgery

If an experimental nerve injury is preceded by another lesion (conditioning lesion) by days to weeks the regenerating axons grow faster than if such a conditioning lesion is not applied (McQuarrie and Grafstein 1973). The most pronounced effect is seen on the so-called initial delay, that is a calculated value of time from repair to when the axons approach the distal nerve segment. The conditioning lesion effect is probably due to changes in the distal nerve segment (such as proliferation of Schwann cells) and to alterations in the nerve cell bodies of the neurons. It seems that even a short conditioning interval such as as 2–3 days is sufficient to improve regeneration (Danielsen et al 1994). Clinically, such a phenomenon is possible when a delayed primary repair or a secondary nerve repair of the nerve injury is carried out. However, a primary nerve suture is still certainly an advantage for technical reasons (Birch and Raji 1991). Furthermore, there are indications that the neuronal cell loss can be diminished if the repair is not delayed (Liss et al 1994). The reconnection of severed nerve segments in combination with treatment with factors to reduce the cell death may be an important aspect of the treatment of nerve injuries in the future, especially if the nerve injury is located proximally close to the spinal cord and DRG (Novikov et al 1995, Novikova et al 1997). In this context it should be stressed that the number of reinnervating motor neurons is strongly correlated to the return of force in the reinnervated muscle (Scherman et al 2000). A delay in performing reconstructive surgery may seriously impair the ability of the Schwann cells to proliferate in an optimal way, because of the observed decrease in expression of the low affinity NGF receptor (p75) in such cells during long-term denervation (You et al 1997). This, in connection with the knowledge about the neuronal loss after nerve injury, implies that nerve repair and reconstruction should not be delayed.

The tube concept in clinical practice

Tubes have been used for a long time to examine the basic mechanism of nerve regeneration. Many different models have been published (Fields et al 1989) and one such model is the silicone tube model (Danielsen 1990, Dahlin and Lundborg 2000). The interior milieu of the tube has been varied, the tube has been filled with plasma, laminin, testosterone, hyaluronic acid and cultured Schwann cells (for example Lundborg 2000a, Dahlin and Lundborg 2001). In clinical practice a prospective randomized study has been performed where repair using the silicone tube model was compared with primary nerve repair (Lundborg et al 1997). The results at follow-up at 1 year (Lundborg et al 1997) and 4–5 years after repair (Lundborg et al 2000) of median or ulnar nerves in the forearm showed no difference between the two methods. At re-exploration of the tube after 1–4 years it was not possible to identify the exact location of the intentionally left gap of 2–3 mm between the nerve segments – a new nerve trunk had formed (Dahlin et al 2001). Furthermore, there was no compression of the new nerve trunk by the tube and the thin capsule observed around the tube mainly contained no inflammatory reaction (Dahlin et al 2001), which is different to single previous reported cases (Merle et al 1989). A silicone tube with a diameter exceeding the diameter of the nerve trunk by about 30% can be used to bridge short gaps, but is not an alternative if longer defects have to be bridged (Braga-Silva 1999). In a multicentre study, Weber et al (2000) used a PGA conduit (polyglycolic acid; bioresorbable) as an alternative to end-to-end repair or nerve graft to treat digital nerve injuries in the hand. They concluded that repair/reconstruction with such a conduit improved the sensation compared with an end-to-end repair technique and the use of nerve grafts (defects <4 mm and >8 mm) – a statement which has been discussed elsewhere (Lundborg 2000c).

Reconstruction of segmental nerve defects

If the nerve injury is severe there may be a segmental defect between the proximal and distal segments, thereby making a direct repair impossible. The basis for such a clinical reconstruction of the peripheral nerve trunk and brachial plexus using autologous nerve grafts was introduced by Millesi 20 years ago (Millesi et al 1972, 1976, Millesi 2000). These principles are still clinically the method of choice. However, knowledge about the mechanism(s) behind nerve regeneration in such nerve grafts has increased substantially during recent years, and new alternatives have been used (Doolabh et al 1996, Chamberlain et al 1998, Dahlin and Lundborg 1998, Hadlock et al 1998, 1999, Rodrigues et al 1999). New strategies and alternatives have been introduced which hypothetically can also be applied in the central nervous sysem (Olson 1997). In many of conduits used, a basal lamina of allo- or xeno-nerves, freeze-thawed muscles or teased tendons is created, but living cells are missing (Ide et al 1983, Glasby et al 1986, Gulati 1988, Sondell et al 1998, Brandt et al 1999b). Therefore insufficient regeneration occurs in such conduits. The gold standard is still the autologous nerve graft. The deposition of Schwann cells in such conduits or along continuously applied sutures ('stepping stones') improves the outgrowth of axons markedly, thereby making it possible to bridge long nerve gaps (Guénard et al 1992, Ansselin et al 1997, Francel et al 1997, Levi et al 1997, Rodrigues et al 1999, Rodriguez et al 2000, Scherman et al 2000, Nishiura et al 2001). In the future, methods have to be improved to harvest and dissociate Schwann cells rapidly, which will make the use of such cells possible in clinical practice. Furthermore, the introduction of monoclonal antibodies to cell surface adhesion molecules to induce antigen tolerance in allografts, together with immunosuppressants like FK-506, may have a potential value in the future (Evans et al 1994, Nakao and Mackinnon 1995). A simple method to improve regeneration in autologous nerve grafts is predegeneration of the donor nerve, which can be carried out by various methods (Kerns et al 1993, Danielsen et al 1994).

Various types of synthetic grafts have been used experimentally (Dahlin and Lundborg 1998, Lundborg 2000a) and recently clinically (Weber et al 2000) to bridge nerve defects. The PGA conduit has recently been suggested to be an alternative to autologous nerve grafts for defects of certain distances in the repair/reconstruction of digital nerves in humans (see above) (Weber et al 2000).

The end-to-side anastomosis of the peripheral nerve has been suggested (Rowan et al 2000), in which a distal nerve segment is used to approach an intact (or with a small perineurial window) nerve trunk when the appropriate proximal segment is not available (Viterbo et al 1992, Lundborg et al 1994b, Tarasidis et al 1998). The detailed mechanisms have not yet been solved, although a double-labelling technique indicates that collateral sprouting from intact axons may occur resulting in axonal growth out into the distal nerve segment and later reinnervation of targets (Zhang et al 1999, Kanje et al 2000). Clinical reports indicate that this method may have a potential value in selected cases at specific locations (Viterbo et al 1993, Frey et al 1999).

Future prospects

We have probably reached the limit of what we can do technically to repair transected nerve trunks. During recent years we have learned a lot about the mechanisms in the extremely complicated cell machinery of nerve regeneration. By the use and application of the new knowledge and possibilities in tissue engineering, gene technology, immunosuppression and neurotrophic factors we may improve clinical results in the future. Understanding of the functional reorganization in the brain is an important part of the treatment of peripheral nerve injuries (Lundborg 2000b), and that aspect would require a chapter of its own. A thorough collaboration is required between clinicians and neuroscientists to improve the treatment of peripheral nerve injuries. Properly designed prospective randomized clinical studies are also needed to perform appropriate evaluations of new methods. An improved protocol designed for the evaluation of the outcome of repair of specific injured nerves is therefore required and has recently become available for the results of repair of ulnar and median nerves in the forearm (Rosén, 2000).

Acknowledgements

The studies from the Malmö group were supported by grants from the Swedish Medical Research Council (5188), the University of Lund, Thelma Zoéga's Fund for Medical Research, the Royal Physiographic Society and the University Hospital, Malmö, Sweden.

References

Agius E, Cochard P (1998) Comparison of neurite outgrowth induced by intact and injured sciatic nerves: a confocal and functional analysis, *J Neurosci* **18**: 328–38.

Allan CH (2000) Functional results of primary nerve repair, *Hand Clin* **16**: 67–72.

Angermann P, Lohmann M (1993) Injuries to the hand and wrist. A study of 50,272 injuries, *J Hand Surg* **18B**: 642–4.

Ansselin AD, Fink T, Davey DF (1997) Peripheral nerve regeneration through nerve guides seeded with adult Schwann cells, *Neuropathol Appl Neurobiol* **23**: 387–98.

Averill S, McMahon SB, Clary DO et al (1995) Immunocytochemical localization of trkA receptors in chemically identified subgroups of adult rat sensory neurons, *Eur J Neurosci* **7**: 1484–94.

Barakat-Walter I (1999) Role of thyroid hormones and their receptors in peripheral nerve regeneration, *J Neurobiol* **40**: 541–59.

Barbacid M (1995) Neurotrophic factors and their receptors, *Curr Opin Cell Biol* **7**: 148–55.

Beaton AA, Williams L, Moseley LG (1994) Handedness and hand injuries, *J Hand Surg* **19B**: 158–61.

Beuche W, Friede RL (1984) The role of non-resident cells in Wallerian degeneration, *J Neurocytol* **13**: 767–96.

Birch R, Raji A (1991) Repair of median and ulnar nerves – primary suture is best, *J Bone Joint Surg* **73B**: 154–7.

Bisby MA, Keen P (1986) Regeneration of primary afferent neurons containing substance P-like immunoreactivity, *Brain Res* **365**: 85–95.

Braga-Silva J (1999) The use of silicone tubing in the late repair of the median and ulnar nerves in the forearm, *J Hand Surg* **24B**: 703–6.

Brandt J, Dahlin LB, Kanje M et al (1999a) Spatiotemporal progress of nerve regeneration in a tendon autograft used for bridging a peripheral nerve defect, *Exp Neurol* **160**: 386–93.

Brandt J, Dahlin LB, Lundborg G (1999b) Autologous tendons used as grafts for bridging peripheral nerve defects, *J Hand Surg* **24B**: 284–90.

Brown MC, Perry VH, Lunn ER et al (1991) Macrophage dependence of peripheral sensory nerve regeneration: possible involvement of nerve growth factors, *Neuron* **6**: 359–70.

Brushart TME (1998) Trophic and tropic influences on peripheral nerve regeneration. In: Omer G, Spinner M, Van Beak A, eds, *Management of Peripheral Nerve Problems* 2nd edn (WB Saunders: Philadelphia) 235–42.

Brushart TME, Seiler WA (1987) Selective reinnervation of distal motor stumps by peripheral motor axons, *Exp Neurol* **97**: 289–300.

Cajal RS (1928) *Degeneration and Regeneration of the Nervous System* (Oxford University Press: London).

Canossa M, Twiss JL, Versity AN et al (1996) p75(NGFR) and TrkA receptors collaborate to rapidly activate a p75(NGFR)-associated protein kinase, *Embo J* **15**: 3369–76

Chamberlain LJ, Yannas IV, Hsu P et al (1998) Collagen-GAG substrate enhances the quality of nerve regeneration through collagen tubes up to level of autograft, *Exp Neurol* **154**: 315–29.

Chen H, He Z, Tessier-Lavigne M (1998) Axon guidance mechanisms: semaphorins as simultaneous repellents and anti-repellents, *Nature Neuroscience* **1**: 436–9.

Dahlin LB (1995) Prevention of macrophage invasion impairs regeneration in nerve grafts, *Brain Res* **679**: 274–80.

Dahlin LB, Lundborg G (1998) Experimental nerve grafting – towards future solutions of a clinical problem, *J Hand Surg* **3**: 165–73.

Dahlin LB, Lundborg G (2001) The use of tubes in peripheral nerve repair. In: Kliot M, ed., *Neurosurg Clin of North Am* **12**(2): 341–52.

Dahlin LB, Nordborg C, Lundborg G (1987) Morphological changes in nerve cell bodies induced by experimental graded nerve compression, *Exp Neurol* **95**: 611–21.

Dahlin LB, Zhao Q, Bjursten LM (1995) Nerve regeneration in silicone tubes: distribution of macrophages and interleukin-1β in the formed fibrin matrix, *Restor Neurol Neurosci* **8**: 199–203.

Dahlin LB, Anagnostaki L, Lundborg G (2001) Tissue response close to silicone tubes used to repair human nerves, *Scand J Plast Reconstr Surg Hand Surg* **35**: 29–34.

Danielsen N (1990) Regeneration of the rat sciatic nerve in the silicone chamber model, *Restor Neurol Neurosci* **1**: 253–9.

Danielsen N, Dahlin LB, Ericson LE et al (1986) Experimental hyperthyroidism stimulates axonal growth in mesothelial chambers, *Exp Neurol* **94**: 54–65.

Danielsen N, Dahlin LB, Thomsen P (1993) Inflammatory cells and mediators in the silicone chamber model for nerve regeneration, *Biomaterials* **14**: 1180–5.

Danielsen N, Kerns JM, Holmquist B et al (1994) Predegenerated nerve grafts enhance regeneration by shortening the initial delay period, *Brain Res* **666**: 250–4.

Davis GE, Engvall E, Varon S et al (1987) Human amnion membrane as a substratum for cultured peripheral and central nervous system neurons, *Dev Brain Res* **33**: 1–10.

Degn J, Tandrup T, Jakobsen J (1999) Effect of nerve crush on perikaryal number and volume of neurons in adult rat dorsal root ganglion, *J Comp Neurol* **412**: 186–92.

Dobretsov M, Dobretsov A, Kuffler DP (1994) Influence of factors released from sciatic nerve on adult dorsal root ganglion neurons, *J Neurobiol* **25**: 1249–66.

Doolabh V, Hertl MC, Mackinnon SE (1996) The role of conduits in nerve repair: a review, *Rev Neurosci* **7**: 47–84.

Dubernard JM, Owen E, Herzberg G et al (1999) Human hand allograft: report on first 6 months, *Lancet* **353**: 1315–20.

Eriksson PL (1997) The effects of neurotrophic substances on primary sensory neurons following peripheral nerve injury, Doctoral thesis, Stockholm, Sweden.

Evans PJ, Midha R, Mackinnon SE (1994) The peripheral nerve

allograft: a comprehensive review of regeneration and neuroimmunology, *Pro Neurobiol* **43**: 187–233.

Fields RD, Le Beau JM, Longo FM et al (1989) Nerve regeneration through artificial tubular implants, *Progr Neurobiol* **33**: 87.

Francel PC, Francel TJ, Mackinnon SE et al (1997) Enhancing nerve regeneration across a silicone tube conduit by using interposed short-segment nerve grafts, *J Neurosurg* **87**: 887–92.

Frey M, Giovanoli P, Girsch W (1999) Clinical application of end-to-side nerve coaptation for sensory or motor reinnervation, *J Hand Surg* **24B** (Suppl 1): 9.

Friedman WJ, Greene LA (1999) Neurotrophin signaling via Trks and p75, *Exp Cell Res* **253**: 131–42.

Gehrmann J, Kreutzberg GW (1993) Monoclonal antibodies against macrophages/microglia: immunocytochemical studies of early microglial activation in experimental neuropathology, *Clin Neuropathol* **12**:301–6.

Gibson JD (1979) The origin of the neural macrophage: a quantitative ultrastructural study of cell population changes during Wallerian degeneration, *J Anat* **129**: 1–19.

Glasby MA, Gschmeissner SE, Huang C-H et al (1986) Degenerated muscle grafts used for peripheral nerve repair in primate, *J Hand Surg* **11B**: 347–51.

Gold BG, Katoh K, Storm-Dickerson T (1995) The immunosuppressant FK506 increases the rate of axonal regeneration in rat sciatic nerve, *J Neurosci* **15**:7509–16.

Guénard V, Kleitman N, Morrissey TK et al (1992) Syngeneic Schwann cells derived from adult nerves seeded in semipermeable guidance channels enhance peripheral nerve regeneration, *J Neurosci* **12**: 3310–20.

Gulati AK (1988) Evaluation of acellular and cellular nerve grafts in repair of rat peripheral nerve, *J Neurosurg* **69**: 117–23.

Gulati AK, Rai DR, Ali AM (1995) The influence of cultured Schwann cells on regeneration through acellular basal lamina grafts, *Brain Res* **705**: 118–24.

Haapaniemi T, Nylander G, Kanje M et al (1998) Hyperbaric oxygen treatment enhances regeneration of the rat sciatic nerve, *Exp Neurol* **149**: 433–8.

Hadlock T, Elisseeff J, Langer R et al (1998) A tissue-engineered conduit for peripheral nerve repair, *Arch Otolarynaol Head Neck Surg* **124**: 1081–6.

Hadlock T, Sundback C, Koka R et al (1999) A novel, biodegradable polymer conduit delivers neurotrophins and promotes nerve regeneration, *Laryngoscope* **109**: 1412–16.

Henken DB, Battisti WP, Chesselet MF et al (1990) Expression of beta-preprotachykinin mRNA and tachykinins in rat dorsal root ganglion cells following peripheral or central axotomy, *Neuroscience* **39**: 733–42.

Heumann R, Lindholm D, Bandtlow C et al (1987) Differential regulation of mRNA encoding nerve growth factor and its receptor in rat sciatic nerve during development, degeneration, and regeneration: role of macrophages, *Proc Natl Acad Sci USA* **84**: 8735–9.

Himes BT, Tessler A (1989) Death of some dorsal root ganglion neurons and plasticity of others following sciatic nerve section in adult and neonatal rats, *J Comp Neurol* **284**: 215–30.

Hökfelt T, Wiesenfeld-Hallin Z, Villar M et al (1987) Increase of galanin-like immunoreactivity in rat dorsal root ganglion cells after peripheral axotomy, *Neurosci Lett* **83**: 217–20.

Hökfelt T, Zhang X, Wiesenfeldt-Hallin H (1994) Messenger plasticity in primary sensory neurons following axotomy and its functional implications, *Trends Neurosci* **17**: 22–30.

Hou XE, Lundmark K, Dahlstrom AB (1998) Cellular reactions to axotomy superior cervical ganglia includes apoptotic cell death, *J Neurocytol* **27**: 441–51.

Ide C, Tohyama K, Yokota R et al (1983) Schwann cell basal lamina and nerve regeneration, *Brain Res* **288**: 61–75.

Iwabuchi Y, Maki Y, Yoshizu T et al (1999) Lack of topographical specificity in peripheral nerve regeneration in rats, *Scand J Plast Reconstr Surg Hand Surg* **33**: 181–5.

Jones JW, Gruber SA, Barker JH et al (2000) Successful hand transplantation. One-year follow-up. Louisville Hand Transplant Team, *N Engl J Med* **343**: 468–73.

Jongsma H, Danielsen N, Grotto KA et al (1999) Exogenous NT-3 & NGF differentially modulate PACAP expression in adult sensory neurons, suggesting distinct roles in injury and inflammation. 29th Annual Meeting Society for Neuroscience. Miami Beach, Florida, USA: Society for Neuroscience Abstracts: 512.

Jongsma H, Danielsen N, Sundler F et al (2000) Alteration of PACAP distribution and PACAP receptor binding in the rat sensory nervous system following sciatic nerve transection, *Brain Res* **853**: 186–96.

Kanje M, Skottner A, Lundborg G (1988) Effects of growth hormone treatment on the regeneration of rat sciatic nerve, *Brain Res* **475**: 254–8.

Kanje M, Arai T, Lundborg G (2000) Collateral sprouting from sensory and motor axons into an end to side attached nerve segment, *Neuroreport* **11**: 2455–9.

Kerns JM, Danielsen N, Holmquist B et al (1993) The influence of predegeneration on regeneration through peripheral nerve grafts in the rat, *Exp Neurol* **122**: 28–36.

Keynes R, Cook G (1990) Cell–cell repulsion: clues from the growth cone? *Cell* **62**: 609–10.

Kline DG, Tiel R, Kim D et al (1998) Lower extremity nerve injuries. In: Omer G, Spinner M, Van Beak A, eds, *Management of Peripheral Nerve Problems*, 2nd edn (WB Saunders: Philadelphia) 420–30.

Koistinaho J, Pelto-Huikko M, Sagar SM et al (1993) Injury-induced long-term expression of immediate early genes in the rat superior cervical ganglion, *Neuroreport* **4**: 37–40.

Kuffler DF (1994) Promoting and directing axon outgrowth, *Mol Neurobiol* **9**: 233–43.

Kuffler DP (1996) Chemotropic factors direct regenerating axons, *News Physiol Sci* **11**: 21–3.

Kuffler DP, Magwinoff O (1994) Neurotrophic influence of denervated sciatic nerve on adult dorsal root ganglion neurons. *J Neurobiol* **25**: 1267–82.

Kvist Reimer M (2000) Neuropeptides during peripheral nerve regeneration. Special reference to galanin and pituitary adenylate cyclase-activating polypeptide, Medical thesis, Lund University, Sweden.

Letourneau PC, Kater SB, Macagno ER (1991) *The Nerve Growth Cone* (Raven Press: New York).

Levi AD, Sonntag VK, Dickman C et al (1997) The role of cultured Schwann cell grafts in the repair of gaps within the peripheral nervous system of primates, *Exp Neurol* **143**: 25–36.

Li L, Oppenheim RW, Lei M et al (1994) Neurotrophic agents prevent motoneuron death following sciatic nerve section in the neonatal mouse, *J Neurobiol* **25**: 759–66.

Li L, Wu W, Lin LF et al (1995) Rescue of adult mouse motoneurons from injury-induced cell death by glial cell line-derived neurotrophic factor, *Proc Natl Acad Sci USA* **92**: 9771–5.

Li L, Houenou LJ, Wu W et al (1998) Characterization of spinal motoneuron degeneration following different types of peripheral nerve injury in neonatal and adult mice, *J Comp Neurol* **396**: 158–68.

Lieberman AR (1971) The axon reaction: a review of the principal features of perikaryal responses to axonal injury, *Int Rev Neurobiol* **14**: 99–124.

Lindholm D, Heumann R, Meyer M et al (1987) Interleukin-1 regulates synthesis of nerve growth factor in non-neuronal cells of rat sciatic nerves, *Nature* **330**: 658–9.

Liss AG, af Ekenstam FW, Wiberg M (1994) Cell loss in sensory ganglia following peripheral nerve injury. An anatomical study in the cat, *Scand J Plast Reconstr Hand Surg* **28**: 177–87.

Ljungberg C, Novikov L, Kellerth JO et al (1999) The neurotrophins NGF and NT-3 reduce sensory neuronal loss in adult rat after peripheral nerve lesion, *Neurosci Lett* **262**: 29–32.

Lu X, Richardson PM (1991) Inflammation near the nerve cell body enhances axonal regeneration, *J Neurosci* **11**: 972–8.

Lundborg G (2000a) A 25–year perspective of peripheral nerve surgery: evolving neuroscientific concepts and clinical significance, *J Hand Surg* **25A**: 391–414.
Lundborg G (2000b) Brain plasticity and hand surgery: an overview, *J Hand Surg* **25B**: 2422–252.
Lundborg G (2000c) A randomized prospective study of polyglycolic acid conduits for digital nerve reconstruction in humans, *Plast Reconstr Surg* **106**: 1046–8.
Lundborg G (2000d) *Nerve Injury and Repair* (Churchill Livingstone: Edinburgh).
Lundborg G, Dahlin L, Danielsen N et al (1994a) Trophism, tropism and specificity in nerve regeneration, *J Reconstr Microsurg* **25**: 345–54.
Lundborg G, Zhao Q, Kanje M et al (1994b) Can sensory and motor collateral sprouting be induced from intact peripheral nerve by end-to-side anastomosis? *J Hand Surg* **19B**: 277–82.
Lundborg G, Rosén B, Dahlin L et al (1997) Tubular versus conventional repair of median and ulnar nerves in the human forearm: early results from a prospective, randomized, clinical study, *J Hand Surg* **22A**: 1–8.
Lundborg G, Dahlin L, Holmberg J et al (2000) Tubular vs conventional repair of median or ulnar nerves in the human forearm – five year follow-up. Scandinavian/Hungarian Hand Society Meeting, Kuopio, Finland.
McQuarrie IG, Grafstein B (1973) Axonal outgrowth enhanced by a previous nerve injury, *Arch Neurol* **29**: 53–5.
Maki Y, Yoshizu T, Tajima T et al (1996a) The selectivity of motor axons during regeneration with sensory axons, *J Reconstr Microsurg* **12**: 553–7.
Maki Y, Yoshizu T, Tajima T et al (1996b) The selectivity of regenerating motor and sensory axons, *J Reconstr Microsurg* **12**: 547–51.
Manthorpe M, Engvall E, Rouslathi et al (1983) Laminin promotes neuritic regeneration from cultured peripheral and central neuron, *J Cell Biol* **97**: 1882–90.
Martin LJ, Kaiser A, Price AC (1999) Motor neuron degeneration after sciatic nerve avulsion in adult rat evolves with oxidative stress and is apoptosis, *J Neurobiol* **40**: 185–201.
Martini R, Schachner M (1988) Immunoelectron microscopic localization of neural cell adhesion molecules (L1, N-CAM, and myelin-associated glycoprotein) in regenerating adult mouse sciatic nerve, *J Cell Biol* **106**: 1735–46.
Martini R, Xin Y, Schmitz B et al (1992) The L2/HNK-1 carbohydrate epitope is involved in the preferential outgrowth of motor neurons on ventral roots and motor nerves, *Eur J Neurosci* **4**: 628–39.
Menei P, Montero-Menei C, Whittemore SR et al (1998) Schwann cells genetically modified to secrete human BDNF promote enhanced axonal regrowth across transected adult rat spinal cord, *Eur J Neurosci* **10**: 607–21.
Merle M, Dellon A, Campbell YN et al (1989) Complications from silicon-polymer intubulation of nerves, *Microsurgery* **10**: 130.
Merzenich MM, Sameshima K (1993) Cortical plasticity and memory, *Curr Opin Neurobiol* **3**: 187–96.
Merzenich MM, Kaas JH, Wall JT et al (1983) Topographic reorganization of somatosensory cortical areas 3b and 1 in adult monkeys following restricted deafferentation, *Neuroscience* **8**: 33–55.
Meyer M, Matsuoka I, Wetrose C et al (1992) Enhanced synthesis of Brain-Derived Neurotropic Factor in the lesioned peripheral nerve: different mechanisms are responsible for the regulation of BDNF and NGFmRNA, *J Cell Biol* **119**: 45–54.
Millesi H (2000) Techniques for nerve grafting, *Hand Clin* **16**: 73–91.
Millesi H, Meissl G, Berger A (1972) The interfascicular nerve grafting of the median and ulnar nerves, *J Bone Joint Surg* **54A**: 727–50.
Millesi H, Meissl G, Berger A (1976) Further experience with interfascicular grafting of the median, ulnar and radial nerves, *J Bone Joint Surg* **58A**: 209–17.
Miyauchi A, Kanje M, Danielsen N et al (1997) Role of macrophages in the stimulation and regeneration of sensory nerves by transposed granulation tissue and temporal aspects of the response, *Scand J Plast Reconstr Surg Hand* **31**: 17–23.
Monaco S, Gehrmann J, Raivich G et al (1992) MHC-positive, ramified macrophages in the normal and injured rat peripheral nervous system, *J Neurocytol* **21**: 623–34.
Mu X, Silos-Santiago I, Carroll SL et al (1993) Neurotrophin receptor genes are expressed in distinct patterns in developing dorsal root ganglia, *J Neurosci* **13**: 4029–41.
Müller HW, Stoll G (1998) Nerve injury and regeneration: basic insights and therapeutic interventions, *Curr Opin Neurol* **11**: 557–62.
Nachemson AK (1988) Axonal regeneration and growth direction in square-shaped mesothelial chambers, *Scand J Plast Reconstr Surg* **22**: 199–206.
Nakao Y, Mackinnon SE (1995) Reconstruction of peripheral nerve gap with allogeneic nerve graft using MAb therapy. In: Vastamaki E, ed., *Current Trends in Hand Surgery* (Elsevier Science: Amsterdam) 235–42.
Nishiura Y, Kanje M, Lundborg G et al (2001) Addition of Schwann cells to teased tendon grafts and cellular muscle grafts improves nerve regeneration. San Diego, California, USA: Society for Neuroscience Abstracts.
Noguchi K, De Leon M, Nahin RL et al (1993) Quantification of axotomy-induced alteration of neuropeptide mRNAs in dorsal root ganglion neurons with special reference to neuropeptide Y mRNA and the effects of neonatal capsaicin treatment, *J Neurosci Res* **35**: 54–66.
Novikov LN (1999) Brain-derived neurotrophic factor in the survival and regeneration of injured spinal motorneurons. Doctoral thesis, Umeå University, Sweden.
Novikov L, Novikova L, Kellerth JO (1995) Brain-derived neurotrophic factor promotes survival and blocks nitric oxide synthase expression in adult rat spinal motoneurons after ventral root avulsion, *Neurosci Lett* **200**: 45–8.
Novikova L, Novikov L, Kellerth JO (1996) Brain-derived neurotrophic factor reduces necrotic zone and supports neuronal survival after spinal cord hemisection in adult rats, *Neurosci Lett* **220**: 203–6.
Novikova L, Novikov L, Kellerth JO (1997) Effects of neurotransplants and BDNF on the survival and regeneration of injured adult spinal motoneurons, *Eur J Neurosci* **9**: 2774–7.
Oblinger MM, Lasek RJ (1988) Axotomy-induced alterations in the synthesis and transport of neurofilaments and microtubules in dorsal root ganglion cell, *J Neurosci* **8**: 1747–58.
Olson L (1997) Regeneration in the adult central nervous system: experimental repair strategies, *Nature Med* **3**: 1329–35.
Olsson Y (1966) Studies on vascular permeability in peripheral nerves. 1. Distribution of circulating fluorescent serum albumin in normal, crushed and sectioned rat sciatic nerves, *Acta Neuropathol Berlin* **7**: 1–15.
Purves D, Njå A (1978) Trophic maintenance of synaptic connections in autonomic ganglia. In: Cotman CW, ed., *Neuronal Plasticity* (Raven Press: New York) 27–47.
Raivich U, Hellweg R, Kreutzberg GW (1991) NGF receptor-mediated reduction in axonal NGF uptake and retrograde transport following sciatic nerve injury and during regeneration, *Neuron* **7**: 151–64.
Reimer M, Kanje M (1999) Peripheral but not central axotomy promotes axonal outgrowth and induces alterations in neuropeptide synthesis in the nodose ganglion of the rat, *Eur J Neurosci* **11**: 3415–23.
Rodrigues FJ, Gomez N, Perego G et al (1999) Highly permeable polyactide-caprolactone nerve guides enhance peripheral nerve regeneration thorugh long gaps, *Biomaterials* **29**: 1489–500.
Rodriguez FJ, Verdu E, Ceballos D et al (2000) Nerve guides seeded with autologous Schwann cells improve nerve regeneration, *Exp Neurol* **161**: 571–84.
Rosén B (2000) The sensational hand. Clinical assessment after nerve repair. Doctoral thesis, Lund, Sweden.
Rowan PR, Chen LE, Urbaniak JR (2000) End-to-side nerve repair. A review, *Hand Clin* **16**: 151–9.

Sastry PS, Rao KS (2000) Apoptosis and the nervous system, *J Neurochem* **74**: 1–20.

Scherman P, Kanje M, Lundborg G et al (2000) Continuous longitudinal sutures – a new and simple approach to repair nerve defects, *J Hand Surg* **25B** (Suppl 1): 44.

Schreyer DJ, Skene JH (1991) Fate of GAP-43 in ascending spinal axons of DRG neurons after peripheral nerve injury: delayed accumulation and correlation with regenerative potential, *J Neurosci* **11**: 3738–51.

Schreyer DJ, Skene JH (1993) Injury-associated induction of GAP-43 expression displays axon branch specificity in rat dorsal root ganglion neurons, *J Neurobiol* **24**: 959–70.

Siironen J, Collan Y, Roytta M (1994) Axonal reinnervation does not influence Schwann cell proliferation after rat sciatic nerve transection, *Brain Res* **654**: 303–11.

Sisken BF, Kanje M, Lundborg G et al (1989) Stimulation of rat sciatic nerve regeneration with pulsed electromagnetic field, *Brain Res* **485**: 309–16.

Sondell M, Lundborg G, Kanje M (1998) Regeneration of the rat sciatic nerve into allografts made acellular through chemical extraction, *Brain Res* **795**: 44–54.

Sorensen J, Haase G, Krarup C et al (1998) Gene transfer to Schwann cells after peripheral nerve injury: a delivery system for therapeutic agents, *Ann Neurol* **43**: 205–11.

Stoll G, Griffin JW, Li CY et al (1989) Wallerian degeneration in the peripheral nervous system: participation of both Schwann cells and macrophages in myelin degradation, *J Neurocytol* **18**: 671–83.

Sun Y, Zigmond RE (1996) Involvement of leukemia inhibitory factor in the increases in galanin and vasoactive intestinal peptide mRNA and the decreases in neuropeptide Y and tyrosine hydroxylase mRNA in sympathetic neurons after axotomy, *J Neurochem* **67**: 1751–60.

Sundler F, Ekblad E, Hannibal J et al (1996) Pituitary adenylate cyclase-activating peptide in sensory and autonomic ganglia: localization and regulation, *Ann NY Acad Sci* **805**: 410–26.

Tanelian DL, Barry MA, Johnston SA et al (1997) Semaphorin Ill can repulse and inhibit adult sensory afferents in vivo, *Nat Med* **3**: 1398–401.

Taniuchi M, Clark HB, Johnson JEM (1986) Induction of nerve growth factor receptor in Schwann cells after axotomy, *Proc Natl Acad Sci USA* **83**: 4094–8.

Taniuchi M, Clark HB, Schweitzer JB et al (1988) Expression of nerve growth factor receptors by Schwann cells of axotomized peripheral nerves: ultrastructural location, suppression by axonal contact and binding properties, *J Neurosci* **8**: 664–81.

Tarasidis G, Watanabe O, MacKinnon SE et al (1998) End-to-side neurography: a long-term study of neural regeneration in a rat model, *Otolaryngol Head Neck Surg* **119**: 337–41.

Terenghi G (1999) Peripheral nerve regeneration and neurotrophic factors, *J Anat* **194**: 1–14.

Thoenen H, Bandtlow C, Heumann R et al (1988) Nerve growth factor: cellular localization and regulation of synthesis, *Cell Mol Neurobiol* **8**: 35–40.

Torigoe K, Tanaka HF, Takahashi A et al (1996) Basic behavior of migratory Schwann cells in peripheral nerve regeneration, *Exp Neurol* **137**: 301–8.

Trumble T, Vanderhooft E (1994) Nerve grafting for lower-extremity injuries, *J Pediatr Orthop* **14**: 161–5.

Trumble TE, Vanderhooft E, Khan U (1995) Sural nerve grafting for lower extremity nerve injuries, *J Orthop Trauma* **9**: 158–63.

Verdu E, Rodriguez FJ, Gudino-Cabrera G et al (2000) Expansion of adult Schwann cells from mouse predegenerated peripheral nerves, *J Neurosci Methods* **99**: 111–17.

Viterbo F, Trindade JC, Hoshini K et al (1992) Latero-terminal neurorrhaphy without removal of the epineural sheath. Experimental study in rats, *Rev Paul Med* **110**: 267.

Viterbo F, Palhares A, Franciosi LF (1993) Restoration of sensitivity after removal of the sural nerve – a new application of lateral-terminal neurorraphy, *Rev Soc Bras Cir Plast Est Reconstr* **8**: 85–7.

Voinesco F, Glauser L, Kraftsik R et al (1998) Local administration of thyroid hormones in silicone chamber increases regeneration of rat transected sciatic nerve, *Exp Neurol* **150**: 69–81.

Wakisaka S, Kajander KC, Bennett GJ (1991) Increased neuropeptide Y (NPY)-like immunoreactivity in rat sensory neurons following peripheral axotomy, *Neurosci Lett* **124**: 200–3.

Wall JT, Kaas JH (1986) Long-term cortical consequences of reinnervation errors after nerve regeneration in monkeys, *Brain Res* **372**: 400–4.

Wall JT, Kaas JH, Sur M et al (1986) Functional reorganization in somatosensory cortical areas 3b and 1 of adult monkeys after median nerve repair: possible relationships to sensory recovery in humans, *J Neurosci* **6**: 218–33.

Walsh FS, Doherty P (1996) Cell adhesion molecules and neuronal regeneration, *Curr Opin Cell Biol* **8**: 707–13.

Weber A, Breidenbach WC, Brown RE et al (2000) A randomized prospective study of polyglycolic acid conduits for digital nerve reconstruction in humans, *Plast Reconstr Surg* **106**: 1036–45.

Weisenhorn DM, Roback J, Young AN et al (1999) Cellular aspects of trophic actions in the nervous system, *Int Rev Cytol* **189**: 177–265.

Wiberg M, Ljungberg C, O'Byrne A et al (1999) Primary sensory neuron survival following target administration of NGF to an injured nerve, *Scand J Plast Reconstr Hand Surg* **33**: 387–92.

Wiklund P (1999) Regeneration of peripheral nerves. The protein kinases, with emphasis on neurotrophic factor stimulation. Thesis, Lund, Sweden.

Williams PL, Hall SM (1971) Chronic Wallerian degeneration – an in vivo and ultrastructural study, *J Anat* **109**: 487–503.

Ygge J (1989) Neuronal loss in lumbar dorsal root ganglia after proximal compared to distal sciatic nerve resection: a quantitative study in the rat, *Brain Res* **478**: 193–5.

You S, Petrov T, Chung PH et al (1997) The expression of the low affinity nerve growth factor receptor in long-term denervated Schwann cells, *Glia* **20**: 87–100.

Zhang Z, Soucacos PN, Bo J et al (1999) Evaluation of collateral sprouting after end-to-side nerve coaptation using a fluorescent double-labeling technique, *Microsurgery* **19**: 281–6.

Zhao Q, Dahlin LB, Kanje M et al (1993) Repair of the transected rat sciatic nerve: matrix formation within silicone tubes, *Restor Neurol Neurosci* **5**:197–204.

Zheng M, Kuffler DP (2000) Guidance of regenerating motor axons in vivo by gradients of diffusible peripheral nerve-derived factors, *J Neurobiol* **42**: 212–19.

7 Peripheral nerve repair: techniques and results

H. Millesi

Introduction

Rational surgery on peripheral nerves started with the description of the epineurial nerve suture by Hueter in 1873. An enormous development started and if one looks into the early literature one realizes that more or less all the ideas we discuss today had already been put forward in the late nineteenth and early twentieth centuries. Tubulization with different materials including veins was recommended. Langley and Hashimoto (1917) suggested performing perineurial (fascicular) nerve repair. Albert (1876) used autologous nerve grafts and Foerster (1915) harvested cutaneous nerves as donors for nerve grafting. Seddon (1947) described the cable graft. Strange (1947) anticipated the vascularized nerve graft by transplanting nerves as pedicled grafts. Different types of end-to-side coaptations were suggested.

This was the environment when I became involved in peripheral nerve surgery. In this chapter I aim to give a survey of my personal experience over the past 50 years and to present what I have learned.

Mechanical versus biological thinking

The outcome of peripheral nerve repair depends to a great extent on factors like age, time interval, etc., which are independent of surgical activities.

Basically the potential for nerve regeneration is very good. Therefore, under favourable conditions favourable results can be achieved in some cases whatever technique is used. Apart from such favourable cases, the overall results in the 1950s were very poor, in spite of the above-mentioned intellectual input. Even an experienced surgeon such as Seddon (Nicholson and Seddon 1957) reported only 70% M3 or plus results in clean median nerve transections at the wrist, a value which dropped to 50% if there was a 'defect' of more than 2.5 cm. Note that it is not clear whether he meant a real defect (loss of nerve tissue) or the distance between the two stumps produced merely by retraction.

The standard technique to restore continuity was a watertight, dense epineurial repair to prevent a dehiscence and to prevent the escaping of axon sprouts. The discussion as to whether an epineurial or a perineurial (fascicular) repair offers better chances was started and still continues today. If there was a distance between the two stumps, the distance was overcome by stretching the adjacent segments of the nerve, supported by vast mobilization in both directions. To avoid disruption or dehiscence, the adjacent joints were maximally flexed for temporary relief of the site of repair, and immobilized in this position for several weeks. By this technique, it was hoped to overcome a so-called 'critical length' (15 cm in the 1920s, and 10 cm in the 1950s). Alternatives were bone resection from the humerus shaft for the radial nerve; essentially transfer to the palmar side of the elbow joint with flexion of this joint for the ulnar nerve. Nerve grafts were regarded as inferior to neurorrhaphy, yielding maximally 50% of an end-to-end repair.

But short grafts have better chances. In all my nerve grafts longer than 3 cm I had to resect the distal site of coaptation, because a dense scar had developed until the axon sprouts had arrived, which prevented them from entering the distal stump (Bsteh and Millesi 1960). It is understandable that surgeons tried to approximate the two stumps as much as possible, to be able to use a short graft (Seddon 1972).

To overcome the calibre difference between a cutaneous nerve and the nerve trunk to be repaired, several segments of a cutaneous nerve were sutured or glued together to form a cable of the diameter of the nerve to be repaired, not considering that a free graft should have a maximal area of contact with the recipient site, and not with another free graft. Proper resection of the two stumps of a transected nerve was not always performed, for fear of increasing the defect.

Owing to irregular protrusion of the endoneurial tissue the surface of the cross-section of a transected nerve is never smooth. As a highlight of mechanical thinking nearly everyone followed Edshage's suggestion (1964) to perform the resection of the stumps using special devices to achieve a smooth surface. It was forgotten that the protrusion depends on the intrafascicular pressure, which will increase by traction in a longitudinal direction.

In retrospect it can be stated that the philosophy of the period was dominated by thinking in terms of mechanics rather than biology. A more biological approach was necessary.

An analysis of failed nerve repairs produced the following conclusions.

(1) The potential of the *axons* to sprout is independent of the surgical technique. The axons will follow neurotropic signals towards the distal stump (Lundborg and Hansson 1979), if they are allowed to do so. A watertight epineurial or perineurial suture is unnecessary and even harmful. Obstacles that interfere with the progress of axons are frequently the result of an inappropriate technique.

(2) *Epineurial and perineurial fibroblasts* divide faster than Schwann cells. There is a danger that they will predominate in the space between the two stumps. In cases with a high percentage of non-neural tissue in the cross-section, resection of a strip of epineurium helps. This fact favours fascicular repair. But fascicular repair makes sense only in a case of a polyfascicular pattern with a limited number of rather large fascicles, and not with an oligofascicular pattern (it is not necessary) or a polyfascicular pattern with many small fascicles (it is not possible). This underlines the importance of the actual fascicular pattern in surgical decision-making.

(3) *Epineurial and perineurial connective tissue proliferation* tends to circumvent obstacles on their outer surface and to shift them towards the centre. This is why stitches are frequently met in the central part of the nerve, and not at the epineurial level where they were originally located.

(4) *Proper resection* of the stumps is of extreme importance even if the defect is increased and eventually a graft is necessary.

(5) *Tension at the site of coaptation* should be minimized. It is acceptable to overcome the distance between the two stumps produced by elastic retraction with primary repair. It is questionable if there is a distance without defect produced by fibrotic retraction in case of a secondary repair.

    If there is a defect, an end-to-end coaptation is possible only if the defect is compensated by elongation of the normal nerve tissue of the proximal and distal stumps. The stumps must not be fibrotic. There must be a long segment of nerve free of branches on either side, and the patient should have rather lax connective tissues. In case of doubt, a graft is a better solution.

    At the coaptation sites of a free graft, tension should be absolutely avoided, because the free graft survives by adhesions. It is not movable and any tension is focused at the sites of coaptation. After grafting, the involved limb should be immobilized for 8 days in an extended position, to avoid forming the adhesions in a flexed state.

    What is wrong with tension at the site of repair?

    - *High tension* carries the danger of dehiscence, which has to be avoided by the use of many strong stitches (this in itself is undesirable) and a prolonged period of immobilization.
    - *No tension* reduces the surgical trauma and the application of stitches as well as of other foreign materials (relief plates, etc.).
    - *Moderate tension* causes a higher degree of connective tissue proliferation and collagenization and produces an elongation of the scar between the stumps.
    - *No tension* may lead to primary healing without a zone of scar tissue.
    - The consequences of tension appear even after a prolonged period of immobilization when the patient starts to move the limb. At this point axons that have already crossed to the distal stump may suffer as a result of the connective tissue changes and may degenerate.

(6) *A free nerve graft* survives completely, including the Schwann cells and the delicate endoneurial framework, if it is small enough to be spontaneously vascularized in a very short time. Under this condition it is a conduit for axon sprouts which just have to cross to the graft to find everything they need, including Schwann cells. An ulnar nerve does not survive a free grafting procedure. It does not become necrotic, because the undifferentiated connective tissue survives, but the Schwann cells and the endoneurial and perineurial framework will get lost. It can be neurotized to a certain degree and a certain length by the advancement of minifascicles (axon sprouts, Schwann cells, capillaries, perineurial fibroblasts). It is a conduit for minifascicles. The same is true for cable grafts and any other alternative to nerve grafts.

If we want to use the ulnar nerve as a graft donor, we have to use it as a vascularized graft by preserving the vascular pedicle by restoring blood circulation via microvascular anastomosis with vessels of the recipient site (Taylor and Ham 1976).

Vascularized grafts have the advantage of being independent from the conditions of the recipient site. They must not form adhesions to survive and are, therefore, less sensitive to tension. The big disadvantage – apart from the fact that a major nerve has to be sacrificed – is that the surgeon has no control whatsoever as to where, after entering the graft at a certain point, the axon sprouts will leave the nerve. An aimed coaptation is impossible.

Under favourable conditions a nerve graft yields as good a result as an end-to-end nerve repair. With increasing length of the defect the graft becomes significantly better. Long distances have been bridged successfully by nerve grafts (> 30 cm).

Within certain limits the length of the graft does not influence the result. It is therefore not necessary to minimize a distance. This would rather combine the disadvantage of a graft – having two sites of coaptation – with the disadvantage of a coaptation under tension. The result is certainly influenced by the length of the defect of a given nerve. It will make a difference if, for example, 5 or 15 cm of the median nerve have been lost, but this has nothing to do with nerve grafting as such.

Nerve lesions

Lesions of peripheral nerves can be of different kinds. In order to be able to analyse our own cases and to compare results, we need a classification system that allows us to sort the cases into comparable groups. The aim of our surgery is to improve the functional loss of the patient. Consequently we also need a classification which describes the functional loss for each particular case and which in the follow-up can serve as a scale to measure the quality of functional return.

Classification of nerve lesions

The classification of nerve lesions by Seddon (1943) into neurapraxia, axonotmesis and neurotmesis is not satisfactory.

Sunderland's system (1951) (degree I = neurapraxia, degree II = axonotmesis, degree III = lesion in continuity with preserved fascicular pattern, degree IV = lesion in continuity with lost fascicular pattern, degree V = loss of continuity) is very useful to describe the siuation as far as continuity of different structures is concerned, but it lacks information about the reaction of different tissues after the trauma.

Millesi (1992) developed a system which is based on the degrees of Sunderland but provides additional information as far as the fibrotic reaction and the formation of neuroma tissue is concerned.

By definition, neurapraxia (degree I) should allow functional return in a very short time because the axons were not interrupted and there was no Wallerian degeneration. It is not common knowledge that the return of function can be prevented if the endoneurial tissue is under constant pressure. Relief of pressure provokes immediate return of conductivity. The same is true for axonotmesis (degree II).

The compression is usually due to a fibrosis of the connective tissue components of a nerve, and can be located at different sites with different consequences. If the fibrosis is located in the epifascicular epineurium, an epineuriotomy would be the adequate treatment. This is fibrosis of type A.

Around the epineurium the nerve trunks are enveloped in a gliding tissue, the paraneurium; this can also develop fibrosis. In this case the paraneurium and epineurium usually merge and cannot be distinguished. This is why the paraneurium is not very well known among surgeons. However, there are, lesions, especially in brachial plexus cases, in which the paraneurium alone is fibrotic. This is fibrosis of type A*.

In these cases a paraneuriotomy is sufficient, and the epineurium can be left alone. If the fibrosis involves the interfascicular epineurium as well, an epineuriectomy is indicated. This is fibrosis of type B.

Fibrosis of type A*, A and B can be accompanied by damage of degree I, II or III.

If the fibrosis has developed in the endoneural space and has replaced the endoneurial tissue, the chances of recovery are nil. This situation is called fibrosis of type C. It can be accompanied by damage of degree III only, because lesions of degree I or II have an intact endoneurium by definition.

A lesion of degree IIIC is treated by resection of the involved fascicles with restoration of continuity by nerve grafting.

A lesion of degree IV means that the fascicular pattern has been lost and the continuity is maintained by connective tissue only. However, it makes, a difference whether there is connective tissue only linking the two stumps, or whether a neuroma has grown across. Consequently we differentiate between a lesion of degree IV N (N = neuroma) and a lesion of IV S (S = scar).

Evaluation of function

We treat nerve lesions in order to improve the functional loss which the lesion has produced. So far surgeons apply schemes which allow them to classify the return of the function by classifying the patient in ranks according to the functional value after surgery. For median and ulnar nerve lesions the Highet scheme with graduation from M0 to M5 for motor, and from S0 to S4 for sensory function is most frequently applied. This system is much too crude to detect minor differences between individual techniques and it is completely unsuited for scientific studies. On the other hand it is extremely useful for presenting the excellent results the surgeon has achieved. The ranks are too few to represent the whole scale of functional return. It is taken for granted that all nerve lesions start with function 0, and consequently there is no space for partial lesions, innervation anomalies and mixed innervation.

Global hand function as a basis for evaluation of median, ulnar and radial nerve lesions

For many years I have been using an evaluation system for the median and ulnar nerves, which is based on the evaluation of hand function in general, by using a points

Table 7.1 *Level 1: anatomy, 1250 points*

Structure	*Points*
Thumb	400
Index finger	200
Medius	200
Ring finger	100
Little finger	100
Wrist	250

system. We start with the assumption that the normal hand has a value of 10,000 points. The scores are calculated at three levels; as described below. These values are assigned if all the structures are present and function normally.

Level 1: anatomy 1250 scores (Table 7.1)
If there is a functional loss, a certain number of scores are deducted:

- Decreased amount of active flexion or extension according to the angle.
- Passive restriction of movement according to the angle.
- Presence of hyperextension.
- Decrease of abduction or adduction.
- Reduction or lack of opposition of the thumb.
- Lack or reduction of extension of the wrist.
- Lack or reduction of flexion of the wrist.
- Lack or reduction of ulnarduction or radialduction.
- Lack or reduction of pronation or supination.

The distribution of the points is such that, for example, lack of active and passive motion in a joint causes a minor loss of points, if the ankylosis is in a position of function.

In summary, the anatomical value of hand function can be between 0 – in case of amputation – and 1250 with a normal anatomy. Additional information, such as the presence of pain, oedema, etc., is given, but not counted.

Level 2: sensibility (Table 7.2)
Sensibility comes in as a factor. The value of any anatomical unit is multiplied by 2, if sensibility is normal. Intact sensibility doubles the anatomical value, producing a total value of 2500 points.

In a case of complete loss of sensibility of both hemipulps of the thumb, the anatomical value (400) is to be multiplied by 1 – therefore remaining at 400.

If only one digital nerve of the thumb does not function, and one hemipulp would be anaesthetic, the anatomical value is multiplied by 1.5 (loss of factor 0.5 for one hemipulp). A further graduation for each hemipulp is possible. It is certainly cumbersome to investigate these values for each hemipulp in case of reduced sensibility, but the functional importance of sensibility justifies these efforts.

In order to get an idea of the handiness, a pick-up test is performed with both hands and the time is defined. If there is a strong difference between right and left hand, or the contralateral hand cannot be used for various reasons, standard values corrected for age and prominent hand are utilized. If the patient cannot perform the pick-up test, the 250 points for the wrist joint are multiplied by 1. If the time taken for the pick-up test is comparable to the contralateral hand, or to the standard hand, the 250 points for the wrist joint are multiplied by 2. Between these two extremes, the factor for the multiplication of the wrist scores is calculated according to the percentage difference.

Level 3: force
The functional value of a hand also depends on the force the patient can apply. The evaluation of the available force comes in as a factor of 4. If the available force corresponds to the corrected value of the contralateral hand, or to a corrected standard, the 2500 points of level 1 and 2 are multiplied by 4, giving a final value of 10,000.

If there is no force at all, the multiplication is done by 1, leaving the scores of level 1 and 2 unchanged. We have, therefore, a factor range of 3 to distribute. We measure by standard dynamometers:

- The power grip: yielding if comparable to corrected normal side, or corrected standard.
- The pinch grip.
- The key grip.

Measuring the force is of enormous value to evaluate a result. This measurement is also the weak point of the system, because we are completely dependent on the patient's cooperation. If the patient does not cooperate, we have to omit level 3.

Table 7.2 *Sensibility as a factor in various situations*

Pain sensibility (pinprick)	= loss of factor 0.4	multiply by 1.6
Protective sensibility (touch and temperature)	= loss of factor 0.3	multiply by 1.7
Static two-point discrimination >11 mm	= loss of factor 0.2	multiply by 1.8
Static two-point discrimination 7–11 mm	= loss of factor 0.1	multiply by 1.9
Sensibility like contralateral side 6 mm	= no loss of factor	multiply by 2

On the other hand, measuring the force provides a realistic feature. At the end of a period of intense physiotherapy, the values for force might be better than at a follow-up study when the patient has stopped doing daily exercises.

No evaluation system can be perfect. It always has to be a compromise between the invested time and the desired exactness. The main point is that the system can be followed in retrospect by studying the chart to see how the values were produced. It should be realistic by giving a global value and not a fictive rank. Here we arrive at the weak point of the system. As it refers to global hand function, it is influenced by other lesions (tendon, vessels, bone) as well and it might be difficult to sort out the functional loss produced by the nerve lesion as such. For scientific studies comparing techniques, cases with pure nerve lesions only should be eligible.

Armamentarium of peripheral nerve surgery

Loss of continuity without defect

The recommended technique is the end-to-end nerve repair (neurorrhaphy).

In the past the terminology described the main procedure of the repair, i.e. the tissue where the stitches were anchored (epineural nerve suture, perineural nerve suture, epi-perineural nerve suture, etc.). Today many different techniques are in use, but all methods can be reduced by the definition of how the four basic procedures are handled:

(1) Preparation of the two stumps

It is extremely important to remove all the damaged tissues and prepare the stumps in a such a way that the cross-section consists mainly of fascicular tissue and contains a small amount of non-fascicular connective tissue. This can be achieved by segmental resection or by interfascicular dissection, to separate fascicles or fascicle groups, and to resect the damaged part for each fascicle or fascicle group separately. Segmental resection is the technique of choice, with stumps showing a mono- or oligo-fascicular pattern, with two to four fascicles. If there are a few larger, manageable fascicles or fascicle groups, the interfascicular dissection is preferable. With many small fascicles without group arrangement we have no other choice than to perform a segmental resection, because isolation of the many small fascicles causes too much surgical trauma and does not make sense.

(2) Approximation

The two stumps are now approximated, using fine stitches. For this procedure I prefer the adjacent joints to be in an extended position, which should be possible with minimal tension. If this is proven, one can flex the joints a little bit, to facilitate the surgical steps. Some surgeons enhance the approximation by flexing the adjacent joint. If this is done, it should be mentioned in the report, noting the degrees of flexion.

(3) Coaptation

This is the most important step. The surgeon has to try to coapt fasicular tissues of the two stumps with fascicular tissue and prevent wrong coaptation. This is easy, if the cross-section consists of one or four fasicles performing a trunk-to-trunk coaptation.

It becomes more difficult if there are 5 or 10 fascicles or fascicle groups. It is certainly easier under such conditions to coapt fascicles or fascicle groups isolated by interfascicular dissection, in the manner of a fascicular, or a group fascicular coaptation. In a polyfascicular pattern without group arrangement, a trunk-to-trunk coaptation is the only reasonable solution. An 'exact' coaptation in the true sense of the word, as we are used to reading it in surgical reports, is impossible in the majority of cases, because in the case of group fascicular coaptation the number of fasicles in the group no longer corresponds owing to the resection. Nevertheless, fortunately a good result can be achieved. Neurotropism and neurotrophism help the axons to get in the correct distal pathway.

Some authors (Lundborg et al 1991) go a step further and not only do a loose coaptation, but leave a gap on purpose, protected by a tube, to give the axon sprouts a better chance to follow neurotropic influences.

(4) Maintaining the coaptation

The coaptation is maintained by very few stitches. Frequently the stitches that have been used to approximate the stumps are sufficient, if there is minimal tension. The stitches are anchored in the interfascicular or in the epifascicular epineurium, or in the perineurium. The site of placing the stitches does not play a role, as long as good coaptation of the fascicular tissue is provided.

Fibrin glue combined with a few stitches has proven its value. With increasing tension more stitches have to be applied, and the surgical trauma is increased. The use of resorbable tension relief plates and tubes of different kinds is occasionally recommended. These recommendations still have to stand the test of time.

Restoration of continuity if there is a defect

Defect and distance

In literature these two terms are not exactly distinguished. After clean transection of a nerve, the nerve tissue retracts because of its elasticity, resulting in a distance between the two stumps. At a primary repair, just the force of elasticity has to be overcome and the two stumps can be coapted.

If the loss of continuity was caused by a blunt trauma, nerve tissue has been damaged and has to be resected in order to coapt sound tissue. This causes a defect, and the final distance between the two stumps which has to be overcome consists of the distance caused by elastic retraction, and of the defect caused by resection of damaged tissue. As far as the elastic contraction is concerned, we have to deal with elastic forces, but the loss of some nerve substance has to be compensated by elongation of the adjacent segments of the nerve. If the original trauma has destroyed a segment of a nerve, we have to deal with the defect caused by the trauma, the defect caused by resection of the nerve stumps to get into sound nerve tissue, and the distance caused by elastic retraction.

Things are complicated by the occurrence of fibrosis. If the two stumps stay for a certain period of time in a position caused by elastic retraction, fibrosis of the connective tissue of the nerve may cause loss of the ability of nerve tissue to elongate. In this situation the distance caused by elastic retraction has to be dealt with like a defect. This is especially the case with late secondary repairs.

Frequently the argument is put forward that with elongation osteotomies, nerve tissue can be elongated to a considerable percentage. This is a completely different situation. In elongation osteotomy we have to elongate a nerve with normal elasticity and normal gliding function. The necessary elongation is distributed over a very long segment of the nerve, and for each particular segment remains below a damaging value. Apart from this, the elongation is performed slowly; if the elongation is done too rapidly, irreversible damage has been observed.

Management of long defects of important nerves

The 'gold standard' in the management of long defects of important nerves is free autologous nerve grafting.

If we have to deal with a nerve with a certain number of large manageable fascicles, or a polyfascicular nerve structure with group arrangement, the two nerve stumps are prepared by interfascicular dissection. This interfascicular dissection follows the spaces between the fascicle groups and it divides the nerve into its minor units, which are not the result of artificial dissection, but of dissection following preformed spaces. The isolated fascicles, or fascicle groups, are resected at different lengths. Nerve grafts are harvested and cut into segments significantly longer than the distance between the two stumps, so that they can be placed individually into the recipient site and have optimal contact with the surrounding tissues for rapid spontaneous revascularization.

It is certainly a problem to identify the corresponding fascicle groups of the two stumps, and it is also evident that this becomes more difficult the longer the defect produced by the trauma. Each nerve graft is approximated by a 9.0 or 10.0 stitch to the elected fascicle group of the proximal, or the distal stump, to avoid touching the nerve tissue. By manipulation with a stitch, the graft is then coapted to the fascicle, or fascicle group. As the fascicles, or fascicle groups, are of different lengths, an interdentation is created in such a way that grafts connected to a shorter fascicle group are in side-by-side contact with longer fascicle groups, which provides excellent stability. It is usually not necessary to add further stitches to maintain the coaptation; normal fibrin coagulation is sufficient to do this. As this process will take some time, it is important to carefully avoid any shearing or longitudinally acting forces during the wound closure and the immediate postoperative phase. If we have to deal with a fascicular pattern with one, two, three or four large fascicles, interfascicular dissection does not bring any advantage, and we perform a resection of the two stumps and coapt the grafts according to the sectors of a monofascicular stump, or the fascicles of an oligofascicular stump.

If there is a polyfascicular pattern without group arrangement, again the operation of the stumps is done by resection, and the grafts are coapted according to the sectors of the cross-section.

Histochemical staining to identify motor or sensory fascicles has been recommended. It plays a certain role in distal segments of a nerve where the nerve fibres are already arranged according to the pending ramification.

At distal levels, one can rely on retrograde tracing. For instance, a median lesion close to the wrist joint poses the problem that we do not know where the fascicles containing the motor fibres for the motor thenar branch are located. It is easy to follow the median nerve across the carpal tunnel and to identify the motor thenar branch. On the surface of the distal stump one can follow the fascicles forming the motor thenar branch to the distal stump, and can identify the exact location. By comparing the fascicular pattern of both stumps, a good guess can be made as to which fascicles of the proximal stump contain the motor fibres. This is not difficult as long as the defect is limited. In a long defect, the motor fibres in the proximal stump are distributed diffusely anyway. In a similar way the location of the motor fibres of the radial nerve can be traced in the distal segment of the radial nerve if one explores the ramification of the radial nerve into the superficial branch and the deep branch, and then follows the deep branch to identify the location in the far section of the distal stump. The same is true for the ulnar nerve to define the fascicle groups carrying the motor fibres for the deep branch.

Some surgeons recommend glueing the ends of a bundle of grafts together, to be able to deal with them as an entity, and to avoid individual coaptation. This technique may be justified, for example, at the brachial plexus level, but with peripheral nerves one loses the main advantage of using interfascicular nerve grafting, the so-called 'aimed connection', connecting an elected point of the proximal stump with another elected point of the distal stump by a single nerve graft.

The length of the graft should be elected according to the maximal distance between the two stumps in extreme position of the joints. This means that early motion can be started after a few days or 1 week. When the limb is moved, the graft is relieved and not extended. If we elect the graft according to the minimal distance, we combine the disadvantage of a nerve graft with two sites of coaptation, and the disadvantage of a suture under tension.

Nerve grafting has proven its value now for over 35 years. Free grafting is performed in different ways and it is certainly not appropriate to talk about 'conventional' nerve grafts if a new technique is compared with an established one.

When Taylor and Ham (1976) published the so-called 'vascularized nerve graft', many surgeons were convinced that now a new era of nerve repair had begun. An enormous amount of effort has been invested in proving the superiority of vascularized nerve grafts over free grafts. The advantages have been listed (see earlier), but there are also disadvantages. Vascularized nerve grafts are a useful tool in very selected cases, but cannot be regarded as a standard technique.

Donor grafts are cutaneous nerves with a small diameter, to be able to survive free grafting well. They usually correspond with the size of major fascicles or fascicle groups in peripheral nerves. Potential donor nerves are:

- sural nerve
- cutaneous antibrachii medialis nerve
- cutaneous femoralis lateralis nerve
- cutaneous antibrachii lateralis nerve
- superficial branch of radial nerve
- saphenus nerve.

Nerve trunks can be used as free grafts after splitting them into minor units.

Vascularized nerve grafts, ulnar nerve based on the superficial collateral ulnar artery and vein – according to Julia Terzis (Breidenbach and Terzis 1984) are: peroneus nerve and saphenus nerve.

Origin of nerve grafts

If autografts are used, the clinician will not have to face immunological problems. Autografts are certainly the 'gold standard'. For the majority of nerve lesions there are enough donors available. Special problems arise in brachial plexus cases and in long lesions of the sciatic nerve. In such cases the use or additional use of allografts would be an advantage; encouraging results have been reported for long sciatic nerve defects (Mackinnon et al 1984). It is an advantage that immunosuppressive drugs like FK504 should have a favourable influence on nerve regeneration. Certainly the day will come when the problem of allografting is solved, but so far it still remains in some ways experimental surgery.

Alternatives to nerve grafting

To avoid having to sacrifice a donor nerve, alternative techniques to nerve grafting have been developed, like the use of autologous veins (Chiu 1980), which have proven their value in limited defects. Silicone tubes, millipore tubes, collagen tubes, absorbable polyglycol tubes and many other materials have been used, including freeze-dried muscle. Battiston et al (2003) now recommend using a vein stuffed with freeze-dried muscle. All these techniques have in common that the tissue is neurotized by minifascicles which advance from the proximal stump along the tube or the graft to reach the distal stump, and all have a limited length which can be bridged in a satisfying fashion.

Alternative techniques have a place in limited defects of less important nerves, such as digital nerves on the ulnar side of the hand, for example, or to provide a space for outgrowth of axons in case of a painful neuroma, etc.

As already mentioned, with autologous nerve grafts there is a possibility of a block at the distal side of coaptation, which can be recognized by a halt of the advancement of the Tinel sign at this level. If the Tinel sign does not advance within a reasonable time, one has to explore the distal site of coaptation, resect it and perform an end-to-end nerve repair.

Management of small nerve defects

In a longer defect, autologous nerve grafting is the technique of choice. What about short nerve defects? In this situation surgeons might be tempted to mobilize the two stumps and perform a nerve repair under tension. Nicholson and Seddon (1957) reported 50% M3 results for median nerves at the wrist, if the defect was > 2.5 cm. This means that in certain patients under certain conditions a suture under tension may yield a satisfactory result. But what about the other 50%? It is certainly not possible to provide a guideline, like for instance: a nerve graft should be done if the distance is more than 1 or 2, or 3 cm, etc. Each surgeon has to make up their own mind and elect the technique which according to their personal experience promises the best result. In case of doubt, I would prefer to do a nerve graft rather than perform a neurorrhaphy under tension. But I would respect the different decision of another surgeon, provided that they follow up the patient and do not hesitate to do a re-exploration if the result does not meet expectations. It is very sad to meet patients who have been operated by nerve repair under tension 2 years previously, who do not show any recovery and now have no chance for a re-exploration owing to the long time interval elapsed and the atrophy of the paralysed muscles.

In some cases, the tension at the site of coaptation can be relieved by transposition of the nerve in a shorter bed. This is especially true for the ulnar nerve. By antepositioning of the ulnar nerve one can gain about 2 cm in length, as long as the elbow joint remains in extension. The gain is limited. Of course, if the elbow joint is flexed one can manage much longer defects, but this would cause all the consequences of a repair under tension.

Another way to deal with small defects would be the pre-operative application of an expander to elongate the nerve before doing the nerve repair (Van Beek, 1989).

What do we do if the proximal stump is lacking?

This is especially the case in brachial plexus lesions, with an avulsion, or a lesion of the route nerve complex. In this case we have to transfer nerve fibres from the proximal segment of another nerve to neurotize the denervated distal stump of the avulsed nerve. In surgical jargon the term 'neurotization' is widely utilized for such a procedure. This is not really correct, because under 'neurotization' we understand the ingrowth of nerve fibres in a denervated tissue – e.g. if performing a neurorrhaphy the distal stump is neurotized from the proximal stump. In case of nerve grafting, the graft is neurotized by advancement of axons from the proximal stump into the graft. If we put the proximal ends of a nerve into a denervated muscle, the muscle is neurotized directly from the proximal stump (nerve–muscle neurotization). If two muscles are brought side-by-side, one innervated and one denervated, without perimysium inbetween, the denervated muscle gets neurotized from the innervated muscle by muscle-to-muscle neurotization. There is even a muscle–nerve–muscle neurotization, when nerve fibres from the innervated side of the orbicularis oris grow along a graft and across the midline to the denervated side of the orbicularis oris, in case of face paralysis.

Neurotization by nerve transfer plays an important role in brachial plexus surgery. Motor branches of the cervical plexus, the phrenic nerve and the dorsalis scapulae nerve have been used, as well as the hypoglossus nerve and others. A very common donor is the accessory nerve, or motor branches of the plexus cervicalis, according to Brunelli (Brunelli and Monini 1984). A nerve transfer can also be performed between innervated and denervated parts of the plexus. However, it soon turned out that nerve transfers at the proximal level do not work very well owing to the dilution of the transferred nerve fibres. The result is very limited if, for example, the accessory nerve is transferred by nerve grafts to the lateral cord. The results are much better if the transfer goes directly to an elected target, e.g. the musculocutaneous nerve, in order to achieve elbow flexion. Oberlin et al (1994) have performed nerve transfer at a medium level, utilizing in upper brachial plexus lesion motor fibre carrying fascicles of the median nerve, to innervate the denervated musculocutaneous nerve, or from the ulnar nerve to the denervated musculocutaneous nerve. This method was modified by Mackinnon (2003), by performing the nerve transfer directly to the biceps and the brachialis muscle with good results. A common factor in all these transfers is that the fascicle with the donor fibres has to be transected; this means that a certain loss of function will occur. This may be important for the accessory nerve if the main trunk is used and if there is no additional innervation of the trapezius muscle by a ramus trapezius from the cervical plexus. We have learned to save the first branch of the accessory nerve to maintain a certain innervation by fibres from the accessory nerve, which prevents a loss of function by intramuscular neurotization. A functional loss of the phrenic nerve should not be underestimated.

If the fascicles of median or ulnar nerve are used as axon donors, the functional loss is nil, because sufficient motor fibres remain to maintain normal function. A successful nerve fibre transfer by end-to-side coaptation would offer functional recovery without transecting functioning nerve fibres (see below: 'End-to-side coaptation').

What do we do if the distal stump is lacking?

If the distal stump of a motor nerve was destroyed, and no recipient nerve is available to perform a restoration of continuity, the proximal stump is divided by interfascicular dissection into minor units, and each of these fascicles, or fascicle groups, is buried into the denervated muscle, if possible at the level where the majority of motor endplates can be expected. By this manoeuvre a nerve-to-muscle neurotization is stimulated and in many cases a very good muscle function can be achieved (Brunelli 1981).

End-to-side coaptation

Putting a denervated nerve stump end-to-side to a normal nerve was suggested long ago, without much success and without eliciting attention. It was, therefore, a great surprise, when Viterbo (1994) published experiments and clinical cases in which a denervated nerve coapted end-to-side to an innervated nerve was successfully neurotized, producing a functional result. It is obvious that this technique, if it works, would open enormous applications at different levels. Experiments proved that the end-to-side coaptation works even if the exact mechanism of the stimulation of the axon proliferation is not yet completely clear. There is, however, great controversy as far as the clinical value is concerned. There are some reports of favourable results, whereas other surgeons have published disappointing results (Battiston 2003). A. Gilbert (2003, personal communication) told me that he did not see positive results when using end-to-side coaptation in brachial plexus cases in adults; however, he had some spectacular results in obstetric brachial plexus lesions in an unpredictable way.

I personally was first confronted with cases of end-to-side coaptation in brachial plexus surgery performed by other surgeons. It is obvious that if avulsion of a spinal nerve is encountered, it is much easier for the surgeon to put the distal stump of the avulsed spinal nerve end-to-side to an innervated one, instead of performing cumbersome dissections to provide axon donors of nerves outside the plexus. In none of the cases was there a functional recovery. As we do not know any mechanism that may influence the quality of the axons that start to proliferate, we have to assume that this follows a random pattern. A neurotropic factor can be excluded, because we know that tubes not containing nerve material stimulate the outgrowth of axons, albeit in a less important way than an autologous nerve graft. If a mixed nerve is used as an axon donor, we have no way to stimulate preferentially the outgrowth of motor fibres or sensory fibres. We will have a random pattern outgrowth, and this might not be sufficient to bring enough fibers to the target organ to produce a functional recovery. The consequence of this consideration is that for end-to-side coaptation we may use pure motor nerves as donors, and pure motor nerves as recipients, as in this case only motor nerve fibres can proliferate.

The stimulus to cause axon sprouting in an end-to-side procedure has to act on the endoneurium of the nerve, and the sprouts have to traverse the sheaths of the nerve. Therefore, from the beginning there have been suggestions to open an epineurial window in the nerve trunk, and to open a perineurial window in the fascicle where the end-to-side coaptation was planned. Opening a perineurial window causes a kind of herniation of endoneurial tissue, as described by Spencer et al (1975). In the long term this does not cause significant damage, but for the moment it is certainly an unfavourable factor. Creating the windows is less important in very thin nerves with tiny epifascicular epineurium and a tiny perineurium. I decided, therefore, to use end-to-side procedures in brachial plexus surgery, following these principles. I was surprised how good results could be obtained and how quickly the recovery occurred. I gave a preliminary report as a discussional remark at the meeting of the ASPEN in Vancouver in 1998.

We used an end-to-side neurorrhaphy for neurotization of the long thoracic nerve, with the dorsalis scapula nerve as donor. We used it to reinnervate the major pectoralis nerve, with the phrenic nerve as donor, putting a nerve graft end-to-side to the phrenic nerve, and performing an end-to-end coaptation with the medial or the lateral pectoralis nerve, with good results. We also used it with success for the suprascapular nerve (Millesi 2003).

Recently we have achieved another step forward. We went to the extreme periphery using rami musculares as donors, and other muscle branches as recipients, performing the proximal coaptation of the graft end-to-side to the donor, and the distal coaptation end-to-end to the recipient. This was successfully performed in a case with a partial brachial plexus lesion, damaging the median nerve but leaving the ulnar nerve intact.

In this case a motor branch to the deep head of the flexor pollicis brevis innervated by the ulnar nerve was used as a donor for a nerve graft coapted end-to-side. The distal end of the graft was coapted end-to-end to the motor thenar branch (see Case report 1). Other clinical indications for this extremely distal nerve transfer are cases in whom, for example, in a lesion of C8 and T1 in the median and ulnar nerve, innervated muscles are paralysed, except for the pronator teres and the flexor carpi radialis, which frequently receive nerve fibres from C7. Nerve grafts can be coapted end-to-side to the motor branches of these two muscles on the one side, and to rami musculares of the ulnar and the median nerve innervated forearm muscles on the other side, to achieve finger flexion.

A further application of similar techniques would be in a high median nerve lesion, to perform a nerve transfer from a motor branch of the deep branch of the ulnar nerve end-to-side distal coaptation and end-to-side to the motor thenar branch, bringing in axons to re-establish the innervation of the median-innervated thenar muscles, to preserve these muscles and prevent degeneration. If median nerve axons arrive, they could take over, because the motor thenar branch was not transected.

Case report 1

The patient, M.M. (born 6 June 1977), suffered a motorcycle accident on 21 May 2000. Among several fractures of the right and left upper extremity, a craniocerebral trauma and a rupture of the liver, the patient suffered a partial brachial plexus lesion with involvement of the spinal nerves C5, C6 and C7. Initially the patient had a complete paralysis of the median nerve-innervated muscles with a corresponding sensory loss. The ulnar nerve-innervated muscles, however, were functioning.

The patient was operated upon on 21 October 2000. The spinal nerve C6 was avulsed. C7 was interrupted, C5 was interrupted as well; C8 and T1 were in continuity. Nerve grafts were performed from C5 to the posterior cord, from C7 to the lateral cord, from the phrenic nerve end-to-side to the superscapular nerve. The superscapular nerve was compressed at the scapular notch and a neurolysis was performed. There was a significant improvement of the muscles of the shoulder and the biceps. There was no recovery as far as wrist and finger extension were concerned. There was function of the pronator teres. This muscle was transferred to the extensor carpi radialis brevis for wrist extension. The patient had a good intrinsic function, he could adduct the thumb, there was no opposition of the thumb. Mixed innervation from the ulnar to the median nerve could be excluded. The patient had a typical median nerve paralysis with no opposition, atrophy of the thenar muscles and reduced flexion of the index finger.

On 23 April 2003 the following procedure was performed. The profundus tendon of the middle finger was sutured side-to-side to the profundus tendon of the index finger. The deep branch of the ulnar nerve was explored and followed until its division into a branch to the adductor pollicis and to the caput profundum of the flexor pollicis brevis. A nerve graft deriving from the superficial radial nerve was harvested. This nerve graft was coapted end-to-side to the motor branches of the deep ulnar nerve. The distal end of the graft was coapted end-to-end to the thenar muscles. Three months after the operation the patient started to actively innervate the thenar muscles. Six months after the accident the patient could perform opposition. An electromyelographic study was performed. The thenar muscles could not be stimulated by stimulation of the median nerve; however, stimulus of the ulnar nerve produced action potentials of a good quality.

This case shows that very peripheral muscle branches can be used as donors of axons, which can be transported via end-to-side coaptation along a graft to another muscle branch.

Surgical procedures to manage lesions with preserved continuity

Each nerve has to be able to move against the surrounding tissues, in order to adapt to the movements of an extremity. The ability to move is provided by several layers of loose tissue which surround a nerve externally to the epineurium and link it to the surrounding tissues. Lang (1962) has described this tissue extensively and called it 'conjunctiva nervorum'. For clinical use the term 'paraneurium' seems more adequate. Many descriptions of the anatomy of peripheral nerves do not mention this tissue, or they regard it as a part of the epineurium. If a nerve joins the vascular bundle, the outer layers of the paraneurium merge with the adventitia of the vessels to a common neurovascular sheeth. The paraneurium, due to its loose organisation, provides space for a nerve to change volume. According to the position of the limb, if all the joints are extended, the nerve becomes elongated and thinner, with flexed joints the nerve becomes shorter and thicker, like a harmonica, without any change of pressure in the endoneurium within the fascicles (H. Millesi, unpublished observations).

The second level of passive motion is located between the fascicles within the nerve trunk. The fascicles of a nerve trunk are embedded in interfascicular epineurium, which is also a loose connective tissue containing vessels and fat lobules. This loose connective tissue allows the fascicles to move against each other and to change place. In this way the nerve trunk can be externally deformed to a certain degree without any change of pressure within the fascicles. The nerve trunk as such is surrounded by a more dense epineurial tissue, the epifascicular epineurium. On top of this is the paraneurium. After trauma or due to internal reasons, especially at the site of an entrapment, the nerve may become adherent and may loose its passive motility. The nerve might be compressed externally by scar tissue, bony fragments or any other external factor. This would provide an indication for an external neurolysis.

Historically, surgeons had noticed the fibrotic thickening that may occur within a nerve, but they did not dare to enter a nerve with the crude techniques then available. With the development of microsurgery surgeons became more courageous and the so-called 'internal neurolysis' or 'endoneurolysis' technique was adopted.

Curtis and Eversman (1973) suggested performing such an internal neurolysis in more severe cases of carpal tunnel syndrome. The idea was to remove the connective tissue around the fascicles of a compressed nerve, to give the nerve the chance to expand again to normal size. In many instances this was unnecessary because without collagenization the connective tissue would allow expansion in time. In contrast, manipulation within the nerve might stimulate collagenization.

Consequently, internal neurolysis got a bad reputation and many surgeons regard internal neurolysis as contraindicated. This has led to developments at the other extreme, i.e. if there is a fibrosis with shrinkage, it has to be treated. Because of the many misunderstandings surrounding it, the term internal neurolysis should be dropped. The following section describes procedures that should be applied step-by-step if there is fibrosis of a nerve with shrinkage.

The fibrosis may involve the paraneurium. If shrinkage occurs, the tissue shrinks in a longitudinal direction in such a way that the fascicles become longer than the nerve and consequently they follow a snake-like or wavy course. If the shrinkage evolves in the epineurium, it develops in a transverse direction and causes tightening of the nerve, like a too-tight stocking. Earlier, in this chapter, these situations were described as type A* and A fibrosis.

If the fibrosis involves the interfascicular epineurium, the fascicles are compressed. Vessels in the fibrotic area are compressed and obliterated as well. Operation in this fibrotic area does not diminish the blood supply of the fascicles, provided that other areas are not fibrotic and will remain intact. This will be fibrosis of type B.

Finally, the endoneural tissue may become collagenized – and this would be fibrosis of type C.

What are the surgical procedures to deal with these situations?

- Adhesions of the paraneurium: neurolysis (external).
- Fibrosis of the paraneurium (type A*): paraneuriotomy or paraneuriectomy.
- Fibrosis of the epifascicular epineurium (type A): epineuriotomy.
- Fibrosis of the epifascicular and interfascicular tissues (type B): epifascicular epineuriectomy, or in extreme cases, partial interfascicular epineuriectomy.
- Fibrosis of type C: resection of the involved fascicles and restoration of continuity by nerve graft.
- If the dissection within the nerve reveals the loss of the fascicular pattern (degree 4), the best approach is also a resection and restoration of continuity, independently of whether there is a neuroma formation (4 N) or just scar tissue (4 S).
- Admittedly the differentiation between degree 3C and degree 4 is difficult, but this does not matter because in both cases a resection is indicated.
- The real clinical problem is a mixture of a lesion of degree 3 and degree 4. Then the experienced surgeon has to make up his mind whether he would rather regard it as degree 3 or degree 4.

Muscle transposition to improve nerve regeneration

There is a mutual influence between nerve regeneration and muscle function. A typical example of this situation is the peroneus nerve. The prognosis for peroneus nerve lesions is generally regarded as very poor. In a majority of cases muscle recovery occurs, but the regenerating muscles do not achieve a functional value. The patient continues to develop a pes equinovarus and has to wear a splint. It is not the peroneus nerve which is responsible for this situation, but the fact that the peroneus nerve-innervated muscles have to work against overwhelming antagonists. The gastrocnemii and the soleus, eventually accompanied by a contracture of the Achilles tendon, and the deep muscles of the calf are much stronger than the peroneus-innervated muscles of the anterior compartment. It is not by a random chance that patients with chronic diseases and long bed-rest develop a pes equinovarus without a nerve lesion. What we have to do in this case is to lengthen the Achilles tendon, to weaken the dorsal muscles and to strengthen the muscles performing dorsiflexion. This can be done by a tibialis posterior tendon transfer across the interosseus space to the dorsum of the foot. A typical example is given as a case report. After achieving a better equilibrium between the muscle antagonists, the nerve regeneration improves significantly and the muscles of the anterior compartment become strong enough to eventually perform their task. In a similar way the radialis regeneration may be enhanced by pronator teres transfer to the extensor carpi radialis brevis, to give the patient an immediate dorsiflexion, and to avoid overextension of the regenerating muscles (see Case report 2). In ulnar nerve regeneration, the interossei may regenerate much better if they are protected against elongation by a Zancolli capsulodesis (H. Millesi, unpublished observations).

Case report 2

The patient, O.T. (born 4 May 1984), was operated upon in August 1996 because of an exostosis at the fibula. On this occasion the deep branch of the peroneus nerve was transected and the patient had a complete paralysis of the muscles of the anterior compartment.

The patient was operated upon on 12 November 1996. A neurolysis of the common peroneal nerve and the superficial peroneal nerve was performed. The deep peroneal nerve had a defect which was covered by four nerve grafts. There was motor recovery of the muscles of the anterior compartment of the right leg. The recovery was, however, too weak to be of functional value. The patient had to continue to wear a peroneus splint. Based on the experience, that change of the muscle balance stimulates nerve regeneration, the patient was operated again on 7 April 1998. The Achilles tendon was lengthened, the tibialis posterior was freed and transferred across the interosseous membrane to the dorsum of the foot. The tendon was fixed at the skeleton. The tendons of the extensor hallucis longus and the extensor digitorum longus were sutured side-to-side to the tibialis posterior tendon in order to transmit some force to the toes as well.

In the following months there was a dramatic improvement of function. The patient could walk without a splint, he could resume sporting activities. This was not only due to the transfer of the tibialis posterior tendon, but to a significant improvement in the efficiency of the originally paralysed and reinnervated muscles of the anterior compartment. The function of the extensor hallucis longus was, however, weaker than the extensor digitorum longus. The shortening of the extensor hallucis longus tendon to provide more efficiency was performed on 5 September 2000. At the follow-up examination on 7 November 2003 the function was close to normal.

Muscle transposition to improve the function in case of partial regeneration

Such procedures have to be carried out especially during the treatment of brachial plexus lesions. During regeneration after a brachial plexus repair co-contractures may develop, for instance, between biceps and triceps. Both muscles then act at the same time and neutralize each other. By injection of botox the triceps can be paralysed for about 3 months so as to strengthen the biceps in the meantime, to give the biceps a surplus of power for flexion until the triceps recovers. The same can be achieved by lengthening of the triceps tendon, which also weakens the triceps. But if the biceps itself is weak, a transfer of the triceps to the biceps or to the radius directly helps to restore elbow flexion of functional value. Such a procedure may even strengthen the biceps according to the principle previously outlined. The disadvantage of a triceps transfer is the loss of active elbow extension, which under otherwise normal conditions is a severe handicap. In cases of brachial plexus lesion with weakness of the shoulder joint and lack of abduction, active elbow extension is not so important and extension by gravity may be sufficient.

Reconstructive surgery with irreversible nerve lesions

I have added this segment to this chapter in spite of the fact that a complete description of all reconstructive procedures would expand the size of this chapter, because I want to demonstrate that peripheral nerve surgeons treat not just nerves, but nerve lesions and their consequences. Reconstructive surgery is an important part of the whole entity, and every surgeon dealing with peripheral nerves should also be an expert in reconstructive surgery.

Management of pain syndromes caused by peripheral nerve damage

In this chapter we are not dealing with typical entrapment syndromes, etc. We want to discuss pain syndromes that have developed spontaneously, or as a consequence of a surgical procedure or a trauma. The common feature of this group of patients is the fact that there are adhesions of the nerve, and a fibrosis has developed to various degrees. This offers the opportunity for surgery to change the environment of the nerve and to break a vicious cycle. With all these patients there is the danger of central fixation of the pain, which may persist even if the local cause has been controlled.

This means that surgery should be done rather quickly without a lengthy delay. The incision to explore such a nerve should be done apart from the localization of the nerve, by lifting a flap or by several transverse incisions. Under certain conditions endoscopic visualization of the nerve might be helpful. We have to distinguish two different situations: lesion with transection of the nerve and lesion with preserved continuity.

Lesion with transection of the nerve

In this case the proximal stump has formed a neuroma which has to be resected. The proximal stump after resection is destroyed by diathermy. There are many different techniques described to deal with a nerve stump after the resection of a neuroma, including putting the nerve into a bone marrow cavity, putting the nerve into muscle, capping the nerve with different tubes, laser treatment of the stump, and putting a nerve into a long vein graft which might allow the axons to grow until the potential for growing has been used up. I have obtained the best results by transferring the nerve into a soft tissue in a region that is not exposed to external irritation. Nerves of the plexus lumbalis (ileohypogastric nerve, ileolingual nerve, genitofemoral nerve, cutaneous femoris lateralis) are best treated by intra-pelvic high osteotomy. If there is a distal stump, the best way to treat a painful neuroma is to restore continuity, or by nerve graft, or by vein graft to avoid the sacrifice of an autologous nerve.

Lesions with preserved continuity

The following situations may be encountered:

(1) The nerve is located in a bony channel and is compressed. Such a pain syndrome may involve the inferior alveolar nerve and may cause a very severe pain syndrome. The mental nerve at the mental foramen is explored, the bony channel is opened by removal of the bone layer by layer, until normal tissue is reached and the nerve is decompressed. In severe cases the nerve is identified before it enters the bony canal, the nerve is transected and connected to a nerve graft which continues outside the bone to the peripheral stump of the mentalis nerve.
(2) The nerve is located in the subfascial space under increased pressure. There are adhesions. This is the situation of a compartment syndrome. The fascia is removed to relieve the pressure from the compartment. An external neurolysis is performed. If the nerve has remained intact so far, the operation can be completed. If not, the different techniques of neurolysis are applied.
(3) The nerve is located in fibrous tissue at the level of a potential entrapment syndrome. There are

adhesions with other structures, like tendons, which cause a constant irritation. A neurolysis is then performed. In such patients the neurolysis alone is not sufficient, because the patient will again develop adhesions and a vicious cycle will start. It is, therefore, necessary after sufficient decompression to envelop the nerve in gliding tissue. For the median nerve in the carpal tunnel, with short segments of fibrosis, a local transposition (e.g. of the palmaris brevis) will provide sufficient cover with soft tissue, or mobilization of synovial tissues from the tendon sheath. For long segments we have successfully transferred the gliding tissue flap from underneath the major pectoralis muscle based on the arteria and vena thoracodorsalis as a free microvascular flap. Other surgeons have recommended the transfer of the omentum majus. In these cases it is extremely important to enlarge the integument as well, because an integument that is too tight may cause elevated pressure (Millesi et al 1989). The whole area is explored from a mid-lateral incision on the ulnar side. At the end of the operation this wound is closed by a split-thickness skin graft, to achieve enlargement of the integumental circumference.

If the pain syndrome developed after surgery because of a thoracic outlet syndrome, an envelopment of the brachial plexus by transferring the gliding tissue from underneath the major pectoralis muscle provides a better environment for the nerve. Of special importance is the enlargement of the integumental circumference in the area of the tarsal canal, if the pain syndrome developed after tarsal tunnel surgery. The typical scar created over the tarsal tunnel during exploration may become adherent to the tibialis nerve, and cause a particular pain syndrome that is very difficult to treat. We therefore prefer a bow-like incision dorsal to the tarsal tunnel, elevating a flap for access to the tunnel, and covering it by the flap again. If necessary, a skin graft may be applied to enlarge the circumference.

Results

Median nerve

Case report 3

This case illustrates the management of a patient with a distal median nerve lesion and provides details about the surgical technique used and an evaluation of the results.

The patient, B.M., is an 18-year-old boy. During skating, he was injured by the skate of another person, and this caused a transverse wound at the distal forearm of the right hand. The wound was primarily sutured, and 4 weeks later the patient was admitted for median nerve repair. The repair was performed on 31 January 1980 (see Figure 7.1). The patient could not perform opposition and lost 150 points at the anatomical level. He had complete loss of sensibility in the median nerve territory and could not perform the pick-up test adequately. The value of anatomy times sensibility was 1250 points, as compared with a normal value of 2500 points.

At a follow-up examination 6 months after the repair, opposition has improved, the value at the anatomical level is 1240 points, i.e. a gain of 140 points. There is some improvement of sensibility at the thumb level, providing a factor of 1.6 (against the original of 1.0), and at the ring finger of 1.6 (against the original 1.5). The pick-up test has improved, leading to a factor of 1.62 (against 2.0 as a normal value). The value for power grip was 1.5 instead of 1.8, pinch grip 0.689 (instead of 1.0) and T-grip 0.125 (instead of 0.2) – altogether the factor for force was 3.229 (instead of 4.0). Altogether the functional value was calculated as 5400 points (against 10,000), which means that there is still a loss of 46%.

According to the Hyatt scale, the patient might have achieved M4.

Nine months after the repair, anatomical functions, i.e. the opposition, have further improved and the patient has gained the normal value of 1250 points. The sensibility has improved. The patient has a factor of 1.8 for the thumb, the index and the middle finger, and of 2.0 for the ring finger. The pick-up test has marginally improved (blindfold 1.35). At the level of anatomy times sensibility, the patient now has 2122.5 points of a normal value of 2500 points. The force has not changed much, and provided an overall factor of 3.296. Altogether the patient had 7160 points at this point in time, which is roughly 72% of the normal value. This can be regarded as a satisfactory result.

The patient continued to improve. At a follow-up 2 years later he achieved more than 9000 points (see Figures 7.2A and 7.2B).

The results of 20 consecutive cases of median nerve lesions are presented. Five of the 20 cases achieved a recovery of the pick-up test of 80–95%, 6 cases achieved 60–80%, 2 cases achieved 40–60%, and 7 cases remained below 40% (see Table 7.3).

Table 7.3 *Median nerve, pick-up test (n = 20 participants; grey column in Figure 7.3)*

Recovery (%)	*Number of cases*	*Case running numbers*
80–95	5	1, 2, 12, 14, 17
60–80	6	3, 5, 6, 8, 11, 13
40–60	2	10, 13
40	5	4, 7, 9, 15, 16
0	2	19, 20

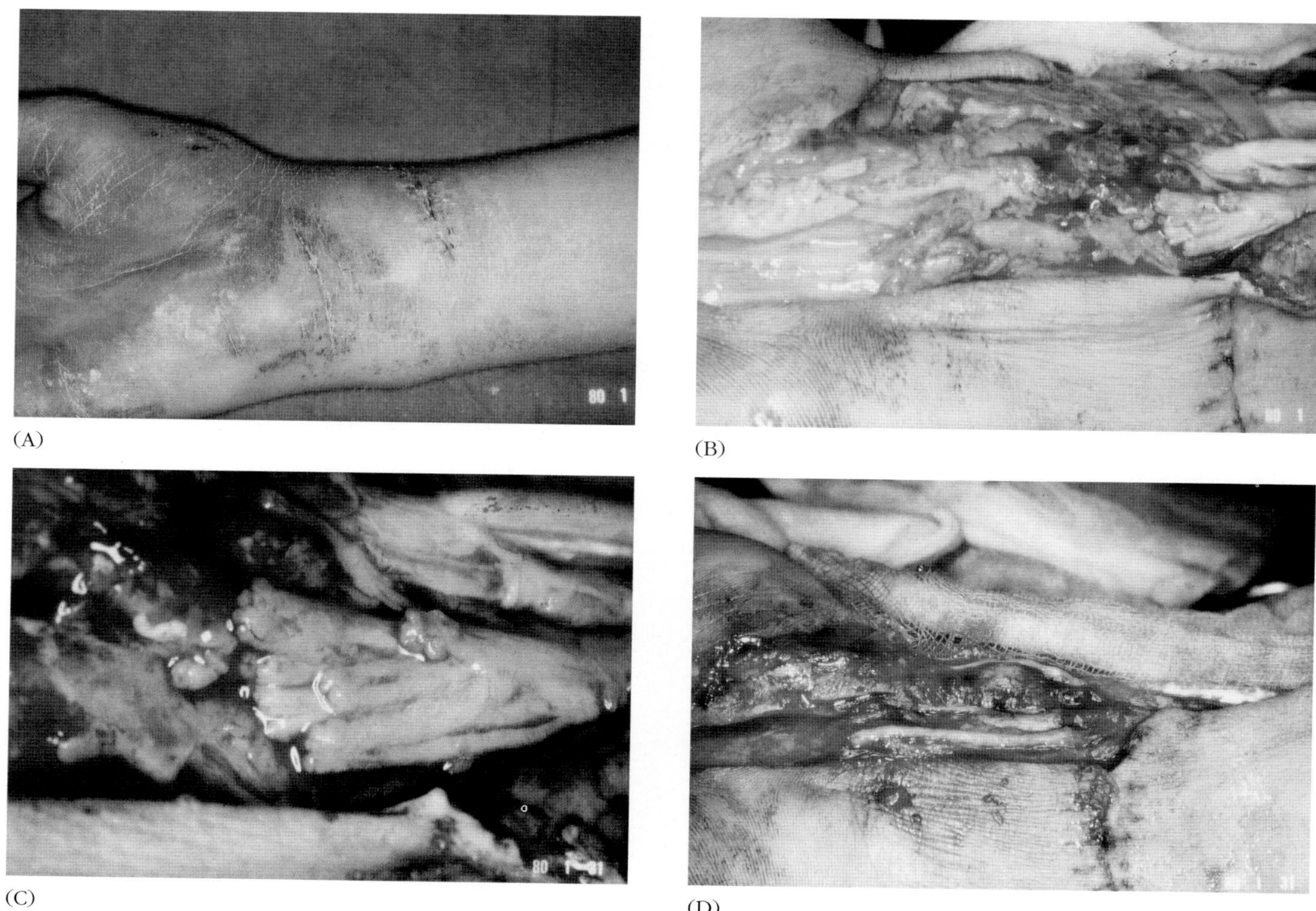

Figure 7.1

Patient B.M., male, 18 years old. (A) Injury: the palmar aspect of the right forearm close to the wrist joint. Four weeks before this photograph was taken the original wound was sutured and it has already healed. There was a complete lesion of the median nerve distal to the wound. On 31 January 1980, an exploration was performed which revealed a complete blunt transection of the median nerve by a skate. The two stumps were prepared by interfascicular dissection as described in the text. (B) The two stumps after interfascicular dissection; left, the distal stump; right, the proximal stump. The carpal tunnel was opened, the motor thenar branch was defined and followed in retrograde direction to localize it at the distal stump. (C) A close-up view of the proximal stump. Note the fascicle groups isolated by interfascicular dissection and transected at different levels. (D) The nerve grafts in place. Note the interdentation.

As far as the force is concerned, 4 of the 20 cases recovered more than 90%; 5 cases recovered between 80 and 90%, 5 cases between 70 and 80%, and 6 cases remained below 70% (see Table 7.4).

As far as the anatomy is concerned, 18 patients improved to about 90% of the normal value; 2 cases did not improve. The evaluation of anatomy times sensibility revealed a recovery of 6 cases to more than 80%, 8 cases between 70 and 80%, 4 cases between 60 and 70%, and 2 cases between 50 and 60% (see Table 7.5).

The final results are shown in Table 7.6.

Figure 7.3 represents the final results of this series of 20 cases. One can see at a glance that the anatomical value (full rhomboids) is very good in 18 of the 20 cases. However, the return of sensibility (open squares) is less good. The overall result follows the line of the sensibility, which reflects that for the median nerve recovery, the return of sensibility plays the most important role.

Ulnar nerve

To illustrate the results of ulnar nerve repair, a group of 24 cases is analysed; 12 of the 24 cases recovered more than 80% of their normal force, 4 cases between 70 and

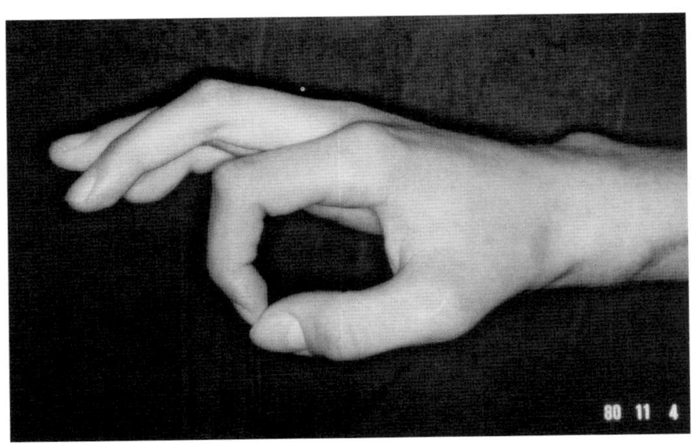

(A)

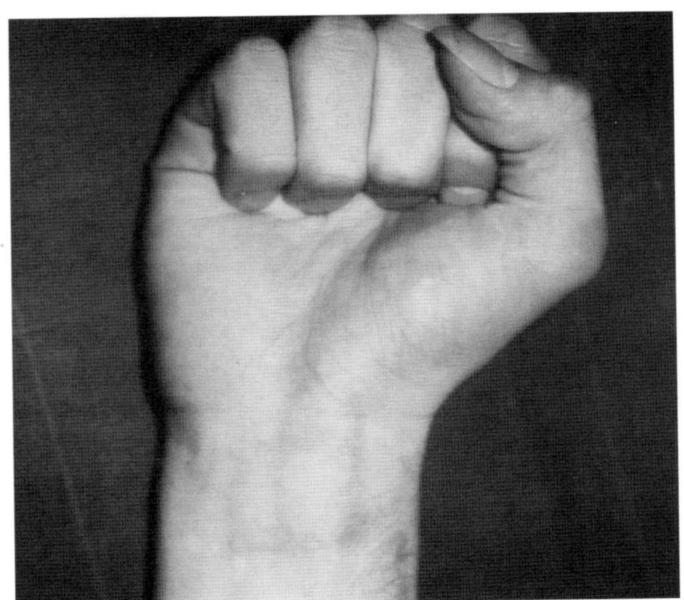

(B)

Figure 7.2
Patient B.M. follow-up. (A) The hand function 9 months after the repair. Opposition has returned. (B) No atrophy of the thenar muscles, and satisfactory healing of the surgical wound. For sensibility and handiness and force, see text.

Table 7.4 *Median nerve, force (n = 20 participants; empty column in Figure 7.3)*

Recovery (%)	*Number of cases*	*Case running numbers*
>90	4	1, 2, 3, 4
80–90	5	5, 7, 9, 16, 19
70–80	5	6, 8, 11, 12, 15
<70	6	10, 13, 14, 17, 18, 20

Table 7.5 *Anatomy multiplied by sensibility (empty dots in Figure 7.3)*

Recovery (%)	*Number of cases*	*Case running numbers*
>90	1	1
80–90	5	2, 3, 4, 6, 8
70–80	8	5, 7, 10, 11, 12, 13, 14, 17
60–70	4	9, 13, 16, 18
50–60	2	19, 20

80%, 6 cases between 60 and 70%, 1 case between 50 and 60%, and 1 case remained below 40% (see Table 7.7).

As far as anatomy is concerned, 22 cases did well, and only 2 cases did not show satisfactory recovery.

If we look at the value of anatomy times sensibility, we see that 1 case has reached 2375 points out of 2500, 21

Table 7.6 *Final results (full squares in Figure 7.3)*

Postoperative status of scores	*Gains*	*Cases in group (out of 20 participants)*	*Percentage of cases*
>9000 points	5500 points	1	5
>8000 points	4500 points	3	15
>7000 points	3500 points	2	10
>6000 points	>2500 points	6	30
>5000 points	1500 points	6	30
>4000 points	500 points	1	5
>3500 points	0	1	5

cases reached 2250 points out of 2500, 2 cases reached only 1750 points out of 2500 (see Tables 7.7 and 7.8)

If we consider anatomy times sensibility and force, 2 cases achieved more than 9000 points, 11 cases achieved more than 8000 points, 9 cases achieved more than 7000 points, 1 case achieved more than 5000 points, and 1 case achieved only more than 4000 points (see Table 7.9).

Figure 7.4 shows the summary of the 24 cases. Again we see at a glance that the line for anatomy is quite high, with only the last 2 cases dropping.

The points for sensibility recovery are also quite high, but the decisive factor is the force (open columns) and we see that the line of the overall result follows the values of the force, indicating that for the ulnar nerve the force is the decisive factor, if we evaluate the result (Figure 7.4).

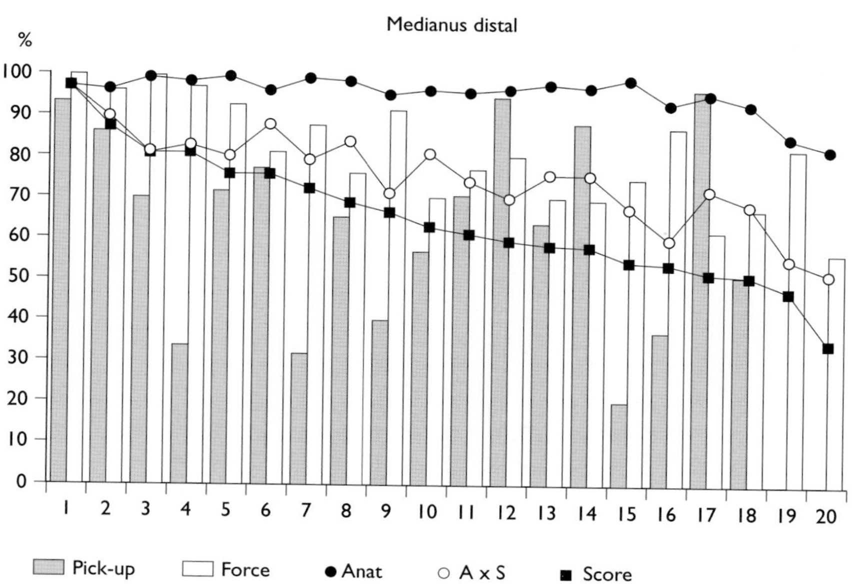

Figure 7.3

This figure represents the final evaluation of 20 cases with median nerve repairs. The patients are listed in the horizontal line, for each patient there is a 'grey column' representing the pick-up test, and an 'empty column' representing the force. Each patient has a 'full dot' indicating the value of anatomy, and an 'empty dot' representing the points for anatomy multiplied by the factor for sensibility, and a 'full square' representing the total number of points. The vertical axis indicates the percentage. At a glance it can be seen that the values for the pick-up test vary a great deal. The values for force are more uniform, but again there are higher and lower values. The line connecting the full dots is the majority of >90%, and case nos 19 and 20 represent lower values. In contrast, the line connecting the 'open dots' shows a descending curve from left to right, which means that the patients on the right side have a rather poor recovery of sensibility. The line connecting the full squares gives the real value for each patient – and here we have very good cases on the left side, the medium cases in the middle and poor cases on the right side. The striking fact is that for the median nerve the line of the final values follows roughly the line of sensibility return, indicating that sensibility is the main indicator of a satisfactory result for a median nerve lesion.

Table 7.7 *Recovery of force in 24 cases of ulnar nerve lesions*

Recovery of force (%)	*Number of cases*	*Running case numbers*
<40	1	24
50–60	1	23
60–70	6	17, 18, 19, 20, 21, 22
70–80	4	13, 14, 15, 16
80–90	10	3, 4, 5, 6, 7, 8, 9, 10, 11, 12
>90	2	1, 2

Figure 7.5 demonstrates the results of 2 cases of ulnar nerve lesions at intermedial level. In 3 cases a neurorrhaphy was carried out. In 17 cases a distance (defect by the trauma, elastic retraction and resection of the two stumps) had been bridged by grafts. Three of the cases with a nerve graft of 0.5–4.5 cm had a result of 3000 points or more, as compared to 1 case with a neurorrhaphy. Six nerve grafts between 2 and 14.5 cm in length

Table 7.8 *Anatomy multiplied by sensibility (values are shown as empty dots in Figure 7.4)*

Score	*Residual loss*	*Number of cases*
2375 points	125 points	1
2250 points	250 points = 10%	21
1750 points		2

Table 7.9 *Final result, anatomy multiplied by sensibility multiplied by force (full squares in Figure 7.4)*

Postoperative scores	*Gains*	*Number of cases*
>9000 points	Approx. 6700 points	2
>8000 points	Approx. 5700 points	11
>7000 points	Approx. 4700 points	9
>5000 points	Approx. 2700 points	1
>4000 points	Approx. 1700 points	1

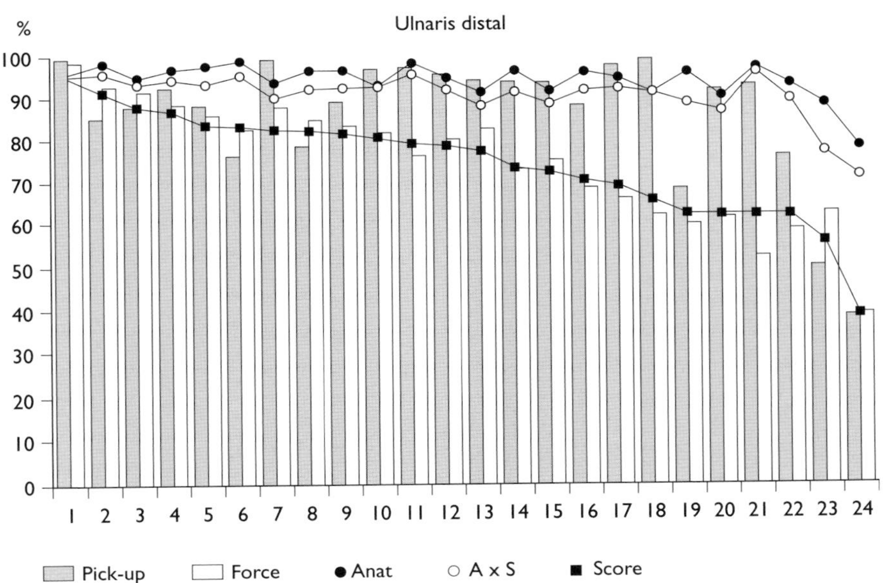

Figure 7.4

This represents the global results of 24 cases of ulnar nerve lesions. As with Figure 7.3, the grey column represents the pick-up test, which in the majority of the cases is rather good, depending more on median nerve function than on ulnar nerve function. However, the value for the force increases significantly from left to right, and there are cases with a rather poor force value. The line for anatomy (connecting the full dots), again is more or less horizontal and only the last two cases drop significantly. The line for sensibility (connecting the empty dots) again is more or less horizontal, only the last two cases drop. The line representing the percentage of the global function (connecting the full squares) is reasonably good for the cases in the left half, but drops significantly for the cases in the right half of the figure. It is striking that this line more or less follows the percentage of force recovery, indicating that for an ulnar nerve lesion, the recovery of force is the main goal.

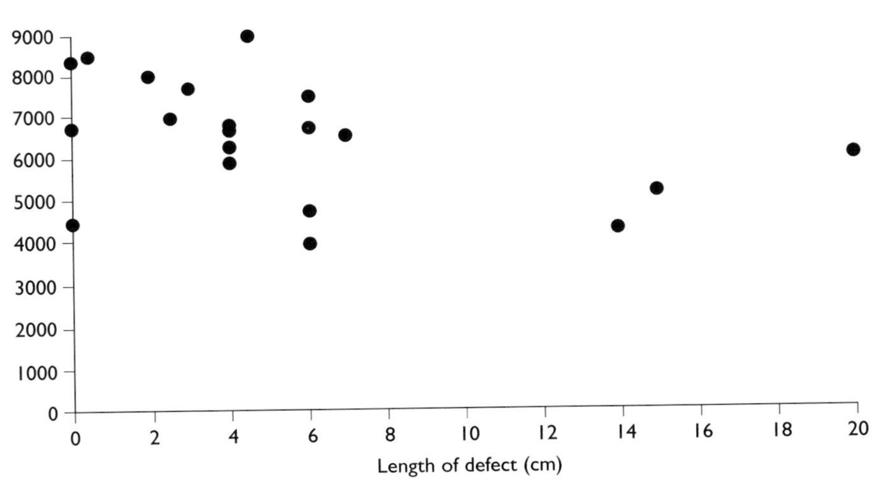

Figure 7.5

Results of 2 cases of ulnar nerve lesions at intermediate level.

had a recovery of more than 6000 points, as compared to 1 of the neurorrhaphy cases. In the group of cases of nerve grafts between 0.5 and 4.5 cm there was no case below 6000 points. But there was 1 case with a neurorrhaphy who had a recovery of 4000 to 5000 points only.

There were 5 cases with nerve grafts of about 6 cm length; 1 case had more than 7000, 2 cases had more than 6000, 1 case between 4000 and 5000, and 1 case remained below 4000 points. There were 3 cases with extremely long defects – between 14 and 20 cm. Of these, 1 case had 5000–6000, 1 case had about 5000, and 1 case about 4000 points. From these values we may conclude that the length of the defect, respective to the length of the graft, does not play an important role if

Box 7.1 *Follow-up of 30 cases of radial nerve lesions*

During this period of time 38 cases of radial nerve lesions have been operated upon. In two cases the radial nerve repair was part of a replantation procedure, and these cannot be compared with cases that are solely the consequence of a trauma. In six cases no follow-up was available. A total of 30 cases remained for evaluation. The evaluation was performed according to the force scale M0–M5. The length of the defect is represented in centimetres, as an average plus standard deviation, with the range indicated in parentheses. The age is presented in years as an average with standard deviation, and the range in parentheses. The interval between trauma and repair is given in months, as an average with standard deviation, and the range. From this table it can be seen that 13 of the 30 patients reached level M5. These patients had a defect of 6.8 cm, ranging between 1 and 15 cm. The age of this group averages 32 years, ranging between 11 and 64 years. The interval is 5.7 months, ranging between 1 and 18 months. Twelve cases reached level M4. The length of the defect is 8.2 cm (range 4–12 cm), a little bit longer than in the M5 group. The age of 28.8 years (range 8–69 years) is quite similar. The interval of 8.3 months (range 0–29 months) is longer. The four patients who achieved an M3 result have a defect length of 10.3 cm – again longer than the foregoing groups – and range between 6 and 14 cm. The age of 22 years is rather lower than the age of the other patients, but the interval of 12.7 months (range 3–29 months) is significantly longer. There was only one case with a defect of 10 cm, with an interval of 3 months and an age of 62 years, who did not reach an M3 level. The radial nerve is known as 'the nerve with the best results'. Statistical evaluation shows clearly that the length of the defect and the interval play an important role – more than the age. But even if this becomes clear by statistics, we see that in the M5 group there is a case with a length of defect of 15 cm, and another case with an interval of 18 months. So even long defects and long intervals do not preclude a good functional outcome.

the distances are between 2 and 4 cm. There is some deterioration in distances of 6 cm. And, of course, distances of more than 14 cm do less well, but still satisfactory results could be achieved.

The end-to-end nerve repairs did no better than the grafts.

Radial nerve

The results of radial nerve repair are given in Box 7.1. They are listed according to the M0–M5 scale, which is adequate for radial nerve lesions.

Sciatic nerve

For an evaluation of the results of sciatic nerve repairs we have developed the following system: the results are divided into four levels (0, 1, 2 and 3) according to the criteria shown in Table 7.10.

Level 3 needs more differentiation. It can be due to three different situations:

1. Recovery of tibialis and peroneus nerve-innervated muscles = 3 T + P.
2. Recovery of tibialis nerve-innervated muscles, including tibialis posterior muscle. Transfer of this muscle to provide active extension of the ankle and stabilization against eversion and inversion = 3 T.

Table 7.10 *Evaluation of functional recovery after sciatic nerve lesions*

Level	*Criteria*
0	• No nerve regeneration • The patient cannot stabilize the ankle, he has no active help when lifting the foot (no flexion of the ankle) and promoting the foot (no extension of the ankle) • There are circulatory disturbances when bringing the leg into vertical position • Lack of protective sensibility favours pressure sores
1	• Return of vasomotor function and protective sensibility, the circulatory problems disappear, or are at least tolerable • The danger of pressure sores is avoided • The patient can walk without complaints, using an orthopaedic shoe
2	• Return of active flexion of the ankle (M. triceps surae), walking is improved, the patient can actively press the foot against the ground, they still need an orthopaedic device to provide extension of the ankle and stabilization • At this level patients can usually resume prior activities
3	• Return of active extension and stabilization of the ankle; the patient can walk without an orthopaedic device

Table 7.11 *Analysis of 15 cases of sciatic nerve repairs*

Age of patient (years)	*Length of graft (cm)*	*Time interval elapsed before operation*
Level 0, no cases		
Level 1, 3 cases		
34	13	11 months after accident
34	15	15 months after accident
21	18	10 months after accident
Level 2, 3 cases		
19	8	3 months after accident
30	12	Interval not known
51	7	11 months after accident
Level 3 T, 7 cases		
37	20	4 months after accident
20	5.5	4 months after accident
17	8	4 months after accident
22	10	5 months after accident
18	9	3 months after accident
8	6	No interval; there was a complete paralysis; however, 20% of the nerve was not transected
25	8	7 months after the accident; there was a complete paralysis; however, the nerve was, not completely transected, but only by 80%
Level 3 T + P, 2 patients		
7	9	4 months after accident
18	13	7 months after accident; there was a complete paralysis; however, the nerve was not completely transected, but only by 80%

3. Recovery of tibial nerve-innervated muscles occurs, tibialis posterior transfer for active extension of the ankle and subtalar arthrodesis to provide stability against eversion and inversion = 3 T + A.

Table 7.11 shows the results of analysis of 15 cases of sciatic nerve repairs.

Table 7.11 demonstrates that only 2 cases had a full recovery of peroneus and tibialis innervated muscles: 1 case was a boy of 9 years, and in the other case the sciatic nerve was not completely transected. Seven of the 15 cases achieved a level of 3T, which means that after tibialis posterior transfer, they could walk without splint. Three cases had level 2, and 3 cases had level 1; this means that even with long defects (between 5.5 and 20 cm) satisfactory recovery of the tibialis-innervated muscles can be achieved in at least 50% of the cases. The tibialis posterior transfer provides a satisfactory final result. In 13 cases we achieved only level 1. These cases had very poor chances. The interval between accident and surgery was 10, 11 and 15 months, respectively. The length of the grafts was between 15 and 18 cm.

References

Albert E (1876) Einige Operationen an Nerven, *Wiener Medizinische Presse* **26**: 1285.

Battiston B et al (2003) Communication. II. Congress of the WSRM, Heidelberg, June 11–14, 2003.

Battiston B (2003) *New techniques in brachial plexus repair.* II. Congress of the WSRM, Heidelberg, 11–14 June, 2003.

Breidenbach WB, Terzis JK (1984) The anatomy of free vascularised nerve grafts, *Clin Plast Surg* **11**: 65–71.

Brunelli G (1981) *Direct neurotization of severely damaged muscles.* 36th Annual Meeting of the American Society for Surgery of the Hand, Las Vegas, 23–25 February, 1981.

Brunelli G, Monini L (1984) Neurotization of avulsed roots of brachial plexus by means of anterior nerves of cervicle plexus, *Clin Plast Surg* **11**: 149–52.

Bsteh FX, Millesi H (1960) Zur Kenntnis der zweiseitigen Nerveninterplantation bei ausgedehnten peripheren Nervendefekten, *Klin Med* **12**: 571–8.

Chiu DTW (1980) Autogenous vein graft as a conduit for nerve regeneration, *Surg Forum* **31**: 550.

Curtis RM, Eversman WW Jr (1973) Internal neurolysis as an adjunct to the treatment of the carpal tunnel syndrome, *J Bone Joint Surg* **55A**: 733–40.

Edshage S (1964) Peripheral nerve suture, *Acta Chir Scand* **33**: 1.

Foerster O (1915) Die Schussverletzungen der peripheren Nerven und ihre Behandlung; Report to Ausserord Tagung d Deutsch Orthopäd Ges Berlin, 2–9 February 1916, *Wiener Med Wochenschr* **63**: 283.

Hueter K (1873) *Die Allgemeine Chirurgie* (Verlag Vogel: Leipzig).

Lang J (1962) Über das Bindegewebe und die Gefässe der Nerven, *Anat Embryol* **123**: 61–79.

Langley JN, Hashimoto M (1917) On the suture of separate nerve bundles in a nerve trunk and on internal plexuses, *J Physiol (Lond)* **51**: 318.

Lundborg G, Hansson HA (1979) Regeneration of a peripheral nerve through a preformed tissue space, *Brain Res* **178**: 573.

Lundborg G, Dahlin LB, Danielsen N (1991) Ulnar nerve repair by the silicone chamber technique – case report, *Scand J Plast Reconstr Surg* **25**: 79–82.

Mackinnon SE, Hudson AR, Falk RE et al (1984) The nerve allograft response, an experimental model in the rat, *Ann Plast Surg* **14**: 334–9.

Mackinnon SE (2003) Nerve repair and reconstruction – surgical decision making and technique. American Society for Surgery of the Hand, Chicago, Illinois, September, 2003.

Millesi H (1968) Zum Problem der Überbrückung von Defekten peripherer Nerven, *Wien Med Wochenschr* **118**: 182–97.

Millesi H (1992) *Chirurgie der Peripheren Nerven* (Urban & Schwarzenberg: Munich).

Millesi H (1998) Discussion, Meeting of the Am Soc Periph Nerve, ASPEN, Vancouver, 22–23 May 1998.

Millesi H (2003) *Läsionen peripherer Nerven und radikuläre Syndrome,* Mumenthaler M, Stöhr M, Müller-Vahl H, eds, 8th edn (Thieme Verlag: Stuttgart).

Millesi H, Zoech G, Balogh B (1989) Relation between integumental circumference and subcutaneous pressure in the upper extremity. 6th Congr. Int Soc Plast Reconstr Surg, Istanbul, 3–6 September, 1989.

Nicholson HR, Seddon HJ (1957) Nerve repair in civil practice. Results of treatment of median and ulnar lesions, *BMJ* **II**: 1065.

Oberlin C, Beal D, Leechavengvongs S, Salon A, Dauge MC, Scarcy JJ (1994) Nerve transfer to biceps muscle using a part of ulnar nerve for C5-C6 avulsion of the brachial plexus: anatomical study and report of four cases, *J Hand Surg* **19A**: 232–7.
Seddon HJ (1943) Three types of nerve injury, *Brain* **66**: 237.
Seddon HJ (1947) The use of autogenous grafts for the repair of large gaps in peripheral nerves, *Br J Surg* **35**: 151.
Seddon HJ (1972) *Surgical Disorders of the Peripheral Nerves* (Churchill Livingstone: Edinburgh).
Spencer PS, Weinberg HJ, Raine CS et al (1975) The perineurial window – a new model of focal demyelination and myelination, *Brain Res* **96**: 323–9.
Strange FGStC (1947) An operation for nerve pedicle grafting, preliminary communication, *Br J Surg* **34**: 423.
Sunderland S (1951) A classification of peripheral nerve injuries producing loss of function, *Brain* **74**: 491.
Taylor GI, Ham FJ (1976) The free vascularized nerve graft, *Plast Reconstr Surg* **57**: 413–26.
Van Beek A (1989) Communication: Making up a gap in a major nerve defect. 5th Annual Meeting of the American Society for Reconstructive Microsurgery, Seattle, Washington, 11–12 September 1989.
Viterbo F (1994) Two end-to-side neurorrhaphies and nerve graft with removal of the epineural sheath: experimental study in rats *Br J Plast Surg* **47**: 75–80.

8 Tendon transfers: general considerations

François Moutet

Introduction

Tendon transfer was first used by Nicoladoni in 1880 in Vienna, then Codovilla (1899) and Lange in 1900 introduced this type of surgical treatment for motor paralysis of the upper limb. The general principles have been gradually set down through the works of Biesalski and Mayer (1916), Steindler (1939), Bunnell (1948), Boyes (1960, 1970), Tubiana (1969) and Brand (1985).

Nowadays, the need for tendon transfers is less frequently due to lack of postoperative regrowth and poor surgical results, because of constant improvements in the quality of nerve sutures. However, the increased occurrence of traumatic avulsions and ballistic lesions has led to the same levels of requirement for restoration of function as before. These procedures have to be adapted for each patient according to the remaining motor muscles.

It must be borne in mind that a tendon transfer can only achieve limited goals, because one muscle is required to replace the function of several. In fact, 39 muscles are required to ensure wrist and hand movements and it is clear that a limited amount of transfers cannot achieve complete restoration of these complex movements. Regarding the level of the lesion, tendon transfers have to restore function that has been lost and not the function of one paralyzed muscle. Obviously several goals require several sophisticated tendon transfers. In the case of isolated nerve palsy, many transferable muscles are available, as well as a choice of techniques.

Indications

The opportune time to carry out a tendon transfer depends on the cause, level and evolution of the lesion. The results of successful nerve repair are far superior to tendon transfers. However, in traumatic conditions, tendon transfers are indicated after 18 months if no clinical and electrical reinnervation occurs after suture, or when nerve repair has failed or when the nerve is irreparable.

The average speed of nerve growth is 1 mm per day. Thus recovery of a middle arm lesion will need 200–300 days (approximately 6 months to 1 year) to reach the motor end plates of the extrinsic muscle at the forearm level and 500–600 days (2 years) to reach the intrinsic musculature at the palm level. However, isolated nerve lesions may produce surprising results and reinnervation may occur 12–18 months after suture. Therefore, it is worthwhile delaying tendon transfer surgery in the early stages after injury. Furthermore, external splinting may be useful and well accepted by the patient, and allows time for nerve regeneration.

Some authors have proposed early palliative surgery, arguing the value of the internal splinting effect of the tendon transfers while waiting for reinnervation. This is a valid option for the opposition palsy as regards the delay in intrinsic muscle recuperation in cases of proximal nerve lesion, but it is not always useful. For example, in radial palsy it seems not to be worthwhile. Furthermore if reinnervation occurs, it may lead to problematic imbalance in finger and wrist motion due to conflict between tendon transfers and reinnervated muscles. This may lead to a poor functional result.

In the case of chronic neurological diseases, transfers will be performed only after evaluation of prognosis and evolution. In others, like leprosy, they will be performed after medical treatment and stabilization.

There are no hard and fast rules, and the needs of the patient must be considered. Profession, age, the use of a partially paralyzed dominant hand, functional substitutes, associated lesions and the cause of the palsy are important. Each element of the procedure as regards the motor muscle, tendon path, and tendon fixation must be adapted to each case. Variations in muscle innervation patterns, individual joint mechanics, muscle anatomy, and patients' abilities have to be considered.

When several functions need to be restored, it is preferable to restore movements from proximal to distal and plan as many operations as necessary.

Sensation of the hand must also be evaluated before operation. In fact, the best restoration will remain unused if the patient has no sensation, and the hand will stay protected and hidden in the pocket.

Once the program is established, the surgeon must communicate it to the patient in simple comprehensive terms and also to the physiotherapist in order to maximize rehabilitation potential.

General technical considerations

The operative technique is of great importance and considerably influences the results. For all tendon transfer procedures some basic rules must be respected and may be summarized in the 'Ten Commandments', as in Table 8.1. General rules regarding hemostasis, asepsis and care while stowing the tendons to be transferred are well known and must be carefully followed. The tendon has to be manipulated with a traction suture. Whenever possible, it is passed through a tunnel created by blunt forceps. The tension given to the transferred tendons must provide the optimal correction in the passive position: if it is too loose there will be no function, if it is too tight function will be impossible and the muscle may become non-functional.

It is essential to minimize the creation of adhesions, which will limit the tendon excursion. The surgical technique should be as kind as possible to the tissues, avoiding traumatic dissection. The tendon should be passed through natural cleavage planes or in subcutaneous fat whenever possible, and contact between the transferred muscle and cut fascia surfaces or bone denuded of periosteum must be avoided.

The skin incision should be judiciously planned so that the scar will not hinder the gliding of the tendon transfer. Bulky sutures should be avoided and suture lines should preferably be located at a distance from fixed fibrous formation.

During the operative procedure, muscular relaxation must be optimal and general anesthesia may be preferred to incomplete local plexus anesthesia. Peridural injection can be used for a tetraplegic patient; this allows voluntary control of the muscular function at the end of the surgical procedure.

Complications may occur in tendon transfer surgery during the postoperative period – particularly hematoma, ruptures, and adhesions. These must be avoided by the use of a very non-traumatic and careful technique during the operative procedure as noted above. A rupture is difficult to diagnose during immobilization and not easy to repair, but repair must be achieved. Adhesions may be treated by tenolysis, but never before the sixth month postoperatively, and they need very skilful and careful rehabilitation.

Table 8.1 The 'Ten Commandments'

1	Do not be prejudicial
2	Take great care of soft tissue equilibrium
3	Choose a motor muscle with the right strength
4	Choose a motor muscle with the right amplitude
5	Forget agonism/antagonism
6	Choose a muscle of grade 4+ or more for transfer
7	Choose the straightest trajectory
8	Avoid sharp angles in the path of the transfer
9	Obtain adequate function by adequate distal fixation
10	Be very attentive to rehabilitation

Specific practical considerations

The main problem in carrying out tendon transfers is to obtain active harmonious hand function and not a simple tenodesis effect. The 'Ten Commandments' (Table 8.1) summarize practical considerations for tendon transfers. The surgeon must always keep in mind the fact that the simpler the action of a tendon transfer, the more likely it is to succeed.

1. Do not be prejudicial

The consequences of removing the motor muscle and the compensation required for the newly created deficit must be anticipated. The gain must obviously outweigh the created deficit.

Sometimes technical points have to be discussed. For example, flexor digitorum superficialis of the fourth finger (FDS IV) is the most versatile motor muscle and is often used, especially for restoration of the thumb while preserving a certain amount of digital independence. However, the harvesting of two FDS (third and fourth) following Boyes (1960, 1970) for radial palsy restoration, may be damaging for grasp and grip strength in manual workers. It must be remembered that 'the closer to the normal you are, the less normal you feel'. This is especially true with tendon transfers.

2. Take great care of soft tissue equilibrium

Unfortunately this problem is not emphasized enough. The soft tissue equilibrium is one of the main conditions to look after regarding tendon transfers. The clinician must always verify that the desired movements are possible passively. If they are limited, a transfer cannot restore them entirely. Indeed, the strongest transfer will not be able to move a stiffened joint or a retracted first web space. Thus, the state of the joints must be evaluated – not only their passive ROM, but also their stability – and they must be treated first.

An undermined tunnel in a scar zone will not provide appropriate gliding surfaces for the transfer. So, resurfacing the scar surfaces with cutaneous flaps, restoring passive motion by arthrolysis of a stiffened joint or freeing a retracted first web space, are sometimes the first steps to restoration of any function. Even bone fixation or osteotomy may be needed at this stage. At the thumb level the need for TMC joint mobility and MCP joint stability must be emphasized. This is of great importance to restoration of opposition

3. Choose a motor muscle with the right strength

Choice of the motor muscle must take into consideration strength and amplitude. When planning a tendon transfer, the strength of the muscle proposed for transfer and the strength of the paralyzed muscle must be compared. Moreover, this factor has to be adapted to obtain the final function required.

An electrical examination of the muscles available for transfer can be useful, especially when the muscles have been affected by palsy and have subsequently recovered.

Regarding strength and excursion of the transferable muscles, the classical values as proposed by Brand et al (1981) may be retained.

When not enough muscles are available (traumatic loss of substance of the forearm, gunshot wound etc.), a simplified method has to be chosen. For example, in radial palsy a simplified method for restoration of finger function when not enough muscles are usable consists of the transfer of FDS IV to extensor digitorum communis (EDC) without transferring a second muscle to restore active wrist extension. This is sufficient to restore passive wrist extension, which follows digit extension and leads to a useful function.

When there is no suitable transferable material at all, the utility of free muscle transfers as proposed by Tamai in 1970 and well demonstrated in clinical cases by Manktelow (1986) may be considered.

4. Choose a motor muscle with the right amplitude

The choice of the motor muscle must take into consideration length and amplitude. The ideal motor muscle should have good length and great amplitude, be powerful, and be long enough to reach the desired distal insertion regarding the final function wanted. A tendon graft may be used as an extension if necessary, but all sutures are sources of adhesion. Furthermore, it must be remembered that most of the vascularization of the transferred tendon is destroyed; thus the transfer will behave like a graft and must have sufficient nutrition from the bed to survive. Once again, the condition of the soft tissue is of great importance.

5. Forget agonism/antagonism

The old rule that an antagonist muscle should not be chosen for transfer may be forgotten if all the other conditions are fulfilled. In fact, cerebral plasticity allows motor reintegration regardless of the original muscle function.

6. Choose a muscle of grade 4+ or more for transfer

A list should be made of the muscles of the limb, rating their strength according to the international five-grade classification established by the Medical Research Council. This allows compilation of a list of muscles available for transfer. It is usually better not to transfer a muscle rated <4+ in this classification.

The old dogma – which stated that one degree was systematically lost when a muscle was transferred – must be forgotten. Loss of strength is only due to the mechanical conditions of the transfer trajectory and gliding. At high pressure levels, such as those produced by sharp angles and pulleys, a lot of strength may be lost.

7. Choose the straightest trajectory

The direction of a transfer must be as straight as possible. Any angulation reduces the power conveyed and this reduction will be proportional to the degree of the angle. However, these changes in direction are sometimes essential (opponenplasties) and are made around a pulley.

For a long time transfer trajectories were only subcutaneous, even around ulna or radius borders. Then transfers always had to be long and might have the disadvantage of crossing scarred zones. Duparc et al (1971) emphasized the benefit of direct trajectory through the interosseous membrane. With this straighter trajectory, the transfer gains in length and strength. This path has to be carefully realized. When traversing the interosseous membrane in the forearm the orifice must be proximal enough (proximal border of the pronator quadratus) to avoid marked angulation. The window must be large enough (and not just a hole) so that the motor muscle belly and its tendon can glide freely without any torsion, avoiding loss of strength and then loss of function. This is even more important when two or three muscle bellies (Boyes 1960) have to pass through it and must have a perfect gliding space at the proximal border of the pronator quadratus. Injury to the interosseous pedicles should be avoided.

It is always better to use the interosseous membrane trajectory when harvesting a tendon from one aspect of the forearm to transfer it to another. As noted above, it produces increased strength, usually avoids the need for grafting, and allows much more choice in pulley location if needed. Thus it allows a better attack angle and diminishes the area of high pressure and the loss of strength and function of all transfers.

8. Avoid sharp angles in the path of the transfer

As stated earlier, pulleys are sometimes needed. They must be designed to minimize the localized area of high pressure. If they are too narrow or create a sharp bend, they may break or stretch or cause obstruction to tendon gliding. They have to be strong, stable, sufficiently wide, and must not create sharp angles in the path of the transfers. They have to be far enough from the distal insertion of the transfer so that it can glide on a sufficient length to obtain a good range of motion. Obviously, the ideal pulley does not exist, but it is needed as soon as the motor muscle does not pull in the right direction to restore function – which is a rather frequent condition. Then the pulley will give the pulling direction and the attack angle of the transfer. Pulleys have to be in the optimal location to improve this attack angle and facilitate the goal of the transfer.

Thus the attack angle of the transfer to its distal fixation depends on the trajectory given to the tendon by the pulley location. This is especially important as regards opponensplasty, and is discussed in Chapter 11. The more proximal and radial the transfer, the more important the anteposition will be; the more distal and medial, the more adduction will be obtained.

9. Obtain adequate function by adequate distal fixation

Regardless of what type of palsy is treated, the distal fixation of the transfer actually creates the motion. This movement has to be as close as possible to the physiological one; thus, distal fixation of the transfer must be very precisely done.

If a monoarticular tendon becomes biarticular through its transfer, it first acts on the proximal joint. If the joint is not stabilized by an antagonist muscle, it is only after achieving the entire range of motion that this tendon can act on the more distal joint, providing sufficient amplitude.

Evaluation of the level of the tension to give to the transfer in this part of the procedure is a delicate technical point; usually it comes from experience. Insufficient tension will lead to an ineffective transfer. Too taut tension is harmful and can even cause fibrous degeneration of the motor muscle. Littler (1977) emphasized the ability of the transferred muscle to find good tension, provided the transferred muscle is not too stretched. Zancolli (1979) evaluated the tension given to a transfer in a very pragmatic way and Brand and Hollister (1999) clarified the evaluation. Arriving at harmonious tension in the transfer of a tendon is a delicate matter. For example, what about one to four or five as in the case of restoration of digital extension? This is certainly one of the trickiest parts of the procedure. It must be done with regard to wrist flexion or extension, aiming to reproduce the physiological extension balance of the digits.

Changing the distal insertion site and the attack angle of the transfer may also mitigate some insufficiencies in length or excursion. Then the moment arm value must be changed to reinforce function. A short tendon must be powerful and have a great attack angle. A weak transfer has to be fixed as distally as possible. A short excursion transfer has to be powerful and have a great attack angle (Figure 8.1).

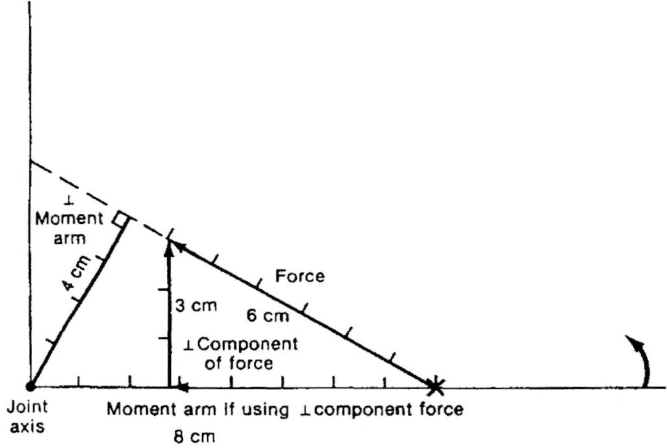

Figure 8.1

Force is divided into two components. The vertical component is perpendicular to the lever arm to be moved. The point of application of force is marked with an X. Either of the two methods indicated can be used to determine the moment of force around the joint axis. Then, the clinician can modify the moment arm and reinforce function. (From Tubiana R, ed., *The Hand*, Vol. III. WB Saunders: Philadelphia, 1988, p. 86.)

At the end of the procedure the clinician must aim to achieve an optimal position for reproducing the desired function. The length of the transfer sometimes dictates the wrist position.

10. Be very attentive to rehabilitation

The postoperative period of rigid immobilization is 1 month in a forearm cast or even in a dynamic splint maintaining the joints in the optimal corrected position, and the wrist in functional or neutral position.

It is very useful to encourage slight motion of the restored limb during the period of immobilization, and of the sound side, to activate the cortical reintegration of the transferred muscles. This biofeedback mechanism is often efficient.

Free active mobilization is started on day 30 after surgery; after the period of immobilization this is carried out without any movements against resistance before day 45 after surgery. Rehabilitation has to recover and reinforce articular motion, soft tissue trophicity and function integration. It must be carried out by a specialized physical therapist as often as possible. The final result may be appreciated around the third month after surgery. The sensorimotor rehabilitation must be done daily for as long as necessary.

Special circumstances

When associated nervous lesions have to be treated, after an upper arm level injury, this is a severe condition and it is sometimes necessary to carry out wrist arthrodesis and then use the liberated tendons for transfer. High level three trunks palsy is a very severe condition close to that of the tetraplegic hand, and the process of restoration will use the remaining possibilities – which are very few – but 'when you have nothing, a little is a lot'.

Results

Results may be appreciated in grip strength; wrist, fingers and thumb function; functional ability and natural synchronism of wrist; fingers and thumb mobility. Sometimes what appears to be a good functional result according to the patient may be viewed differently in physiological terms by the surgeon; particularly when a tenodesis effect is observed in wrist flexion at the extensor digitorum level.

Analysis of the final result is obtained around the third month postoperatively, but is usually useful around the sixth month. A good technique performed in good conditions will be maintained over time, and not only in adults but equally in children.

Conclusions

Whatever motor muscle has been chosen, as regards the remaining motor muscles and the whole therapeutic project, it has to contribute to optimal trajectory and distal fixation. Its choice has only to follow the general principles of tendon transfers according to the 'Ten Commandments' outlined above.

Thus it could be said that motor muscle choice is the least important part of the problem of tendon transfers: distal fixation, attack angle, and gliding are the crucially important factors.

References

Biesalski K, Mayer L (1916) *Die Physiologische Sehnerverpflanzung* (Springer: Berlin) 330.

Boyes JH (1960) Tendon transfer for radial paralysis. *Bull Hosp Joint Dis* **21**: 97–105.

Boyes JH (1970) *Bunnell's Surgery of the Hand*, 5th edn. (JB Lippincott: Philadelphia) 409.

Brand PW (1985) *Clinical Mechanics of the Hand* (CV Mosby: St Louis).

Brand PW, Beach RB, Thomsen DE (1981) Relative tension and potential excursion of muscles in the forearm and hand, *J Hand Surg* **6**: 209.

Brand PW, Hollister AM (1999) *Clinical Mechanics of the Hand* (CV Mosby: St Louis).

Bunnell S (1948) *Surgery of the Hand*, 2nd edn (JB Lippincott: Philadelphia).

Codovilla A (1899) Sui trapienti tendinei nella practica orthopedia, *Archivo d'Orthopedia* **16**: 225.

Duparc J, Caffiniére de la JY, Roux JP (1971) Les plasties d'ópposition par le transplantation tendineuse à travers la membrane interosseuse, *Rev Chir Orthop* **57**: 29.

Littler JW (1977) Restoration of power and stability in the partially paralyzed hand. In: Converse JM, ed., *Reconstructive Surgery*, 2nd edn (WB Saunders: Philadelphia) 32–66

Macktelow RT (1986) Functional muscle transplantation. In: *Microvascular Reconstruction* (Springer: Berlin) 151–64.

Nicoladoni C (1880) Em Vorschlag zur Sehnennaht, *Wien Med Wochenschr* **30**: 144.

Steindler A (1939) Tendon transplantation in the upper extremity, *Am J Surg* **44**: 260.

Tubiana R (1969) Anatomic and physiologic basis for the surgical treatment of paralysis of the hand, *J Bone Joint Surg* **51A**: 643.

Tubiana R, Brockman R (1988) Tendon transfers: theoretical and practical considerations. In: Tubiana R, ed., *The Hand*, Vol. III. (WB Saunders: Philadelphia) 79.

Zancolli E (1979) *Structural and Dynamic Basis of Hand Surgery*, 2nd edn. (JB Lippincott: Philadelphia) 238.

9 Paralysis of flexion and extension of the elbow

P Raimondi and M Del Bene

Deficit of elbow function has a great impact, especially on elbow flexion. An upper arm with good shoulder function and a normal hand but with deficit of elbow flexion is severely impaired to the point that even the hand loses a great amount of its use. On the contrary, deficit of elbow extension is often considered a minor loss thanks to the compensating action of gravity that allows a spontaneous passive extension. This fact is not always true and the specific conditions in which even elbow extension is of paramount importance will be described in this article.

The most frequently utilized muscle and tendon transfers will be reviewed, with particular regard to those that have been used systematically by the authors over the years and have proved to be effective in their personal experience.

As in all palliative surgery it is important to evaluate the cause of paralysis and assess which motors are available to compensate for the deficit. Thus it is not a matter of the surgeon's choice but rather a balanced evaluation of all the different available motors and the patient's needs. The cosmetic effects must also be taken into consideration when choosing the muscle transfer, especially in young female patients.

Another crucial point is the timing of these palliative operations. It is a general rule to wait for a complete assessment after neurosurgical repair, which means at least 2 years. In children it is better to wait until they are 3–4 years old so as to achieve a greater degree of cooperation for the rehabilitation programme.

Transfers for elbow flexion

Among the various techniques for restoring elbow flexion that have been described only those that have proved to be the most suitable in terms of functional results either in the literature or in the authors' own experience will be selected.

Latissimus dorsi transfer

The indication for this transfer is classically described mainly in sequelae of brachial plexus lesions in which the function of latissimus dorsi (LD) has been spared. Nevertheless, depending on its innervation (usually from C6,C7,C8), this muscle is not always completely normal and cannot be utilized safely for transfer in upper palsy of the plexus. The frequent anatomical variation of C7 sometimes makes this muscle weak and the results of transfer are often disappointing. It is therefore of paramount importance to evaluate its strength correctly before indicating a transfer. The sequelae of obstetric paralysis can give rise to a different situation: spontaneous reinnervation may lead to a strong muscle even in upper root involvement and therefore its use may be more effective.

Schottstaedt et al in 1955 and Hovnanian in 1956 described the LD transfer and later Zancolli and Mitre (1973) contributed to its popularity. This transfer can be performed in two different ways: either the muscle can be transferred while maintaining its bony insertion to the humerus (monopolar transfer) or the whole muscle can be detached while maintaining its neurovascular pedicle and transferred by performing two new insertions to the arm (bipolar transfer). A bipolar transfer is suggested by the authors whenever possible. This can reproduce the anatomical axis of the biceps, thus improving the functional result and avoiding the adduction effect of a monopolar transfer. But sometimes, especially with a poor pectoralis function, a monopolar transfer of LD can maintain a certain degree of adduction together with elbow flexion that can be useful in severe cases. To avoid unnecessary compression on the muscle once it has been transferred to the arm, it is sometimes useful to raise the muscular flap together with a cutaneous island flap.

Technique (Figures 9.1 and 9.2)

The patient lies in supine position and their hemithorax is elevated using a rolled up sheet as a support: this makes the access to the posterior part of the muscle easier. If a cutaneous island flap is taken with the muscle, it must be drawn on the anterior part of the muscle, centred on the main vascular axis, towards the posterior iliac spine. The entrance of the neurovascular pedicle into the muscle is approximately 9–10 cm distal to the bony insertion onto the humerus and this must be taken into account.

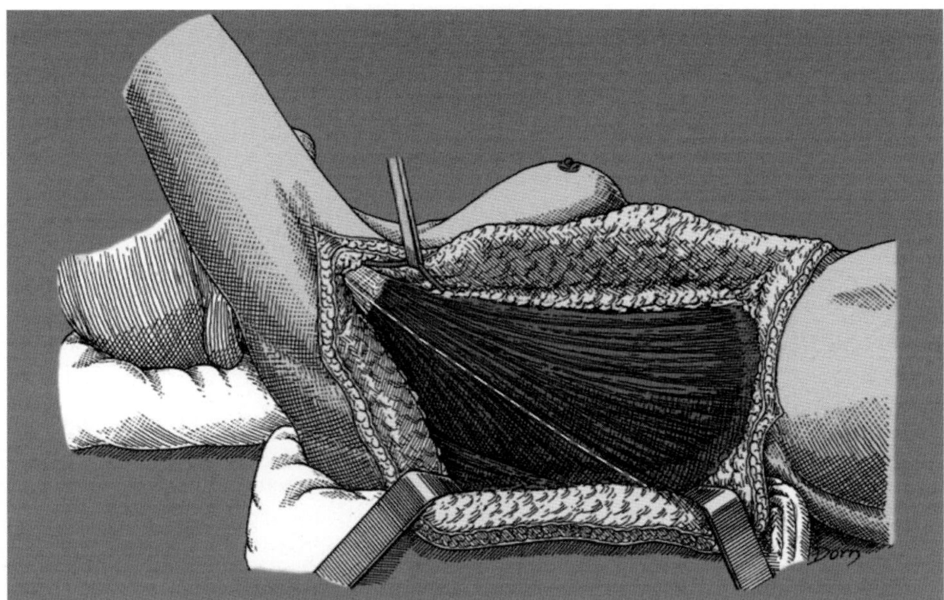

(A)

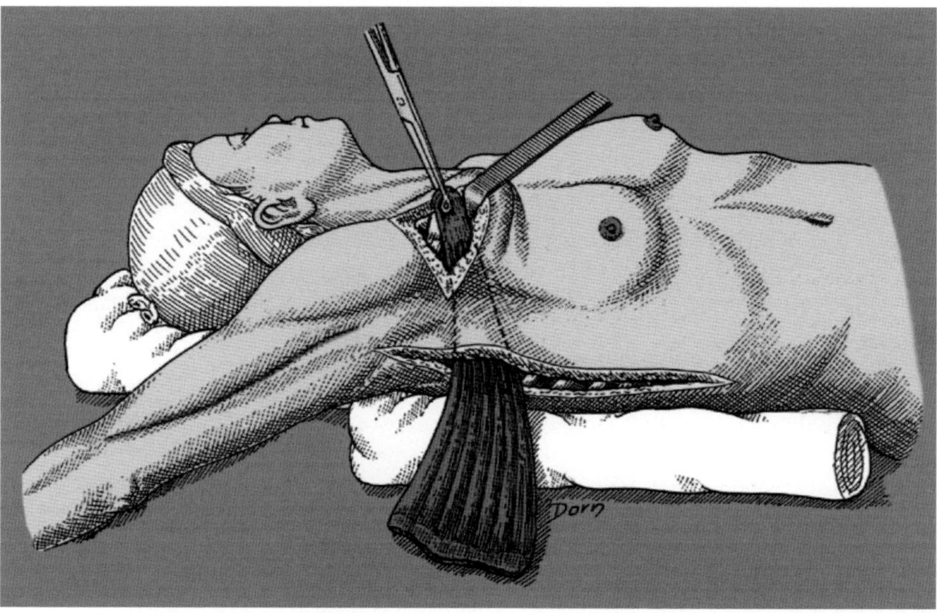

(B)

Figure 9.1

(A) The LD and the vascular pedicle have been exposed.

(B) The humeral tendon and the caudal insertion have been detached. The muscle is in continuity only by its neurovascular pedicle and its caudal part is passed through a subcutaneous tunnel.

A straight incision is traced along the anterior margin of the LD muscle from the posterior axillary fold, so as to reach the tendon insertion to the humerus and the distal muscular insertion to the thorax. The muscle is totally exposed by means of a wide subcutaneous dissection, leaving the skin island in place. The thin fascia of LD muscle must be spared. The subcutaneous margins of the island are secured to the muscular fascia with sutures, to avoid damaging perforating vessels. The posterior superior margin of LD is then separated at the angle of the scapula from the teres major muscle. Remember that these two muscles have a common tendon that can easily be split to maintain both the teres major muscle and its insertion intact.

At this point the whole muscle is exposed with the neurovascular bundle under control. As the muscle is longer than the biceps that it is going to substitute, the muscle does not necessarily have to be completely raised caudally before sectioning the tendon and raising the muscle. For this purpose it is useful to measure the length of the arm (from the coracoid process to the biceps tendon) to raise the LD in such a way that the

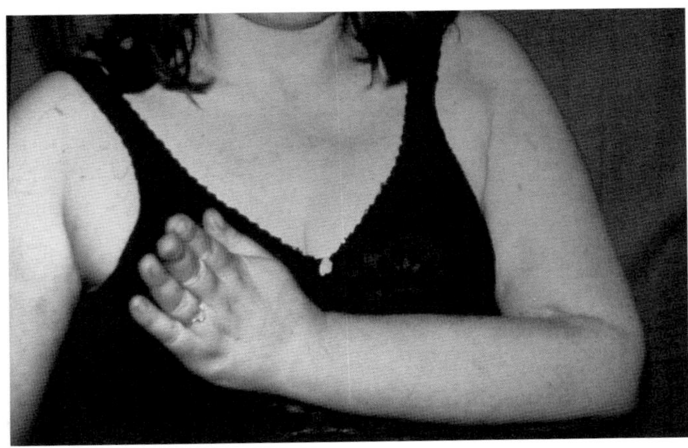

(A)

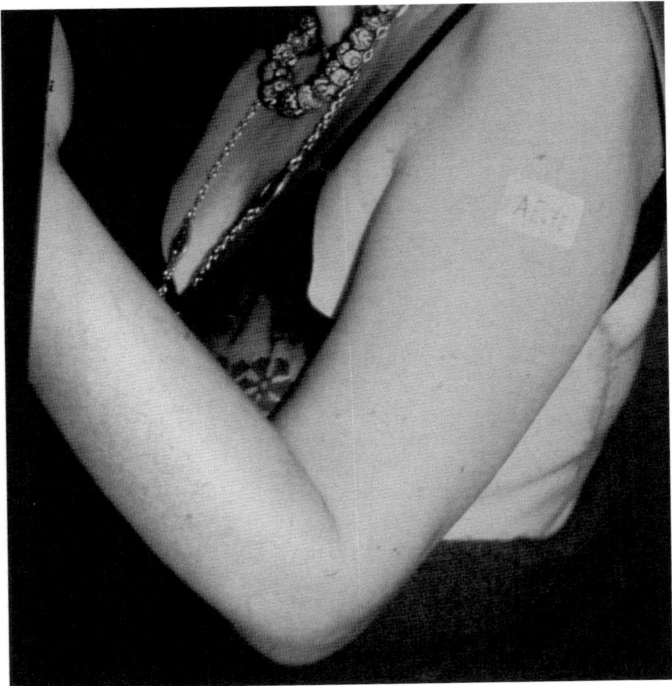

(B)

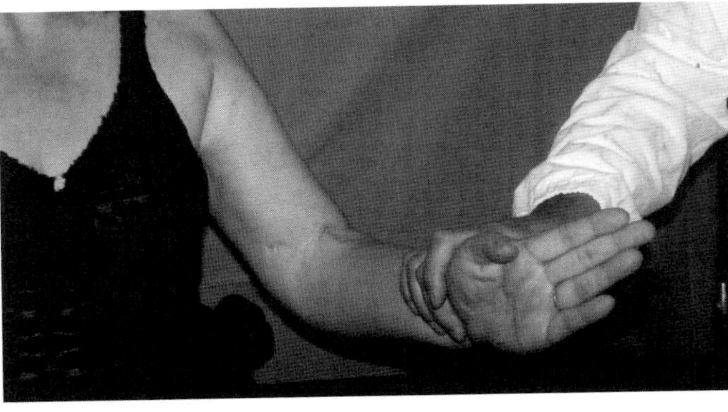

(C)

Figure 9.2

(A–C) The result of monopolar LD transfer to biceps in a female patient: a posterior scar is far more acceptable than a pectoral one: the force is 8 kg.

transfer will fit well in the arm. This is a crucial point: on some occasions reduced function of the transfer has been observed owing to the excessive length of the muscle, thus requiring secondary shortening of the transfer.

Before sectioning the tendon and completely raising the muscle the authors suggest that a subcutaneous tunnel is prepared under the axillary region to allow the tendon to reach its new insertion to the coracoid process. This will prevent unnecessary tension on the neurovascular pedicle. The detachment of the LD from the posterior insertion to the thoracic wall and the lumbodorsal fascia produces bleeding owing to the perforators to the intercostal vessels; therefore careful haemostasis must be performed to avoid possible haematomas or seromas in this wide undermined area. Anteriorly the LD is separated from the serratus anterior muscle. The inferior border is then detached taking into account that it is useless to reach the iliac crest, as already mentioned.

The distal part of the muscle is then rolled up to form a tendon that will be inserted to the biceps tendon. The muscle is rolled up and its margins are sutured up to the entrance point of the neurovascular bundle, and care is taken not to compress it. A flat muscle has therefore been transformed into a cylindrical-shaped muscle.

At this point a skin incision on the delto-pectoral groove exposes the coracoid process and completes the subcutaneous tunnel under which the tendon of the LD will be passed to be reinserted onto the bone with a strong non-resorbable suture. On the anterior aspect of the arm a straight incision goes from the anterior margin of the axilla to the biceps tendon. If possible the three incisions should not communicate with each other, so as to prevent unnecessary scar retractions. A slight subcutaneous undermining of the margins is performed until it is felt that the LD transfer fits into the arm without tension. Special care must be taken with the distal insertion, as we are dealing with a pseudo-tendon of the LD which does not have the same consistency and resistance as a normal tendon. Reinforced non-absorbable sutures will fix not only its tendon to the biceps tendon but even more proximally will fix the transfer to the musculotendinous portion of the biceps.

The authors suggest that the distal reinsertion is performed first, which will allow better closure of the skin wound and final adjustment of the correct tension at the time of the proximal bony reinsertion to the coracoid. Apart from a more practical closure of the wide surgical wounds, this will protect the pedicle, which will be loose rather than stretched at the time the final tension for the reinsertion is determined.

At the end of the operation a good tension of the transfer must be proved: resistance must be recorded in the attempt to extend the elbow that must maintain itself in flexion against gravity.

Suction drains are inserted, one in the arm and two in the donor area due to the wide exposure.

The arm is then immobilized in a plaster cast in adduction with the elbow flexed at 50° for 5 weeks.

Pectoralis major transfer

Pectoralis major (PM) is a wide muscle innervated by two different nerves – the lateral pectoral nerve which innervates the clavicular part and the medial pectoral nerve which innervates the sternocostal part. The two nerves are formed by different roots; the lateral pectoral nerve comes from C5,C6,C7 while the medial pectoral nerve comes from C8 and T1. This means that apart from very few circumstances, in brachial plexus lesions the PM muscle is nearly always involved at least partially in the paralysis. In upper plexus palsies, which are the case with lack of elbow flexion, the upper part of the PM is also paralysed. Therefore the transfer will make use only of the sternocostal portion.

Clark (1946) first described the transfer of the sternocostal portion on the biceps. Brooks and Seddon (1959) described the transfer of the long head of the biceps (the muscle belly of which is split from the short head) on the PM tendon sectioned at its insertion. Merle d'Aubigné (1956) was the first to describe a bipolar transfer of the sternocostal portion of PM to the coracoid proximally and to the biceps tendon distally. Dautry et al (1977) described the transfer of nearly the whole muscle, leaving only a thin external part of the clavicular portion; moreover, they lengthened the muscle, elevating a segment of rectus abdominis sheath to obtain a distal tendon that could easily and strongly attach the transfer to the biceps tendon. This suggestion had already been decribed by Seddon (1947). One year later Carrol and Kleinman (1979) wrote an article that popularized this technique, utilizing the whole PM with the advantage of utilizing both neurovascular pedicles. Some other changes have been described, such as the cephalad fixation to the acromion instead of the coracoid process. Tsai et al (1983) suggested the associated transfer of PM and pectoralis minor. The bipolar transfer has an unquestionable biomechanical advantage due to the more physiological position of the transfer on the appropriate axis of the biceps and moreover helps to stabilize the glenohumeral joint.

Therefore the indication for PM transfer would be ideal in pure lack of elbow flexion with a normal PM. This happens very rarely, as in sequelae of an isolated musculocutaneous lesion or in arthrogryposis, while in brachial plexus lesions as already mentioned the PM hardly ever is completely functioning. Moreover, in severe brachial plexus lesions with incomplete recovery of arm adductors, the lack of function of PM transferred for elbow flexion deprives the arm of the only adductor left. For this reason in these circumstances the authors prefer to utilize the transfer in a monopolar way, leaving the entire clavicular insertion in situ to obtain flexion of the elbow together with arm adduction. In the authors' opinion another contraindication is in female patients, because the scars are in a very visible area. Whenever possible a LD transfer will be indicated in female patients.

Technique (Figures 9.3–9.6)

The Carrol technique consists of a curved incision extending from the 7th sternocostal joint directed upward and laterally towards the lateral half of the clavicle, 2 cm under it. The incision is then continued to the deltopectoral groove until the insertion of the tendon of PM to the humerus. The entire muscle is exposed together with the margin of the acromion; the PM is then totally detached from the clavicular and sternocostal insertions. Caudally the muscle is detached together with a strip of anterior rectus abdominis fascia approximately 8–10 cm long and 4 cm wide. Then the humeral tendon is completely divided.

Care must be taken throughout the operation to avoid stretching or damaging the neurovascular pedicles, as both are maintained in place. The muscle (the distal part of which has been rolled into a tube) is now rotated 90° on its pedicles and the distal part of the muscle with its new prolonged tendon is passed through a subcutaneous tunnel to insert to the distal tendon of the biceps at the elbow. The cranial tendon crossing the anterior glenohumeral capsule is then fixed under relative tension by means of non-resorbable sutures to the anterior border of the acromion.

After careful haemostasis, suction drains are applied and skin closure is performed. Thoracobrachial immobilization with elbow flexed at 50° in plaster will be maintained for 6 weeks.

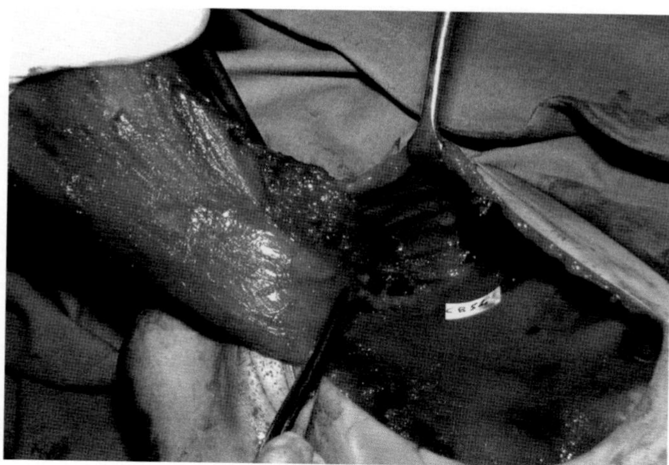

Figure 9.3
The vascular pedicle has been isolated.

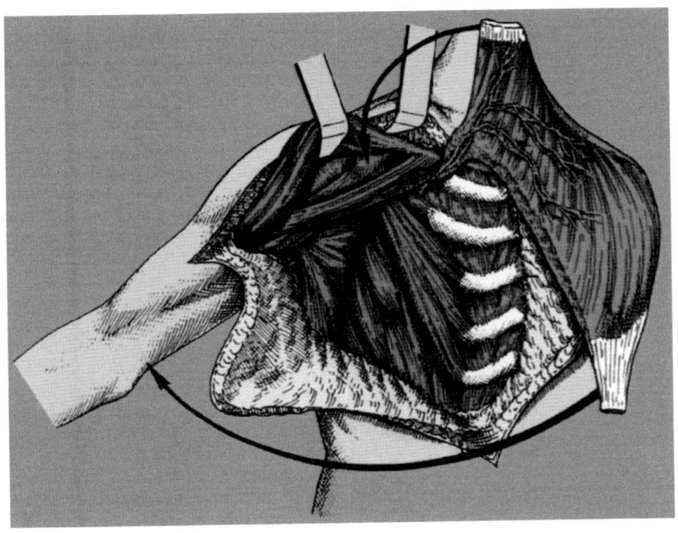

(A)

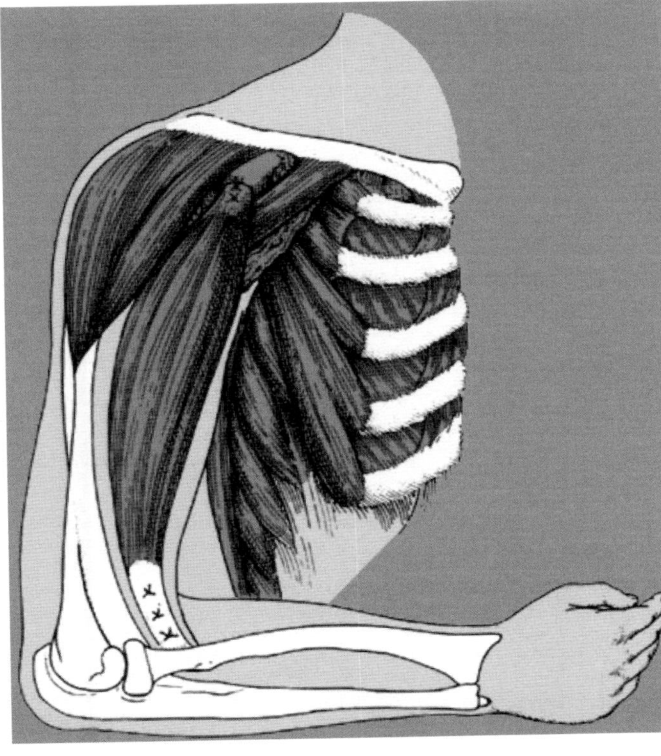

(B)

Figure 9.4

(A) The muscle is completely detached except for its lateral portion, to protect the vascular pedicle.

(B) The muscle in its new position with the distal suture to the biceps and the proximal insertion to the coracoid.

We have utilized a variation of this technique as described by Dautry et al (1977) on some occasions with good results. The lateral third of PM is left in place and the cranial tendon is fixed to the coracoid instead of the acromion.

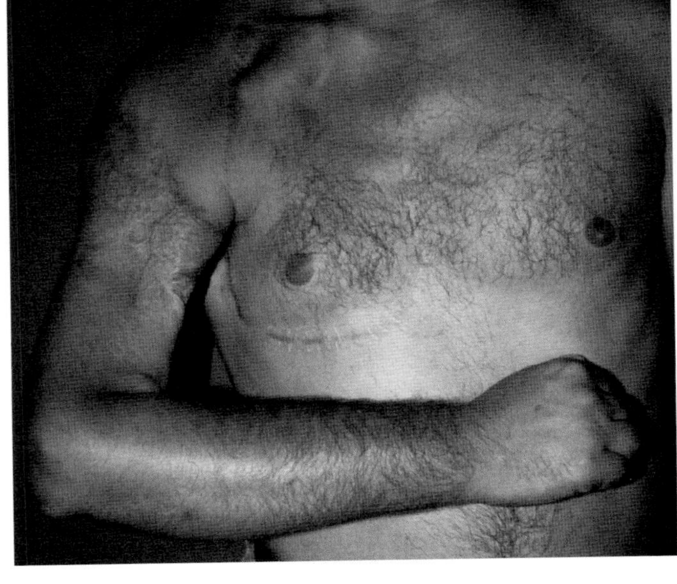

(A)

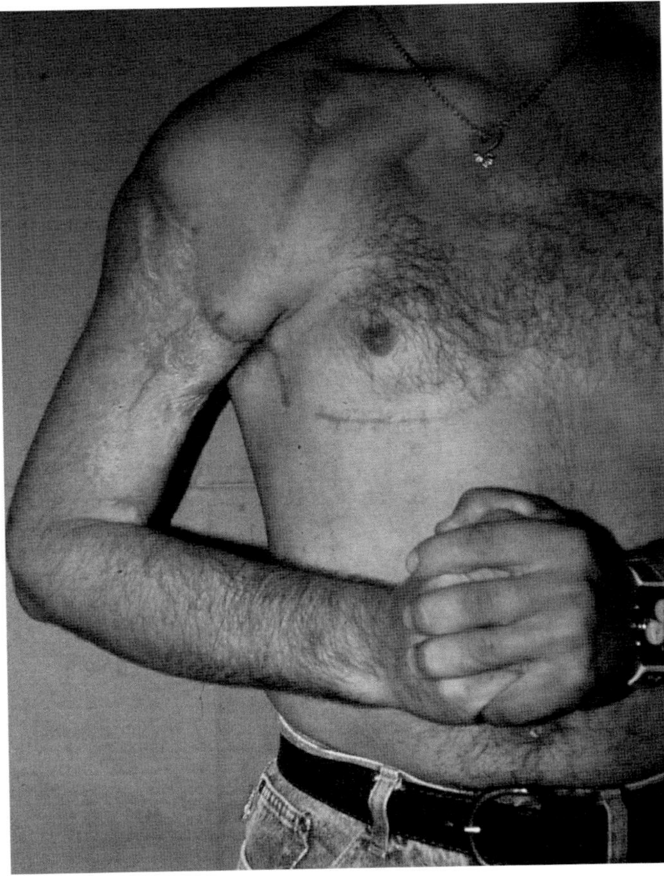

(B)

Figure 9.5

(A) Result after a bipolar transfer of pectoralis major, the incisions have been modified utilizing the deltopectoral incision to detach the clavicular portion of the muscle.

(B) Flexion of the elbow against a strong resistance (6 kg).

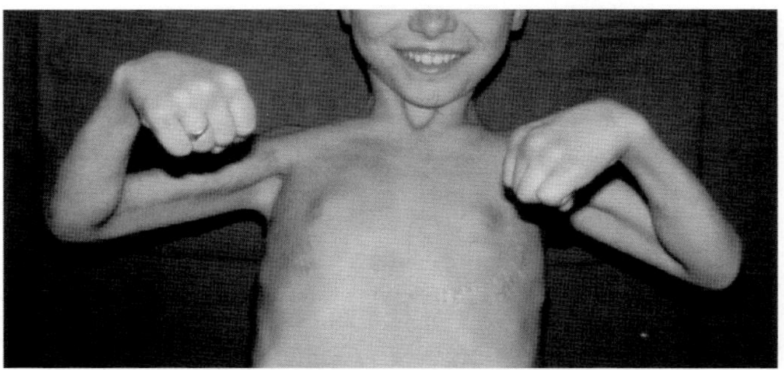

Figure 9.6
Result of a double pectoralis major transfer in arthrogryposis.

A similar technique has been described by Tsai et al (1983). A variation comprises the utilization of both pectoralis major and minor muscles with the aim of reducing the possible damage to both neurovascular bundles which are located laterally to the middle portion of the clavicle and at the same time to reinforce the strength of PM by adding the action of pectoralis minor, the coracoid insertion of which is maintained intact. In this particular technique a wide strip of fascia attached to the coracoid (actually a part of the coracobrachialis) has been woven into the PM insertion. The distal insertion is not very different from the one described above. This variation seems logical as it provides a stronger elbow flexion, assuring better protection of the neurovascular bundles.

Pectoralis minor transfer

This transfer was described by Le Coeur in 1953, 1956; it has the advantage of not harming the function of PM and not interfering with the aesthetic aspect of the pectoral area, which is very important in young females. However, it has the defect of giving a limited flexion strength; therefore it is indicated in cases in which a certain degree of weak elbow flexion is still present, so that it can integrate the existing weak function. In some instances it can be associated with a Steindler operation.

One problem can be the functional assessment of this muscle to evaluate its suitability for transfer. Being a depressor of the scapulae this muscle is tested by placing a hand under the coracoid process, asking the patient to push their shoulder down against resistance. In this way the active contraction and strength of pectoralis minor can be evaluated. Because the innnervation is similar to that of the PM this muscle will not be suitable for transfer with a lack of function of this muscle.

Technique

The skin incision follows the inferior margin of the PM muscle to the axilla. The pectoralis minor muscle is exposed under the PM and its origins from the 3rd, 4th

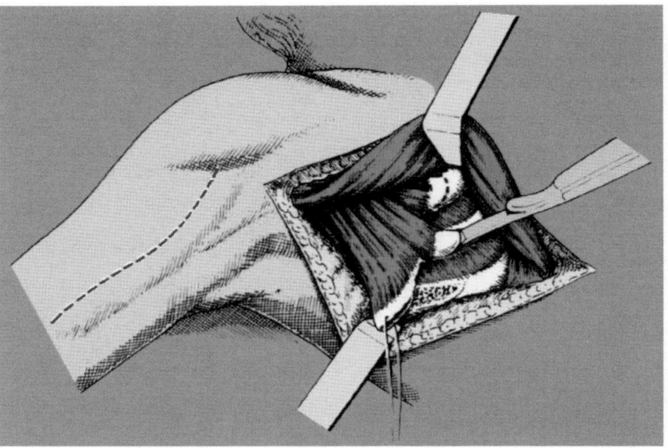

(A)

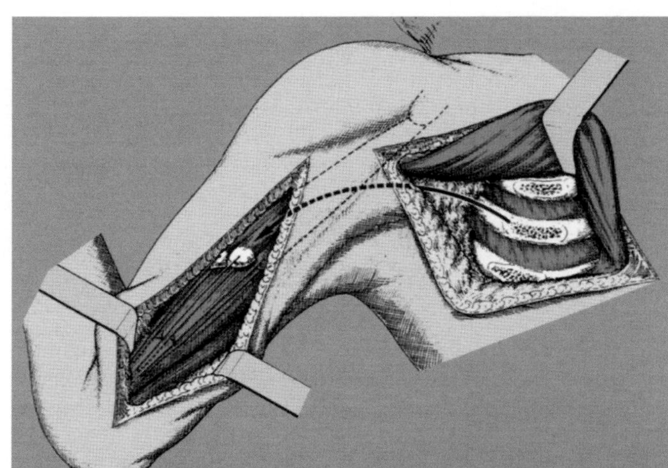

(B)

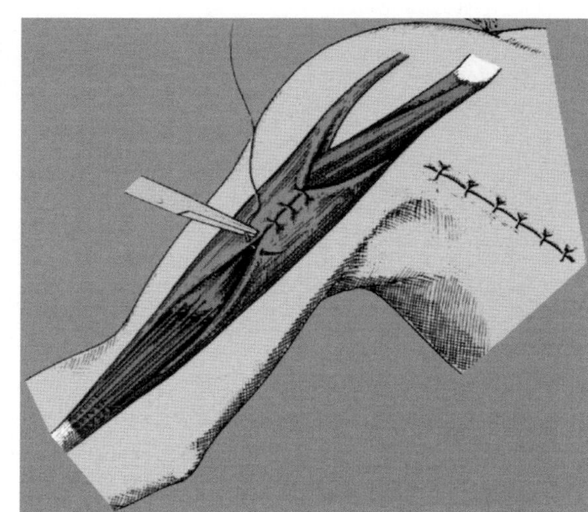

(C)

Figure 9.7
(A) Detaching the pectoralis minor from its origins.
(B) The muscle has been passed through a tunnel and to reach the biceps each origin is woven by strong sutures that are fixed to the biceps tendon.
(C) The paralysed biceps is overlapped over the sutures to reinforce the fixation (Alnot and Abols 1984; Alnot and Oberlin 1994).

and 5th ribs are detached together with strips of periosteum; at every origin it is woven by strong non-resorbable sutures to facilitate the distal suture to the biceps. Care must be taken to avoid damaging the neurovascular bundle (which penetrates the muscle in its anterior proximal aspect) while dissecting the muscle to the coracoid.

By means of a separate incision on the internal aspect of the arm the biceps is exposed to its middle portion. As the pectoralis minor is short it does not reach the biceps tendon and therefore must be fixed to the biceps at its middle third, but sutures are passed from every origin distally into the biceps tendon to ensure a good fixation. The paralysed muscle is overlapped longitudinally over the reinforced sutures (Alnot and Oberlin 1994). This transfer is actually a substitution of the coracobrachial muscle rather than the biceps itself. The postoperative immobilization in plaster is as usual with flexion of the elbow at 50° and the shoulder immobilized with the arm adducted for 5 weeks.

Triceps transfer

Transfer of triceps to biceps, described by Bunnel (1951), is generally considered a great sacrifice and is utilized on very few occasions. Elbow extension may be fundamental, for instance in patients who have to use crutches or wheelchairs, in brachial plexus lesions in cases in which a recovery of shoulder abduction can elevate the arm more than 90°. Therefore this transfer is used only in severe complete paralysis of the plexus in which a triceps recovered at M4 in the presence of a poor or absent biceps and with a poor shoulder in which gravity can help spontaneous elbow extension. In the authors' experience this transfer has always functioned well, with good strength, providing that the indications have been properly assessed. Another ideal indication will be in cases in which a co-contraction of biceps/triceps will ruin elbow flexion function. In these cases a weak elbow flexion will be strongly improved by the contemporary function of the triceps (Birch et al 1998).

Technique (Figure 9.8)

A longitudinal median posterior incision at the arm runs from the olecranon to the middle third of the arm. Isolation of the ulnar nerve (which is located medially) is suggested as a first step: after that the triceps muscle is detached medially and laterally and from the humerus

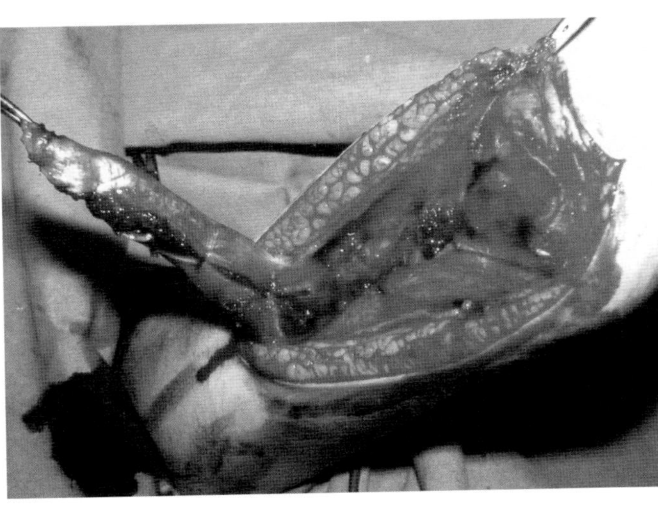

(A)

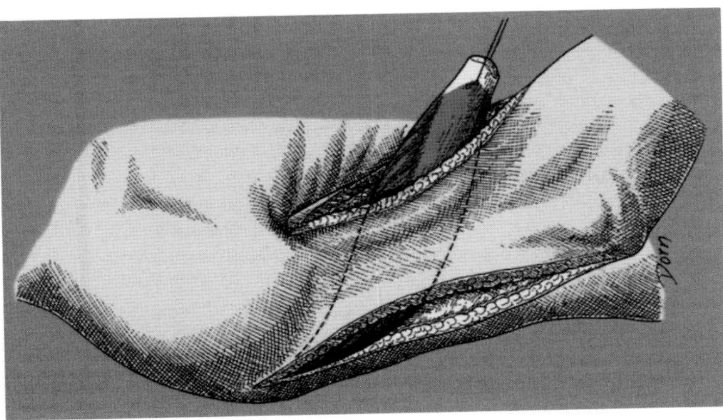

(B)

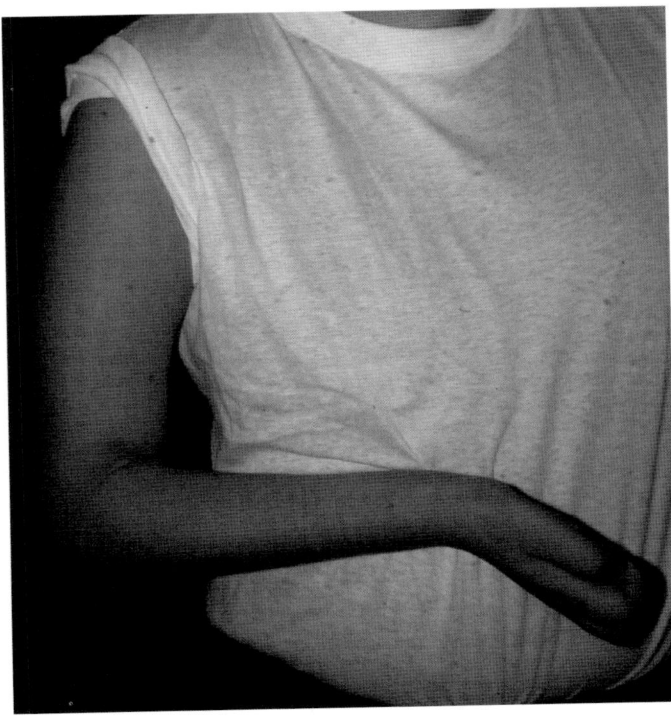

(C)

Figure 9.8

(A) The triceps with its tendon detached.

(B) The muscle is passed anteriorly around the lateral aspect of the arm.

(C) Result in a case of total plexus paralysis; the strength is 3 kg.

until the distal insertion to the olecranon, where it is detached with a strip of periosteum to facilitate the reinsertion to the biceps. The muscle is detached proximally up to the radial groove (taking special care not to damage the radial nerve).

The medial part of the triceps is detached further proximally than the lateral part to facilitate its rotation around the external (radial) aspect of the arm to reach the anterior aspect so that it can be reinserted to the biceps tendon. A subcutaneous tunnel is prepared radially for the passage of the muscle and its tendon. At the volar aspect of the elbow the biceps tendon is exposed and the tendon of the triceps muscle is sutured in flexion to it. As usual the correct tension is crucial to obtain a good functional result. It is a general rule to perform the transfer in such a way that at the end of the transfer the elbow must maintain a flexion of approximately 30–35°.

As usual a plaster will maintain the elbow flexed at 60° for 5 weeks.

Epitrochlear muscle transfer (Steindler operation)

Steindler (1918) had the idea or transferring the origin of the flexor pronator muscles more proximally, in this way changing their lever arm and allowing flexion of a paralysed elbow. The original technique included the transfer of the flexor muscles to the medial intermuscular septum of the arm 3–4 cm more proximally.

Mayer and Green (1954) modified the technique by transferring the pronator flexor muscles with a bony segment of epitrochlea which was then reattached to the humerus by means of a screw. Other more recent variations have been described by Brunelli et al (1995) and Comptet et al (1999). In order to minimize the so-called Steindler effect (pronation of the hand and finger flexion when the elbow is flexed) Brunelli et al suggested leaving the flexor digitorum superficialis (FDS) insertion in place; they transfer the medial epicondyle 5 cm higher on the anterior aspect of the humerus. To obtain a stronger flexion Comptet et al suggested reinserting the olecranic portion of the flexor carpi ulnaris (FCU) to the humerus.

The result of this transfer in brachial plexus palsies is better in C5, C6 than in C5, C6, C7 palsies. It seems (Comptet et al 1999) that the weak function of the supinator and extensors of the wrist (that is when the C7 root is also involved) is more likely to lead to a Steindler effect. All authors agree that the best results of this operation are achieved when flexion of the elbow is already present with an M1-M2 force at least. It must be remembered that both in C5, C6 and in C5, C6, C7 palsies in which no recovery occurs after surgery, a Steindler transfer will necessarily be weak; the reason is that in these palsies pronator teres and flexor carpi radialis are also paralysed, together with the biceps

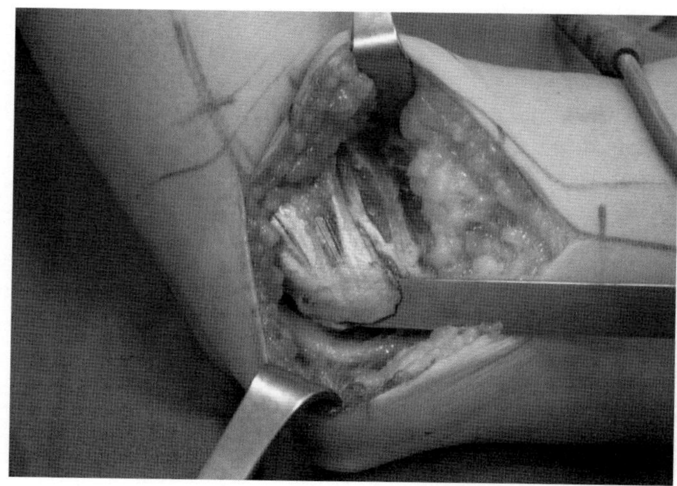

(A)

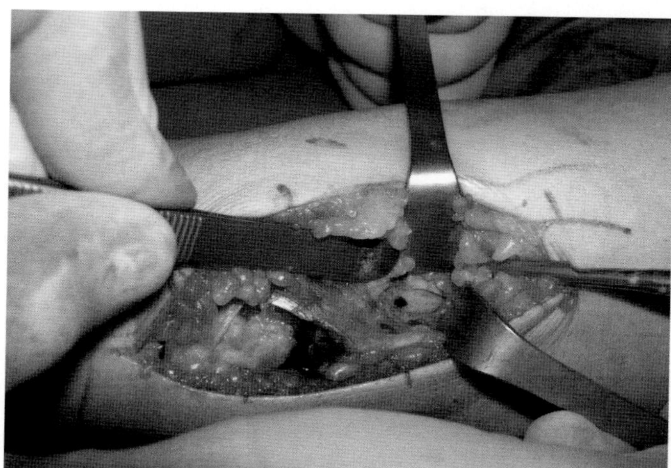

(B)

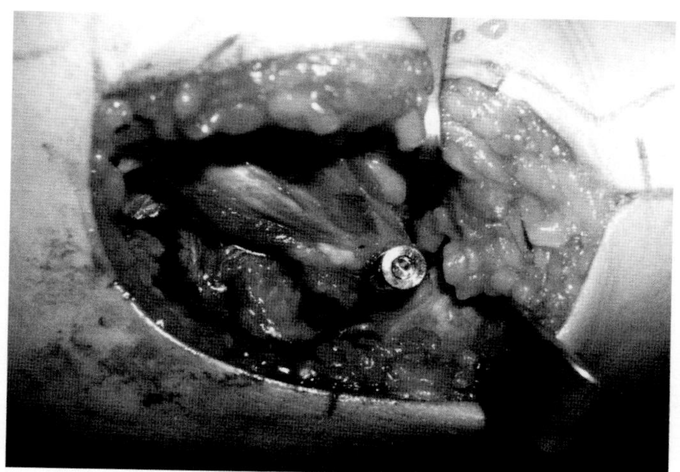

(C)

Figure 9.9

(A) Detaching the epitrochlea after exposure of the ulnar nerve.

(B) Preparing the hole in the humerus for the reinsertion.

(C) The segment of epitrochlea will be screwed to the humerus.

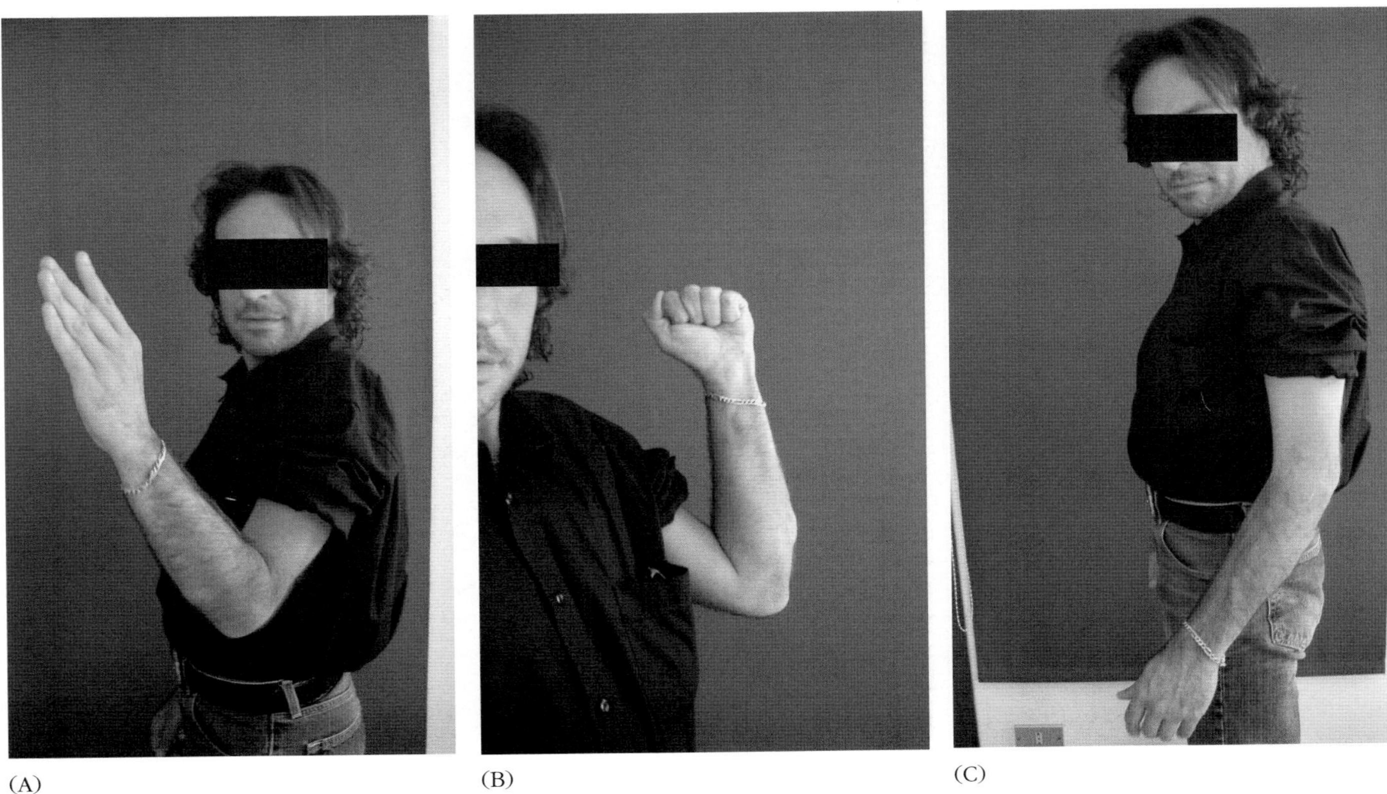

(A) (B) (C)

Figure 9.10
(A) Result after a Steindler operation in C5, C6 root avulsion; flexion of the elbow is present even with finger and wrist extension.
(B) Powerful flexion (5 kg); note the empty space at the epitrochlear region.
(C) Lack of elbow extension of about 30°.

muscle. In fact, for the Steindler operation the only muscle that has normal strength is the FCU. The indication for this transfer would be in cases in which a certain amount of weak active flexion has been recovered. It is fundamental to have an active wrist extension (Hentz 2001). On the contrary, a tendon transfer for wrist extension should be performed before a Steindler operation. In children great cautioun should be exercised when sectioning a segment of epitrochlea, to avoid severe varus deformation with growth due to destruction of the growth plate.

Technique (Figures 9.9 and 9.10)

A curved incision runs from distal to proximal from the middle line of the proximal forearm, passes over the epitrochlea and then again towards the middle anterior part of the distal arm 6–7 cm over the elbow crease. The first step is to isolate the ulnar nerve and medially the median nerve: the ulnar nerve is isolated up to the two branches for the epitrochlear and olecranian part of the FCU, whereas with the median nerve it is important to isolate the branches for pronator teres and flexor carpi radialis (FCR). When control of both nerves has been obtained the mass of flexor pronator is isolated.

A bony segment of the epitrochlea is detached, including the insertion point of the flexor pronator muscles, with the help of an electric saw. The FDS is left in place to reduce the so-called Steindler effect. The olecranic part of the FCU is usually left in place, while some authors suggest detaching this segment too and reinserting it to the humerus to reinforce the strength of the transfer. The bony segment must be sufficiently large to include the muscles and to allow perforation and to be subsequently screwed to the humerus. In fact, the muscles transposed are FCU (epitrochlear head), FCR and pronator teres. The point of fixation to the humerus is approximately 5–6 cm proximal to the elbow joint. As already mentioned, some authors have suggested fixing the epitrochlea more proximally and more anteriorly to reduce the pronation effect during flexion of the elbow.

After placing of subcutaneous and cutaneous sutures the elbow is immobilized at 60° of flexion with a plaster for 5 weeks while the arm is maintained in adduction.

Functional free muscle transfers

The idea of substituting a destroyed muscle with a newly revascularized and reinnervated muscle is due to Manktelow (Manktelow and McKee 1978) who applied it in a severe Volkmann's contracture. Later Berger et al (1990), Akasaka et al (1991), Doi et al (1991, 2000) and Chung et al (1993) described its use in reconstruction of severe brachial plexus paralysis and a double free muscle transfer to restore elbow flexion and finger flexo-extension.

When the elbow paralysis is long-standing (no possibility of direct nerve repair) and when no muscles are available to perform palliative surgery, the only possibility of restoring a functional flexion of the elbow is a free muscle transfer. In fact this situation is very frequent in total traumatic plexus lesions rather than in obstetric palsies where the elbow flexion-extension is almost always achieved, even if not completely, either spontaneously or after microsurgical repair. As a free muscle flap needs to be revascularized to suitable vessels by microsurgical sutures and reinnervated by suitable nerves some limitations in its indications may arise. The occlusion of the subclavian artery, a situation quite frequent in traumatic brachial plexus lesions, represents a contraindication for a free muscle transfer. The lack of suitable donor nerves may represent a limitation in indications. As the majority of these cases have already been operated on with multiple neurotizations (with spinal accessory and intercostal nerves) sometimes the only possibility of achieving a donor nerve to reinnervate the transfer comes from the healthy contralateral side (C7 or PM branches). As a muscle transfer can give one function, great efforts have been made by Doi et al (1991, 2001) to achieve two functions (elbow flexion and finger extension) with one transfer and in a second stage a new free transfer to achieve finger flexion.

Free transfers may be considered as a rescue operation for failed plexus surgery, generally recovering elbow flexion; or they may represent primary surgery as for the strategy suggested by Doi et al (1991, 2001), which includes a two-stage free muscle transfer associated with neurotization of triceps rami with intercostals to achieve stabilization of the elbow; this is the key point in achieving good function of the hand. Another prerequisite is to have a stable shoulder, which can be achieved either by microsurgical repair or with a secondary shoulder arthrodesis.

Different muscles have been utilized in the past, such as LD, rectus femoris and gracilis. Nowadays the gracilis muscle is the most frequently used muscle for this purpose.

Technique (Figures 9.11 and 9.12)

The gracilis muscle is harvested from the contralateral limb, as the direction of its vessels is better oriented to allow a good anastomosis without tension and narrowing. The authors prefer to harvest the muscle with an incision that allows them to take it together with an island of skin as a probe for the vascularization of the flap. The vascular pedicle comes from the deep femoral artery and enters into the muscle 8 cm below the pubic tubercle; its length is approximately 6 cm with a diameter of 1.2–1.8 mm for the artery and slightly more for the vein. The innervation of the gracilis muscle is an anterior branch of the obturator nerve. The calibre is between 1 and 2 mm, so it can be sutured to two to three intercostal nerves depending on their calibre. The cutaneous island must be drawn centred at the level of the entrance of the vessels and its dimensions are 10 × 12 cm maximum. The size of the skin flap is not a problem, as the aim is to use it as a means of good vascularization and not to provide a large amount of tissue coverage, as the muscle is quite thin and there is sufficient room to fit it in the arm. Once the neurovascular pedicle has been identified the muscle is harvested and detached from its insertion to the pubis and from the medial tibia by cutting its distal tendon.

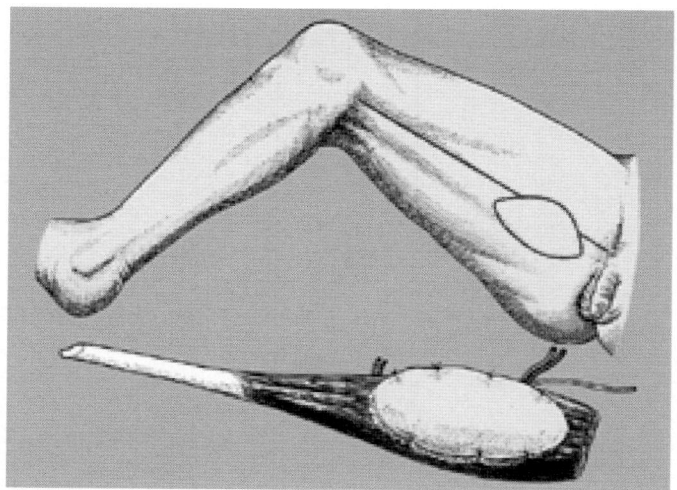

Figure 9.11
Diagram of the myocutaneous flap and the raised flap.

The proximal part of the gracilis is reinserted onto the acromion and onto the lateral part of the clavicle, with the distal tendon to the distal insertion of the biceps. As the muscle is generally longer than a normal biceps the difficulty is to adapt it to the new position. This adaptation is done both in the proximal and in the distal reinsertion. If the muscle must supply not only elbow flexion but even finger extension the whole length of the muscle will be utilized. In this case the brachioradialis muscle and wrist extensors will provide the pulley for the transfer that will be reinserted distally directly to the extensor digitorum communis. The tension of the transferred muscle is a crucial point; the common rule is to mark the muscle with stitches at 5 cm distance from one another before harvesting it from the thigh and to

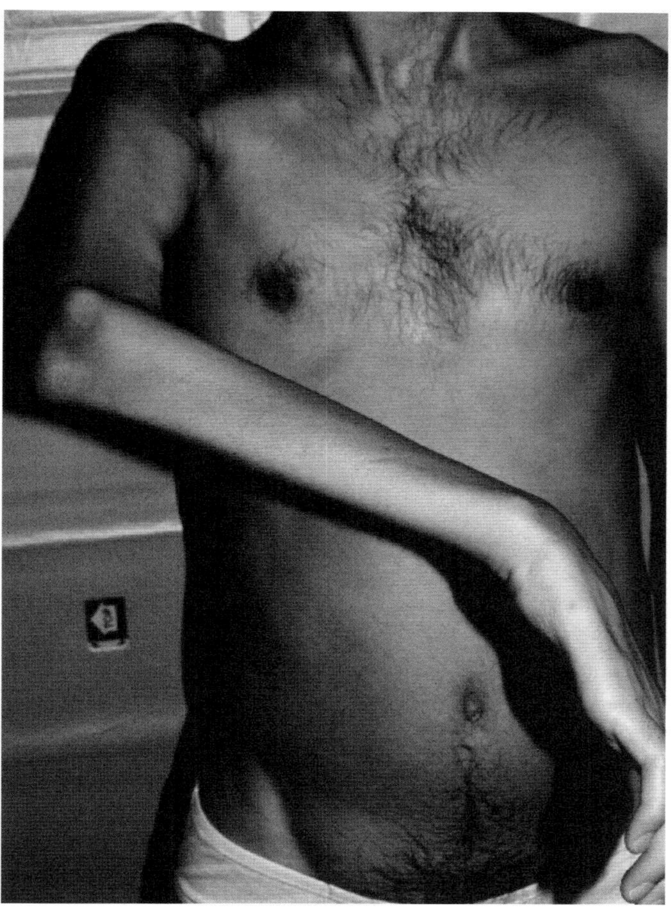

(A)

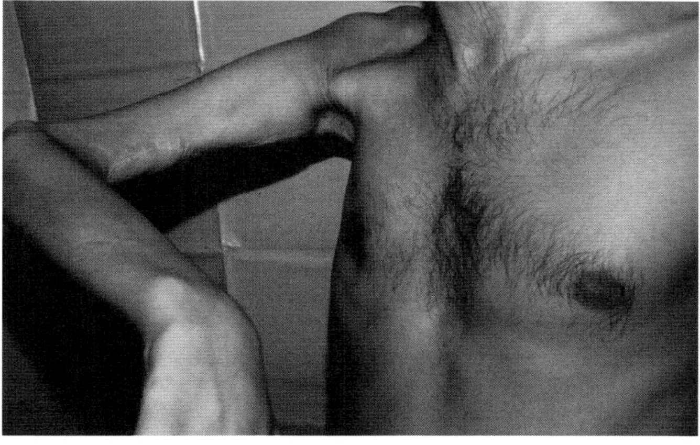

(B)

Figure 9.12

(A, B) A functional result with gracilis free transfer to restore elbow flexion. The patient recovered sufficient active control of the shoulder and weak elbow extension by primary surgery. The strength of the recovered flexion is no more than 1 kg.

restore the same distance when placing the muscle in the recipient area. When utilizing the transfer solely for elbow flexion the authors fix the muscle so as to obtain the correct tension with the elbow flexed at 80°. The difficulty in calculating suitable tension arises when the transfer must take on two functions, i.e. elbow flexion and finger extension.

Another problem, as already mentioned, is selecting the donor nerves, as in many instances they have already been utilized in the primary repair of the plexus. Usually the authors utilize two to three intercostal nerves that can generally adapt perfectly to the calibre of the nerve of the gracilis. Other authors utilize the spinal accessory nerve if it is available. In severe cases, in which despite multiple neurotizations no recovery occurred, in presence of complete lack of donor nerves the only source will be the contralateral plexus. In this case the anterior portion of the contralateral C7 root or a branch for the PM muscle can be utilized. As grafts are obviously necessary to bypass the chest, another problem will be to find enough grafts when dealing with previously operated cases in which both sural nerves and internal cutaneous nerves of the arm have already been utilized.

The recipient vessels may be the thoracoacromial artery and the cephalic vein; the authors have utilized a posterior branch of the humeral artery and collateral veins. As already mentioned, contraindications to this transfer may be an occlusion of the subclavian artery and the lack of suitable vessels for the revascularization of the transplant.

After revascularization of the myocutaneous transfer the elbow will be immobilized in 70° of flexion for 4 weeks. After that an orthosis will be used to maintain the elbow flexed for at least one more month.

Unlike classic palliative surgery, in which an active contracture of the transferred muscles is always present and must only be reinforced by means of rehabilitation, free muscle transfers are paralysed muscles that must be reinnervated. Therefore, for at least 6–10 months, which is the mean period necessary for reinnervation in a case of neurotization by direct suture with intercostal nerves or spinal nerve, electrical stimulation of the gracilis muscle must be employed from the moment that plaster is removed. Passive mobilization in flexion is performed for the first month after the removal of plaster and progressive extension of the elbow is gradually started only from the second month.

Transfer for elbow extension

The deficit of elbow extension is a clinical situation that is more frequent in tetraplegic patients and in some sequelae of obstetric paralysis. Elbow extension can easily be compensated by gravity and therefore indications for transfer to restore extension are very limited in traumatic lesions of the brachial plexus. In tetraplegic patients with spared C5, C6 function a good shoulder function is present together with elbow flexion but with an absent or weak elbow extension. Elbow extension is crucial for patients who have to lie in bed in a supine position to move their arm over their head and to control elbow flexion. For patients in a wheelchair, recovery of elbow extension is of paramount importance to allow transfer from bed to wheelchair and to make pushing on the wheel easier. Recovery of active elbow extension will allow a subsequent programme of more distal transfer for the hand.

The other clinical situation which would require elbow extension is obstetric paralysis, mainly in cases of spontaneous recovery for avulsion of C7, C8 roots in which reasonable shoulder function and elbow flexion have recovered in the absence of functional elbow extension. Unfortunately tendon transfer in obstetric patients does not offer the same useful results as in tetraplegic patients, in whom the motors to be transferred are usually very powerful.

The muscles that are suitable for transfer for elbow extension are LD, brachioradialis, deltoid and biceps.

Latissimus dorsi to triceps transfer

Indications for this transfer are very rare (poliomyelitis patients or some particular cases with isolated lack of elbow extension in the presence of a good LD muscle). In children with obstetric paralysis LD is the preferred transfer for shoulder reconstruction, therefore its transfer for extension of the elbow is very rarely indicated. The technique for harvesting LD has already been described for elbow flexion transfer. It must be underlined that it is not necessary to perform a bipolar transfer but a simple monopolar transfer will suffice to achieve elbow extension.

The idea of utilizing a LD transfer to triceps to restore elbow extension came from Harmon in 1949; he transferred the conjoint tendon of LD and teres major (TM) to triceps while in 1956 Hovnanian described his modified technique of complete transfer of LD both for extension and flexion of the elbow.

Deltoid to triceps transfer

Moberg described this technique in 1975, for restoration of elbow extension in tetraplegic patients. The indication is mainly for patients (mainly group 1, or flexion of the elbow group) who maintain shoulder function and elbow flexion with or without brachioradialis muscle.

Technique (Figures 9.13–9.15)

An incision on the posterior border of the deltoid runs from the middle third of the spine of the scapula to the middle third of the arm. The posterior third of the deltoid muscle is isolated and detached from its insertion on the humerus. As this muscle has a short belly and does not reach the tendinous portion of the triceps many variations of the technique have been described to overcome this problem. The original technique described by Moberg utilized finger extensor tendons in the foot (in tetraplegic patients) to connect the deltoid tendon to the triceps tendon. For this purpose a second incision on the dorsal aspect of the elbow allows exposure of the distal part of the triceps at its musculotendinous junction, while a subcutaneous tunnel will allow the two structures to be connected.

Hentz et al (1983) suggested a variation for the musculotendinous connection utilizing a graft of fascia lata which is more resistant and can be divided distally to be passed through a hole in the olecranon. As usual in these types of transfer the problem of junction is twofold, not only the distal but mainly the proximal suture may have a dehiscence. For this purpose the technical variation described by Castro-Sierra and Lopez-Pita (1983) is very interesting: he detached the posterior deltoid with a fragment of humeral bone and the triceps tendon is detached distally with a fragment of olecranon; the slip of triceps is then turned upward 180° and fixed bone to bone with the posterior deltoid tendon. In this way the junction is more resistant. Moreover, a loop with a Dacron strip reinforces the triceps tendon to avoid it detaching from the humerus under tension. Allieu et al (1985) described using fascia lata reinforced with a strip of Dacron inside. Landi et al (1998) suggested utilizing the tibialis anterior tendon, whose distal passage into the triceps tendon is blocked with two stay-sutures to make it strong and secure. Moreover, they perform two to three transverse aponeurotomies of deltoid muscle to enhance the excursion of the muscle.

These variations progressively reduced the immobilization period in plaster (from the shoulder to the wrist with elbow in complete extension) from the 6 weeks initially suggested by Moberg to 3 weeks as suggested by Allieu et al, so that physiotherapy can be started early.

Biceps to triceps transfer

The indication for this transfer (described by Friedenberg in 1954) is only in tetraplegic patients grade 2,3,4, i.e. patients with wrist extension. The presence of an active and strong brachioradialis muscle is crucial for this transfer, in addition to the presence of a brachialis anterior muscle. In fact if we utilize the biceps for triceps with a weak or absent short supinator, we will lose the only possibility of supinating the forearm.

It can be calculated that when transferring biceps to triceps, elbow flexion loses 30% of its strength. It has been demonstrated that in these patients the loss is highly compensated by the extension recovery at the elbow. Another interesting indication for this transfer is for patients in whom the elbow has a strong spastic component in flexion.

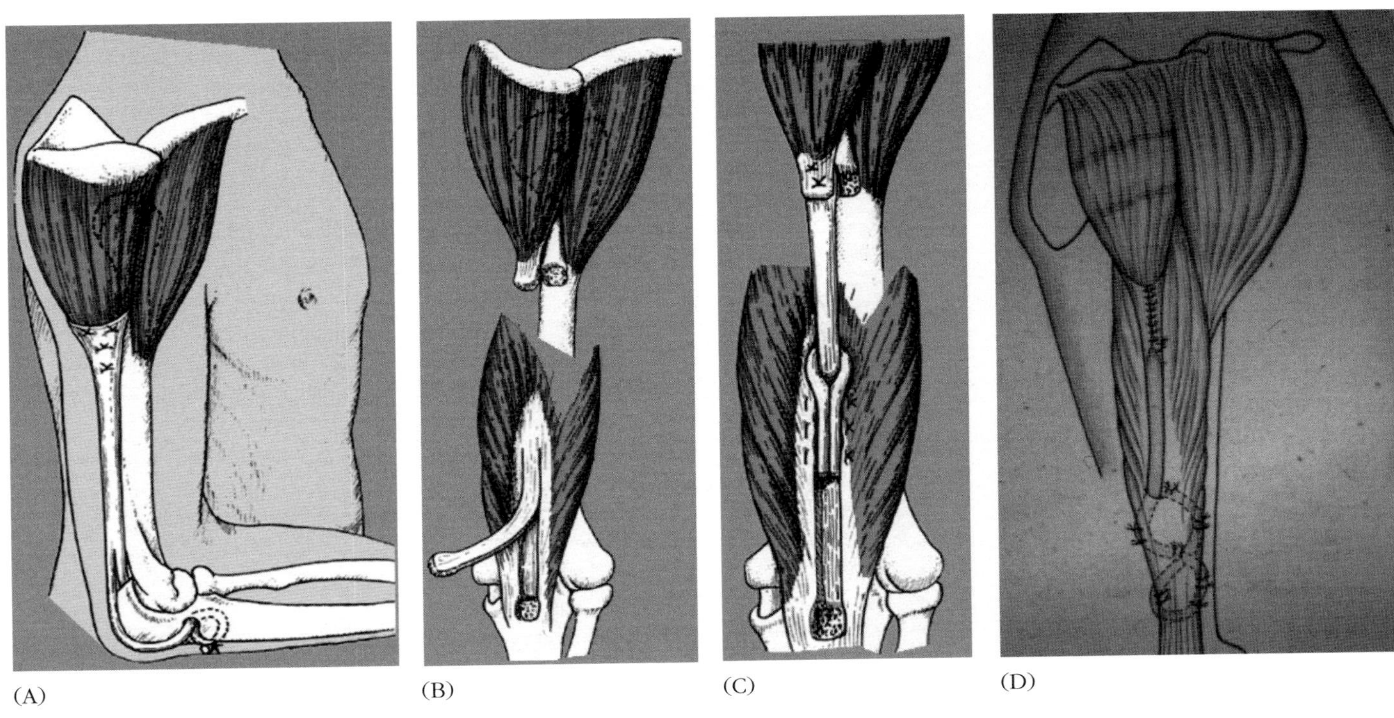

(A) (B) (C) (D)

Figure 9.13
(A) Hentz variation of the Moberg technique.
(B, C) Castro Sierra variation.
(D) Landi variation.

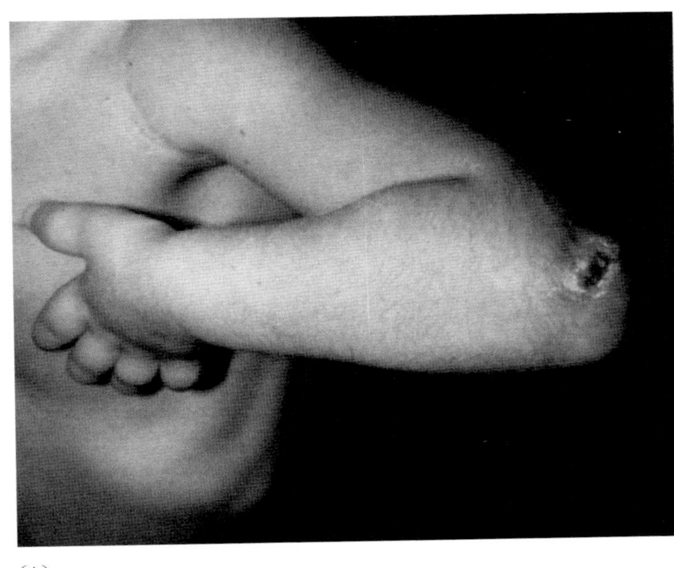

(A)

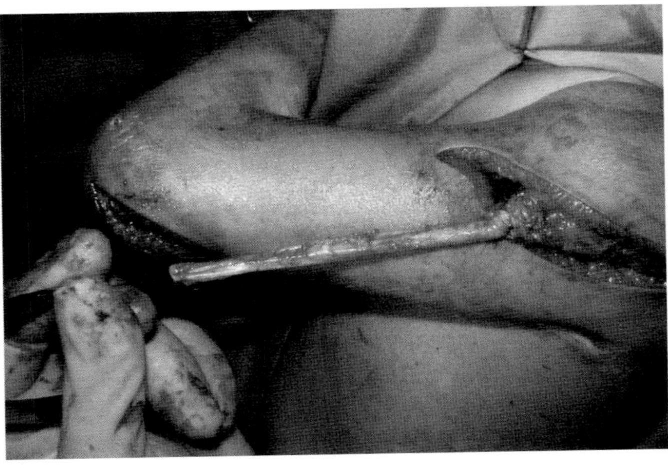

(B)

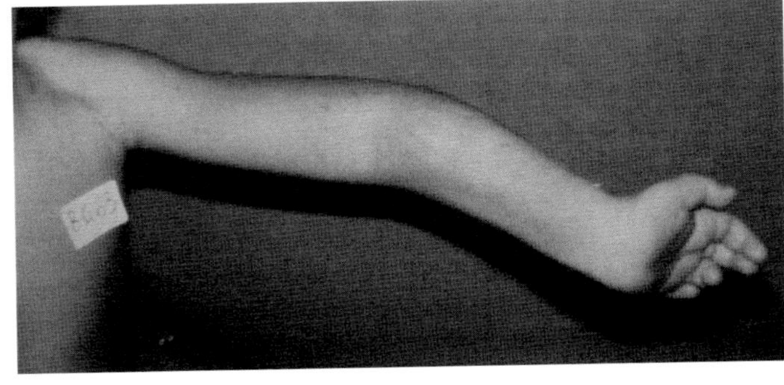

(C)

Figure 9.14
(A) In obstetric palsies a transfer for elbow extension may be indicated in severe cases; note the unstable scar at the elbow.
(B) A Moberg operation has been performed utilizing fascia lata.
(C) Functional result with a strong active extension. A 'flexum' contracture is present, as in many obstetric palsies.

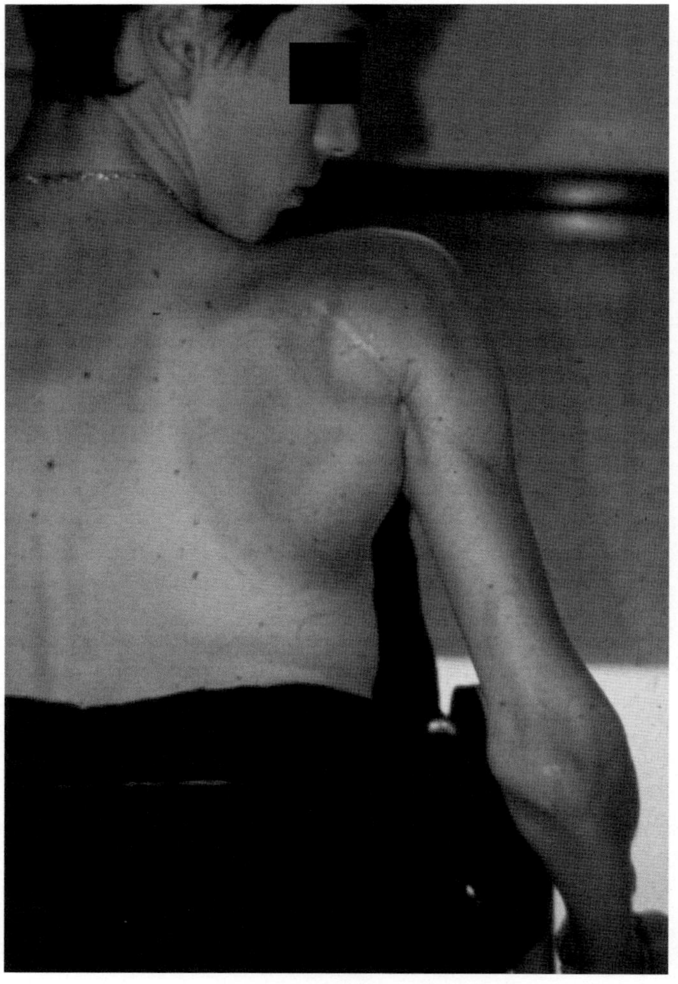

(A)

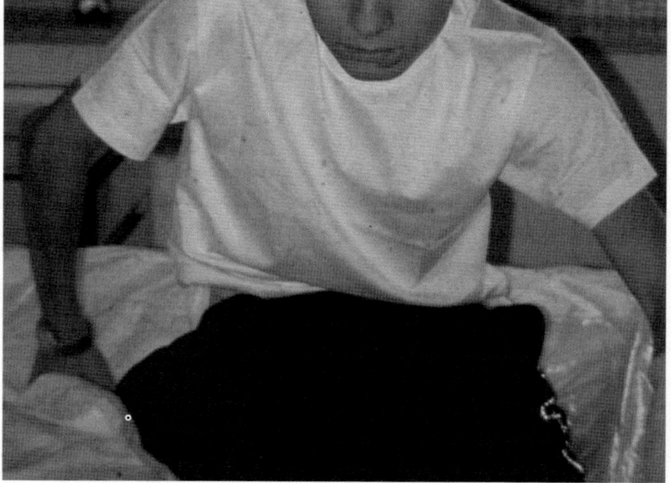

(B)

Figure 9.15

(A) A good result after deltoid to triceps transfer (Moberg operation with Landi's technical variation). The patient is able to push his wheelchair.

(B) The patient had improved the strength needed for changing position from bed to wheelchair.

Technique

An incision is made from the radial aspect of the distal third of the arm curved medially at the elbow crease to reach the insertion of the biceps tendon to the radius. The biceps is isolated and its tendon is detached from the radius. The biceps is then detached proximally enough to allow its transfer in a straight manner, through a subcutaneous tunnel to reach the triceps tendon (exposed with a separate incision in the olecranic region). The best way to fix the biceps tendon to the triceps is through an intraosseous passage into the olecranon of the biceps tendon divided into two strips, as suggested by Zancolli. The suture must be under maximum tension with the elbow flexed at 10°. Care must be taken not to compress or damage the radial nerve, as wrist extension in tetraplegic patients provides the only possibility of developing some function of the hand. The elbow is then immobilized in extension with plaster for 1 month.

Brachioradialis transfer to triceps

This technique was described by Ober and Barr in 1938 and it is described here even if its utilization is really limited to some sequelae of traumatic lesions of the posterior cord or isolated lesions of the triceps rami. It is not indicated in tetraplegic patients, as the brachioradialis muscle is generally utilized as a transfer to recover thumb pinch or finger flexion. The rationale of the technique is to partially detach the brachioradialis that is an elbow flexor transforming it into an elbow extensor. We have utilized this technique on three occasions with a reasonable result in post-traumatic cases. A strong brachioradialis is necessary in the absence of a triceps to obtain a functional result and it is not easy to find in sequelae of brachial plexus lesions.

Technique

A skin incision runs on the radial aspect of the distal third of the arm and over the belly of the brachioradialis muscle. The medial border of the muscle is identified and isolated along all its muscle belly. The muscle is isolated proximally, taking care to isolate its nerve branch to avoid any damage. The bone insertion at the humerus is left intact as well as the distal tendon. The muscle, free on its medial aspect, is then turned forwards like the page of a book and the medial border of the muscle becomes lateral. The free margin of the turned muscle is fixed with non-resorbable sutures to the triceps aponeurosis and the epicondylar muscle near the olecranon. The more dorsally the muscle is moved, the more active extension of the elbow will be achieved. During the whole muscle fixation procedure the motor branch must be checked and any tension must be avoided.

Conclusions

Palliative surgery for distal paralysis in the upper arm, i.e. for median, radial or ulnar paralysis, is quite standardized and, even if sometimes technically demanding, almost always offers a good functional solution. For more proximal paralysis, i.e. usually for brachial plexus lesions, the situation is quite different; the motors at our disposal are limited, sometimes only partially reinnervated and as in obstetrical cases with the problem of co-contractions. It is not a matter of choice of a preferred technique, but rather a problem to be forced to utilize the only motor at our disposal with limited chances of achieving a functional result. This is why only short series of cases have been published in the literature, probably because of the limitations in indicating such surgical procedures.

Therefore, while in tetraplegic patients we can always turn to a Moberg operation (with the many technical variations) to recover useful elbow extension, as the deltoid is always in good condition, in palliative surgery for elbow flexion the question is still open.

On the basis of their experience, the authors offer the following suggestions:

- In totally paralysed elbow flexors, if a good LD is available this will be the authors' first choice in adults (Petrolati and Raimondi 1987). In children, due to the frequent problems at the shoulder level, the authors prefer to devote this muscle to external rotation transfer. The results for flexion are usually good and this transfer is actually the strongest (in the best cases between 5 and 8 kg) (Catalano et al 1987).
- If LD is not available, the PM muscle will be used in totally paralysed elbow flexors, the bipolar method as a preferred choice; but in severe traumatic plexus cases, with a poor shoulder, it is preferable to use the monopolar method, being aware of the adduction component that in this case will be functionally useful. There is obviously a limitation in indications in female patients due to the unaesthetic scarring produced.
- In cases of partial elbow flexor paralysis, for incomplete recovery after plexus repair in the presence of good forearm flexors, the authors' first choice is the Steindler operation. They do not have experience in pectoralis minor transfer, which could be another option in these cases.
- Triceps to biceps transfer will be indicated only in severe cases of traumatic brachial plexus lesions with poor recovery of elbow flexors and with a certain active control of shoulder that cannot reach 60–70° of abduction. Another indication could be the presence of co-contraction biceps-triceps, always with a poor shoulder in which gravity will always compensate the lack of elbow extension due to the deficit in shoulder abduction.

A separate comment must be made regarding free muscle transfer. It is certain that microsurgery offers a brilliant possibility to substitute a long-standing paralysed muscle with a new vascularized and reinnervated muscle. The authors' experience in this field has always been limited to a rescue technique in the hopeless cases where no transfers at all were possible. In fact their experience is limited to the pure transfer for elbow flexors. The results obtained have involved seven cases; one M3, two M2 and four useless results. In the Doi series, which seems to be the largest for this specific indication, the following results were reported for 24 cases: two M4; four M3; eight M2; five M1; five M0. In the authors' opinion this means that this technique must not be utilized as a first choice; it is of paramount importance to give the patient the chance of a primary brachial plexus repair even with multiple extraplexal neurotization. In a second stage, microvascular free muscle transfer can integrate the results obtained by primary nerve reconstruction, adding some functional results at the hand.

References

Allieu JY, Teissier J, Triki F et al (1985) Réanimation de l'extension du coude chez le tétraplégique par transplantation du deltoïde postérieur. Etude de 21 cas, *Rev Chir Orthop* **71**: 195–200.

Alnot JY, Abols Y (1984) Réanimation de la flexion du coude par transferts tendineux dans les paralysies traumatiques du plexus brachial de l'adulte. A propos de 44 blessés, *Rev Chir Orthop* **70**: 313–23.

Alnot JY, Oberlin C (1994) Transferts musculaires dans les paralysies de la flexion et de l'extension du coude. Technique chirurgicale. In: Tubiana R, ed, *Traité de Chirurgie de la Main*, Vol 4 (Masson: Paris) 162–75.

Akasaka Y, Hara T, Takahashi M (1991) Free muscle transplantation combined with intercostal nerve crossing for reconstruction of elbow flexion and wrist extension in brachial plexus injuries, *Microsurgery* **12**: 346–51.

Berger A, Flory PJ, Schaller E (1990) Muscle transfers in brachial plexus lesions, *J Reconstr Microsurg* **6**: 113–16.

Birch R, Bonney G, Wynn Parry CB (1998) Reconstruction. In: Birch, Bonney, Winn Parry, eds, *Surgical Disorders of the Peripheral Nerves* (Churchill Livingstone: London) 431–7.

Brooks DM, Seddon HI (1959) Pectoral transplantation for paralysis of the flexors of the elbow. A new technique, *J Bone Joint Surg* **41B**: 36–43.

Brunelli GA, Vigasio A, Brunelli GR (1995) Modified Steindler procedure for elbow flexion restoration, *J Hand Surg* **20A**: 743–6.

Bunnel S (1951) Restoring flexion to the paralytic elbow, *J Bone Joint Surg* **33A**: 566–71.

Carrol RE, Kleinman WB (1979) Pectoralis major transplantation to restore elbow flexion of the paralytic limb, *J Hand Surg* **4**: 501–7.

Castro-Sierra A, Lopez-Pita A (1983) A new surgical technique to correct triceps paralysis. *Hand* **15**: 42–6.

Catalano F, Fanfani F, Pagliei et al (1987) Surgical techniques to restore active flexion of the elbow in patients with brachial plexus sequelae, *Chirurgia della Mano* **24**: 403–11.

Chung DC, Wei FC, Noordhoff MS (1993) Cross chest C7 nerve grafting followed by free muscle transplantation for the treatment of total avulsed brachial plexus injuries: a preliminary report, *Plast Reconstr Surg* **92**: 717–25.

Clark JMP (1946) Reconstruction of the biceps brachii by pectoral muscle transplantation, *Br J Surg* **34**: 180–1.

Comtet JJ, Fredenucci JF, Pham E et al (1999) L'effet parasite de pronation, flexion des doigts et du poignet après opération de Steindler n'est pas inéluctable, *La Main* **4**: 15–26.

Dautry F, Apoil A, Moinet F et al (1977) Paralysie radiculaire supérieure du plexus brachial, traitement par transpositions musculaires associées, *Rev Chir Orthop* **63**: 399–407.

Doi K, Sakai K, Kuwata N et al (1991) Reconstruction of finger and elbow function after complete avulsion of the brachial plexus, *J Hand Surg* **16A**: 796–803.

Doi K, Muramatsu K, Hattori Y et al (2000) Restoration of prehension with the double free muscle technique following complete avulsion of the brachial plexus, *J Bone Joint Surg* **82A**: 652–66.

Freidenberg ZB (1954) Transposition du biceps brachial pour faiblesse du triceps, *J Bone Joint Surg* **36A**: 656–8.

Harmon PH (1949) Muscle transplantation for triceps palsy, *J Bone Joint Surg* **31A**: 409–12.

Hentz VR (2001) Obstetrical paralysis. Palliative surgery: elbow paralysis. In: Gilbert A, ed, *Brachial Plexus Injuries* (Martin Dunitz: London) 261–74.

Hentz VR, Brown M, Keosian LA (1983) Upper limb reconstruction in quadriplegia; functional assessment and proposed treatment modifications, *J Hand Surg* **8**: 119–31.

Hovnanian P (1956) Latissimus dorsi transplantation for loss of flexion or extension at the elbow, *Ann Surg* **143**: 493–9.

Landi A, Caserta G, Della Rosa N (1998) Patologia neurologica: il gomito nella tetraplegia. In: Monografia SICM, *La Patologia Non Traumatica del Gomito* (Mattioli: Fidenza), 91–100.

Le Coeur P (1953) Procedé de restauration de la flexion du coude paralytique, *Rev Chir Orthop* **39**: 655–6.

Le Coeur P (1956) Paralysies du coude. Transplantations musculaires, *Semaine des Hôpitaux* **32**: 1943–8.

Manktelow RT, McKee NH (1978) Free muscle transplantation to provide active finger flexion, *J Hand Surg* **3**: 416–26.

Mayer L, Green W (1954) Experience with the Steindler flexor-plasty at the elbow, *J Bone Joint Surg* **36A**: 775–89.

Merle D'Aubigné R (1956) *Chirurgie Orthopédique des Paralysies* (Masson: Paris) 122–39.

Moberg E (1975) Surgical treatment for absent single hand grip and elbow extension in quadriplegia, *J Bone Joint Surg* **57A**: 196–205.

Ober FR, Barr JS (1938) Brachioradialis muscle transposition for triceps weakness, *Surg Gynecol Obstet* **67**: 105–7.

Petrolati M, Raimondi PL (1987) Palliative surgery in the sequelae of brachial plexus lesions, *Chirurgia della Mano* **24**: 389–401.

Schottstaedt ER, Larsen LJ, Bost FC (1955) Complete muscle transposition, *J Bone Joint Surg* **37A**: 897–919.

Seddon HJ (1947) Transplantation of pectoralis major for paralysis of the flexors of the elbow, *Proc R Soc Med* **42**: 837.

Spira E (1957) Replacement of biceps brachii by pectoralis minor transplant, *J Bone Surg* **39B**: 126.

Steindler A (1918) A muscle plasty for the relief of flail elbow in infantile paralysis, *Interstate Med J* **35**: 235–41.

Tsai TM, Kalisman M, Burns J et al (1983) Restoration of elbow flexion by pectoralis major and pectoralis minor transfer, *J Hand Surg* **8**: 186–90.

Zancolli E, Mitre H (1973) Latissimus dorsi transfer to restore elbow flexion, *J Bone Joint Surg* **55A**: 1265–75.

10 Paralysis of the radial nerve

Raoul Tubiana

Paralysis of the extensors of the wrist and digits is classified according to the level of the neurologic lesion. Lesions of the cervical spinal cord and of the brachial plexus are discussed in the relevant chapters; here, it is important to emphasize that restoration of wrist extension is a fundamental step in the treatment of extensive paralyses of the hand. This chapter will cover radial nerve paralyses. Fracture of the humerus is the most frequent cause; however, these paralyses may also be the result of nerve compression or of various neurologic diseases.

Anatomy

The radial nerve is a continuation of the posterior cord. Its roots emerge at the C6, C7, C8, and T1 levels. Initially lying behind the axillary artery, it runs distally in the arm by winding around the posterior aspect of the humerus from medial to lateral. It continues in the lateral bicipital groove. In the arm the radial nerve successively gives branches to the triceps, the brachioradialis and the extensor carpi radialis longus (ECRL) (Figure 10.1).

As it reaches the humero-radial joint line, the radial nerve divides into two terminal branches, the anterior sensory branch (which runs into the forearm under the brachioradialis, lateral to the radial artery), and a posterior motor branch, the posterior interosseous nerve (which penetrates the supinator muscle by passing under the arcade of Frohse). This arcade is fibrous in about one-third of cases and may compress the nerve. The nerve winds around the neck of the radius between the two heads of the supinator. In 25% of cases it lies against the periosteum for about 3 cm (bare area) when the forearm is supinated; it is more vulnerable at this level (Spinner 1978). The nerve then emerges from the supinator in the posterior compartment; it runs along the posterior aspect of the interosseous membrane and sends sensory branches to the wrist and carpometacarpal joint.

The radial nerve supplies all the extensors of the elbow, the wrist, and the fingers. By contrast, its sensory territory is relatively limited (the lateral half of the dorsum of the hand), and the autonomous zone is restricted to the dorsal aspect of the first interosseous space, so that sensory nerve palsy is functionally insignif-

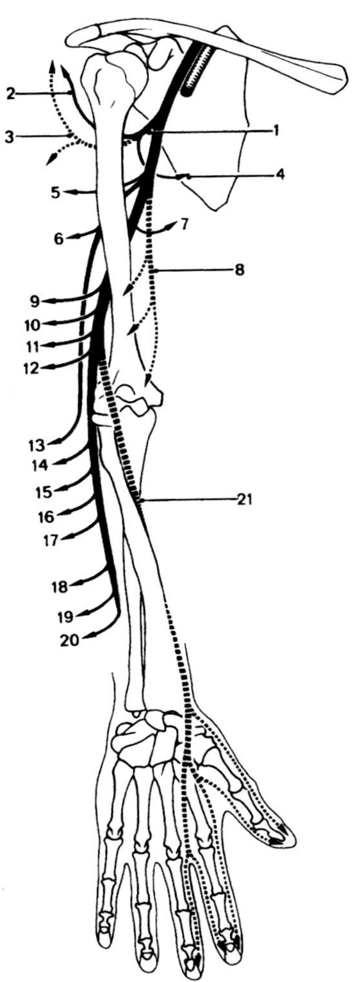

Figure 10.1

The radial and axillary nerves; muscles supplied and cutaneous distribution. The forearm is pronated. (1) Axillary nerve; (2) deltoid; (3) cutaneous branch to shoulder; (4) teres minor; (5) triceps (long); (6) triceps (lateral); (7) triceps (medial); (8) medial cutaneous branch; (9) brachioradialis; (10) extensor carpi radialis longus; (11) extensor carpi radialis brevis; (12) supinator; (13) anconeus; (14) extensor digitorum communis; (15) extensor digitorum to fifth digit; (16) extensor carpi ulnaris; (17) abductor pollicis longus; (18) extensor pollicis brevis; (19) extensor pollicis longus; (20) extensor indicis proprius; (21) anterior sensory branch. The sensory branches are shown as dotted lines.

icant. However, sectioning of the small sensory branches of the radial nerve at the wrist can give rise to painful neuromas.

Clinical aspects

Radial palsy results in paralysis of the triceps, the supinator muscle, and the brachioradialis, and paralysis of the extensors of the wrist, the thumb, and the proximal phalanges of the fingers.

Paralysis of the triceps is uncommon, because the site of the trauma is usually distal to the branches that innervate this muscle. Therefore, triceps paralysis is usually seen in more proximal lesions, including brachial plexus or medullary lesions. With the arm hanging at the side, gravity provides extension of the elbow. The deficit of extension becomes evident either when the arm is elevated or when an attempt is made to actively extend the elbow. It may be necessary to eliminate this deficit, particularly in tetraplegics, in order to allow these patients to straighten up while supporting themselves on their upper limb. Transfers of the posterior third of the deltoid (Moberg 1978) or of the biceps (Friedenberg 1954, Zancolli 1975) are indicated in certain circumstances, which are described in the chapter on Tetraplegia. In paralysis of the supinator muscle, the loss of supination is compensated for by the biceps and by the movements of the shoulder. Likewise paralysis of the brachioradialis, which is essentially an elbow flexor, is compensated for by the biceps.

By contrast, three movements that are essential to hand function are lost and cannot be compensated for: extension of the wrist (all three wrist extensors are supplied by the radial nerve), extension and retroposition of the thumb (brought about by the extensor pollicis longus (EPL), abductor pollicis longus, and extensor pollicis brevis), and extension of the metacarpophalangeal (MP) joints of the fingers.

Radial nerve injuries and fractures of the humerus

The close anatomical relationship of the radial nerve with the humeral shaft accounts for the high incidence of radial nerve injuries in fractures of the humerus. As it crosses the spiral groove on the posterior aspect of the humerus, the nerve is not in contact with the bone; they are kept apart by thin sheets of muscle, and come into direct contact only at the lateral supracondylar border of the bone. At this level the nerve crosses the inextensible posterior intermuscular septum to enter the lateral bicipital groove; it is somewhat stretched at this point, and lack of mobility accounts for its vulnerability in humeral fractures (Holstein and Lewis 1963).

Early treatment of radial nerve palsy associated with fractures of the humerus

These fractures are usually characterized by lateral angulation and overriding of the distal fragment. Seddon (1975) demonstrated that actual division of the nerve is rare and that the initial signs of motor recovery may not appear until 4–5 months. Thus emergency treatment should be directed at proper closed management of the fracture with evaluation of the status of the nerve injury before any operative intervention is undertaken. This conservative approach is now being reconsidered. Vichard et al (1982) found that in >25% of their cases of radial nerve palsy associated with a humeral fracture, there was either complete disruption or significant entrapment of the nerve. The advantage of early operative intervention in these cases is obvious. It is possible that this increase in the severity of the radial nerve lesions is a result of the now frequent association of severe multisystem trauma with this injury.

Iatrogenic radial nerve palsy is a separate problem. It results from the technique of closed reduction or surgical exposure and fixation.

Paralysis of the extension of the wrist

Extension of the wrist is dependent on three muscles: the extensor carpi radialis longus (ECRL), the extensor carpi radialis brevis (ECRB), and the extensor carpi ulnaris (ECU) (Figure 10.2). The ECRL, which inserts on the base of the second metacarpal, extends the wrist and draws it into radial deviation. The ECRB inserts on the base of the third metacarpal; this more medial location makes it the primary wrist extensor, but it also acts in radial deviation. The ECU inserts on the base of the fifth metacarpal and crosses the wrist at the level of the ulna, in contrast to the ECRB and ECRL tendons, which cross at the level of the radius. Furthermore, the ECU tendon rotates around the ulnar head: when the forearm is in pronation, its tendon is situated on the ulnar side of the styloid process, whereas in supination it is on the radial side in a dorsal position closer to the radius (Figure 10.3). Thus the ECU is an extensor of the wrist in supination and primarily causes ulnar deviation of the wrist in pronation.

It is common to consider both the ECRB and the ECRL as similar muscles, but in fact they differ in many respects. The ECRL takes its origin at the supracondylar ridge of the humerus, about 4–5 cm proximal to the epicondyle. It plays a role in elbow flexion and loses a part of its wrist action when the elbow is flexed. In contrast, the ECRB has its origin on the epicondyle and is not affected by the position of the elbow, all of its

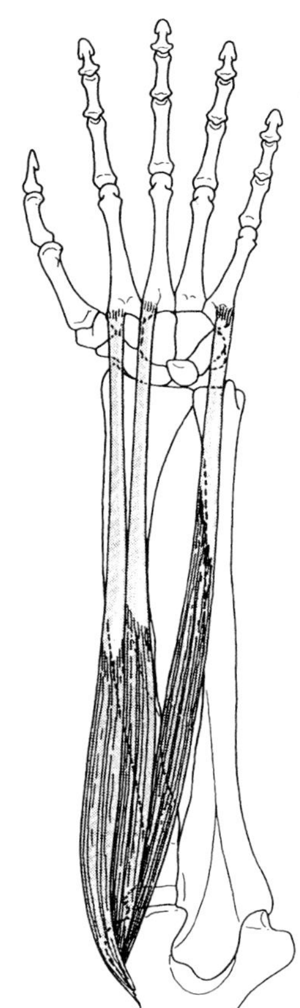

Figure 10.2

The extensors of the wrist. From radial to ulnar: ECRL, ECRB and ECU.

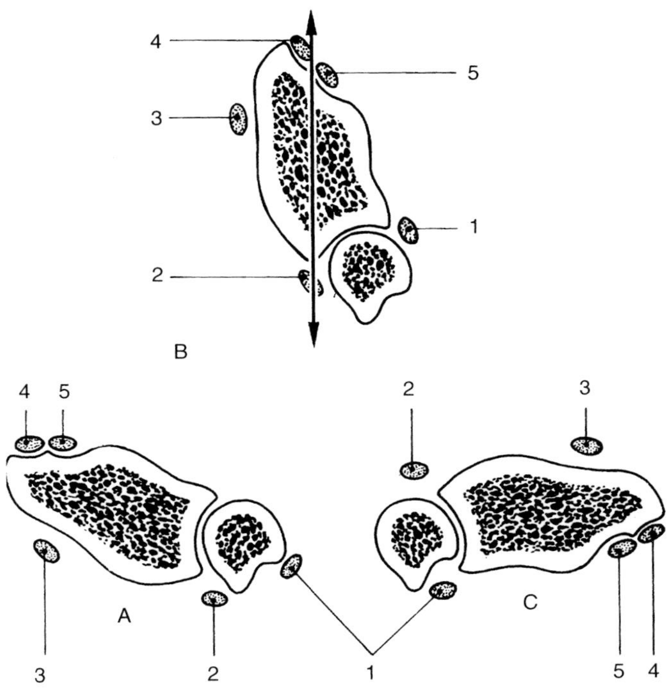

Figure 10.3

Position of the wrist extensor and flexor tendons during pronation/supination (right wrist)

1 ECU, 2 FCU, 3 FCR, 4 ECRL, 5 ECRB

(A) Pronation. ECR (4 and 5) are extensors and FCU is a flexor

(B) Semipronation. The axis of wrist movement is oblique between the ECR and the FCU

(C) Supination. The ECR and ECU are extensors, the FCU and FCR are flexors

action is on the wrist. These two tendons are congruent along most of their length in the forearm and often have tendinous connections. However, they diverge at the wrist level so that at their insertions the ECRL tendon is about 1.5 cm lateral to the ECRB.

The moment arms for extension of the wrist are 16.30 mm for the ECRB and only 12.50 mm for the ECRL (Ketchum et al 1978). In the ECRL the moment arm for elbow flexion and radial deviation is more important than that for wrist extension; the ECRL only becomes a wrist extensor after radial deviation is balanced against the ulnar forces of the ECU. The ECU has the weakest moment of extension (6.3 mm in supination), which becomes zero when the wrist is in complete pronation. Thus the three wrist extensors have very different moment arms of extension. The ECRB is the most effective extensor of the wrist.

Remember that the most frequently used wrist movements are not those in the axis of flexion-extension, but those in semi-pronation. The axis of the movements is oblique between the ECRL and ECRB (which produce extension and radial deviation of the wrist), and the flexor carpi ulnarus (FCU) (which produces flexion and ulnar deviation of the wrist), thus explaining the essential importance of this muscle (see Figure 10.3).

Neither the flexors nor the extensors of the fingers are long enough to allow simultaneous, maximal movements at the wrist and the fingers. The restraining action of the antagonistic extrinsic muscles explains why complete flexion of the fingers is possible only if the wrist is in slight extension of approximately 15°.

As the wrist position changes, the functional lengths of the digital flexor tendons change, and the resultant forces in finger flexion vary. Studies by Hazelton et al (1975) have evaluated the influence of wrist position on the forces generated at the middle and distal phalanges; the greatest force is exerted in slight ulnar deviation and extension; the least force is generated in radial deviation and flexion.

In full flexion of the wrist, the grip strength of the hand is less than the third of its maximum in extension (Napier 1955).

Loss of active extension in the wrist has serious repercussions on the action of the extrinsic muscles in the hand: flexor action in the thumb and fingers is normally reinforced by extension of the wrist, and therefore, palsy

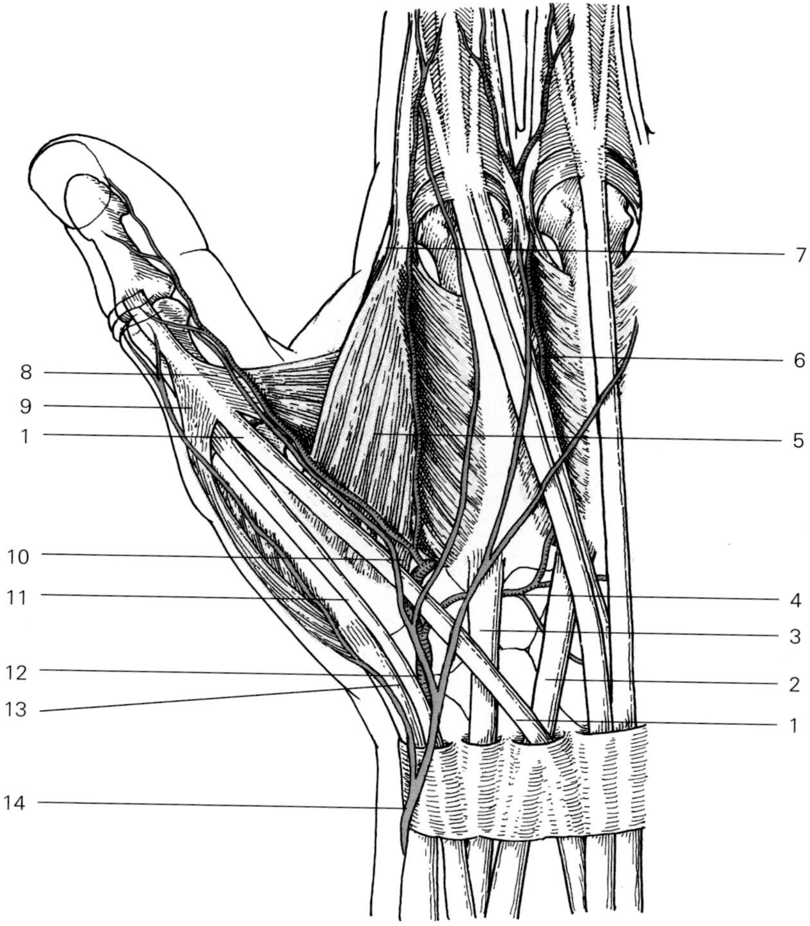

Figure 10.4

Extensor tendons of the thumb.

1 EPL
2 ECRB
3 ECRL
4 Dorsal carpal branch of radial artery
5 First dorsal interosseous
6 Second MC artery
7 First lumbrical muscle
8 Expansion of AP to EPL tendon
9 Expansion of APB to EPL tendon
10 First dorsal artery
11 EPB
12 Radial artery
13 APL
14 Radial nerve (sensory branch)

of the extensors in the wrist involves a great loss of grip strength. In certain cases this can be the most serious sequela of these palsies. Permanent flexion of the wrist exerts tension on the extensor tendons of the fingers, resulting in passive extension of the MP joints of the fingers. In extension the lateral collateral ligaments of these joints contract; thus paradoxically, one of the most common complications of poorly supervised radial paralysis is an extension contracture of the MP joints.

Paralysis of the extensor muscles of the fingers

The extensor muscles of the fingers that are innervated by the radial nerve are the extensor digitorum, the extensir indicis proprius (EIP) and the extensor digiti minimi (EDM). These extrinsic muscles extend the proximal phalanx but are unable to completely extend the distal phalanges, because their action is limited to the level of their proximal insertions. These proximal insertions are on the volar plate of the MP joints via the sagittal bands and at the base of the proximal phalanx. Extension of the distal phalanges is ensured by the intrinsic muscles.

Paralysis of the extensor muscles of the thumb

These muscles include the extensor pollicis longus (EPL), the extensor pollicis brevis (EPB), and the abductor pollicis longus (APL) (Figure 10.4). It is important to recall that:

1. The excursion of the EPL is 5 cm and the excursion of the EPB and APL is only 2.5 cm. The same transfer should not be used on the three tendons whose excursions differ greatly (Merle d'Aubigné 1946).
2. The intrinsic muscles of the thumb contribute to the extension of the distal phalanx. In radial palsy, the distal phalanx of the thumb can be extended when the proximal phalanx remains flexed.

Reconstructive treatment

It is commonly agreed that reconstructive treatment is indicated after peripheral nerve palsy in the upper extremity once it is certain that nerve recuperation is impossible. In fact, the problem is complex after radial nerve injury because it is difficult to determine precisely the likelihood and quality of potential nerve regeneration; and because early reconstructive treatment can be useful, even when there is later nerve recovery, provided that the treatment itself does not constitute a source of complications and adverse sequelae.

Although reconstructive surgery is now performed less frequently for radial nerve palsy because of the better results after nerve repair, it still has good indications, which will be discussed later.

History of tendon transfers for radial palsy

The history of tendon transfers for radial palsy has been reviewed by Saikku (1947), Boyes (1962), and Ueba (1986). Boyes compiled a list of 58 transfers described up until 1960; this list has lengthened since that period.

In a first stage, surgeons attempted to obtain only finger and thumb extension, using transfer of the ECRL (Drobnik 1897), of the ECU (Rochet 1897), or of the FCU (Capellen 1899, Francke 1899). Paralysis of the wrist extensors was treated mainly by arthrodesis of the wrist (Perthes 1918) or by tenodesis of the ECR to the radius (Fioro 1907).

Robert Jones (1916) is credited with re-establishing extension of the wrist by the transfer of the pronator teres (PT) to the ECR. This classic transfer has proved its value over the years and continues to be the procedure of choice. The choice of transfers he advised were as follows:

- PT transfer to ECRB and ECRL.
- FCU transfer to the EDC of the third, fourth, and fifth fingers.
- FCR transfer to the EPL, EDC of the index finger, and EIP.

In 1921, Jones extended the transfer of the flexor carpi radialis (FCR) to include the APL and the EPB. Other choices of transfers have been used as follows. Biesalski and Mayer (1916) transferred a flexor superficialis to the ECR, whereas Stoffel (1919) used the FCR. Dunn (1918) advocated transfer of the palmaris longus (PL) to the EPL for extension of the thumb. Scuderi (1949) improved this technique by rerouting the EPL outside Lister's tubercle, thus giving a more direct angular path toward its anastomosis with the palmaris longus.

Starr (1922) seems to be the first to mention the danger of using all the wrist flexors as transfers. He retained the FCU and transferred the FCR and PL.

Zachary (1946), using a system of coding that allowed him to analyse the results of transfers performed in the Wingfield-Morris Hospital during World War II, demonstrated that it was necessary to retain one powerful active wrist flexor in order to stabilize the joint. In 18 cases in which the FCU and FCR were both transferred but the PL remained intact, the results, expressed as a percentage according to the code, averaged 57%. In five cases within this group in which the PL was not present, the percentage fell to an average of 26%; these results were unacceptable, for no patient could completely extend the fingers or the thumb. In 29 cases in which the FCU and PL (when it existed) were transferred and the FCR was preserved, the results were obviously better, as the percentage increased to an average of 91%. This study showed that conservation of the PL is not always sufficient to stabilize the wrist.

The use of the FCU, which is the strongest flexor of the wrist, as a transfer remains debated. Boyes (1960), Tsuge and Adachi (1969), and Brand (1975) recommend other combinations of transfers that leave the FCU in place. Biomechanical studies (Brand 1985) have further analysed these different types of transfer.

Principles of reconstructive surgery for radial palsy

A single transfer cannot act effectively on the tendon of five different muscles, as used by Jones. A transferred tendon can act on different tendons of the same muscle, such as the EDC, but its action is dispersed or even cancelled if it is fixed on the tendons of different muscles that each have a specific function.

A tendon transfer used to extend the fingers will also extend the wrist if the latter is not stabilized. If the amplitude of movement has already been used to extend the wrist, the tendon will not have sufficient action left to extend the fingers. Therefore, the main lines of treatment are established in the following manner:

- Re-establish, by separate transfers (1), wrist extension; (2) extension of the proximal phalanges of the fingers; and (3) extension, spreading, and retropositioning of the thumb.
- Conserve a muscle that will ensure stability of the wrist.

For each tendon transfer, the surgeon must consider the three basic elements of technique: the choice of the motor muscle, the path of the transferred tendon, and the site of fixation.

Re-establishment of wrist extension

Arthrodesis

For a long time, orthopedic surgeons who treated these lesions often arthrodesed the wrist, because this then freed the muscles of the wrist for transfer. Now, there is widespread agreement that a transfer to re-establish extension of the wrist – rather than an arthrodesis, because arthrodesis destroys the active tenodesis effect of wrist extension – is necessary for complete movement of the extrinsic tendons of the hand.

Motor muscles for transfer

The surgeon attempts to adapt the strength and the excursion of the motor muscle to those of the paralysed muscles. According to Fick (1911), the three extensors of the wrist comprise a force totaling 3.1 kg (ECRL, 1.1 kg; ECRB, 0.9 kg; ECU, 1.1 kg). Evaluations with the aid of electronic techniques (Ketchum et al 1978; Freehafer et al 1979) have produced different results, but the ratios are similar to those of Fick.

The excursion of the ECR tendons, according to Bunnell and Boyes (1964), is approximately 3.7 cm, excursion of the ECU is minimal in wrist extension.

Various transfers are possible, including the PT, a finger flexor, a wrist flexor, or even the brachioradialis when its enervation is preserved. The PT presents the greatest number of advantages, because (1) its force (1.2 kg) is somewhat superior to that of the ECRB or the ECRL alone; (2) its excursion (5 cm) is slightly greater in extension of the wrist, making rehabilitation easy; and (3) the pronator quadratus, innervated by the median nerve, continues to ensure pronation of the forearm after the removal of the PT. Furthermore the PT, inserted on the ECR tendons, keeps the same direction with the same obliquity and therefore continues to play a role in pronation of the forearm. Although the PT provides good wrist extension, it does not compensate for the loss of power caused by paralysis of the three wrist extensors.

Path of the transferred tendon

This differs with the motor muscle used for transfer.

Site of fixation

This important point is still debated. The ECRL and ECRB tendons run together in the middle third of the forearm and diverge more distally. It is tempting to fix the transfer on both tendons, but this should not be done, as it accentuates radial deviation and diminishes extension of the wrist (Brand 1985). Because the ECRL has a smaller moment arm than the ECRB for wrist extension and because its moment arm of radial deviation is greater than its moment arm of wrist extension, the patient's wrist is forced into radial deviation when extended.

Said (1974) has proposed a transfer of the PT on the three extensors of the wrist. This is even more objectionable because the extension moment arm of the ECU is even smaller than that of the ECRL and varies with rotation of the forearm; in pronation the ECU exerts an action opposite to that of the radial wrist extensors. Fixation solely to the ECRB offers the best extension to the wrist; however, this always allows some radial deviation. We have adopted another technique, as described later in the chapter.

Re-establishment of extension in the proximal phalanges of the fingers

The motor muscles

Although there is general agreement regarding the use of the PT as a transfer for extension of the wrist, the choice for the fingers is still disputed. The FCU, the FCR, or one or more flexors digitorum superficialis (FDS) may be chosen. The FCU has a force of 2 kg, close to that of the extensors in the fingers. Its excursion (3.3 cm) is less than that of the EDC (4.5 cm). The FCR is clearly weaker (0.8 kg), and its excursion (4 cm) is also less than that of the EDC. Thus if a wrist flexor is transferred to the EDC, complete extension of the fingers can only be obtained by simultaneous flexion of the wrist, which has an active tenodesis effect. For this reason, Boyes (1960) advocated using the flexor digitorum superficialis tendons, whose amplitude of 6.5 cm is clearly greater than that of the finger extensors. He used two FDS tendons (Chuinard et al 1978). The transfer scheme was the following: PT → ECRL + ECRB; FCR → APL + EPB; FDS (IV) → EPL + EIP; FDS (III) → EDL

Path of the transferred tendon

The path of the transfer must be as direct as possible. If the FCU is used, the tendon and muscle body must be freed to the upper third of the forearm so that they may pass around the medial border of the ulna. Some authors pass the FCU through the interosseous membrane (Cappelen 1899, Axhausen 1916).

The tendons of the FDS can also be transferred through the interosseous membrane (Boyes 1960), as can the FCR (Tsuge and Adachi 1969). Passage through the interosseous membrane provides the most direct course for the tendon and an increased action on the extension of the wrist. The interosseous neurovascular pedicles must be spared. The opening in the membrane should not be placed too proximal or it will create an acute angle in the path of the transfer; it must be placed just above the pronator quadratus muscle and should be made large enough to permit easy passage of the muscular body. Other authors pass these tendons around the radial or ulnar borders of the forearm.

Fixation

Most authors individually transfix the tendons of the EDC with the motor tendon. Some use the same transfer for the EIP and EDM; others recommend not including the

EDM, fearing that its flexion will be diminished. Still others prefer to use a distinct motor unit in order to ensure independence of the index finger. In these cases, they often use the same motor unit for the EIP and EDM. Others recommend not including the EDM, fearing that its flexion will be diminished. Still others prefer to use a distinct motor unit in order to ensure independence of the index finger. In these cases, they often use the same motor unit for the EIP and the EPL, following the initial scheme of Jones.

The tension extending from the index to the little finger must be calculated with care. Moberg and Nachemson (1967), as well as Brand (1975), recommend end-to-end rather than end-to-side suture transfixion, as it permits more direct traction.

Re-establishment of thumb extension, abduction, and retroposition

The motor muscle

The three long posterior muscles of the thumb column are the APL, the EPB, and the EPL, all of which are relatively weak. Their role is to open the hand, not to grasp. These muscles are divided into two groups whose axes of traction diverge and whose courses differ. Thus it is preferable not to use the same transfer for all of these tendons. The usual motor muscles chosen are the wrist flexors or an FDS.

All the possible combinations of transfers have been described. The action of these different muscles must be kept in mind, along with the objective of the procedure. The APL stabilizes the trapeziometacarpal joint and causes abduction of the first metacarpal in the radial plane, explaining its ancient name, 'extensor ossei metacarpi pollicis'. Its action is synergistic to that of the ECU, which opposes radial deviation of the wrist when the thumb is abducted. As noted by Duchenne (1867), in the case of paralysis of the ECU, abduction of the first metacarpal cannot occur without also causing radial deviation of the hand. Thus it is necessary to be aware of the action of an overly powerful transfer to the APL, especially if the FCU is also used for a transfer.

The EPB inserts more distally than the APL and runs parallel to it. It produces isolated extension of the proximal phalanx. The EPL, whose amplitude is much greater, has a different course, as it travels around Lister's tubercle. It not only contributes to the extension of the thumb, but it also brings the first ray in adduction and retroposition.

Path and fixation of the transferred tendon

When these three muscles are paralysed, the individual action of each is not required; rather the extension, abduction, and retroposition of the thumb column are required, while avoiding radial deviation of the wrist.

It is possible to make use of the same transfer for the EDC and the EPL. However, the thumb loses all independence of movement and, although good retroposition of the thumb can be obtained, separation of the first commissure remains limited. Another transfer is necessary on the APL and EPB.

Another solution is Scuderi's procedure (1949), which consists of transferring the palmaris longus to the EPL, having rerouted the EPL tendon lateral to Lister's tubercle to diminish adduction. In this manner, abduction and extension of the thumb are obtained. However, the lateral location of the transfer prevents it from benefiting from the active tenodesis effect provided by wrist movements. Retroposition is not complete and will only worsen with the tendon's tendency toward volar subluxation.

In any case, the thumb MP joint must be stable, because if the joint is lax, the transfer can exert a primary force on the proximal phalanx, rather than the first metacarpal, thereby causing hyperextension of the MP joint instead of extension and abduction of the first metacarpal.

The author's preferred techniques

None of the techniques described above is completely satisfactory. We have progressively modified these techniques (Tubiana 1985, Tubiana et al 1989). The choice of transfers is not original; the main changes made to the classic techniques consist of operative modifications. The following transfers are used:

- PT to the ECRB and to the rerouted ECRL
- FCU to the EDC and the EIP
- PL to the EPL.

The transfer for extension of the wrist is fixed after the transfer on the digits, as the passive movements of the wrist are used to adjust the tension of the transfers.

Incisions

Rather than several small incisions, an extensive approach is made on both sides of the forearm (Figure 10.5), which allows freeing of the motor muscles and of the recipient tendons. It offers the possibility of adapting the operative plan to individual cases and eventually passing a tendon through the interosseous membrane. It facilitates the adjustment of different tendon sutures that are placed within the same operative field.

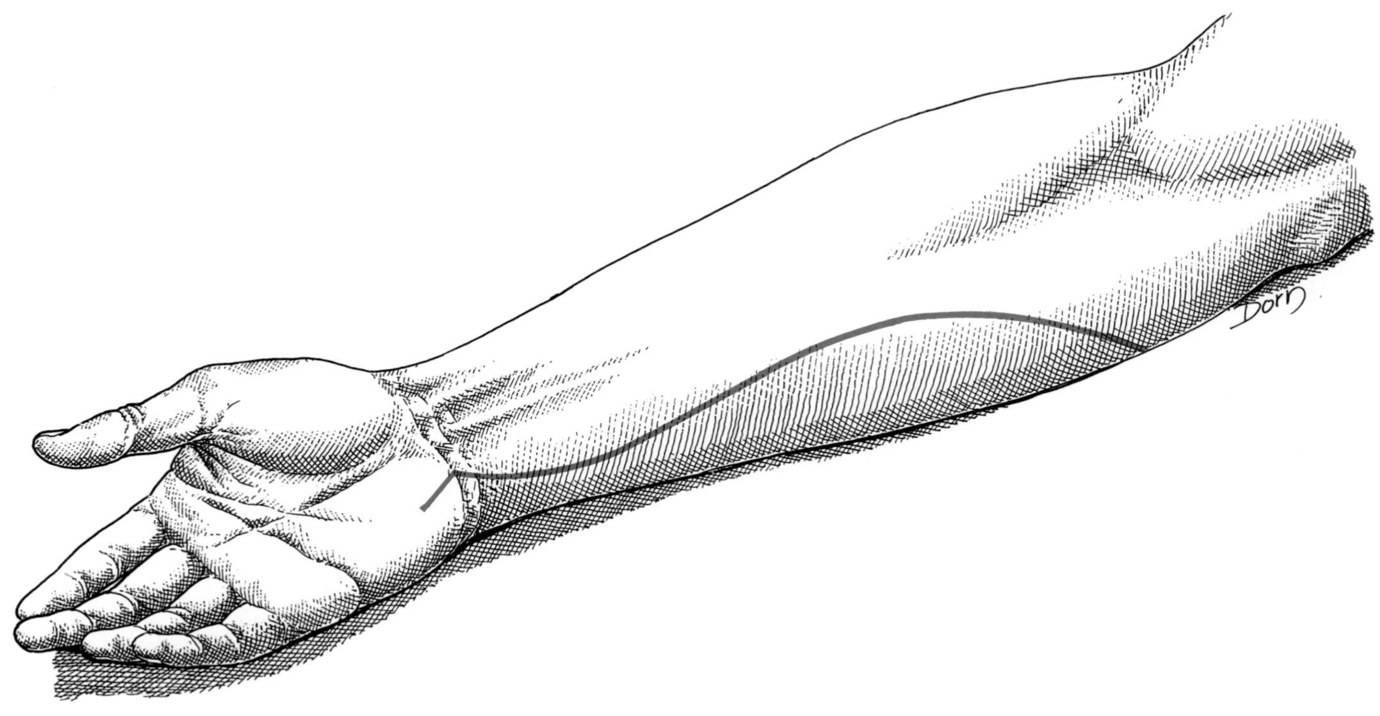

(A)

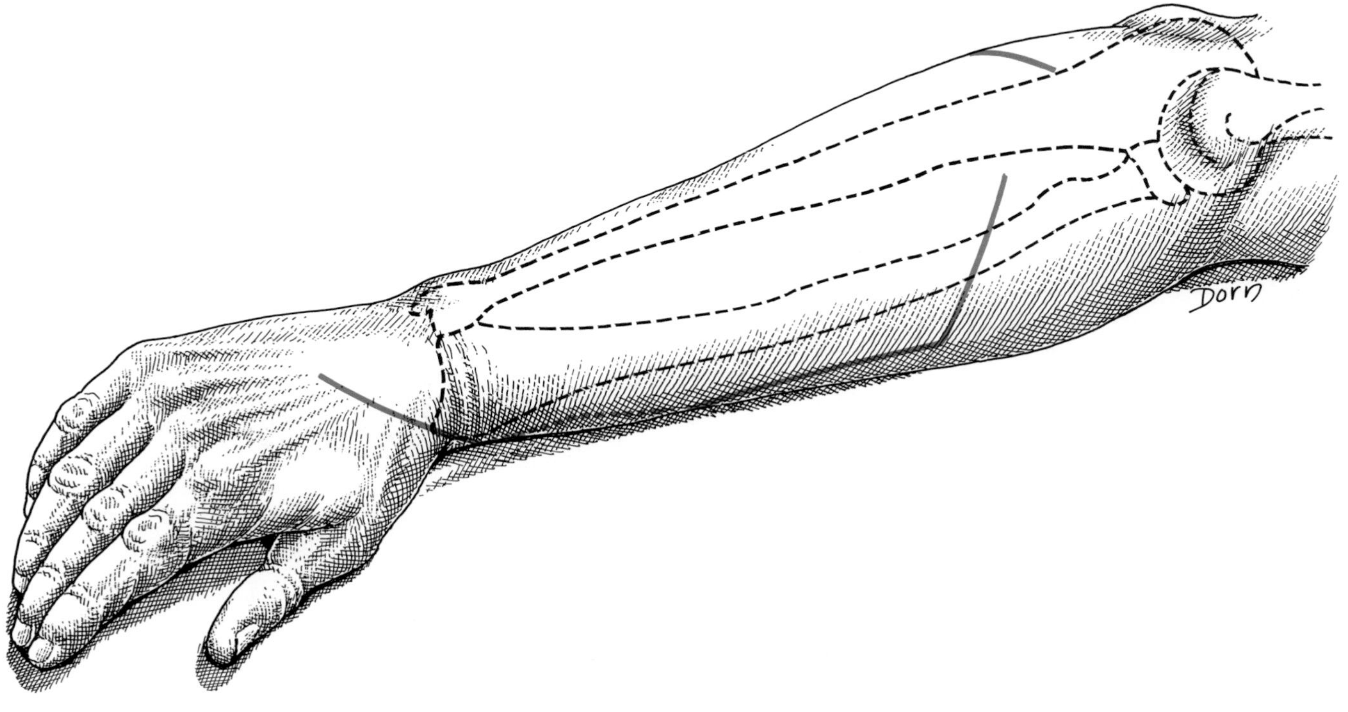

(B)

Figure 10.5
Incisions: (A) anterior approach; (B) posterior approach.

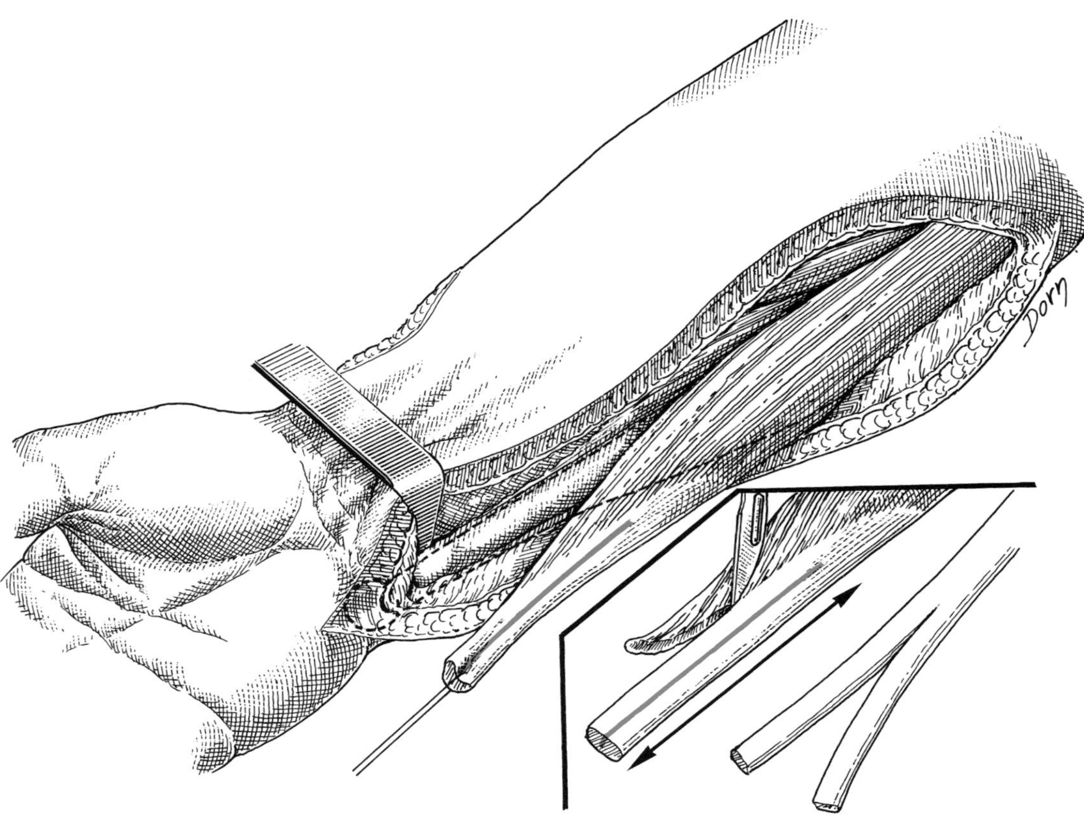

Figure 10.6

The FCU is divided and freed; the excess distal fleshy fibers are removed; the tendon is split into two strips, each approximately 6 cm long.

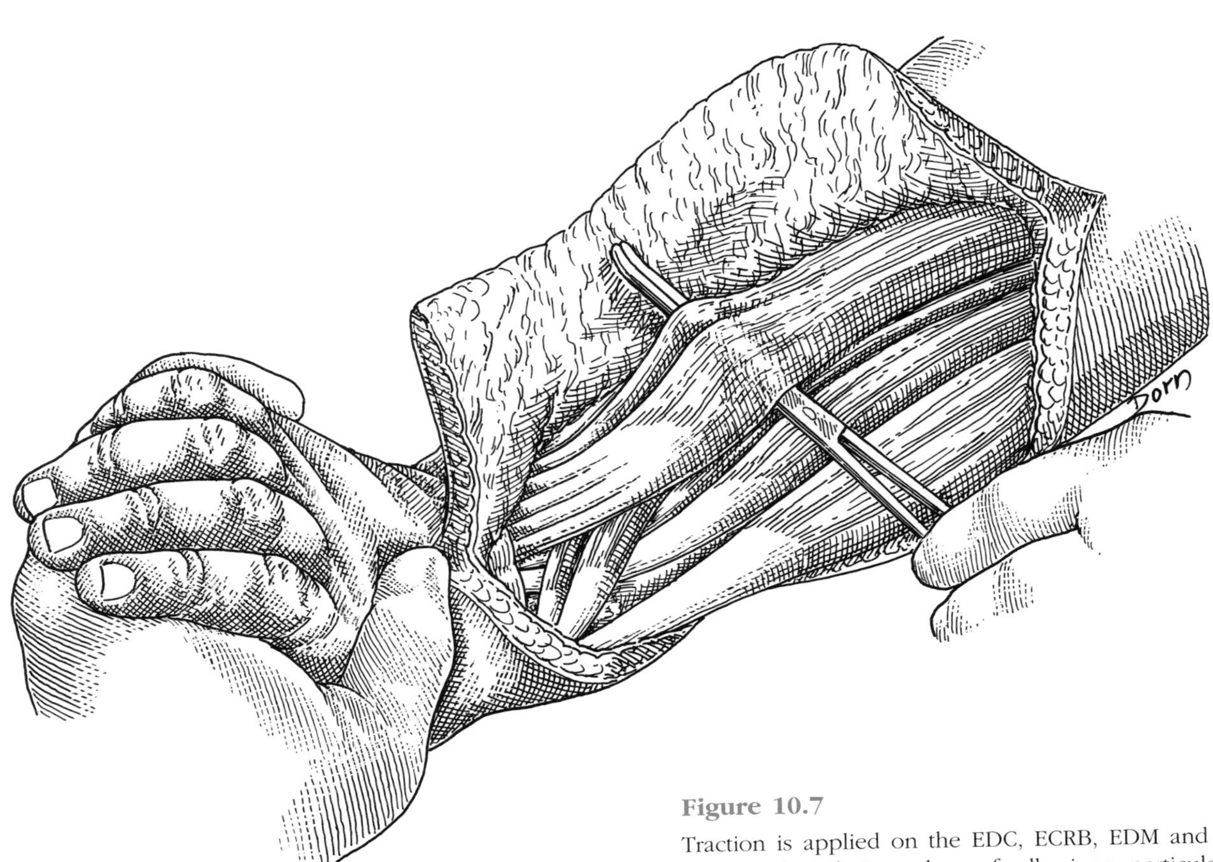

Figure 10.7

Traction is applied on the EDC, ECRB, EDM and EPL, in order to free their tendons of adhesions, particularly within the osteofibrous tunnels.

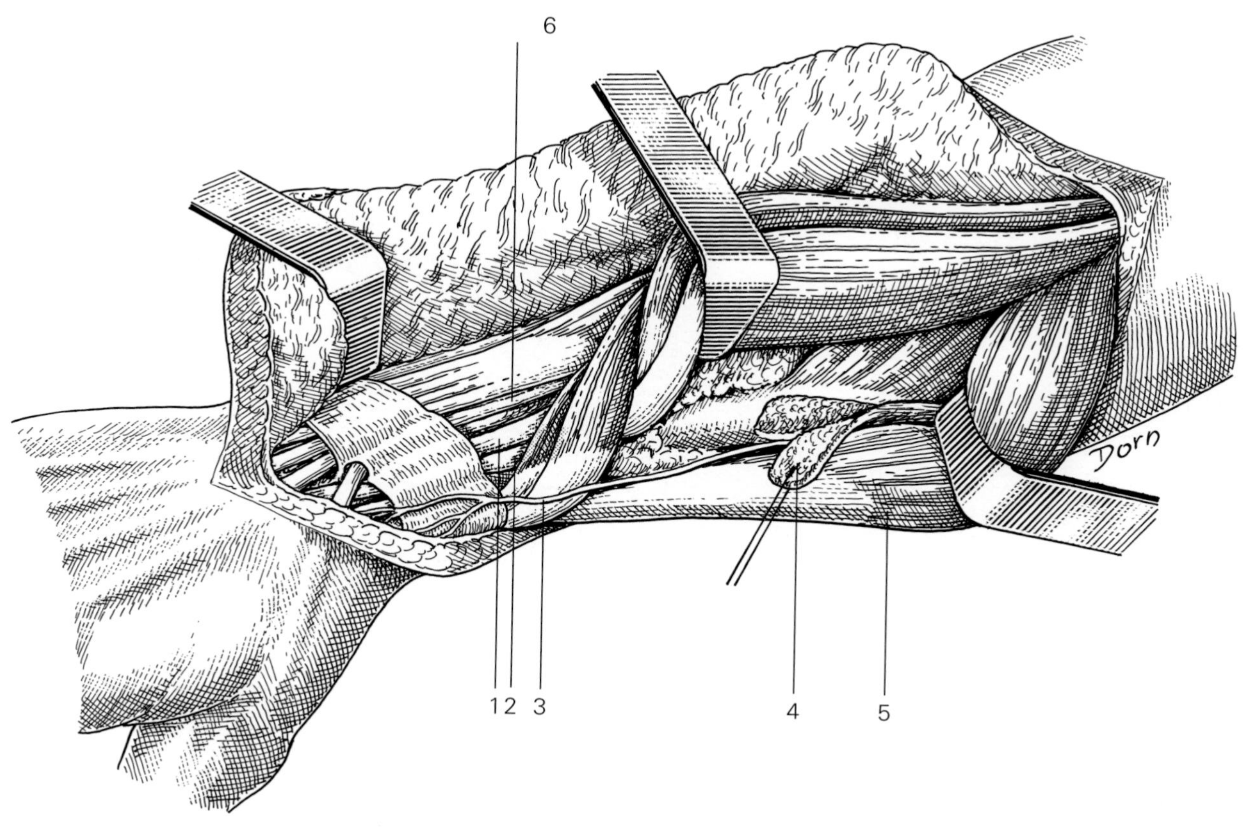

Figure 10.8

Elevation of the PT tendon with a strip of periosteum

1 ECRB, 2 ECRL, 3 sensory branch of the radial nerve, 4 tendon prolonged with a strip of periosteum, 5 BR, 6 site of division of the EPL tendon

Elevation of the transferred tendons

Elevation of the FCU and PL tendons

The FCU tendon is divided at the level of the distal flexion crease of the wrist. The muscle is freed throughout the length of the incision from its aponeurotic attachments with a periosteal elevator. Occasionally a small neurovascular pedicle joins the muscle distally, so it must be divided. The main pedicle is located proximally, joining the muscle at its deep surface about 6 cm from its origin from the epicondyle. The medial fascia is resected as necessary so that the FCU can pass from the volar to the posterior aspect of the forearm without angulation. Because the muscle body attaches low on the tendon, it is preferable to strip the excess distal fleshy fibers, conserving only 5 cm of the exposed tendon (Figure 10.6). This reduces the cosmetically unattractive bulge of the transfer beneath the wrist and facilitates suturing.

The PL tendon is sectioned at its distal end. The sinuous anterior incision permits it to be freed throughout its length.

Freeing the extensor tendons

The large veins on the posterior aspect of the forearm are preserved. The dorsal fascia is thick distally; it is dissected so that the sutured tendons are able to glide readily in the subcutaneous tissues.

The EDC, EIP, EDM, and ECR are exposed. Traction is applied to these tendons in order to free them of adhesions within the osteofibrous tunnels (Figure 10.7).

Complete passive extension of the wrist and of each finger is essential.

Elevation of the PT

The antebrachial fascia is incised between the brachioradialis and ECRL. The tendon of the PT arises from the volar aspect of the forearm and curves round the lateral border of the radial diaphysis beneath the brachioradialis. The muscle is dissected and detached with a 2-cm strip of periosteum to make its insertion in the recipient tendons easier (Figure 10.8). A traction suture is placed in the end of the tendon, allowing traction on the PT, which must be completely freed. At this point, the three motor muscles are ready for transfer.

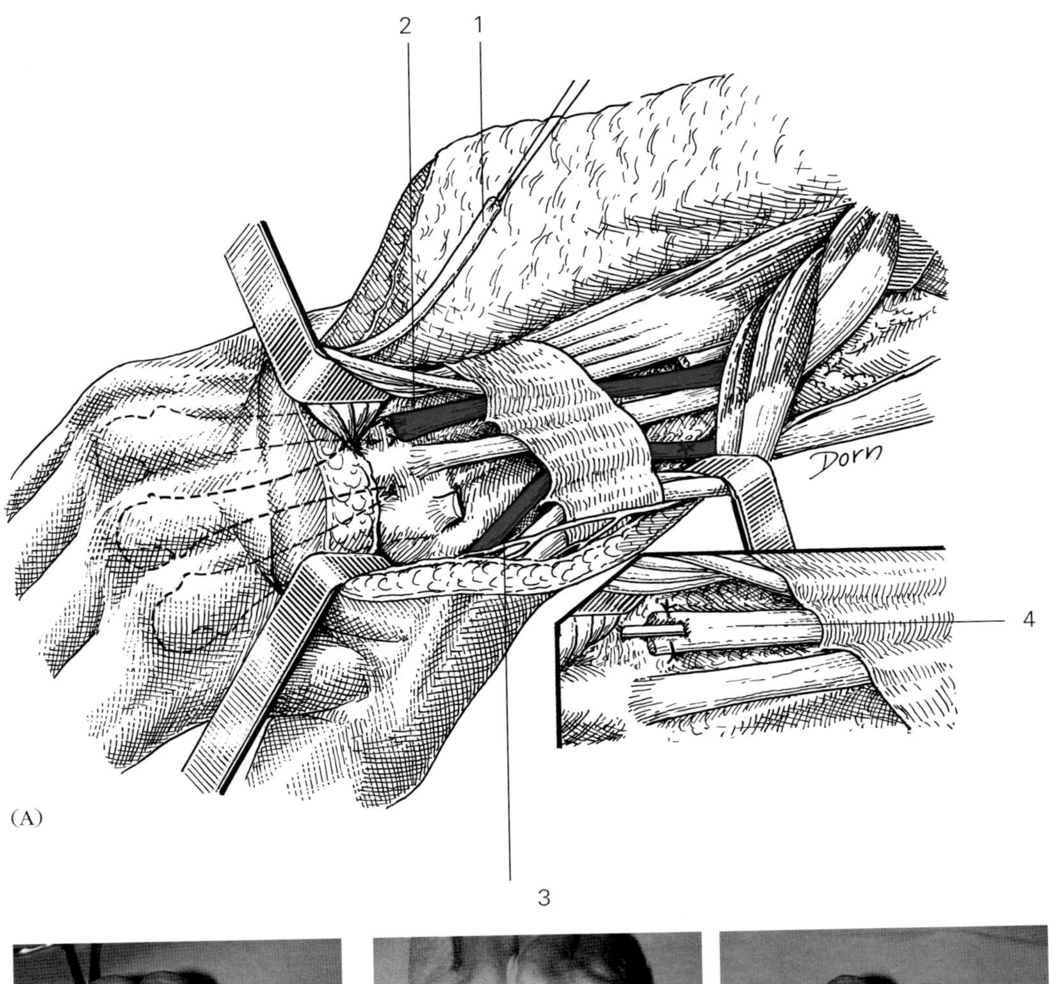

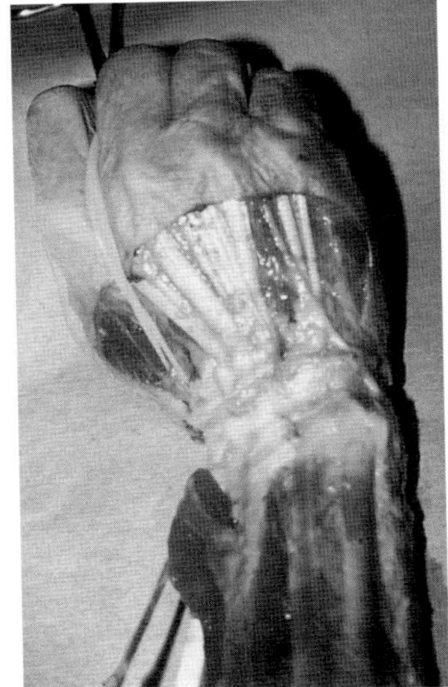
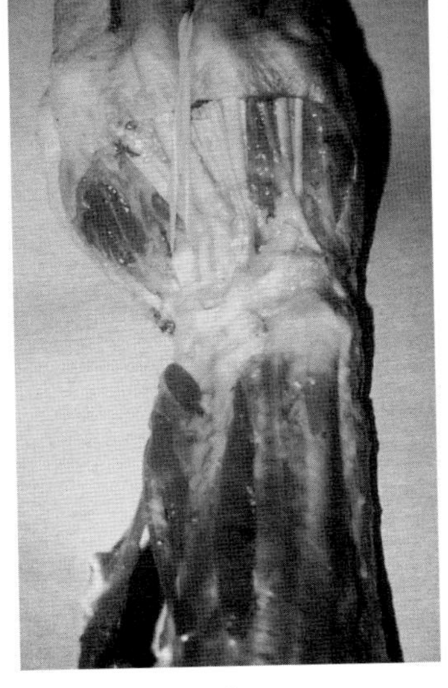
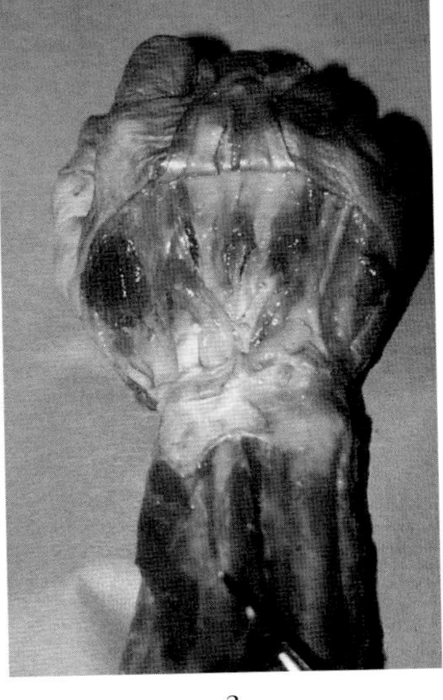

Figure 10.9

(A) Centralization of the ECRL tendon.

1 The ECRL tendon has been divided at the site of its insertion on the base of the second metacarpal and rerouted through the EDC tendon compartment

2 The EIP tendon is divided in the forearm at its musculotendinous junction and pulled out distally to make more room in the EDC tendon compartment

3 The EPL tendon is also rerouted in the second compartment, in place of the ECRL tendon to be sutured with the PL

4 The ECRL is fixed on the ulnar side of the base of the third metacarpal

(B) Action of the centralization of the ECRL tendon

1 In a normal wrist, traction of the ECRL causes marked radial deviation

2 Traction on the ECRB also causes radial deviation of the wrist, although it is less pronounced

3 Traction on the centralized extension of the wrist without deviation

Centralization of the ECRL tendon

To eliminate radial deviation of the wrist, several different techniques were tried. First the PT was transferred to the ECRB only. Then, to avoid the possibility of new adhesions between the two ECR tendons (which might create recurrent radial deviation), the ECRL tendon was divided distally and sutured to the ECRB. The correction of radial deviation still remained incomplete.

In 1985 we described the centralization of the insertion of the insertion of the ECRL tendon (Figure 10.9). The tendon of the ECRL is divided at the second

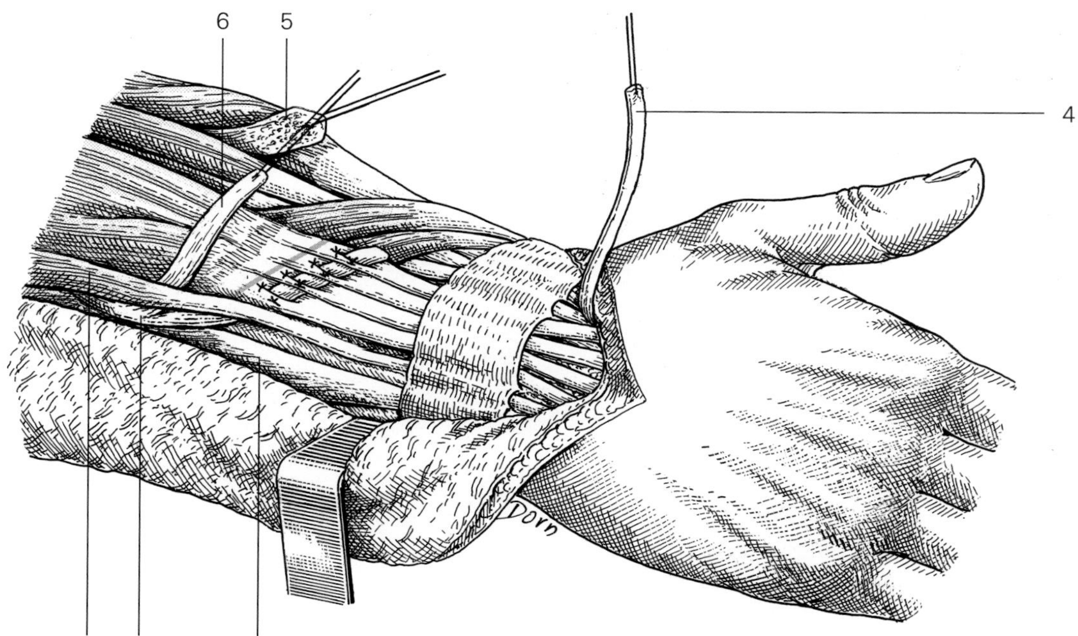

Figure 10.10

Fixation of the FCU to the EDC. One strip of the FCU is passed through each EDC tendon. Note the proximally placed suture on each EDC tendon to prevent it spreading open at the fixation site. The wrist and fingers are in extension. The EDC will be divided proximal to the transfer.

1 EDM
2 FCU
3 ECU
4 EIP
5 PT
6 Second strip of FCU tendon

metacarpal. It is pulled out of the dorsal retinaculum and freed up to the level of its musculotendinous junction. It is passed again under the retinaculum, but through the EDC tendon compartment. To make more room in this compartment, the EIP tendon is divided in the forearm and pulled out distally and then passed over the retinaculum. The rerouted ECRL tendon is fixed to the ulnar side of the base of the third metacarpal with sutures and staples, medial to the insertion of the ECRB tendon, symmetrical to the ECRB with respect to the longitudinal axis of the wrist. This centralization is completed before any transfer to the thumb and fingers is performed.

Releasing the tourniquet

It is important to release the tourniquet and secure hemostasis after the dissection, before fixation of the transfers, to set appropriate tension on the different transfers.

Fixation of the transfers

Fixation of the FCU on the EDC

The FCU is passed to the posterior aspect of the forearm. As the tendon of the FCU is somewhat bulky, it is splinted into two strips, each approximately 6 cm long. One slip is passed through the tendons of the EDC, and the other, at the end of the procedure will reinforce and adjust the sutures.

The suture is situated approximately 5 cm above the proximal edge of the dorsal retinaculum when the wrist is in a neutral position. When the wrist is completely flexed, the sutures must remain proximal to the retinaculum.

With an assistant holding the wrist in 40° of extension and the thumb and the fingers extended, the little, ring, long, and index finger tendons of the EDC are successively perforated with a sharp tendon clamp. These perforations are made in the oblique, dorsal, and radial directions. One strand of the split end of the FCU is pulled through the perforations. The tendons of the EDC are fixed to each other above the transfixation line with non-absorbable suture material, which prevents the hole from enlarging (Figure 10.10).

Then 2 cm of the paralysed EDC muscle are resected proximal to this suture, to avoid an angulation at the level of fixation of the transfer (Moberg and Nachemson 1967). Each perforated tendon is sutured independently to the motor slip. By varying the site of the suture of each tendon, it is possible to adjust the tension for each finger. Tension is more important for the radial fingers than for the ulnar ones. Motion in the wrist facilitates this adjustment. Secondary relaxation always takes place. Complete extension of the proximal phalanges should be possible when the wrist is in 30° of flexion.

Fixation of the PL to the EPL

The tendon of the EPL is sectioned at its musculotendinous junction in the lower third of the forearm and drawn distally out of its osteofibrous groove.

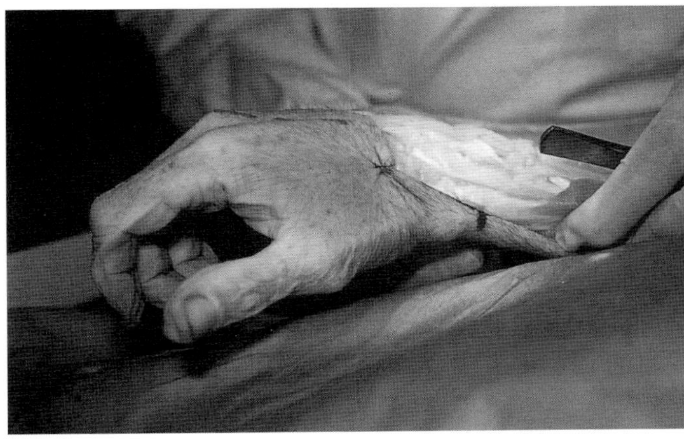
(A)

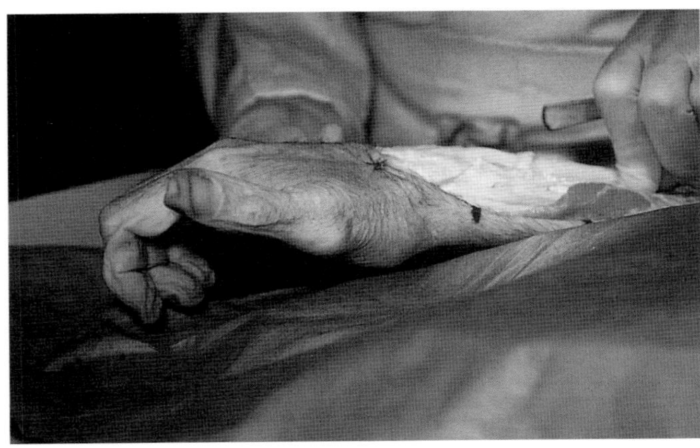
(B)

Figure 10.11
Transfer of the PL to the EPL tendon.
(A) Scuderi's procedure: the EPL tendon is rerouted lateral to Lister's tubercle
(B) Tubiana's modification: the EPL is rerouted through the ECRL compartment, showing better retroposition of the thumb column

Scuderi's technique has been modified. The EPL tendon is passed under the extensor retinaculum but in the ECR compartment in place of the ECRL, which is first rerouted. Thus, the EPL is in a more radical location and its new pulley prevents volar subluxation (see Figures 10.9 and 10.11).

The PL, approached by the volar anterior incision, is also freed, so that it takes a straight course to meet the EPL. The two tendons are sutured on the radial side of the forearm, above the wrist; with the thumb in radial abduction, complete extension, and retroposition; the wrist in neutral position; and the PL under maximum tension. Reactivation of the EPL by the PL is sufficient to produce extension and abduction of the thumb column, making it unnecessary to perform another transfer to the APL, as its antagonist, the ECU, is paralysed.

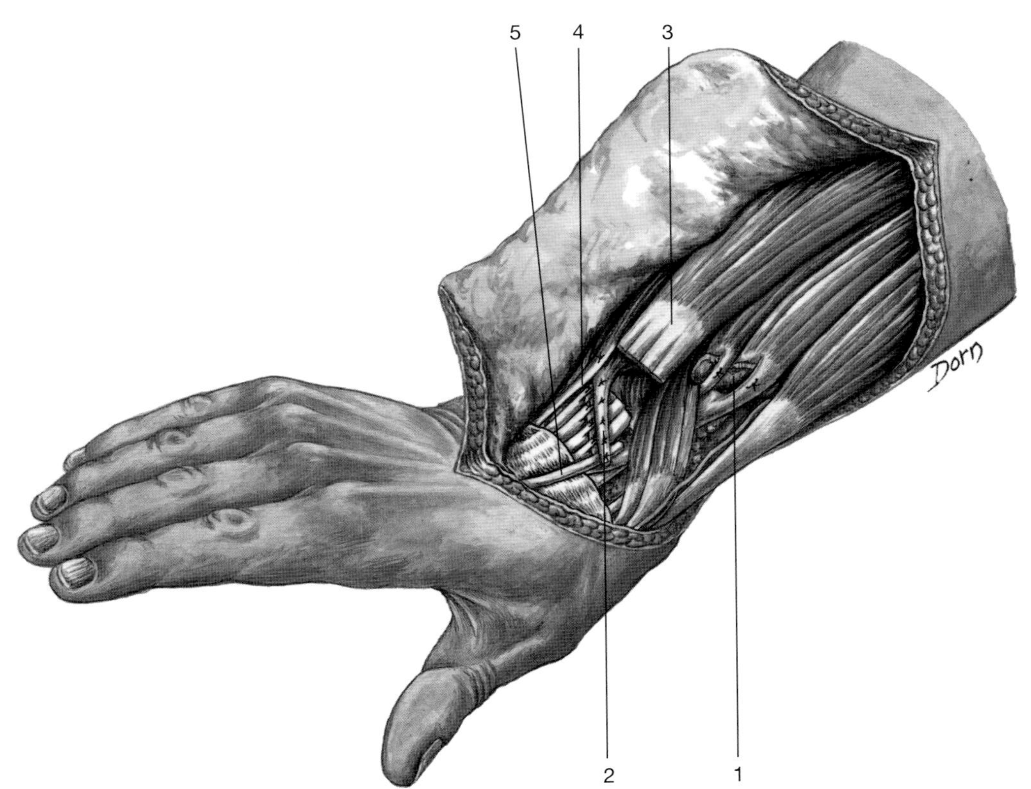

Figure 10.12
Fixation of the PT and EIP tendons and of the superficial slip of the FCU tendon.
1 The PT tendon is fixed on the ECRB and on the rerouted ECRL
2 Fixation of the superficial slip of the FCU tendon on each EDC tendon
3 Proximal part of the EDL
4 The EDM tendon may be fixed to the FCU
5 The EIP tendon is passed superficial to the extensor retinaculum and fixed to the superficial slip of the FCU

Fixation of the PT

The PT is passed subcutaneously for its new attachment into the extensor carpi radialis muscles. The periosteal strip of the PT is fixed through the ECRB and the rerouted ECRL tendons just distal to their musculotendinous junction (Figure 10.12); the transferred muscle is under tension. An assistant maintains the wrist in 40° extension, the MP joints of the four fingers slightly flexed at 15°, and the interphalangeal joints in extension.

Fixation of the superficial slip of the FCU tendon

Adjustment of the tension of the FCU transfer on the digits is probably the most delicate part of the operation, which is why we prefer to fix the second slip of the FCU tendon last of all. Tension should be adjusted individually for each finger. The EIP tendon, still unsutured, is now fixed to the FCU (Figure 10.11).

The EDM

The EDM is left free unless complete extension by the EDC to the little finger alone is incomplete. This may be tested by pulling on the common extensor. If extension is incomplete, the EDM tendon should be tacked onto the transfer, but without excessive tension.

Technique maintaining the FCU in place and transferring one flexor superficialis

In some cases, it seems appropriate to maintain the FCU in place. When the patient is engaged in heavy manual labor without requiring great digital dexterity, one would tend to reinforce wrist extension by using a transfer of the flexor superficialis (FS), especially in the dominant hand (see Indications section, later in chapter).

The following choices of transfer have been adopted:

- PT → ECRB and rerouted ECRL
- FDS of IV → EDC of II, III, IV, and little fingers
- FCR → EPL + EIP
- PL → APL + EPB

Incisions

The same approach as in the previous procedure is used on the posterior aspect of the forearm. On the volar aspect, a transverse incision is made at the base of the ring finger for the division of the FDS tendon proximal to the chiasma. The longitudinal sinuous incision in the forearm is more central than in the previous procedure.

On the dorsal aspect of the forearm

1. Elevation of the EIP, EPL, EPB, and APL. All these tendons are divided at the level of their musculotendinous junction and are extracted from their respective osteofibrous compartments (Figure 10.13).

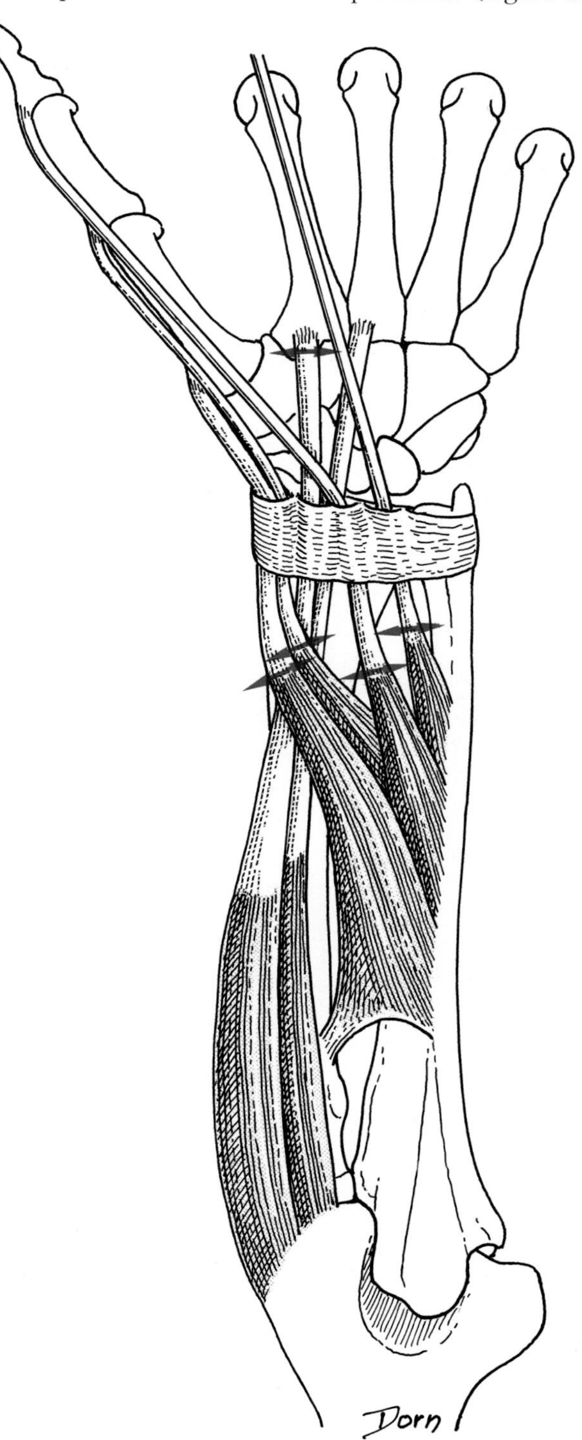

Figure 10.13

Transfers of the FS tendon to the EDC tendons of the FCR to the rerouted EPL and EIP tendons and of the PL to the APL and EPB. Site of the tendon divisions on the dorsal aspect of the forearm.

2. Centralization of the ECRL tendon, as in the preceding technique.

On the volar aspect of the forearm

1. The muscular belly of the FS of the ring finger is freed and the muscle is passed medially to the FDP. The volar interosseous pedicle is located and retracted. A large window is made in the interosseous membrane at the proximal edge of the pronator quadratus with fibrous removal performed deep to the muscle (Figure 10.14). If the orifice is too proximal, the tendon will not have a direct route and may be caught on the distal edge of the window.
2. The FCR tendon is divided at the level of the wrist, the FCR is freed up to the middle third of the forearm and passed posteriorly around the radius.
3. Elevation of the PL and PT.

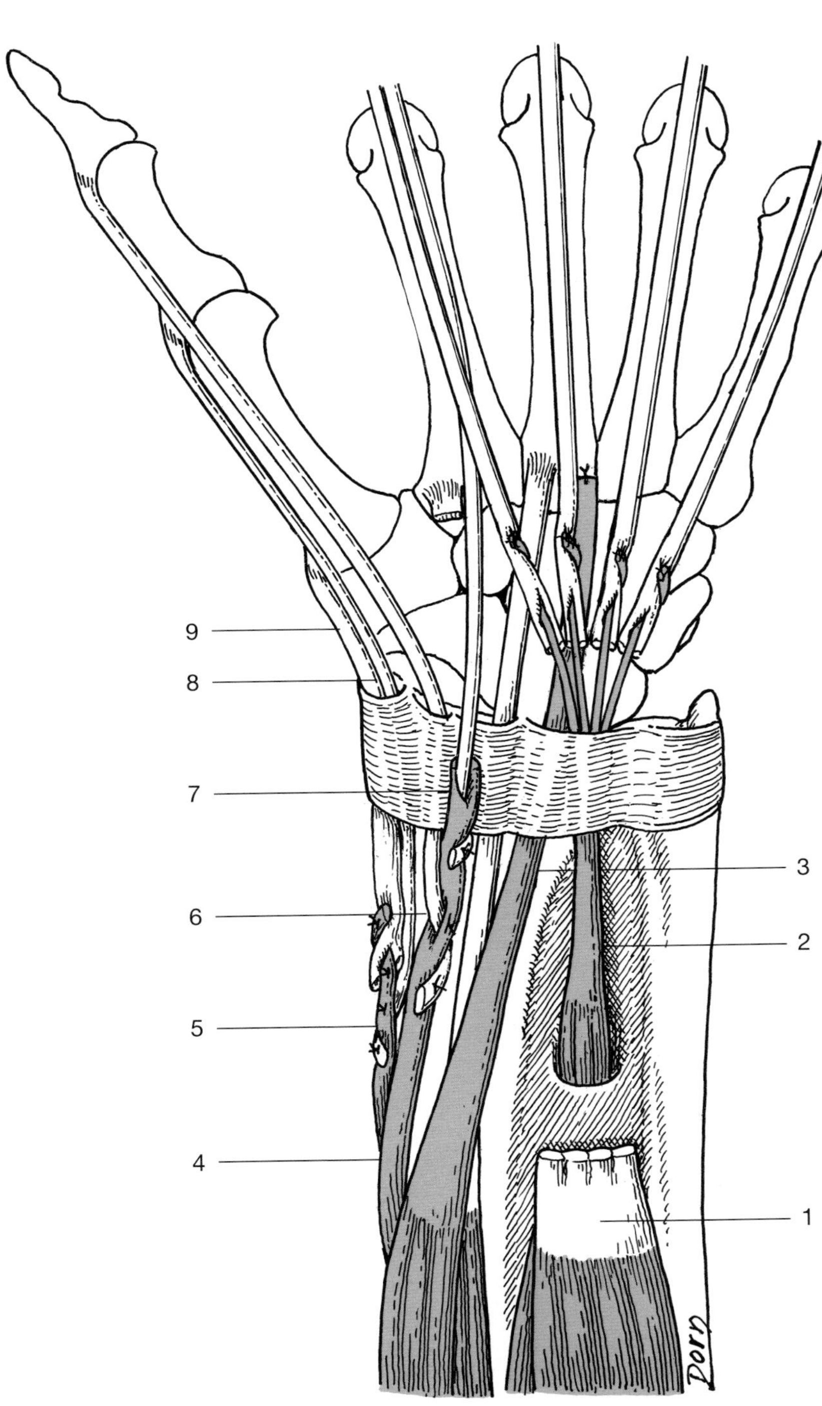

Figure 10.14

1, EDC proximal part; 2, FDS; 3, rerouted ECRL; 4, FCR; 5, PL; 6, EPL; 7, EIP.

The FDS of the ring finger (2) is passed through the interosseous membrane window and sutured to the EDC tendons distal to the retinaculum

The ECRL tendon (3) has been rerouted through the fourth compartment

The FCR (4) is fixed on the EPL and EIP tendons

The EPL tendon (6) has been rerouted through the second compartment

The EIP tendon (7) is passed over the retinaculum

The PL (5) is fixed on the EPB (8) and APL (9) tendons

Transfer of the FS tendon to the EDC tendons

The FS tendon is rerouted through the interosseous membrane in the posterior compartment and is then passed under the extensor retinaculum at the site of the extensor digitorum tendons, which have been largely resected. The FS tendon is divided into four bands, which are sutured to the four EDC tendons on the dorsal aspect of the hand, distal to the extensor retinaculum, with the fingers passively in extension as in the preceding technique and the wrist in 40° extension (Figure 10.14).

Transfer of the FCR to the rerouted EPL and EIP (see Figure 10.14)

The FCR tendon is fixed both to the EPL and to the EIP. The EPL tendon is rerouted through the second compartment as before and transfixed into the larger FCR tendon. This suture should be as proximal as possible, in order to prevent the limitation of gliding under the retinaculum. The EIP fixation can be more distal because its tendon is passed superficial to the retinaculum.

Transfer of the PL to the APL and EPB (see Figure 10.13)

When the PL is missing, a tenodesis is possible. The APL and EPB tendons are divided at their musculotendinous junction about 6 cm above the radial styloid process. These tendons circle the styloid insertion of the brachioradialis and are then sutured back to themselves under strong tension.

Transfer of the PT to the ECRL and ECRB

The periosteal strip of the PT transfixes the ECRL and ECRB at the level of their musculotendinous junction as in the preceding technique.

Postoperative care

A volar splint, prepared before the operation, is applied to maintain the wrist in 50° of extension and 10° of ulnar deviation, the interphalangeal joints in extension, and the MP joints in 15° of flexion; the thumb in extension, abduction, and complete retroposition; and the forearm in full pronation. The splint should never place the wrist and fingers in complete extension and should extend above the elbow so that pronation and supination are avoided. This splint is worn continually for 2 weeks, after which the interphalangeal joints only are freed. The support is removed after 3 weeks and is replaced by a dynamic splint composed of a dorsal antebrachial support on which is fixed a system of dynamic elastic appendages with harnesses placed on the volar aspect of the phalanges. Almost the entire palmar aspect of the hand is free.

Progressively, starting with the fifth postoperative week, active extension and complete flexion of the fingers are allowed. It is important to move the fingers and the wrist separately.

Indications

Indications for reconstructive surgery in radial palsy must take into account:

1. the time elapsed since the injury;
2. the nature of the nerve lesions;
3. the extent of the lesions;
4. the associated lesions;
5. the characteristics of each patient.

Time elapsed since the injury

Bevin (1976), because of good results attained after tendon transfers for radial palsy, abstained from nerve repair. On the other hand, some surgeons, struck by the possibility of very late recovery, now have the tendency to delay reconstructive surgery; waiting 3 years after brachial plexus repair, 2 years after repair of radial nerve in the arm, or 18 months if the lesion is in the forearm or at the wrist (Sedel and Mériaux 1985).

In appropriate cases early reconstructive surgery permits a functional recovery and prevents the development of deformities and trick movements that are difficult to eliminate. It also renders cumbersome and constraining external splints useless. It is for this reason that these operations have been referred to as internal splints. Also, because all the tissues are still supple at this early stage, less powerful transfers are necessary than in late reconstructive surgery.

On the other hand, there are two kinds of risk. First, harvesting of active muscles for use as transfers will increase the motor deficit unnecessarily if nerve recuperation eventually occurs. Second, deformities may develop because of excessive force after nerve recuperation.

Indications for early reconstructive surgery

The indications for these operations are thus limited to instances in which (1) for any reason, nerve repair cannot be done; and (2) the theoretical chance of recuperation is remote or projected to be very late.

The decision for early reconstructive surgery after a radial nerve suture is theoretically guided by the time required for reinnervation of the paralysed muscles. An estimate is made by adding the time that has elapsed before nerve repair to the time necessary for axonal regeneration to the paralysed muscles, approximately 1 mm per day. If the total is >1 year, it may sometimes be wise to combine nerve repair with reconstructvie surgery that will not compromise function in the case of reinnervation.

Unfavorable prognosis after a nerve repair is another reason in favor of early reconstructive surgery: poor technical repair, proximal lesion site, delayed repair, and elderly patients are factors that militate against successful recovery.

However, one should be cautious in recommending early reconstructive surgery after radial nerve repair because recovery is more frequent than for the median or ulnar nerves owing to the great proportion of motor fibers and the proximal location of the muscles innervated by this nerve. However, transfer of the PT to the ECRB can be performed early in some cases: this transfer re-establishes wrist extension, and the PT conserves its pronating action on the forearm. Regeneration of the wrist extensors reinforces the action of the PT transfer and does not hinder hand function if the wrist flexors are conserved. On the contrary, transfers to the finger and thumb extensors become too powerful after nerve regeneration, causing a constraint to finger flexion and to opposition that is harmful for function. The handicap is magnified if the FDS or FCU is used for the transfer.

I have secondarily treated a patient who suffered an open fracture of the humerus, with section and crush injury of the radial nerve that had been sutured. Tendon transfers had been performed early for wrist and finger extension, because the chance of reinnervation seemed remote and the patient was a pianist. The radial nerve recovered more than had been anticipated, and the patient had his fingers and wrist fixed in hyperextension, so that I was obliged to operate to take down the transfers.

Nature of nerve lesions

Compression neuropathies of the radial nerve have been described at different levels. Disturbances of sensibility are most often related to a compression of the superficial branch to the wrist (see Chapter 23, Radial nerve compression).

Compression proximal to the elbow or at the level of the elbow results in muscle weakness or even in incomplete or complete paralysis. These paralyses usually recover after conservative treatment or surgical decompression; reconstructive surgery is rarely indicated.

Extent of the paralysis

The extent of the paralysis depends on several factors:

- the nerve lesions,
- the site of the lesion,
- the amount of recuperation.

Partial lesion of the radial nerve causes paralysis of only some extensor muscles and the treatment must be adapted according to the extent of the paralysis.

Posterior interosseous nerve palsy

In distal palsy, affecting only the posterior interosseous nerve, innervation of the brachioradialis and ECRL is retained and thus active wrist extension persists. The origin of the branch for the ECRB is variable, and it may be clinically difficult to confirm whether one or two wrist extensors are active. Persistent innervation of the ECR muscles causes severe radial deviation. In this case, removal of the FCU results in an uncompensated disequilibrium.

In these distal paralyses, the transfer of the FCR to the EDC seems particularly indicated. The ECRB and FCU must always be preserved.

When a severe radial deviation persists, one solution is to suture the FCU tendon to the ECU tendon; this technique makes the FCU into a pure ulnar deviator (Brand 1985).

Incomplete recovery

With the amelioration of nerve repair techniques, it has become more common to treat patients with incompletely recovered radial nerve repairs or a loss of wrist or digit extension associated with a more proximal nerve lesion, rather than only those with a pure radial nerve palsy.

Association with other peripheral nerve injuries

In such cases, the choice of transfers is limited. It is necessary first to re-establish active wrist extension, as this movement provides flexion of the fingers when combined with tenodesis of the finger flexors. When the PT is paralysed a flexor of the fingers or wrist, or even the brachioradialis (if it still has its innervation), can be utilized. The brachioradialis is also innervated by the radial nerve, but its branches are more proximal than those of the ECR. Similarly, its nerve origins in the cervical cord are higher, so this muscle is sometimes the only one that can be transferred (Freehafer and Mast 1967). Brachioradialis originates on the distal third of the

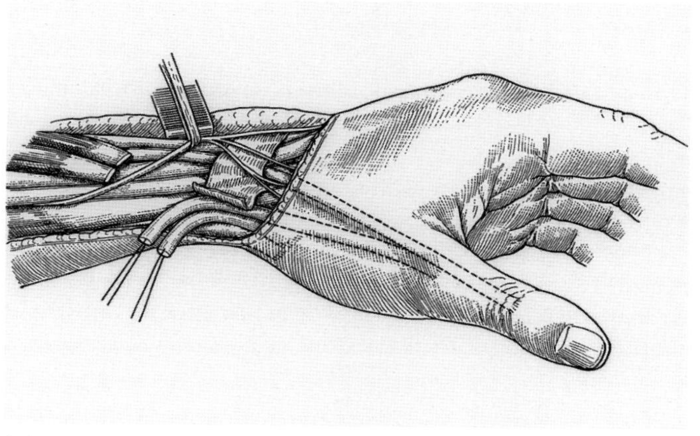
(A)

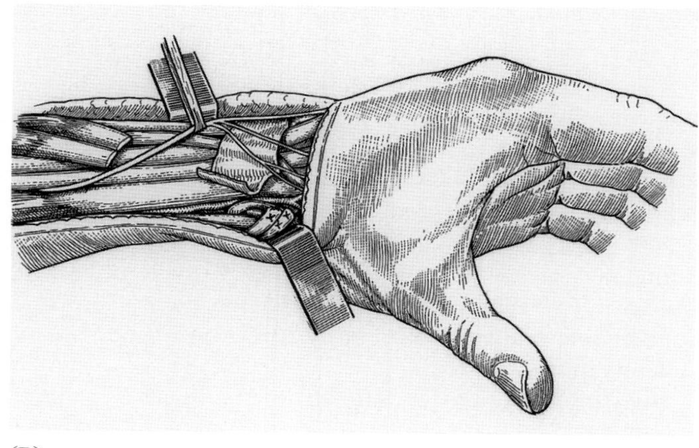
(B)

Figure 10.15
Tenodesis of the APL and EPB. (A) The APL and EPB tendons are divided at their musculotendinous junction. (B) These two tendons are wrapped around the insertion of the brachioradialis tendon.

humerus and is essentially an elbow flexor. An active elbow extensor is required to allow the brachioradialis to be used as a wrist extensor. Although the brachioradialis is one of the most powerful muscles of the forearm, its excursion is very limited (1.3 cm). However, this can be considerably augmented by freeing all of its proximal forearm connections and disinserting its proximal portion on the humerus (Tubiana et al 1989).

Characteristics of each patient

When the patient is engaged in heavy manual labor without requiring great digital dexterity, one would tend to reinforce wrist extension by using a transfer of the FS, especially in the dominant hand, and leave the FCU intact. There is now a greater tendency to conserve the FCU; however, the technique utilizing the FS is more delicate and the rehabilitation takes longer. Therefore, we only transfer the FS in young and cooperative patients. Removal of FS tendons is avoided if independence of individual fingers is desired, especially in those occupations utilizing keyboards.

In the absence of the PL we prefer to use an FCR type of transfer. A tenodesis of the APL and EPB tendons wrapped around the insertion of the BR tendon is possible (Figure 10.15).

Conclusion

Although palliative treatment for radial nerve palsy poses fewer problems than that for median or ulnar nerve paralyses, numerous factors determine the choice of transfer and the surgical technique.

References

Axhausen (1916) *Berliner Klin Wochenschr* **7**.

Bevin AG (1976) Early tendon transfer for radial nerve transsection, *Hand* **8**: 134–6.

Biesalski K, Mayer L (1916) *Die Physiologische Schnerverps Flanzung* (Berlin: Springer) 330.

Boyes JH (1960) Tendon transfers for radial palsy, *Bull Hosp Joint Dis* **21**: 97.

Boyes JH (1962) Selection of a donor muscle for tendon transfer, *Bull Hosp Joint Dis* **23**: 1–4.

Boyes JH (1964) *Bunnell's Surgery of the Hand*, 4th edn (JB Lippincott: Philadelphia).

Brand PW (1975) Tendon transfers in the forearm. In: Flynn JE, ed, *Hand Surgery*, 2nd edn (Williams & Wilkins: Baltimore).

Brand PW (1985) *Clinical Mechanisms of the Hand* (CV Mosby: St Louis).

Capellen (1899) Centralblatt für Chirurgie, 1335.

Chuinard RG, Boyes JH, Stark HH, Ashworth CR (1978) Tendon transfers for radial nerve palsy: use of superficialis tendons for digital extension, *J Hand Surg* **3**: 560–70.

Duchenne GB (1867) *Physiologie des Mouvements* (GB Baillière: Paris). Translated and edited by EB Kaplan (WB Saunders: Philadelphia, 1959).

Dunn N (1918) Treatment of lesion of the musculo-spinal nerve in military surgery, *Am J Orthop Surg* **16**: 258–65.

Fick R (1911) *Handbuch der Anatomie und Mechanik der Gelenke* Vol 3 (G Fischer: Iena).

Fiori (1907) *Clin Chirurg* **7**.

Francke (1899) *Archiv Klin Chir* **LVII**(Suppl): 763.

Freehafer AA, Mast WA (1967) Transfer of the brachio-radialis to improve wrist extension in high spinal cord injury, *J Bone Joint Surg* **49A**: 648–52.

Freehafer AA, Peckham PH, Keith MW (1979) Determination of muscle-tendon unit properties during tendon transfer, *J Hand Surg* **4**: 331.

Friedenberg B (1954) Transposition of the biceps brachii for triceps weakness, *J Bone Joint Surg* **36A**: 656.

Hazelton FT, Smidt GL, Flatt AE, Stephens RL (1975) The influence of wrist position on the force produced by the flexors, *J Biomechanics* **8**: 301–6.

Holstein A, Lewis GB (1963) Fractures of the humerus with radial nerve paralysis, *J Bone Joint Surg* **45A**: 1382–8.

Jones R (1916) On suture of nerves, and alternative methods of treatment by transplantation of tendon, *BMJ* **1**: 641–3, 679–82.

Jones R (1921) Tendon transplantation in cases of musculospinal injuries not amenable to suture, *Am J Surg* **35**: 333–5.

Ketchum LD, Thomson D, Pocock GS (1978) The determination of moments for extension of the wrist generated by muscles of the forearm, *J Hand Surg* **3**: 205–10.

Merle d'Aubigné R, Lance P (1946) Transplantations tendineuses dans le traitement des paralysies radiales post-traumatiques, *Semin Hop Paris* **22**: 1666–80.

Moberg E (1978) *The Upper Limb in Tetraplegia* (Georg Thieme: Stuttgart).

Moberg E, Nachemson A (1967) Tendon transfers for defective long extensors of the wrist and fingers, *Acta Chir Scand* **133**: 31–4.

Napier JR (1955) Prehensile movements of the human hand, *J Anat* **89**: 564.

Perthes G (1918) Über Schnenoperationen bei irreparabler Radialislähmung Bruns', *Beitr Klin Chir* **113**: 289.

Rochet (1897) *Lyon Med J* **34**: 379.

Said GZ (1974) A modified tendon transference for radial nerve paralysis, *J Bone Joint Surg* **56B**: 320–2.

Saikku LA (1947) Tendon transplantation for radial paralysis. Factors influencing the results of tendon transplantation, *Acta Chir Scand* **96**(suppl 132): 7–100.

Scuderi C (1949) Tendon transplants for irreparable radial nerve paralysis, *Surg Gynecol Obstet* **88**: 643–51.

Seddon H (1975) *Surgical Disorders of the Peripheral Nerves*, 2nd edn (Churchill Livingstone: Edinburgh) 31.

Sedel L, Mériaux JL (1985) *La Main Paralytique, Les Opérations Palliatives* (Encyclopédie Médico-Chirurgicale, Techniques Chir: Paris).

Spinner M (1998) The radial nerve. In: *Injuries of the Major Branches of Peripheral Nerves of the Forearm*, 2nd edn, p. 79 (WB Saunders: Philadelphia).

Starr CL (1922) Army experiences with tendon transference, *J Bone Joint Surg* **4**: 321.

Stoffel (1919) *Zentralbl Chir* **8**: 148.

Tsuge K (1969) Tendon transfer for extensor palsy of forearm, *Hiroshima J Med Sci* **18**: 219–32.

Tubiana R (1985) Notre expérience des transfers tendineux pour paralysie radiale, *Ann Chir Main* **4**: 197–210.

Tubiana R (1999) Radial nerve paralysis. In: Tubiana R, Gilbert A, Masquelet A, eds, *An Atlas of Surgical Techniques of the Hand and Wrist* (Martin Dunitz: London) 307–20.

Tubiana R, Miller HW, Reed S (1989) Restoration of wrist extension after paralysis, *Hand Clin* **5**: 53–67.

Ueba Y (1986) Tendon transfer for radial nerve palsy, *J Jpn Soc Surg Hand* **2**: 876–83.

Vichard P, Tropet Y, Laudecy G et al (1982) Paralysies radiales contemporaines des fractures de la diaphyse humerale, *Chirurgie* **108**: 791–5.

Zachary RB (1946) Tendon transplantation for radial paralysis, *Br J Surg* **33**: 358–64.

Zancolli EA (1975) Surgery for the quadriplegic hand with active strong wrist extension preserved. A. Study of 97 cases, *Clin Orthop* **112**: 101.

11 Paralysis of the thumb

François Moutet

Introduction

The importance of the opposition of the thumb in the abilities of the human hand has often been emphasized. Opposition is not specific to mankind, as all primates have an opposable thumb, even lemurs. However, erect posture on lower limbs permitted the opposition of the thumb to be developed while the first toe lost this ability. The features specific to mankind are the conjunction of length of the first column, density of tactile pulp receptors and opposition amplitude. This gave mankind supremacy in hunting, gathering and tool production, while the erect posture allowed skull volume to increase.

Motor paralyses of the thumb are a heterogeneous group and it is difficult to establish indications for surgery. First, it is necessary to classify and analyse these paralyses precisely.

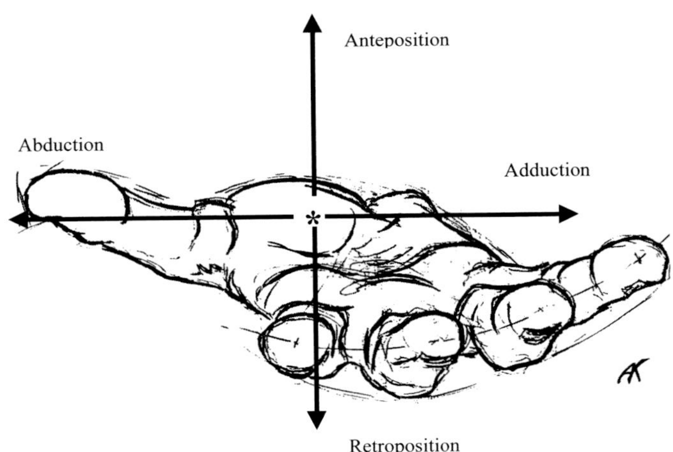

Figure 11.1

Terminology for movements of the first column. Anteposition and retroposition in sagittal plane, and adduction and abduction in the coronal plane. From Kapandji (1988) with permission.

What is opposition?

Opposition is the ability of the human thumb to ensure extensive contact between the pulp of the long fingers and the pulp of the thumb; i.e. the ability to execute a termino-terminal pinch. In 1867, Duchenne de Boulogne effectively demonstrated the specific action of abductor pollicis longus (APB), opponens pollicis (OP) and flexor pollicis brevis (FPB). APB is the main motor of the opposition movements as regards strength and amplitude.

The movements that take place during opposition may be summarized in four components. These movements will be described by the terminology presented in Figure 11.1. They are created by nine muscles and three joints, coordination of which is needed to create the physiological function.

1. First web space opening is due to extrinsic muscles extensor pollicis brevis (EPB) and abductor pollicis longus (APL) innervated by the posterior motor branch of the radial nerve.
2. Anteposition of the first web space is due to the lateral thenar muscles (APB, OP and FPB superficial head). They are innervated by the median nerve thenar motor branch.
3. Adduction is due to the medial thenar muscles: adductor pollicis (AP), first palmar interosseous (PIO) and FPB deep head. They are innervated by the ulnar nerve motor branch.
4. An automatically axial rotation of the thumb is combined with anteposition. This automatic movement is needed to bring the pulp of the thumb in front of the pulp of the long fingers. This movement is due to the connected action of the opposing muscles, the saddle configuration of the trapeziometacarpal (TMC) joint and the dorsal TMC joint ligament.

Thus, it must be kept in mind that full opposition will be obtained only if the thumb adduction and anteposition are present and if the TMC joint is not stiff. Also, it

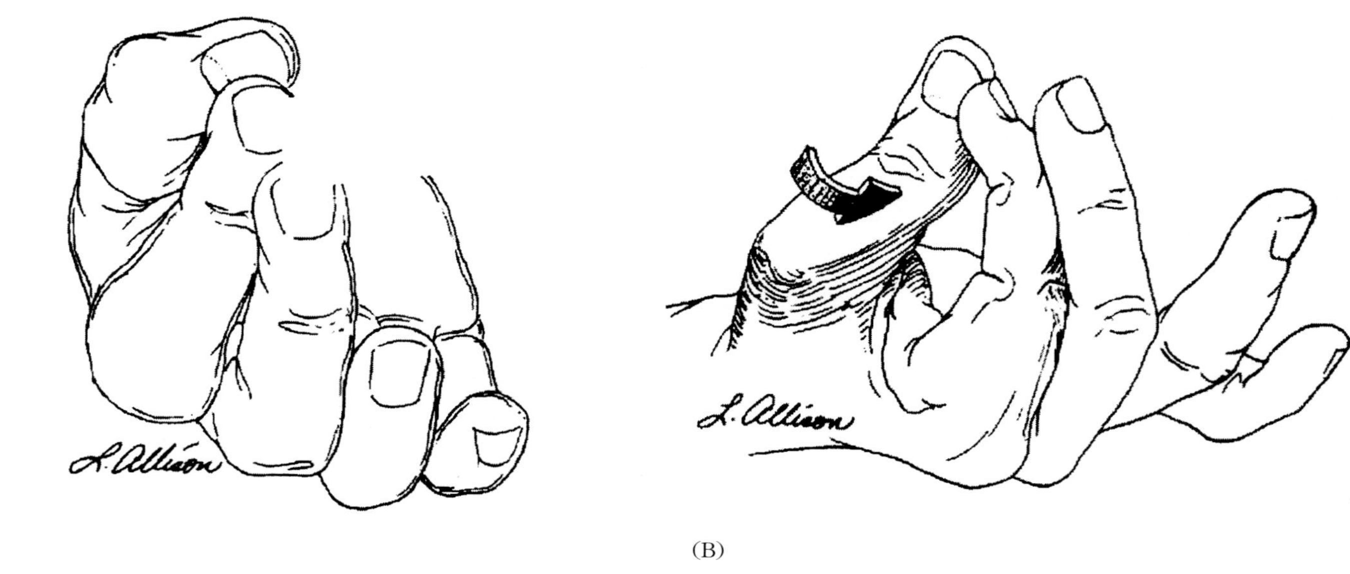

(A) (B)

Figure 11.2

The crank-handle effect (Brand 1985). (A) With hyperflexion of the IP joint of the thumb, a moment for supination of the thumb occurs if the index finger contacts the thumb with power. (B) With a flexed thumb MCP joint, the index finger exerts a powerful supinatory effect on the thumb. The moment arm is the entire length of the distal and proximal phalanges of the thumb. It is also a crank-handle effect, but with a longer moment arm. Adapted from Burkhalter (1993).

should be noted that the three upper limb motor nerves (median, ulnar and radial) are involved in complete opposition function.

It is also common to see thumb paralyses caused by more proximally located nerve root or spinal cord lesions. The problems created by three complex opposition palsies are very difficult to solve.

An isolated median nerve lesion at the wrist will theoretically jeopardize anteposition only (lateral thenar muscles palsy). In fact there are many neurological and anatomical variations. If the two heads of the FPB are totally innervated by the ulnar nerve full opposition (anteposition and adduction) will remain intact and surgical restoration will not be needed. In contrast, should this same group of patients have a paralysis of the ulnar nerve, the reduction of grip strength in the thumb caused by paralysis of the adductor would be aggravated by the associated paralysis of the FPB.

According to Burkhalter (1993), the main role of FPB in stabilizing the pinch must be emphasized. In fact this muscle is simultaneously a light metacarpophalangeal (MCP) joint flexor and a pronator of the first column. Without this light flexion long fingers will push the thumb in supination during the pinch. Then flexor pollicis longus (FPL) will create a hyperflexion of the interphalangeal (IP) joint. This creates the 'crank-handle action' described by Brand (1985) (Figure 11.2A). This effect will also happen if a strong MCP joint flexion is created by a wrong distal insertion of the transfer. Without EPB action a similar effect will be noticed (Figure 11.2B); it is also a thumb MCP joint stabilizer.

An ulnar nerve lesion at the wrist level only precludes adduction, and so just requires its correction.

As regards median–ulnar nerve lesions, the whole function has to be restored whatever the level of the lesion. MCP joint instability is maximal without AP and FPB actions, which is why Tubiana first suggested ligamentoplasty or fusion of the MCP joint of the thumb. This creates a functional unit made up of the proximal phalanx and the first metacarpal bone on which the tendon transfer will act.

If there is no radial traction due to abductor pollicis longus (APL) and EPB, this will have to be compensated by restoration of the APL. Failure to do so will jeopardize the full anteposition of the thumb.

As stated by Tubiana (1969) and Alnot (1993), it must be emphasized that it is necessary to aim for clinical diagnosis of paralysed muscles and global functional goals for restoration, rather than to apply systematic formulae. It appears preferable to classify thumb paralyses according to the muscles involved and to the function lost, and not according to the nerve lesion. Each hand is a specific problem and the strategy for restoration depends on the remaining motor muscles, associated palsy and other potential restoration needed.

Finally, it must be kept in mind that tendon transfers use the available forces on the limb. It is not possible to restore with one or two tendon transfers, however skilful they may be, the physiological function previously created by nine muscles. Once again the surgeon can perform a reconstructive role, but he is not a creator. His main goal is to restore a functional pinch between thumb and long fingers and not to produce a poor imitation of the complexity of nature.

Opponenplasty: historical background

Steindler (1918) first performed an opponenplasty by splitting the FPL longitudinally into two from its distal insertion and severing the radial half of this tendon. This lateral part was pulled around the external edge of the first metacarpal bone and fixed at the dorsal aspect of the base of the proximal phalanx.

Spitzy (1919) suggested that the loss of opposition be treated by a TMC joint fusion.

Ney (1921) severed the EPB above the extensor retinacular ligament at the wrist level and brought the distal part forwards subcutaneously. He fixed it to the flexor carpi radialis (FCR) or the palmaris longus (PL), which acted as motors.

Lyle in 1924 combined these two procedures to obtain sufficient strength and function.

Silfverskiold in 1920 severed the whole FPL, carried it around the radial and the posterior aspect of the first metacarpal bone and fixed it back to the dorsal aspect of the proximal phalanx. Withchurch did the same but sutured the FPL back to itself.

Von Bayer in 1925 severed the FPL at its distal insertion level, routed it subcutaneously along the radial aspect of the thumb and fixed it back to its primal insertion.

Some authors used flexor tendons as motors. Krukenberg (1922) split the flexor digitorum superficialis (FDS) of the third finger (III) into two and fixed it on the lateral aspect of the first metacarpal bone. Similarly, Roeren used the FDS of the fourth (IV) finger.

Other authors used several other motors. Huber (1921) and Nicolaysen (1922) transferred the abductor of the fifth finger (ADQ) and fixed it to the first metacarpal. This idea was used again by Littler and Cooley (1963).

In 1924 Bunnell described his first attempt at restoring opposition of the thumb. The evolution of this technique was to lead to his introduction of the pulley procedure 14 years later.

Jahn in 1929 routed the extensor communis of the third finger (EDC III) tendon graft subcutaneously, extended it around the ulnar border of the hand and fixed it to the first metacarpal bone. Cook (1921) had done the same using extensor indicis proprius (EIP) or extensor digiti quinti (EDQ).

Camitz (1929) used palmaris longus, palmar aponeurosis extended, which was fixed at the lateral aspect of the MCP joint of the thumb.

Again Bunnell changed the thinking about tendon transfer. In January 1938, the *Journal of Bone and Joint Surgery* published his classic paper on opponenplasties. It described 14 years' experience using FDS IV, flexor carpi ulnaris (FCU) or PL. Dissatisfied with his preliminary results, he decided to construct a pulley near the pisiform. So Bunnell's pulley operation developed gradually until he laid out its principles in this classic paper. Bunnell gave two main principles that are still useful today.

1. The distal fixation of the transfer has to be done at the medio-dorsal aspect of the proximal phalanx of the thumb to obtain axial rotation of the first column.
2. The transfer must always be routed subcutaneously from the pisiform area. This last condition requires construction of a pulley. Bunnell suggested four types, which have been more or less copied by all authors since that time.

All or nearly all that needs to be said about the opponenplasty technique can be found in Bunnell's writings. Some interesting observations were made later, particularly by Royle (1938), Thompson (1942), Littler (1949), Goldner and Irwin (1950), Le Cœur (1953), Merle d'Aubignée et al (1956), Riordan (1964), White (1960), Brand (1970, 1975), Ramselaar (1970) and Tsuge (1974).

After a rather long period of indifference, opponenplasty has had a great 'comeback', which has led to the development of more than 50 different operative procedures to date. Often these procedures are only variations of a few basic principles. Among the main contemporary authors are Burkhalter (1974), Tubiana (1969, 1974, 1979, 1987), Tubiana and Valentin (1968), and Zancolli (1961, 1965, 1975, 1979). These authors have all really worked on opponenplasty and brought some worthwhile technical improvements.

However, each case is unique and a routine pulley operation for restoring opposition will not satisfy all the needs of the different clinical varieties of thumb paralyses.

Theoretical and practical considerations of restoration of function

General principles

The general principles are discussed in Chapter 8; however, some special considerations regarding opponenplasty must be emphasized.

Distal fixation of the transfer (no matter what form of palsy was previously present) actually creates the final movement and has to be able to emulate the physiological function as closely as possible.

The attack angle of the transfer on its distal fixation is due to the pulley location; as regards opponenplasty, it is the cornerstone of the final result. The more proximal and radial the transfer, the greater the importance of anteposition; the more distal and medial the transfer, the more adduction is obtained. Thus a mid-location pulley around the pisiform area will be the ideal location for restoration of opposition following median–ulnar palsy.

Whichever motor is used, it must satisfy distal fixation and trajectory requirements. Ultimately, the choice of motor mainly has to satisfy the general principles of tendon transfer described in Chapter 8. All other considerations have to be analysed for each patient individually, taking into account the level and type of lesion that needs to be treated.

Timing of the opponenplasty

The opportune time to carry out an opponenplasty depends on the cause, level and evolution of the lesion. A successful nerve repair result is obviously far superior to tendon transfer. However, in traumatic conditions, opponenplasty may be indicated after 6 months if no clinical and electrical reinnervation occurs after suture, or when nerve repair has failed or has been impossible. The average speed of nerve regeneration is about 1 mm a day. Thus recovery of a middle arm lesion will need 500–600 days (2 years) to reach the intrinsic musculature at the palm level.

With regard to the opposition and the major role it plays in the human hand, it may be worthwhile indicating tendon transfer surgery quite soon after injury if there are no clinical and electrical signs of nerve regeneration. Indeed, restoring sensation or at least protective sensation may be possible with a late nerve repair made years after division of the nerve. This does not apply to the motor power, for which chances of recovery are markedly reduced after 6 months. Keeping in mind the level of lesion and the age of the patient, it seems justifiable to consider palliative treatment before the induction of compensatory movements restoring a thumb index pinch in retroposition because of the action of the EPL. One cannot afford to be inactive during this waiting period; contractures and stiffness must be prevented by physical therapy and splinting in opposition.

Some authors even propose early palliative surgery, arguing the value of the internal splinting effect of the tendon transfers while waiting for reinnervation. As stated above, this is a valid option for opposition palsy as regards the delay for intrinsic muscle recuperation in cases of proximal nerve lesions.

In chronic neurological diseases, transfers will be performed only after evaluation of the prognosis and evolution. In certain conditions such as poliomyelitis, in which considerable improvement follows the acute phase, it is safer to wait in order to evaluate prognosis before performing reconstructive surgery. However, in children especially, fixed deformities may affect the skeleton and render the restoration of opposition impossible, as emphasized by Goldner and Irwin (1950). Thus it is important to prevent fixed deformities from the onset of the disease. In other conditions such as Charcot–Marie disease, the patient may benefit from surgery if the progress is very slow. Lastly in others, like leprosy, surgery will be performed after medical treatment and stabilization.

Methodology

Soft tissue equilibrium

Once again, the importance of soft tissue equilibrium for the success of tendon transfers has to be emphasized. It is especially important for restoration of opposition. Soft tissue equilibrium has to be achieved carefully before any opponenplasty procedure. Indeed, scarred tissue will not allow a perfect gliding of a subcutaneously transferred tendon. The strongest muscle will not be able to move a stiffened joint or a retracted first web space. Thus resurfacing scarred surfaces with flaps, freeing stiffened joints by arthrolysis and opening the first web space by means of local or island flaps, may be the first steps in some restoration procedures. The importance of TMC joint mobility and MP joint stability for the function of the whole first column has already been emphasized.

Distal fixation of the transfer

Royle (1938) and Thompson (1942), then White (1960) split the distal portion of the motor tendon into two parts. One is fixed on the first metacarpal bone, the other on the base of the proximal phalanx through the bone. Bunnell preferred to use the radio-dorsal part of the proximal phalanx. Littler (1949) fixed the transfer to the APB terminal tendon up to the EPB. He emphasized that every force restoring APB action restores opposition, which is exactly what Duchenne de Boulogne stated in 1867.

Riordan (1953) proposed fixing the transfer to the APB terminal tendon and to its extension to the EPL to obtain a better proximal phalanx control. That approach became the gold standard.

Brand (1985) improved Riordan's procedure. He brought one part of the divided transfer by the radial side to the medial sesamoid. The other part was pulled by the medial side of the first metacarpal and fixed to the terminal APB tendon. This produced a kind of yoke, which gives supplementary axial rotation to the first column.

Tubiana (1969) disregarded the transosseous fixation to the first metacarpal bone; this does not create the axial rotation of the proximal phalanx needed to restore functional opposition. Even if used at the base of the

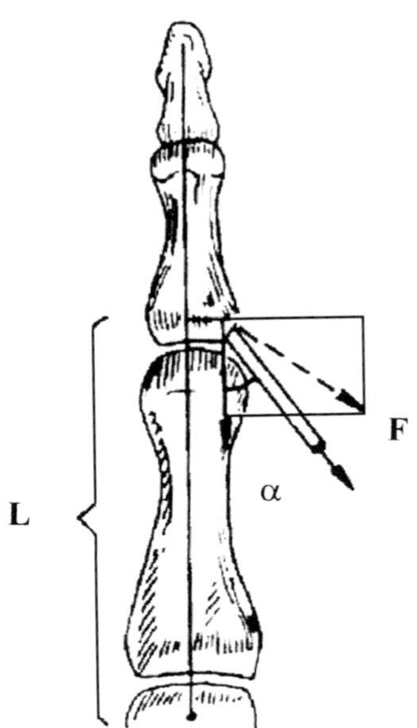

Figure 11.3

Fixation of the transfer. The strength (**F**) is acting as a first grade lever. The longer the lever arm (**A**) between the carpometacarpal joint and the wider the angle of insertion (α), the more displacement is produced. Adapted from Tubiana 1993.

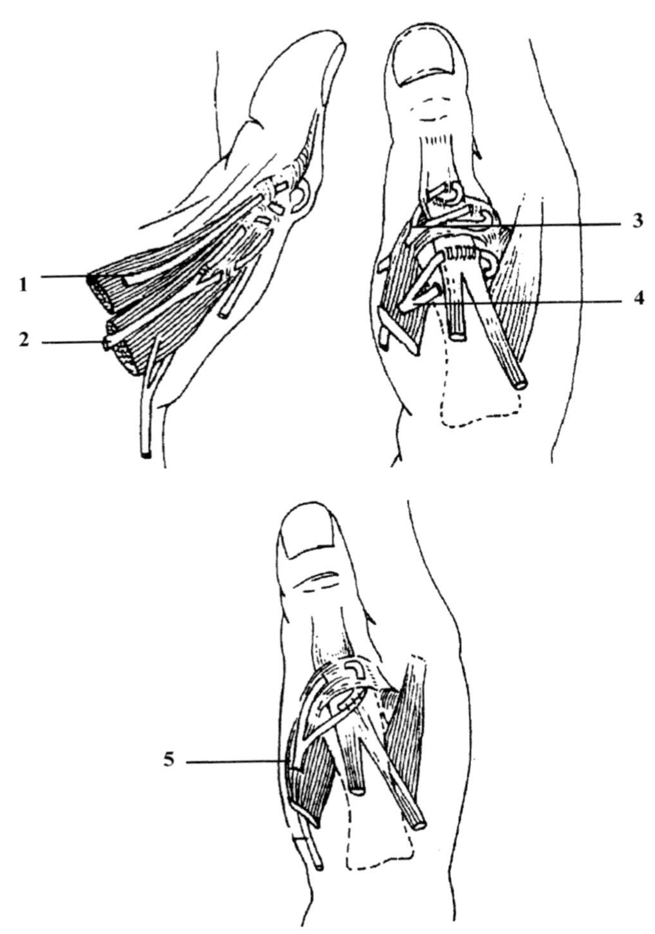

Figure 11.4

Tendon distal fixation techniques. (1) On distal APB tendon (Littler). (2) On FPB and the dorsal hood (Camitz). (3) On APB, EPL and dorsal hood (Riordan, Tubiana). (4) On APB and through the first metacarpal neck (Thompson). (5) On APB and EPL combined (Brand and Riordan). Adapted from Cooney WP et al 1984.

proximal phalanx level, it may cause MCP joint flexion if the transfer is not exactly positioned at the real rotation axis of the MCP joint. Thus, according to Tubiana, if a dynamic stabilization of the MCP joint of the thumb cannot be obtained, it has to be fused.

Mayer in 1939 emphasized the value of the first metacarpal bone osteotomy as an adjuvant procedure; for him it was an obligation if the MCP joint was stiff.

Zancolli (1979) fixed the distal insertion of the transferred tendon into the radial sesamoid, which is the FPB distal insertion; thus the MCP joint of the thumb is stabilized by the dorsal expansion of the lateral thenar muscles when stretching.

It must be remembered that force applied to the first metacarpal bone works like a simple lever. The longer the distance between transfer distal insertion and the centre of rotation of the TMC joint, the greater the attack angle of the transfer. So the movement of the first metacarpal and the first column will be greater (Figure 11.3). On the other hand, strength applied on the distal insertion automatically works out at this first fixation level. Therefore, two different fixation locations to restore two different functions with one motor at the same time (according to some authors) need a perfect constant isometric tension during movement (in space and time). This is unrealistic and seems totally ineffective and hazardous.

To obtain internal rotation with pronation of the thumb, a proximal transfer must be attached to the thumb column on its radial aspect. If it is attached on the ulnar side it produces an external rotation with supination of the thumb contrary to opposition. So, under certain conditions, all opponenplasties have to be inserted on the distal part of the APB and to its expansion to the EPL, according to Riordan. The transfer has to be fixed to the EPL proximally to the axis of rotation of the MCP joint, otherwise it will become a MCP joint flexor. Furthermore, this assumes the availability of an innervated FPL; if this is not the case IP joint hyperextension will be produced. This is one of the crank-handle actions emphasized by Brand (Figure 11.2B). Nevertheless, when well-executed this type of fixation, whichever motor is used, and wherever it is taken from, will create anteposition with axial rotation of the thumb. This will lead to the most physiologically appropriate opposition (Figure 11.4).

If the transfer is too short, permitting only a proximal attachment, this disadvantage must be compensated for by extra strength; increasing the angle of insertion augments the transfer power. If the transfer lacks strength, the insertion must be more distal (the longer the excursion, the better the result). A muscle with short excursion must be powerful and have a significant angle of insertion. In conclusion, the mode of fixation should be adapted to the individual needs of each patient, keeping in mind the characteristics of the muscle transferred, the type of palsy and the conditions of the joints.

Attack angle and pulley

It could be said 'give me a perfect pulley and I will restore you a perfect opposition'. A pulley is needed as soon as the motor does not pull spontaneously in the axis of the movement to be restored. Of course, the usual conditions apply in this situation. This pulley gives the transfer trajectory, then its attack angle. It has to be in the best possible situation to improve its attack angle and to be useful for the function required. The pulley has to be much more proximal and lateral (radial) when anteposition is sought. It has to be much more distal and medial (ulnar) when the goal is adduction (Figure 11.5). It has to be stable, strong, wide enough not to create a high pressure area. It must not create sharp angles, which lead to loss of strength and function of the transfer. If the transferred tendon has to be lengthened with a tendon graft, contact of the suture zone with the pulley must be avoided. At the very least, the pulley has to be

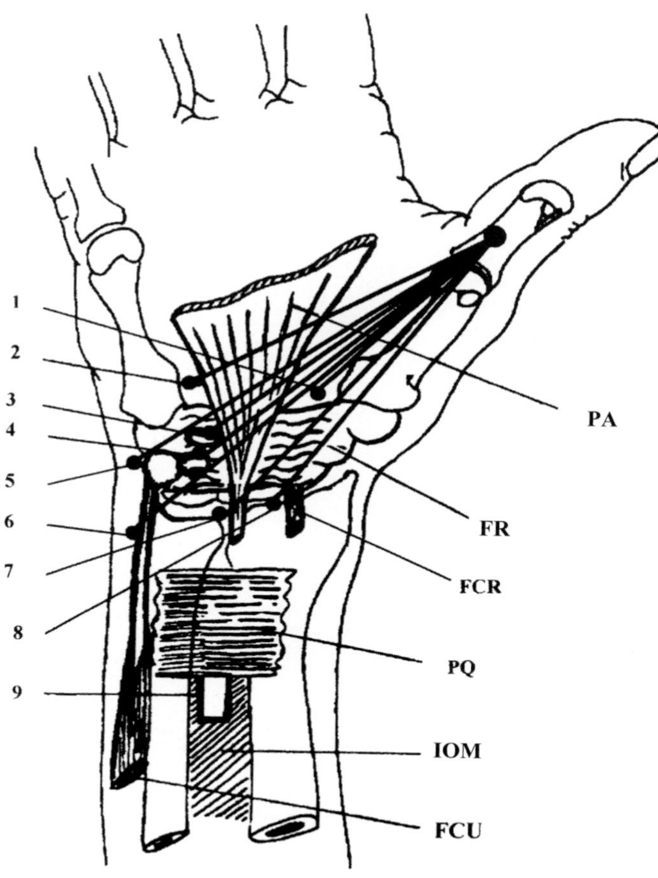

Figure 11.5

Location and pulley mechanism. (1) Distal edge of the flexor retinaculum (Ney, Williams). (2) Ulnar side of the palmar aponeurosis (Thompson). (3) Distal window in the flexor retinaculum (Roeren). (4) Around the pisiform (Palazzi). (5) A tendon construction in the pisiform area (Bunnell). (6) Around FCU distal tendon (Bunnell). (7) Around PL (Edgerton and Brand). (8) Around FCR. PA = palmar aponeurosis, FR = flexor retinaculum, FCR = flexor carpi radialis, PQ = pronator quadratus, IOM = interosseous membrane, FCU = flexor carpi ulnaris. It should be borne in mind that the more distal and ulnar the more adduction, the more proximal and radial the more anteposition. From Chammas et al (1999) with permission.

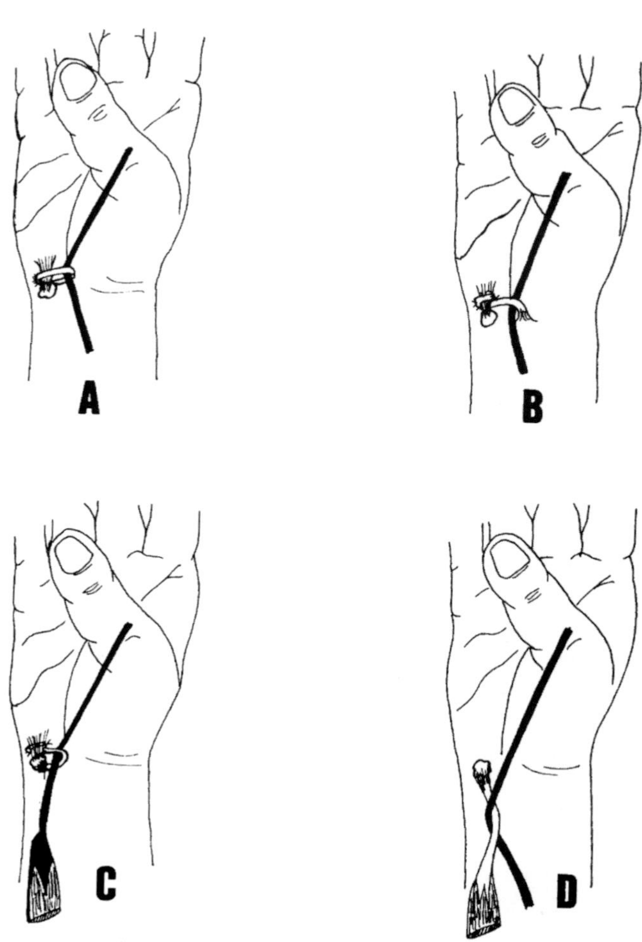

Figure 11.6

Pulley construction following Bunnell. (A) Using a tendon graft around the pisiform. (B) Using the PL tendon as a dynamic pulley. (C) Using a distal part of the FCU to build the pulley. (D) Using the distal FCU tendon as a dynamic pulley. From Chammas et al (1999) with permission.

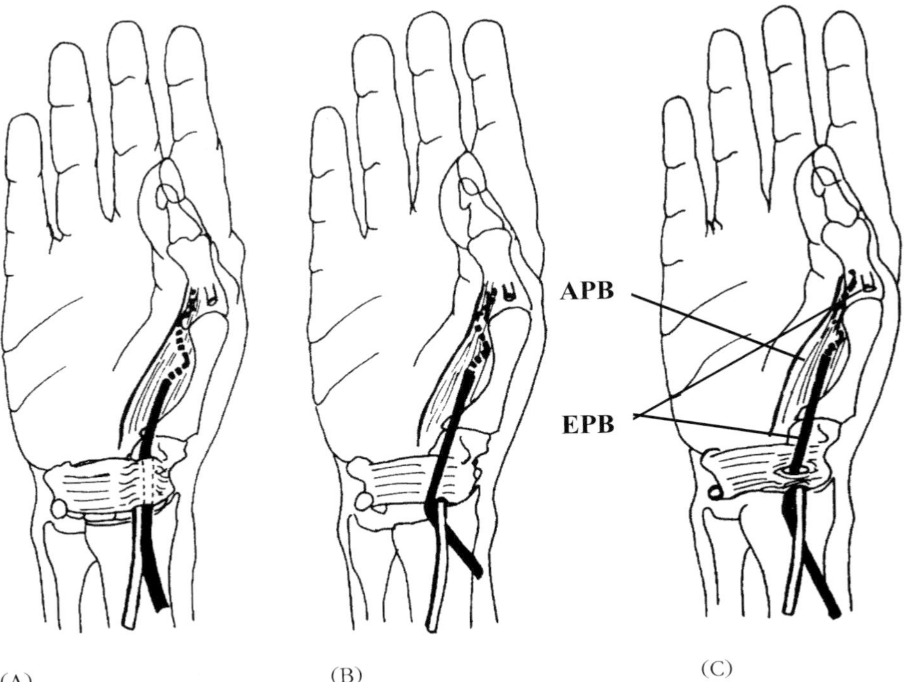

Figure 11.7

Pulley construction using the FCR tendon. (A) Using the FCR canal (Zancolli). (B) Around the FCR distal tendon used as a dynamic pulley (Tubiana). (C) Using a window at the proximal part of the FCR canal (Zancolli). From Chammas et al (1999) with permission.

located at a sufficient distance from the thumb to allow sufficient excursion to the transfer. Of course, the ideal pulley does not exist.

Cadaveric experiments have shown the importance of depth level in pulley location. This factor may change the attack angle, which is why Le Cœur (1953) proposed the use of a bony wedge between the distal fixation of the transfer and the metacarpal bone, which pushed the transfer attack angle forward while trying to avoid a pulley construction.

According to Bunnell the best location for a pulley is the pisiform area (Figure 11.6). It could be argued that this does not allow differentiation between true anteposition needs (isolated median nerve palsy) and anteposition adduction necessities (median–ulnar palsy).

Zancolli primarily proposed a rather lateral pulley, closer to the centre of the wrist, using a hole in the flexor carpi radialis (FCR) canal retinaculum at the flexor retinaculum level. After passing through it, the transfer follows the direction of the APB fibres. In this situation anteposition is great and adduction is weak. The radial opposition force (APL and EPB) gives more anteposition and, as regards the adduction and axial rotation, the ulnar force is combined to obtain opposition. Later, Zancolli (like Tubiana) used the terminal tendon of the FCR as a pulley, but used the transverse fibres of the FCR canal to build a fixed pulley and create a stable pulley location.

Tubiana routes the transfer around the FCR tendon, proximal to its canal. The distal FCR tendon is then the dynamic pulley. This pulley has a tendency to lose its effect during wrist flexion or if the FCR is paralysed. Furthermore, it does not allow restoration of adduction (Figure 11.7).

The most likely complications must be borne in mind: stretching of the pulley, displacement from the point of reflection when the pulley is not fixed (thus altering the course of the transfer, as stated above) and finally formation of adhesions between pulley and transfer. This last complication is most common when a pulley is constructed from a split tendon or lies in a scarred area. In a case in which adhesions are feared, it is preferable to construct the pulley around a silicone rod 2 or 3 months before the transfer, which allows the pulley to be placed in a good position.

Overall, the distal portion of the FCU tendon seems to be the best location for a pulley as regards combined restoration of anteposition and adduction. The distal FCR tendon is a good location for isolated restoration of anteposition. Distal to the pisiform or at the ulnar border of the palmar aponeurosis, following Thompson (1942), will be the best location for the pulley in the case of an isolated adduction restoration.

Course of the transfer

The course of the transfer must be as direct as possible. Any angulation reduces the power conveyed and this reduction will be proportional to the degree of the angle. However, these changes in direction around a pulley are essential regarding opponenplasties as noted earlier.

For a long time transfer trajectories were only subcutaneous around ulna or radius borders. Then transfers always had to be long and might have the disadvantage of crossing scarred zones.

Duparc et al (1971) emphasized the value of a direct trajectory through the interosseous membrane (IOM) when using a posterior forearm muscle. With this straighter trajectory, the transfer gains in length and strength. This path has to be carefully executed. When traversing the interosseous membrane at the forearm, the orifice must be proximal enough (proximal border of the pronator quadratus) to avoid marked angulation. The window must be large enough (and not just a hole) so that the motor muscle belly and its tendon can glide freely without any torsion, avoiding loss of strength and then loss of function. Injury to the interosseous pedicle should be avoided.

It is always better to use the interosseous membrane trajectory when harvesting a transfer from one aspect of the forearm to transfer it to another. As already stated, it gains in strength, it avoids grafting and allows much more choice in pulley location. Thus it allows a better attack angle and diminishes the area of high pressure and the loss of strength and function of all transfers. This is why every time it is possible it is the preferred method of the author.

Choice of the motor and tension of the transfer

These two points have been developed in Chapter 12. An ideal motor is a muscle whose removal causes no serious functional loss; the tendon is long enough to be fixed directly to the thumb in order to avoid intermediate anastomosis (a source of adhesion); the tendon does not have to be removed from its normal course for too great a length, so that its blood supply is not compromised; power and amplitude are adapted to the paralysed muscle that it has to replace; rehabilitation is as easy as possible. Changing distal insertion and its attack angle can incorporate all these components working on the moment arm as noted earlier (Figure 11.3). However, caution must be exercised. Power needed to restore anteposition is less than that required for a flexion adduction grip. Inappropriately strong adduction hinders anteposition and rotation of the thumb into pronation. Conversely, too much anteposition interferes with adduction. To balance these forces, both the choice of motor muscle and the direction of transfer must be considered. Of course a number of muscles may be used, each with its own advantages and disadvantages.

Evaluation of the level of tension to give to the transfer in this part of the procedure is a delicate technical point; usually it comes through experience. Insufficient tension will lead to an ineffective transfer. Too taut tension is harmful and can even cause fibrous degeneration of the motor muscle. Littler emphasizes the ability of the transferred muscle to find its optimal tension and recommends that the transferred muscle is not stretched too much. It must be done with regard to wrist flexion or extension, aiming to reproduce the physiological extension balance of the digits.

Postoperative care

Postoperative rigid immobilization is carried out for 1 month in a forearm cast or even in a dynamic splint, maintaining the joints in the optimal corrected position. This most often means that the pulp of the thumb is in front of the pulp of the third or fourth finger, with the MCP joint of the thumb in light flexion (20°) and the IP joint extended. The wrist is in functional or neutral position, or even in light flexion if the insufficient length of the transferred tendon requires this position.

It is very useful to encourage slight motion of the restored thumb during immobilization, and also of the sound side, to activate the cortical reintegration of the transferred muscles and so restore function. This biofeedback mechanism is often effective.

Active mobilization is started on the 30th day after surgery (after immobilization removal) with no movements against resistance before the 45th day post surgery. Rehabilitation has to recover and reinforce articular motion, soft tissue trophicity and function integration. This must be done by a specialized physical therapist as often as possible. The final result may be evaluated around the third month post surgery. Sensitomotor rehabilitation must be carried out daily for as long as necessary.

The role of rehabilitation must be strongly emphasized even before surgery. One cannot afford to be inactive during the nervous recuperation period. Contractures and stiffness must be prevented by physical therapy and splinting in opposition. If it is carefully performed, rehabilitation can improve the condition of the hand before surgery takes place.

Use of various transfers

First of all, the attack angle and distal fixation of the transferred tendon will give function, whatever motor is chosen. So theoretically the clinician can restore one of the two main functions of opposition – anteposition or adduction – or both together.

As noted above, sensitivity is still an important part of the success of the treatment. If there is no tactile sensation in the hand, as in median–ulnar palsy, there may be a total functional failure of the most perfectly executed surgical procedure. So a nerve graft must be carried out, even at a late stage, in order to obtain even a partial sensory recovery.

Flexor digitorum tendons

FDS IV (Bunnell 1938)

This classic transfer uses FDS IV as a motor. Several incisions are necessary in this procedure. An incision at the base of the ring finger allows removal of the tendon.

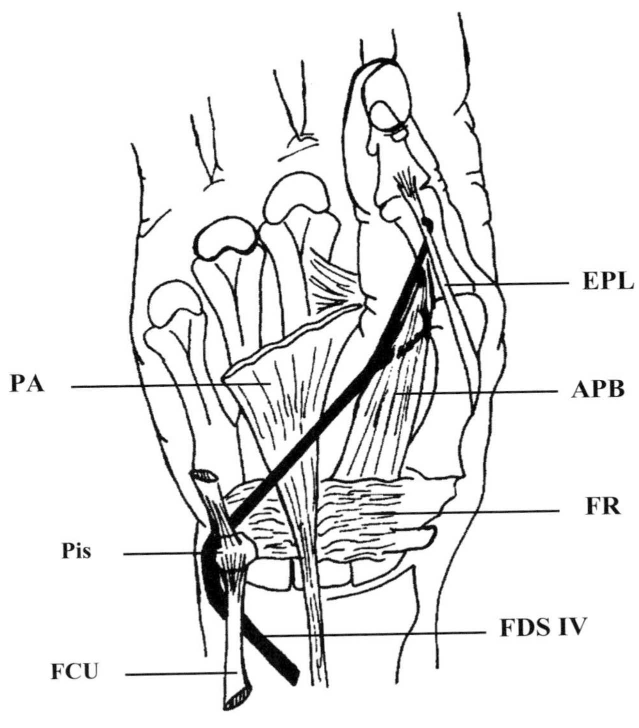

Figure 11.8
The Bunnell procedure using FDS IV. The original Bunnell operation, here modified by Merle d'Aubignée, uses the pisiform as a pulley. EPL = extensor pollicis longus, APB = abductor pollicis brevis, PA = palmar aponeurosis, FR = flexor retinaculum, Pis. = pisiform, FCU = flexor carpi ulnaris, FDS IV = flexor digitorum superficialis.

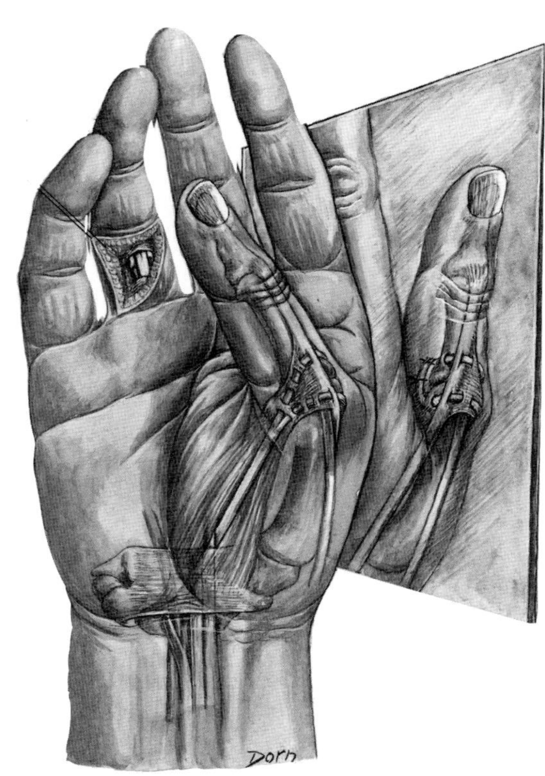

Figure 11.9
Distal fixation. (1) Mirror. (2) The two terminal slips of the FDS passed on either side of the MCP joint. Each slip transfixes the EPL tendon, the distal phalanx is maintained in complete extension. (3) Each slip passes through the capsuloligamentous tissue from posterior to anterior in contact with the bone. The two tendon ends are then fastened to one another under tension on the ulnar volar aspect of the joint to prevent MCP joint hyperextension, with the proximal phalanx held in slight flexion (10°) and the distal phalanx in complete extension. (4) FDS transfer. From Tubiana et al 1999.

A second in the palm distal to the flexor retinaculum is necessary if the chosen pulley will be located in this area. A third above the wrist allows the FDS IV to be pulled out. The last is a sigmoid incision at the MCP joint of the thumb area, according to the distal fixation procedure one has chosen. The layout of these incisions is modified if the transfer to the thumb is associated with transfers to the fingers. The tendon is divided proximal to the Camper's chiasma and is pulled out proximal to the wrist.

In the original procedure, the tendon was passed around the distal part of the FCU tendon, which was used like a dynamic pulley. Passing around the pisiform, as suggested by Merle d'Aubigné, allows a more stable and fixed pulley. The result may be more constant with time; but in this situation the pulley is rather distal and medial and the anteposition gain is rather poor (Figure 11.8). Also, this pulley has to be wide enough not to create a high pressure area.

The tension of the transfer is adjusted while the wrist is held straight, the first metacarpal is in mid-anteposition and the MCP and IP joints are also straight. If there is a marked laxity in the MCP joint, the fixation of the transfer can be use to stabilize the articulation; indeed it is long enough to do so. An S-shaped dorsal incision centred over the dorsal aspect of the MCP joint gives a perfect exposition. The two terminal slips of the FDS IV, after being woven through the tendon of the APB, are fixed on either side of the joint and act as a tenoplasty. The two tendon ends are fastened to one another under tension with the proximal phalanx held in slight flexion around 10º (Figure 11.9). The resultant stability allows a certain amount of play in the MCP joint and it is preferable to arthrodesis in patients whose paralyses are limited and non-complicated.

The versatility of the FDS IV and its ease of harvest made these transfers one of the gold standards, and a lot of variations of this procedure have been described. Nevertheless, it be borne in mind that some pitfalls may occur after severing FDS IV. Swan-neck deformity, loss of flexion of the PIP joint, loss of strength in grasp in manual workers may be observed. These pitfalls may be minimized by a careful harvesting technique, but cannot always be avoided.

Other flexor superficialis tendons

Jacobs and Thompson (1978) used FDS III or FDS IV in equal proportions. Gobell and Freudenberg used FDS V. Pallazzi (1962) advocated the use of any FDS as far as the proximal insertion of the ADQ, at the pisiform level, it is used as a pulley. Nevertheless, FDS IV remains the best choice among the FDS. In fact, the FDS V is rarely strong enough, FDS III is less versatile than FDS IV and sometimes needs a muscle belly reduction to pass through a constructed pulley.

Steindler (1930), and Williams after him, advocated the use of FPL split into two, subcutaneously rerouted through the palm and fixed at the base of the two phalanges of the thumb. A flexor digitorum profundus (FDP) may be used in the same way, but only when the donor digit arises from an amputation procedure – otherwise the sequelae are too severe.

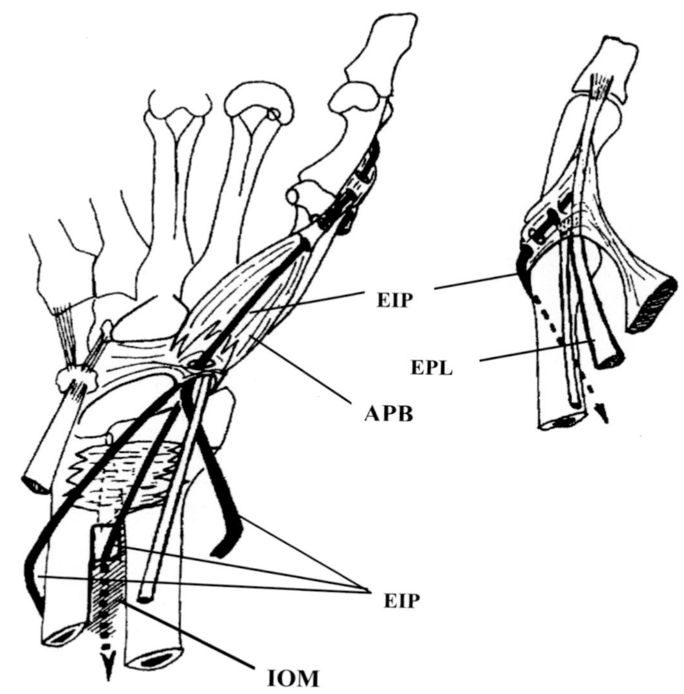

Figure 11.10

The EIP transfer and its variations. (A) Around the radius. (B) Through the IOM. (C) Around the ulna. (D) Distal fixation following Riordan.

Flexor carpi tendons

FCU

Bunnell (1938) and Phalen and Miller (1947) proposed the use of the FCU tendon prolonged by a tendon graft. The tendon is subcutaneously routed through the palm, using the pisiform as a pulley. With this same motor, Iselin and Prudet (1984) used the palmar aponeurosis as a pulley and Kessler (1979) did the same, but fixed the transfer to the EPB severed at the proximal phalanx level.

As noted by Brand, the FCU is of great importance; it is the main wrist stabilizer. Therefore, it is not always wise to use it, furthermore its strength and excursion are not always appropriate. Finally, lengthening by a tendon graft increases the adhesion phenomena.

Palmaris longus

Camitz (1929) used the palmaris longus by the central pretendinous band of the superficialis palmar fascia. The transfer is routed subcutaneously straight to its distal fixation. This easy, direct but weak transfer may be used to restore anteposition only in flexible hands in cases of severe carpal tunnel syndrome. Distally fixed on the APB tendon it gives a good cosmetic aspect to the thenar eminence and is rather useful in these conditions.

Extensor tendons

EIP

First described by Chouy-Aguirre and Kaplan (1956), this procedure has been developed by Zancolli (1965), Price (1968) and Burkhalter (1993), and uses an independent tendon of adequate length and strength. The routing is easy to perform and does not lead to any damaging consequences. This is actually one of the best choices for opponenplasty (Figure 11.10).

A curve-shaped incision at the proximal portion of the MCP joint of the index allows the elevation of the EIP from its ulnar aspect. This does not lead to any sequelae if the interosseous muscle hood is perfectly respected or reconstructed. The distal cut end of the EIP has only to be fixed to the tendon of the EDC of the index. EIP is then elevated back at the wrist level through a curve-shaped incision at the distal third of the forearm above the proximal border of the extensor retinaculum. A short incision at the metacarpal base level may be necessary to avoid too strong a traction on the tendon while pulling it back to the wrist. Failure to do so may risk an avulsion at the musculotendinous junction. The muscle belly must be dissected far enough proximally to obtain the best excursion possible. The tendon is routed either subcutaneously around the ulna or straight through the interosseous membrane. Some authors advocate routing

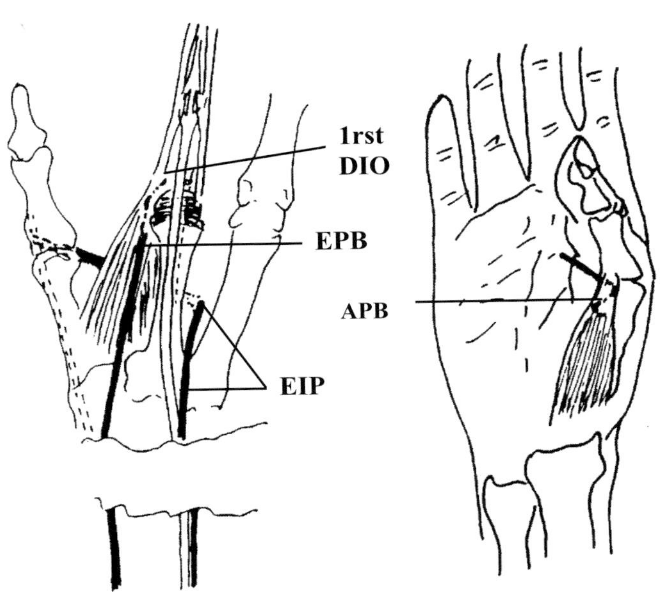

Figure 11.11

Transferring EIP for correction of Froment's sign. EPB is directly fixed on the first IOD muscle. EIP is routed around the ulnar border of the second metacarpal bone and then transversally to be fixed at the ends of the terminal tendon of the APB. EIP = extensor indicis proprius, EPB = extensor pollicis brevis, APB = abductor pollicis brevis, first DIO = first dorsal interosseous muscle.

around the radial side of the forearm; but this seems to produce too sharp an angle, causing a very high pressure area. The original fixation was done to the APB terminal tendon with a light wrist flexion. The direct path of the transfer, which crosses the wrist longitudinally, allows maximal advantage to be taken of the active tenodesis effect provided by flexion and extension of the wrist. This effect reinforces its action. Passive intraoperative extension of the wrist should produce complete opposition of the thumb, and flexion should bring the first column into retroposition.

It may be noticed that the EIP is also the best transfer to use for correcting Froment's sign during isolated ulnar palsy. This needs a double tendon transfer. In fact, EPB will restore the first dorsal interosseous (DIO) muscle function by a straight transfer using its good attack angle and its compatible strength and excursion. The EIP will restore the adductor pollicis (AP) function. It needs to use the ulnar edge of the palmar aponeurosis at the second metacarpal level as a pulley, according to Thompson. The EIP is fixed not to the AP, but to the APB, which (using a very distal and horizontal excursion) allows a better restoration of adduction (Figure 11.11). Use of the FDS IV would be the wrong option for this particular purpose because it is too strong a muscle for this function.

EDQ

Cook (1921), then Schneider (1969), advocated the use of EDQ subcutaneously routed around the ulna. Some pitfalls must be emphasized. EDQ may be the only fifth finger extensor tendon and so has to be respected; it is often not long enough and needs to be prolonged by a tendon graft. Also, its strength is rather poor.

EPL

Bureau et al (1981) advocated the use of EPL. This radial innervated muscle, like EIP, has a good excursion and is strong. Its length remains available if it is routed through the IOM (Figure 11.12). However, care must be taken to fix it back to itself proximally to the rotation axis of the MCP joint of the thumb after its fixation to the APB. Failure to do so will run the risk of losing thumb extension and producing a permanent flexion of

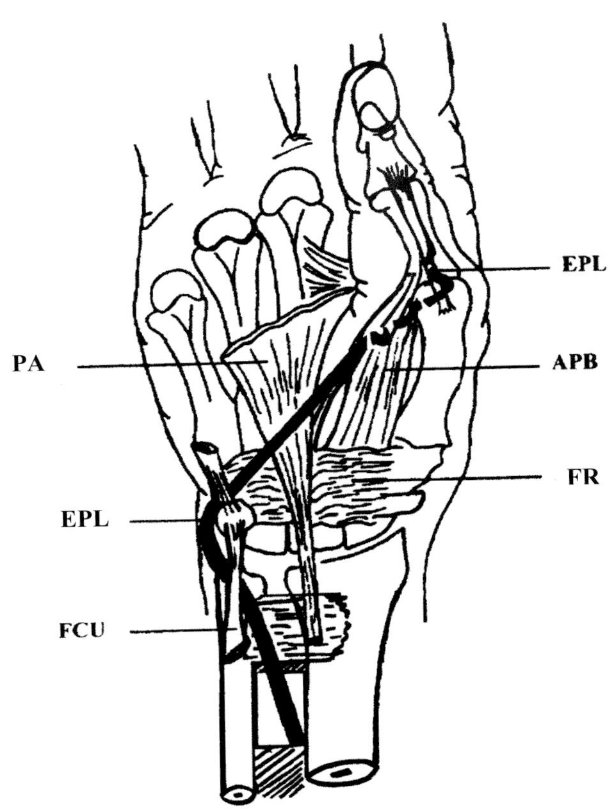

Figure 11.12

The EPL transfer following Bureau et Decaillet. The EPL is routed through the IOM and then turned around the FCU terminal tendon, which is the dynamic pulley. Then it is routed subcutaneously through the palm. The distal fixation is just proximal to the centre of flexion of the joint. EPL = extensor pollicis longus, APB = abductor pollicis brevis, PA = palmar aponeurosis, FR = flexor retinaculum, FCU= flexor carpi ulnaris.

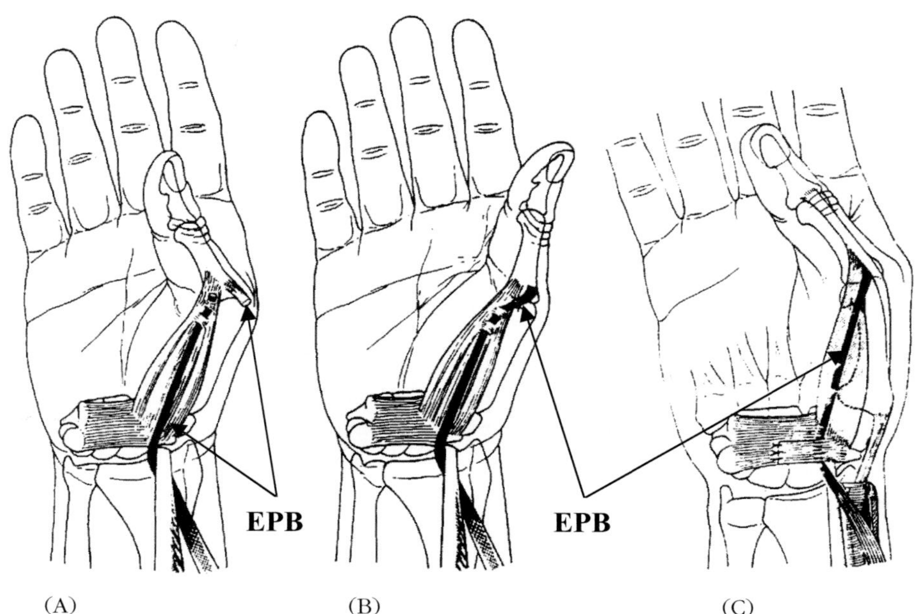

Figure 11.13

The EPB transfer following Tubiana. Tubiana and others have described many variations utilizing the EBP. (A) The transfer is fixed to the APB tendon using the FCR as a dynamic pulley, but it will not restore extension of the MCP joint. (B) It is much better to suture the EPB back to itself after passing through the APB fibres, thus the MCP extension and stabilization are re-established. (C) Matev proposed leaving the EPB tendon undivided, and just relocating it out of the first extensor dorsal compartment. The EPB tendon is rerouted under a flexor retinaculum slip used as a pulley (radial and proximally located).

the MCP joint. Of course, retroposition of the first column is always diminished due to the change of excursion of the EPL. This technique provides an alternative choice to other methods. It is a consistently effective procedure and the results are maintained over time. It seems to be a valuable technique for restoring opposition in high median and ulnar nerve palsy, but it must not be used for an isolated palsy of one of the components of the opposition mechanism.

EPB

Zancolli (1965) proposed the use of the EPB and the procedure has been improved by Tubiana in several ways.

A longitudinal dorsal incision slightly curved to the radial side of the MCP joint exposes the distal insertions of the EPB and APB, and the tendon of the EPL. It allows the presence of the EPB tendon to be confirmed. Sometimes it is too slender to be transferred. A second incision is made on the radial side of the wrist: often it is sectioned distally and the EPB is pulled proximally out of the osteofibrous tunnel. The tendon is then brought anterior to the wrist. This tendon is long enough to avoid grafting, it does not necessarily need a pulley construction if a trajectory around the radial side of the forearm is chosen for restoration of anteposition alone, and its strength is sufficient. Its distal insertion at the dorsal aspect of the proximal phalanx is very well located.

As regards distal fixation, severing the EPB removes an important MCP stabilizer, so the mode of distal fixation has evolved. Rather than inserting it onto the APB tendon and its dorsal expansion – thus re-establishing the APB function but losing that of the EPB – it is preferable to fix it back to its own insertion. Thus extension of the MCP joint is re-established, independent of the of the IP joint (Figure 11.13).

APL

Edgerton and Brand (1965) advocated the advancement of the APL distal insertion after rerouting the tendon around the radial aspect of the forearm. This increases the attack angle and the lever arm of abduction, but it is not very selective as it acts only on the metacarpal bone. Furthermore this tendon is too short and needs a tendon graft extension; which leads to the usual pitfalls of this approach. The frequent existence of several APL distal tendons may allow the elevation of one of them. However, the specific action of the transfer is then lost and what was gained in tendinous material is lost in function. This procedure should only be used in median and ulnar nerve palsies and with an adduction transfer technique.

Extensor carpi tendons

Extensor carpi radialis longus and brevis (ECRL and ECRB)

Bunnell advocated the use of ECRB, but argued that it was too weak and too short as a motor. A tendon graft is needed to prolong the ECRB and this creates adhesions. Kaplan et al (1976) proposed the use of the

ECRL routed around the ulna and fixed to the EPL, which avoids grafting and gives sufficient length.

Extensor carpi ulnaris (ECU)

This may be used by following Verdan's method in two ways. The first one is to use the ECU prolonged by a tendon graft and fixed at the APB after a subcutaneous route around the ulnar aspect of the wrist. The second one is to use ECU sutured at the EPB severed at its musculotendinous junction, which is routed subcutaneously to the hypothenar region. Unfortunately the ECU suppression leads to a disabling radial inclination of the wrist.

Use of intrisic muscles

ADQ

The idea of using ADQ was first proposed by Huber (1921) and Nicolaysen (1922). It was then 'popularized' by Littler and Cooley (1963). This procedure is performed without a pulley transfer, using ADQ fixed on the APB (Figure 11.14). The trajectory is direct, the strength is appropriate and this transfer has the advantage of replacing one intrinsic muscle by another one. The resulting opposition is very close to the original physiological status. Furthermore, this excellent opponenplasty, despite its rather distal and horizontal excursion, gives much more anteposition than would be expected. This requires a very careful operative technique, freeing the proximal part of the ADQ very proximally up to the FCU terminal tendon without damaging the neurovascular bundle. This transfer is innervated by the ulnar nerve so is only used for isolated median nerve palsy. It is an excellent choice for children and/or congenital hand disabilities. It is also utilized to reinforce opposition in a pollicized thumb. Finally it restores some volume to the thenar eminence and improves the appearance of the emaciated paralysed hand. In adults, especially in manual workers, it is not the best solution as regards the transverse and subcutaneous excursion across the palm. In this situation the transferred muscle is in the direct path of impacts and this may damage its muscle belly. Furthermore, in severing the ADQ, the cylindrical grip strength of the ulnar border of the hand may be jeopardized.

Flexor digiti minimi (FDM)

Pallazi Duarte in 1964 proposed the use of the FDM using the same principles as the ADQ. When severing the FDM, great care must be taken in freeing the FDM from the ADQ, which lies over it, and in freeing it up to the hamatum carefully so not to damage its neurovascular bundle. The transfer is routed in the same way transversely subcutaneously through the palm and fixed to

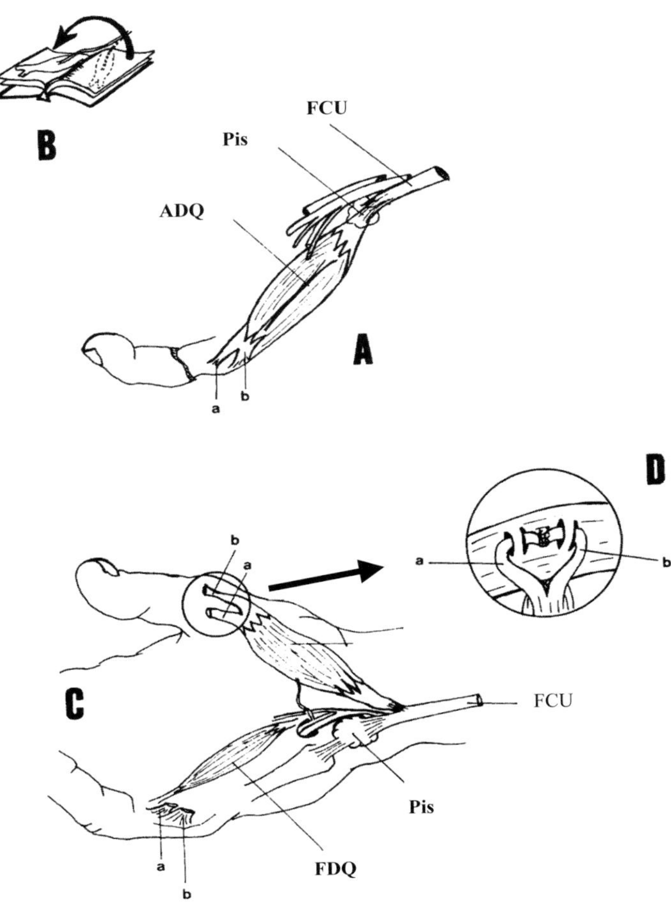

Figure 11.14
The ADQ transfer following Littler. (A) The muscle has to be freed from its fascial attachments to the other hypothenar muscle and freed very proximally over the pisiform and on the FCU terminal tendon. (B) Then the muscle tendon unit is rotated 180° on its long axis and turned round its pedicle, like opening a book. (C) The ADQ is routed subcutaneously through the palm transversally. Care must be taken to avoid traction on its neurovascular pedicle. (D) The distal fixation on the terminal tendon of the APB tendon uses the two heads of the transferred muscle. ADQ = abductor digiti quinti, FDQ = flexor digiti quinti, APB = abductor pollicis brevis, Pis. = pisiform, FCU= flexor carpi ulnaris.

APB. This is technically a more tricky transfer than the ADQ, but it is supposed to have the advantage of creating an attack angle close to the FPB. Also, it is unlikely to damage little finger abduction, which is useful in the cylindrical grip of the ulnar hand, noted above.

AP

De Vecchi (1961) proposed the use of the Add I. transferred to the APB. In fact this is not a real opponenplasty, but this transfer reinforces the deep head of the

FPB and leads to a rather satisfying pinch in hands affected by poliomyelitis which have no extrinsic muscles (flexor or extensor) available for transfer.

The deep head of the FPB

Makin and Silfverkiold first proposed this idea, followed by Bunnell and Howell; then Orticochea (1971) updated it. The deep head of the FPB is transferred on the medial part of the base of the proximal phalanx. The distal fixation is made back to the flexion axis of the MCP joint. Thus the action of the transfer is IP joint flexion, anteposition and some adduction; but amplitude is poor and it is a weak transfer.

Discussion

Choice of approach

In the case of incomplete palsy after nerve repair, anteposition of the thumb is sometimes limited and can be reinforced with a transfer; but in fact it is the lack of power in the thumb–finger pinch that plagues the patients. The transfer of the FDS seems excessive or this tendon may not be available, so a radial nerve-innervated motor may be used after careful consideration.

The problem is rather complicated when all intrinsic muscles are paralysed (median–ulnar palsy). In these cases, the clinician seeks to re-establish:

1. anteposition of the thumb, enabling its separation from the front of the palm;
2. the power of the thumb grip in flexion adduction;
3. extension of the distal phalanx for greater pulpar contact;
4. pronation of the thumb column;
5. stabilization of the MCP joint, whose stabilizing muscles have been paralysed.

As stated esrlier, one transfer cannot hope to satisfy all these demands.

One or two transfers?

By using two transfers it is possible to approximate, more closely than a single transfer could, the normal physiology of opposition of the thumb. One transfer restores anteposition, as a preliminary to the second transfer, which allows closure of the grip. A double transfer also allows better stabilization of the MCP joint and more effectively prevents flexion of the distal phalanx. Obviously it requires more tendon material and the availability of a sufficient amount of motors.

When using only a single transfer the motor should be powerful, have good excursion and should satisfy the basic principles emphasized in Chapter 12 regarding theoretical and practical considerations. As noted, the pulley situation governs the attack angle, and the distal fixation governs the moment arm of the transfer. These are the two main considerations that require care. Furthermore, the patient must have an active extension of the wrist, which reinforces the action of the transfer, and must not have a MCP joint of the thumb that is too unstable.

Author's preferred methods

With regard to the availability of remaining muscles and other planned restorative procedures on the same limb, the first choice is usually the EIP transfer, then the FDS IV. We always use a trajectory through the IOM for all the reasons noted above. EPL is used only for median and ulnar nerves combined palsy when the two other preferred motors are needed for other aspects of restoration. ADQ is only used in children in congenital conditions or if no extrinsic muscles are available (e.g. crush injury of the forearm).

Bureau et al (1981) noticed that restoration of opposition was only needed in 15% of all cases of isolated median nerve palsy, perhaps less: either the nerve regrowth is functionally sufficient and remaining muscles can achieve opposition or the ulnar nerve innervates the two heads of the FPB. It may be noted that in low isolated ulnar palsy, patients do not usually ask for isolated restoration of adduction. Therefore, indications for opponenplasty are more often seen in median–ulnar combined distal or proximal palsy conditions.

Transfers in proximal palsies

These conditions concern the lesion proximal to the elbow or the proximal third of the forearm. It must be kept in mind that, in these conditions, a radial palsy may be associated with median and/or ulnar palsy, which obviously makes the restoration more complicated regarding the motors available for use. The overall upper limb restoration problem has to be evaluated, according to the remaining possibilities and the patient's abilities. The general principles of tendon transfers remain reliable, but a lot of variations are posible.

Isolated proximal palsy of the median nerve

Pronation of the forearm, wrist flexors, thumb, index and long finger is affected. Most often nerve regeneration allows restoration of extrinsic muscles; therefore, the problem is the restoration of lateral thenar muscles, as noted above. As regards local conditions it is certainly the best indication for early opponenplasty in many cases. If the extrinsic palsy does not recover, thumb flexion must be restored first, then finger flexion (see Chapter 8), then the opposition. The best motor choice for opponenplasty is then a radial or ulnar innervated muscle. Usually EIP is chosen, and EPL is also a reliable technique.

Isolated proximal palsy of the ulnar nerve

FCU and FDP of the fourth and fifth fingers are paralysed, in addition to all the medial intrinsic muscles of the thumb. Tendon transfers, then, will have to correct the claw hand deformity, the Jeanne's sign and the Froment's sign. It seems valuable to use the FDS IV to correct the claw hand deformity and the EIP and EPB to restore thumb–index pinch as shown earlier (Figure 11.11). Fusion of the IP joint of the thumb with a slight pronation and flexion allows stabilization of the IP joint and gives the FPL an adduction effect on the whole first column.

Proximal median–ulnar palsy

Disability is then maximum in this condition and the remaining muscles, which are few, have to be shared. EIP opponenplasty is the best choice, while stabilizing the MCP joint of the thumb. It may be achieved by using distal fixation (Figure 11.9) as suggested by Tubiana or it may require MCP joint fusion.

Proximal median–radial palsy

At the upper arm level this is a very severe condition. A wrist arthrodesis can be performed and then the FCU can be used for restoration of the finger extension. The thumb may need to be fixed by a carpometacarpal arthrodesis.

It maybe better to use the Groves and Goldner procedure (1975). The FCU is used as a motor to restore the FCS IV paralysed muscle. The FDS IV is then used exactly as usual to restore opposition. It can be argued that this procedure withdraws the only remaining wrist flexor. Actually the authors prefer to restore sufficient wrist flexion when the MCP joint is stabilized. Restored opposition is strong and increased by the tenodesis effect between wrist extensor and thumb opposition (Figure 11.15).

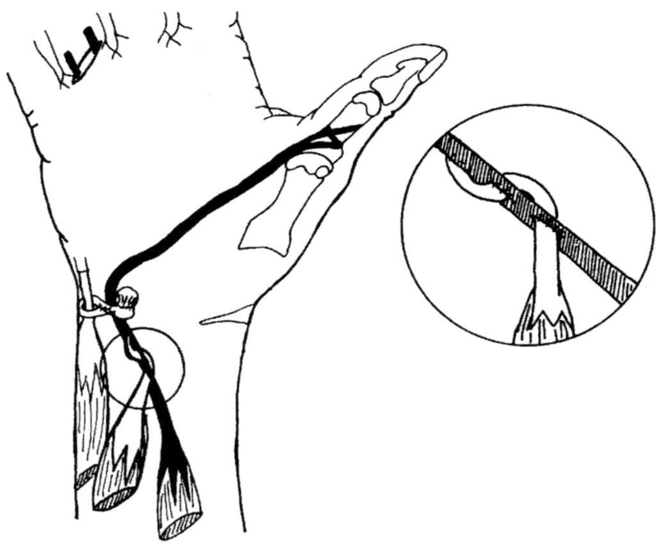

Figure 11.15
Groves and Goldner (1975) procedure for proximal median–radial palsy. Transferring the FCU (ulnar nerve innervated) restores the FDS IV. Then the FDS (motorized by the FCU) may be transferred in the usual manner to restore opposition (FCU = flexor carpi ulnaris, FDS IV = flexor digitorum superficialis).

Associated palsies

Associated median ulnar and radial nerve palsy (three trunks palsy), is almost the same condition as distal brachial plexus palsy; the surgical possibilities are the same and will use the remaining motors, which are very few. Thereafter, a lot of additive techniques become essential (see below). The surgeon may be obliged to use less desirable tendon transfers, in which case all tendons of the forearm can serve if needed. Some, such as FPL or EPL, have a tendon of sufficient length to fix directly to the thumb. A graft or a tendon must prolong other transfers and they must be inserted on to the thumb. Then the distal end of the EPB provides a suitable means of prolonging an opposition transfer that is too short. In fact, its distal insertion in the mid-dorsal aspect of the base of the proximal phalanx makes an ideal place for fixation if the MCP joint is stable. However, this tendon can slip laterally over the side of the MCP joint and become a flexor. To avoid this complication Kaplan et al (1976) recommended wrapping the tendon of EPB from radial to medial side, around that of the EPL, before suturing it to the motor tendon.

Additive techniques

Many techniques have been advocated for treatment of severe conditions following thumb paralyses. Some are

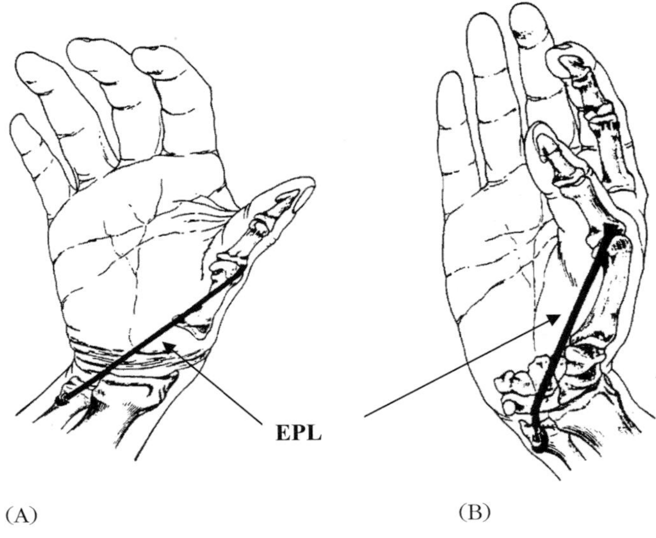

Figure 11.16
Restoring thumb anteposition according to Brooks. The proximally severed EPL is fixed at the head of the ulna. (A) During the wrist flexion the first web space opens. (B) The wrist extension leads the thumb to anteposition and allows the pinch with long fingers.

for mobilization to create or reinforce movement. Some are active, such as all the tendon transfers, and some are more or less passive, such as tenodesis. Other techniques aim to stabilize a joint or correct deformity (capsulodeses, ligamentoplasties, arthrodesis and osteotomies). In severe conditions (such as spinal cord lesions, brachial plexus palsy and associated proximal multiple nerve lesions or Volkmann's syndrome) these additive techniques become useful. The goal here is more limited than that in isolated opposition palsy. The aim is no longer to re-establish the opposition of the thumb and the various thumb–finger pinches. The goal is to produce a useful pinch, often lateral. It is a modest goal, but can represent a significant improvement for the patient. Bunnell used to say: 'When you have nothing a little is a lot'.

Active tenodeses

Tenodesis may allow restoration of a pinch between thumb and fingers, utilizing the wrist movement. It is necessary for the wrist to have active extension of at least 30°. One wrist extensor can be sufficient even in the absence of wrist flexors; in fact gravity allows passive flexion when the forearm is pronated.

This type of operation is indicated for very extensive paralyses or in spinal cord injury (tetraplegic hand). The EPL tendon may be used, according to Brooks (1966), fixed to the ulnar head (Figure 11.16) or the FPL fixed to the radius according to Moberg (1978). Allieu et al (1993) improved the Moberg's procedure by fixing EPL to the stump of the FPL through the radius (Figure 11.17). Active extension of the wrist produces closure of

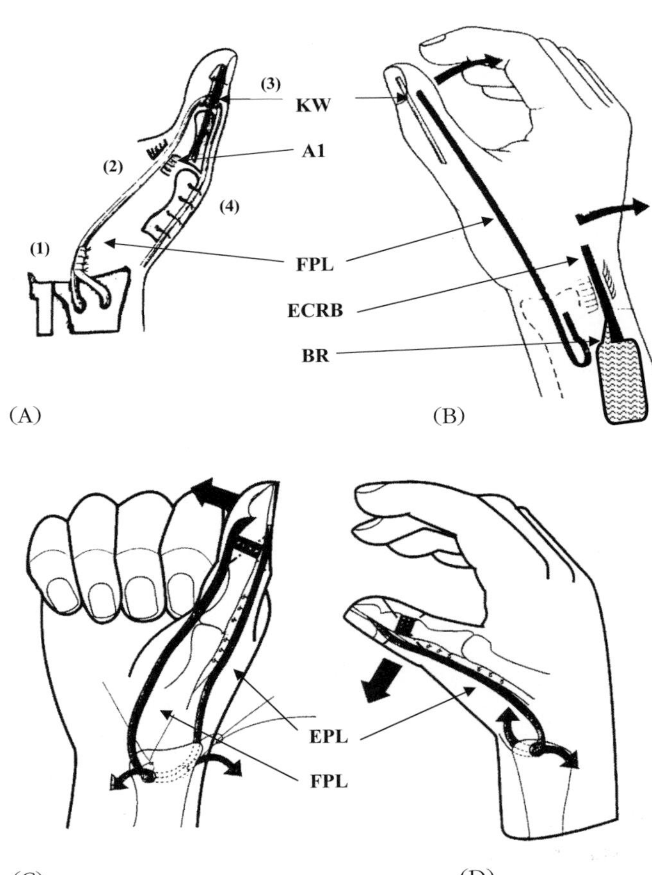

Figure 11.17
Moberg's key grip procedure. (A–B) Basic procedure to restore a lateral pinch (key grip) following Moberg (1975). (A) (1) The flexor pollicis longus (FPL) is tenodesed to the volar surface of the radius through the bone. (2) The A1 pulley at the metacarpophalangeal (MCP) joint level is resected to permit the tendon to bowstring and increase the strength of the key grip. (3) The thumb interphalangeal (IP) joint is stabilized with a Kirschner wire (KW) to prevent flexion and to maintain a broad contact surface. (4) If too much flexion of the MCP joint is possible extensor tendons are tenodesed to the first metacarpal dorsal aspect. (B) If wrist extension is weak the brachioradialis (BR) is transferred to extensor carpi radialis brevis (ECRB). Wrist extension brings the thumb to the index pulp, performing a strong 'key grip'. (C–D) Modifications of the key grip operation following Allieu et al (1993). (C) The FPL is tenodesed to the extensor pollicis longus through the radius distal extremity to adjust the key pinch precisely. All the other steps remain identical. (D) Extension to open the first web space and abduct the thumb passively.

the pinch; flexion due to gravity results in its opening. It should be emphasized that a tenodesis relying on the activity of one muscle is a procedure of last resort. Obviously the pinch is better restored if two active muscles are disposable below the elbow whose action can oppose one another.

It should be noted that the activity of this type of tenodesis is related to the existing amount of wrist movement; so the amount of wrist flexion and extension increases above the minimal requisite of 30°. Furthermore, the tenodesis will respond better to wrist movement if the tendon is positioned centrally and not laterally.

Stabilizing operations

The thumb is a pluriarticular chain, so after extensive paralyses, articular laxity is frequent. At the TMC joint level it can cause radial subluxation accompanied by supination of the thumb. This is an indication for stabilizing operations such tenoplasties, capsulodeses or arthrodeses. At the MCP joint level the most frequent deformation is hyperextension accompanied by lateral laxity pushing in the head of the first metacarpal and then closing the first web space.

Stabilizing operations without articular fusion

At the TMC joint level, a ligamentoplasty using a slip of the FCR tendon following Eaton and Littler (1973) can be used, as can all the other ligamentoplasties described after this procedure, which restore the radial ligament of the TMC joint.

At the MCP joint level, anterior tenodeses and capsulodeses may prevent it from hyperextending. Several techniques of capsulodesis have been described, but do not appear to be very reliable and always lead to loosening with time. It may be better to use a tendon graft following Adams (1959); the EPB tendon following Kessler (1979); a strip of the distal half of the FPL tendon fixed in the base of the proximal phalanx, following Tsuge (1974); the palmaris longus severed proximally and fixed at the base of the proximal phalanx, following Eiken (1981); or advancing the distal conjoined tendon of APB and FPB into the proximal phalanx following Posner et al (1988). Zancolli (1968) fixes the lateral sesamoid to the metacarpal neck, with the MCP joint slightly flexed at 10–15°.

At the IP joint level, hyperextension of the IP joint can be corrected by a tenodesis of the FPL tendon fixed to the bone in 15º of flexion, according to Littler (1971).

Stabilizing operations with articular fusion

At the TMC joint level arthrodesis fixes the thumb in opposition to the fingers and permits pinch through finger movement. It cannot prevent the mobility that can develop around the trapezium, so it may be preferable to carry out an intermetacarpal arthrodesis between the first and second metacarpal bones following Foerster (1930). Actually the indication for this procedure is much more for tetraplegia. Following Zancolli the fixation of the joint has to be from 40 to 45º of anteposition and 20–25º of radial abduction.

At the MCP joint level, fusion has been strongly advocated by Tubiana (1993) and in practice it achieves several goals. (1) It treats the instability of the joint, which is very common in extensive palsy. (2) It enables the thumb to be in a position of pronation and optimal angulation. (3) It allows correction of the stiffness of the MCP joint in defective position, which often occurs. (4) It may improve distal joint extension. (5) It permits the use of EPB, EPL and FPL as transfers if needed and so is a very economical solution as regards availability of transferable tendons. (6) It allows secondary improvement of a transfer whose result is poor because of MCP joint instability, or an unfavourable thumb position.

At the IP joint level, fusion in a straight position allows correction of the frequent pronounced stiffness of the IP joint in flexion. It also reinforces flexion of the MCP joint by the FPL.

Following Tubiana (1993), some authors prefer to perform fusion of the MCP joint rather than the IP joint, because movement of the MCP joint has less amplitude and is not as useful. Actually the problem is not the choice between two fusions: the two thumb phalanges create a functional unit and so instability of the MCP joint must in any case be corrected.

Osteotomy of the first metacarpal

Makin (1967) and later Comtet and Bemelmans (1979) outlined the indication for osteotomy at the base of the first metacarpal. It can allow accentuation of anteposition and pronation of the first column when transfers are insufficient, but only when the MCP joint is stable.

Additive techniques for complex pluritissular lesions

Severe conditions affecting thumb movements are often caused by crush or blast injuries, Volkman or severe ischaemic conditions or severe burn injury sequelae. Soft

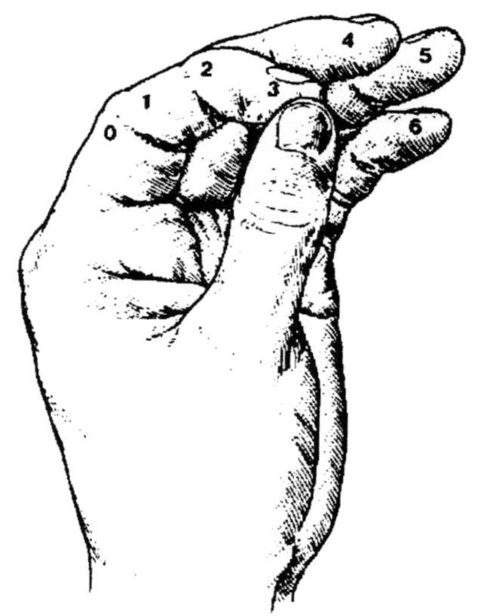

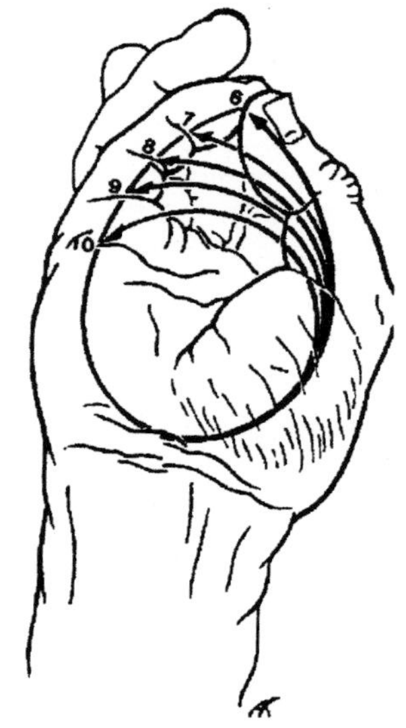

Figure 11.18

Kapandji's assessment of thumb opposition in 10 points (1992). During opposition the thumb has to pass one after another on each point from 0 to 10. 0 is lateral proximal pinch (radial side of the proximal phalanx); 1 is lateral middle pinch (intermediate phalanx); 2 is lateral distal pinch (DIP joint); 1 and 2 achieved the key pinch; 3 is the terminoterminal pinch between the thumb and index (IP joint flexed); 4, 5 and 6 are pinch between the thumb and the pulp of the third, fourth and fifth fingers. From stages 7 to 10 the thumb moves on the palm crossing the DIP (7) joint crease, the PIP joint crease (8), the proximal finger crease (9) and finally the distal palmar crease (10). From Kapandji (1988) with permission.

tissue lesions may be more problematical than nervous lesions. Scanning of the remaining motors will lead to the surgical approach, usually as a second procedure. All the soft tissue reconstruction problems are present and have to be managed. These conditions seem to be the main indications for intrinsic muscle transfers in adults, if they are still innervated. There is also a place for Makin's procedure (1967), rerouting the FPL through a proximal phalanx osteotomy. In fact there is no need to sever a tendon, perfect gliding course conditions are not essential and it is useful for the replanted thumb, for example.

When no transferable material at all is useable, the utility of free muscle transfers may be considered, as proposed by Tamai in 1970 and effectively demonstrated in clinical cases by Manktelow (1986).

Clinical results

The final result may be evaluated around the third month after surgery, but usually real functional and useful utilization is obtained around the sixth month. A good technique performed in good conditions will be maintained after time, not only in adults, but equally in children.

The evaluation of opponenplasties must be based on a complete functional examination. Opposition may be easily and globally scored by the Kapandji scale from 0 to 10 (Figure 11.18). However, pinch grasp and grip strength must be evaluated precisely. The final results must be correlated with the clinical conditions present before surgery.

Conclusions

The first problem in restoration of movement in a paralysed thumb should take into account the muscles available for transfer; then a decision can be made as to which varieties of pinch may be restored. Numbers are severely limited in extensive paralyses, and the movements of the wrist must also be considered. Depending on the extent of paralyses, thumb paralysis are classified as follows (Tubiana 1993):

- Group I: Paralysis of the intrinsic muscles.
- Group II: Paralysis of the intrinsic muscles associated with partial paralysis of the extrinsic muscles and conservation of > 30° of active wrist extension.
- Group III: Paralysis of the intrinsic muscles associated with partial paralysis of the extrinsic muscles, without active wrist extension. This group can be subdivided according to whether or not the wrist extension can be recovered with a transfer.

The clinician must take into consideration the associated lesions, stiffness, contractures, instabilities and sensory disorders. As stated earlier, sensory factors have an important influence on the use of the restored thumb and can sometimes render the re-established pinch ineffective. Tubiana (1974) demonstrated effectively that the results show a correlation between sensory problems and the quality of recuperation. So, when it is feasible, neurosensory island flaps can be used to obtain, at the very least, sensitive protection for the thumb pulp.

Finally, the definitive importance of clinical analysis must be emphasized and palliative treatment must be adapted to each individual patient.

References

Adams JP (1959) Correction of chronic dorsal subluxation of the proximal interphalangeal joint by means of a crisscross volar grail, *J Bone Joint Surg* **41A**: 111.

Allieu Y, Benichoud M, Ohanna F et al (1993) Chirargie fonctionnelle du membre supérieur chez le tétraplégique. Orientation actuelle après 10 ans d'expérience du centre PROPARA, *Rev Chir Orthop* **79**: 79–88.

Alnot JY (1993) La main plexique, atteinte du poignet et de la main dans les paralysies traumatiques du plexus de l'adulte. In: *Cahier d'Enseignement de la Société Française de Chirurgie de la Main*, no. 5 (Expansion Scientifique Française: Paris) 129–43.

Brand PW (1970) Tendon transfer for median and ulnar nerve paralysis. *Orthop Clin North Am* **1**: 447.

Brand PW (1975) Tendon transfers in the forearm. In: Flynn JE, ed., *Hand Surgery*, 2nd edn (Williams & Wilkins: Baltimore) 189.

Brand PW (1985) *Clinical Mechanics of the Hand* (CV Mosby: St Louis).

Brooks DM (1966) Treatment of the paralytic band. In: Pulvertaft EG, ed., *Clinical Surgery. The Hand* (Butterworths: London).

Bunnell S (1924) Reconstructive surgery of the hand, *Surg Gynecol Obstet* **39**: 259.

Bunnell S (1938) Opposition of the thumb, *J Bone Joint Surg* **20**: 269.

Bureau H, Decaillet JM, MaGalon G et al (1981) La restauration de l'opposition par le muscle long extenseur du pouce, *Ann Chir* **25**: 281.

Burkhalter WE (1974) Early tendon transfer in upper extremity peripheral nerve injury, *Clin Orthop* **104**: 68.

Burkhalter WE (1993) Median nerve palsy. In: Green DP, ed., *Operative Hand Surgery*, 3rd edn (Churchill Livingstone: New York) 1419–48.

Burkhalter WE, Christensen RC, Brown PW (1973) Extensor indicis proprius opponensplasty. *J Bone Joint Surg* **55A:** 725.

Camitz H (1929) Über die Behandlung der Oppositionslähmung. *Acta Orthop Scand* **65**: 77.

Chammas M, Chiesa G, Dimeglio A et al (1999) *Cahier d'enseignment de la Société Française de Chirurgie de la Main*, no. 11 (Expansion Scientifique Publications: Paris).

Chouy A, Kaplan S (1956) Sobre secuelas de lesion alta e irreparable de nervious mediano y cubital y su tratarniento, *Prensa Med Argent* **43**: 2431.

Comtet N, Bemelmans D (1979) The palmar abduction–pronation osteotomy of the first metacarpal bone combined with tendon transfer for lateral thenar muscle paralysis, *Hand* **11**: 191.

Cook (1921) Reconstruction of the hand. A new technique in tenoplasty, *Surg Gynecol Obstet* **32**: 237.

Cooney WP. Linseheid RL, An K-N (1984) Opposition of the thumb: an anatomic and biomechanical study of tendon transfers, *J Hand Surg* **9A**: 777–85.

De Vecchi J (1961) Oposicion del pulgar fisiopatologia una nueva operacion transplante del aductor, *Bol Soc Cir Uruguay* **32**: 432.

Duchenne GB (1867) *Physiologie des Mouvements* (JB Baillière: Paris).

Duparc J, Caffinière de la JY, Roux JP (1971) Les plasties d'opposition par la transplantation tendineuse à travers la membrane interosseuse, *Rev Chir Orthop* **57**: 29.

Eaton RG, Littler JW (1973) Ligament reconstruction for the painful thumb carpometacarpal joint, *J Bone Joint Surg* **55A**: 1655.

Edgerton MT, Brand PW (1965) Restoration of abduction and adduction to the unstable thumb in median and ulnar paralysis, *Plast Reconstr Surg* **36**: 150.

Eiken O (1981) Palmaris longus tenodesis for hyperextension of the thumb metacarpophalangeal joint, *Scand J Plast Reconstr Surg* **15**: 149.

Foerster O (1930) Beitrag zum Werte Fixierender Orthopadiseher Operationen bei Nervenlcrankheiten, *Acta Chir Scand* **67**: 351.

Goldner JL, Irwin CE (1950) An analysis of paralytic thumb deformities, *J Bone Joint Surg* **32A**: 627.

Groves RJ, Goldner JL (1975) Restoration of strong opposition after median nerve or brachial plexus paralysis, *J Bone Joint Surg* **57**: 112.

Huber E (1921) Hilfsoperation bei median Usläliumg, *Dtsch Arch Klin Med* **136**: 271.

Iselin F, Pradet G (1984) Transfert de l'abducteur dii 5e doigt, palliatif de la paralysie des thénariens externes, *Ann Chir Main* **3**: 207.

Jacobs G, Thompson TC (1978) Opposition of the thumb and its restoration, *J Bone Joint Surg* **42A**: 1015.

Kapandji IA (1988) *Dessins de Mains* (Malone: Paris).

Kapandji IA (1992) Clinical evaluation of the thumb's opposition, *J Hand Ther* **5**: 102.

Kaplan I, Dinner M, Chait L (1976) Use of extensor pollicis longus tendon as a distal extension for an opponens transfer, *Plast Reconstr Surg* **57**: 186.

Kessler I (1979) A simplifled technique to correct hyperextension deformities of the metacarpophalangeal joint of the thumb, *J Bone Joint Surg* **61A** 905

Krukenberg H (1922) Uber Ersatz des M. opponens pollicis, *Z Orthop Chir* **12**: 178.

LeCoeur P (1953) Procedé de restauration de l'opposition du pouce par transplantation sur chevalet, *Rev Orthop* **39**: 655.

Littler JW (1949) Tendon transfers and arthrodesis in combined median and ulnar nerve paralysis, *J Bone Joint Surg* **31A**: 225.

Littler JW (1971) Restoration of digital joint stability. In: Cramer LM, Chase RA, eds, *Symposium on the Hand* (CV Mosby: St Loius).

Littler JW, Cooley SGE (1963) Opposition of the thumb and its restoration by abductor digiti quinti transfer, *J Bone Joint Surg* **45A**: 389.

Makin M (1967) Translocation of the flexor pollicis longus tendon to restore opposition, *J Bone Joint Surg* **49B**: 458.

Manktelow RT (1986) Functional muscle transplantation. In: *Microvascular Reconstruction* (Springer: Berlin) 151–64.

Merle d'Aubigné R, Benassy J, RamadierJ (1956) *Chirurgie Orthopédique des Paralysie* (Masson: Paris).

Moberg E (1975) Surgical treatment for absent single-hand grip and elbow extension in quadriplegia, *J Bone Joint Surg* **57A**: 196.

Moberg E (1978) *The Upper Limb in Tetraplegia* (Georg Thieme: Stuttgart).

Ney KW (1921) A tendon transplant for intrinsic hand muscle paralysis, *Surg Gynecol Obstet* **33**: 342.

Nicolaysen J (1922) Transplantation des M. abductor dig. V. bie Fehlender Oppositions Fahigkeit des Daurnens, *Dtsch Z Chir* **168**: 133.

Orticochea M (1971) Use of the deep bundie of the flexor pollicis brevis to restore opposition of the thumb, *Plast Reconstr Surg* **47**: 22O.

Palazzi AS (1962) On the treatment of the lost opposition, *Acta Orthop Scand* **32**: 396.

Phalen GS, Miller RC (1947) Transfer of wrist extensor muscles to restore or reinforce flexion of fingers and opposition of thumb, *J Bone Joint Surg* **29**: 993.

Posner M, Langa V, Ambrose L (1988) Intrinsic muscle advancement to treat chronic palmar instability of the metacarpophalangeal joint of the thumb, *J Hand Surg* **13A**: 10.

Price EW (1968) A two-tendon transplant for low median–ulnar palsy of the thumb in leprosy, *Proc R Soc Med* **61**: 22O.

Ramselaar JM (1970) *Tendon Transfers to Restore Opposition of the Thumb* (Stenfert Kroese NV: Leiden).

Riordan DC (1953) Tendon transplantation in median nerve and ulnar nerve paralysis, *J Bone Joint Surg* **35A**: 312–320, 386.

Riordan DE (1964) Tendon transfers for nerve paralysis of the hand and wrist, *Curr Pract Orthoo Surg* **2**: 17.

Royle ND (1938) An operation for paralysis of the intrinsic muscles of the thumb, *JAMA* **111**: 612.

Schneider LH (1969) Opponensplasty using the extensor digiti minimi, *J Bone Joint Surg* **51A**: 1297.

Spitzy H (1919) Hand und Fingerpiastiken (14 Orthop. Congress, Vienna 1918). *Vern Dtsch Orthop Gesellsch* **14**: 120.

Steindler A (1918) Orthopaedic operations on the hands, *JAMA* **71**: 1288.

Steindler A (1930) Flexorplasty of the thumb in thenar plasy, *Surg Gynecol Obstet* **50**: 1005.

Thompson TC (1942) A modified operation for opponens paralysis, *J Bone Joint Surg* **24**: 632.

Tsuge K (1974) Reconstruction of opposition in the paralyzed hand. In: McDoweil F, Enna CD, eds, *Surgical Rehabilitation in Leprosy* (Williams & Wilkins: Baltimore) 185.

Tubiana R (1969) Anatomic and physiologic basis for the surgical treatment of paralysis of the hand, *J Bone Joint Surg* **51A**: 643.

Tubiana R (1974) Indications thérapeutiqucs dans les paralysies étendues et conpliquées du pouce, *Ann Chir* **28**: 25.

Tubiana R (1979) La rétablissement de l'opposition du pouce après paralyse, *Chirurgie* **105**: 920.

Tubiana R (1987) Tendon transfers for restoration of opposition. In: Hunter J, Schneider LH, Mackin E, eds., *Tendon Surgery in the Hand* (CV Mosby: St Louis) 419.

Tubiana R (1993) Paralyses of the thumb. In: Tubiana R, ed., *The Hand*, vol. lV (Saunders: Philadelphia) 182–253.

Tubiana R, Valentin P (1968) Opposition of the thumb, *Surg Clin North Am* **48**: 967.

Tubiana R, Gilbert A, Marquelet AC (1999) *An Atlas of Surgical Techniques of the Hand and Wrist* (Martin Dunitz: London).

White WL (1960) Restoration of function and balance of the wrist and hand by tendon transfers, *Surg Clin North Am* **40**: 427.

Zancolli EA (1961) Cirurgia de le mano. Correccion de las contracturas en adduccion y supinacion del pulgar, *Bol Trab Soc Argent Orthop Traum* **26**: 199.

Zancolli EA (1965) Transfers after ischemic contracture of the forearm, *Am J Surg* **109**: 356.

Zancolli EA (1968) *Structural and Dynamic Bases of Hand Surgery* (JP Lippincott: Philadelphia).

Zancolli EA (1975) Surgery for the quadriplegic hand with active strong wrist extension preserved–study of 97 cases, *Clin Orthop* **112**: 101.

Zancolli EA (1979) *Structural and Dynamic Bases of Hand Surgery* 2nd edn (JP Lippincott: Philadelphia).

12 Paralysis of the ulnar nerve

Raoul Tubiana

Ulnar nerve paralyses result from nerve lesions of diverse causes occurring at different levels of the nerve.

The deformity considered characteristic of ulnar nerve palsy is the claw hand. In fact, this deformity is not always present and ulnar nerve paralyses are responsible for many other functional disabilities.

Anatomy

The ulnar nerve arises from the medial cord of the brachial plexus (Figure 12.1). Its fibers come from the C7, C8, and T1 roots. It runs medial to the humeral artery, goes through the medial intermuscular septum, and passes between the medial epicondyle of the humerus and the olecranon (Figure 12.2). It enters the forearm between the humeral and ulnar origins of the flexor carpi ulnaris (FCU) and descends within the anteromedial compartment of the forearm under cover of the FCU. At the wrist, lying on the medial side of the ulnar artery, it runs with the latter, in the so-called Guyon osseofibrous canal (distinct from the carpal tunnel). Just distal to the pisiform it divides into its two terminal branches: the superficial sensory branch, which supplies the medial skin of the hand, and the deep motor branch, which winds around the hook of the hamate, crosses the sharp lower border of the opponens digiti minimi muscle and, under cover of the deep flexor tendons, reaches the adductor pollicis (AP) and flexor pollicis brevis (FPB) muscles on the lateral side of the hand (Figure 12.3)

The ulnar nerve supplies the FCU and the ulnar head of the flexor digitorum profundus (FDP). In the lower third of the forearm it gives off the dorsal cutaneous branch, which supplies the skin of the ulnar half of the dorsum of the hand. Between them the median and ulnar nerves supply all the intrinsic muscles of the hand: the deep terminal branch of the ulnar nerve sends fibers to all the intrinsic muscles of the long fingers (except the two lateral lumbricals), to the AP, and to the deep head of the FPB. In fact the respective territories of the median and ulnar nerves are poorly defined. Anastomoses occur in the forearm (Martin-Gruber

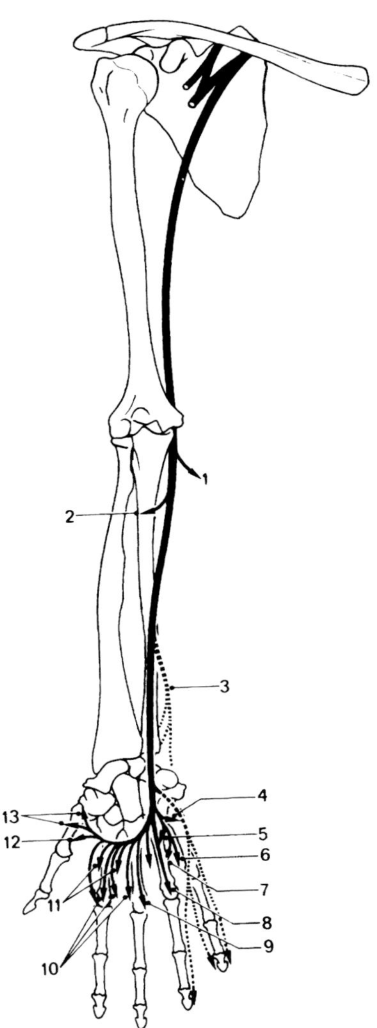

Figure 12.1

The ulnar nerve, muscles supplied and cutaneous distribution. (1) Branch to flexor carpi ulnaris; (2) branch to flexor digitorum profundus supplying fourth and fifth digits; (3) dorsal cutaneous branch; (4) palmar cutaneous branch; (5) branch to abductor digiti minimi; (6) branch to opponens digiti minimi; (7) branch to flexor digiti minimi; (8) fourth lumbrical branch; (9) third lumbrical branch; (10) branch to palmar interosseous muscles; (11) branch to dorsal interosseous muscles; (12) deep branch to flexor pollicis brevis; (13) branch to adductor pollicis. The sensory branches are shown as dotted lines.

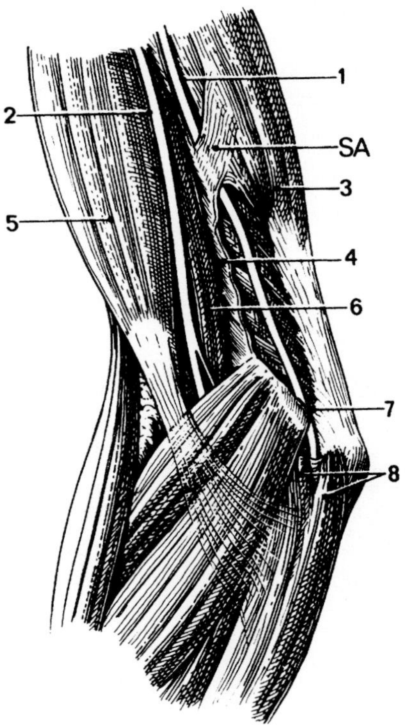

Figure 12.2.

The ulnar nerve at the elbow. 1. Ulnar nerve; 2. Median nerve; 3. Triceps; 4. Medial intermuscular septum; 5. Biceps; 6. Brachialis; 7. Medial epicondylar groove; 8. The two heads of FCU; SA = Struthers arcade

anastomosis) in 15% of cases according to Mannerfelt (1966) and also occur in the palm (anastomosis of Riche (1897) and Cannieu (1897)), which explains the frequent anomalies of distribution (Figure 12.4).

The ulnar nerve is most vulnerable at the elbow and the wrist.

Etiology

Ulnar nerve motor deficits in Western countries most often result from direct trauma to the nerve or from long-standing nerve compression. However, ulnar nerve paralyses secondary to leprosy or poliomyelitis are frequent in Asia and Africa.

Ulnar nerve compression

The ulnar nerve can be compressed at several sites.

In the lower third of the arm

The nerve enters the posterior compartment by passing through an osseofibrous foramen. This is formed laterally by the medial intermuscular septum which is attached to the humerus, above by a fibrous expansion

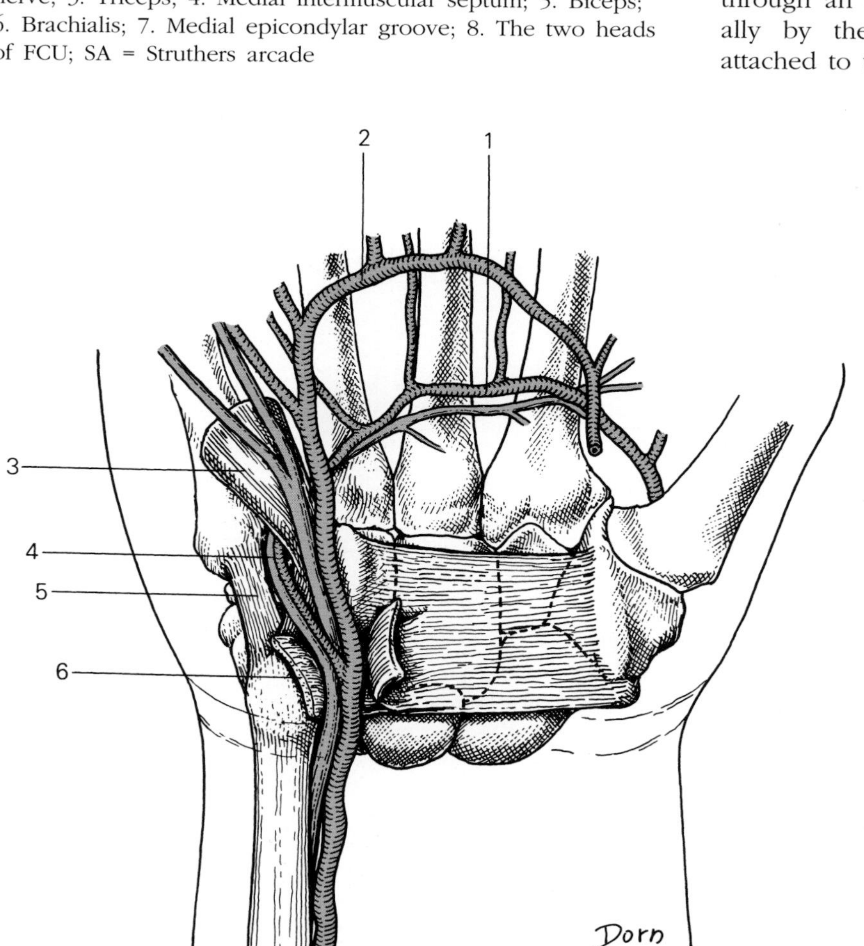

Figure 12.3

The terminal branches of the ulnar nerve.

1 Ulnar nerve
2 Ulnar artery
3 FCU
4 Deep motor branch of ulnar nerve
5 Pisometacarpal ligament
6 Volar carpal ligament (incised)
7 Digital branches of ulnar nerve
8 Flexor digiti minimi
9 Superficial palmar arch
10 Deep palmar arch

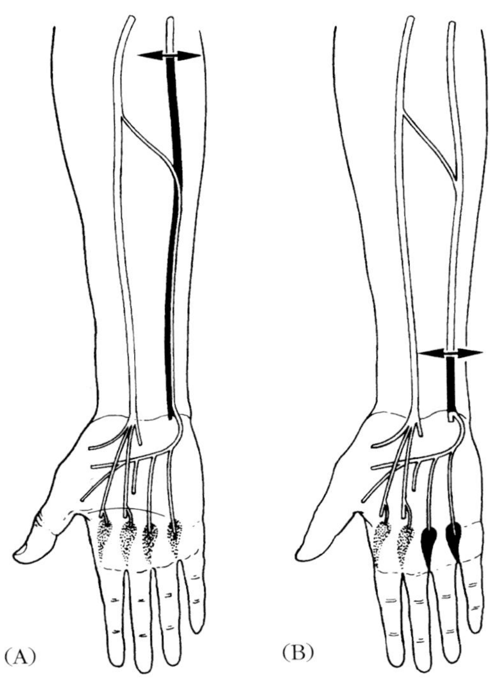

Figure 12.4

Martin–Gruber anastomosis between the median and ulnar nerves in the forearm. In high lesions of the ulnar nerve (A), the anastomosis from the median nerve can result in prevention of paralysis of the ulnar innervated intrinsic muscles. In lesions of the ulnar nerve distal to the anastomosis (B), this will not occur.

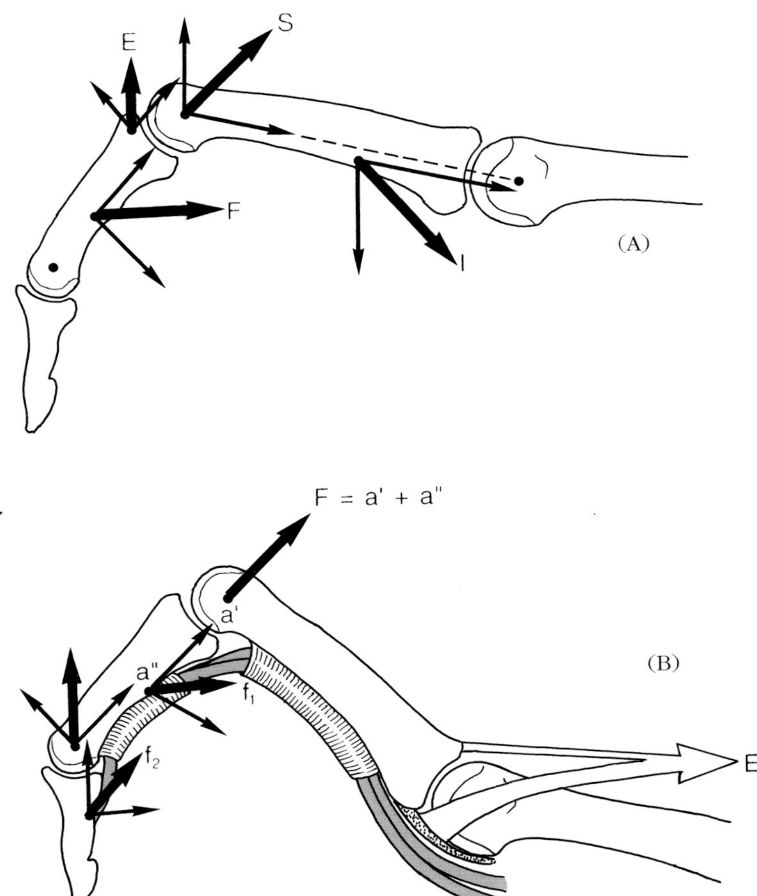

Figure 12.5

The claw hand deformity.

(A) Mechanical explanation of the claw-hand deformity. Force (E) of the EDC contributes to carrying the proximal phalanx into hyperextension. The force of the flexors also produces extension in the proximal phalanx. Force (F) of the FDS has an axial component (a'). Force (f_2) of the flexor profundus has an axial component that, as it is transmitted to the head of the middle phalanx, can be broken down into an axial force (a"), and an extension force on the middle phalanx counteracted by the flexion component of (f_1). The sum of (a') and (a") represents the total force of extension acting on the middle phalanx (F). Force (E) of the EDC and force (F) of the FDS each has an axial component the sum (S) of these is applied to the head of the proximal phalanx over which it is extended. Force (I) of the intrinsic muscles counteracts this extension force at the proximal phalanx.

(B) When the intrinsic muscles are paralysed, no force exists to prevent the proximal phalanx from swinging into hyperextension. The EDC, which exhausts its baction at the level of its proximal insertion (E), has no effect on the distal phalanges. Note that hyperextension of the MP joint is only seen if the EDC and FD are active.

of the coracobrachialis, and medially by the medial head of the triceps. Distally the foramen may be narrowed by inconstant insertions of the triceps, which form 'Struthers' arcade' (Struthers 1854) (Figure 12.2).

At the elbow

The nerve passes through a narrow channel between the epicondyle and the olecranon, where it may be compressed or elongated (see Chapter 26, Upper limb nerve compression in musicians). Next the nerve runs between the humeral and ulnar heads of the FCU under a fibrous arcade, which must be divided to relieve compression at that level (Osborne 1970).

In the wrist

The nerve can be compressed in Guyon's canal, the floor of which is formed by the flexor retinaculum and the roof by an expansion of the FCU.

In the hand

The deep motor branch arises from the medial side of the nerve, passes under the fibrous band between the pisiform and the hook of the hamate and dives between abductor digiti minimi and flexor digiti minimi (see Figure 12.3).

Clinical features

Clinical features of ulnar nerve palsy include sensory and motor manifestations.

Sensory ulnar palsy

This affects both the palmar and the dorsal aspects of the ulnar half of the hand. The autonomous zone of the ulnar nerve is limited to the skin of the distal two phalanges of the little finger.

Motor ulnar palsy

Motor ulnar palsy, by contrast, has far more functional consequences (Table 12.1). Distal ulnar nerve lesions produce the classic claw deformity. The claw consists of hyperextension of the proximal phalanx while the two distal phalanges are in flexion (Figure 12.5). It is important to be aware that every ulnar paralysis does not result in a claw hand. This deformity is caused by the paralysis of the intrinsic muscles, when the extrinsic muscles, i.e. the long flexors and the long extensors of the fingers, are active. This deformity is present in varying degrees, depending on the extent of the paralysis and the supple-

Table 12.1 *Symptoms and signs in ulnar nerve paralysis (adapted from Mannerfeit, 1966)*

Original description by	*Year*	*Symptoms and signs*
Duchenne	1867	Clawing of the ring and little fingers The little finger cannot be adducted to the ring finger; inability to play high notes on the violin because the flexor carpi ulnaris and opponens digiti quinti are paralysed and there is loss of sensibility of the little finger
Jeanne	1915	Hyperextension of the metacarpophalangeal joint of the thumb in pinch grip (Jeanne's sign)
Froment	1915	Pronounced flexion of the interphalangeal joint of the thumb during adduction toward the index finger (Froment's sign)
Masse	1916	Flattening of the metacarpal arch
André-Thomas	1917	The wrist tends to fall into volar flexion during action of the extensors of the middle finger
Pollock	1919	Inability to flex the distal phalanx of the fifth finger
Pitres-Testut	1925	The transverse diameter of the hand is decreased Radial-ulnar abduction of the metacarpophalangeal joint of the middle finger is impossible Inability to shape the hand to a cone
Wartenberg	1939	Inability to adduct the extended little finger to the extended ring finger (Wartenberg's sign)
Sunderland	1944	Inability to rotate, oppose, or supinate the little finger toward the thumb (Sunderland's sign)
Fay	1954	Inability of the thumb to reach the little finger in true opposition (probably a misinterpretation of the author because the little finger cannot always reach the thumb in cases of paralysis of the opponens of the little finger)
Bunnell	1956	The thumb no longer pinches against the index finger to make a full circle
Egawa	1959	Inability of the flexed middle finger to abduct radially and ulnarly and to rotate at the metacarpophalangeal joint
Mumenthaler	1961	On abduction of the little finger against resistance, no normal dimple appears in the hypothenar region because of paresis of the palmaris brevis musculature
Mannerfelt	1966	Hyperflexion sign Thumb: Interphalangeal joint flexed; metacarpophalangeal joint slightly hyperextended; the thumb is markedly supinated Index finger: With increasing force in the collapsed pinching grip, a flexion position (often more than 90°) of the proximal interphalangeal joint is seen; the distal interphalangeal joint is hyperextended, and the radial part of the pulp slides in a proximal direction along the ulnar part of the thumb

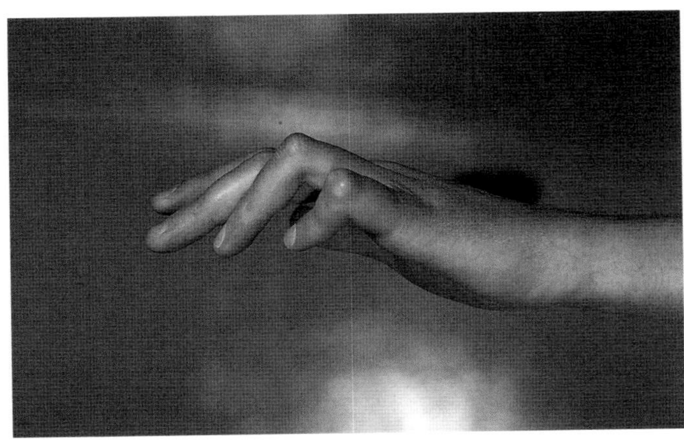
(A)

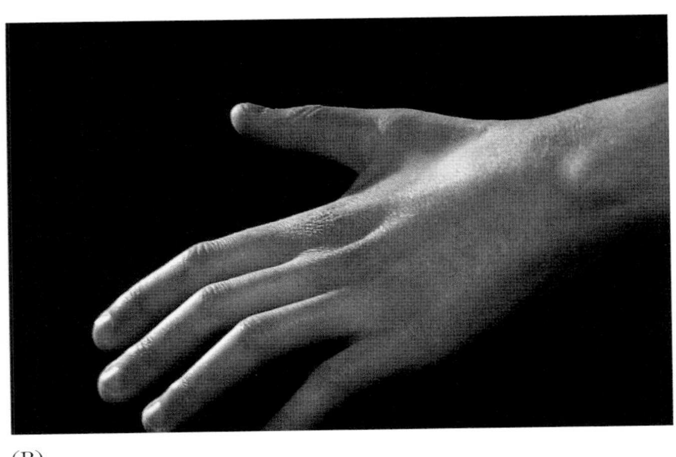
(B)

Figure 12.6.
Claw hand. (A) Distal ulnar palsy. (B) Proximal ulnar palsy. The long flexors are paralysed, the claw deformity is minimized.

ness of the digits. It involves only the ring and small fingers in cases of isolated ulnar paralysis, because the two radial lumbricals, innervated by the median nerve, prevent deformity of the index and long fingers when the hand is at rest. The third lumbrical may be innervated by both the median and ulnar nerves, and clawing is more severe in the little finger than in the ring finger (Kaplan and Spinner 1980). The deformity is more marked when the nerve lesion is distal and the long flexors are intact (Figure 12.6). It involves the four fingers (Figure 12.7) in cases of associated paralysis of the ulnar and median nerves.

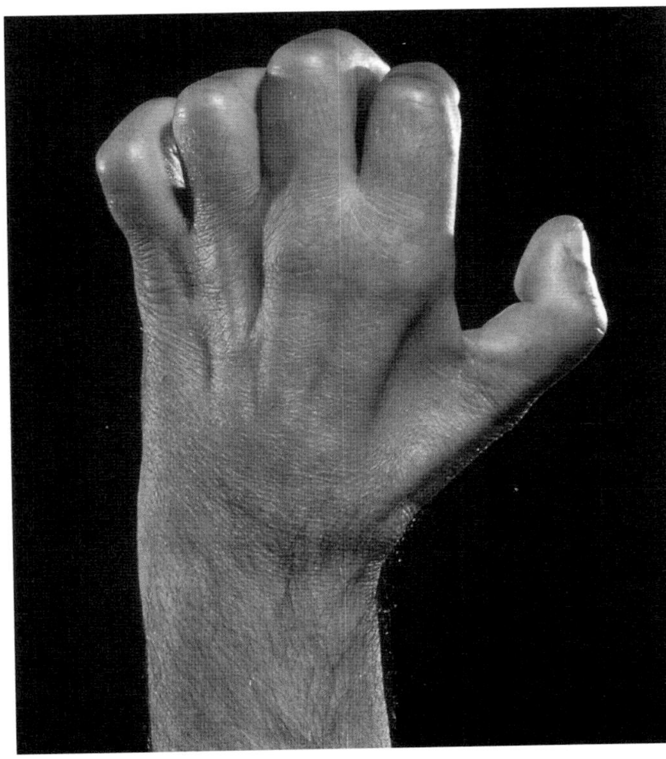

Figure 12.7
Associated paralysis of the ulnar and median nerves with claw deformity of the four fingers. Note the depression at the first commissure.

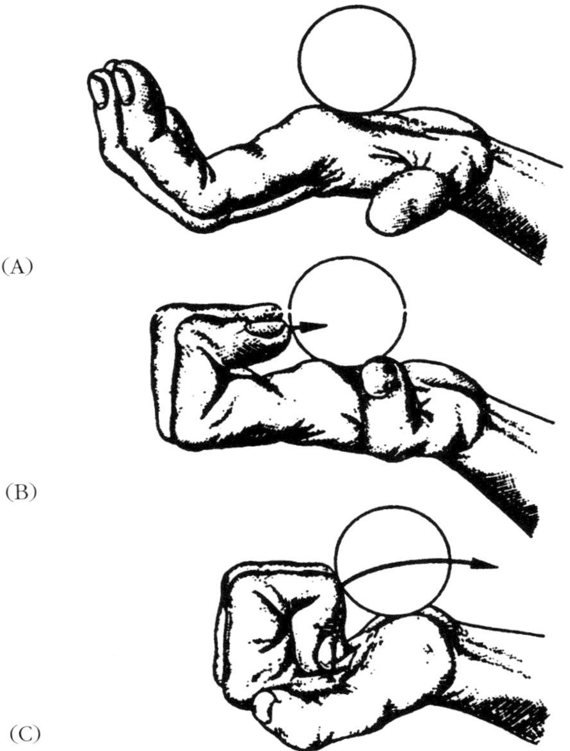

Figure 12.8
Inversion of the sequence of phalangeal flexion
(A) Intrinsic muscle paralysis
(B) Finger flexion is accomplished by the longer flexors and begins with the distal phalanges
(C) The hand cannot grasp large objects

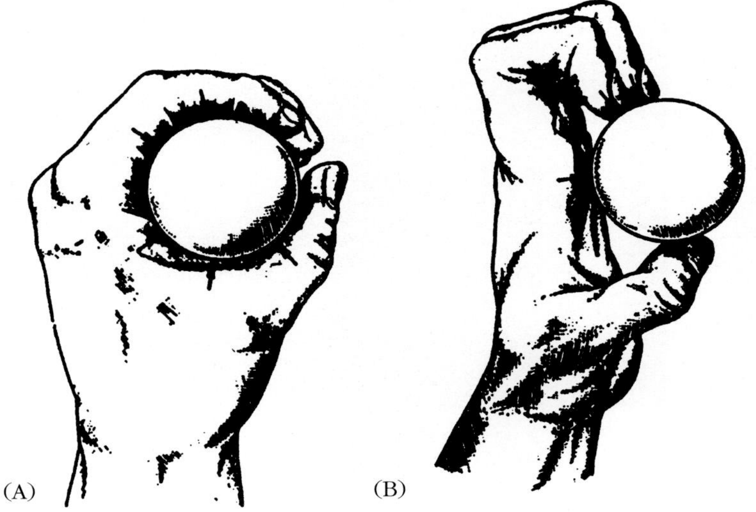

Figure 12.9
Location of pressure zones.
(A) Normal grasp. The zone of pressure is widely distributed
(B) Grasp in a hand with intrinsic paralysis. The pressure on the extremities of the flexed fingers is considerable

Dynamic problems producing troubles of prehension are far more bothersome than the claw hand itself.

Grasp is disturbed for several reasons.

1. Lack of extension of the distal phalanges, which prevents the grasping of large objects.
2. Inversion of the sequence of phalangeal flexion. Normally, finger flexion begins at the level of the proximal interphalangeal (PIP) and metacarpophalangeal (MP) joints and is followed by distal interphalangeal (DIP) joint flexion. In cases of interosseous paralysis, the sequence of flexion is altered (Figure 12.8). Finger flexion is accomplished by the long flexors alone, which act first on the distal phalanges. The MP joint flexes last. With flexion, the pulps of the fingers shave the palm, and the hand cannot grasp large objects. This 'dyskinetic finger flexion' is one of the most awkward functional consequences of these paralyses.
3. For a long time, intrinsic muscle strength has been underestimated. This strength is far from negligible, especially in the peripheral digits. The more proximal the ulnar paralysis, the more marked is the deficit of the strength of finger flexion, because the flexor profundus paralysis of the ring and little finger is added to the intrinsic paralysis. When there is concomitant proximal median nerve paralysis, all the digital flexors, intrinsics and extrinsics, are paralysed.
4. The disturbance in finger flexion causes a modification of the location of pressure zones during grasp. Normally during grasp the pressure over the zone of contact is widely distributed on the palmar aspect of the fingers, on the metacarpal heads, and on the thenar and hypothenar eminences. When an ulnar-paralysed hand grasps an object, it is the extremities of the flexed fingers that do the grasping, and the pressure on these limited zones of contact is considerable (Figure 12.9). This can cause ulceration of the fingertips, especially when problems of pressure distribution are associated with a sensory disturbance.
5. Flattening of the palmar arch considerably weakens the power to grasp large objects and may need to be corrected for certain manual laborers.
6. A considerable lack of thumb strength is always added to the lack of finger strength, because the AP and often the FBP, are paralysed. Measurements performed by Mannerfelt (1966) showed that the residual strength of thumb adduction in ulnar palsy is only 20% of normal. The lack of hand strength is a major complaint of patients with ulnar palsy.

Thumb–finger grip

All the pinch grip modalities are disturbed by intrinsic muscle paralysis. Precision pinch between the thumb and fingers becomes extremely difficult, because the patient is unable to adapt the position of the distal phalanges, which are deprived of active extension. The thumb also presents with flexion of its distal phalanx during pinch: this is Froment's sign. This deformity is not fixed (at least not initially); it is dynamic, and the degree of flexion augments with increasing effort. It is caused by the paralysis of the AP, which is the extensor of the distal phalanx of the thumb. This difference in position of the distal phalanx between median and ulnar nerve paralysis is explained by the predominance of muscles innervated by the ulnar nerve.

For Bunnell (1942), flexion of the distal phalanx is due to the collapse of the thumb column and is secondary to the hyperextension of the MP joint (Jeanne's sign) that causes tension of the flexor pollicis longus (FPL). It is, in effect, sometimes possible to diminish the flexion of the distal joint by stabilizing the MP joint in slight flexion. However, effort-induced flexion of the distal phalanx of the thumb unaccompanied by hyperextension of the proximal phalanx can be observed when the FPB is not paralysed.

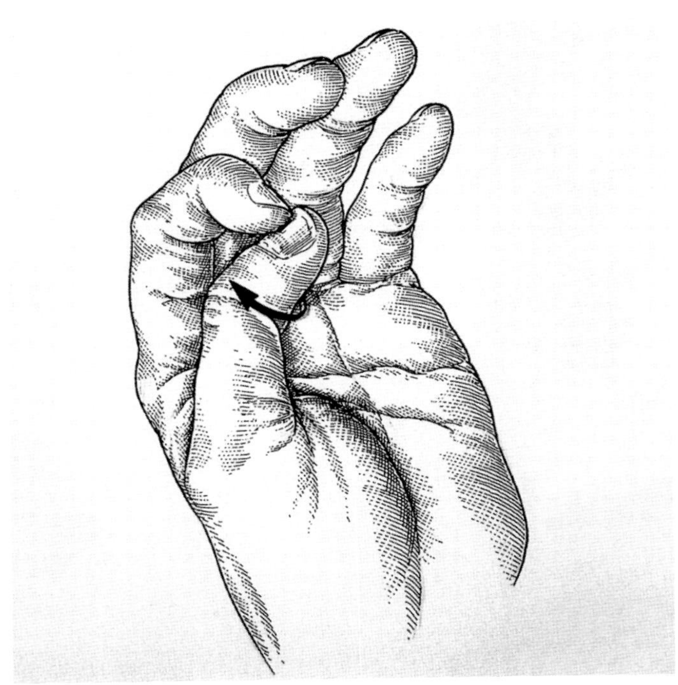

Figure 12.10
The 'crank-handle' effect.

The flexion deformity of the distal phalanx of the thumb is functionally disabling because it hinders the most useful type of pinch. Furthermore, during finger–thumb pinch, pressure from the index is exerted on the dorso-ulnar aspect of the distal phalanx of the thumb, forcing the thumb into supination (the 'crank-handle' effect; Brand, 1985) (Figure 12.10).

Differential diagnosis

Weakness and atrophy in the thenar and hypothenar musculature may be caused by more proximal nerve lesions or compression at the level of the cervical spine, particularly impingement of the lower cervical nerve roots or lesions of the lower elements of the brachial plexus. The ulnar nerve supplies no sensation in the forearm and if there is sensory loss on the ulnar side of the forearm, the cause may well be found at the thoracic outlet.

Intrinsic atrophy may be seen in more generalized nerve disorders.

In all cases nerve conduction velocity and electromyography studies may be very helpful.

Treatment

Reconstructive treatment of ulnar nerve palsy seeks to restore two essential functions of the hand: normal finger grip and thumb–index lateral pinch.

Several options are possible according to the level of the ulnar nerve lesion, the age and expectations of the patient, and the availability of donor tendons for transfers.

In a proximal lesion (high ulnar palsy), in addition to the loss of 80% of the intrinsic muscles, there is paralysis of the FCU and the ring and little finger FDP muscles.

It should be remembered that superficialis tendons from the ring and little fingers cannot be used in high ulnar palsy because this would deprive these digits of an active flexor. In cases of injury to the ulnar nerve at the forearm or wrist, the flexor tendons are often lacerated and repaired at the time of injury. These repaired flexors do not make ideal transfers because of the risk of adhesions.

The clinician should also try to avoid using the flexor carpi radialis (FCR) tendon as a donor because of the absence of a functional FCU muscle.

In a proximal lesion, it is difficult to obtain useful functional recovery of the intrinsic muscles, especially in patients over the age of 40, because of the distal location of these muscles. In this situation, early reconstructive surgery may be indicated.

Preoperative care

Physical therapy is essential. Exercises are directed at maintaining mobility of the finger joints.

A lumbrical bar splint that fits over the dorsum of the metacarpal heads and proximal phalanges of the ring and little fingers is particularly useful. This splint prevents the MP joints from hyperextension without impeding finger flexion. This splint will not improve grip strength; it will allow the extrinsic extensor tendons to extend the interphalangeal joints and will diminish the likelihood of fixed contractures.

Also, in ulnar nerve palsy, the strength of the thumb is much diminished because of the adductor paralysis, to which is often added paralysis of the FPB. The patient compensates for the loss of the adductor by using the adducting action of the extensor pollicis longus (EPL), which brings the thumb column into retroposition and supination. If this deforming posture is not resisted early, the patient will have difficulty restoring opposition of the thumb if the nerve recovers or after a late transfer. Thus the assistance of a hand therapist is necessary for the prevention of this deformity.

Timing of reconstructive surgery

Early reconstructive surgery is indicated when the nerve lesion is proximal and recovery of distal motor function will be very delayed. Early surgery attempts to prevent deformity by providing an internal splint.

Simple stabilization of the MP joints in slight flexion is sufficient to ensure extension of the distal phalanges and prevent joint stiffness. This stabilization can be achieved by tenodeses, capsulodeses, or tendon transfers. In this situation procedures that do not require borrowing a tendon from the hand, tenodesis using a tendon graft (such as a Parkes tenodesis), or a capsuloraphy are preferable.

Surgical treatment

Many surgical procedures have been described for the treatment of ulnar nerve palsy. They seek to:

1. improve synchronous finger motion and correct clawing;
2. correct the claw deformity;
3. increase grip strength;
4. restore thumb adduction and thumb–index pinch;
5. in high level ulnar nerve lesion, to restore flexion of the distal phalanges of the ring and small fingers.

Correction of functional deficits resulting from intrinsic muscle paralysis of the fingers

Correction of the claw hand deformity can be achieved by any procedure preventing hyperextension of the MP joints using tenodesis, capsulodesis, or finger tendon transfers. However, only the addition of a tendon transfer from the wrist motor muscles or from a more proximal muscle can increase grip strength.

The following section describes tendon transfers, tenodesis, and capsulodeses used for the correction of the long finger disabilities.

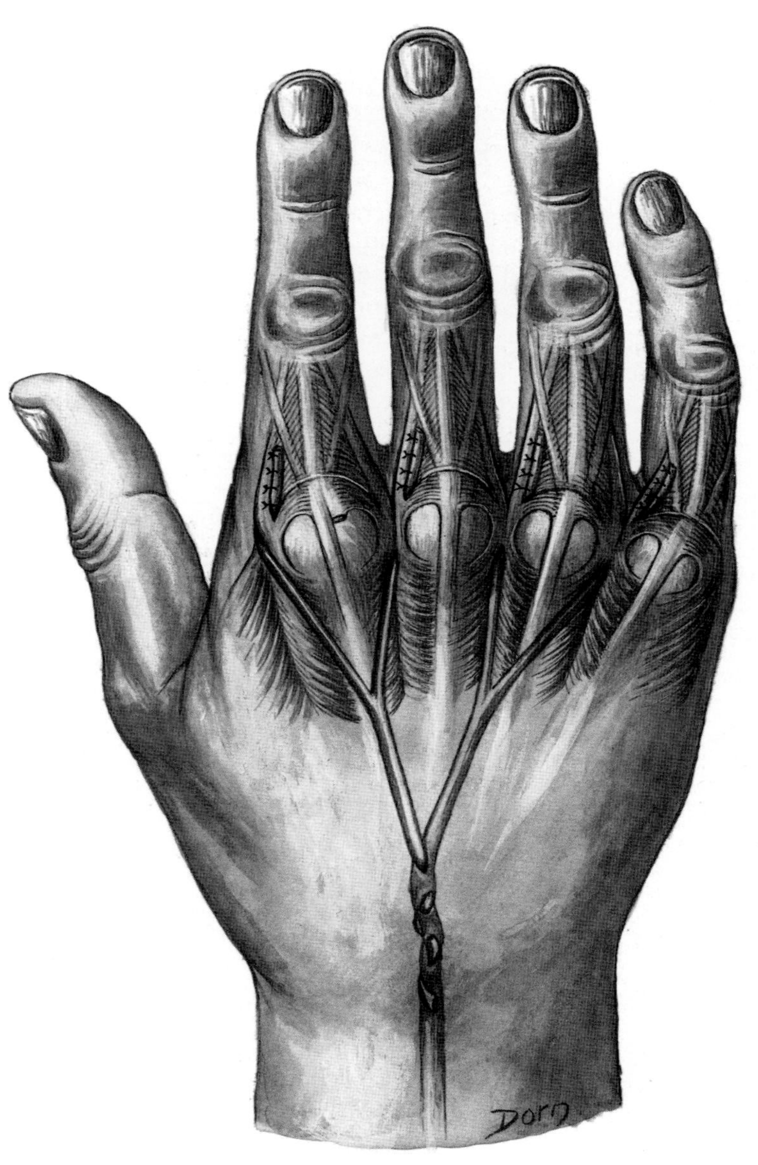

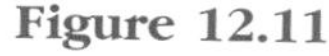

Figure 12.11

Transfer of the EIP, Riordan's modification of the Fowler procedure. The EIP tendon is transferred to the two ulnar fingers, passing dorsal to the wrist and palmar to the deep, transverse metacarpal ligament. A tendon graft is fixed to the transfer for the two radial fingers.

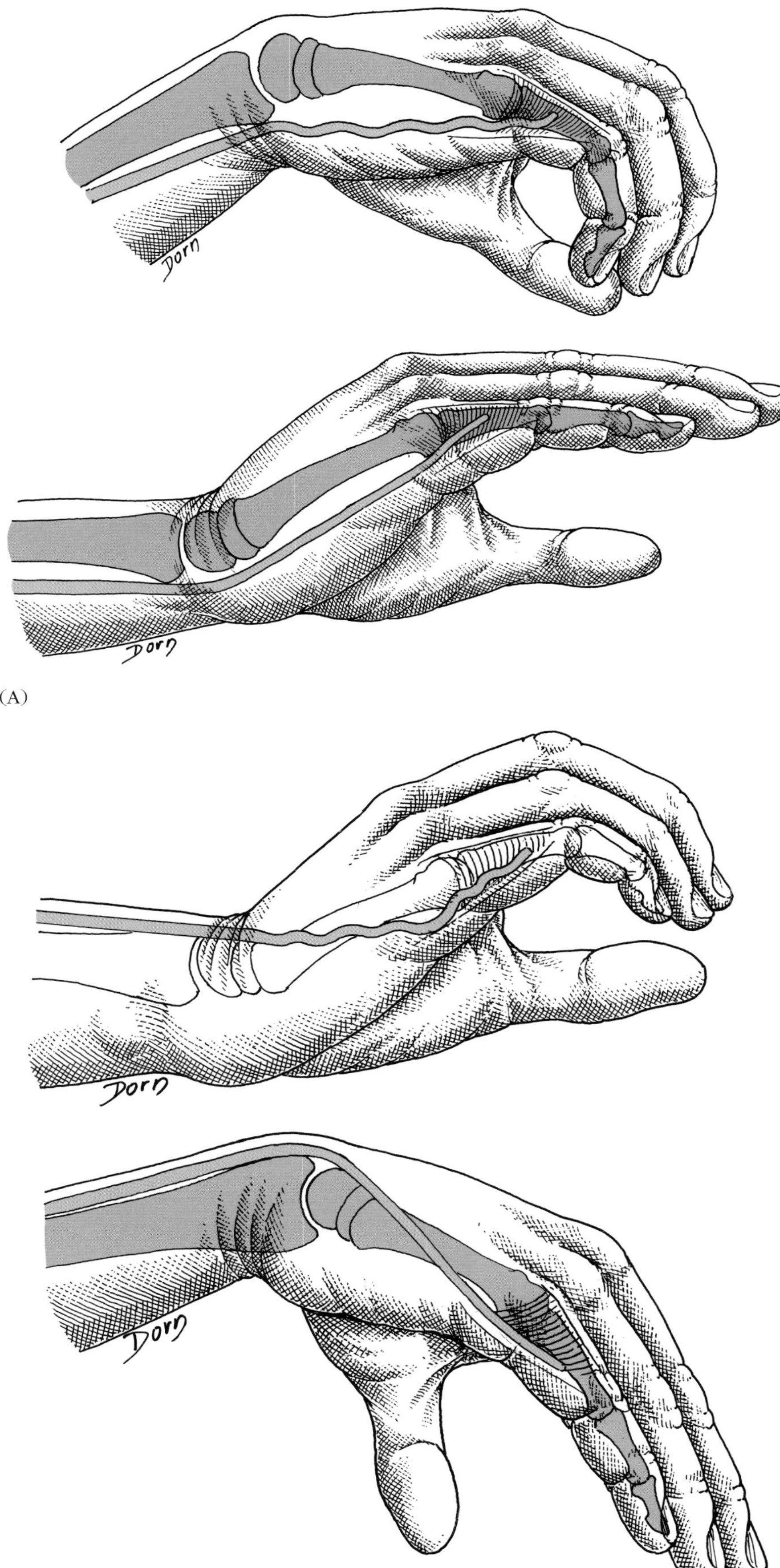

Figure 12.12

Path of the transfer at the wrist.

(A) A transfer volar to the wrist is tightened with wrist extension

(B) A transfer dorsal to the wrist is tightened with wrist flexion and becomes lax with extension of the wrist

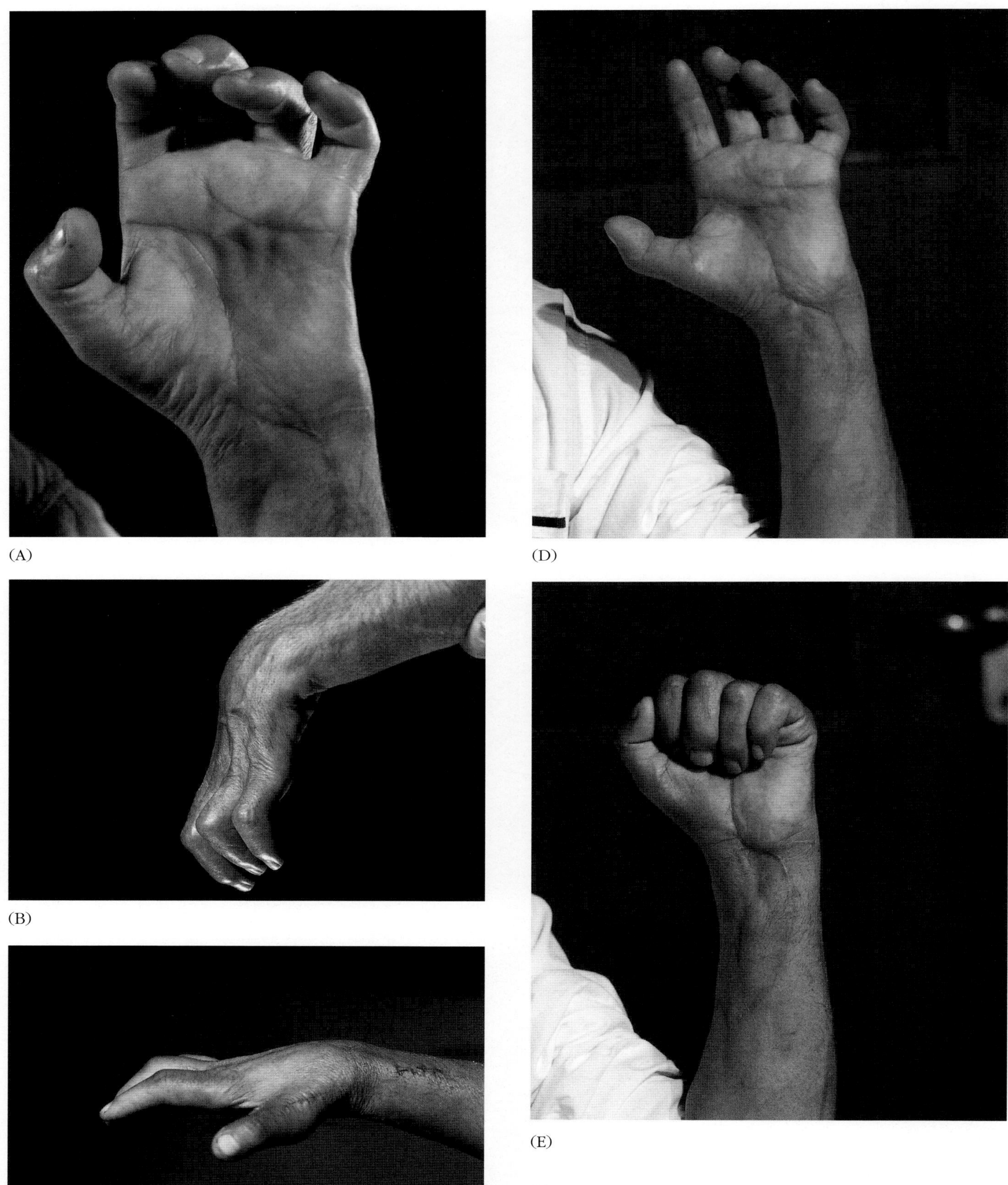

(A)

(D)

(B)

(E)

(c)

Figure 12.13

Severe long-standing median ulnar paralysis. The patient had acquired the habit of flexing the wrist. (A, B) Preoperative views. (C, D, E) Postoperative views after a wrist extensor transfer dorsal to the wrist.

Tendon transfers

Several techniques of tendon transfers are used. Factors to be considered for the transfer include the choice of the motor, the course of the transfer, and the site of insertion.

Choice of motor muscle

The strength of the motor should be adapted to the deficit. The more commonly performed procedures include transfer of a wrist motor and transfer of an extrinsic muscle of the fingers (flexor or extensor).

Only wrist motors will increase grip strength but they must be lengthened by tendon grafts – Brand (1961) uses the ECRL. We are reluctant to use the ECRB which is the main extensor of the wrist. Other authors, rather than weaken wrist extension, prefer to transfer a wrist flexor. Riordan (1953) suggested transferring the FCR. Even the slender palmaris longus has been used (Antia 1969, Palende 1976, Fritschi 1984), prolonged by grafts.

Flexor digitorum superficialis (FDS) transfers do not require lengthening by a graft, but their displacement results in a deficit in the power and independence of the donor finger. Nevertheless FDS transfer (Stiles–Bunnell), is still commonly used. However, rather than borrowing four superficialis tendons like Bunnell (1942), most surgeons now use only one flexor superficialis tendon, from either the index or middle finger, divided into bands and inserted on one side of each finger. Fowler (1949) described transfer of the extensor indicis proprius (EIP) and extensor digiti minimi (EDM), each divided into two terminal strips. It seems preferable, however, not to use the EDM, which is often the only active extensor of the little finger. Riordan (1953) transferred the EIP to the ring and little fingers and augmented this with a tendon graft whose distal extremity was split into two terminal strips, one for the index and one for the middle finger (Figure 12.11). The EIP is a very convenient transfer, its displacement causes insignificant deficit and it is the first choice for Zancolli (1979) for the correction of clawing on the two ulnar fingers.

In summary, there has been an increasing tendency to use a single motor for the correction of the clawing, whose transfer will cause minimal morbidity. However, it is sometimes necessary to increase grip strength in proximal level ulnar palsy or for persons with higher functional demands; in these situations a wrist motor is indicated.

Path of the transfer

According to Bunnell (1944), the transfer (or graft) should run along the lumbrical canal and pass volar to the deep transverse intermetacarpal ligament. The clinician should decide whether the transfer should pass volar or dorsal to the wrist. While a dorsal transfer becomes lax with extension of the wrist, a volar transfer may be expected to restore a more physiologic grip with the wrist extended (Figure 12.12). When the deformity is long-standing, the patient will have developed the habit of flexing the wrist to extend the fingers: this habit is very hard to discard. In these cases a dorsal approach is preferable (Figure 12.13).

Point of insertion

Side of insertion on the finger

Bunnell (1944) inserted the transfers to reproduce intrinsic-like action on both sides of each finger. Later authors advocated unilateral insertions.

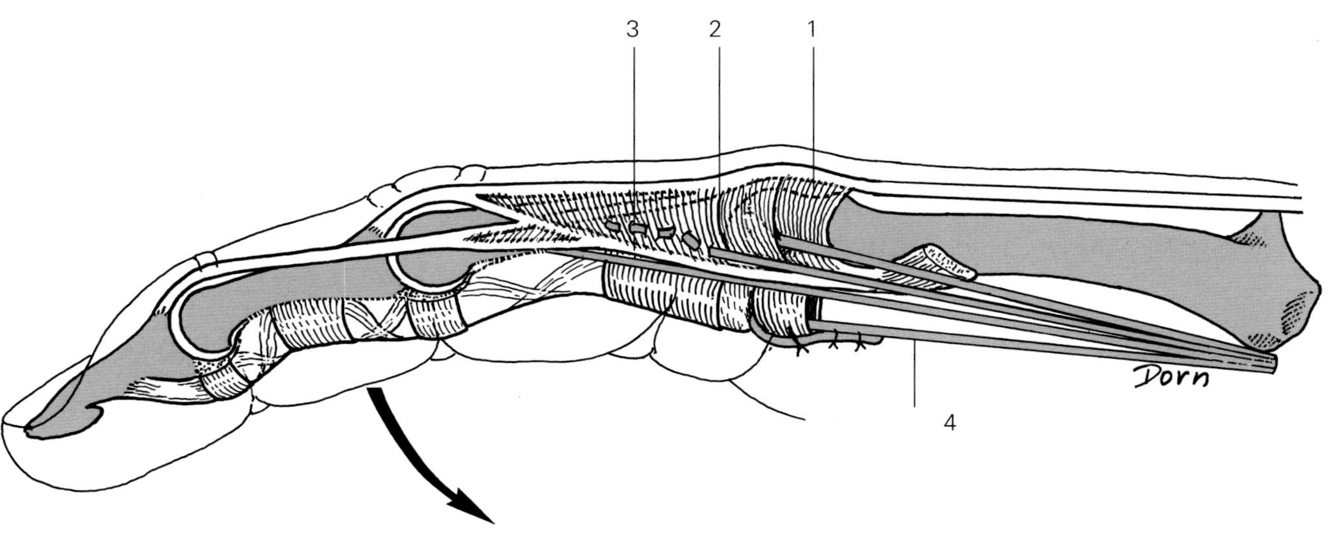

Figure 12.14

How far palmar to place the insertion. 1. On the interosseous tendon; 2. on the interosseous hood; 3. through the proximal phalanx; 4. on the flexor tendon sheath.

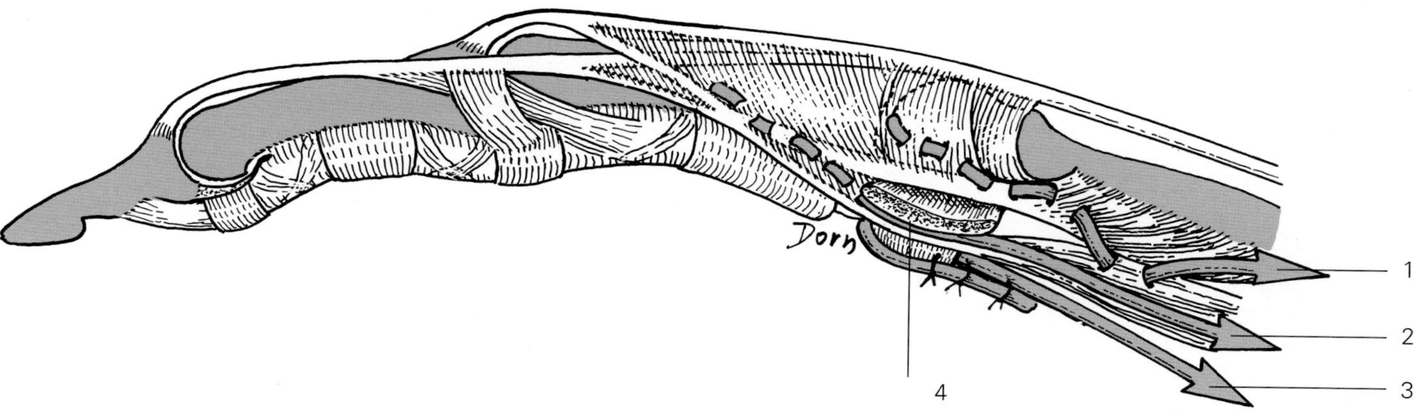

Figure 12.15

How far distal to place the insertion. 1. On the interosseous tendon; 2. on the interosseous hood; 3. on the flexor tendon sheath; 4. deep transverse intermetacarpal ligament.

Fowler (1949) at first inserted his transfers on the radial borders of the index and middle fingers, and the ulnar borders of the ring and little fingers, so as to obtain maximal spread of the fingers. However, it soon became obvious that ulnar deviation was best avoided by attaching all transfers on the radial side.

Brand (1970) still prefers an ulnar side insertion for the index finger to avoid separation of index and middle fingers, which allows small objects to slip through. He also believes that an ulnar insertion for the index facilitates its rotation in supination toward the thumb. Most authors still advocate a radial insertion for the index finger to restore the action of the first dorsal interosseous and to reinforce the resistance of the index finger against the pressure of the thumb.

How far palmar to place the insertion (Figure 12.14)
The more palmar the insertion of the transfer with regard to the axis of rotation of the MP joint the more marked will be the flexion of the joint. A transfer passing dorsal to the deep transverse MC ligament and fixed to the tendon of the interosseous muscle has a moment of flexion less than that of a transfer passed volar to the ligament and fixed to the interosseous hood, the proximal phalanx, or the flexor tendon sheath.

How far distal to place the insertion (Figure 12.15)
In Bunnell's technique, the transfer was inserted into the oblique fibers to the interosseous hood, the MP joint being kept in flexion and the IP joints in extension. The dangers of transforming the claw deformity into a swan neck by an overpowerful transfer are well known. These dangers are magnified if the flexor superficialis is sacrificed and the IP joints are lax. A distal insertion of the transfer into the interosseous aponeurosis is only useful if it is difficult to achieve active extension of the distal phalanges with the MP joints stabilized in slight flexion; an active transfer inserted into the dorsal apparatuses will then make up for insufficient central tendons. When stabilization of the MP joint in flexion allows the IP joints to extend, it is functionally more useful to reinforce proximal phalangeal flexion than distal phalangeal extension. The transfer will then be fixed more proximally to the interosseous tendon, into the proximal phalanx or in the fibrous flexor sheath.

How many fingers should be rebalanced?
Although clawing of the index and long fingers is usually absent in low ulnar nerve palsy, inclusion of all four fingers in the transfer is recommended for improved asynchronous finger motion and dexterity.

Surgical technique

It is not possible to mention the many tendon transfer procedures devised for the treatment of intrinsic muscle paralysis. Three procedures using different motor transfers will be described:

- transfer of a wrist motor,
- transfer of an FDS,
- transfer of the EIP.

Transfer of the extensor carpi radialis longus (ECRL)
Brand (1958) started by transferring the ECRL, prolonged by four dorsal tendon grafts fixed on the interosseous hood. Later (Brand 1975) the wrist extensor and the grafts were passed through the carpal tunnel (Figure 12.16).

Four slips of tendon graft are required to prolong the ECAL for insertion into the proximal phalanges. The plantaris tendons graft is usually long enough to be fixed to the ECRL in its centre, each extremity is divided into two slips (Figure 12.17). The plantaris graft is harvested through limited incisions using a tendon-stripping instrument. The long toe extensors may be used if the plantaris tendons are absent or of insufficient size.

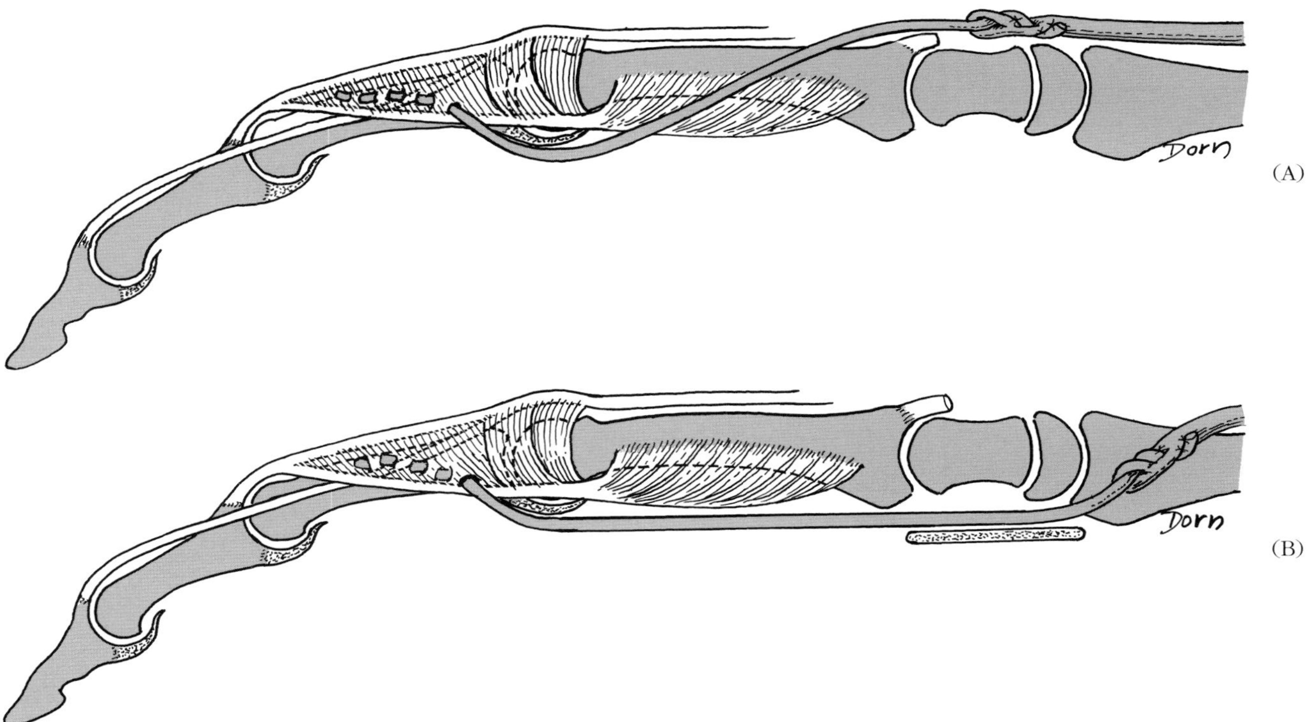

Figure 12.16

Brand's procedure. Transfer of an ECR prolonged by a tendon graft. The ECRL or the ECRB can be used. It seems preferable to avoid transferring the ECRB, which is the more efficient extensor of the wrist, but if it is necessary, it must be left within the second dorsal compartment. (A) The transfer is dorsal to the wrist; (B) the transfer is passed through the carpal tunnel.

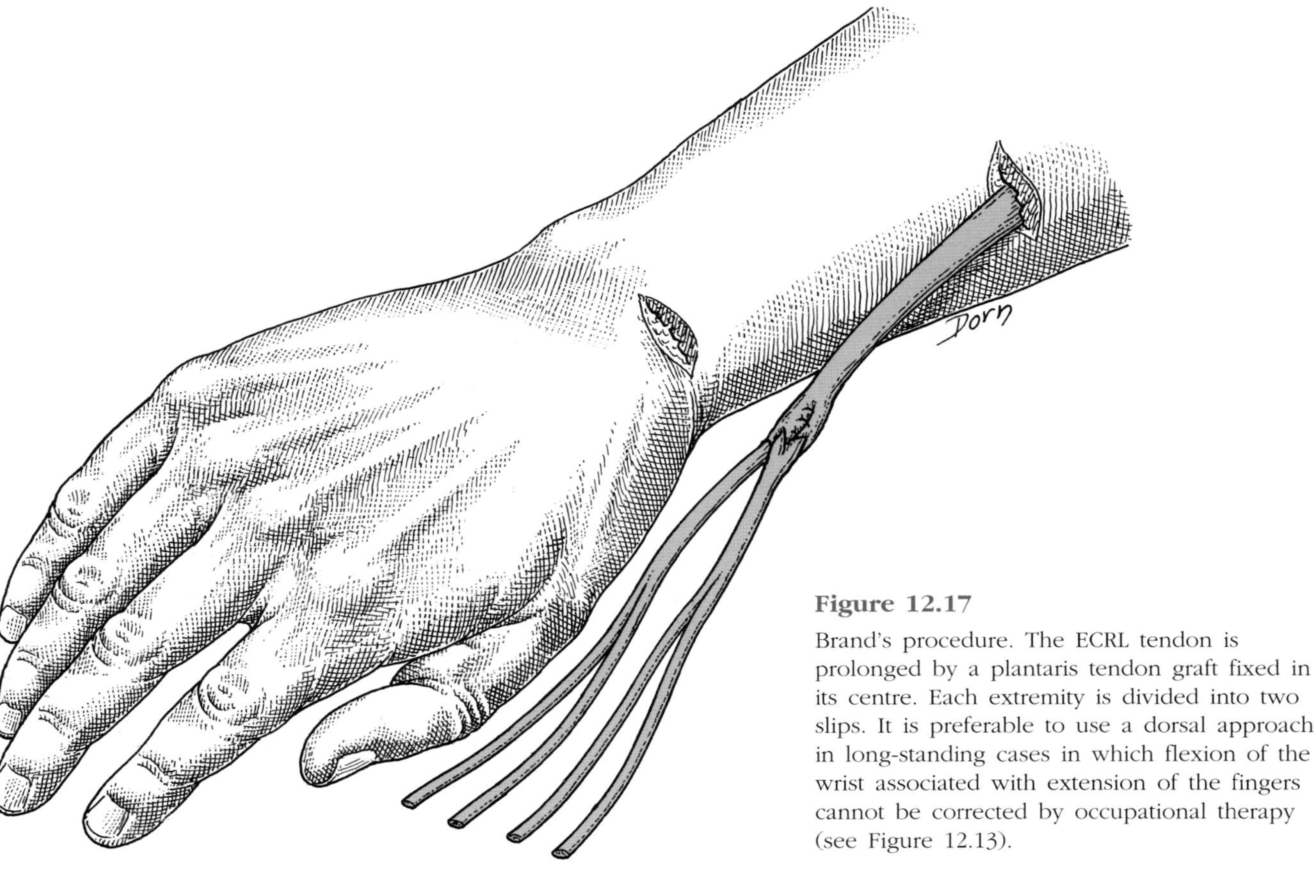

Figure 12.17

Brand's procedure. The ECRL tendon is prolonged by a plantaris tendon graft fixed in its centre. Each extremity is divided into two slips. It is preferable to use a dorsal approach in long-standing cases in which flexion of the wrist associated with extension of the fingers cannot be corrected by occupational therapy (see Figure 12.13).

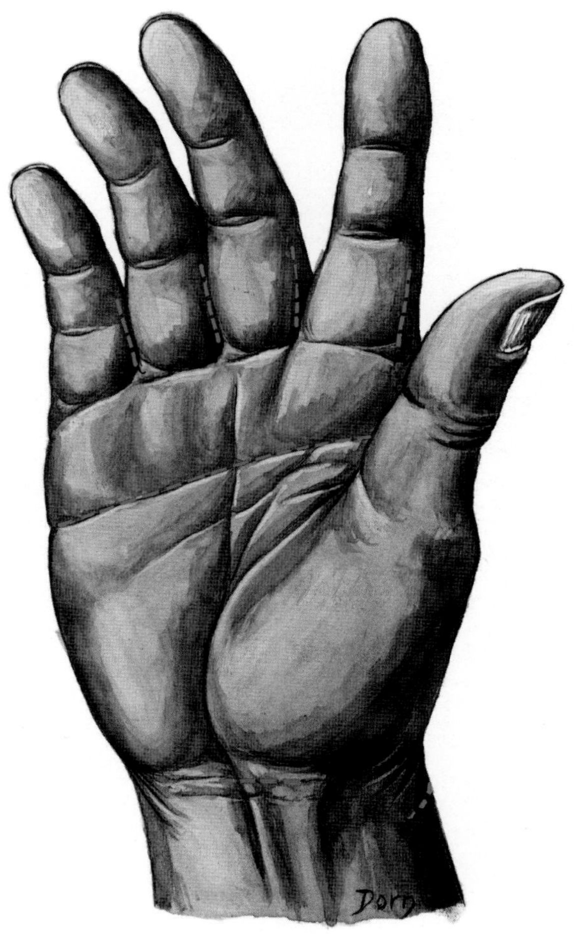

Figure 12.18

Incision needed for a Brand palmar approach. Most authors attach all transfers on the radial side of the fingers. However, Brand prefers an ulnar side insertion for the index finger, which facilitates its rotation in supination toward the thumb.

The division of terminal slips must be in the proximal palm, so that their course is not interrupted by the vertical septa of the palmar aponeurosis. A palmar incision is used to provide good exposure (Figure 12.18).

The superficial palmar aponeurosis is divided. Short lateral incisions are made on the base of the fingers. A curved tendon passer is placed through the lumbrical canal from distal to proximal to help deliver the transfer to the proximal phalanx of each finger. The slips are pulled together so that their progression is symmetrical and none regresses as its neighbor is pulled distally. Such a regression indicates that an obstacle is impeding the tendon's progression or that the division of the tendon into slips is not proximal enough.

Some surgeons (Burkhalter 1976) prefer a bone distal insertion of the grafts rather than in the extensor aponeurosis. The lateral extensor bands are identified and retracted dorsally, exposing the proximal phalanges. A 2.0-mm transverse drill hole is made through each proximal phalanx at a point in the mid-axis corresponding to the second annular pulley. The near cortices are enlarged to accommodate insertion of the tendon grafts. The tendons are seated securely by passing the attached sutures through the bone tunnels with Keith needles. Correct tensioning is achieved with the wrist held in full extension and the finger MP joints in maximum flexion. The wrist is immobilized postoperatively in slight extension, with the MP joints flexed 60° and the IP joints extended.

The FCR can be substituted if the ECRL is required for another procedure.

Transfer of the FDS

In Bunnell's procedure (1942) all four FDS tendons were transferred. Borrowing all the superficialis not only is wasteful but inevitably influences the movements and grip strength of the fingers. As a result, several authors such as Littler (1949) and Goldner (1974), suggested alternative methods whereby only one or two superficialis flexor tendons were taken, divided into bands, and inserted on one side only (usually the radial) of each finger (Figure 12.19).

Zancolli (1974) described an ingenious technique called 'the lasso'. He uses a superficial flexor tendon. The tendon is harvested through a hole made in the tendon sheath at a level proximal to the PIP joint, care being taken to be proximal to the chiasma (Figure 12.15). One band of insertion of the FS is cut, and tension is applied, delivering the second band into the hole in the tendon sheath, which is cut in turn. The two bands are pulled into the palm. Each one is divided into two slips, each sutured to itself after a loop (lasso) has been made around the proximal A_1 pulley (Figure 12.20). Thus, it becomes a flexor of the proximal phalanx and stabilizer of the MP joint during extension of the finger.

The tension placed on the transfer depends on the laxity of the finger joints, because even a lasso procedure can cause a swan neck deformity if there is too much tension on a flexed MP joint or if the PIP joints are too lax, although it has no direct insertion on the extension aponeurosis. Zancolli recommended fixation of the lasso with the MP joints extended and maximum tension on the transfer.

The loop is sutured back to itself by three sutures, with the most distal suture on the proximal border of the A1 pulley (Figure 12.21).

Transfer of the EIP

The EIP tendon is slightly short. To avoid a suture under tension, Zancolli (1987) passed the tendon through the interosseous membrane of the forearm distal to the pronator quadratus, and then through the carpal tunnel. It is split and the two slips are fixed with the lasso technique (Figure 12.22).

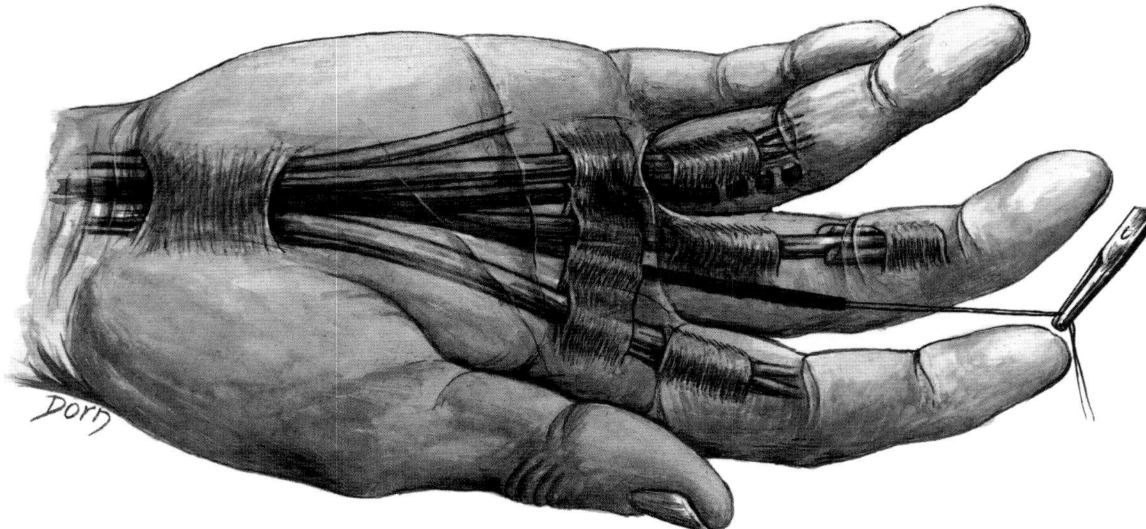

Figure 12.19

Bunnell's procedure. One or two FDS tendons are divided into bands. Each band is passed through the lumbrical canal under the intermetacarpal ligament and is fixed dorsally on the interosseous hood.

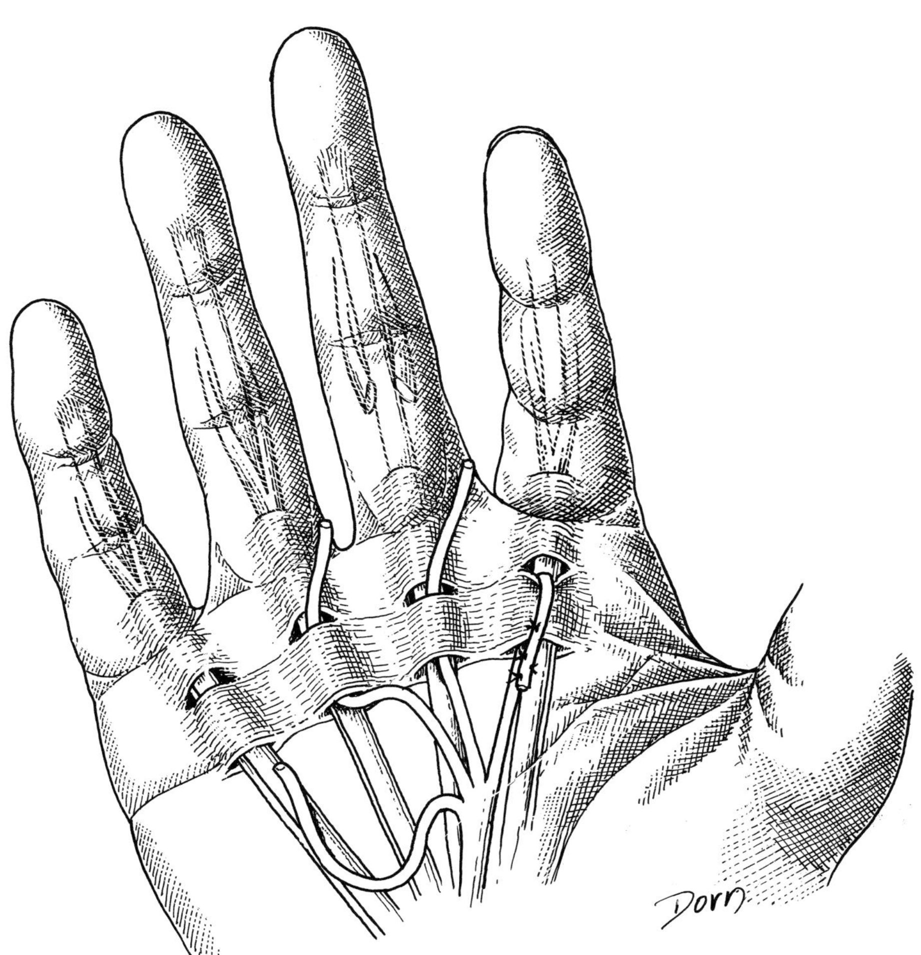

Figure 12.20

Zancolli's lasso procedure.

The FS tendon of the long finger is harvested proximal to its chiasma. It is divided into four bands. Each band is inserted at the base of each respective finger using the lasso procedure around the A_1 pulley of the flexor tendon sheath.

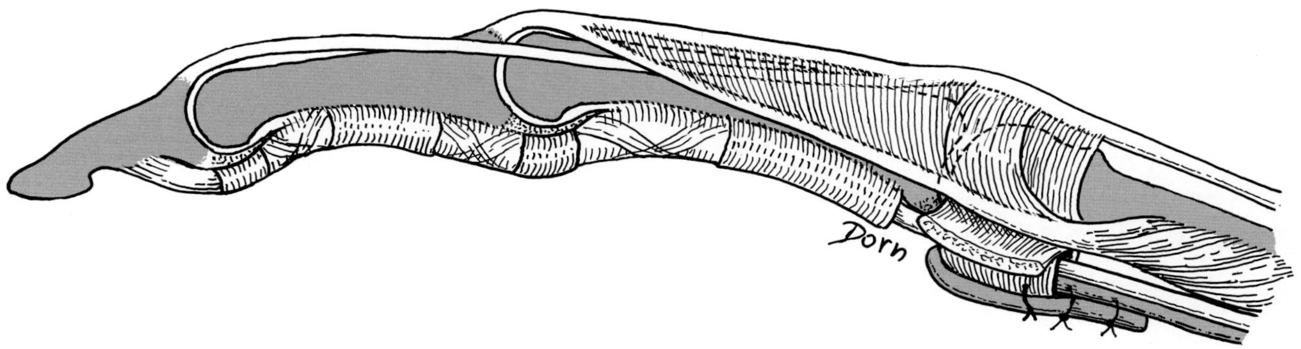

Figure 12.21

Zancolli's lasso procedure. The most distal suture on the loop around the A_1 pulley is fixed on the proximal border of the pulley.

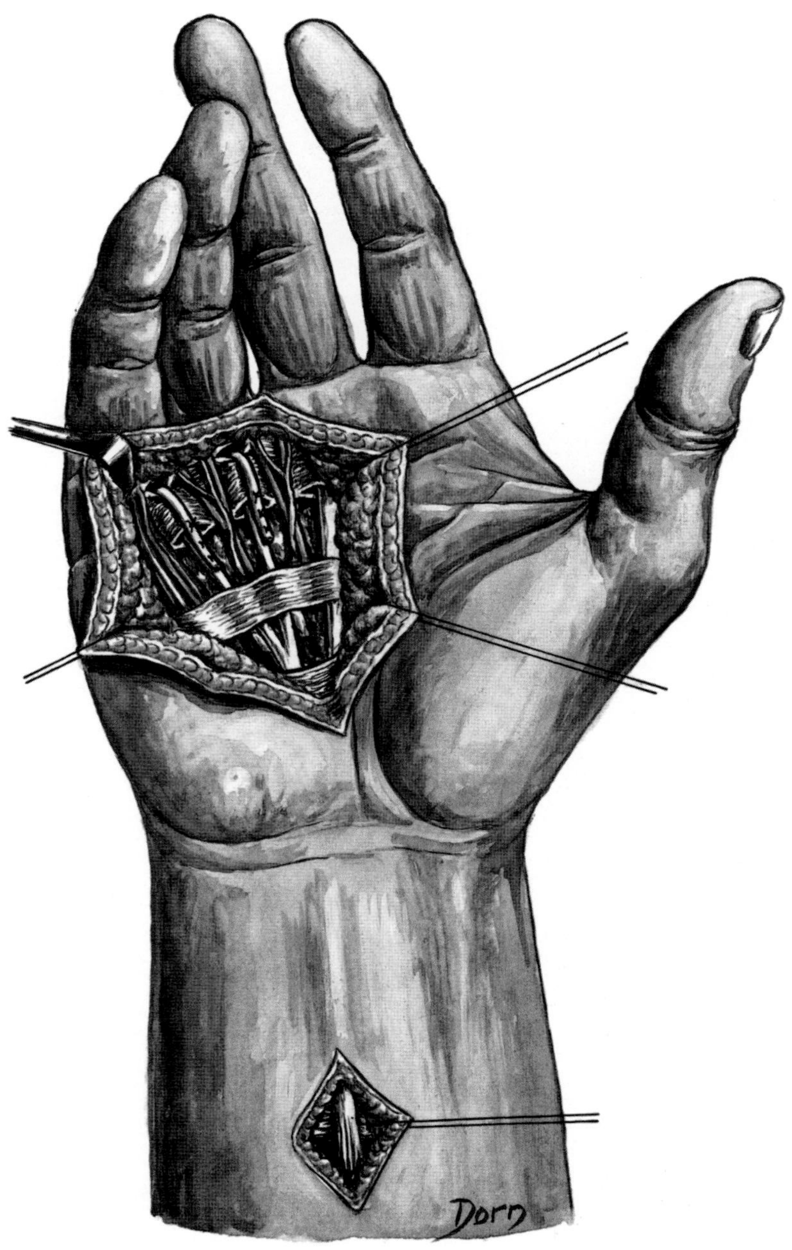

Figure 12.22

Zancolli's transfer of the EIP. The EIP tendon is passed through the interosseous membrane of the forearm and through the carpal tunnel. It is split and the two slips are fixed with the lasso technique.

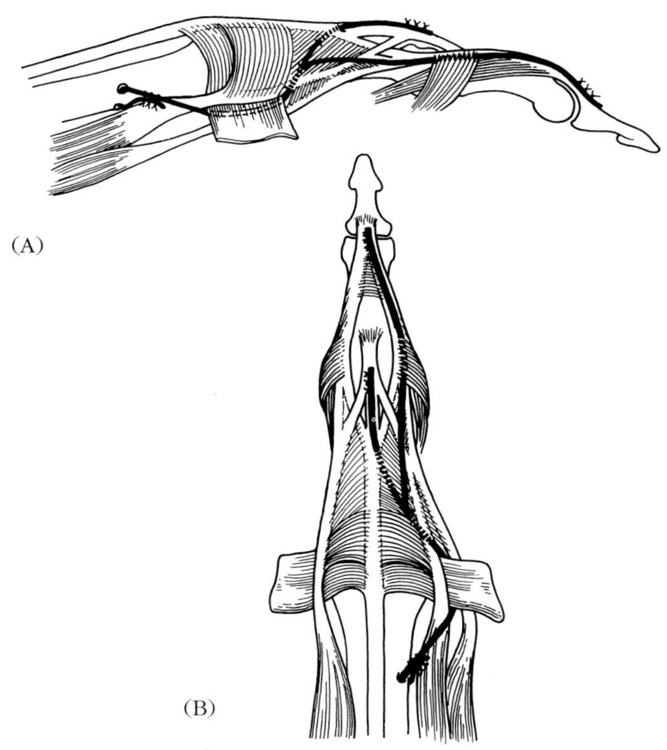

Figure 12.23
Dynamic tenodesis of the intrinsic muscles.
(A) Tendon graft fixed at one end of the metacarpal is passed volar to the deep transverse metacarpal ligament
(B) It is split into two strips and each is sutured on the dorsal aspect of the bases of the middle and of the distal phalanges. They are activated by the long extensors and flexors

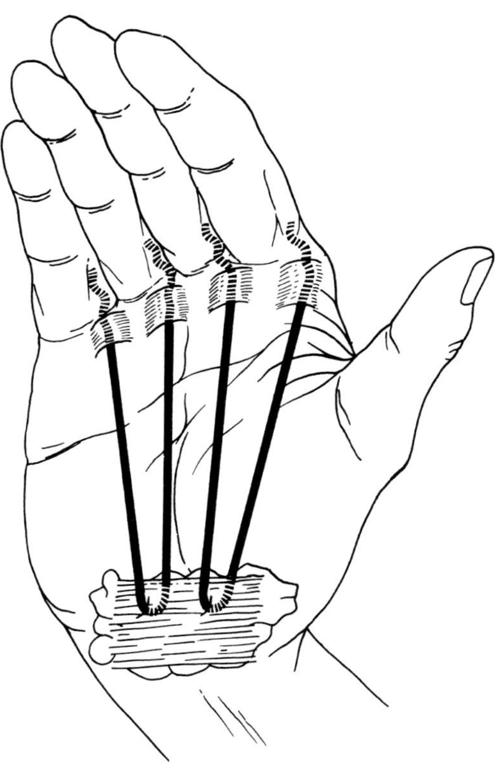

Figure 12.24
Parkes' tenodesis. A tendon graft is fixed proximally in the wrist flexor retinaculum, passed through the lumbrical canal and fixed distally to the interosseous hood.

Postoperative care

When the transfer is fixed on the extensor aponeurosis, the immobilization includes the wrist in slight extension, the MP joints in flexion, and the interphalangeal joints in extension. After 2 weeks the IP joints are mobilized while the MP joints remain in flexion for a further 2 weeks.

The category of transfers which aim only at active flexion of the MP joints without direct extension of the IP joints allows early mobilization of the IP joints. It is sufficient to maintain immobilization of the MP joints in 30° of flexion for 1 month.

Tenodeses

These procedures aim only at preventing hyperextension of the MP joints, thus allowing the long extensors to extend the distal phalanges. Many techniques of tenodesis have been described for the treatment of paralysis of the intrinsic muscles of the fingers. When the tendon fixed at its two extremities crosses one joint, it simply limits that joint's range of motion. When it crosses two joints, it can transmit the movement of one joint to that of the other joint; it becomes a 'dynamic tenodesis' (Figure 12.23).

All the tenodesis procedures used for correction of the claw hand cannot be described here. The simplest involves a tendon graft fixed to the metacarpal, passed through the lumbrical canal in front of the deep transverse metacarpal ligament and then fixed to the interosseous hood (Zancolli 1957).

A modification of this procedure used on leprous patients fixes the graft proximally to the extensor tendon itself (Schinivasan 1977).

In Parkes' tenodesis (1973), a plantaris tendon graft is passed through the lumbrical canal. It is fixed distally to the interosseous hood and proximally in the flexor retinaculum (Figure 12.24); its tension maintains graduated MP flexion between 45° in the little finger and 30°

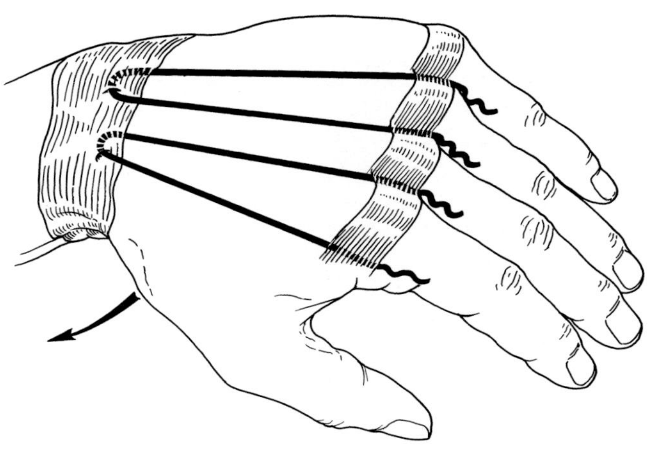

Figure 12.25

Fowler's tenodesis. The graft is fixed proximally in the wrist dorsal retinaculum, passed through the lumbrical canal and fixed distally to the interosseous hood.

for the index finger with IP joints in extension. These grafts are activated by the extrinsic muscles of the fingers.

If the proximal end of the tenodesis is attached above the wrist, movements of the wrist may result in activation of the tenodesis. For example, in Fowler's technique (Fowler 1949, Enna and Riordan 1973) a graft is fixed to the extensor retinaculum (Figure 12.25) or in Tsuge's technique (1967) the transfer is the tendon of the brachioradialis split into four strips, each of which is fixed in the interosseous hood (Figure 12.26).

Capsulodesis

Zancolli (1957) advocated the use of capsulodeses to prevent MP joint hyperextension. A transverse incision in the distal palmar crease provides access to the MP joints. The radial side of the A1 pulley is opened and the flexor tendons are retracted laterally (Figure 12.27).

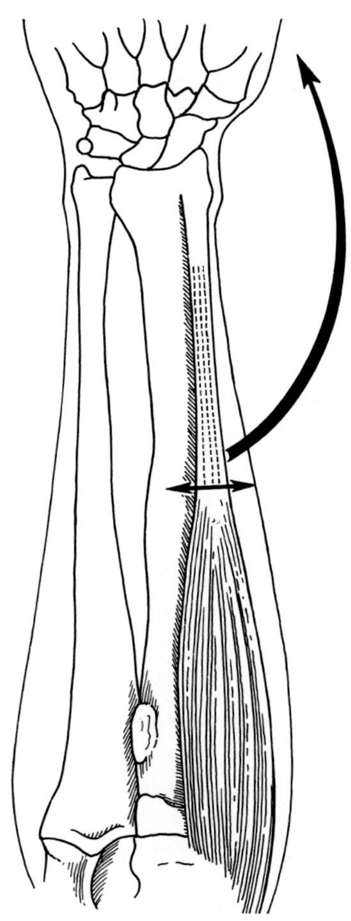

(A)

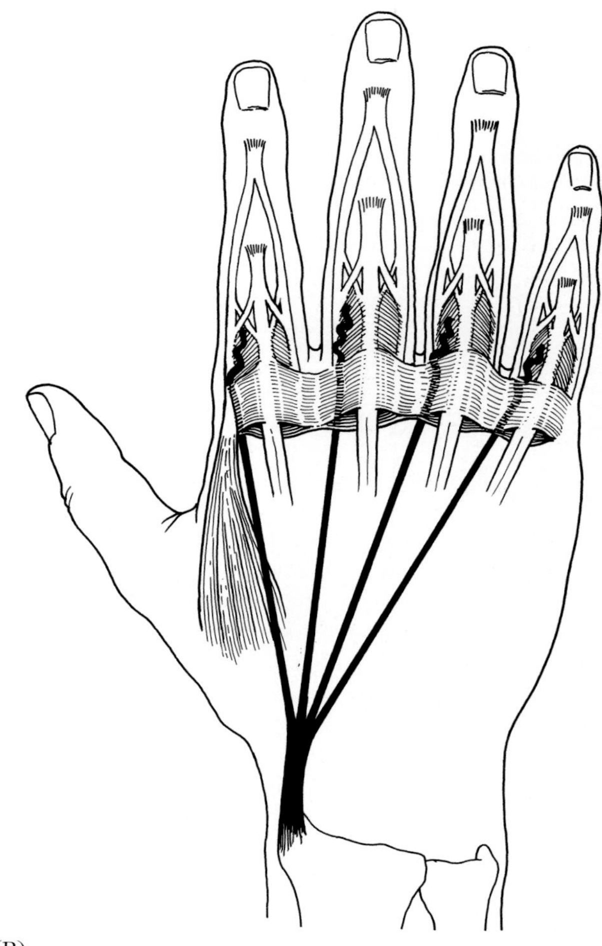

(B)

Figure 12.26

Tsuge's tenodesis. (A) The brachioradialis tendon is divided and reflected. (B) The tendon is split into four strips, each of which is passed through the lumbrical canal and fixed in the interosseous hood.

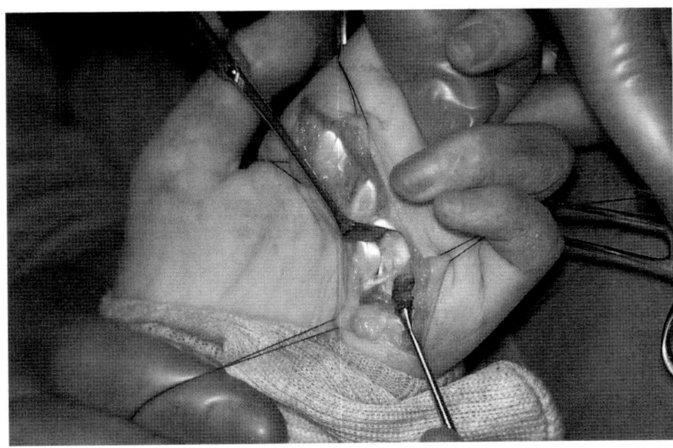

Figure 12.27
Capsulodesis. The flexor tendons are retracted laterally.

Zancolli makes a longitudinal division in the volar plate and advances the two sides to be sutured through drill holes in the metacarpal neck, creating slight MP flexion (between 15 and 30°) (Figure 12.28). The MP joints are immobilized in flexion for a month, while the IP joints are left free.

Fixation to bone introduces a degree of technical difficulty but appears to strengthen the capsulodesis (Figure 12.29).

Bourrel (1986) has devised an H-shaped capsular incision to simplify the procedure for 'surgery en masse' in leprosy. This defines two capsular flaps, one based proximally and the other distally. A transverse resection of 6 mm from one or the other of the H flaps is made as required and the edges are approximated.

One of the advantages of capsulodeses is that they do not necessitate the plundering of an already handicapped hand for tendon grafts. Also, they can correct the claw deformity whatever the position of the wrist, and they can be redone in cases of failure.

In fact, to approach the volar aspect of the MP joints in capsulodesis procedures, one must retract the flexor tendons and divide the A1 pulley. This in itself constitutes a pulley advancement as advocated by Bunnell (1944) (Figure 12.30). The effect of this advancement is to increase flexion of the MP joint. By thus altering the points of application of the flexion forces, some improvement in the sequence of phalangeal flexion is obtained. The disadvantage of pulley advancement is that it favors ulnar drift of the fingers.

Indications

Treatment of intrinsic muscle paralysis of the long fingers

Surgical indications are governed by the claw deformity and the severity of the functional problems. It must be

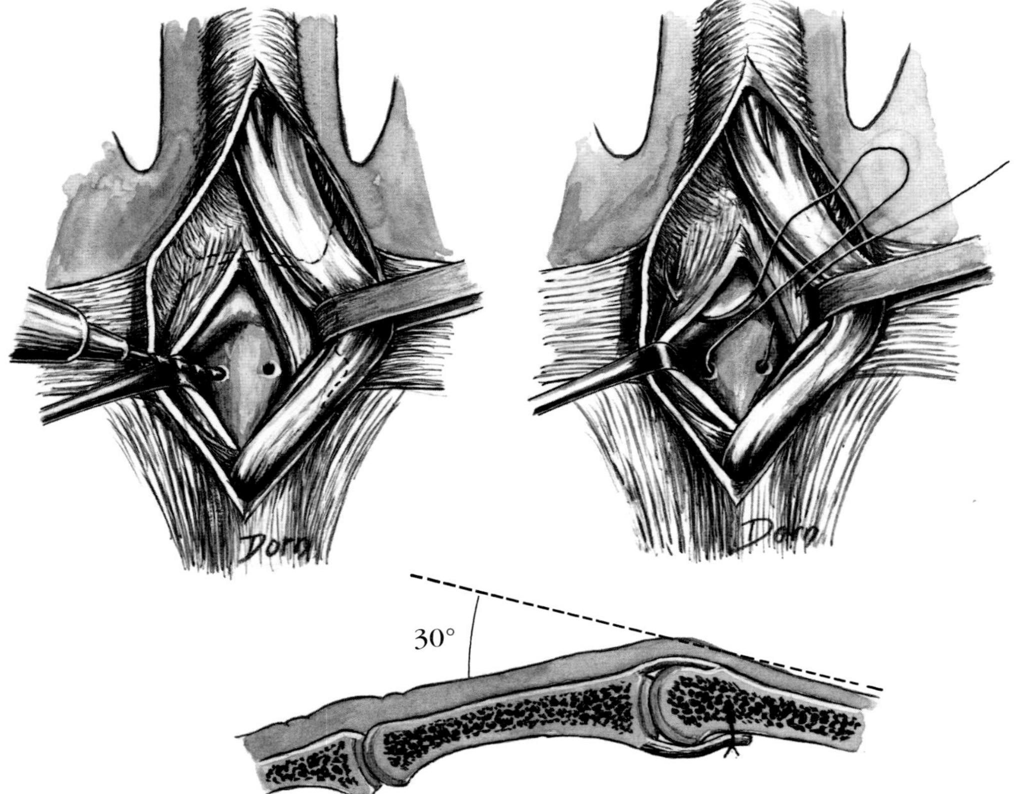

Figure 12.28
Capsulodesis. Zancolli's procedure of transosseous fixation.

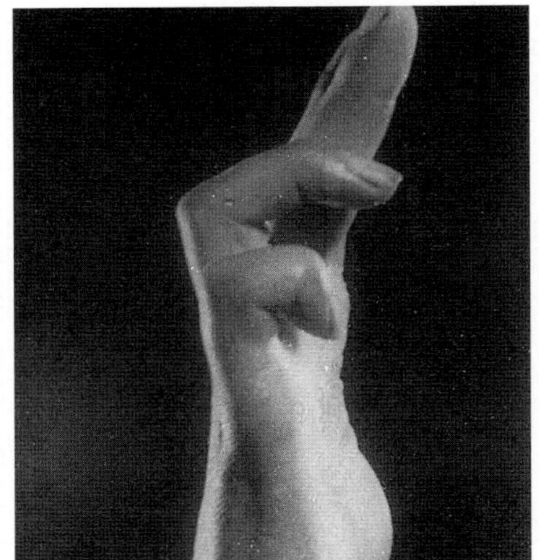

(A)

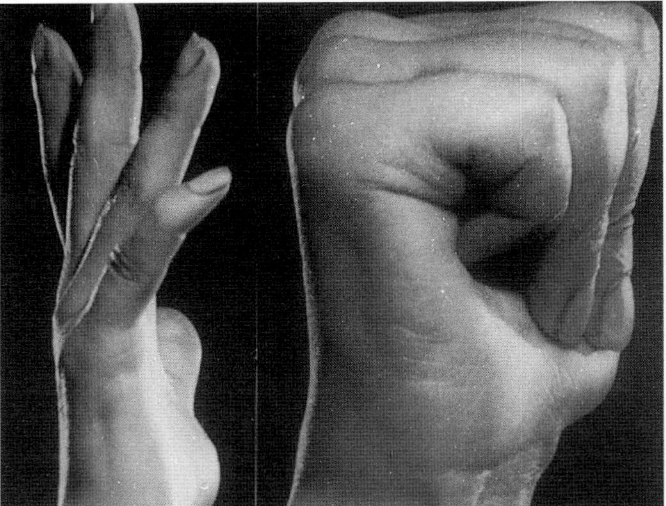

(B)

Figure 12.29
Capsulodesis. Clinical example. (A) Ulnar paralysis; (B) treated by capsulodesis; postoperative result.

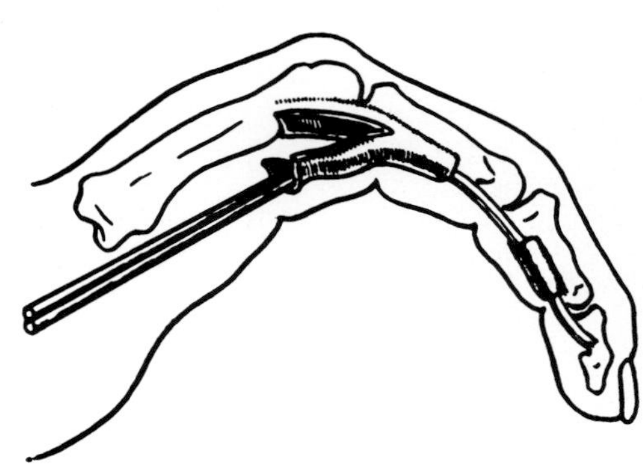

Figure 12.30
Pulley advancement.

determined whether the claw can be actively corrected by Bouvier's test (Figure 12.31), and if not whether passive correction is possible.

Functional problems alone may justify surgery. An abnormal flexion sequence, beginning distally, is often a greater problem than the claw. The weakness of grip is determined by the level and extent of the paralysis. It is important to increase the strength of finger flexion when paralysis of the long flexors is added to paralysis of the intrinsics.

When the claw is actively correctable

In these cases, MP hyperextension can be prevented by tendon transfer, tenodesis, or capsulodesis. All these methods can correct the deformity.

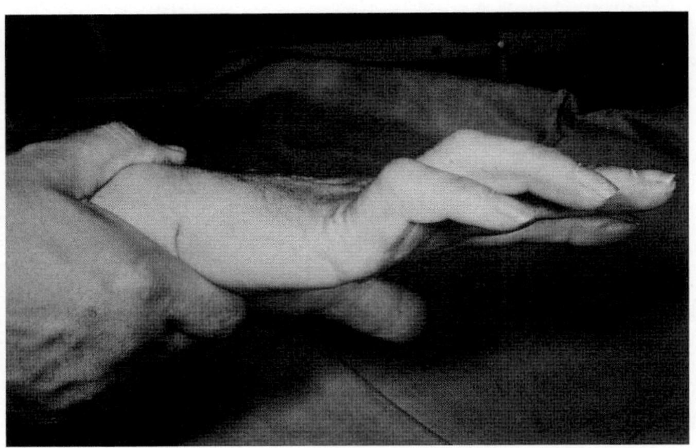

(A)

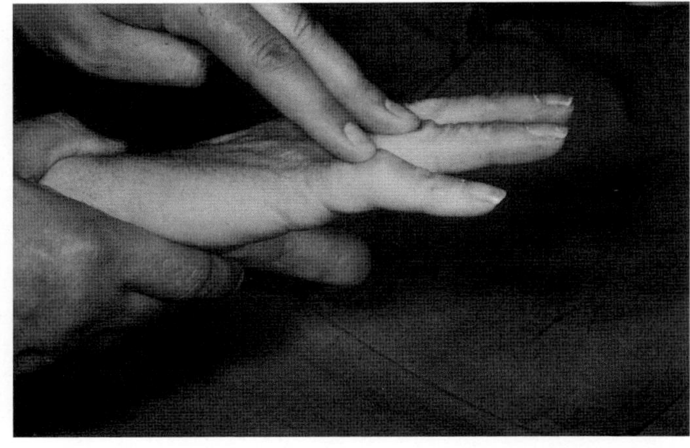

(B)

Figure 12.31
Bouvier's test. (A) Claw hand; (B) correction of MP joints hyperextension. The claw is reducible.

Passive techniques have essentially only one effect, i.e. correction of the deformity. Their use should be limited to the following conditions:

- When transfers are not available, because of extensive paralysis.
- When there is a possibility of intrinsic muscle recovery after long delays.
- When conditions for surgery are unfavorable.

These easy procedures allow surgery 'en masse' in developing countries.

Tendon transfers in all other conditions

Their choice is influenced by the age and expectations of the patient, the level and extent of paralysis, and also eventually on associated lesions (such as injury to the volar wrist structure), on the laxity of finger joints, and on the particular needs of each patient. The clinician must distinguish between distal paralysis, in which FDP strength is maintained, and proximal paralysis, in which the FDP is lost. It is important to remember that superficialis tendons from the ring and little fingers cannot be used in high ulnar palsy, because this would deprive these digits of an active flexor.

Use of a finger flexor for transfer simply redistributes balance within the hand but diminishes grip strength if it is inserted into the interosseous hood. Transfer of a wrist flexor or extensor muscle–tendon unit will enhance grip strength and is preferable in proximal paralysis and even in distal paralysis for young patients with high functional demands. For other cases, a weak transfer such as that of the EIP (or even the PL (Antia 1969)) will sufficiently stabilize the MP joint, correct the claw, and restore physiologic flexion of the finger.

It must be remembered that restoration of thumb strength and reinforcement of the thumb–index lateral pinch will also require another transfer.

When the claw is not actively correctable (Figure 12.32)

In this case, passive procedures that aim to prevent hyperextension of the MP joint are not adequate. The clinician should look for the cause of this problem and try to correct it.

When passive motion of the three finger joints is conserved, a deficit of the extension of the distal phalanges (despite the maintenance of the MP joints in flexion), in most cases indicates a lesion of the extensor apparatus. An extension deficit greater than 30° is an indication for a transfer fixed on the interosseous to provide distal extension. In long-standing flexion deformity of the PIP joint, the extensor apparatus distends and the lateral extensor tendons sublux to either side of the joint, resulting in a boutonnière deformity. The boutonnière may be corrected by a trident graft, which reinforces the central extensor tendon and corrects the palmar subluxation of the lateral extensor tendons (Figure 12.33).

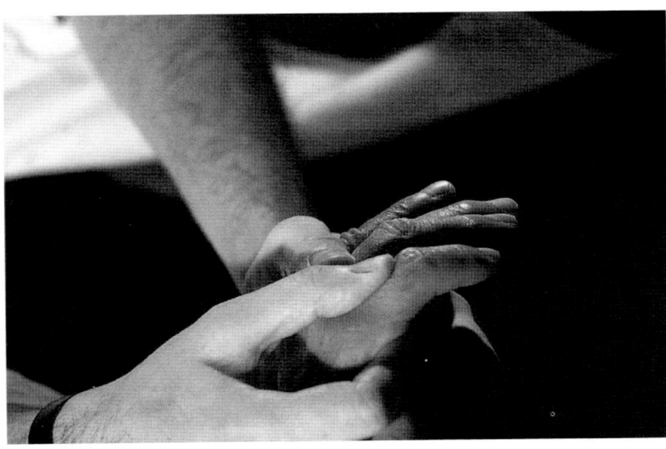

Figure 12.32
The claw is not actively correctable.

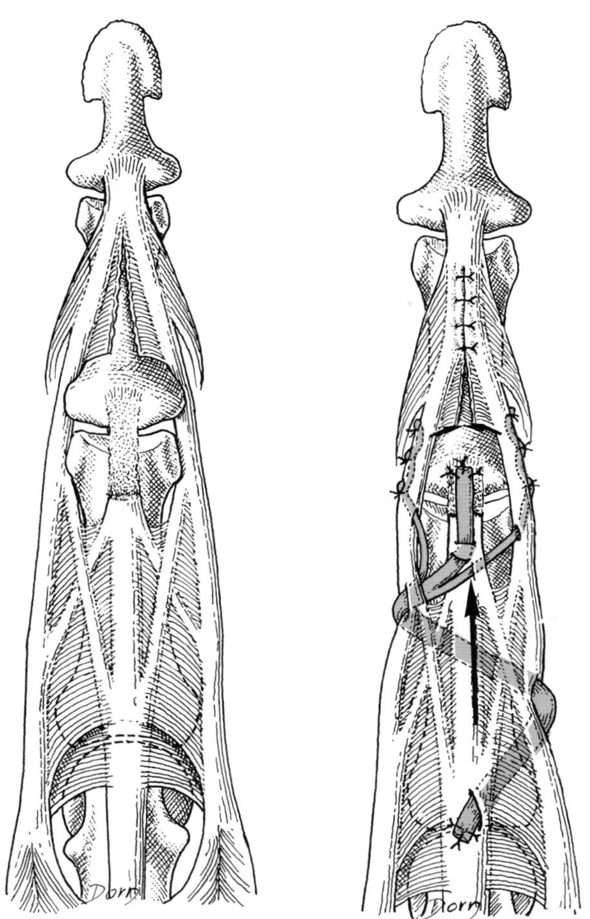

Figure 12.33
The trident graft (Tubiana 1968). A tendon graft is fixed proximally on the EDC at the MP joint level, then through the lateral extensor tendons; the graft is then divided into three strips. The central strip is fixed to the central extensor tendon at the base of the middle phalanx, the two remaining strips are fixed to the lateral extensor tendons and correct their palmar subluxation.

A number of other factors can prevent active correction of the claw deformity: skin contracture, flexor or extensor tendon adhesions, and articular stiffness. These should be analysed and treated before any transfer (Figures 12.34 and 12.35).

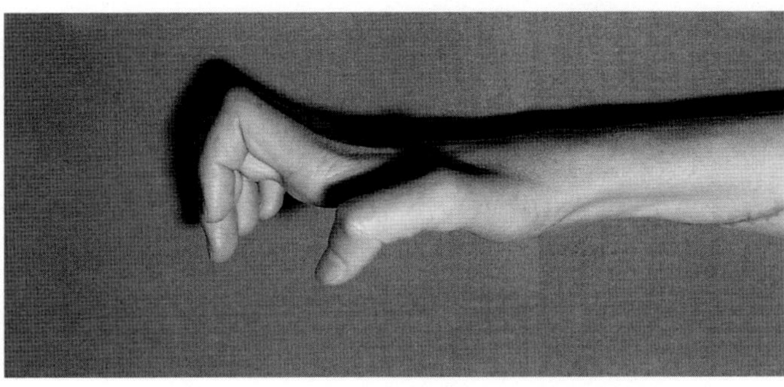

(A)

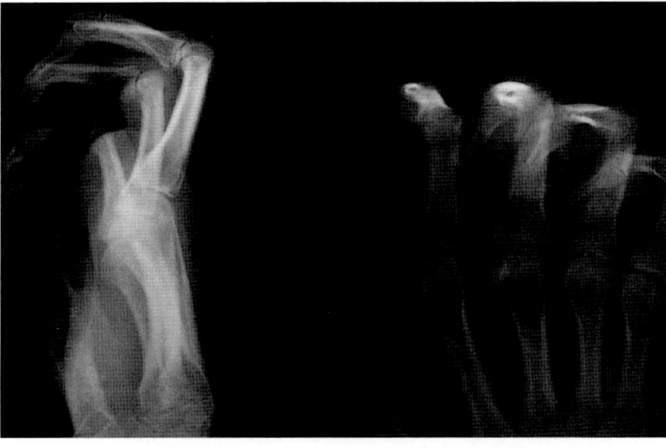

(B)

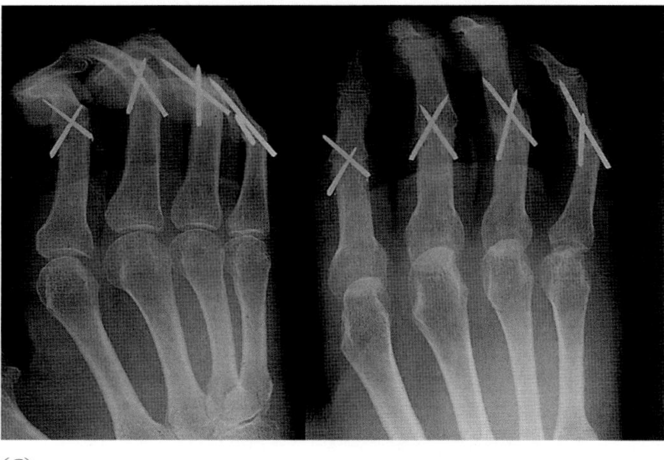

(C)

Figure 12.34

(A) and (B) Claw hand with marked stiffness of the PIP joints. (C) Arthrodesis of the PIP joints in functional position.

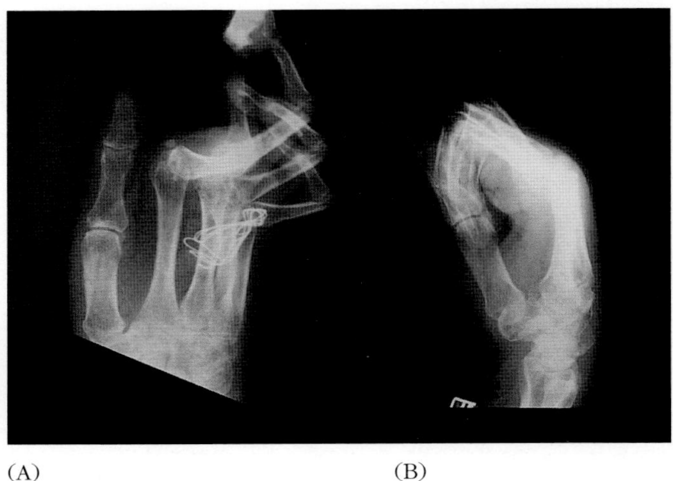

(A) (B)

Figure 12.35

(A) Fixed claw deformity, the MP joints in hyperextension and PIP joints in flexion. (B) MP arthroplasty associated with FDS transfer, PIP joint arthrodeses will be done at a second stage.

Restoration of thumb pinch

The thumb pinch is always seriously weakened by AP paralysis. When a paralysis of the FPB is added, stability of the MP joint is lost, the MP joint is hyperextended, and flexion of the distal phalanx is accentuated. If the lumbrical muscles of the index and long fingers are also paralysed in a median ulnar paralysis, both the index and thumb column are destabilized (Figure 12.36).

Many procedures have been described to restore thumb adduction, most of them do not restore the strength of the thumb lateral pinch, which necessitates a strong adduction of the thumb and an active resistance of the index finger.

Thumb adductorplasty

Choice of motor muscle

The EIP, an FDS, or the ECRL can be used. The EIP and a FDS are long enough; however, the ECRL requires lengthening by a graft. We are reluctant to use the ECRB, the main extensor of the wrist, although it has been used by several authors with good results on the thumb pinch strength (Smith 1983, Jebson and Steyers 1996, Kalainov 2002).

Of course, the choice of the motor for thumb adductor plasty is influenced by the technique used for the correction of the intrinsic muscle paralysis of the long fingers.

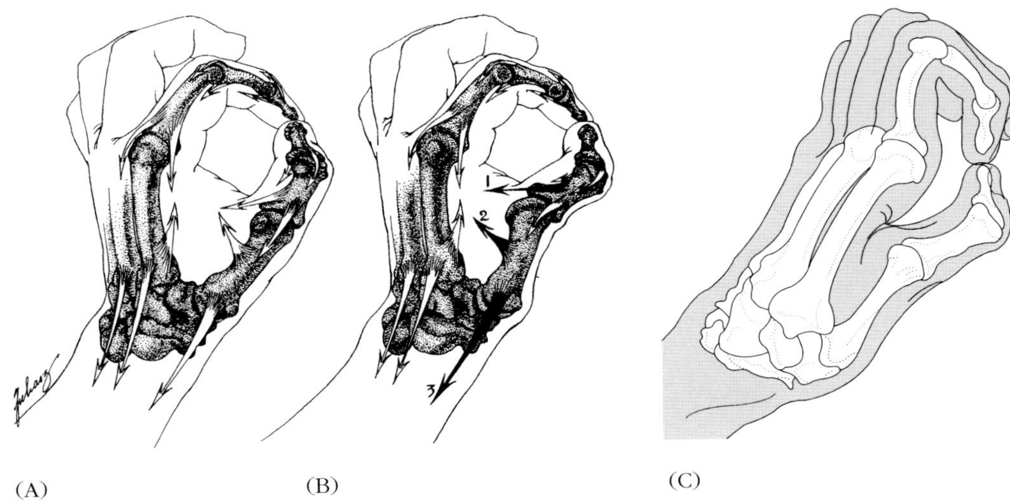

Figure 12.36

The thumb–index pinch.

(A) Normal terminal pinch (regular-shaped O)

(B) Ulnar nerve paralysis with AP and FPB paralysis. The first lumbrical maintains the balance of the index finger

(C) Median and ulnar nerve palsy. All intrinsic muscles are paralyzed, causing loss of balance of the articular chains of the thumb fingers

Path and site of insertion of the transfer

The path depends on the motor chosen. The EIP could be rerouted subcutaneously towards the AP insertion; this would bring the thumb in retroposition and impede opposition. It seems preferable to reroute the EIP through the interosseous membrane and deep in the carpal tunnel.

The FDS of the ring or the long fingers is rerouted after its passage through the carpal tunnel.

The ECRL, prolonged by a graft (palmaris longus), is passed in a subcutaneous tunnel created with a curved clamp connecting the dorsal wrist and the MP joint of the thumb, in the interval between the AP and the first dorsal interosseous muscle.

Whatever the motor used, it is necessary to take into account the condition of the FPB. The predominance of the ulnar innervation of the FPB can be estimated if, when Froment's sign is elicited, contraction of the FPB does not prevent hyperextension of the MP joint (Jeanne's sign). In this case, the opponens and the APB would be unable to counterbalance the effect of a powerful deep transfer re-established in the path of the transverse fibers of the adductor, rather it is the action of the FPB that must be restored. The path of the transfer should be deep and oblique and it should approach the thumb from its radial side (Figures 12.37 and 12.38).

In cases of ulnar palsy in which the MP joint of the thumb is put in slight flexion when the patient is requested to produce a pinch, it may be assumed that the FPB is producing an effective contraction. The transfer may be given the path of the oblique head of the AP, or a more transverse course. The ulnar side of the superficial palmar fascia, distal to the flexor retinaculum, may be used as a pulley (Royle 1938, Thompson 1942). In this type of procedure, the transfer may also be inserted onto the tendon of the adductor and its dorsal expansions up to the tendon of the EPL. The adduction action of the transfer will be more marked than in the previous procedure, but supination of the thumb will be reinforced.

Stability of the thumb MP joint is essential to ensure a strong grip. In cases of joint laxity, different techniques for stabilizing the MP joint should be used. The EIP is not sufficient to stabilize the thumb MP joint if it is lax, a concomitant fusion of the thumb MP joint is considered to augment pinch strength and improve longitudinal stability of the thumb.

Stabilization of the index finger

Transfer of the EIP to the tendon of the first dorsal interosseous was proposed by Bunnell (1944). In this procedure the course of the EIP is changed to the radial aspect of the index. Because of the angle of approach, stabilization of the MP joint, but not abduction, is provided. Solonen and Bakalim (1976) improved this technique by passing the EIP around the EPL, which acts like a dynamic pulley (Figure 12.39). A transfer of the EPB (Bruner 1948) has a better angle of approach, but its transfer leaves a deficit of extension of the thumb MP joint. However, this transfer is recommended when the thumb MP joint is fused. The FDS was proposed by Graham and Riordan (1947); the tendon was removed from the carpal tunnel, passed radially and subcutaneously in the 'snuffbox' area, and then sutured to the first dorsal interosseous. It seems inappropriate to use such a powerful and precious tendon for this function. In a more economical fashion, a strip of the ring FDS can be transferred across the palm and sutured to the first dorsal interosseous tendon, and the other strips are used for the correction of the other fingers.

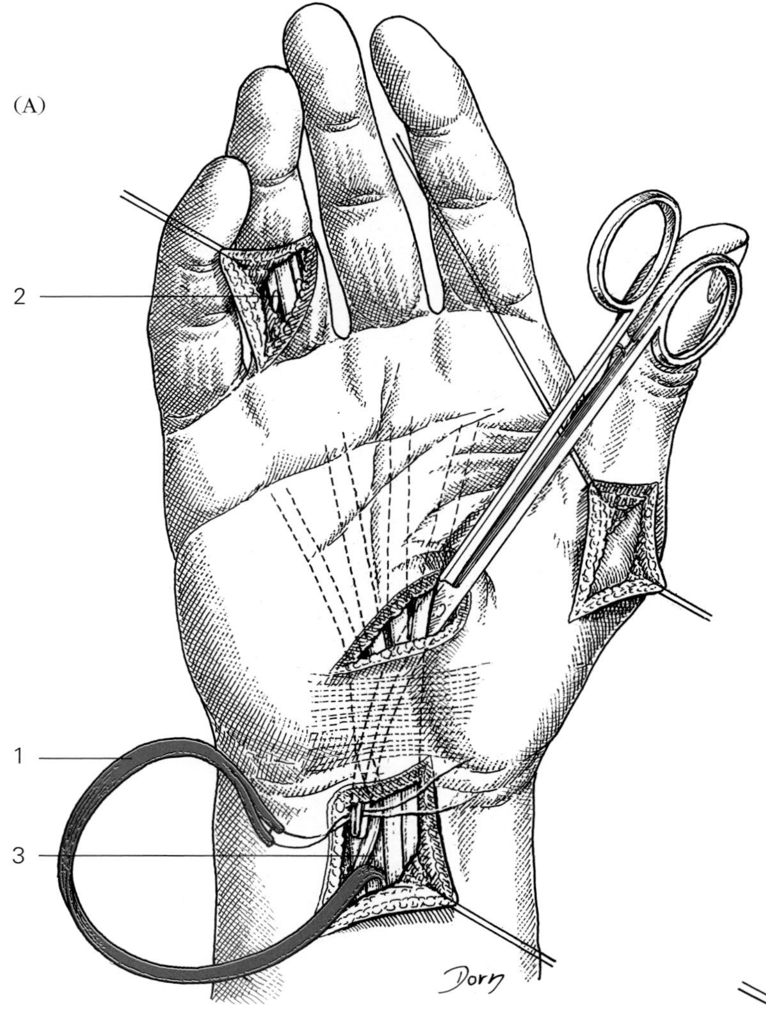

Figure 12.37

FDS transfer of the ring finger (in a distal ulnar palsy) used when the flexor pollicis brevis is also paralysed.

(A) The FDS of the ring finger is passed around the ulnar border of the flexor tendons, at the wrist level and then deep to them in the carpal tunnel.

1 FDS of the ring finger
2 FDP of the ring finger
3 FDS of the little finger

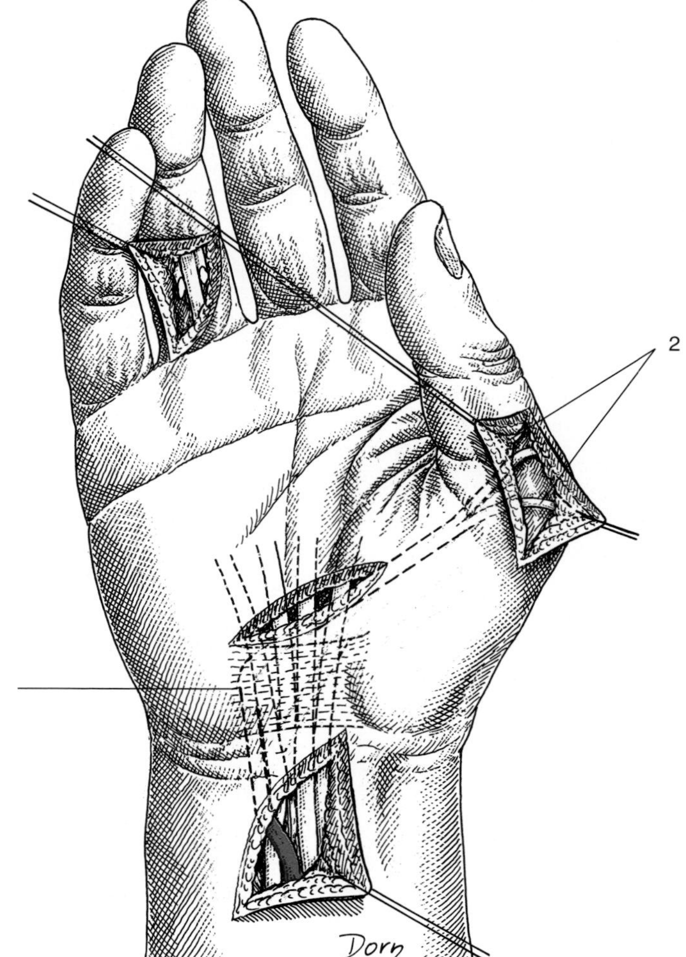

(B)

(B)

1 The rerouted FDS tendon follows the direction of the FPB toward the radial side of the MP joint of the thumb
2 The two terminal slips of the FDS are passed on either side of the thumb MP joint. Each slip transfixes the EPL tendon, the distal phalanx maintained in extension, then they are passed through the capsuloligamentous tissue from posterior to anterior in contact with the bone. The ends of the two slips are then fastened to one another on the ulnar volar aspect of the joint, to prevent MP joint hyperextension, with the proximal phalanx held in slight flexion (10°)

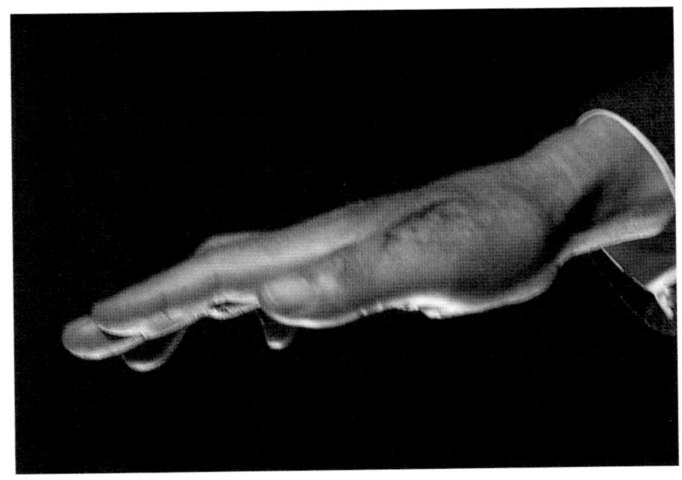

(A)

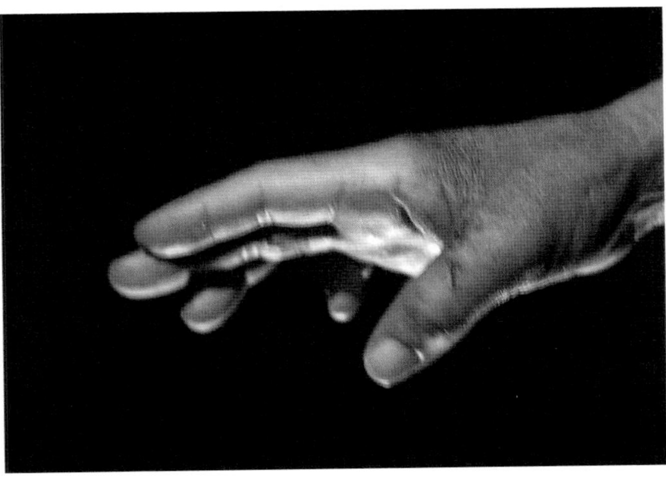

(B)

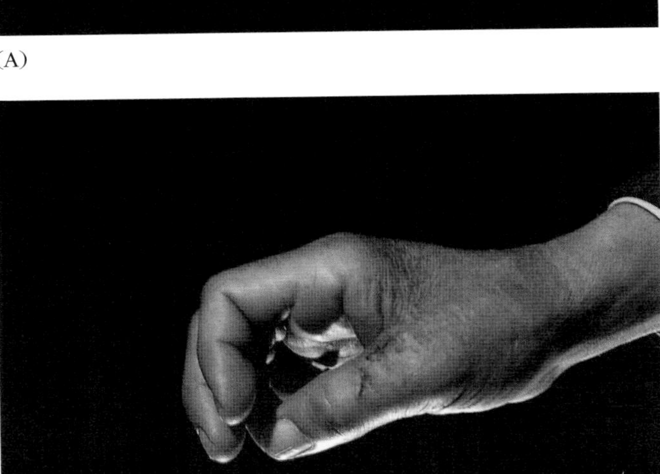

(C)

Figure 12.38

Distal ulnar nerve paralysis. (A, B, C) Transfer of a FDS inserted on the radial aspect of the joint of the thumb.

Neviaser et al (1980) described the abductor pollicis longus (APL) transfer; several tendons from the APL occur in over 96% of patients. The direction is also favorable but the excursion is short, and extension by a graft is mandatory.

We have used the Hirayama procedure with satisfactory results (Hirayama et al 1986). The PL prolonged by the palmar fascia (as in the Camitz procedure), is transferred around the radial aspect of the wrist and sutured to the first dorsal interosseous (Figure 12.40). Fixation is performed with the wrist in 10° of extension, and the index MP joint at 30° of flexion and 20° of radial deviation. The direction of the resultant transfer is parallel to the first dorsal interosseous, and its course palmar to the joint stabilizes the MP joint in flexion. A drain split longitudinally in the second web space provides a convenient splint during the postoperative period (Figure 12.41).

Indications for restoration of thumb pinch

Not all patients with ulnar nerve palsy are appropriate candidates for restoration of a strong thumb pinch necessitating powerful tendon transfers. Here also, indications depend on the age and expectations of the patient, the availability of donor tendons, and the extent of the paralysis.

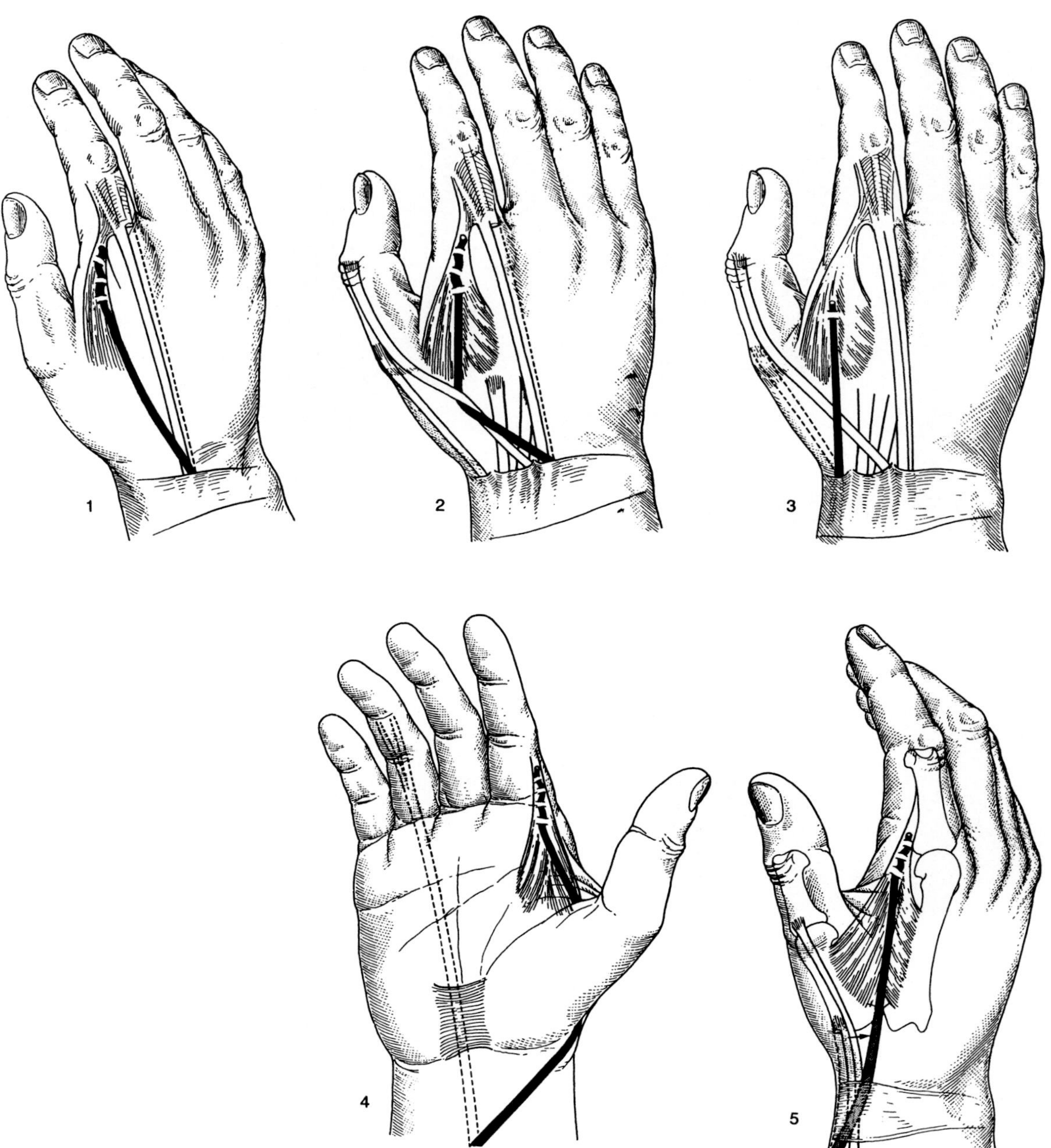

Figure 12.39

Stabilization of the index finger.

1 Bunnell
2 Solonen and Bakalim
3 Bruner
4 Graham and Riordan
5 Neviaser, Wilson and Gardner

References

Antia NH (1969) The palmaris longus motor for lumbrical replacement, *Hand* **1**: 139.

Bourrel P (1986) Interventions palliates pour correction des griffes des doigts. *Ann Chir Main* **5**: 230.

Bourrel P, Carayon A, Languillon J (1982) Deux nouvelles techniques de traitement des paralysies des muscles intrinsèques de la main, *Ann Chir* **16**: 81.

Bouvier M (1851) Note sur un cas de paralysie de la main, *Bull Acad Med* **27**: 125.

Brand PW (1961) Tendon grafting illustrated by a new operation for intrinsic paralysis of the fingers, *J Bone Joint Surg* **43B**: 444.

Brand PW (1970) Tendon transfers for median and ulnar nerves paralysis, *Orthop Clin North Am* **1**: 477.

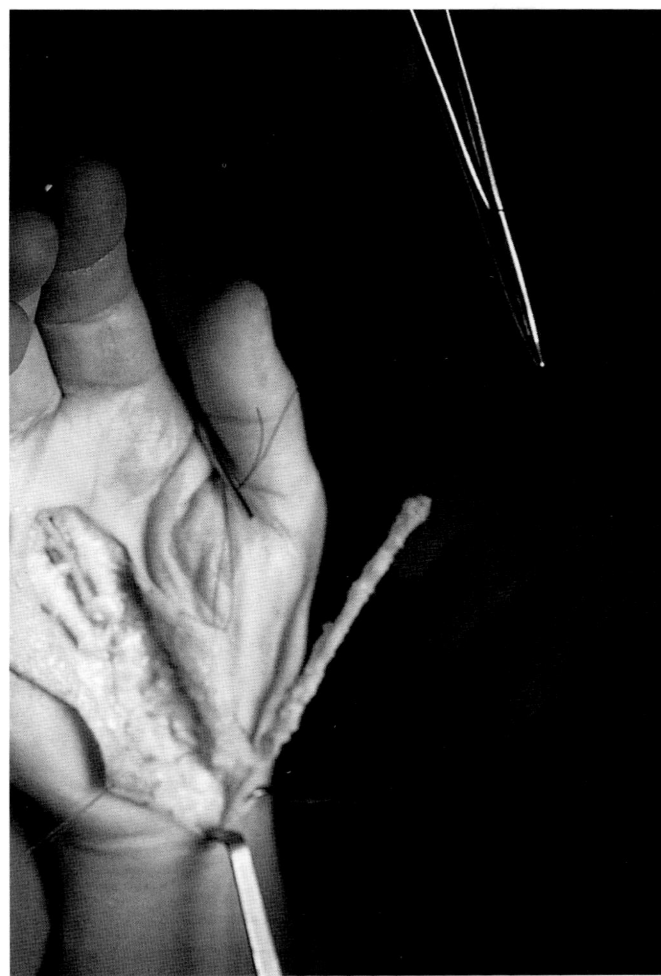

Figure 12.40

Harvesting of the palmaris longus tendon prolonged by a strip of the superficial palmar aponeurosis.

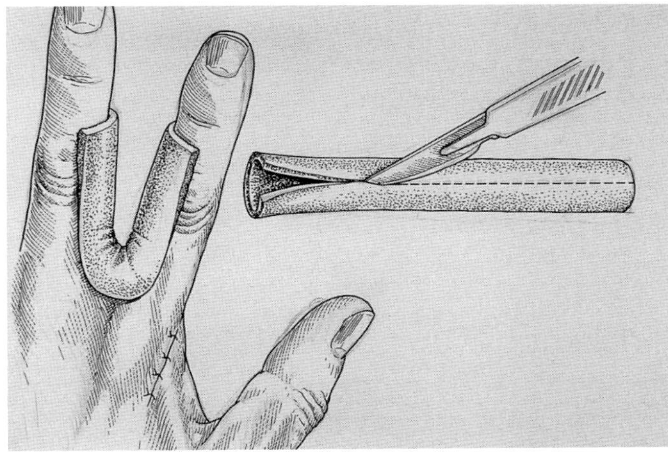

Figure 12.41

Maintenance of abduction of the index finger by a drain split longitudinally and placed in the second web space.

Brand PW (1985) *Clinical Mechanics of the Hand* (CV Mosby: St Louis).

Bruner JM (1948) Tendon transfer to restore abduction of the index finger using extensor pollicis brevis, *Plast Reconstr Surg* **3**: 197.

Bunnell S (1942) Surgery of the intrinsic muscles of the hand other than those producing opposition of the thumb, *J Bone Joint Surg* **24**: 1.

Bunnell S (1944) *Surgery of the Hand* (JB Lippincott: Philadelphia).

Burkhalter WE (1974) Early tendon transfer in upper extremity peripheral nerve injury, *Clin Orthop* **104**: 68.

Burkhalter WE, Strait JL (1976) Metacarpophalangeal flexor replacement for intrinsic muscle paralysis, *J Bone Joint Surg* **A**: 1667.

Camitz H (1929) Surgical treatment of paralysis of the opponens of the thumb, *Acta Chir Scand* **65**: 77.

Cannieu JM (1897) Recherche sur une anastomose entre la branche profonde du cubital et le median, *Bull Soc Anat Physiol Bordeaux* **18**: 339-360.

Enna CD, Riordan DC (1973) The Fowler procedure for correction of the paralytic claw hand, *Plast Reconstr Surg* **52**: 352.

Fowler SB (1949) Extensor for correction of the paralytic claw hand, *Plast Reconstr Surg* **31B**: 447.

Fritschi EP (1984) *Surgical Reconstruction and Rehabilitation in Leprosy*, 2nd edn. Director for Southern Asia. The Leprosy Mission, New Delhi.

Froment J (1915) La prehension dans les paralysies du nerf cubital et le signe du pouce. *Presse Med* **21**: 409.

Gaisne E, Palende DD (1986) Chirurgie reconstructive des paralysies des muscles intrinsèques des doigts. Etude de 100 cas, *Ann Chir Main* **5**: 12.

Giraudeau P (1971) Traitement palliatif des paralysies des intrinsèques des doigts par le grand plamaire prolongés par quatre bandelettes de fascia lata, *Rev Chir Orthop* **57**: 145.

Goldner JL (1967) Replacement of the function of the paralyzed adductor pollicis with the flexor digitorum sublimis: A ten year review. Proceedings of American Society for Surgery of the Hand, *J Bone Joint Surg* **49A**: 583.

Goldner JL (1974) Tendon transfers for irreparable peripheral nerve injuries of the upper extremity, *Orthop Clin North Am* **5**: 343–75.

Graham WC, Riordan DC (1947) Sublimis transplant to restore abduction of the index finger, *Plast Reconstr Surg* **2**: 459.

Gruber W (1870) Uber die Verbindung Nervus Medianus mit dem nervus ulnaris am Unterarme des Menschen und der Sängethiere, *Arck Anat Physiol* **37**: 501–22.

Hastings H II, Davidson S (1988) Tendon transfers for ulnar nerve palsy: Evaluation of results and practical treatment considerations, *Hand Clin* **4**: 167–78.

Hirayama T, Atsuta Y, Takemitsu Y (1986) Palmaris longus transfer for replacement of the first dorsal interosseous, *J Hand Surg* **11B**: 84.

Jebson PJL, Steyers CM (1996) Adductorplasty with the extensor carpi radialis brevis. In: Blair WF, ed, *Techniques in Hand Surgery* (Williams and Wilkins: Baltimore) 682–7.

Kaplan EB, Spinner M (1980) Normal and anomalous innervation patterns in the upper extremity. In: Omer GE, Spinner M, eds, *Management of Peripheral Nerve Problems* (WB Saunders: Philadelphia).

Littler JW (1949) Tendon transfer and arthrodesis in combined median and ulnar nerves paralysis, *J Bone Joint Surg* **31A**: 225.

Mannerfelt L (1966) Studies on the hand in ulnar nerve paralysis. A clinical experimental investigation in normal and anomalous innervation, *Acta Orthop Scand* **(Suppl)** 87.

Martin R (1887) *Tal om Nervus allmana Egenskaper* (Mannsikans Kropp Lars Salvius Stockolm).

Neviaser RJ, Wilson JN, Gardner MM (1980) Abductor pollicis longus transfer for replacement of first dorsal interosseous, *J Hand Surg* **5**: 53.

Omer GE Jr (1980) Tendon transfers for reconstruction of the forearm and hand following peripheral nerve injuries. In: Omer GE Jr, Spinner M, eds, *Management of Peripheral Nerve Problems* (WB Saunders: Philadelphia) 817.

Omer GE Jr (1999) Ulnar nerve palsy. In: Green DP, Hotchkiss RN, Pederson WC, eds, *Green's Operative Hand Surgery*, 4th edn (Churchill Livingstone: Philadelphia) 1526–41.

Osborne G (1970) Compression neuritis of the ulnar nerve at the elbow, *Hand* **2**: 10–12.

Palende DD (1976) Correction of paralytic claw-finger in leprosy by capsulorrhaphy and pulley advancement, *J Bone Joint Surg* **58A**: 59.

Parkes A (1973) Paralytic claw finger – a graft tenodesis operation, *Hand* **5**: 192.

Riche P (1897) Le nerf cubital et les muscles de l'éminence thenar, *Bull Mem Soc Anat Paris* 251–2.

Riordan DC (1953) Tendon transplantation in median nerve and ulnar nerve paralysis, *J Bone Joint Surg* **35A**: 312, 396.

Royle ND (1938) An operation for paralysis of the thumb intrinsic muscles, *JAMA* **III**: 612–12.

Schrinivasan H (1977) Movement patterns of intrinsic minus finger, *Ann R Coll Surg Engl* **59**: 33.

Smith RJ (1983) ECRB tendon transfer for thumb adduction: A study of power pinch, *J Hand Surg* **8**: 4–15.

Smith RJ (1987) Tendons transfers to restore intrinsic muscle function to the fingers. In: *Tendon Transfers of the Hand and Forearm* (Little Brown: Boston) 103–33.

Solonen KA, Bakalim GE (1976) Restoration of pinch grip in traumatic ulnar palsy, *Hand* **8**: 39.

Stiles HJ, Forrester-Brown MF (1922) *Treatment of Injuries of the Peripheral Spinal Nerves* (Stoughton, Frowde and Hodder) 166.

Struthers S (1854) On some points in the abnormal anatomy of the arm, *Br For Med Chir Rev* **14**: 224.

Thompson TC (1942) A modified operation for opponens paralysies, *J Bone Joint Surg* **26**: 632–40.

Tsuge K (1967) Tendon transfers in median and ulnar nerve paralysis, *Hiroshima J Med Sci* **16**: 29.

Tubiana R, Malek R (1968) Paralysis of the intrinsic muscles of the fingers, *Surg Clin North Am* **48**: 1140.

Tubiana R (1969) Anatomic and physiologic basis for the surgical treatment of paralysis of the hand, *J Bone Joint Surg* **51A**: 643.

Tubiana R (1993) Paralyses of the intrinsic muscles of the fingers. In: Tubiana R, ed, *The Hand*, vol 4 (Philadelphia: WB Saunders) 254–98.

Zancolli EA (1957) Claw hand caused by paralysis of the intrinsic muscles. A simple procedure for its correction, *J Bone Joint Surg* **39A**: 1076.

Zancolli EA (1974) Correction de la garra digital por paralisis intrinseca. La operacion del 'Lazo', *Acta Orthop Latina Am* **1**: 65.

Zancolli EA (1979) *Structural and Dynamic Bases of Hand Surgery*, 2nd edn (Philadelphia: JB Lippincott).

Zancolli EA (1987) Symposium on Reconstructive Procedures for the Paralytic Upper Limb. Conferences of Zancolli EA. Paris.

13 Associated paralysis

Ph Valenti

Combined nerve lesions in the upper limb result in severe functional loss. Direct sutures or nerve grafts generally give partial results at the level of the hand.

This chapter describes the choice of palliative procedures to improve the function of the hand in low and high combined nerve paralysis. The paralysis of the shoulder and elbow that occurs with brachial plexus injury or proximal nerve injury (axillary, subscapularis, musculocutaneous) has been excluded: direct suture or more frequently nerve graft of these proximal nerves gives quite good results because the motor units are close and their function is essentially muscular.

Assessment of the deficit in functions, the muscles spared and the patient's individual needs is the first step in selecting appropriate procedures in combined nerve injuries.

Principles of palliative surgery in associated paralysis

A careful evaluation and examination of each patient is essential in planning the reconstruction of the upper limb (Masquelet 1989). Proximal nerve injuries are frequently associated with vascular and soft tissue lesions: oedema, swelling and secondary scarred tissue and stiff joints with fibrosis contraindicate reconstructive surgery. The use of upper limb physiotherapy, with special splinting and active exercises with pressure techniques to control the oedema and fibrosis are very helpful. If full passive motion is not obtained after meticulous splinting and rehabilitation, then arthrolysis and tenolysis should be performed. Sometimes it is necessary to use a flap to resurface a retractile scar and to improve vascularization of soft tissue (frequently at the level of the wrist).

The second stage is to evaluate the functional loss of the upper limb. This evaluation should be accurate if the functional loss is stable and not evolving. Each muscle should be tested but with the aim of restoring function. Several muscles can be involved in a motion, but as the number of tendons that can be transferred is limited in combined nerve paralysis, more than one tendon transfer cannot be used to achieve the same motion. In severe proximal nerve injuries, many functions are repaired but these are not sufficient muscles available to restore each function of the upper limb. Therefore, arthrodesis of the wrist should be avoided to preserve the possibility of the tenodesis effect on fingers; for example, the mobility of the wrist can improve the function of a tendon transfer, which can be used to rehabilitate the flexion of the fingers.

The surgeon should respect a hierarchy of function to restore elbow flexion, wrist extension, finger flexion, finger extension and thumb opposition, and secondarily, the intrinsic function of the thumb and the fingers. The goals of palliative surgery in combined nerve injury must of necessity be lower and weaker than the results of nerve microsurgery or palliative surgery with a single nerve injury.

The selection of the muscle for use in tendon transfer is limited, and it is not recommended that a reinnervated muscle is used as a tendon transfer for reconstruction because it did not regain full normal strength (Moheb et al 1986). Restoration of sensibility is essential to improve the rehabilitation of tendon transfer. A secondary nerve graft can allow recovery of a protective sensibility. Therefore, an anaesthetic hand may be better after a tendon transfer that optimizes the function of the fingers.

These surgical techniques must respect the usual principles of tendon transfer reconstruction: the severity of the lesion didn't miss simplicity and no complexity of this palliative surgery (Omer 1974, 1982a).

Several degrees of paralysis can occur in combined nerve lesions but, to simplify the choice of tendon transfer, this chapter discusses cases of complete paralysis arising from high and low nerve lesions.

Low median and low ulnar nerve paralysis (Table 13.1, Figures 13.1, 13.2)

This is the most common combined nerve paralysis. It is characterized by a sensory loss on the volar aspect of all digits and a complete intrinsic motor loss. Often,

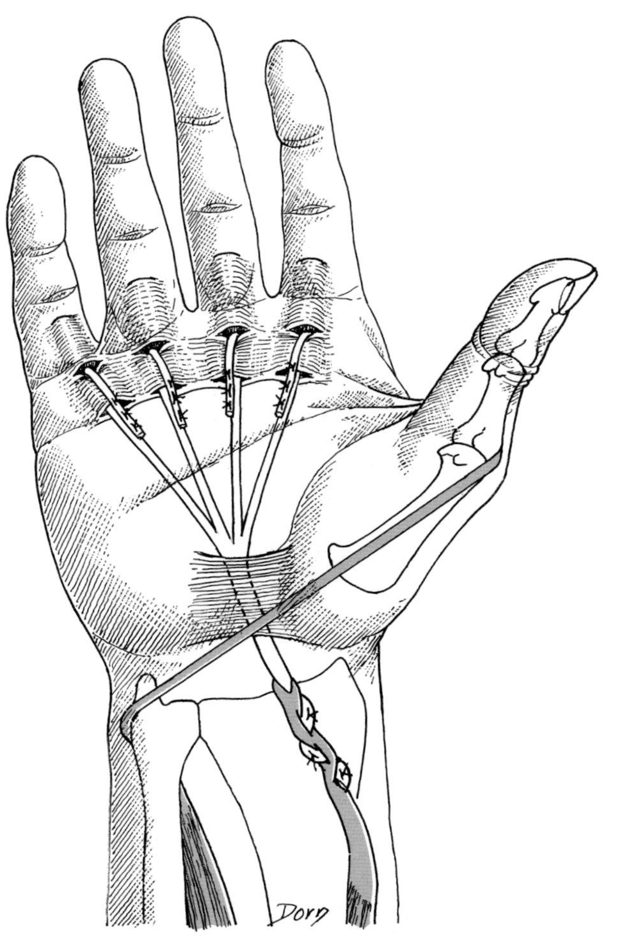

Figure 13.1

Low median and ulnar nerve paralysis in a manual worker. Transfer of the ECRL to the fingers and transfer of the EIP to the thumb.

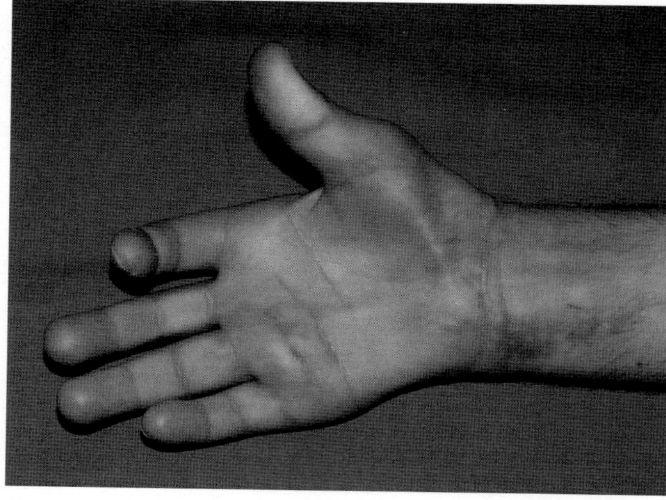

(A)

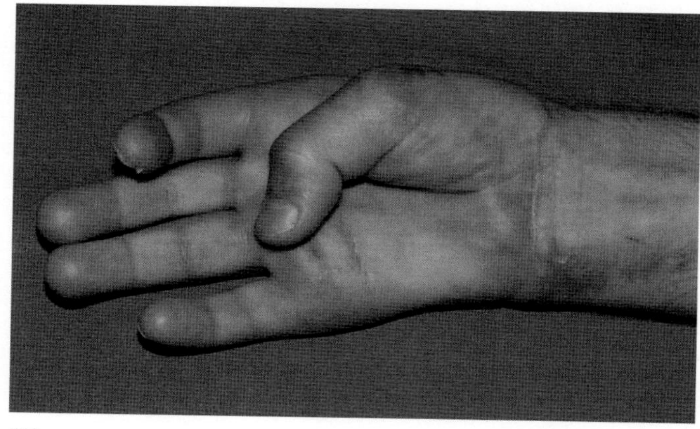

(B)

Figure 13.2

Results of EIP transfer to restore opposition of the thumb in low median and low ulnar palsy.

multiple tendons are also transected during the trauma and are not always available for tendon transfer. Sometimes the course of the tendon repaired is limited by adherence and it is preferable to use a tendon from the radial territory. Examination of the hand shows a thumb in the same plane as the metacarpal with a hyperextension at the metacarpophalangeal (MP) joint and flexion at the proximal interphalangeal (PIP) joints (claw deformity). The absence of first web space contracture, and the passive motion of the PIP joint and MP joint must be evaluated before any transfer. Physiotherapy, splinting and sometimes articular arthrolysis and tenolysis represent the first surgical stage.

The goals of palliative procedures are to restore sensibility of the ulnar pulp of the thumb and radial pulp of the index and middle finger, with a strong key pinch and a strong grasp.

Sometimes, a long time after the injury, a secondary nerve suture or more frequently a graft of the median nerve is indicated to restore the essential sensibility of the volar aspect of the radial fingers. A resurfacing of the palmar aspect of the wrist with a pedicled flap is sometimes necessary during or before this operation.

Thumb abduction is restored by transfer of the extensor indicis proprius (EIP) around the ulnar border of the hand and across the thenar eminence to insert on the abductor pollicis (Chouhy-Aguirre 1956, Burkhalter 1973, Mehta et al 1996). A fusion of the MP joint can be performed to increase the stability of the thumb (Omer 1985), but if the EIP is long enough, a loop around the extensor pollicis longus (EPL) provides stability of the MP joint.

Thumb adduction is restored by transfer of the extensor carpi radialis brevis (ECRB) prolonged with a tendon graft and then passed through the third metacarpal space to the insertion of the adductor pollicis on the thumb (Smith 1987). Another possibility is to use the flexor superficialis of the ring finger with a pulley at the level of the distal palmar crease to follow the same direction of the adductus muscle of the thumb (Goldner 1974).

Table 13.1 *Low median and low ulnar paralysis*

Function restored	*Author's preferred transfer*
Thumb abduction	EIP to APB (arthrodesis of MCP joint I)
Thumb adduction	ECRB + graft to AP thumb FDS IV to AP thumb
Radial stabilization of the index	EPB to first dorsal interosseous muscle PL to first dorsal interosseous muscle
Claw deformity: four fingers	Bouvier test positive: capsulodesis of MP joint lasso procedure Bouvier test negative: ECRL + graft to interossei Flexion contracture of PIP: arthrodesis
Adduction of little finger	EDM to radial collateral ligament of MP
Volar sensibility I/II, V	Neurovascular island flap from dorsum of index finger Neurotization by sensitive radial nerve to digital nerve (I, II, III, V) End-to-side nerve repair (radial sensory nerve) + graft to digital nerve (I, II, III, V)

Table 13.2 *High median and high ulnar paralysis*

Function restored	*Author's preferred transfer*
Wrist pronation	Rerouting of the biceps tendon Rotation osteotomy of the radius
Finger flexion	ECRL to FDP Tenodesis of DIP joint
Thumb	
Flexion IP	BR to FPL
Abduction	EIP to APB Arthrodesis of MP joint
Adduction/abduction (other procedure)	EIP + graft to APB EPL (Revol and Servant 1987)
Radial stabilization of the index	EPB to first dorsal introsseous
Claw deformity	Capsulodesis of MP joint Tenodesis with a free tendon graft
Wrist flexion	ECU to FCU
Volar sensibility	Neurovascular island flap from dorsum of index finger Neurotization by sensitive radial nerve to digital nerve (I, II, III, V) End-to-side nerve repair (radial sensory nerve) + graft to digital nerve (I, II, III, V)

Key pinch can be improved by providing radial stability to the index finger with transfer of the extensor pollicis brevis (EPB) to the first dorsal interosseous muscle (Bruner 1948).

If the palmaris longus (PL) has been repaired in emergency, it can be used as a tendon transfer to reinforce the first dorsal interosseous muscle (Hirayama 1986).

The procedure to restore intrinsic function of the fingers depends on the result of Bouvier's test (Bourrel 1985) and the passive mobility of the PIP joints. If the claw hand deformity is actively correctable by flexion of the MP joints, a capsulodesis of the MP joint (Zancolli 1957) or a lasso procedure (Zancolli 1979) can be performed if the flexor superficialis of the ring finger is available. If the claw hand deformity is not correctable or if the PIP joint is stiff, it is preferable to harvest the extensor carpi radialis longus (ECRL) (prolonged with a graft), pass through under the intermetacarpal ligament and fix to the interosseous band (Brand 1970). This procedure is particularly useful for a manual worker to provide grasp strength. But, if the flexion contracture of the PIP joint is irreducible (after failure of physiotherapy or if there has been a long delay after the trauma), arthrodesis of the PIP joint is the last alternative.

Transferring the extensor digiti minimi (EDM) to the radial collateral ligament of the MP joint (Blacker et al 1976) restores adduction of the little finger.

Restoration of volar sensibility

All the procedures described above are based on the intact sensibility of the radial territory. The goal is to obtain a protective sensibility for the pulp of the radial fingers and the ulnar pulp of the little finger. A neurovascular island flap from the dorsum aspect of the index can provide the sensibility of the pulp of the thumb (Foucher and Braun 1979). The procedure of neurotization of the sensitive branches of the radial nerve to the digital nerve of the radial fingers or the little finger provides a protective sensibility (Bedeschi 1984, Ozkan et al 2001). An end-to-side nerve suture of the sensitive branches of the radial nerve to the digital nerve can provide a protective sensibility without deficiency of the radial territory (Rowan et al 2000).

High median and high ulnar nerve paralysis (Table 13.2, Figures 13.3, 13.4)

Functional loss is severe in this combined paralysis. The goals of palliative surgery are to restore the sensibility of the volar aspect of the hand and a simple grasp and pinch and mostly a key type of pinch.

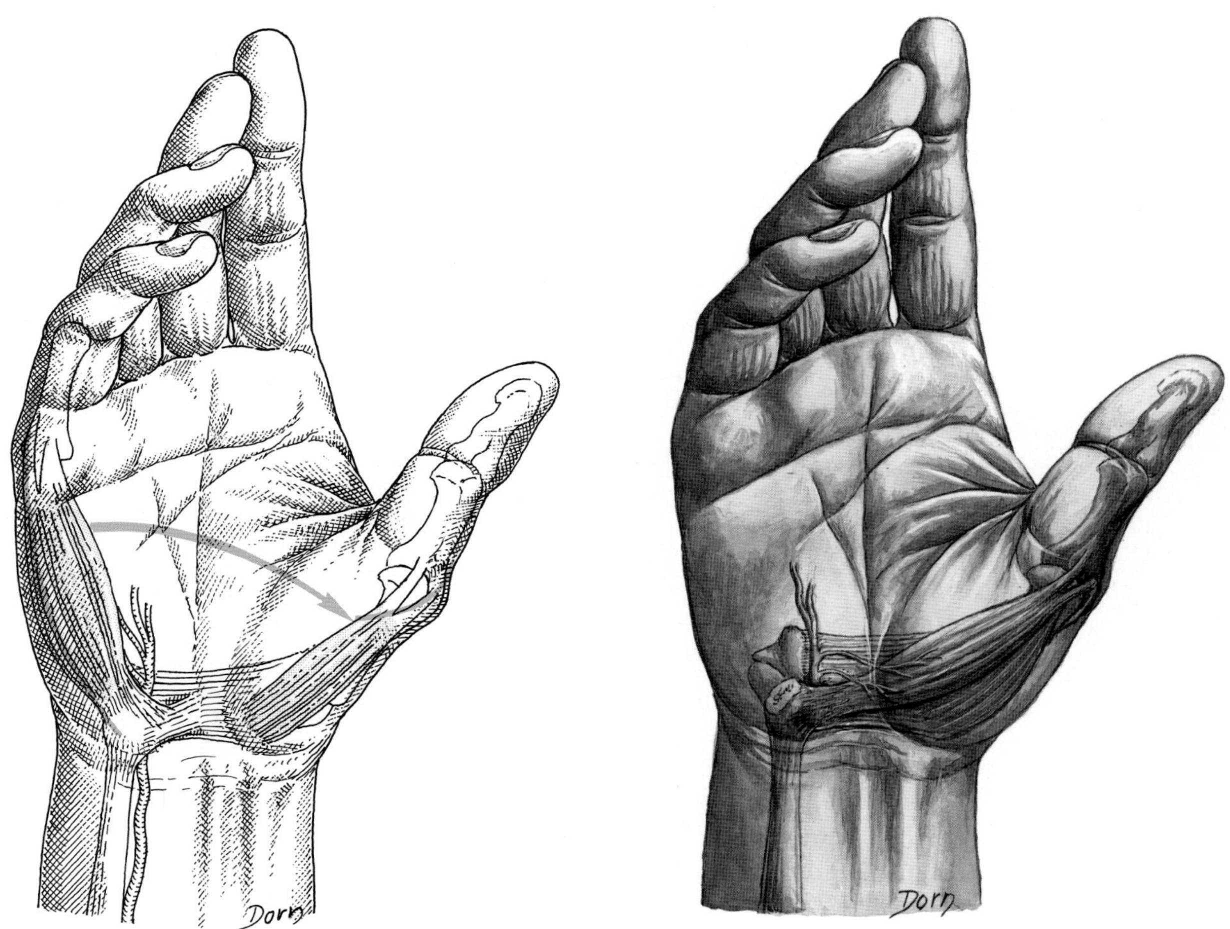

Figure 13.3
Transfer of the abductor digiti minimi in high median and high radial paralysis to restore abduction of the thumb.

The tendons available for transfer depend on the radial nerve.

Wrist pronation can be restored by a rerouting of the biceps brachii around the radius (Zancolli 1967). If the passive range motion of the forearm is limited, we prefer an osteotomy of the radius, which allows correction of the fixed supination of the forearm. The extrinsic loss of the flexor tendon can be restored by ECRL transfer to the flexor digitorum profundus (FDP) routed along the radial side of the forearm and with a tenodesis of the distal interphalangeal joints (DIP) (Brand 1970, Omer 1974).

Wrist flexion is restored by transfer of the extensor carpi ulnaris (ECU) tendon to the insertion of the flexor carpi ulnaris (FCU) tendon around the ulnar border of the forearm.

For thumb flexion, and to restore a strong key pinch, the transfer of the brachioradialis tendon (BR) to the flexor pollicis longus (FPL) seems to be the best approach (Riordan 1983, Omer 1985). Many transfers have been reported to restore thumb opposition.

Thumb abduction is restored by transfer of the EIP around the ulnar border of the hand and across the thenar eminence to insert on the abductor pollicis brevis (APB) (Chouhy-Aguirre 1956, Burkhalter et al 1973). To increase the stability of the thumb, we can perform a fusion of the MP joint (Omer 1968). However, if the EIP is long enough, a loop around the extensor pollicis longus (EPL) can provide stability of the MP joint.

Other alternatives are the EPB around the flexor carpi radialis (FCR) (Tubiana 1969) or EPL (Revol and Servant 1987) around the ulnar border of the forearm.

If we use the EPL to restore the abduction, the EIP prolonged with a graft can be transferred through the second intermetacarpal space to restore thumb adduction (Brown 1974).

Key pinch can be improved by providing radial stability to the index finger with transfer of the EPB to the first dorsal interosseous muscle.

Correction of claw hand deformity is possible with a capsulodesis of the MP joint or with tenodesis of the

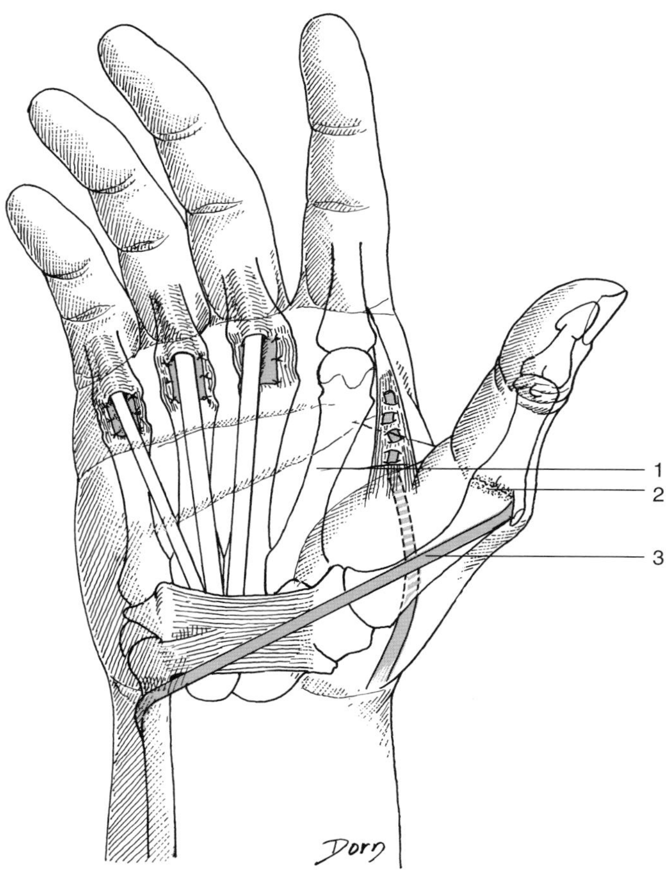

Figure 13.4

Transfer of the EIP around the ulnar border to the thumb. Capsulodesis of MP joints and transfer of the EPB to the first dorsal interosseous muscle in high median and high ulnar paralysis.

interosseous with a free graft (Parkes 1973, Burkhalter et al 1973). To provide protective sensibility to the pinch, we use procedures based on the intact sensibility of the radial territory. Three procedures (that can also be used in low ulnar and low median paralysis) are useful: neurovascular island flap from the dorsum of the index, neurotization and end-to-side nerve repair of sensitive branches of the radial nerve.

High median and high radial paralysis (Table 13.3)

Reconstructive surgery in this type of paralysis is difficult because the available transfers are limited. Only the FCU and the abductor digiti minimi (ADM) can be used. Some authors (Omer 1974, Riordan 1974, Eversmann 1988) have proposed a wrist arthrodesis. We prefer to stabilize the wrist with transfer of the latissimus dorsi to the ECRB: the latissimus dorsi is harvested with the fascia from the posterior crest of the ileum, and without dividing the neurovascular pedicle, it is able to reach the extensor tendon (or flexor tendon) at the level of the forearm (Doi et al 1985). So, the active extension of the wrist increases the flexion of the fourth and fifth fingers and the strength of the grasp (tenodesis principle). Finger extension and thumb extension are restored by transfer of the FCU around the ulnar border to the extensor digitorum communis (EDC) and the EPL. The suture is performed obliquely and proximally to the dorsal carpal ligament. The suture tension should be adjusted when the tendon transfer for flexion of the fingers has been performed.

Table 13.3 *High median and high radial paralysis*

Function restored	*Author's preferred transfer*
Wrist pronation	Rerouting of the biceps tendon Rotation osteotomy of the radius
Wrist extension	Latissimus dorsi pedicled flap to ECR
Finger extension	FCU to EDC and EPL
Finger flexion	Tenodesis of FDP (II/III) to FDP (IV/V)
Thumb abduction	ADM to APB and tenodesis of FPL
Thumb opposition	Arthrodesis of IP joint
Volar sensibility	Neurovascular island pedicled flap from IV to ulnar pulp I
Key pinch I/II	Neurotization or end-to-side from sensitive ulnar nerve Common digital nerve IV space to digital nerve II/III

Flexion of the fingers will be obtained by side-to-side suture of the tendon of the index and middle fingers to the ring and little fingers.

The choice of transfer to restore the opposition of the thumb depends on the ulnar nerve. Frequently the function of the flexor pollicis will be preserved. The reconstruction of the thumb requires a transfer of the ADM to the APB (Littler and Cooley 1963). A tenodesis of the FPL (Omer 1985) or an arthrodesis of the interphalangeal joint is preferable when the flexor pollicis brevis (FPB) is functional.

Forearm pronation is restored by rerouting the biceps brachii tendon around the proximal radius to improve key pinch.

The sensibility of the ulnar pulp of the thumb benefits from the transfer of a neurovascular cutaneous island pedicle flap from the ring finger. The procedures of neurotization or end-to-side suture from the ulnar sensitive branches can restore a protective sensibility of the index and middle finger.

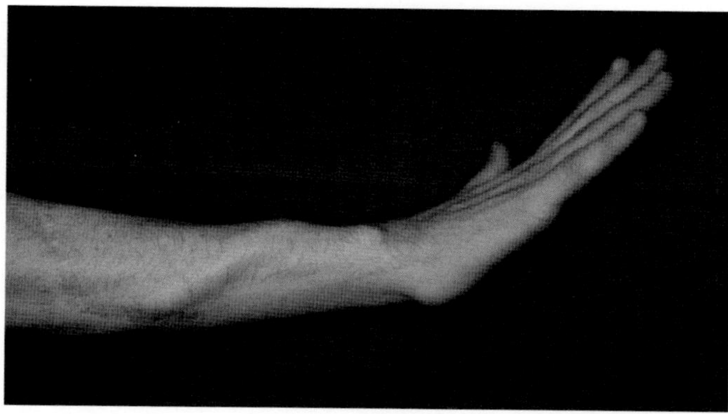

(A)

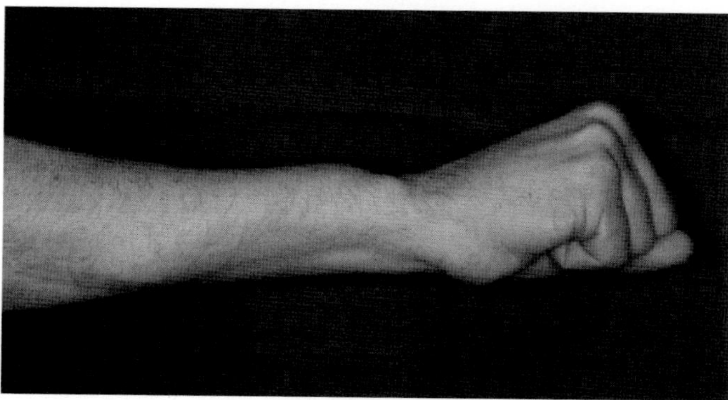

(B)

Figure 13.5

Results of reanimation of the wrist and finger extensions with Tubiana's procedure in high radial palsy.

Table 13.4 *High ulnar and high radial paralysis*

Function restored	*Author's preferred transfer*
Wrist extension	PT to ECRB (transferred to M4)
Finger extension Thumb extension	FDS III to ECD and EPL
Finger flexion (IV/V)	Tenodesis of FDP (IV/V) to FDP (II/III) Tenodesis of DIP joints
Claw deformity (IV/V)	Capsulodesis of MP joints Tenodesis with a free tendon graft
Radial stabilization of the index	PL to first dorsal interosseous muscle
Sensibility of ulnar V	Neurotization or end-to-side from common digital nerve third space to ulnar digital nerve Neurovascular island pedicled flap from III

High ulnar and high radial paralysis (Table 13.4, Figure 13.5)

Volar sensibility of the three radial fingers is respected and the main action for the hand surgeon should be to restore wrist, finger and thumb extension. Secondary, palliative surgery will correct the intrinsic function of the fingers.

Transfer of the pronator teres (PT) to extensor carpi radialis (ECR) (Jones 1916) is the basic transfer to restore wrist extension. However, two points should be respected to avoid a radial deviation of the wrist (Tubiana 1985): the ECRL should be freed from its connecting tendon with the ECRB; the distal insertion of the ECRB is replaced more medially (on the base of the fourth metacarpal).

Extension of the fingers and thumb can be gained by tendon transfer of the flexor digitorum superficialis (FDS) of the middle finger, through the interosseous membrane, to the EPL.

Flexion of the ring and little fingers is obtained by side-to-side suture of the FDP tendon to the index and middle fingers (Eversmann 1988).

To prevent a claw deformity and to allow active extension at the PIP joint, we perform a capsulodesis of the MP volar capsule (Zancolli 1979) or a tenodesis of the interosseous with a free tendon graft (Parkes 1973).

Flexor pollicis and abductor pollicis are spared and thumb abduction does not always need to be restored. Therefore, to improve the strength of the pinch (I/II), the radial stabilization of the index finger can be increased by transfer of the PL to the first interosseous muscle (Hirayama et al 1986). The ulnar sensibility of the little finger can be supplied by a neurovascular cutaneous island flap from the median nerve territory (ulnar middle finger)).

Other procedures such as neurotization and end-to-side nerve sutures from the common digital nerve of the third space can be used for the ring and little finger.

High combined median, ulnar and radial paralysis (Table 13.5, Figure 13.6)

High three-nerve palsy is characterized by a flail hand with a paralytic elbow. Functional loss is dramatically severe and clinical aspects can be compared to a complete avulsion of the brachial plexus or to a proximal amputation of the upper limb. The goals of palliative procedures are to restore simple prehension with sensibility of the median territory.

Table 13.5 *High combined median, radial and ulnar paralysis*

Function restored	*Author's preferred transfer*
Elbow flexion	Latissimus dorsi pedicled or gracilis free
Wrist stabilization Thumb extension	Tenodesis of ECR and EPL to radius
Finger flexion	Latissimus dorsi pedicled flap to FDP Gracilis muscle free flap (intercostal nerve)
Finger extension	Gracilis muscle free flap (intercostal nerve or pectoralis nerve + graft)
Volar sensibility	Tendon transfer + rehabilitation Intercostal nerve (sensitive part) to median nerve

If the biceps is functional, Gousheh (1999) used it to restore finger flexion; the distal part of the tendon of the biceps is detached completely from the radius. A graft (fasci lata, local) is sutured distally to the flexor profundus at the level of the musculotendinous junction. The suture should be done with elbow in extension and fingers in flexion. The flexor profundus longus is rerouted subcutaneously and fixed to the graft. Doi in 1984 and Gousheh et al (2000) more recently, reported a procedure used in Volkman's contracture with the latissimus dorsi muscle. Elbow flexion and finger flexion are restored by transfer of the latissimus dorsi pedicled flap: harvest of the latissimus dorsi muscle with the fascial origin from the iliac crest of the Ilium, without dividing the neurovascular pedicle, makes it possible to reach the flexor tendons on the distal forearm. This procedure is safe and restores the function immediately.

If the latissimus dorsi muscle is denervated, as in complete avulsion of the brachial plexus, a double free muscle transfer technique can be used to restore simple prehension (Chuang 1995, Doi et al 1999). Free muscle transfer (gracilis medialis), with reinnervation by a terminal branch of the plexus (proximal amputation) can be used to restore elbow flexion and finger extension. Free muscle transfer (gracilis or latissimus dorsi) with reinnervation by the fifth and sixth intercostal nerves can be used to restore finger flexion.

Tenodesis of thumb extensors and fixation to the radius of the FPL can restore a lateral pinch with an active extension of the wrist of at least 30° (Moberg 1978).

Intrinsic hand function cannot be actively corrected (no available transfer) and it is preferable to perform a capsulodesis of the MP joints and an arthrodesis of the thumb MP joint.

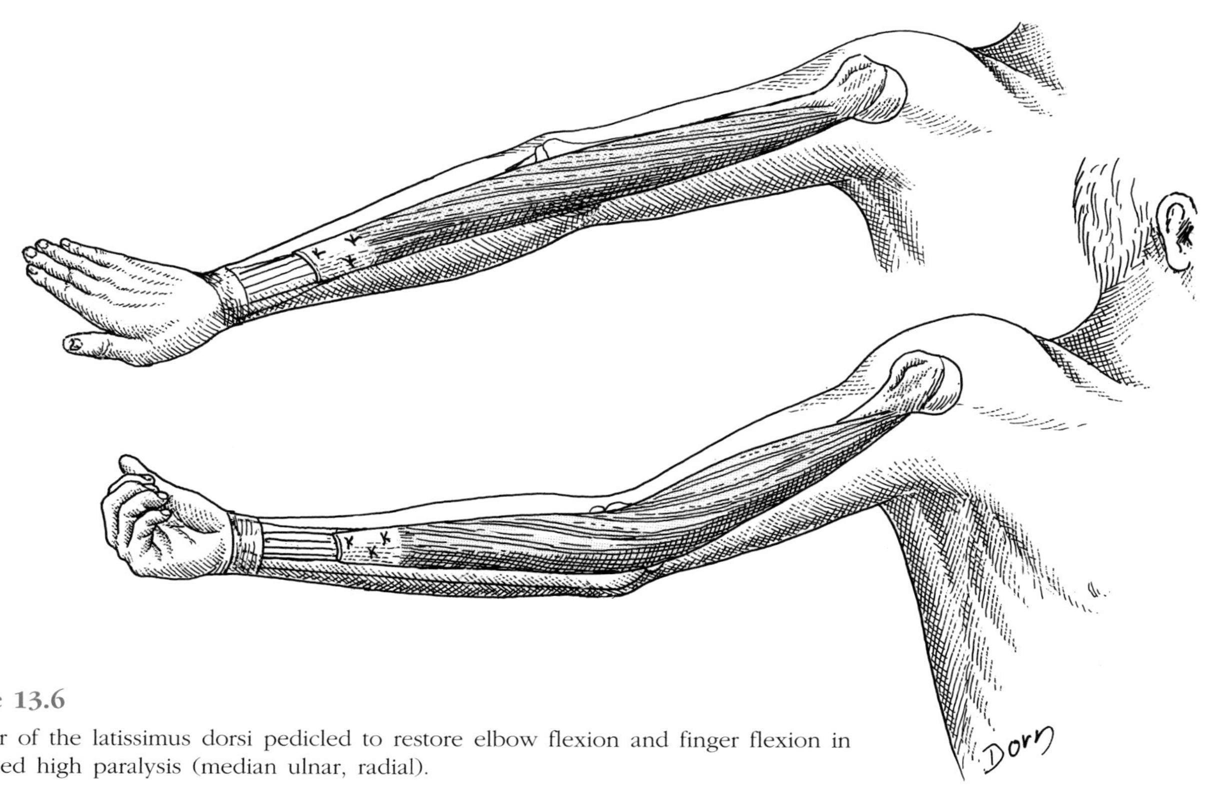

Figure 13.6

Transfer of the latissimus dorsi pedicled to restore elbow flexion and finger flexion in combined high paralysis (median ulnar, radial).

When there is a high ulnar and radial palsy with a low median palsy, as seen in leprous palsy (Sundararaj and Mani 1984), we can use extrinsic muscles innervated by the median nerve which are spared. The opposition can be restored by a Makin's procedure (Makin 1967) with an arthrodesis of the MP joint or a winch procedure as reported by Levasoy (1981) with a tenodesis of the EPL to the ulna.

Sensibilility of the volar aspect of the three radial fingers can be achieved by neurotization of the median nerve with sensitive branches from the intercostal nerve. However, loss of sensibility of the hand is not a contraindication for the transfer of tendons, because the improvement of motion facilitates the return of a protective sensibility.

Conclusion

Reconstruction of the main functions of the upper limb after combined nerve injuries requires a thorough assessment of the functional loss and an adapted choice of the functions to be restored, depending on the number of available muscles (these are frequently limited). Surgical procedures will be simply to restore elbow flexion, wrist extension, finger flexion and thumb adduction. The functional goals depend on the gravity of the combined nerve lesions, but the patient should be informed that the best procedure cannot create a normally functional hand.

References

Bedeschi P, Celli L, Balli A (1984) Transfer of sensory nerves in hand surgery, *J Hand Surg* **9B**: 46.

Blacker GJ, Lister GD, Kleinert HE (1976) The abducted little finger in low ulnar nerve palsy, *J Hand Surg [Br]* **1**: 190–6.

Bourrel P (1985) The metacarpophalangeal stabilization test beevor or bouvier?, *Ann Chir Main* **4**: 31–5.

Boyes JH (1960) Tendon transfers for radial palsy, *Bull Hosp Joint Dis* **21**: 97.

Brand PW (1970) Tendon transfer for median and ulnar nerve paralysis, *Clin Orthop North Am* **1**: 447–54.

Brown P (1974) Reconstruction for pinch in ulnar palsy, *Clin Orthop North Am* **5**: 323–41.

Bruner JM (1948) Tendon transfer to restore abduction of the index using the extensor pollicis brevis, *Plast Reconstr Surg* **3**: 197–201.

Burkhalter W, Christensen RC, Brown P (1973) Extensor indicis proprius opponensplasty, *J Bone Joint Surg Am* **55**: 725–32.

Chouhy-Aguirre S, Caplan S (1956) Sobre secuelas de lesion alta e irreparable de nervios mediano y cubital y su tratimiento, *Prensa Med Argentina* **43**: 2341–6.

Chuang DCC (1995) Functioning free muscle transplantation for brachial plexus injury, *Clin Orthop Rel Res* **314**: 1004.

Doi K, Ihara K, Sakamoto T, Kawai S (1985) Functional latissimus dorsi island pedicle musculocutaneous flap to restore finger flexion, *J Hand Surg* **10**: 678.

Doi K, Kuwata N, Muramatsu K, Hottori Y, Kawai S (1999) Double muscle transfer for upper extremity reconstruction following complete avulsion of the brachial plexus, *Hand Clin* **15**: 757–67.

Eversmann WW Jr (1988) Tendon transfers for combined nerve injuries, *Hand Clin* **4**: 187–99.

Foucher G, Braun JB (1979) A new island flap transfer from the dorsum of the index to the thumb, *Plast Reconstr Surg* **63**: 344.

Goldner JL (1974) Tendon transfers for irreparable peripheral nerve injuries of the upper extremity, *Orthop Clin North Am* **5**: 343–75.

Gousheh J, Arab H, Gilbert A (2000). The extended latissimus dorsi muscle island flap for flexion or extension of fingers, *J Hand Surg [Br]* **25**: 160–5.

Gousheh J (1999) Biceps transfer to finger flexion. In: Tubiana R, Gilbert A, Masquelet AC, eds, *Atlas of Surgical Techniques of the Hand and Wrist* (London: Martin Dunitz) 351–2.

Hirayama T, Atsuta Y, Takemitsu Y (1986) Palmaris longus transfer for replacement of the first dorsal interosseous, *J Hand Surg [Br]* **11**: 84–6.

Jones R (1916) On suture of nerves, and alternative methods of treatment by transplantation of tendon, *BMJ* **i**: 641.

Lesavoy MA (1981) A new "puppet procedure" for functional movement of totally deanimated tri-nerve paralysis below the elbow, *Plast Reconstr Surg* **67**: 240–5.

Littler JW, Cooley SGE (1963) Opposition of the thumb and restoration by abductor digiti transfer, *J Bone Joint Surg* **45A**: 1389–96.

Makin M (1967) Translocation of the flexor pollicis longus tendon to restore opposition, *J Bone Joint Surg* **49B**: 458–61.

Masquelet A (1989) Proximal combined nerve paralysis, *Hand Clin* **5**: 43–52.

Mehta R, Malaviya GN, Husain S (1996) Extensor indicis opposition transfer in the ulnar and median palsied thumb in leprosy, *J Hand Surg [Br]* **21**: 617–21.

Moberg E (1978) *The Upper Limb in Tetraplegia* (Stuttgart: Georg Thieme).

Moheb S, Moneim MS, Omer GE Jr (1986) Latissimus dorsi muscle transfer for restoration of elbow flexion after brachial plexus disruption, *J Hand Surg [Am]* **11**: 135–9.

Omer GE Jr (1974) Tendon transfers in combined nerve lesions, *Orthop Clin North Am* **5**: 377–87.

Omer GE (1982a) Early tendon transfers in the rehabilitation of median, radial, and ulnar palsies, *Ann Chir Main* **1**: 187–90.

Omer GE Jr (1982b) Reconstructive procedures for extremities with peripheral nerve defects, *Clin Orthop* **163**: 80–91.

Omer GE Jr (1985) Reconstruction of a balanced thumb through tendon transfers, *Clin Orthop* **195**: 104–16.

Omer GE Jr (1986) Acute management of peripheral nerve injuries, *Hand Clin* **2**: 193–206.

Omer GE (1992) Tendon transfers for combined traumatic nerve palsies of the forearm and hand, *J Hand Surg [Br]* **17**: 603–10.

Ozkan T, Ozer K, Gulgonen A (2001) Restoration of sensibility in irreparable ulnar and median nerve lesions with use of sensory nerve transfer: long-term follow-up of 20 cases, *J Hand Surg [Am]* **26**: 44–51.

Parkes A (1973) Paralytic claw fingers: a graft tenodesis operation, *Hand* **5**: 192–9.

Revol M, Servant JM (1987) Paralysies médio-cubitales hautes. In: *Paralysies de la Main et du Membre Supérieur* (Paris: Medsi).

Riordan DC (1974) Radial nerve paralysis, *Orthop Clin North Am* **5**: 283–7.

Riordan DC (1983) Tendon transfers in hand surgery, *J Hand Surg [Am]* **8**: 748–53.

Rowan PR, Chen LE, Urbaniak JR (2000) End to side nerve repair: a review, *Hand Clin* **16**: 151–9.

Smith RJ (1987) *Tendon Transfer of the Hand and Forearm* (Boston: Little Brown).

Sundararaj GD, Mani K (1984) Surgical reconstruction of the hand with triple nerve palsy, *J Bone Joint Surg [Br]* **66**: 260–4.

Tubiana R (1969) Anatomic and physiologic basis for the surgical treatment of paralysis of the hand, *J Bone Joint Surg* **51A**: 643.

Tubiana R (1985) Notre expérience des transferts tendineux pour paralysie radiale, *Ann Chir Main* **4**: 197–210.

Zancolli EA (1957) Claw hand caused by paralysis of the intrinsic muscles. A simple procedure for its correction, *J Bone Joint Surg* **39A**: 1076–80.

Zancolli EA (1967) Paralytic supination contracture of the forearm, *J Bone Joint Surg* **49A**: 1275–84.

Zancolli EA (1979) *Structural and Dynamic Bases of Hand Surgery*, 2nd edn (Philadelphia: JB Lippincott) 174.

14 Trauma of the adult brachial plexus

Jean-Yves Alnot

Lesions can be situated at any level from the base of the nerve roots to the division of the brachial plexus in the axillary region and several types of lesions can be differentiated:

- Supraclavicular lesions at root or primary trunk level (75% of cases).
- Infra- and retro-clavicular lesions of secondary trunks (10% of cases).
- Terminal branches (15% of cases).

A better comprehension of pathological lesions (Sunderland 1978, Millesi 1984, Alnot et al 1996) leads to a clearer classification of injuries, because classifications are essential for evaluation of the results, particularly after nerve repair; and the use of charts and diagrams describing the nerve injuries and the type of repair is a great help for further follow-up.

Diagnosis and treatment

The traumatic brachial plexus injuries present numerous problems. They are characteristic of young adults aged 18–20 years who have sustained a motorcycle or car accident.

Whatever the clinical presentation (Figure 14.1) a patient showing no recovery at 4 or 6 weeks after a

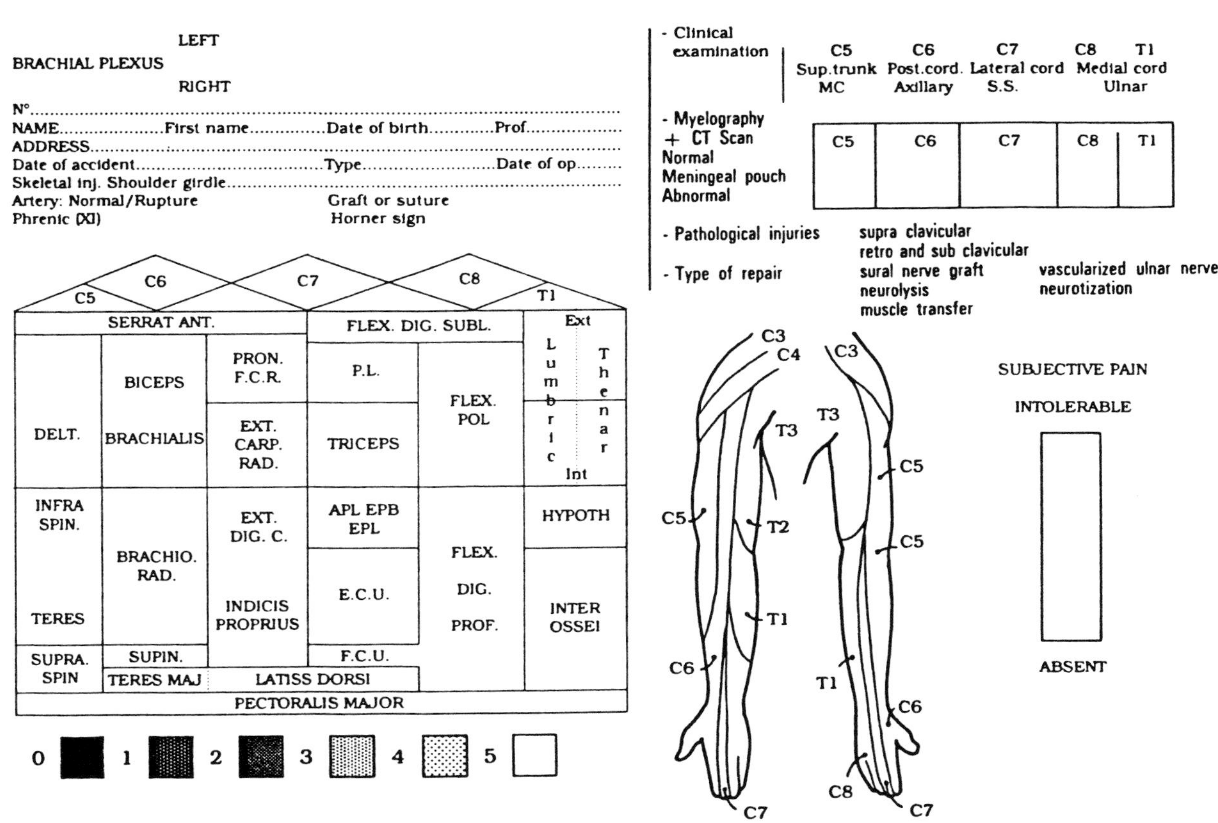

Figure 14.1

Chart for recording clinical and paraclinical findings.

traumatic palsy must undergo investigation (myelography combined with CTS and EMG) in order to identify the surgical indications at an early stage.

Our experience at Bichat Hospital includes >1200 cases operated between 1975 and 1998; the results have been published in several papers (Alnot et al 1989, 1993, 1996, 1998, Alnot 1993, 1995, Alnot and Oberlin 1993, Alnot and Narakas 1996). Many other authors have also published their experience (Narakas 1978, Brunelli and Manini 1984, Miltesi 1984, Sedel 1986, Ferzis 1987, Allieu et al 1997).

Palsies due to supraclavicular lesions

Among these lesions, which account for 75% of all cases, and which occur at two levels in 15%, the following can be distinguished:

- C5–C6 or C5–C6–C7 palsies which occur in 20–25% of cases;
- C8–T1, which occur in 2–3% of cases;
- C5–C6–C7–C8–T1 lesions, which are the most frequent, occurring in 75–80% of cases.

It is important to determine the exact site of the lesions as this will greatly influence the prognosis and the future of the patient.

Careful clinical and paraclinical examinations should be undertaken rapidly in order to obtain an exact diagnosis and permit intervention within a period of 6 weeks to 3 months after trauma.

Clinical examination, supported by paraclinical investigations, permits evaluation of nerve lesions according to the roots which have been affected, after which therapeutic indications and a prognosis can be made.

Some factors can be considered favourable – for example, a patient with a brachial plexus palsy secondary to dislocation of the shoulder due to a minor trauma has a 90% chance of recovery (Sunderland grades 1–3) – but in some cases there are ruptures at the level of the terminal branches with indications for repair.

In contrast, the following factors carry a poor prognosis:

- Violent trauma involving the upper limb as well as the plexus. Multiple bone fractures and other traumatic lesions are frequent in the upper limb that has been injured (21% of all cases), bone lesions are found in 58% of these cases and vascular lesions in 11%.
- Serratus anterior involvement and the presence of Horner's syndrome, both of which indicate a proximal lesion.
- Presence of pain and medullary signs suggesting injury to the cord.

Repeated clinical examination shows the evolution over time, and if there is no clinical recovery within a period of 30 days, paraclinical investigations such as CT scan-myelography and electromyography should be done. The value of CT scan-myelography is to establish the existence of root lesions and especially root avulsion with pseudomeningocele (rupture of the dura sheath and rootlets).

In peripheral mechanisms, depending on the direction of traction, the forces have an action on anterior and posterior rootlets.

Avulsion is a very specific injury at the level of spinal rootlets, and is beyond surgical possibilities for repair. The rootlets are avulsed from the spinal cord, notably C7 and mostly C8 and T1, which become horizontal with abduction of the arm. Superior C5 and C6 roots, because of their oblique route, are often ruptured more distally in the scalenic region. Nerve injury can also be located immediately next to the transverse canal, with frequent longitudinal disruption injuries and staged ruptures of the nerve fascicular groups, from the transverse canal to the interscalenic space. Nerve repair remains possible in some cases, but the proximal stump may have lost its possibility of axonal regeneration to some extent. In addition, damage to the fascicular groups in the transverse canal can cause retrograde degeneration of nerve fibres, involving the motor cell in the ventral horn or the sensory cell in the posterior ganglion, which is equivalent to avulsion.

Rupture can be more distal in the supraclavicular area, between the scalene muscles and beyond, preserving a proximal stump of root or of trunks of variable length and quality, possibly available for nerve repair.

Electromyography is also a part of the assessment and is particulary useful in C5–C6 and C5–C6–C7 palsies.

The surgical indications depend on the clinical evolution and the indications for surgery can be decided on the basis of all the factors discussed above. In our experience there is no indication for immediate nerve repair; the palsy is assessed by repeated motor and sensory examination and CT scan-myelography must be done if there is no clinical and electrical recovery after 4–8 weeks, depending on the general condition of the patient.

The prognosis depends on the anatomy and type of lesions and the early therapeutic indications (1–3 months) also depend on knowledge of the anatomical lesions.

Surgical procedure

The operation is carried out through a long zigzag cervico-axillary incision and the whole plexus must be explored.

Two types of skin incision are preferred by the author. The first comprises a large Z incision including a vertical cervical incision at the posterior border of the sternocleidomastoid (SCM) muscle; a horizontal subclavicular incision, and a vertical incision in the deltopectoral groove. The second comprises a multiple zigzag incision at the level of the cervical area to avoid a retractile scar and open V incisions in the subclavicular area and in the deltopectoral groove.

The key to the cervical approach is the omohyoid muscle. It must be located at the beginning of the dissection and must be transsected in the middle and retracted laterally in order to expose the supraclavicular plexus. The approach is done at the posterior border of the SCM; the external jugular vein must be preserved with the posterior SCM muscle belly. The lateral transverse branches must be ligated, but the nerve branches of the superficial cervical plexus must be preserved.

At the upper part of the triangle made by the SCM and the trapezius muscle, the C4 loop must be preserved onto the SCM muscle belly, this represents an important topographic landmark.

Then, the scalene outlet must be exposed and the phrenic nerve – at the anterior aspect of the anterior scalenus muscle – must be located and stimulated. The transverse cervical artery and vein must be ligated to complete the exposure of the plexus.

The suprascapular nerve is an essential landmark, as there is no nerve element lateral to it. It is also important to locate the Charles Bell nerve which must be preserved.

Finally, the spinal accessory nerve must be dissected if a neurotization is scheduled. It is important not to dissect it too proximally in order not to destroy the branches for the upper and mid trapezium. If neurotization must be done with the distal accessory spinal nerve, the section can be performed after the departure of the branches for the upper trapezius muscle.

The key to the subclavicular and axillary approach is the pectoralis minor muscle. The approach in the deltopectoral groove must be wide and must respect the cephalic vein.

De-insertion of the lateral part of the clavicular insertion of the anterior pectoralis major can be convenient.

The pectoralis minor must then be dissected and exposed and in certain cases, it may be necessary to divide it.

Communication between the cervical area and the axillary area is then established under the clavicle using a sponge held with a clamp. In the majority of cases, it is not necessary to cut the clavicle; this additional step (which has been recommended systematically by some authors) is now only done in sub- and retro-clavicular brachial plexus palsies.

The musculocutaneous nerve is identified as it enters the coracobiceps muscle. This must be systematic in all explorations in order to avoid a double level lesion.

The other nerves are identified and the dissection is performed distal to proximal and proximal to distal. The axillary artery can be also located.

A complete evaluation of the lesions is made after exploration of the whole plexus. However, if there are meningoceles on C8 and T1 it is not necessary to explore these roots, which are located deep and would entail a dangerous dissection.

At the end of the procedure, depending on the types of exploration and on the repair, closure is done plane by plane without drainage, or in certain cases a superficial drain can be placed at the distal part of the incision, at a distance from the nerve grafts.

In the immediate postoperative period, immobilization with the elbow against the thorax is done for a period of 3 weeks, associated with a cervical collar if nerve grafts have been performed at the level of the roots.

The type of repair depends on the localization of the lesions and in a majority of cases, there is a C7–C8 and T1 avulsion.

C5 and C6 roots are vertical and have lost their oblique direction and they will then be explored in the scalene outlet.

Nerve grafts (sural nerve or more rarely the ulnar nerve as a free or vascularized graft) will be performed depending on the root rupture in the scalenic area.

Neurotizations must be also performed (spinal accessory nerve, intercostal nerves, etc.). For intercostal nerve neurotization, a skin incision is performed below the pectoralis major muscle. Three intercostal nerves (D3-D4-D5) are transected anteriorly to perform a direct suture with the musculocutaneous nerve, for example.

Several clinical pictures can be described for palsies due to supraclavicular lesions, as discussed below.

The complete palsy without recuperation

Total palsies with avulsions of the lower roots

These are seen in 64% of cases. CT scan-myelography shows pseudomeningoceles at C8 and T1 and often at C7. C6 may have an abnormal aspect and C5 is usually normal in the CT scan.

In these total palsies with avulsion of the lower roots (C7–C8–T1), when only one or two roots are ruptured in the scalenic area, it is not possible to graft all the plexus. The surgery must be performed early (6 weeks to 3 months) and our approach is to aim for reinnervation of the proximal territories. Patients must be informed that they will have definitive paralysis of the hand.

The results depend on the anatomopathological lesions. When only one root (C5) can grafted (Figure 14.2A), our choice would be to repair the anterior part of the first trunk with the C5 root and the suprascapular nerve by neurotization (direct suture) with the spinal accessory nerve, which is divided distal to the origin of the branches for the superior and middle parts of the trapezius. The goal is to obtain stabilization of the shoulder, an active pectoralis major to adduct the arm, flexion of the elbow and some palmar sensibility in the forearm and palm.

When there are two roots (C5 + C6) (Figure 14.2B) which can be grafted, it is also possible to graft some parts of the posterior cord for radial or axillary nerve function. Every effort is made to connect the anterior plane of the root grafts with the anterior plane of the plexus and the posterior plane of the root with the

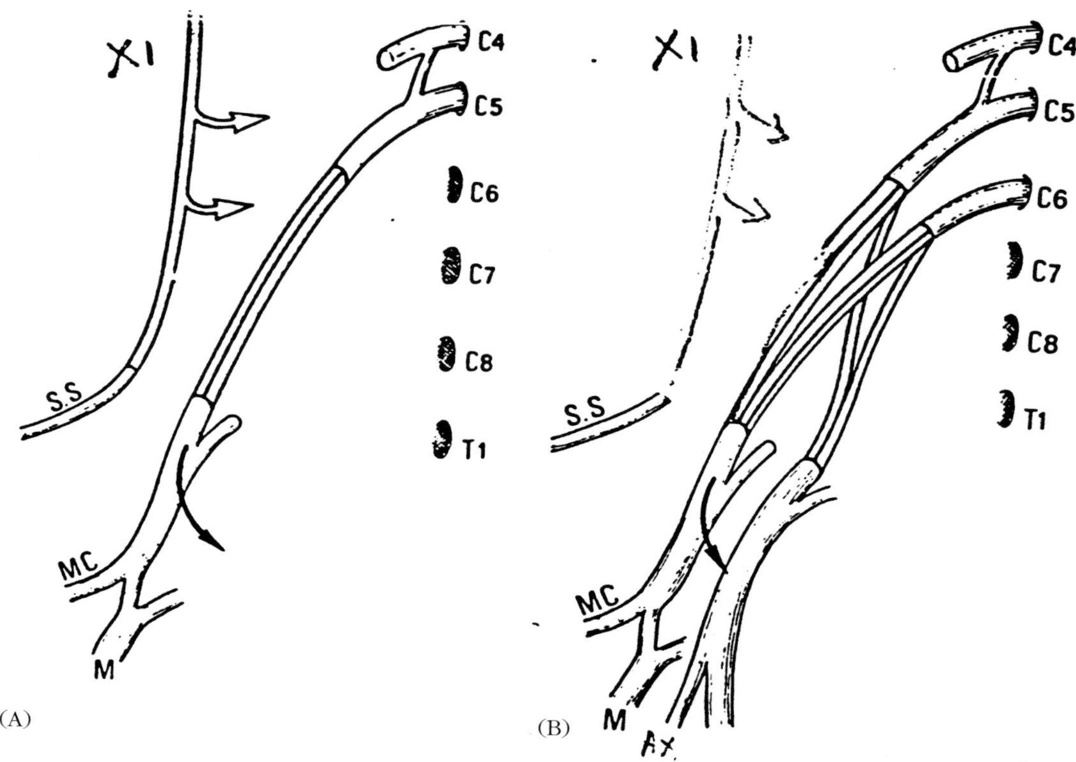

Figure 14.2
Total palsies. (A) Avulsion of C6–C7–C8–T1 with one graftable root. (B) Avulsion of C7–C8–T1 with two graftable roots.

posterior plane of the plexus in order to respect the cortical topography and to avoid co-contractions between antagonist muscles. The surgeon must not try to graft everything and if the roots are thin the technique is similar to that used for one graftable root. From the technical point we most frequently use the sural nerve, but when T1–C8–C7 are proved to be avulsed, it is possible to use a vascularized ulnar nerve graft (either free or pedicled) when the aspect and size of C5 or C5 and C6 are good and when the length of the nerve defect is longer than 15 cm.

The results must be analysed critically with evaluation of motor and sensory function. They can be evaluated only after sufficient time has elapsed, because reinnervation after nerve grafting is always delayed. This requires 2–3 years, depending on the type of lesion and its location (roots, trunks, cords and terminal branches) and the result must be evaluated according to the function of the structures to be repaired and therefore the therapeutic objectives to be achieved.

Finally, the pain syndrome must be considered, and it is important to stress that surgical interventions with nerve repair for any given region considerably modify the afferents originating in the upper limb.

The final functions (Narakas 1977, 1986, Brunelli and Monini 1984, Sedel 1986, Terzis 1987, Alnot et al 1993, Alnot 1995, Rusch et al 1995, Alnot and Narakas 1996, Allieu et al 1997) must be studied according to the nerve repair. They depend on the number of grafted roots, and a useful result means that as a minimum elbow flexion is possible. In our experience 75–80% of the patients have had satisfactory results with good elbow flexion at M3 + M4.

The pectoralis major function is obtained in 60% of cases, making it possible to hold objects against the thorax.

The shoulder poses problems, but it is possible to obtain stabilization of the shoulder, some active abduction and external rotation in 50% of cases by spinal accessory nerve neurotization; some authors perform shoulder arthrodesis.

It is rare to obtain function in the hand, but in the majority of cases, a 'shovel hand' or 'paperweight hand' is still useful to stabilize an object on a table. Finally, some sensation in the forearm and hand is obtained and this may explain why 80% of the patients suffer little or no pain.

Total palsies with avulsions of all roots

These occur in 24% of cases. CT scan-myelography shows meningoceles or lacunae on all the roots and there is no root available for repair. In these cases (Figure 14.3), neurotizations are indicated, utilizing the spinal accessory nerve, the cervical plexus, the intercostal nerves, and more rarely the hypoglossus nerve or the contralateral C7 root (Narakas 1977, Brunelli and

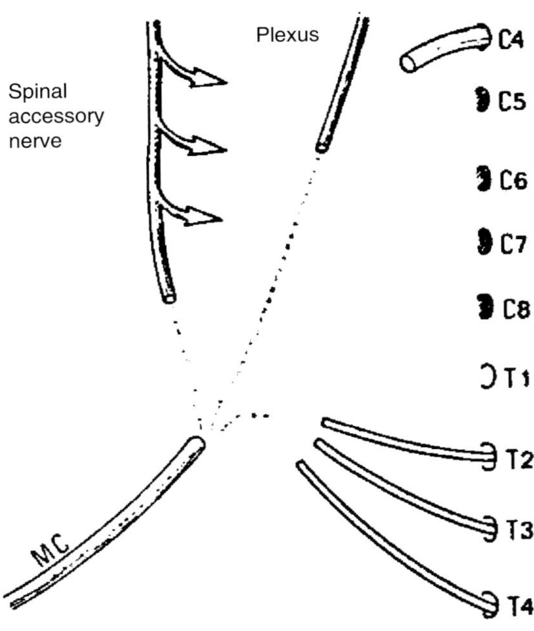

Figure 14.3
Total palsies with avulsion of all the roots, indicating possibilities for neurotizations.

Monini 1984, Alnot et al 1993, Allieu et al 1997). The goal is to provide elbow flexion by neurotization of the musculocutaneous nerve; this can be associated with shoulder arthrodesis.

When using the spinal accessory nerve associated with the superficial cervical plexus, an intervening autograft is necessary with two strands of sural nerve. The spinal motor fibres are connected to the lateral part of the musculocutaneous nerve trunk and we add sensory fibres from the cervical plexus connected to the medial part of the musculocutaneous nerve.

When using intercostal nerves, the neurotization can be performed by direct suture between intercostal nerves 3–4–5 divided in their anterior portion and the musculocutaneous nerve (Hara's technique).

The results are good in 75% of cases, with elbow flexion at M3 + M4 and the main problem is to establish whether other associated neurotizations can produce better results.

Partial palsies C5–C6 or C5–C6–C7

These occur in 25% of cases. The clinical pictures can be either C5–C6 or C5–C6–C7 palsies or an initial total palsy with rapid recovery in C8–T1.

The prognosis is dominated by the fact that the hand appears to be normal or only partially involved, but useful. Surgery must be done early because the lesions are often in the scalenic area on the roots or upper trunk, with a good possibility for nerve repair with a satisfactory result.

As regards the surgical approaches, the musculocutaneous nerve is identified as it enters the coracobiceps muscle and dissection from distal to proximal then allows dissection of the lateral cord and the anterior component of the upper trunk, as well as the posterior trunk, and then the posterior component of the upper trunk.

Then, the lesions must be located and repaired in the scalene space between the anterior and middle scalene muscles.

Lesions of C5–C6 and possibly C7 roots are evaluated and if there are ruptures in the scalenic area it is possible to perform grafts.

On the other hand, in C5–C6 avulsion we carry out a medial approach to the upper arm, approximately 120 mm distally below the acromial process, in order to perform a neurotization of the biceps nerve with a bundle of the ulnar nerve (Oberlin 1994).

Nerve reconstruction and muscular transfer will be studied according to a global scheme (Alnot and Oberlin 1993, Alnot et al 1998, Rostoucher et al 1998) and the indications are derived from the anatomopathological lesions (Figure 14.4).

In C5–C6 palsies when the two roots are disrupted in the scalenic area (Figure 14.4A) it is possible, if they are a good size and aspect, to graft all the lesions. However, if the roots are too small or when only one root is available (Figure 14.4B), the nerve fibres must not be dispersed and the graft must be performed to the anterior part of the first trunk. The addition of neurotization of the spinal accessory nerve on the suprascapular nerve produced better results than those obtained after graft from C5 with one strand of sural nerve. Another alternative is to also perform a graft on the axillary nerve and use ulnar biceps neurotization.

Finally in C5–C6 palsies when no roots are available (Figure 14.4C), we neurotize the spinal accessory nerve to the suprascapular nerve and perform a neurotization at the same operation, using a fascicular group of the ulnar nerve with direct suture on the biceps nerve (Oberlin 1994, Loy et al 1997, Leechavengvongs et al 1998), or perhaps after end-to-side neurorraphy (Viterbo et al 1994, Francoisi et al 1998).

At present the results of this ulnar biceps neurotization are good in C5–C6 palsies, but the results are still uncertain in C5–C6–C7 palsies and muscular transfer must be discussed and performed at the same operating time.

As regards C5–C6–C7 palsies, the overall plan is similar, but is complicated by the severity of the lesions. When all the roots are avulsed and when there are no acceptable possibilities for muscular transfer, we perform associated neurotizations to restore elbow flexion and shoulder stability.

Our results have been published in many papers (Alnot and Oberlin 1993, Alnot and Nakaras 1996, Alnot

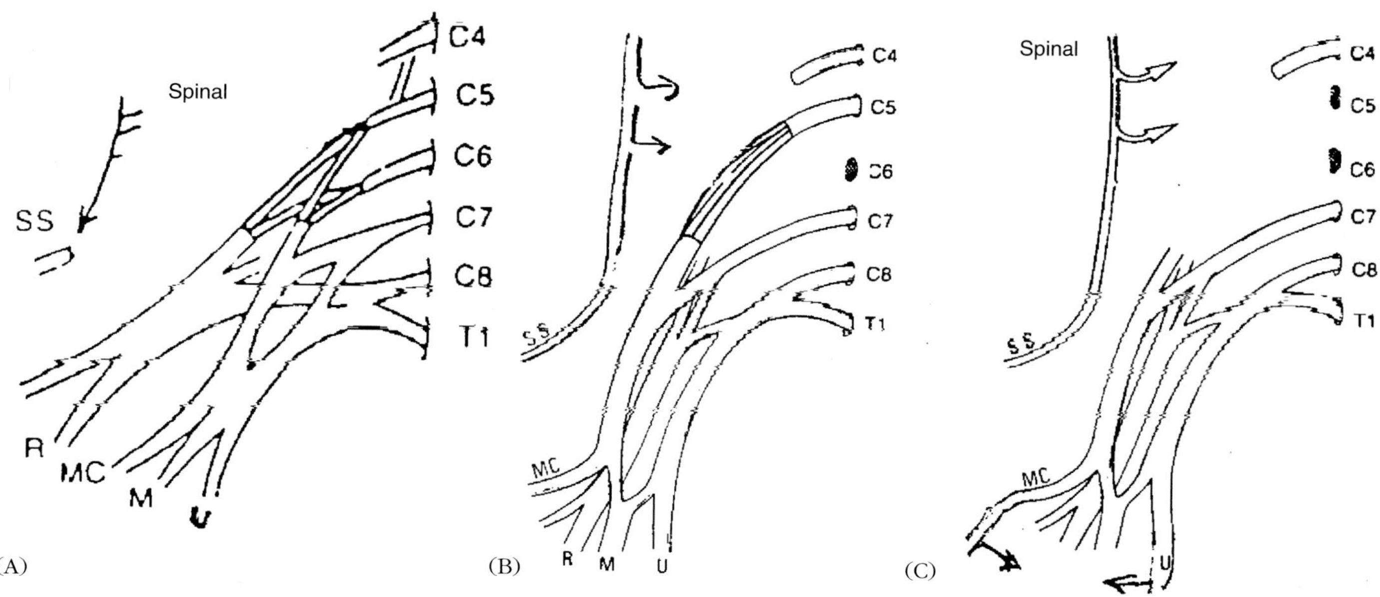

Figure 14.4

C5–C6 palsies. (A) Two graftable roots with good aspect and size: it is possible to graft all the lesions. (B) One graftable root C5 with possibilities for repair associated with accessory nerve neurotization. A similar repair is performed if there are two graftable roots of small size. (C) C5–C6 avulsion. Accessory nerve neurotization and ulnar biceps neurotization. Muscular transfers are also possible in C5–C6–C7 palsies.

et al 1996, Rostoucher et al 1998), they depend upon correct indications.

In C5–C6 palsies, active elbow flexion must be obtained in all cases by nerve surgery or muscular transfer.

The shoulder can be stabilized after accessory nerve neurotization, with recovery active anteposition and active external rotation are essential in order to allow more functional elbow flexion. However, the shoulder remains the main problem, with 73% of good results in C5–C6 cases and only 49% in C5–C6–C7 cases, because of the greater severity of the lesions.

Rotation osteotomy of the humerus, ligamentoplasty and arthrodesis can all be used. As regards the axillary nerve, an end-to-side neurorraphy is a possible new approach (Viterbo et al 1994, Francoisi et al 1998). Finally, with regard to the wrist and the hand in C5–C6–C7 palsies, there is always the possibility of muscular transfers, which can be decided at an early stage.

Partial palsies C8–T1

In these cases a decision regarding surgery will be based upon the results of the clinical examination and other diagnostic studies. Here again, the prognosis is determined by the degree of hand function and the severity of the nerve lesions. Myelography will reveal the presence or absence of pseudomeningoceles, and based on the degree of diagnostic certainty of the existence of avulsion of different roots, the clinical status should be re-evaluated and a decision made regarding surgical exploration.

If pseudomeningoceles involve the lower roots, exploration is not justified and muscle transfers are the next step (Alnot 1993, Alnot and Narakas 1996). However, if the myelograms are normal but spontaneous regeneration has not occurred, surgery is appropriate for assessment and possibly for nerve repair. It is important to remember that if C8 and Tl roots or even some more distal lesions of the trunk and cords can be repaired by nerve grafts, the distance between the nerve lesions and hand precludes reinnervation of the intrinsic muscles.

Palsies due to retro- and infra-clavicular lesions

Retro- and infra-clavicular lesions represent 25% of cases, and the nerve lesions are frequently associated with bone and vascular lesions (Alnot and Narakas 1996). The diagnosis and prognosis are based on the results of clinical examination. CT scan-myelography is normal and electromyography often shows diffuse signs that are difficult to evaluate.

The patients can be schematically divided in two groups. The first group comprises those with lesions affecting the secondary trunks behind and under the clavicle. In these cases the diagnosis is most difficult, with frequent associated bone and vascular lesions. The treatment is complex and a clavicle osteotomy is necessary in order to make an adequate assessment. The associated vascular lesions increase the problem and it appears judicious to repair not only the nerves but also the vessels, even if there is an adequate vascular supply. This gives a better chance for nerve regeneration. In our experience of brachial plexus palsies with vascular ruptures, the nerve lesions are severe and two situations may arise. One is a severe ischaemic syndrome in which emergency vascular repair is necessary, and very difficult technical problems can be expected during secondary nerve repair. In the other situation there is no acute ischaemia and it is judicious to carry out secondary repair of nerves and vessels at the same operation.

The surgical approaches will require a transection of the pectoralis minor muscle belly and clavicle osteotomy. Before performing the osteotomy, the fixation plate must be contoured on to the anterior edge of the clavicle and used for predrilling the screw holes. The nerve lesions are very important. Posterior cord injuries are the most frequent and can either be isolated or associated with concomitant lesions (posterior + lateral + medial cord); they may account for a more complex clinical picture and treatment. The exploration is long and difficult, and because of multiple and diffuse lesions repair presents problems owing to the length of the lesions and limited stock of nerve graft (Alnot and Narakas 1996).

The results are difficult to judge because of the very varied anatomopathological lesions (from the first to the fifth Sunderland degree of gravity), which are complicated by proximal nerve trunk lesions. The main problems concern the median and the ulnar nerves.

The second group of patients in this category comprises those with distal lesions affecting the terminal branches of the plexus (Alnot and Narakas 1996, Alnot et al 1996). Clinically, the sensory and motor signs are established and in the majority of cases the lesions involve the axillary nerve. In typical cases the clinical picture is characterized by a paralytic shoulder, but the diagnosis can be difficult because a complete palsy of the deltoid muscle may exist without any functional loss except loss of power. This is due to the compensatory action of the rotator cuff muscles and explains the frequent delay in diagnosis and treatment.

In these injuries, which are caused by stretching, the nerve lesion is usually located at a level of relative fixation (quadrilateral space for the axillary nerve, coracoid notch for the suprascapular nerve and entry into the coracobrachialis muscle for the musculocutaneous nerve). There may be a Sunderland grade one or two lesion which recovers spontaneously, but the nerve is ruptured in about 20% of cases and operation is indicated if there is no clinical and electrical recovery at 4–6 months.

Surgical approach in the deltopectoral groove makes it possible to locate the proximal stump of the axillary nerve posteriorly and the musculocutaneous nerve anteriorly. An additional posterior approach is then necessary at the posterior edge of the posterior deltoid in order to dissect the distal stump. The nerve graft, generally done with two strands, is pulled out anteriorly from the posterior approach through the quadrilateral space using a strong nylon. The distal microsuture is performed first and the posterior approach is closed immediately; proximal suture is performed as a secondary procedure.

Axillary nerve injury is often associated with lesions of other terminal branches. The musculocutaneous nerve lesion is easy to expose through the anterior approach, but the problem is much more difficult in the case of suprascapular nerve injury. In some cases, it will be necessary to dissect the nerve distally until it crosses the coracoid fossa, which represents a fixed level where rupture can occur. In those cases, it is very difficult or even impossible to expose the distal stump, and an additional posterior approach is required at the level of the scapular spine and of the supraspinatus fossa.

The results (Alnot and Narakas 1996, Alnot et al 1996) after graft are good on the whole because of the proximity of the muscle, and we obtain 90% recovery at M3 + M4 after axillary or musculocutaneous repair.

Conclusions

An update of this problem was published in a monograph by Alnot and Narakas in 1996, with many contributors. Preoperative diagnosis is fundamental, and clinical evaluation and other investigations (CT scan-myelography, electromyography) must be used to arrive at coherent therapeutic indications.

If surgery is indicated, the preoperative assessment must anticipate any pathological lesions that may be encountered, in order to form a specific surgical plan. Early surgical exploration (6 weeks to 3 months) will permit evaluation of these lesions and determination of the possibilities for neurolysis, nerve grafts or neurotization.

The best results evidently occur in the upper root partial palsies involving C5–C6 supraclavicular lesions and also in terminal branch lesions. However, in total root paralysis, the increasing percentage of useful return of function – depending upon the roots grafted and the structures repaired – suggests that this type of surgery must be carried out with precise and early indications.

References

Allieu Y, Chammas M, Picot MC (1997) Paralysie du plexus brachial par lesions supraclaviculaires chez l'adulte. Résultats comparatifs à long terme des greffes nerveuses et des transferts nerveux, *Rev Chir Orthop* **83**: 51–9.

Alnot JY (1993) *La Main Plexique.* Atteinte du poignet et de la main dans les paralysies traumatiques du plexus brachial de l'adulte. Presented at Cahier des Conferences d'Enseignement de la Sociéte Française de Chirurgie de la Main (GEM), Expansion Scientifique Française, 1993, pp. 129–43.

Alnot JY (1995) Traumatic brachial plexus lesions in the adult. Indications and results, *Hand Clin* **11**: 623–33.

Alnot JY, Narakas A eds, (1989) *Les Paralysies du Plexus Brachial,* 1st and 2nd edn. (Monographie du GEM, Expansion Scientifique, Paris); (1989 and 1995) *Traumatic Brachial Plexus Injuries,* (English edn) (Monographie du GEM, Expansion Scientifique: Paris).

Alnot JY, Oberlin C (1993) Tendon transfers in palsies of flexion and extension of the elbow. In: Tubiana R, ed., *The Hand,* Vol IV. (WB Saunders: Philadelphia) 134–46.

Alnot JY, Daunois O, Oberlin C et al (1993) Total palsy of brachial plexus by supra-clavicular Iesions, *J Orthop Surg* **7**: 58–66.

Alnot JY, Liverneaux PH, Silberman O (1996) Les lésions du nerf axillaire, *Rev Chir Orthop* **82**: 579–90.

Alnot JY, Rostoucher P, Oberlin C, Touam C (1998) Les paralysies traumatiques C5–C6 et C5–C6–C7 du plexus brachial de l'adulte par lésions supraclaviculaires, *Rev Chir Orthop* **84**: 113–23.

Brunelli G, Monini L (1984) Neurotization of avulsed roots of brachial plexus by means of anterior nerves of cervical plexus, *Clin Plast Surg* **11**: 144–53.

Franciosi LF, Modestti C, Mueller SF (1998) Neurotization of the biceps muscle by end to side neurorraphy between ulnar and musculocutaneous nerves. A series of five cases, *Ann Chir Main* **17**: 362–7.

Leechavengvongs S, Witoonchart K, Uepairojkit Ch et al (1998) Nerve transfer to biceps muscle using a part of the ulnar nerve in brachial plexus injury (upper arm type): a report of 32 cases, *J Hand Surg* **23A**: 711–16.

Loy S, Bhatia A, Asfazadourian H, Oberlin C (1997) Ulnar nerve fascicle transfer on the biceps motor nerve in C5–C6 or C5–C6–C7 avulsion of the brachial plexus based on a series of 18 cases, *Ann Hand Upper Limb Surg* **16**: 275–84.

Millesi H (1984) Brachial plexus injuries. Management and results, *Clin Plast Surg* **11**: 115–21.

Narakas A (1977) The surgical management of brachial plexus injuries. In: Daniel RK, Terzis IK, eds, *Reconstructive Surgery.* (Little Brown: Boston).

Narakas A (1978) Surgical treatment of traction injuries of the brachial plexus, *Clin Orthop* **133**: 71–90.

Narakas A (1986) Les neurotisations ou transferts nerveux dans le traitement des lesions traumatiques du plexus brachial. In: Tubiana R, ed., *Traité de Chirurgie de la Main. Chirurgie des Tendons, des Nerfs et des Vaisseaux,* Vol. 3. (Masson: Paris) 542–68.

Oberlin C (1994) Nerve transfer to biceps muscle using a part of ulnar nerve for C5–C6. Avulsion of the brachial plexus. Anatomical studies and report of four cases, *J Hand Surg* **19A**: 232–7.

Rostoucher P, Alnot JY, Oberlin C, Touam C (1998) Tendon tranfers to restore elbow flexion after traumatic paralysis of the brachial plexus in adults, *Int Orthop* **22**: 255–63.

Rusch DS, Friedman A, Nunley JA (1995) The restoration of elbow flexion with intecostal nerve transfer, *Clin Orthop* **314**: 95–103.

Sedel L (1986) Resultats des reparations microchirurgicales du plexus brachial. A propos d'une serie de 170 cas. In: Tubiana R, ed., *Traite de Chirurgie de la Main. Chirurgie des Tendons, des Nerfs et des Vaisseaux,* Vol. 3 (Masson: Paris) 568–71.

Sunderland S (1978) *Nerves and Nerve Injuries,* 2nd edn. (Churchill Livingstone: Edinburgh) 854–900.

Terzis J (1987) *Microreconstruction of Nerve Injuries.* (WB Saunders: Philadelphia).

Viterbo F, Trindade JCS, Hoschino K, Mazzoni Nito A (1994) End to side neurorraphy with removal of the epineural sheath. Experimental study in rat, *Plast Reconstr Surg* **94**: 1038–47.

15 Paralysis of terminal branches of the brachial plexus

Rolfe Birch, William Williams and Robert J Spinner

Introduction

Ruptures of the cords and of the terminal branches of the brachial plexus are usually caused by violent injury. They are often complicated by fractures or fracture/dislocations of the shoulder girdle. The incidence of injury to the axial vessels is high. Penetrating missile injuries cause extensive damage to skin and muscle. Closed traction lesions result in extensive longitudinal injury to the nerve trunks which retract widely if ruptured. Nerves are particularly vulnerable to the activities of surgeons working on the shoulder joint or humerus. The prognosis for restoration of hand function after repair of the long nerves, the radial, median and ulnar, is compromised by the level of injury. Diagnosis and treatment is urgent and in the presence of an arterial injury, it is an emergency. The operating surgeon needs to be able to treat the vascular and the skeletal injuries as well as the neurological injury. The prognosis for the lesion in continuity of the nerve trunk, commonly seen after penetrating missile injuries or after stretching injury, is particularly perplexing.

Three significant nerves pass from the brachial plexus in the posterior triangle of the neck. The nerve to serratus anterior (C5, C6, C7), the dorsal scapular nerve (C5) and the suprascapular nerve (C5, upper trunk).

The divisions of the brachial plexus lie deep to the clavicle and their display in a scarred field can be particularly tedious. The posterior division of the upper and the middle trunk is consistently larger than the anterior division. In perhaps 10% of cases there is no posterior division of the lower trunk. The formation and relations of the three cords are variable. Immediately inferior to the clavicle the posterior cord lies lateral to the axillary artery; the medial cord behind and the lateral cord in front. The cords assume their appropriate relations about the axillary artery deep to pectoralis minor. Miller (1939) found considerable variation in 9% of 480 dissections of the neurovascular axis. In the most common variation the axillary artery lies anterior to the three cords and the median nerve.

The branches of the posterior cord, the largest of the three trunks, are consistent: in sequence they are the subscapular, the thoraco-dorsal and the circumflex nerves. The branches of the medial cord are usually predictable. First the medial pectoral nerve, the medial cutaneous nerve of forearm, then the division into the medial root of the median nerve and the ulnar nerve. Not infrequently, the ulnar nerve arises as two or three branches.

The greatest variation in formation of trunk nerves is found within the lateral cord. In about 10% of cases the musculocutaneous nerve arises more distally than usual, springing directly from the lateral cord as two or three branches or even from the median nerve itself. The lateral root of the median nerve may arise as two or three branches, in some cases it appears as a branch of the musculocutaneous nerve. These variations of formation of the terminal branches of the plexus and their variation to the great vessels are important because they can cause difficulty during urgent exploration.

The clinical material which forms the basis of this chapter is set out in Table 15.1. We also relate our experience of the 11th cranial nerve, the spinal accessory nerve, because damage to this has such severe

Table 15.1 *Operations for injuries to the infraclavicular brachial plexus and terminal branches showing incidence of vascular injuries, 1970–2000*

Injuries	*Total*	*Vascular*
Involving supraclavicular and circumflex nerves	176	16
From dislocation of shoulder without nerve rupture	52	5
From shoulder dislocation with vascular injury but no nerve rupture in patients aged over 55 years	14	14
Multiple nerve ruptures, open and closed traction	314	104
Penetrating missile injuries	71	32
Spinal accessory nerve	148	4
Nerve to serratus anterior	20	1
Total	795	176

Table 15.2 *Vascular injuries encountered in lesions of the brachial plexus and terminal branches, 1975–2000*

	Closed Total	*Repaired*	*Open Total*	*Repaired*
Subclavian	82	40	9	9
Axillary	63	54	31	27
Brachial	7	6	35	31

Traumatic false aneurysms and arteriovenous fistulae with associated nerve injuries

	Aneurysm	*Arteriovenous fistula*
Axillary	20	4
Brachial	4	2

consequences for function and for the upper limb as a whole. Important patterns of injury will be discussed before we turn to individual nerve trunks. These include:

1. The infraclavicular injury from closed traction injury.
2. Nerves injured by fractures or fracture/dislocations.
3. Penetrating missile injuries.

We shall also refer to the significance of the associated arterial injury and the requirement for adequate exposure in dealing with this (Table 15.2).

The closed infraclavicular traction lesion

We think that this is among the worst of all true peripheral nerve injuries. It is characterized by the violence of the causal lesion and by the high incidence of rupture of the axillary artery (about 25% in our cases). Bonney introduced a policy of primary repair of the neurovascular injury for this group in the 1960s at St Mary's Hospital, London (Birch et al 1998a). This policy has been followed since then in our unit. About one-half of the neurovascular injuries discussed in this chapter have been treated in this way (Figure 15.1).

It is common to find nerve trunks ruptured at different levels up and down the limb and it is not rare to find them avulsed from muscle bellies. Alnot (1988) emphasized the technical difficulty of nerve repair where there had been widespread longitudinal nerve injury in a large series, and noted that two level injury (preganglionic injury of a spinal nerve with peripheral rupture) occurred in 15% of cases (Figure 15.2).

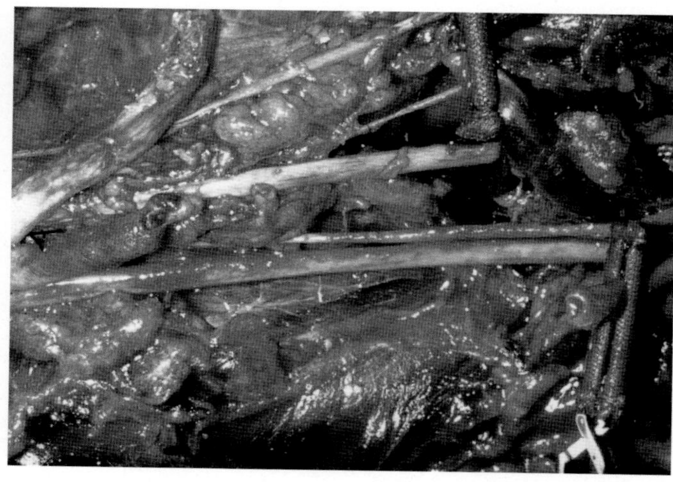

Figure 15.1
A 24-year-old male, following a motorcycle accident. Fracture of the proximal humerus, and rupture of the axillary artery and radial nerve. The arterial stumps are retracted. There is extensive longitudinal damage within the ruptured nerve trunks and also within the distal artery.

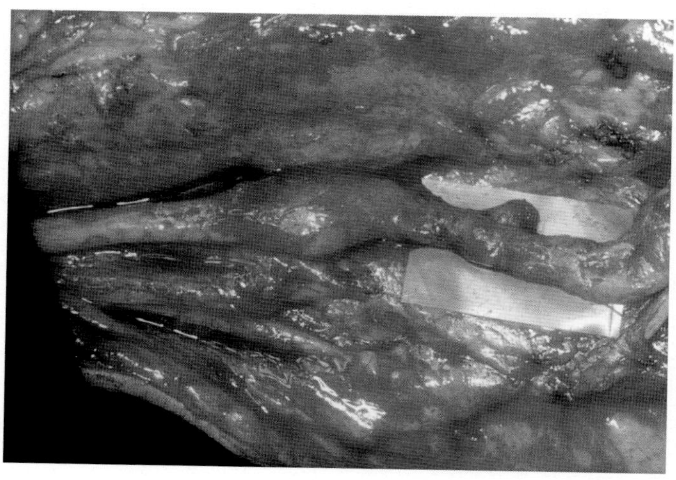

Figure 15.2
A 17-year-old woman. High speed motorcycle accident with fracture/dislocation at shoulder and fracture of distal humerus. The axillary artery was ruptured at the level of the coracoid. The musculocutaneous nerve was torn from the lateral cord at that level. Here, the median nerve is shown just proximal to the elbow, with extensive longitudinal destruction of the trunk.

The advantages of urgent repair of the vessel and the nerves at the same time include: ease of identification of ruptured structures, the use of the nerve stimulator to detect more distal nerve injuries and the ability to diminish the gap between related nerve stumps. The exposure of Fiolle and Delmas (1921) is ideally suited to these cases.

Cavanagh et al (1987) outlined the results of the repair in 89 cases operated over a 10-year period. In 46% there was damage to the subclavian and axillary arteries; in 52% there was bony injury. Indications for operation included signs of arterial injury, evidence of severe local trauma with a deep neural lesion. A good case for primary repair was made out. In some late referred cases nerve repair was abandoned because of technical difficulty or because the state of the tissues was so poor. As might be expected, results were a good deal better for the suprascapular, the circumflex, the radial and the musculocutaneous nerves than they were for the median and ulnar nerves. What was particularly striking was the effect of delay. Results were very much better in nerves repaired within 14 days of injury than in those repaired later. Only one of 22 cases of median and ulnar nerve repairs achieved a good result in that delayed repair group.

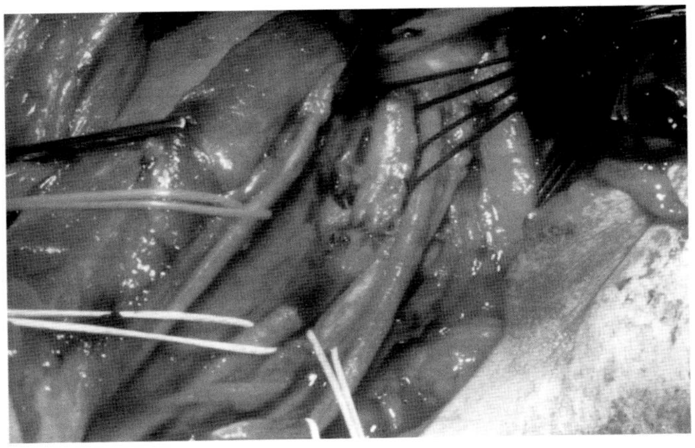

Figure 15.3

Closed traction lesion in a 33-year-old man. The rupture of the intima of the axillary artery is seen as a clear crescent-shaped margin. The adventitia contains a length of thrombus.

The vascular injury

Ligation of axial arteries was widely practised in World Wars I and II. Tinel (1917) described the consequences of ligation of the subclavian artery: intense pain, followed by hypersensitivity, which progressed to complete anaesthesia and paralysis. Makins (1919) observed that lacerations of the subclavian or axillary artery led to general depression of motor and sensory function in the limb.

De Bakey and Simeone (1946, 1955) found that nearly 50% of limbs came to amputation after ligation of an axial vessel in nearly 2500 arterial injuries. Hughes and Bowers (1961) wrote, 'we have been amazed at the lack of interest and knowledge of many surgeons who have no idea as to which vessels may be safely ligated'. Harsh words! Sadly, we have found them applicable today. Eastcott and colleagues (1992) condemned sympathectomy in the treatment of the acute limb ischaemia. Narakas (1987) commented 'vascular prostheses should not be used in young patients with brachial plexus injury. Prostheses cannot adapt to changes in the calibre of the anastomotic site and may leak causing minor or massive haemorrhage which afterwards embeds the nerve trunks in a fibrotic mass'.

Closed traction injury of the vessels causes fracture of the intima, which progresses to rupture of all coats of the vessel. The intimal injury can be seen as a pale crescent-shaped line, the damaged segment of the artery being filled with thrombus. Attempts to restore flow using embolectomy catheters are futile. We found that the length of damage ranged from 3 to 28 cm. The brittle atheromatous vessels of older patients are vulnerable even in low energy injuries (Figure 15.3).

While we have occasionally found vessels lacerated by fractures of the clavicle or proximal humerus, the artery is nearly always ruptured deep to pectoralis minor in an infraclavicular traction lesion. Arteriography, while valuable, should not unduly delay operation. A reasonable circulation of the skin is not the issue: what is important is whether the muscles are perfused. Failure to restore flow through a damaged axillary or common brachial artery within 6 hours of injury is usually followed by, at least, some post-ischaemic fibrosis. In most cases the clinical diagnosis was obvious. The posterior triangle was neither swollen nor deeply bruised; the subclavian pulse was palpable whereas in the infraclavicular fossa there was swelling with bruising of the skin. The brachial pulse was absent.

Repair is by reversed vein graft using interrupted sutures of between 6/0 and 8/0 nylon. The apparent cause of failure of arterial repair in the 32 cases sent to us, which we revised, included:

- The use of embolectomy catheter (4 cases).
- The use of continuous suture leading to stenosis and later thrombosis (20 cases).
- Inadequate resection of the damaged vessel in closed traction lesions (8 cases).

In other referred cases the initial triumph in restoring arterial circulation was lost by failure to decompress the limb. Division of the axillary and brachial sheath and of the deep fascia of the forearm is essential in all cases except those where a simple wound is successfully sutured within 3 hours of injury. Rupture of the axillary or subclavian vein is uncommon in closed lesions (6 cases) but more frequent in open wounds (18 cases). Ischaemic fibrosis was particularly severe in these cases. For a more extensive description of exposure and of techniques in arterial repair, the reader is referred to Birch et al (1998a) and Barros d'Sa (1992).

Nerves injured by fractures and fracture/dislocations

'Compound nerve injuries' are those in which the damage to a nerve or nerves is associated with major damage to other tissues or organs such as skin, muscle, skeleton, viscera and major vessels at the same site (Birch et al 1998b)). Many injuries to the terminal branches fall within this group.

Nerves are injured by damage to the adjacent skeleton by: traction from displacement, laceration by a fragment of bone, entrapment within the dislocated joint or in the fracture, and later entrapment or compression by callus. On the whole, dislocations are more damaging (Figure 15.4). It seems to be widely assumed that the prognosis for nerves injured in this way is good but this is generally not the case. Seddon (1975a), thought that in nerves injured in the arm and at the elbow by fractures or fracture/dislocations recovery could be awaited if two conditions were met: 'the first is reasonable apposition of the bony fragments and the other *is complete certainly that there is no threat of ischaemia of the forearm muscles*'.

Seigel and Gelberman (1991) in an extensive review found 85% of nerve palsies recovering from closed fractures and 65–70% after open fractures. However, of those nerves that went on to recover 90% had done so by 4 months and these cannot have been wholly degenerative lesions; there must have been an element of conduction block. Seigel and Gelberman's indications for intervention include:

- The fracture needs internal fixation.
- There is associated vascular injury.
- Wound exploration of an open fracture is necessary.
- A fracture or dislocation is reducible.

We suggest two more:

- The lesion deepens while it is under observation.
- The lesion occurred during operation for internal fixation.

It is often assumed that the prognosis for radial nerve palsy in closed fractures of the proximal mid-shaft of humerus is good. We are not sure about this, and suggest that the surgeon embarking on an operation of open reduction and internal fixation in a patient with radial nerve palsy should expose that nerve during the operation and that the presence of such a nerve palsy adds weight to the argument for open intervention.

Dislocation of the shoulder

Injury to the infraclavicular plexus associated with anterior dislocation of the shoulder is produced by the pressure of the head of the humerus intruding onto the cords and the terminal branches of the plexus. The medial and posterior cords are predominantly affected. The lesion will become more extensive so long as the humeral head is permitted to stretch the plexus. In a few cases the lesion is permitted to deepen from recoverable axonotmesis to irrecoverable neurotmesis through failure to recognize the

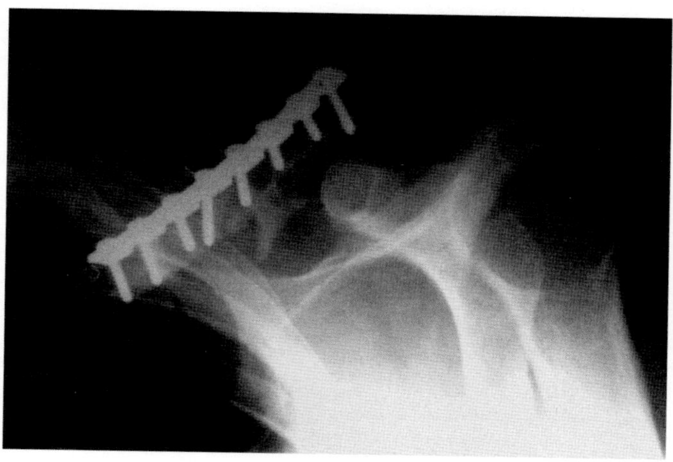

Figure 15.4

A 38-year-old man with a comminuted fracture of the clavicle from a direct blow. The displaced spike of bone had perforated the axillary artery and was embedded within the lateral cord of the brachial plexus. Pain was intense. Closure of the false aneurysm after removal of the bone fragment was followed by rapid relief of pain and complete recovery.

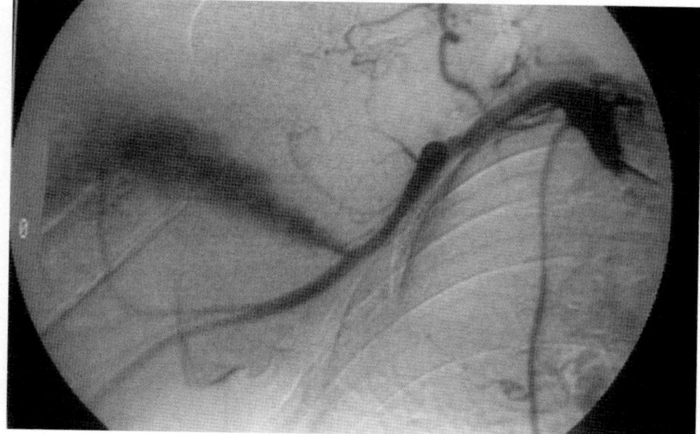

Figure 15.5

An 85-year-old woman with fracture/dislocation of the shoulder. Eight weeks after the injury the false aneurysm burst. There was rapid but painless loss of sensation and of power. Closure of the false aneurysm and evacuation of the haematoma was followed by complete recovery. Operation was done at 6 hours from the onset of neurological symptoms.

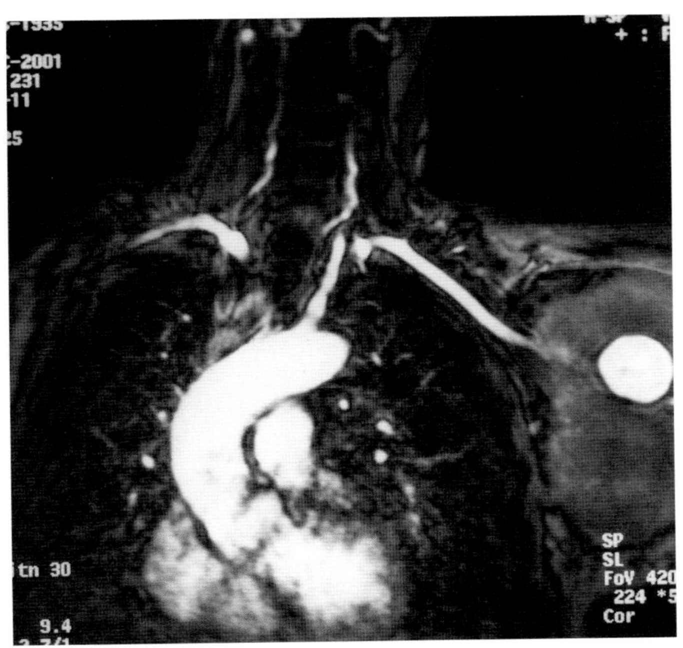

Figure 15.6
A 68-year-old man showing an enormous false aneurysm from damage to circumflex vessels in dislocation of the shoulder. The correct diagnosis was not made for 3 months by which time the patient was nearly moribund. There was complete brachial plexus palsy. The defect in the axillary artery was closed and the haematoma was excised. There was early relief of pain. Neurological recovery was slow and incomplete.

dislocation. Intervention without delay in cases in which unrecognized dislocation has produced a deepening extensive lesion of the infraclavicular part of the plexus is justified. Flaubert's (1827) account of late closed reduction of dislocation of the shoulder by manual traction is salutary. He recorded a Bernard Horner sign long before this was formally described; at necropsy there was rupture of C5, avulsion of C6, C7, C8 and T1. The subclavian artery was ruptured. Radicular vessels had been ruptured leading to a haematoma within the spinal canal.

Bigliani et al (1991) found that ruptures of the axillary artery, secondary to shoulder fractures or dislocations, accounted for 7% of all arterial injuries. We have seen 14 cases, in older patients, who suffered damage to the axillary artery from fractures of the proximal humerus in low energy injuries. The nerves are injured by ischaemia or compression by an expanding haematoma or aneurysm (Figures 15.5 and 15.6).

Penetrating missile injuries

Delorme (1915), then Inspector General of the Medical Services of the armies of France, proposed a method of treatment for shell and bullet wounds based on three principles: resection of scar until a healthy bed was secured; excision of damaged nerve until healthy stumps were reached; and tension-free suture by adequate mobilization and flexion of adjacent joints, or grafting. This work was heavily criticized at the time but his advice was supported by Tinel (1917) who added 'when the distance between the segments of the nerve trunk is too great to permit direct suture *the only legitimate operation is nerve grafting* as recommended by J&A Dejeurine and Mouzon'. Seddon (1975a) thought that 'longitudinal extent of the fibrosis is a reflection of the distortion that the nerve has suffered and in this there is probably an element akin to traction'. In his series of 379 median and ulnar nerves damaged by missiles no less than 70% had been divided or partially divided.

Omer (1974) sutured 83 nerves, finding useful recovery in 40%. His worst group were the above-elbow high velocity missile injuries. Brown (1970) sutured 135 nerves in the upper limb; 44% regained useful function, and the ulnar nerve fared worst. Omer confirmed the findings of Woodhall and Beebe (1956) who said, on the basis of more than 3000 nerve sutures following war wounds, that: 'delay in suture involves a loss of, on average, about 1% of maximal performance for every six days of delay'. Gousheh (1995) described great experience in the treatment of 369 war injuries of the brachial plexus. Major arterial injury complicated 74 of these. Results were at least useful in 45 from 54 of the repaired roots and in 87% of 107 cord elements. The results from repair in these injuries were better than those for closed traction lesions.

The largest published series of civilian gunshot injuries comes from Kline (1989) – 141 wounds of the brachial plexus (90 operated cases). Arterial injury was found in one-third of the brachial plexus injuries; 125 nerve elements were repaired. Recovery was at least useful for lesions: of C5, C6 and C7 lesions, to the upper and middle trunks and the posterior and lateral cords. The value of recording compound nerve action potentials (CNAPs) across the lesion has been demonstrated (Kline and Hudson 1975a); CNAPs were demonstrated traversing the lesion in 48 of 166 cases. Good or useful results followed neurolysis in 44 of these 48 lesions. In the absence of CNAP the lesion was resected and grafted and histological examination of the resected specimens confirmed neurotmetic changes in each case.

Stewart and Birch (2001) analysed 58 patients with penetrating missile injuries to the brachial plexus. The Red Cross Wound Classification was used to define the extent of tissue damage and indicate the violence of the injury. Grade 1, low energy transfer (LET) wounds were caused by metallic fragments. Grade 2, high energy transfer (HET) were predominantly caused by military rifle bullets. Grade 3, massive energy transfer were caused by close range shotgun blasts or other similar blast injuries. The indications for operation included vascular injury (16), severe persisting pain (35) or

Table 15.3 *Results of repair of 56 elements (36 patients) in penetrating missile wounds*

	Roots/trunks		*Cords/nerves*	
	Number of nerve elements	*Number of patients*	*Number of nerve elements*	*Number of patients*
Good	2	2	1	1
Useful	12	8	20	15
Poor	15	4	4	4
Unknown	0		2	2
Total	29	14	27	22
Results of decompression of 47 lesions in continuity (23 patients)				
Good	13	7	5	4
Useful	11	3	15	7
Poor	0	0	0	0
Unknown	0	9	3	2
Total	24	19	23	13

From Stewart MPM, Birch R (2001) Penetrating missile injuries of the brachial plexus. *J Bone Joint Surg* **83**: 517–24, by kind permission of the Editor.

complete loss of function in the distribution of one or more elements of the brachial plexus. In 36 patients nerve graft of one or more elements of the plexus was done; good or useful results were obtained in 26. Poor results followed repair of the medial cord and the ulnar nerve but especially in patients with the associated injury to the spinal cord (Table 15.3).

The response to treatment of patients with severe pain was striking:

1. Causalgia. This, the most severe of the neuropathic pain states, is usually provoked by a partial transection of the lower roots of the brachial plexus, below a trunk and the medial cord or derivative nerve. It was seen in 10 patients, and characterized by intense burning pain extending beyond the area of the injured nerve, by severe allodynia and by hyperpathia. Disturbance of sympathetic function was obvious. Pain worsened in response to emotional or other physical stimulae. One patient recovered spontaneously. In the other nine patients causalgia was cured by repair of the damaged nerves and correction of the false aneurysm or arteriovenous fistulae seen in seven. Sympathectomy was performed only once. (See Figures 15.7 and 15.8.)
2. Neurostenalgia This pain, caused by persisting compression, distortion or ischaemia of a nerve, was observed in 19 patients. In most of these the nerve trunk was intact and the lesion was neurapraxia or at worst, axonotmesis. In neurostenalgia the nerve is, in some way, irritated, tethered, compressed or ischaemic. Treatment of the cause relieves the pain and in all 10 patients liberation of the nerve trunk from an entrapment in scar tissue or callus or after removal of a missile fragment was complete.
3. Post-traumatic neuralgia occurs after partial nerve injury; it is not sympathetically maintained. It

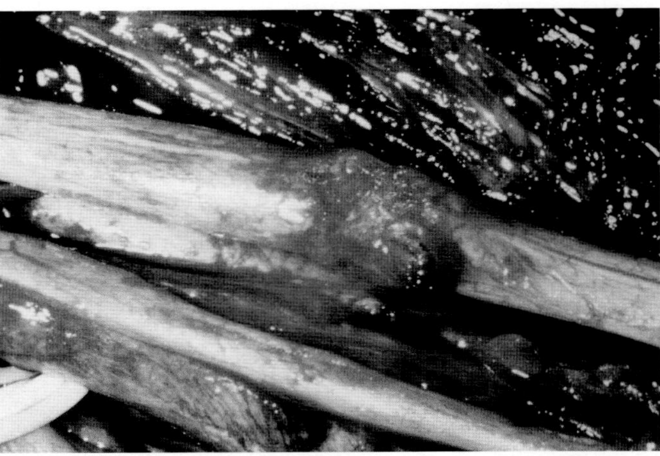

Figure 15.7

Causalgia. Partial transection of the median nerve by a bullet from a handgun. Pain was abolished by sympathectomy. Useful function followed repair of the nerve.

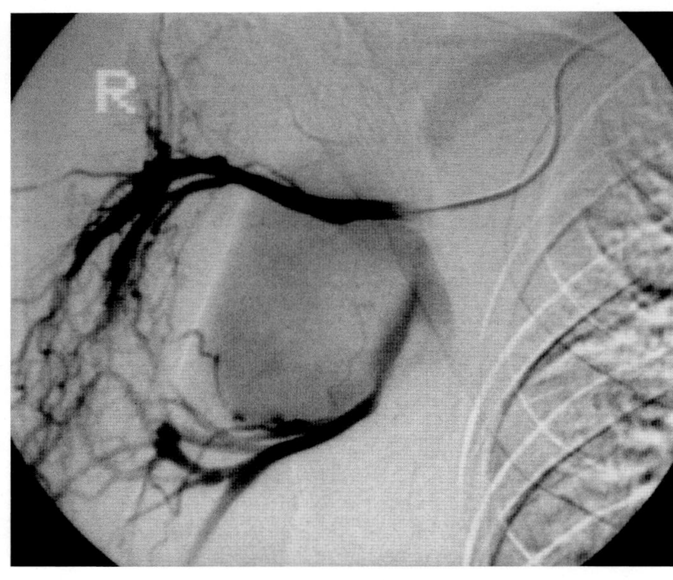

Figure 15.8

Causalgia. Complex arteriovenous fistula of axillary vessels from a military rifle bullet. The patient had a right-sided cardiac failure. Diagnosis was delayed for 10 weeks. Pain was abolished by correction of the fistula and neurolysis of the nerves, which went on to recovery.

responded to local anaesthetic block in four patients. There was some improvement after the transected nerve was repaired.

We think that a vigorous approach is justified in the treatment of nerve damage in penetrating missile injuries. The nerve lesion may be the first sign of a false aneurysm or arteriovenous fistula, as we found in 25% of our cases. Two distinct pain syndromes, causalgia and neurostenalgia, regularly respond to operative treatment. Results of repair are by no means bad, and with the exception of the complete lesion of the brachial plexus associated with damage to the spinal cord, they are better than closed traction ruptures.

Individual nerves

Nerves controlling the shoulder girdle

Bonnell (1989) estimated that one-quarter of the nerves of the brachial plexus pass to this complex of joints, which permits an extraordinary range of movements for the upper limb. One cranial and three peripheral nerves are of particular importance: the spinal accessory (XIth cranial) nerve, the nerve to serratus anterior, and the suprascapular and circumflex nerves. Comtet et al (1993) analysed the biomechanics of the shoulder and the scapulo-thoracic girdle in a particularly enlightening manner: 'elevation of the scapulo-humeral joint can be executed by two different and distinct systems, both capable of performing this movement separately. The deltoid muscle is composed of several parts contracting independently, sometimes antagonistic to one another and providing elevation in different directions'. Exceptionally important observations were made by Narakas (1993) who measured the scapulo-humeral angle (SHA) in 183 patients with various shoulder girdle disorders. The apex of the angle lies at the centre of the humeral head, the sides are formed by the lateral border of the scapula and the longitudinal axis of the humerus. The SHA is greatly reduced in attempting active abduction in isolated rotator cuff rupture, isolated suprascapular nerve palsy, combined injury to circumflex and suprascapular nerves, and combined injury to circumflex nerve and rotator cuff Narakas (1993).

Pain is usual after injury to these nerves, most especially to the accessory and the nerve to serratus anterior. It is a commonly held misconception that the three nerves without a cutaneous sensory component are purely 'motor nerves'. This is quite wrong for all three contain large numbers of A-delta and C fibres. Biopsies of the suprascapular nerve weeks after proven preganglionic injury to the fifth and sixth cervical nerves showed that over 30% of the larger myelinated fibres survived, these presumably being those responsible for proprioception with cells in the dorsal root ganglion (Birch et al 1998c). (See Figures 15.9 and 15.10.)

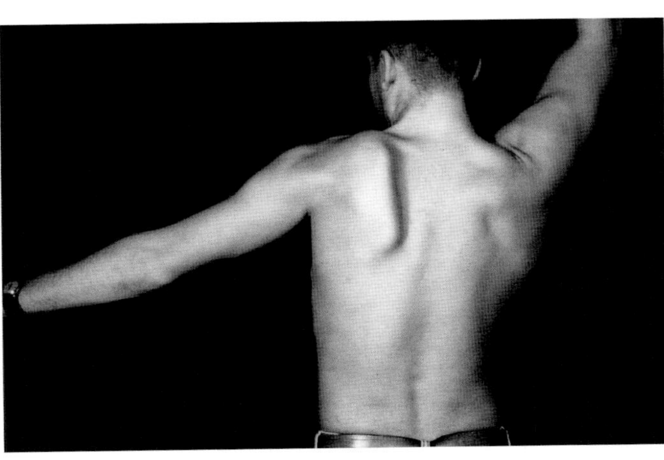

Figure 15.9
Iatropathic lesion of the spinal accessory nerve. Marked winging of the scapula, prominence of the spine of the scapula with wasting of the muscles. An earlier diagnosis of paralysis of the serratus anterior had been made.

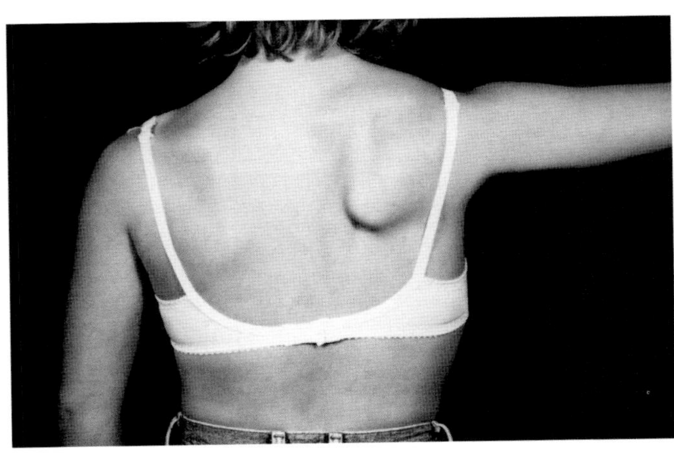

Figure 15.10
Serratus anterior paralysis (neuralgic amyotrophy). The weight of the limb pushes the winged scapula towards the spine and upwards.

Spinal accessory nerve injury

The eleventh cranial nerve innervates the sternocleidomastoid and trapezius muscles. It has no known cutaneous distribution. The nerve is at risk of injury as it crosses the posterior triangle of the neck. This can be intentional during radical neck surgery for carcinoma of the pharynx, accidental during lymph node biopsy or operations in the posterior triangle of the neck, or after trauma, e.g. assault or brachial plexus injury (Hanford 1933, Wulf 1941, Norden 1946, Brown et al 1988). Injury causes a characteristic syndrome (Nahum et al 1961):

1. Pain.
2. Paralysis of trapezius – shoulder droop
   – restricted shoulder movement
   – scapula winging.
3. Facial numbness.

Pain

Most patients experience pain, with over two-thirds experiencing pain at rest and enough to disturb their sleep. This is the most debilitating consequence of the injury. The pain is described as a dragging sensation or ache localized in the shoulder girdle. One explanation for the cause of this pain is the shoulder droop producing traction on the brachial plexus causing a neuritis. In fact, the pain, which is often immediate in onset, is usually neuropathic.

Bremner-Smith et al (1999) demonstrated that the nerve has a composition of ~50% Ad and C fibres, i.e. nocioceptive fibres. Stimulation of muscle nerve fascicles in human mixed nerves produces a distinct cramp-like pain projected over the muscle belly and sometimes to remote parts (Thomas and Ochoa 1993). Michaelis et al (2000) showed that cutting muscle afferent fibres led to continuing and spontaneous firing in dorsal root ganglion neurones. This work is exceptionally important in understanding pain provoked by cutting 'motor' nerves. Patients often report an improvement in their pain, immediately or shortly after surgery (neurolysis or graft) despite still having a paralysed trapezius and a shoulder droop.

Trapezius paralysis

The most obvious sign of trapezius paralysis is a shoulder droop.

Restricted shoulder movement

Few patients can abduct the shoulder more than 90° (Woodhall 1952, Valtonen and Lilius 1974, Gordon 1977, Vastamaki and Solonen, 1984, Osgard et al 1987). Shoulder suspension is provided passively by the deep cervical fascia, and actively by levator scapulae and upper trapezius muscles (Perry 1988). This has been confirmed by EMG studies (Bearn 1961). The loss of active suspension with trapezius paralysis produces the shoulder droop.

To elevate the arm in both flexion and abduction above 80°, the scapula must externally rotate. The muscles responsible are trapezius and serratus anterior (Comtet et al 1993). If the trapezius is paralysed, rotation cannot occur and shoulder elevation above 90° becomes impossible. However, there is a small group of patients who do have normal abduction. This has been explained by the trapezius receiving its motor innervation from the cervical plexus.

Scapula winging

Trapezius paralysis allows the medial border of the scapula to lift off the chest wall. Winging is less than that associated with serratus anterior paralysis (Brown et al 1988), but these two causes are often confused.

Facial numbness

A proportion of patients experience numbness over the angle of the jaw or around the ear, from associated injury to the transverse cervical and great auricular nerves. The accessory nerve emerges deep to the posterior border of sternocleidomastoid a few millimetres cephalad to these nerves, which are often injured as well. This anatomical association is a useful landmark in identification of the accessory nerve when the field is scarred.

Results of surgical intervention

Small series of repairs or neurolysis come from Norden (1946), Woodhall (1952), Vastamaki and Solonen (1984), Osgard et al (1987) and Nakamichi and Tachibana (1998). We described results in 36 patients who underwent surgery, either neurolysis or graft (Williams et al 1996), the outcome is known in 36 and the results are summarized in Table 15.4. The majority of patients were improved, but only four patients regained a normal shoulder with normal power, movement and no pain.

The spinal accessory nerve is particularly vulnerable to the activities of surgeons. Delay in diagnosis is unacceptably frequent. Although useful results have been seen when the nerve has been repaired as long as 2 years after injury, late repair is compromised by intractable neuropathic pain, by traction upon the brachial plexus from the dependent upper limb and by the secondary impingement between the head of the humerus and the overlying acromion. Contracture of the glenohumeral joint is usually seen in such late cases.

Table 15.4 *Results of operations on accessory nerve: 36 cases*

Outcome	*Grade*	*Number*	*Treatment*
A No change	Poor	7	Graft 4, neurolysis 3
B Pain improved Movement improved	Fair	10	Graft 6, neurolysis 4
C Almost normal Difficulty with overhead work	Good	15	Graft 13, neurolysis 2
D Normal from patient's point of view	Excellent	4	Graft 1, neurolysis 3

Reproduced by kind permission of the Editors of the *Annals of the Royal College of Surgeons of England.*

Table 15.5 *Results of repair in 96 wounds of spinal accessory nerve, 1980–2001*

A	Poor	12
B	Fair	40
C	Good	38
D	Excellent	8

Table 15.5 summarizes outcome in repairs of 96 spinal accessory nerve lesions, using the grading system of Williams; 71 of these were iatropathic injuries. We now perform far fewer neurolyses. Neurolysis is reserved for those cases where the nerve is not scarred and where the lesion is proved to be axonotmesis at exposure. Improvement in the defect was seen in 84 cases.

Neurotization of the accessory nerve

The accessory nerve is widely used to reinnervate the suprascapular and musculocutaneous nerves. An important step in utilizing the accessory nerve is to avoid denervating the upper fibres of trapezius (Alnot and Oberlin 1996). Usually the nerve is divided cephalad or caudad to the junction with branches of the cervical plexus at the base of the posterior triangle. However, the branches are not always present. Pereira and Williams (1999) demonstrated that there is always a plexus of veins adjacent to or overlying the nerve at this point. This can be used as a landmark instead.

The nerve to serratus anterior

This nerve is most commonly damaged in lesions of the brachial plexus but it is particularly vulnerable to accidental damage where it crosses the first and second rib. When serratus anterior is paralysed the inferior pole of the scapula does not move forward but slides medially and cranially. Deep aching pain is common and it is sometimes severe. We have been able to repair the nerve in six stab wounds and in seven intraoperative injuries. Results were very good, indeed, better than for almost any other peripheral nerve. Narakas (1995) emphasized to us the importance of the innervation of serratus anterior and suggested the use of deep branches of intercostal nerves in cases of avulsion of the fifth, sixth and seventh cervical nerves. We have used this technique in about 40 cases and in over three-quarters functional power was regained in serratus anterior. We have found this a particularly reliable nerve transfer.

The suprascapular and circumflex nerves

Injuries to these two nerves are often combined. The suprascapular nerve passes away from the upper trunk about 3 cm above the clavicle and it is not unusual to find it arising entirely from the fifth cervical nerve. It passes laterally and posterior to the omohyoid to the suprascapular notch, entering the supraspinous fossa deep to the superior transverse ligament. It traverses the fossa deep to the muscle to wind around the lateral border of the spine of the scapula entering the infraspinous fossa. The nerve contains between 3000 and 4000 myelinated nerve fibres and nearly 50% of these are afferent even though the nerve has no cutaneous distribution. It is particularly vulnerable to traction lesion and it may be injured at its take off from the upper trunk, in its more horizontal course in the posterior triangle, at the supraspinous notch and also within the supra- and infraspinous fossae. The nerve is essential for abduction and lateral rotation at the glenohumeral joint and patients with isolated paralysis of the deltoid with an intact suprascapular nerve and an undamaged rotator cuff are usually able fully to abduct and laterally rotate the shoulder.

The circumflex nerve is the terminal branch of the posterior cord and it contains 6000–7000 nerve fibres which pass to it through the fifth and sixth cervical nerves. The nerve divides into two branches within the quadrilateral tunnel: the anterior division continues round the neck of the humerus to innervate the anterior deltoid; the larger posterior branch innervates the teres minor and the posterior deltoid.

In many cases the nerve is only partially injured. De Laat et al (1994) found electromyographic changes in 45% from 101 cases of nerves injured by shoulder dislocation; nerves did not recover in eight cases.

Three important papers have described the exposure and treatment of combined injuries. Ochiai et al (1988) showed that the suprascapular nerve might be serially damaged in several places and recommended that the nerve be exposed along its entire course. Mikami et al (1997) described results of nerve grafting in 33 cases. In 22 patients both the nerves were ruptured. In other patients both nerves were damaged, at least one sustaining lesion in continuity. On the whole the results were good. Repairs were done within 4 months of injury. Bonnard et al (1999) reported the enormous experience of Narakas (1999) in 121 patients. In 69 the lesion was confined to the circumflex nerve; in 30 more both circumflex and suprascapular nerves were damaged. In 40 cases the two nerves were damaged in combination with other injuries to terminal branches of the brachial plexus. The conclusions from this study are important. First, 85% of useful results followed repair of isolated circumflex nerve injury. Next: 'the dramatic decrease in the rate of success seen with longer delays . . . suggest that surgery should be undertaken within three months of injury'. Other factors depressing outcome included arterial injury (21 cases), tear of rotator cuff, skeletal injury and age. The rotator cuff, was repaired at the same time as the nerve.

This is very good advice, but we think that the only really good results of repair of circumflex nerve are those

Table 15.6 *Grading of results of operation on the circumflex and suprascapular nerves*

Grade	*Description*
Circumflex nerve	
Good	Deltoid MRC 4 or better; abduction, elevation at least 120°
Fair	Deltoid MRC 3+ or better; abduction, elevation 90–120°
Poor or bad	Less than above
Suprascapular nerve	
Good	Abduction, 120° or more; lateral rotation 3° or more
Fair	Abduction, 90–120°; lateral rotation 0–30°
Poor or bad	Less than above

From Birch R, Bonney G, Wynn Parry CB (1998) *Surgical Disorders of the Peripheral Nerves* (Edinburgh: Churchill Livingstone).

Table 15.7 *Results obtained in repairs of the circumflex nerve and suprascapular nerve, 1979–1995*

Result	*Number of cases*
Circumflex nerve	
Good	25
Fair	23
Poor	8
Suprascapular nerve	
Good	20
Fair	2
Poor	2

From Birch R, Bonney G, Wynn Parry CB (1998) *Surgical Disorders of the Peripheral Nerves* (Edinburgh: Churchill Livingstone).

obtained when repair is undertaken within days of injury. The nerve is much more likely to be ruptured in high energy transfer injuries. Rupture of the circumflex humeral vessels causes haematoma and later, severe fibrosis within the quadrilateral space.

Myometric measurements of strength and stamina after repair of the circumflex nerve reveal an unfavourable picture. The stamina of the shoulder with deltoid paralysis is no more than about 30% of the normal side. It lies between 40 and 45% in those cases where there has been some recovery through lesions in continuity. Stamina of the shoulder after successful repair of the suprascapular nerve with an intact circumflex nerve reaches 70% of

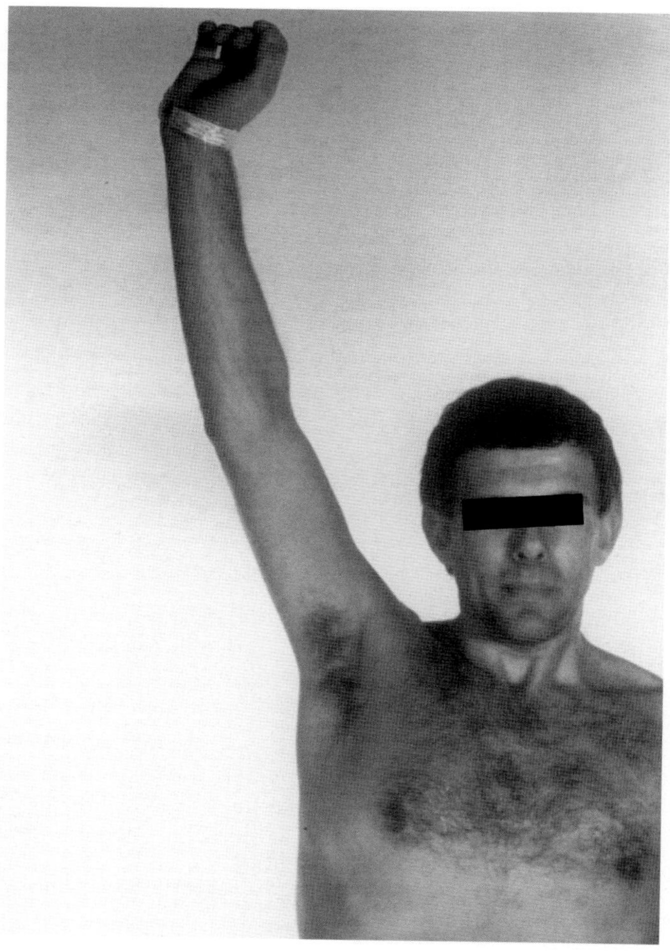

Figure 15.11

A 28-year-old man. Full elevation of the shoulder in the presence of complete paralysis of the deltoid from circumflex rupture.

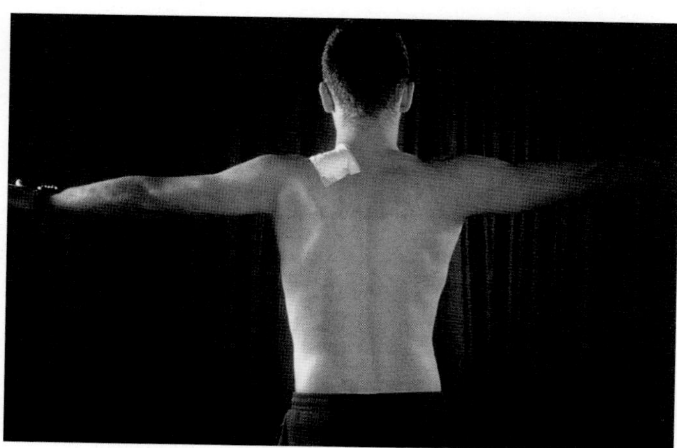

Figure 15.12

Shoulder elevation in a 33-year-old man, seen here at 6 weeks after graft of rupture of the suprascapular nerve. The circumflex nerve and rotator cuff were intact. Function such as this is unusual after rupture of the suprascapular nerve.

normal. When the circumflex nerve has been grafted the shoulder achieves 50% of normal stamina (Spilsbury and Birch 1996) (Tables 15.6 and 15.7).

A more vigorous approach toward palsies of the suprascapular and circumflex nerves ought to be adopted. A patient with obvious circumflex nerve palsy who is unable to abduct the shoulder has damage either to the suprascapular nerve or to the rotator cuff or both. Urgent exploration is justified in an open wound and where there is an associated arterial lesion. Direct implantation of nerve into muscle is a valuable innovation in cases where the distal stump is useless (Brunelli and Monini 1985) (Figures 15.11 and 15.12).

The radial nerve

The radial nerve is the largest terminal branch of the brachial plexus and it was the most commonly injured nerve reported in 16,500 cases of war wounds (Sunderland 1978). The anatomical studies of Sunderland and Bradley (1949) and of blood supply by Ramage (1927) revealed potentially significant features. The long head of triceps is innervated by branches arising in the axilla or brachio-axillary angle, the median head by branches in the brachio-axillary angle and the lateral head by branches arising in the spiral groove. The number of nerve bundles was, on average, 22 in the axilla, 5 in the spiral groove and 9 at the lateral epicondyle. Bundles occupied about 33% of the cross-sectional area of the trunk of the nerve in the axilla, about 50% in the spiral groove and just below 40% at the lateral epicondyle. These findings suggest that nerve repair is likely to be more difficult proximally where the nerve fibres are more dispersed and where the proportion of connective tissue is relatively high.

Between its origin and its entrance into the spiral groove, the nerve receives fewer arteries than elsewhere along its course. The first 8–10 cm of the nerve may not have a nutrient artery. The segment may therefore be wholly supplied by descending intraneural channels which reach it from the posterior cord and consequently it will be relatively avascular if transected at its origin. The profunda brachial artery accompanies and supplies the nerve in the spiral groove and damage to this vessel compromises the circulation to the nerve.

Zachary (1954) studied 113 cases of repair done by direct suture, all within 6 months of injury, mostly wounds. There was a good or fair outcome in 61.5% of the cases. In Seddon's (1975b) own series of 63 sutures of the radial nerve, again where the gap between nerve stumps was relatively short, 77.8% of results were graded fair or poor.

Kline and Hudson (1995b) described their findings in 171 cases of radial nerve injury. Results were better in the more distal lesions, the outcome after repair of lacerated nerves was better than that of nerves damaged by fractures or gunshot wounds. The best results were obtained after primary repair followed by secondary repair; the worst were in cases that required grafting.

Shergill et al (2001) reported on 260 of our radial nerve repairs. Direct suture was done in 31 cases. There were four groups of nerve injuries:

1. Open 'tidy wounds' from glass, knife or scissors (73).
2. Open 'untidy wounds' from penetrating missile injury, open fracture or fracture dislocation and/to contaminated wound (52).
3. Closed traction injury almost always associated with fracture of the shaft of the humerus (62).
4. Injuries which included an associated lesion of the axillary or brachial artery (55).

Overall 30% had good results, 28% were fair, 42% of the repairs failed. The violence of injury was the most important factor in determining outcome: 79% of the open 'tidy' repairs achieved a good or fair result; 36% of cases with arterial injury reached this level. Most repairs failed when the defect in the nerve trunk exceeded 10 cm. When repair was done within 14 days of injury 49% achieved a good result; only 28% of later repairs did so.

Table 15.8 *Grading of results for radial nerve repairs*

	Good	*Fair*	*Poor*
High – above nerves to triceps, 21 cases	Elbow extension M4 Wrist extension M3 or better	Elbow extension M4	Less than results in 'Fair' category
Intermediate – proximal to PIN, 221 cases. Useful triceps function	Wrist extension M4 Finger and thumb extension M3 or better	Wrist extension M3 or better	Less than results in 'Fair' category
PIN, 18 cases	Finger and thumb extension M4	Finger and thumb extension M3	Less than results in 'Fair' category

PIN, posterior interosseous nerve.

Table 15.9 *Results of repairs of 242 radial nerves, by cause*

Cause	*Number of nerves repaired*	*Results (%)*		
		Good	*Fair*	*Poor*
Open tidy	73	28 (38)	30 (41)	15 (21)
Closed traction	62	19 (31)	17 (27)	26 (42)
Open untidy	52	13 (25)	13 (25)	26 (50)
Associated vascular injury	55	12 (22)	8 (14)	35 (64)
Total	242	72 (30)	68 (28)	102 (42)

From Shergill et al (2001) The radial and posterior interosseous nerves: results from 260 repairs, *J Bone Joint Surg* **83B**: 646–9, by kind permission of the Editor.

All repairs undertaken after 12 months failed. Perhaps unsurprisingly, 16 of the 18 repairs of posterior interosseous nerve achieved a good result (Tables 15.8 and 15.9).

This study confirms that the most important influence on the prognosis after repair of the nerve is the violence of the injury and this is closely followed by delay between the injury and the repair. Seventy-seven of these repairs were carried out within 14 days, a higher proportion than in other published series. It is likely that the proportion of severe injuries with combined arterial and multiple nerve ruptures is also higher. Nonetheless, it is remarkable that these results are no better than those reported by Seddon or earlier workers. This might suggest that outcome from repair of this nerve has not improved over last 50 years. One possible explanation is the higher incidence of closed traction injury and associated arterial damage.

We recommend urgent repair of this nerve in 'tidy' wounds and in closed traction ruptures. The radial nerve is not easy to mobilize, direct suture is possible only in the fresh 'tidy' wound. Anterior transposition of the radial nerve will shorten a gap by some 3 cm. Repair by graft is usually required.

The profoundly depressing effect of associated injuries to the axillary or brachial arteries (64% poor results from 65 cases) requires further examination. Mild fibrosis was evident in 18 of these cases, compression and fibrosis of the distal trunk was a common finding. Post-ischaemic fibrosis of muscle and ischaemic compression of the nerve were factors that contributed to the particularly poor results in this group. There is, too, the question of the blood supply to the nerve, described earlier, which may lead to relative ischaemia of the distal stump in high injuries of this nerve. We suggest that early flexor to extensor transfer is indicated when the prognosis for recovery is poor and that a high traction rupture of the radial nerve with a defect between prepared stumps exceeding 10 cm is better treated by musculotendinous transfer. If the interval from injury exceeds 12 months then muscle transfer is more likely to improve function. Brunelli (personal communication) and Sedel (personal communication) have advised us that reinnervation of the wrist extensors, by transfer of intercostal nerves to nerves to extensor carpi radialis longus (ECRL) and extensor carpi radialis brevis (ERCB) using interposed graft, is an important possibility, and we have begun to use this method when the proximal stump is unsuitable.

The musculocutaneous nerve

Brandt and McKinnon (1993) found that there are usually two branches to biceps arising about 18 cm proximal to the medial epicondyle and, usually, one branch to brachialis arising 13.5 cm proximal to that epicondyle. Their detailed analysis of the number of myelinated nerve fibres suggests that less than half of the myelinated fibres within the musculocutaneous nerve pass to the skin. Obviously a significant proportion of the fibres within the nerves to the muscles will be afferent from muscle spindles or nociceptors. This degree of segregation of the muscle branches and the relatively small number of fascicles does help repair.

Kline and Hudson (1995c) found a useful outcome in 29 cases of repairs of rupture and infraclavicular stretch injuries. Seddon (1954), writing about nerve grafting, said that the 'case of division of the musculocutaneous nerve with a large gap was a striking success'.

We have repaired 160 ruptures or transections of musculocutaneous nerve; Osborne et al (2000) studied 85 of these performed between 1968 and 1997. The injuries fell into three groups:

1. Open 'tidy' wounds from glass, knife and scalpel – 13.
2. Open 'untidy' wounds from open fracture or fracture dislocation, contaminated wound or penetrating missile injury – 24.
3. Closed traction injuries – 48.

Table 15.10 *Results of 85 musculocutaneous nerve repairs, by type of injury*

Injury	*Good (%)*	*Fair (%)*	*Poor (%)*	*Total*
Open tidy	12 (92.3)	0 (0)	1 (7.7)	13
Open untidy	15 (62)	7 (29.2)	2 (8.3)	24
Closed traction	30 (62.5)	10 (20.8)	8 (16.7)	48

From Osborne et al (2000) The musculocutaneous nerve: results in 85 repairs, *J Bone Joint Surg* **82B**: 1140–2, by kind permission of the Editor.

Table 15.11 *Methods of grading results of median and ulnar nerve repairs*

Grade	*Motor*	*Sensory*	*Equivalent of Seddon's grading*
Excellent	Power MRC 5. No wasting or deformity. No trophic changes	Function indistinguishable from normal hand. Good stereognosis, no hypersensitivity. 2PD* equivalent to uninjured digits	Good M5 S4
Good	Power MRC 4–5. Abolition of paralytic deformity. Minimal pulp wasting	Accurate speedy localization. Can recognize texture or objects. Minor cold sensitivity and hypersensitivity. 2PD <8 mm at tips of fingers	Good M5 S3+
Fair	MRC 3 or more. Some sweating. Pulp wasted	Accurate localization to digit. No stereognosis. 2PD >8 mm. Significant cold sensitivity and hypersensitivity	Fair M3 S3
Poor or bad	MRC 3 or less. No sweating, trophic changes	No sensation or severe cold sensitivity and hypersensitivity	Bad M01 or 2S 01 or 2

* Two-point discrimination.
From Birch R, Raji A (1991) Repair of median and ulnar nerves, *J Bone Joint Surg* **73B**: 154–7, by kind permission of the Editor.

Thirteen nerves were sutured, the remainder were grafted. The groups were further subdivided according to the presence or absence of associated arterial injuries. The axial artery was ruptured in 43 of these cases. In three cases the nerve was found to be avulsed from the muscle and was re-implanted using the technique of Brunelli and Monini (1985). The results were good in 57 patients (67%), fair in 17 (20%) and poor in 11 (13%).

There was no significant relationship between the level of injury or the age of the patient in clinical outcome. Results were poor in five patients in whom the nerve had been damaged at its point of entry into muscle and in all four with post-ischaemic fibrosis. Results were worse in injuries with greater violence, particularly so when associated with skeletal injury. Ten of the 14 cases with penetrating missile injury achieved a good result. The outcome was rather better in the 21 patients with isolated damage to the musculocutaneous nerve compared with the 64 with multiple nerve palsies. Two useful results were achieved in the three cases of direct implantation of nerve into muscle. Of the 16 repairs performed after 180 days, good results were seen only in seven, and there were four failures (Table 15.10).

The indications for urgent exploration of this nerve are particularly strong in open wounds. We also advise early exploration in closed traction injury with a deep lesion of the musculocutaneous nerve, particularly when linear bruising is noted along the line of the coraco-brachialis. It is important always to bear in mind the possibility of a lesion at two levels. Oberlin's operation (Oberlin et al 1996), developed for suprascapular palsies of C5, C6, C7, is exceptionally valuable for those peripheral injuries where the proximal stump is unsuitable. With an intact radial nerve powerful flexion of elbow is often provided by brachioradialis and sometimes by the lateral part of brachialis but supination is defective.

Table 15.12 *Repair of 165 ulnar nerves in adults (16–65 years) in tidy wounds from distal wrist crease to elbow crease*

	Primary repair	*Delayed suture*	*Graft*	*Total*
Excellent	8	1	2	11
Good	26	7	25	58
Fair	14	19	30	63
Poor or bad	2	10	21	33
Total	50	37	78	165

Note: all except one of the excellent results were seen in patients aged 21 or less.

The median and ulnar nerves

The effects of age and the level of injury are very striking for these two nerves; even more so are the cause of injury and delay between injury and repair.

Tables 15.11, 15.12 and 15.13 set out the method of assessment and outcome in repairs of 289 median and ulnar nerves in tidy wounds in the forearm from the elbow to the wrist crease. The results of repair of high median and ulnar nerves are, on the whole, so much more modest than those following repair of these nerves

Table 15.13 *Repair of 134 median nerves in adults 15–65 years in tidy wounds from wrist to elbow*

	Primary repair	*Delayed suture*	*Graft*	*Total*
Excellent	5	1	0	6
Good	29	11	13	53
Fair	14	16	27	57
Poor or bad	3	8	7	18
Total	51	36	47	134

Note: Five of the six excellent results were seen in patients aged 21 or less.

Table 15.14 *Grading of results in high median and ulnar nerve repair*

Grade	*Description*
Median nerve	
Good	Long flexor muscles, MRC 4 or better Localization to digit without hypersensitivity Return of sweating
Fair	Long flexor muscles, MRC 3 or 3+ 'Protective sensation', moderate or no hypersensitivity Sweating diminished or absent
Poor or bad	Long flexor muscles, MRC 2 or less 'Protective sensation', but severe hypersensitivity or no sensation
Ulnar nerve	
Good	FCU and FDP of little and ring fingers, MRC 4 or better Intrinsic muscles MRC 2 or better Localization to little and ring fingers No hypersensitivity Return of sweating
Fair	FCU and FDP of little and ring fingers, MRC 3 or 3+ No intrinsic muscle function 'Protective' sensation in little and ring fingers Moderate hypersensitivity Little or no sweating
Poor or bad	FCU and FDP of little and ring fingers, MRC 2 No intrinsic muscle function 'Protective' sensation with severe hypersensitivity, *or* no sensation No sweating

FCU, flexor carpi ulnaris; FDP, flexor digitorum profundus. From Birch R, Bonney G, Wynn Parry CB (1998) *Surgical Disorders of the Peripheral Nerves* (Edinburgh: Churchill Livingstone).

Table 15.15 *Results in 117 repairs of median nerve infraclavicular – axilla-arm, in adults and children, by cause*

	Tidy	*Untidy*	*Traction*	*Total*
Good	8	6	3	17
Fair	10	16	22	48
Poor	4	15	33	52
Total	22	37	58	117

This includes 28 repairs of either lateral or medial root of nerve in the axilla; 13 of the 17 good results followed repair within 5 days of injury, 4 of them were in children.

Table 15.16 *Results of 99 repairs of ulnar nerve or medial cord – infraclavicular-axilla-arm, in adults and children, by cause*

	Open	*Untidy*	*Traction*	*Total*
Good	5	5	0	10
Fair	7	16	24	47
Poor	3	14	25	42
Total	15	35	49	99

Seven of the good results followed repair within 48 hours of injury – three in children. Results of repair with delay of 3 months or more were particularly poor in the untidy and traction group.

at the wrist that a less demanding system of assessment is used. Our assessment and results for repairs of 216 median and ulnar nerves in the axilla or arm are shown in Tables 15.14, 15.15 and 15.16. These are a little better than damage to these nerve trunks in the infraclavicular injury but they are poor enough in all regards.

Conclusion

A vigorous approach must be adopted to the severe infraclavicular brachial plexus injury. The clinician must be ready to deal with associated arterial injury and to deal with damage to the joints and the skeleton. The case for urgent repair is strong, overwhelmingly so when there is an associated arterial injury. We hope that growing interest in these complex nerve injuries will lead to improvement in the treatment of patients who are afflicted; we hope that the growing subspecialization of surgical disciplines does not lead to worsening of that treatment.

References

Alnot JY (1988) Traumatic brachial plexus palsy in the adult, *Clin Orthop Rel Res* **237**: 9–16.

Alnot J-Y, Oberlin C (1996) Nerves available for neurotization: the spinal accessory nerve. In: Alnot J-Y, Narakas A, eds, *Traumatic Brachial Plexus Injuries (Paris: Expansion Scientifique Francaise)* 33–8.

Barros d'Sa (1992) Arterial Injuries. In: Eastcott HHG, ed, *Arterial Surgery, 3rd edn* (Edinburgh: Churchill Livingstone) 355–413.

Bearn JG (1961) An EMG study of the trapezius, deltoid, pectoralis major, biceps and triceps muscles, during static loading of the upper limb, *Anat Rec* **140**: 103–6.

Bigliani LU, Craig EV, Butters KP (1991) Fractures of the shoulder. In: Rockwood CA, Green DP, Bucholz RW, eds, *Fractures in Adults, 3rd edn* (Philadelphia: Lippincott) 871–1020.

Birch R, Bonney G, Wynn Parry C (1998a) The vascular injury. In: *Surgical Disorders of the Peripheral Nerves* (London: Churchill Livingstone) 172–81.

Birch R, Bonney G, Wynn Parry C (1998b) Compound nerve injuries. In: *Surgical Disorders of the Peripheral Nerves* (London: Churchill Livingstone) 123–55.

Birch R, Bonney G, Wynn Parry C (1998c) Motor and sensory pathways. In: *Surgical Disorders of the Peripheral Nerves* (London: Churchill Livingstone) 27–36.

Bonnard C, Anastakis DJ, van Melle G, Narakas AO (1999) *J Bone Joint Surg* **81B**: 212–17.

Bonnelt F (1989) Anatomie du plexus brachial chez le nouveau ne et l'adulte. In: Alnot JY, Narakas A, eds, *Les Paralysies du Plexus Brachial. Monographies du Groupe d'Etude de la Main* (Paris: Expansion Scientifique) 3–13.

Brandt KE, MacKinnon SE (1993) A technique for maximising biceps recovery in brachial plexus reconstruction, *J Hand Surg* **18A**: 726–33.

Bremner-Smith AS, Unwin AJ, Williams WW (1999) Sensory pathways in the spinal accessory nerve, *J Bone Joint Surg* **81B**: 226–8.

Brown H, Burns S, Kaiser WC (1988) The spinal accessory nerve plexus, the trapezius muscle, and shoulder stabilisation after radical neck cancer, *Ann Surg* **208**: 654–61.

Brown PW (1970) The time factor in surgery of upper extremity peripheral nerve injury, *Clin Orthop* **68**: 14–21.

Brunelli G, Monini L (1985) Direct muscular neurotisation. Proceedings of the Second Congress of the International Federation of Societies for Surgery of the Hand. *J Hand Surg* **10A**: 993–4.

Cavanagh SP, Birch R, Bonney G (1987) The infraclavicular brachial plexus: the case for primary repair. *J Bone Joint Surg [Br]* **69**: 489.

Comtet JJ, Herzberg G, Alnaasan I (1993) Biomechanics of the shoulder and the scapulothoracic girdle. In: Tubiana R, ed, *The Hand*, Vol IV (Philadelphia: WB Saunders) 99–111.

DeBakey ME, Simeone FA (1946) Battle injuries of the arteries in World War II. *Ann Surg* **123**: 534–79.

DeBakey ME, Simeone FA (1955) Acute battle incurred arterial injury. In: *Surgery and World War Two, Vascular Surgery* (Medical Department US Army, Washington: US Government Printing Office) 60–148.

De Laat EAT, Visser CPJ, Coene LNJEM, Pahplatz PVM, Tavy DLJ (1994) Nerve lesions in primary shoulder dislocations and humeral neck fractures. A prospective clinical and EMG study, *J Bone Joint Surg* **76B**: 381–3.

Delorme E (1915) The treatment of gunshot wounds of nerves, *BMJ* **1**: 853–5.

Eastcott HHG, Blaisdell FW, Silver D (1992) In: Eastcott HHG, ed, *Arterial Surgery, 3rd edn* (Edinburgh: Churchill Livingstone) 31–54.

Fahrer H, Ludin HP, Mumenthaler M, Neiger M (1974) The innervation of the trapezius muscle. An electrophysiological study, *J Neurol* **207**: 183–8.

Fiolle J, Delmas J (1921) In: Cumston CG, trans ed, *The Surgical Exposure of the Deep Seated Blood Vessels* (London: Heinemann) 61–7.

Flaubert AC (1827) Mémoire sur plusiers cas de luxations dans les efforts pour la réduction ont été suivis d'accidents graves, *Répertoire Générale d'Anatomie et de Physiologie Pathologique* **3**: 55–79.

Gordon SL, Graham WP, Black JT, Miller SH (1977) Accessory nerve function after surgical procedures in the posterior triangle, *Arch Surg* **112**: 264–8.

Gousheh J (1995) The treatment of War injuries in the brachial plexus, *J Hand Surg* **20A**: 568–76.

Hanford JM (1933) Surgical excision of tuberculous lymph nodes of the neck. A report of 131 patients with follow-up results, *Surg Clin North Am* **13**: 301–10.

Hughes CW, Bowers WF (1961) *Traumatic Lesions of Peripheral Vessels* (Springfield, IL: CC Thomas).

Kline DG (1989) Civilian gun shot wounds to the brachial plexus, *J Neurosurg* **70**: 166–74.

Kline DG, Hudson AR (1995a) Compound nerve action potential recordings. In: *Nerve Injuries* (Philadelphia: WB Saunders) 87–99.

Kline DG, Hudson AR (1995b) Results: radial nerve. In: *Nerve Injuries* (Philadelphia: WB Saunders) 167–85.

Kline DG, Hudson AR (1995c) Stretch injuries to the brachial plexus. In: *Nerve Injuries* (Philadelphia: WB Saunders) 397–460.

Makins GH (1919) *On Gunshot Injuries to the Blood Vessels: Founded on Experience during the Great War 1914–1918* (London: Wright).

Michaelis M, Lui XG, Janig W (2000) Axotomised and intact muscle afferents but not skin afferents develop ongoing discharges of dorsal root ganglion origin after peripheral nerve lesion, *J Neurosci* **20**: 2724–48.

Mikami Y, Nagano A, Ochiai N, Yamamoto S (1997) Results of nerve grafting for injuries of the axillary and suprascapular nerves, *J Bone Joint Surg* **79B**: 527–31.

Miller RA (1939) Observations upon the arrangement of the axillary artery and brachial plexus, *Am J Anat* **64**: 143–63.

Nahum AM, Mulhally W, Manmoor L (1961) A syndrome resulting from radical neck dissection, *Arch Otolaryngol* **74**: 424–8.

Nakamichi K, Tachibana S (1998) Iatrogenic injury of the spinal accessory nerve. Results of repair, *J Bone Joint Surg* **80A**: 1616–21.

Narakas AO (1987) Thoughts on neurotization of nerve transfers in irreparable nerve lesions. In: Terzis JK, ed, *Microreconstruction of Nerve Injuries* (Philadelphia: WB Saunders) 447–54.

Narakas AO (1993) Paralytic disorders of the shoulder girdle. In: Tubiana R, ed, *The Hand*, Vol. 4, (Philadelphia: WB Saunders) 112–25.

Norden A (1946) Peripheral injuries to the spinal accessory nerve, *Acta Chir Scand* **94**: 515–32.

Oberlin C, Beal D, Bhatia A, Dauge MC (1996) The ulnar nerve. In: Alnot JY, Narakas A, eds, *Traumatic Brachial Plexus Injuries. Monographie de la Societe Française de Chirurgie de la Main* (Paris: Expansion Scientifique Française) 28–32.

Ochiai N, Nagano A, Akinaga S, Murashima R, Tachibana S (1988) Brachial plexus injuries: surgical treatment of combined injuries of the axillary and suprascapular nerves, *J Japanese Soc Surg Hand* **5**: 151–5.

Omer GE (1974) Injuries to nerves of the upper extremity, *J Bone Joint Surg* **56A**: 1615–24.

Osborne AWH, Birch R, Munshi P, Bonney G (2000) The musculocutaneous nerve: results of 85 repairs, *J Bone Joint Surg* **82B**: 1140–2.

Osgard O, Eskesen V, Rosenorn J (1987) Microsurgical repair of iatrogenic accessory nerve lesions in the posterior triangle of the neck, *Acta Chir Scand* **153**: 171–3.

Pereira MT, Williams WW (1999) The spinal accessory nerve distal to the posterior triangle, *J Hand Surg* **24B**: 368–9.

Perry J (1988) Muscle control of the shoulder. In: Rowe CR, ed, *The Shoulder* (New York: Churchill Livingstone) 17–34.

Ramage D (1927) The blood supply to the peripheral nerves of the upper limb in man, *J Anat* **61**: 198.

Seddon HJ (1954) Nerve grafting. In: *Peripheral Nerve Injuries*, London: Medical Research Council Special Report Series no. 282 (HMSO) 402–3.

Seddon HJ (1975a) Common causes of nerve injury. In: *Surgical Disorders of Peripheral Nerves*, 2nd edn (Edinburgh: Churchill Livingstone) 67–8.

Seddon HJ (1975b) Repair of the radial nerve. In: *Surgical Disorders of Peripheral Nerves*, 2nd edn (Edinburgh: Churchill Livingstone) 306–7.

Seigel DB, Gelberman RH (1991) Peripheral nerve injuries associated with fractures and dislocations. In: Gelberman RH, ed, *Operative Nerve Repair and Reconstruction* (Philadelphia: JB Lippincott) 619–33.

Shergill G, Birch R, Bonney G, Munshi P (2001) The radial and posterior interosseous nerves: results of 260 repairs, *J Bone Joint Surg* **83B**: 646–9.

Spilsbury J, Birch R (1996) Some lesions of the circumflex and suprascapular nerves, *J Bone Joint Surg* **73B** (Suppl): 59 (abstract).

Stewart M, Birch R (2001) Penetrating missile injuries, *J Bone Joint Surg* **83B**: 517–24.

Sunderland S (1978) *Nerve and Nerve Injuries*, 2nd edn (Edinburgh: Churchill Livingstone).

Sunderland S, Bradley K (1949) The cross sectional area of peripheral nerve trunks devoted to nerve fibres, *Brain* **72**: 428–49.

Thomas PK, Ochoa J (1993) Diseases of the peripheral nervous system – clinical features and differential diagnosis. In: Dyck PJ, Thomas PK, eds, *Peripheral Neuropathy*, 3rd edn (London: WB Saunders) 760–1.

Tinel (1917) *Nerve Wounds* (revised and edited by Joll CA) (London: Ballière Tindall and Cox).

Valtonen E, Lilius HG (1974) Late sequelae of iatrogenic spinal accessory nerve injury, *Acta Chir Scand* **140**: 453–5.

Vastamaki M, Solonen KO (1984) Accessory nerve injury, *Acta Orthop Scand* **55**: 296–9.

Williams WW, Donell ST, Twyman RS, Birch R (1996) The posterior triangle and the painful shoulder: spinal accessory nerve injury, *Ann R Coll Surg Eng* **78**: 521–5.

Woodhall B (1952) Trapezius paralysis following minor surgical procedures in the posterior cervical triangle, *Ann Surg* **136**: 375–80.

Woodhall B, Beebe GW (1956) *Peripheral Nerve Regeneration, VA Medical Monograph* (Washington, DC: US Government Printing Office).

Wulf HB (1941) Treatment of tuberculous cervical lymphoma. Late results in 230 cases treated partly surgically and partly radiologically, *Acta Chir Scand* **84**: 343–66.

Zachary RB (1954) Results of nerve sutures. In: Seddon HJ, ed, *Peripheral Nerve Injuries, Medical Research Council, Special Report Series no. 282*: 354.

16 Neurotization in brachial plexus injuries

Chantal Bonnard and Dimitri J Anastakis

Definition

The terms neurotization, nerve transfer, and nerve crossover have been used interchangeably. During a neurotization procedure, a healthy donor nerve is divided and its proximal stump is coapted directly or via a nerve graft to the distal stump of an injured non-functioning nerve. The transferred nerve eventually assumes new end-organ specificity. The sacrificed donor nerve must be expendable. The function gained with the transfer must be of greater value than the function lost.

Introduction

Multiple preganglionic root avulsions represent a reconstructive challenge for the surgeon. Attempts at replantation of preganglionic root avulsions into the spinal cord remain experimental (Carlstedt et al 1995). Neurotization or nerve transfer procedures represent the best option for functional reconstruction in this group of patients (Narakas and Hentz 1988).

Neurotization or nerve transfer procedures can be classified as intraplexal or extraplexal (Figure 16.1).

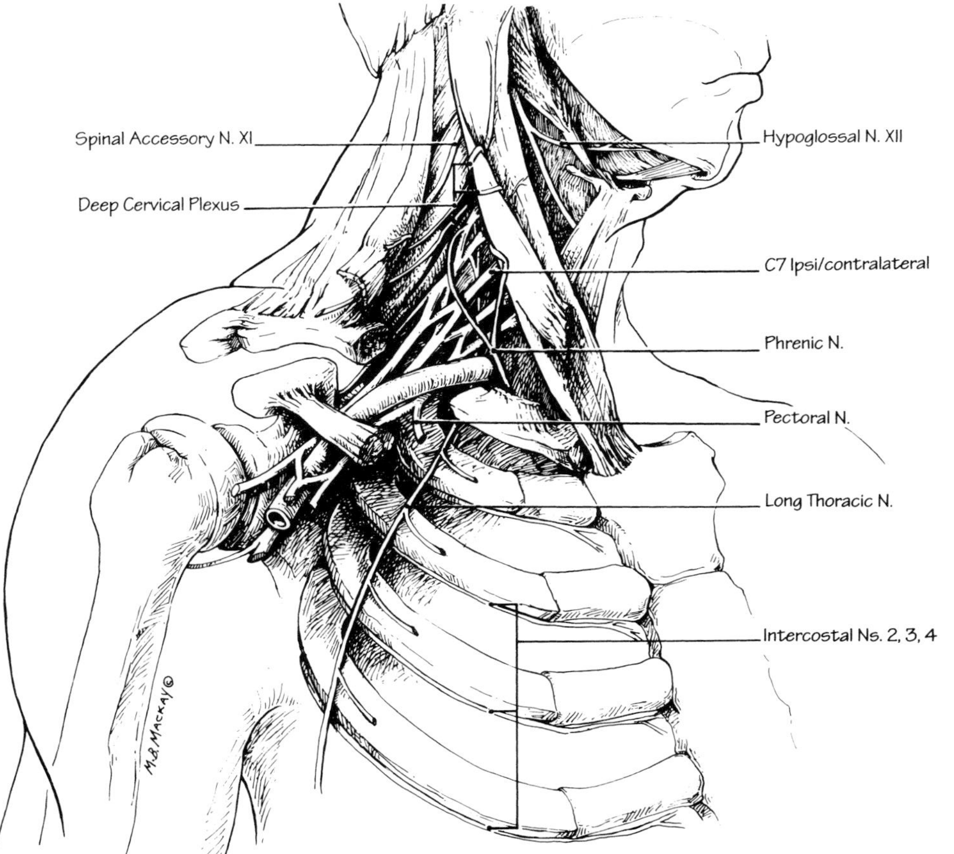

Figure 16.1

Potential nerve transfers for brachial plexus reconstruction. Extraplexal nerve transfers include the intercostal nerves, spinal accessory nerve, cervical plexus, phrenic nerve, contralateral C7 root, contralateral pectoral nerve, and hypoglossal nerve.

Table 16.1 *Potential donor nerves*

Donor nerve	*Myelinated axon count*	*Nerve graft needed*	*Common transfers*
Intercostal nerve	1200–1300	+/–	MCN
Spinal accessory nerve	1300–1600	–	SSN
Deep cervical plexus	740–950	+	SSN, AxN
Phrenic nerve	800	–	MCN, SSN, upper trunk
C7 ipsi- and contralateral	16,000–40,000	+	MCN, median
Long thoracic nerve	1600	–	–
Lateral pectoral (contralateral)	400–600	+	MCN
Hypoglossal nerve	9200	+	MCN, lateral cord

MCN, musculocutaneous nerve; SSN, suprascapular nerve; AxN, axillary nerve.

Intraplexal nerve transfers make use of proximal nerve stumps or motor branches of the brachial plexus in cases of partial or incomplete avulsion injuries. Extraplexal nerve transfers include those donor nerves found outside the injured brachial plexus. Extraplexal nerve transfers include the intercostal nerves, spinal accessory nerve, cervical plexus, phrenic nerve, contralateral C7 root, contralateral pectoral nerve, and hypoglossal nerve. Table 16.1 lists all nerve transfers described in the reconstruction of the brachial plexus.

Factors associated with improved results following neurotization include: a donor nerve with principally motor function and a large number of myelinated axons; a donor nerve that is close to the brachial plexus; direct nerve–nerve coaptation; and, if a bridging graft is needed it should be short.

There is growing evidence of the importance of cortical plasticity as it relates to functional outcomes following reconstructive surgery of the paralysed upper extremity. Recent work by our group has shown that assessment of cortical plasticity in patients who have undergone reconstructive surgery (i.e. free functioning muscle transfer) is feasible using the techniques of functional MRI and transcranial magnetic stimulation. Our preliminary work has shown that there is increased cortical excitability with similar patterns of cortical representation in patients who have had a free functioning muscle transfer for upper extremity paralysis of various etiologies when compared with normal controls. In one particular patient who had biceps function restored with a free functioning muscle transfer neurotized by intercostal nerves, we found an absence of respiratory motor cortex activation during elbow flexion. This finding suggested a shift in motor cortex control following neurotization with intercostal nerves. Changes in cortical excitability and a shift in cortical representation are suggestive of cortical plasticity in this unique patient population (DJ Anastakis 2001, personal communication). Further work is required to better understand the role of cortical plasticity as it relates to functional outcomes in upper extremity reconstruction (i.e. nerve repair, nerve transfers, tendon transfers, and free functioning muscle transfers).

Intercostal nerves

History

Yeoman and Seddon first purposed that the intercostal nerves be used to reconstruct the brachial plexus following complete avulsion injury (Yeoman 1961). In 1963, Seddon transferred the second, third, and fourth intercostal nerves to the distal musculocutaneous nerve in an attempt to reinnervate the biceps and brachialis muscles. Since these early descriptions, several authors have used and perfected intercostal nerve transfers for brachial plexus reconstruction (Millesi 1977, Dolenc 1984, Chuang et al 1992, 1993a, Nagano et al 1992, Ogino and Naito 1995, Mackinnon and Novak 1999, Nath and Mackinnon 2000, Samardzic et al 2000).

Anatomy

Of the 12 thoracic spinal nerves, 10 are actually intercostal nerves. The first thoracic spinal nerve (T1) contributes to the brachial plexus after crossing the first rib and the 12th thoracic spinal nerve (T12) does not travel in an intercostal space. Typically, the second to fourth intercostal nerves are used as nerve transfers for brachial plexus reconstruction.

The intercostal nerves originate from the spinal cord. The upper two intercostal nerves (T1 and T2) also supply the upper extremity and thorax. The intercostal nerves travel in the intercostal space inferior to the intercostal artery and vein. The nerve runs between the intercostalis intimi and the internal intercostal muscles. The nerve divides into a motor branch, a lateral sensory branch to the chest wall, and a collateral branch that travels along the upper border of the rib below. Each intercostal nerve ends in anterior cutaneous branches that supply the anterior thorax or abdomen. The motor branch is usually deep to the sensory branch and can be followed beyond the mid-clavicular line. There can be up to three nerve branches in the intercostal space. Intraoperative nerve stimulation permits motor branch identification.

Motor and sensory function

The intercostal nerves innervate the external, internal, and innermost (i.e. intercostalis intimi) intercostal muscles. The intercostals are muscles of respiration. In addition, the intercostal nerves end in anterior cutaneous branches that supply the anterior thorax or abdomen. Specifically, T2 innervates the axillary skin and gives a branch to the medial brachial cutaneous nerve. T3 contributes to the innervation of the posterior two-thirds of the axilla and contributes to the medial brachial and sometimes the medial antebrachial cutaneous nerves. T4 typically does not contribute to the upper extremity. T5 supplies the nipple.

Motor axon counts

The intercostal nerves contain between 1200 and 1300 myelinated fibers (Freilinger et al 1978, Narakas 1984, Chuang 1995).

Surgical exposure/harvesting

We use an anterior thoracic exposure to facilitate direct suture of the intercostal nerves to the recipient nerve. A semicircular incision is extended from the usual brachial plexus incision at the anterior border of the axilla onto the chest wall. The incision is placed so that access to the second through to fifth intercostal nerves is possible up to the mid-clavicular line. The superficial muscular layer in the intercostal space is incised near the lower border of the rib and then dissection is carried deeper until the nerve is identified. The nerve may be located between the intercostalis intimi and the internal intercostal muscles. The nerve may lie in close relationship to the parietal pleura. Care must be taken not to perforate the pleura during dissection. Intercostal nerves T3–T5 may be directly coapted to recipient nerves in the plexus at the upper arm level. For intercostal nerves from T6 and lower, an intermediate nerve graft is required to reach the plexus. Narakas provides an excellent description of the various exposures and methods for intercostal nerve harvesting (Narakas 1991).

Deficit following harvest

Harvesting of ipsilateral intercostal nerves (T2–T4/T5) when the phrenic nerve intact is not associated with postoperative pulmonary dysfunction (Giddins et al 1995, Waikakul et al 1992). Harvesting of the intercostal nerves when there is an ipsilateral phrenic nerve lesion is considered a relative contraindication by most surgeons because of potential respiratory complications (Giddins et al 1995). Nevertheless, a few surgeons have described harvesting both phrenic and intercostal nerves together (Chuang 1999, Terzis et al 1999). When there is a diaphragmatic paralysis, we do not use the intercostal nerves. We do not use a combined intercostal and phrenic nerve transfer.

Contraindications

- *Relative:* Phrenic nerve palsy is a relative contraindication. Intercostal nerves can be used even when the ribs have been fractured but dissection may be difficult. The sensory branch of T5 should be left to supply a normal sensation of the nipple.
- *Absolute:* Intercostal nerves must not be used when the patient suffers from Brown-Séquard syndrome because they are non-functional. Brown-Séquard syndrome is present in 5% of complete palsy cases (Birch et al 1998).

Common transfers

The intercostal nerves are among the most commonly used nerve transfers in brachial plexus reconstruction. These nerves are typically transferred to the musculocutaneous nerve or lateral cord (Chuang et al 1992, 1993a, Ogino and Naito 1995, Mackinnon and Novak 1999, Nath and Mackinnon 2000, Samardzic et al 2000). The intercostal nerves have also been transferred to the long thoracic, medial pectoral, radial, median, ulnar, and axillary nerves (Millesi 1977, Dolenc 1984, Ogino and Naito 1995, Samardzic et al 2000) and/or to reanimate a free functional muscle transfer (Doi et al 2000).

In 1989, Nagano et al showed that the transfer of three versus two intercostal nerves to the musculocutaneous nerve gave similar results. In 1992, Chuang et al demonstrated that there was no statistical difference in the results following two versus three intercostal nerve transfers to the musculocutaneous nerve. The author prefers to transfer three intercostal nerves to the musculocutaneous nerve.

Intercostal nerves may be coapted to the motor portion or to the entire musculocutaneous nerve. In the first technique, the motor fascicles from the biceps motor branch are dissected up into the axilla and directly sutured to the intercostal nerves. This fascicular dissection may be too traumatic for the musculocutaneous nerve. The second technique avoids a fascicular dissection. The motor branches of the intercostal nerves are sutured with the central part of the musculocutaneous nerve (where the motor fascicles should be located) and the sensory branches of the intercostal nerves are sutured around the periphery of the nerve (Chuang et al 1992). We prefer the first method except when there are frequent interfascicular connections – this makes atraumatic dissection of the musculocutaneous nerve impossible.

Pitfalls/complications

The two most common intraoperative pitfalls/complications include pneumothorax during harvesting and inadequate nerve length requiring interpositional nerve grafting. There may be a limited number of motor axons available from the small intercostal motor nerves, which may contribute to poor functional results. Some patients complain of involuntary motor contraction with coughing, yawning, sneezing, and laughing. Finally, poor functional results are associated with interpositional nerve grafts and following transfer of the intercostal nerves onto the medial cord.

Spinal accessory nerve

History

Tuttle, in 1913, was the first to consider using the spinal accessory nerve to neurotize the upper trunk. In 1963, Kotani reintroduced the idea of using this nerve as a transfer in brachial plexus reconstruction. Kotani used the spinal accessory nerve to neurotize the musculocutaneous nerve, upper trunk, and radial nerve (Kotani et al 1972).

Anatomy

The spinal accessory nerve has cranial and spinal roots. The cranial roots come from the medulla and leave the skull by passing through the jugular foramen. These roots supply the laryngeal muscles. The spinal portion is made up of roots originating from C1 through to C6. The spinal portion rises through the foramen magnum joining the cranial portion and passes out through the jugular foramen. The nerve lies deep to the digastric muscle, travels alongside and then crosses the internal jugular vein, to reach the anterior aspect of the sternocleidomastoid. In most cases, it reaches the upper one-third of the anterior border of the sternocleidomastoid. The nerve may travel through the sternocleidomastoid or along the anterior aspect to enter the posterior triangle of the neck. Connections with the cervical plexus are common – providing the nerve with motor and proprioceptive fibers. In the posterior triangle of the neck the spinal accessory nerve is adjacent to veins, branches of the superficial cervical artery and lymph nodes. Just above the clavicle it gives off muscular branches for the upper trapezius and then travels deep to the trapezius, travelling further caudally and medially to innervate the middle and lower portions of the muscle. The nerve is harvested distal to the motor branch for the upper trapezius.

Motor and sensory function

The spinal accessory nerve innervates both the sternocleidomastoid and trapezius muscles. The trapezius is innervated by the spinal accessory nerve (XI) and several cervical nerves. The nerve usually brings with it some fibers derived from C2, and before it enters the anterior or deep surface of the trapezius, it is joined by C3 and C4 nerves, or these may enter the muscle directly.

The trapezius muscle retracts the scapula and more importantly elevates the lateral angle of the scapula, since it is the only muscle that passes downward to insert on the lateral angle. It is the only muscle that can perform this function. This is an important function with respect to upward rotation of the scapula, especially if abduction of the arm is to be carried out with considerable force.

Together, the upper and lower fibers of the trapezius help in upward rotation of the scapula. Total paralysis of the trapezius results in the superior medial angle of the scapula being higher than normal, although the point of the shoulder is lower than normal. The unopposed levator scapulae and rhomboids elevate the medial border, while the weight of the arm pulls the unsupported lateral angle of the scapula down. These combined actions result in a downward rotation of the scapula.

The other shoulder muscles are able to compensate for a muscle that is paralysed or missing. The serratus anterior muscle is the most active upward rotator of the scapula and can undoubtedly produce this action without the aid of the trapezius if the scapula is sufficiently fixed by other muscles, such as the levator scapulae and the rhomboids.

Motor axon counts

The spinal accessory nerve contains approximately 1300–1700 myelinated fibers distal to the motor branch for the upper trapezius (Narakas 1984, 1991, Chuang 1995).

Surgical exposure/harvesting

To expose the spinal accessory nerve, the cranial end of a typical brachial plexus incision is extended posteriorly. Along the lateral margin of the sternocleidomastoid muscle, the spinal accessory nerve is usually found one finger's breadth above the emergence point of the greater auricular nerve, where multiple divisions of the cervical plexus also emerge from beneath the sternocleidomastoid muscle. This is an important landmark in the dissection of the brachial plexus. With nerve stimulation the spinal accessory nerve is confirmed with concomitant contraction of the trapezius. The nerve is dissected as far distally as possible. The contribution of C4 to the spinal accessory nerve and the superior branch of the spinal accessory nerve are left intact, thereby preserving upper trapezius function. Only the distal branch is divided and used for neurotization of the avulsed brachial plexus.

Deficit following harvest

Harvesting the spinal accessory nerve distal to the branch for the upper trapezius results in partial paralysis of the lower trapezius. In those patients with complete C5T1 avulsion, the lower trapezius paralysis has no functional consequence because of the concomitant serratus anterior paralysis.

Common transfers

The spinal accessory nerve is most commonly transferred to the suprascapular nerve for the restoration of abduction and flexion of the shoulder (Narakas 1987, Allieu and Cenac 1988, Narakas and Hentz 1988, Chuang 1995, Mackinnon and Novak 1999, Terzis et al 1999, Nath and Mackinnon 2000). Transfers to the posterior cord, axillary and radial nerves or the musculocutaneous nerve have been performed (Katoni et al 1972, Allieu et al 1984, Chuang et al 1993a, Bentolila et al 1999, Terzis et al 1999, Samardzic et al 2000). The branches to the upper trapezius (from the spinal accessory nerve or from C4) must be preserved to maintain scapular control and eventually allow for future trapezius muscle transfer.

Neurotization of the suprascapular nerve with the spinal accessory nerve does not require interpositional nerve grafts. In our experience with neurotization of the suprascapular nerve we have been able to achieve 90° of shoulder abduction in 38% of cases and 45–90° abduction in 33% of cases. Results are equivalent whatever the type of C5C6 lesion (rupture or avulsion). Recently, the spinal accessory nerve has been used to reinnervate free muscle transfers for biceps reconstruction.

Contraindications

Harvesting of the spinal accessory nerve in patients with a C4 lesion is contraindicated because of the resulting shoulder instability (Songcharoen et al 1996).

Pitfalls/complications

Intraoperative

Occasionally there may be size discrepancies between the suprascapular and spinal accessory nerve. When this occurs, we have had to use branches of the deep cervical plexus with nerve grafts to accommodate the size difference. Transfer to the musculocutaneous nerve requires interpositional grafts (Allieu et al 1984, Waikakul et al 1999b). The spinal accessory nerve or C4 is injured in one out of five cases of total root avulsion. A C4 injury may be a contraindication to using the spinal accessory nerve, because of the risk of a complete shoulder instability caused by a postoperative trapezius paralysis combined with a paralysis of the levator scapulae and the rhomboids (Songcharoen et al 1996).

Long-term

Use of the spinal accessory nerve means that future use of the trapezius as a muscle transfer for shoulder reanimation is lost. Lower trapezius paralysis contributes to the dysfunction of the scapulothoracic musculature.

Ipsilateral ulnar nerve

History

Oberlin first proposed this technique in 1994. This transfer is used to restore elbow flexion when C5 and C6 roots are avulsed, by transferring a portion of the functional ulnar nerve directly to the nerve to the biceps.

Anatomy

The ulnar nerve is the main continuation of the medial cord and receives contributions from roots C8 and T1. At the upper arm, the ulnar nerve is located between the brachial artery and vein, and behind the median nerve. Above the humeral attachment of the coracobrachialis muscle, the neurovascular bundle including the ulnar nerve is anterior to the medial intermuscular septum. At the level of the humeral attachment of the coracobrachialis, the ulnar nerve leaves the neurovascular bundle and passes posteriorly through the intermuscular septum to reach the posterior compartment of the arm. The ulnar nerve does not give any branches at the arm level.

At the mid-arm level, the ulnar nerve contains between 4 and 15 fascicles, with a mean of 9 fascicles (Sunderland 1978). At this level there are multiple interfascicular communications. As such, no one fascicle is associated with a specific motor function. Harvesting of one or two anterior fascicles is of no clinical consequence.

At the arm level, the musculocutaneous nerve lies between the two heads of the biceps. Its point of entry into the biceps is above the middle of the arm in 20% of cases, about the middle of the arm in 50% of cases and below in 30% of cases (Sunderland 1978). Anatomic variations of the musculocutaneous nerve include the root origins (from C4 and/or C7) and its relation with the muscles of the arm and with the median nerve. A part or the whole musculocutaneous nerve may accompany the median nerve, or fibers of the median nerve may be within the musculocutaneous nerve.

Usually, the musculocutaneous nerve sends a single common branch to the biceps that then further divides into two branches; one to the short and one to the long head of the biceps. In 12–45% of cases, two separated branches come from the musculocutaneous nerve directly to the two heads of the biceps (Oberlin 1997, Leechavengvongs et al 1998).

Motor and sensory function

The ulnar nerve sends branches to the flexor carpi ulnaris and to the flexor digitorum profundus at the forearm level. At the hand, the ulnar nerve innervates the hypothenar muscles, the interossei, and the third and fourth lumbrical muscles. The palmar and dorsal cutaneous branches innervate the little finger, the ulnar side of the ring finger, and the ulnar side of the hand.

Motor axon counts

The ulnar nerve contains 14,161 nerve fibers (Bonnel 1996) at the upper arm level. Comparing the size of the ulnar nerve with the branch to the biceps, Oberlin concluded that the number of nerve fibers innervating the biceps muscle would be 10% of the nerve fibers of the ulnar nerve at the same level (Oberlin 1994).

Surgical exposure/harvesting

The brachial artery and medial intermuscular septum are palpated and marked. A longitudinal skin incision is made on the medial aspect of the upper arm along the intermuscular septum. The deep investing fascia is opened anterior to the intermuscular septum. The musculocutaneous nerve is identified between the two heads of the biceps. The motor branches to the biceps are identified. The ulnar nerve is exposed through the same approach. Under the microscope, a fascicular dissection of the ulnar nerve is performed. Using an electrical nerve stimulator, two fascicles are identified that mainly supply the wrist flexor muscles. These two fascicles are divided and directly sutured to the biceps branches.

Deficit following harvest

In Leechavengvong's series of 32 patients, grip and pinch strength and two-point discrimination on the little finger were unchanged postoperatively following this nerve transfer (Leechavengvong et al 1998). There was no functional loss in the hand after surgery. The authors noted improved grip and pinch strength after surgery; this was probably the result of increased use of the hand. Nine of 32 patients had transient paresthesia in the small finger for 2–3 weeks. Sungpet et al (2000) described the same experience with a series of 36 patients who underwent this transfer.

Common transfers

In this technique, one or two fascicles of the ulnar nerve are transferred to the nerve to the biceps. This nerve transfer allows an M4 biceps in 83–87% of the cases (Leechavengvongs et al 1998, Sungpet et al 2000).

Pitfalls/complications

No complications are described, but traumatic dissection of the ulnar nerve may be followed by an ulnar nerve partial palsy. The main advantages of this technique are the short distance between the donor ulnar nerve and the motor point of the biceps and the possibility of doing a direct suture between the donor ulnar nerve and the motor branches of the biceps without intermediate graft. As in other nerve surgery, delay between trauma and nerve repair and age of the patient are negative factors influencing final outcome.

Deep cervical plexus

History

The first description of using the deep cervical plexus as a nerve transfer in brachial plexus reconstruction is not known. In 1913 Tuttle described using the deep cervical plexus to neurotize the upper trunk. Brunelli has been a major proponent of using the deep cervical plexus in brachial plexus reconstruction (Narakas 1987, 1991, Brunelli 1996).

Anatomy

The cervical plexus is made up of ventral branches of C1, C2, C3, and part of C4, which unite along the origins of the medial scalenus muscle and the levator scapulae muscle. The plexus is covered by the prevertebral laminae of the cervical fascia. The cervical plexus is formed through loop-like anastomoses. The cutaneous branches penetrate the prevertebral lamina of the cervical fascia at Erb's point (junction of the upper and middle third of sternocleidomastoid). Erb's point is a key landmark in the dissection of the cervical plexus. From Erb's point the branches of the cervical plexus spread out over the anterior and lateral aspect of the neck.

Motor and sensory function

According to Brunelli's description, the cervical plexus most often has four motor and four sensory branches (Brunelli 1996). The sensory branches of the cervical plexus include the greater auricular nerve (C3), transverse cervical nerve (C3C4), the supraclavicular nerves (C3C4), and the lesser occipital nerve. There are motor branches for the sternocleidomastoid, trapezius, levator scapulae, and the rhomboid muscles. The deep motor branches of the cervical plexus are situated under the prevertebral lamina of the cervical fascia. These branches supply the prevertebral neck musculature and part of the levator scapulae and the medial scalenus muscle. There are branches going to the trapezius muscle (from C3 and C4) that participate in motor innervation of this muscle and may also contain many proprioceptive fibers.

Motor axon counts

Brunelli has described the number of myelinated axons of motor branches of the cervical plexus. The number of myelinated fibers ranged from 3400 to 4000 (Brunelli 1996).

Surgical exposure/harvesting

The cervical plexus is easily identified in the brachial plexus operative field. The cervical plexus is covered by the prevertebral laminae of the cervical fascia. The cervical plexus can be found by identifying Erb's point at the junction of the upper and middle thirds of the sternocleidomastoid muscle. Erb's point is a key landmark in the dissection of the brachial plexus and should be marked out at the onset of the procedure. From Erb's point the branches of the cervical plexus spread out over the anterior and lateral aspect of the neck and are easily identified. The motor branches of the deep cervical plexus are located between the scalenus anterior and medius muscles. The cervical plexus courses between the C5 spinal nerve and the spinal accessory nerve. While dissecting the phrenic nerve up to the origin of the C4 spinal nerve, two or three branches (innervating the levator scapular, rhomboids or trapezius) can be found. These branches are verified with nerve stimulation.

Deficit following harvest

Harvesting of motor branches of the cervical plexus will result in motor paralysis of the corresponding muscle (i.e. sternocleidomastoid, trapezius, levator scapulae, and rhomboid muscles).

Common transfers

Brunelli has transferred motor branches of the deep cervical plexus to the suprascapular, axillary, and median nerves (Brunelli 1996). Narakas has described augmenting the transfer to spinal accessory nerve to suprascapular nerve with additional input from motor branches of the deep cervical plexus, and has transferred the motor branch to levator scapulae to the long thoracic nerve (Narakas 1991). The cervical plexus has been used for reconstruction of the suprascapular, axillary, musculocutaneous, median, and radial nerves by Terzis et al (1999).

Pitfalls/complications

- Intermediate nerve grafts are required.
- It has been our experience that motor branches of the cervical plexus provide unpredictable results when used as sole nerve transfer.
- Harvesting of all motor branches of the cervical plexus would result in destabilization of the scapula.

Phrenic nerve

History

The phrenic nerve as a potential nerve transfer in brachial plexus reconstruction was first proposed by Lurje (1948). Gu in China has been a major proponent of this nerve transfer (Gu et al 1989, 1990, Gu and Ma 1996); its use by Western surgeons has been limited. The phrenic nerve has been used as a nerve transfer in the avulsed brachial plexus lesion by several authors (Chuang 1995, Terzis et al 1999).

Anatomy

The phrenic nerve is the motor nerve to the diaphragm. The origin of the phrenic nerve is variable. It originates principally from the 4th cervical nerve but may receive contributions from the 3rd and 5th cervical nerves. The phrenic nerve lies anterior to the scalenus anterior muscle. An accessory phrenic nerve usually joins the main trunk distal to the clavicular level and has an individual course down to the diaphragm only in rare cases.

Motor and sensory function

The phrenic nerve innervates the ipsilateral hemi-diaphragm.

Motor axon counts

The phrenic nerve has approximately 800 myelinated axons (Chuang 1995).

Surgical exposure/harvesting

The main trunk of the phrenic nerve is easily identified over the anterolateral margin of the scalenus anterior and descends obliquely over the muscle with an angle of 25–30° toward the clavicle. The nerve can be identified by nerve stimulation. The main trunk of the phrenic nerve passes in front of the subclavian artery and behind the vein. The phrenic nerve is dissected distally to the level of the jugular fossa and divided. The proximal end of the nerve is transposed laterally for neurotization to the brachial plexus.

Deficit following harvest

Harvesting of the phrenic nerve results in ipsilateral hemi-diaphragm paralysis.

Common transfers

The phrenic nerve has been commonly transferred to the musculocutaneous (Terzis et al 1999), median, radial (Terzis et al 1999) or axillary nerves (Gu et al 1989). In 1995 Chuang described phrenic nerve transfer most commonly to the suprascapular or the dorsal one-half of the upper trunk or the axillary nerve for shoulder abduction. In a series of 96 patients, all with a complete avulsion, Waikakul (1999a) transferred the phrenic nerve to the suprascapular nerve to restore shoulder abduction. The author achieved shoulder abduction of more than 60° in 85% of the cases. We do not use the phrenic nerve routinely as a nerve transfer.

Pitfalls/complications

A major drawback to using the phrenic nerve as a nerve transfer lies with concerns surrounding decreased pulmonary function following harvesting. Gu et al (1989) found that pulmonary capacity was reduced owing to limited excursion of the diaphragm for 1 year but then pulmonary capacity recovered to normal values by 2 years postoperatively. Chuang (1995) describes frequent use of the phrenic nerve for neurotization in adults following avulsion of the brachial plexus without any significant respiratory problems. No significant respiratory problems were noted even when harvesting the phrenic nerve with concomitant intercostal nerve transfers (Chuang 1995).

C7 spinal nerve: ipsilateral or contralateral

History

In 1989 Gu et al first reported the use of the contralateral C7 root for neurotization of severe brachial plexus lesions. Since this early description, several authors have used the contralateral and ipsilateral C7 root for brachial plexus reconstruction without major morbidity (Gu et al 1992, 1998, Chuang et al 1993a, 1998, Gu 1994, 1997, Gu and Shen 1994, Liu et al 1997, Bertelli and Ghizoni 1999, Terzis et al 1999, Waikakul et al 1999a).

Anatomy

The C7 root consists of sensory, motor, and autonomic fibers. The C7 spinal nerve contributes to the posterior cord and to the median, pectoral, musculocutaneous, and ulnar nerves. The C7 innervated muscle receives contributions from other roots, mainly C6 and C8, and to a lesser degree C5 and T1. Because of this overlap, isolated C7 harvesting does not usually result in significant loss of any specific motor function (Chuang 1995, Gu et al 1998).

Motor axon counts

The C7 root has 16,000–40,000 myelinated axons (Chuang 1995).

Surgical exposure/harvesting

The C7 root is identified through a transverse incision placed 1 cm above the clavicle. The incision starts medially at the suprasternal area and ends laterally at the distal third of the clavicle. The C7 root is dissected down to the level of where it divides. Motor function is tested with intraoperative nerve stimulation (Holland and Belzberg 1997).

Deficit following harvest

Sensory and motor deficits in the distribution of C7 root are possible; few authors have described permanent defects in the limb. This may be explained by the fact that the adjacent roots overlap the territory of C7 root. After sectioning the C7 root, transient numbness in the index finger (74%), middle finger (58%), and thumb (38%) have been described (Gu 1994, Gu and Shen 1994, Liu 1997).

Electromyography and nerve conduction studies after complete harvesting of C7 (performed 1 week to 51 months postoperatively) showed no statistical difference in radial nerve motor conduction when compared to a control group. Median nerve sensory conduction was slightly lower (statistically significant) than in the control group (Gu 1994, Gu and Shen 1994).

Common transfers

Chuang (1995) has described the use of the ipsilateral C7 plexoplexus neurotization and contralateral C7 transfer to the musculocutaneous and median nerves with vascularized interpositional ulnar nerve grafts. Waikakul et al (1999a) use contralateral C7 to the median nerve only. The contralateral C7 has been transferred to the suprascapular and axillary nerves with good resultant shoulder abduction despite long nerve grafts (Bertelli and Ghizoni 1999).

Pitfalls/complications

A study by Chuang et al (1998) revealed that nearly half of the study group (48%) reported no significant sensory changes and most patients (81%) did not notice any weakness of the limb following C7 transection. Some patients did experience sensory and motor abnormalities that were most frequent during the first postoperative month and in most cases resolved by the third postoperative month. The only long-term abnormality was a weak or absent triceps reflex. Liu et al (1997) described initial weakness in a few muscles after sectioning C7 root.

Long thoracic nerve

History

Narakas (1987) was the first to describe utilization of the long thoracic nerve.

Anatomy

The long thoracic nerve takes its origin from the anterior rami of the C5, C6, and C7 close to the intervertebral foramina. The long thoracic nerve may also receive contributions from C4 and very rarely from C8. The nerve passes down behind the rest of the brachial plexus, and emerges from behind the axillary vessels and the plexus in the upper part of the axilla. It then continues down on the outer (superficial) surface of the serratus anterior to supply it. The long thoracic nerve is relatively well protected in the neck, for after it emerges from the scalenes it lies behind the brachial plexus and the subclavian vessels.

Motor and sensory function

The long thoracic nerve innervates the serratus anterior muscle. The serratus anterior protracts the scapula, especially its inferior angle. With protraction of the inferior angle, it produces upward rotation of the scapula necessary for full abduction of the arm. Owing to its course around the curve of the thorax, the muscle also holds the medial border of the scapula tightly against the thoracic cage.

Upward rotation of the scapula by the serratus is assisted by the upper fibers of the trapezius. The serratus can perform upward rotation of the scapula without the trapezius. Upward rotation and therefore full abduction or flexion of the arm cannot occur when the serratus is paralysed, owing to absence of upward rotation of the scapula.

Motor axon counts

The long thoracic nerve has approximately 1600–1800 myelinated axons (Narakas 1984, Chuang 1995).

Surgical exposure/harvesting

The long thoracic nerve can be found behind the middle trunk and underlying the scalenus medius muscle. Intraoperative nerve stimulation can be used for verification.

Deficit following harvest

Harvesting of the long thoracic nerve is associated with paralysis of the serratus anterior and subsequent winging of the scapula.

Common transfers

The use of this nerve is not recommended because of the high likelihood of injury and the inability to estimate the degree of injury and because of the serratus anterior paralysis and subsequent shoulder dysfunction.

Pitfalls/complications

The likelihood of finding the long thoracic nerve in continuity and functioning following a brachial plexus injury is quite low. Harvesting of the long thoracic nerve results in paralysis of the serratus anterior and major dysfunction of the scapulothoracic joint.

Pectoral nerves

History

Gilbert (1992) described the transfer of an uninjured pectoral nerve from the contralateral side onto the musculocutaneous nerve in a two-stage procedure with a long sural nerve graft. In 1999, Mackinnon and Novak described the use of the ipsilateral medial pectoral nerve for neurotization of the musculocutaneous nerve in upper trunk brachial plexus injuries.

Anatomy

Lateral pectoral nerve

The lateral pectoral nerve is derived from the lateral cord of the brachial plexus and usually contains fibers from C5 to C7; it supplies the clavicular and the upper portion of the sternal parts of the pectoralis major muscle.

Medial pectoral nerve

The medial pectoral nerve is derived from the medial cord, and usually contains fibers from C8 and T1. It supplies the pectoralis minor and then continues through or around the lateral edge of the minor to end in the lower part of the pectoral major. It supplies the lower sternal and abdominal parts of the pectoralis major.

Motor and sensory function

Pectoralis major

Two nerves, the lateral and medial pectoral nerves, innervate the pectoralis major. The pectoralis major is an adductor and internal rotator of the arm; it contracts for internal rotation only against resistance.

Pectoralis minor

The chief action of the pectoralis minor is to depress the lateral angle of the scapula. It thus assists in downward rotation of the scapula. If the shoulder is retracted, the pectoralis minor will help to draw the scapula forward.

Motor axon counts

The ramus to the pectoral muscles has 400–600 myelinated axons per ramus (Narakas 1984, Chuang 1995).

Surgical exposure/harvesting

During exposure of the brachial plexus, the pectoralis major muscle is reflected and the underlying pectoralis minor is divided at its insertion. Branches of the medial pectoral nerve can be identified on the deep surface of the pectoralis minor muscle. Intraoperative nerve stimulation will help to identify these branches. The branches are dissected distally as they make their way to innervate the pectoralis major muscle; this will increase the length of the nerve available for neurotization, facilitating direct coaptation.

Deficit following harvest

Harvesting of the pectoral nerves may result in weak shoulder adduction and flexion. Paralysis of the sternal portion of the pectoralis major will alter the anterior axillary fold; this may result in change in breast position in the female.

Common transfers

Gilbert (1992) transferred healthy lateral pectoral nerves from the contralateral side onto the musculocutaneous nerve on the affected side and obtained M3+ power of elbow flexion (that is the ability to flex the elbow against resistance of gravity). This transfer was performed in two separate procedures via a long cross-chest nerve graft. Mackinnon and Novak (1999) described direct coaptation to the musculocutaneous nerve.

Pitfalls/complications

Transfer of the ipsilateral medial pectoral nerve is possible only in cases where the medial cord is spared, typically in upper trunk lesions. The use of the contralateral pectoral nerves, as described by Gilbert, requires long nerve grafts. Paralysis of the sternal portion of the pectoralis major will alter the anterior axillary fold; this may result in change in breast position in the female.

Hypoglossal nerve

History

There has been limited clinical experience using the hypoglossal nerve as a donor for neurotization of the adult brachial plexus. Narakas (1987) first proposed that the hypoglossal nerve be used as a donor nerve for neurotization of severe adult brachial plexus lesions. In 1992, Romana presented two cases of hypoglossal nerve transfer with promising results. Slooff and Blaauw (1996) later reported their experience of using the hypoglossal nerve in the treatment of severe adult traumatic and obstetric brachial plexus lesions. The authors described the indications for using the hypoglossal nerve as a nerve transfer and several important anatomic and surgical considerations. They suggested that the hypoglossal nerve may be used in cases of multiple root avulsions for the neurotization of the musculocutaneous nerve.

Anatomy

The hypoglossal nerve (cranial nerve XI) arises from the medulla. It passes to the hypoglossal canal where it pierces the dura and leaves the skull. It is a motor nerve to the intrinsic and extrinsic muscles of the tongue. The hypoglossal nerve also carries somatomotor and proprioceptive fibers.

The hypoglossal nerve passes out of the skull along the hypoglossal canal and then runs between the internal jugular vein and the internal carotid artery. It passes forward superficial to the external carotid artery and its branches. The hypoglossal nerve enters the digastric triangle by passing deep to the posterior belly of the digastric muscle or its tendon. The nerve then passes deep through the mylohyoid muscle and runs forward, superficial to the hyoglossus muscle between the hyoid bone and the submandibular duct. It ends by passing deep to the genioglossus muscle. In its course it supplies branches to the intrinsic muscles of the tongue and the styloglossus, genioglossus, hyoglossus, thyrohyoid, and geniohyoid muscles.

Ansa cervicalis

The ansa cervicalis is associated with the hypoglossal nerve. The ansa cervicalis is a loop of nerve tissues supplying the strap muscles. The hypoglossal nerve is joined by fibers from the 1st cervical nerve shortly after it leaves the skull. It then runs forward, superficial to most structures, to supply muscles of the tongue. Before it reaches the tongue, the fibers from the 1st cervical nerve pass inferiorly and join with fibers from the 2nd and 3rd cervical nerves to form the ansa cervicalis. The ansa cervicalis gives branches to the sternohyoid, sternothyroid, and omohyoid muscles.

Motor and sensory function

The hypoglossal nerve is principally a motor nerve to the tongue.

Motor axon counts

This nerve has approximately 9200 myelinated axons (Chuang 1995, Mackinnon and Dellon 1995). The largest number of myelinated axons in a potential donor nerve is found in the contralateral C7 root (16,000–40,000 myelinated axons). This makes the hypoglossal nerve the second largest donor nerve in terms of myelinated axons.

Surgical exposure/harvesting

The hypoglossal nerve is found by extending the brachial plexus incision diagonally below the mandible over the anterior border of the sternocleidomastoid muscle. The underlying platysma and fascia are divided. A key landmark in identifying this nerve is the digastric muscle. The hypoglossal nerve runs deep to the plane of the digastric muscle and superficial to the carotid vessels. Another key landmark is the hyoid horn. The hypoglossal nerve is found in the space separating the hyoid horn from the digastric muscle. Once the posterior belly of the digastric muscle is identified, the hypoglossal nerve is dissected free immediately medial to the intermediate tendon of the digastric muscle. The nerve may be confirmed with electrical stimulation and direct visualization of ipsilateral tongue movement. The ansa hypoglossi may be identified and dissected so that, if desired, it can be sutured to the distal hypoglossal stump for reinnervation of the tongue musculature. The hypoglossal nerve should be transected as far distal as possible to provide maximal length. The nerve is then delivered into the plexus wound, passing deep to the posterior belly of the digastric and deep or superficial to the sternocleidomastoid muscle, where it will be grafted to the recipient nerve.

Deficit following harvest

Harvesting of the hypoglossal nerve is associated with ipsilateral paralysis of the tongue.

Common transfers

Hypoglossal nerve to upper trunk, lateral cord, and musculocutaneous nerve transfers have been associated with favorable functional results. Biceps motor strength was graded as M4 or M3 with a mean active elbow flexion of 109° in five of eight cases. Terzis has used the hypoglossal as a nerve transfer to the musculocutaneous in two cases (Terzis et al 1999).

Pitfalls/complications

Hemiparalysis of the tongue. Patients describe difficulty moving food to the back of the throat – making swallowing difficult. Pronunciation may be difficult immediately after surgery but this recovers quickly. All patients noted easy fatigability after talking for a prolonged period of time. Use of the hypoglossal nerve may not be ideal in patients who need clear speech for their profession. Patients with active elbow motion were able to augment the force of biceps contraction by pressing their tongues onto their palates. In this group of patients, involuntary elbow movements while chewing were noted at the very onset of biceps reinnervation. With time and practice, all patients were able to control these movements with simultaneous co-contraction of the triceps.

Co-contraction of the triceps during chewing was later carried out without conscious effort by all patients. Involuntary elbow movement was not a major complication or problem.

Neurotization procedures

Neurotization is planned along with consideration of future reconstructive procedures (e.g. arthrodesis, tenodesis, musculotendinous and free functioning muscle transfers).

C5 to T1 root avulsion

In cases of total root (C5 to T1) root avulsions, the reconstructive goals are to (1) restore elbow flexion, (2) reconstruct thoracobrachial grasp, (3) stabilize the shoulder, and (4) restore wrist and finger flexion as well as hand sensation.

Nerve transfers for elbow flexion

The third and fourth intercostal nerves are transferred to the musculocutaneous nerve in an effort to restore elbow flexion. When the spinal accessory nerve or the intercostal nerves are not available, the hypoglossal nerve is transferred to the musculocutaneous nerve (Figure 16.2A).

Nerve transfers for thoracobrachial grasp

The second intercostal nerve can be transferred to the medial pectoral nerve to restore function of the lower portion of pectoralis major (Figure 16.2B).

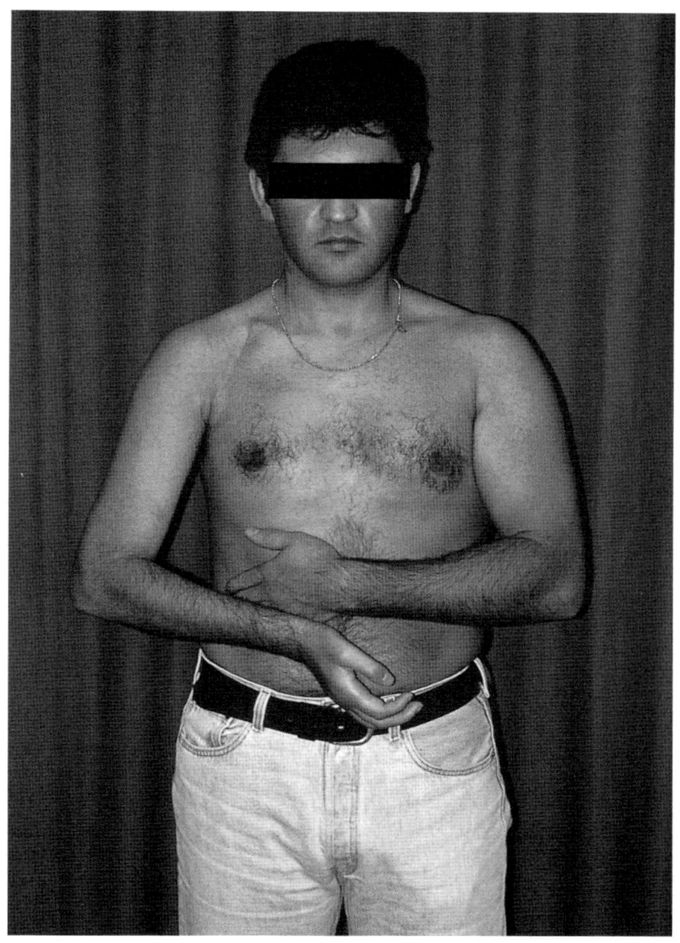

(A)

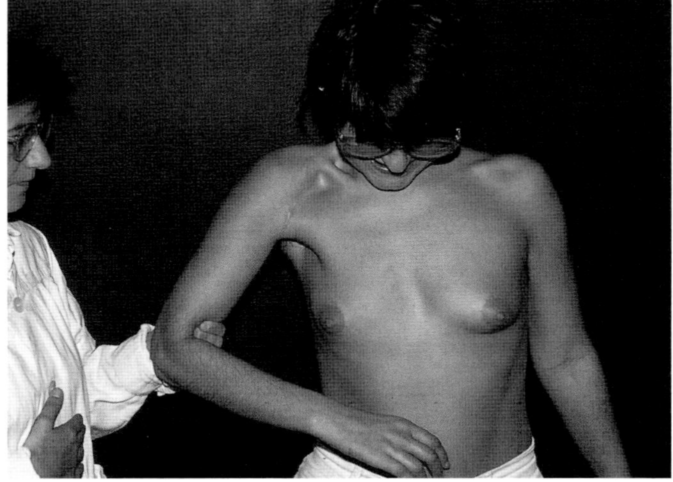

(B)

Figure 16.2
(A) XII to musculocutaneous nerve transfer. Functional results at 2 years after neurotization of the musculocutaneous nerve with the hypoglossal nerve. (B) Intercostal nerve 2 to medial pectoral nerve transfer. Functional results at 2 years after neurotization of the medial pectoral nerve with the second intercostal nerve. The lower part of the pectoralis major has partially recovered.

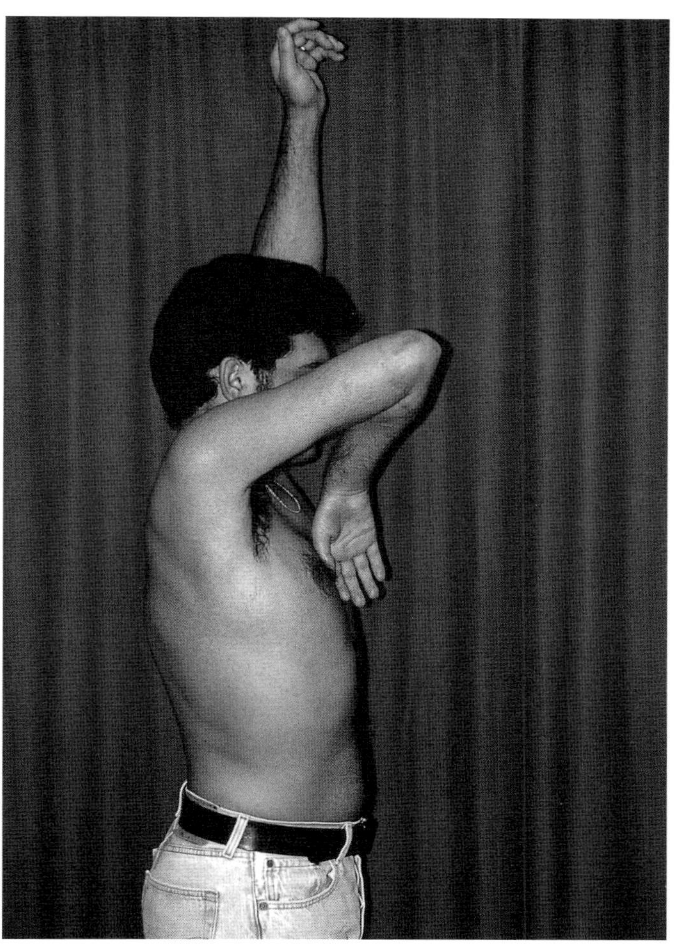

Figure 16.3
Spinal accessory nerve to suprascapular nerve transfer. Result 2 years after neurotization of the suprascapular nerve through the spinal accessory nerve. Full abduction and shoulder flexion with a large opening of the scapulo-humeral angle.

Nerve transfers for shoulder stabilization

In an effort to stabilize the shoulder by reanimating the serratus anterior muscle, the nerve to levator scapulae or the second intercostal nerve is transferred to the long thoracic nerve. In addition, the spinal accessory nerve is transferred to the suprascapular nerve in an effort to reanimate the supraspinatus (Figure 16.3).

Nerve transfers for wrist/finger flexion and hand sensation

Intercostal nerves 5 and 6 are transferred to the median nerve in an effort to restore wrist and finger flexion as well as protective hand sensation.

Conclusions

Neurotization or nerve transfers are used in the treatment of brachial plexus avulsion injuries. The gain in function must be greater than the loss of function that occurs following harvest of a donor nerve. All motor and sensory nerves, within or outside the brachial plexus, are potential nerve transfers. Cortical plasticity as it relates to nerve transfers, particularly extraplexal transfers, is important and may eventually be shown to be an important variable in terms of functional outcomes.

The theoretical advantage of nerve transfers, as opposed to nerve grafts, is the ability to perform direct coaptation between the donor nerve and the recipient (i.e. spinal accessory nerve transferred to the suprascapular nerve versus C5 grafted to the suprascapular nerve). There is no clinical difference between the results of these two types of reconstruction. In several clinical situations, nerve transfers are the only available reconstructive option (i.e. C5–T1 avulsion injuries). The results in this clinical scenario are variable. The following principles should be followed:

- Nerves with predominant motor function recover better (radial better than median).
- When the nerve being reconstructed innervates one or two muscles (e.g. musculocutaneous or suprascapular nerve) the results are better than in neurotization of a nerve with multiple motor functions (median or ulnar nerve). Therefore, nerve transfers to the suprascapular or musculocutaneous nerves work better than neurotization of the median or ulnar nerves.
- The shorter the distance between the nerve coaptation and the motor end plate the better the results.
- Do not transfer intercostal nerves in cases of Brown-Séquard syndrome because the intercostals are nonfunctional.
- Do not use the spinal accessory nerve in cases of C4 avulsion because this will result in destabilization of the shoulder.

Finally, nerve transfers are used in the late reconstruction of brachial plexus lesions. These are being used to motor free functioning muscle transfers, when patients present with a brachial plexus lesion older than 9 months (Doi et al 2000).

References

Allieu Y, Cenac P (1988) Neurotization via the spinal accessory nerve in complete paralysis due to multiple avulsion injuries of the brachial plexus, *Clin Orthop* **237**: 67–74.

Allieu Y, Privat JM, Bonnel F (1984) Paralysis in root avulsion of the brachial plexus. Neurotization by the spinal accessory nerve, *Clin Plast Surg* **11**: 133–6.

Bentolila V, Nizard R, Bizot P, Sedel L. (1999) Complete traumatic brachial plexus palsy. Treatment and outcome after repair, *J Bone Joint Surg* **81A**: 20–8.

Bertelli JA, Ghizoni MF (1999) Selective motor hyperreinnervation by using contralateral C-7 motor rootlets in the reconstruction of an avulsion injury of the brachial plexus. Case report, *J Neurosurg* **90**: 1133–6.

Birch R, Bonney G, Wynn Parry CB (1998) *Surgical Disorders of the Peripheral Nerves* (Churchill Livingstone: Edinburgh).

Bonnel F, Canovas F (1996) Anatomy of the brachial plexus at the newborn and the adult. Macroscopic and histologic structures. In: Alnot JY, Narakas A, eds, *Traumatic Brachial Plexus Injuries* (Expansion Scientifique Française: Paris) 3–13.

Brunelli G (1996) The cervical plexus. In: Alnot JY, Narakas A, eds, *Traumatic Brachial Plexus Injuries* (Expansion Scientifique Française: Paris) 39–42.

Carlstedt T, Grane P, Hallin RG et al (1995) Return of function after spinal cord implantation of avulsed spinal nerve roots, *Lancet* **346**: 1323–5.

Chuang DC (1995) Neurotization procedures for brachial plexus injuries, *Hand Clin* **11**: 633–45.

Chuang DC, Yeh MC, Wei FC (1992) Intercostal nerve transfer of the musculocutaneous nerve in avulsed brachial plexus injuries: evaluation of 66 patients, *J Hand Surg* **17A**: 822–8.

Chuang DC, Epstein MD, Yeh MC, Wei FC (1993a) Functional restoration of elbow flexion in brachial plexus injuries: results in 167 patients (excluding obstetric brachial plexus injury), *J Hand Surg* **18A**: 285–91.

Chuang DC, Wei FC, Noordhoff MS (1993b) Cross-chest C7 nerve grafting followed by free muscle transplantations for the treatment of total avulsed brachial plexus injuries: a preliminary report, *Plast Reconstr Surg* **92**: 717–25

Chuang DC, Cheng SL, Wei FC, Wu CL, Ho YS (1998) Clinical evaluation of C7 spinal nerve transection: 21 patients with at least 2 years' follow-up, *Br J Plast Surg* **51**: 285–90.

Doi K, Muramatsu K, Hattori Y et al (2000) Restoration of prehension with the double free muscle technique following complete avulsion of the brachial plexus, *J Bone Joint Surg* **82A**: 652–66.

Dolenc VV (1984) Intercostal neurotization of the peripheral nerves in avulsion plexus injuries, *Clin Plast Surg* **11**: 143–7.

Freilinger G, Holle J, Sulzbruber S (1978) Distribution of motor and sensory fibers in the intercostal nerves, *Plast Reconstr Surg* **62**: 240.

Giddins GE, Kakkar N, Alltree J, Birch R (1995) The effect of unilateral intercostal nerve transfer upon lung function, *J Hand Surg* **20B**: 675–6.

Gilbert A (1992) Neurotization by contralateral pectoral nerve. Presented at the 10th Symposium on the Brachial Plexus, Lausanne, Switzerland.

Gu YD (1994) Distribution of the sensory endings of the C7 nerve root and its clinic significance, *J Hand Surg* **19B**: 67–8.

Gu YD (1997) Functional motor innervation of brachial plexus roots. An intraoperative electrophysiological study, *J Hand Surg* **22B**: 258–60.

Gu YD, Shen LY (1994) Electrophysiological changes after severance of the C7 nerve root, *J Hand Surg* **19B**: 69–71.

Gu YD, Ma MK (1996) Use of the phrenic nerve for brachial plexus reconstruction, *Clin Orthop* **323**: 119–21.

Gu YD, Wu MM, Zhen YL et al (1989) Phrenic nerve transfer for brachial plexus motor neurotization, *Microsurgery* **10**: 287–9.

Gu YD, Wu MM, Zhen YL et al (1990) Phrenic nerve transfer for treatment of root avulsion of the brachial plexus, *Chin Med J* **103**: 267–70.

Gu YD, Zhang GM, Chen DS, Yan JG, Cheng XM, Chen L (1992) Seventh cervical nerve root transfer from the contralateral healthy side for treatment of brachial plexus root avulsion, *J Hand Surg* **17B**: 518–21.

Gu YD, Chen DS, Zhang GM et al (1998) Long-term functional results of contralateral C7 transfer, *J Reconstr Microsurg* **14**: 57–9.

Holland N, Belzberg A (1997) Intraoperative electrodiagnosis testing during cross-chest C7 nerve root transfer, *Muscle Nerve* **20**: 903–5.

Katoni P, Matsuda H, Suzuk T (1972) Trial surgical procedures of nerve transfer to avulsion injuries of plexus brachialis. In: *Orthopaedic Surgery and Traumatology* (Proceedings of the 12th Congress of the International Society of Orthopaedic Surgery and Traumatology: Tel Aviv) 348–50.

Leechavengvongs S, Witoonchart K, Uerpairojkit C, Thuvasethakul P, Ketmalasiri W (1998) Nerve transfer to biceps muscle using a part of the ulnar nerve in brachial plexus injury (upper arm type): a report of 32 cases, *J Hand Surg* **23A**: 711–16.

Liu J, Pho RW, Kour AK, Zhang AH, Ong BK (1997) Neurologic deficit and recovery in the donor limb following cross-C7 transfer in brachial-plexus injury, *J Reconstr Microsurg* **13**: 237–42.

Loy S, Bhatia A, Asfazadourian H, Oberlin C (1997) Ulnar nerve fascicle transfer on to the biceps muscle nerve in C5–C6 or C5–C6–C7 avulsions of the brachial plexus. Eighteen cases, *Ann Chir Main Memb Super* **16**: 275–84.

Lurje A (1948) Concerning surgical treatment of traumatic injury of the upper division of the brachial plexus (Erb's type), *Ann Surg* **127**: 317–26.

Mackinnon SE, Dellon AL (1995) Fascicular patterns of the hypoglossal nerve, *J Reconstr Microsurg* **11**: 195–8

Mackinnon SE, Novak CB (1999) Nerve transfers. New options for reconstruction following nerve injury, *Hand Clin* **15**: 643–66

Millesi H (1977) Surgical management of brachial plexus injuries, *J Hand Surg* **2A**: 367–78.

Nagano A, Ochiai N, Okinaga S (1992) Restoration of elbow flexion in root lesions of brachial plexus injuries, *J Hand Surg* **17A**: 815–21.

Narakas AO (1984) Thoughts on neurotization or nerve transfers in irreparable nerve lesions, *Clin Plast Surg* **11**: 153–9.

Narakas A (1987) Neurotization or nerve transfer in traumatic brachial plexus lesions. In: Tubiana R, ed, *The Hand* (WB Saunders: Philadelphia) 656–83.

Narakas A (1991) Neurotization in the treatment of brachial plexus injuries. In: Gelberman R, ed, *Operative Nerve Repair and Reconstruction* (Lippincott Company: Philadelphia) 1329–57.

Narakas AO, Hentz VR (1988) Neurotization in brachial plexus injuries. Indication and results, *Clin Orthop* **237**: 43–56.

Nath RK, Mackinnon SE (2000) Nerve transfers in the upper extremity, *Hand Clin* **16**: 131–9.

Ogino T, Naito T (1995) Intercostal nerve crossing to restore elbow flexion and sensibility of the hand for a root avulsion type of brachial plexus injury, *Microsurgery* **16**: 571–7.

Oberlin C, Beal D, Leechavengvongs S, Salon A, Dauge MC, Sarcy JJ (1994) Nerve transfer to biceps muscle using a part of ulnar nerve for C5–C6 avulsion of the brachial plexus: anatomical study and report of four cases, *J Hand Surg* **19A**: 232–7.

Romana C (1992) Communication in the Congress of the European Federation of Microsurgical Societies, Rome.

Samardzic M, Rasulic L, Grujicic D, Milicic B (2000) Results of nerve transfers to the musculocutaneous and axillary nerves, *Neurosurgery* **46**: 93–101.

Seddon HJ (1963) Nerve grafting, *J Bone Joint Surg* **45B**: 446–61.

Slooff ACJ, Blaauw G (1996) The hypoglossal nerve. In: Alnot JY, Narakas A, eds, *Traumatic Brachial Plexus Injuries* (Expansion Scientifique Française: Paris) 50–2.

Songcharoen P, Mahaisavariya B, Chotigavanich C (1996) Spinal accessory neurotization for restoration of elbow flexion in avulsion injuries of the brachial plexus, *J Hand Surg* **21A**: 387–90.

Sunderland S (1978) The ulnar nerve. Anatomical and physiological features. In: Sunderland S, ed, *Nerves and Nerve Injuries*, 2nd edn (Churchill Livingstone: Edinburgh) 728–49.

Sungpet A, Suphachatwong C, Kawinwonggowit V, Patradul A (2000) Transfer of a single fascicle from the ulnar nerve to the biceps muscle after avulsions of upper roots of the brachial plexus, *J Hand Surg* **25B**: 325–8.

Terzis JK, Vekris MD, Soucacos PN (1999) Outcomes of brachial plexus reconstruction in 204 patients with devastating paralysis, *Plast Reconstr Surg* **104**: 1221–40.

Tuttle H (1913) Exposure of the brachial plexus with nerve transplantation, *JAMA* **61**: 15–16.

Waikakul S, Orapin S, Vanadurongwan V (1999a) Clinical results of contralateral C7 root neurotization to the median nerve in brachial plexus injuries with total root avulsions, *J Hand Surg* **24B**: 556–60.

Waikakul S, Wongtragul S, Vanadurongwan V (1999b) Restoration of elbow flexion in brachial plexus avulsion injury: comparing spinal accessory nerve transfer with intercostal nerve transfer, *J Hand Surg* **24A**: 571–7.

Yeoman PMSH (1961) Brachial plexus injuries. Treatment of the flail arm, *J Bone Joint Surg* **43B**: 493–500.

17 Paralytic disorders of the shoulder girdle

Chantal Bonnard and Dimitri J Anastakis

Introduction

Normal mobility of the scapulothoracic and glenohumeral joints is necessary in order to control hand position in three-dimensional space. Stability and movement of the shoulder girdle are accomplished by three joints (i.e. sternoclavicular, acromioclavicular and glenohumeral joints), a gliding plane between the chest wall and scapula, and 19 muscles.

During shoulder abduction, one-third of the movement occurs through the scapulothoracic joint and two-thirds at the glenohumeral joint. During shoulder flexion, the combined action of trapezius and serratus anterior move the center of rotation of the scapula superior. This results in upward and medial displacement of the glenoid fossa and lateral displacement of the scapula's lower angle. The scapulo-humeral angle ranges from 25° at rest to 150° in abduction (Narakas 1993a). Abduction at the glenohumeral joint initially depends on the supraspinatus and then on the deltoid. With the arm adducted, the deltoid draws the humeral head up against the acromion – there is no abduction of the arm. When the glenohumeral angle gradually opens due to the supraspinatus, the deltoid becomes an efficient abductor, while the depressors of the shoulder stabilize the humeral head in front of the glenoid cavity. During full abduction, the humerus must be in a neutral position or in external rotation. This orchestration of shoulder girdle movements is referred to as the humero-scapulo-thoracic rhythm.

The humero-scapulo-thoracic rhythm is broken either by weakness or paralysis of a shoulder girdle muscle or by an underlying orthopedic lesion. The critical muscles required to maintain this rhythm are the trapezius and serratus anterior for scapulothoracic control and the supraspinatus and deltoid for glenohumeral control. This chapter will focus on isolated paralysis of the trapezius and serratus anterior and on lesions of the suprascapular and axillary nerves.

Spinal accessory nerve

Anatomy

The spinal accessory nerve has cranial and spinal roots. The cranial roots come from the medulla and leave the skull by passing through the jugular foramen. These roots supply the laryngeal muscles. The spinal portion is made up of roots originating from C1 to C6. The spinal portion arises through the foramen magnum joining the cranial portion and passes out through the jugular foramen. The nerve lies deep to the digastric muscle, alongside and then crosses the internal jugular vein, to reach the anterior aspect of the sternocleidomastoid.

The nerve may travel through the sternocleidomastoid or along its anterior aspect to enter the posterior triangle of the neck. Connections with the cervical plexus are common – providing the nerve with motor and proprioceptive fibers. The C4 contribution may innervate the upper trapezius directly. In the posterior triangle, the spinal accessory nerve is adjacent to lymph nodes. This anatomic relationship accounts for the high frequency of iatrogenic lesions associated with lymph node biopsy. Above the clavicle it gives off muscular branches for the upper trapezius and then moves deep, travelling further caudal and medial to innervate the middle and lower portions of the muscle. The spinal accessory nerve does not travel through an outlet or tunnel and does not have an entrapment-associated syndrome.

Etiology

The most common cause of a spinal accessory nerve lesion is iatrogenic, following lymph node biopsy (Alnot et al 1994, Bigliani et al 1996, Birch et al 1998). Nerve injury has also been described following rhytidectomy and repair of the carotid artery. This nerve may require resection during a radical neck dissection. The spinal accessory nerve may be injured following a stab or gunshot wound.

Trapezius paralysis may occur following a constant pressure across the shoulder (e.g. a heavy load carried across the shoulder), causing a stretching nerve injury. Trapezius paralysis may also appear spontaneously, resembling Parsonage–Turner syndrome.

Rarely, a neoplasm in the foramen jugulare may affect the ninth, tenth, eleventh, and twelfth nerves in a variety of described syndromes (Newsom-Davis et al 1984). In all these syndromes, the trapezius and sternocleidomastoid muscles are paralyzed. Finally, the spinal accessory nerve along with the entire brachial plexus may be injured following radiation therapy.

Symptomatology

Subjective symptom

Patients with spinal accessory palsy may suffer from pain for several reasons. Firstly, direct trauma (e.g. section, cauterization, or stretching) of the spinal accessory nerve is painful because this nerve contains sensory fibers. Secondly, the abnormally inferior position of the scapula strains the levator scapulae and rhomboids, leading to muscle spasm and pain. Finally, as the shoulder girdle falls impingement of the suprascapular nerve at the scapular notch may occur.

Objective findings

At rest, the shoulder is depressed and laterally translated, so that the distance between the medial side of the scapula and the spine increases. Abduction and flexion are limited because the scapula is incapable of normal rotation. The unopposed action of the serratus anterior pulls the scapula forwards and downwards so that the glenoid cavity cannot be oriented upwards and the scapulohumeral angle never reaches normal values (Narakas 1988).

To assess an isolated lesion of the middle and lower trapezius, the patient is asked to lie prone with the head and upper part of the chest raised off the bed. The patient is asked to raise their outstretched arms. It is easy to identify a trapezius paralysis during this maneuver when compared with the normal side (Figure 17.1). In this position, the last few degrees of shoulder flexion require normal lower trapezius contraction. Atrophy of the trapezius becomes increasingly evident with time as the scapula becomes more visible. Finally, in proximal lesions of the spinal accessory nerve (e.g. neoplasm in the foramen jugulare), both the trapezius and sternocleidomastoid muscles are paralyzed.

The diagnosis of a spinal accessory nerve lesion is often made late. This may be due to the fact that many

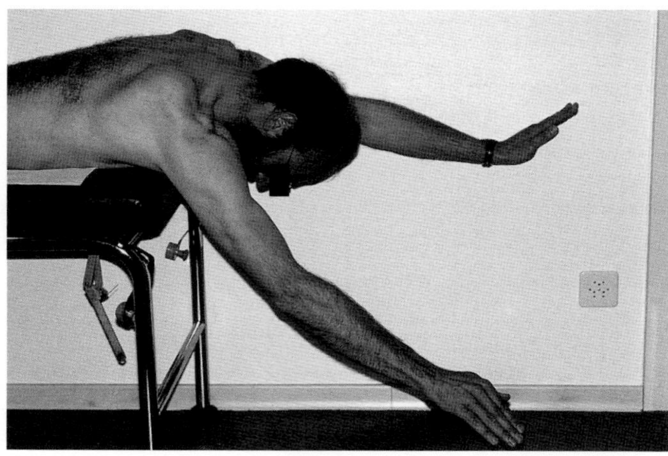

(A)

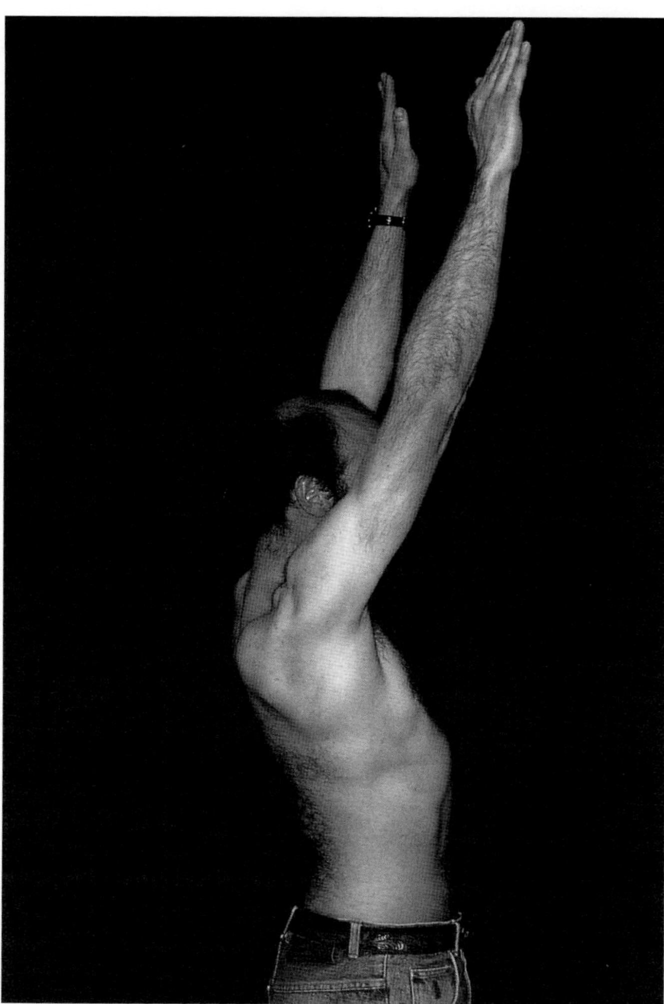

(B)

Figure 17.1

This patient has a complete right-sided trapezius paralysis, and illustrates the position for testing the middle and the lower trapezius. The complete trapezius paralysis is noted when the patient is lying prone (A) rather than when he is standing (B).

patients may still raise their shoulder by using the levator scapulae – masking a trapezius paralysis. Limited shoulder abduction and/or flexion may lead to an incorrect diagnosis of an orthopedic shoulder lesion such as a rotator cuff tear (Matz and Barbaro 1996). In Bigliani's series, the trapezius muscle had not been evaluated in half of the cases that had been referred to a neurologist for EMG studies (Bigliani et al 1996).

Treatment

With early diagnosis and depending on the type of injury, repair of the nerve with neurolysis or grafting is recommended (Alnot et al 1994, Birch et al 1998). Functional recovery is better following stab wounds than iatrogenic injuries. Occasionally, the distal end of the nerve cannot be identified. In such cases, the upper trapezius may then be reinnervated by a direct muscular neurotization (Alnot et al 1994). Following repair of the nerve, pain relief of varying degrees has been described. When the diagnosis of a spinal accessory nerve lesion is made late, reconstructive surgery is recommended.

Reconstructive surgery

In cases where the nerve repair fails or when the diagnosis of a spinal accessory nerve lesion is made late, reconstructive surgery is recommended. Two types of procedures exist for reconstruction of trapezius paralysis: (1) static stabilization of the scapula, or (2) dynamic muscle transfer. Dynamic muscle transfers improve the rotation of the scapula and diminish the lateral and forward translation due to excessive serratus anterior activity.

Static stabilization

This procedure involves stabilization of the medial border of the scapula using fascial slings to secure it to the spinous processes. Unfortunately, this procedure may loosen with time and at present it is not recommended. Spira (1948) described arthrodesis of the scapula to the sixth rib. This procedure severely limits shoulder function and is not indicated in isolated trapezius paralysis.

Dynamic muscle transfers

Dewar and Harris in 1950 first described a combination of static stabilization with a dynamic transfer of the levator scapulae onto the acromion. This procedure is recommended in chronic paralysis where the rhomboid muscles have been stretched over time and cannot be used in a transfer (Coessens and Wood 1995).

Transfer of the levator scapulae and rhomboids

Transfer of the levator scapulae and rhomboids is the most common dynamic muscle transfer for trapezius paralysis (Bigliani et al 1996, Birch et al 1998, Wiater and Bigliani 1999). It was first described by Eden (1924) and later by Lange (1951). The distal insertion of the levator scapula is transferred laterally adjacent to the acromion. The rhomboids major and minor are elevated with a portion of bone from the medial border of the scapula and fixed further laterally onto the spine and wing of the scapula (Figure 17.2). Bigliani et al (1996) transfer the rhomboid minor cephalad to the scapular spine in an attempt to recreate an action similar to that of the middle portion of the trapezius.

The first incision is made along the medial border of the scapula. The trapezius is divided and the levator scapulae and rhomboids are dissected with their pedicles and elevated with their distal bony insertions. The infraspinatus is detached from the scapula, the periostium is elevated, and holes are made in the wing of the scapula 4–5 cm lateral to the medial border. The distal portion of the rhomboids is fixed in its new position with nonabsorbable transosseous sutures. The infraspinatus is reattached. A second incision is made along the spine of the scapula. The plane between trapezius and supraspinatus muscle is dissected. The levator scapulae is passed through this tunnel and fixed on the spine of the scapula at 4–5 cm from the acromion.

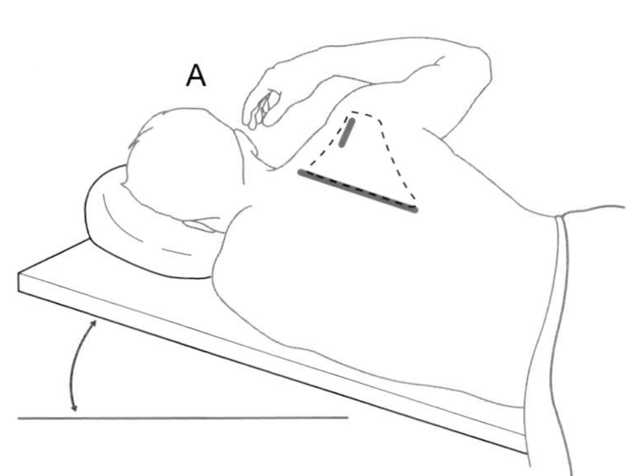

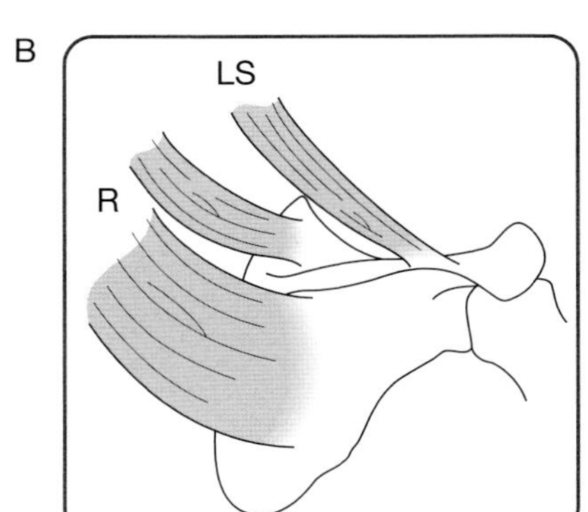

Figure 17.2
Eden–Lange procedure: (A) skin incisions; (B) transfer of levator scapulae near the acromion and transfer of the rhomboids laterally on the scapula.

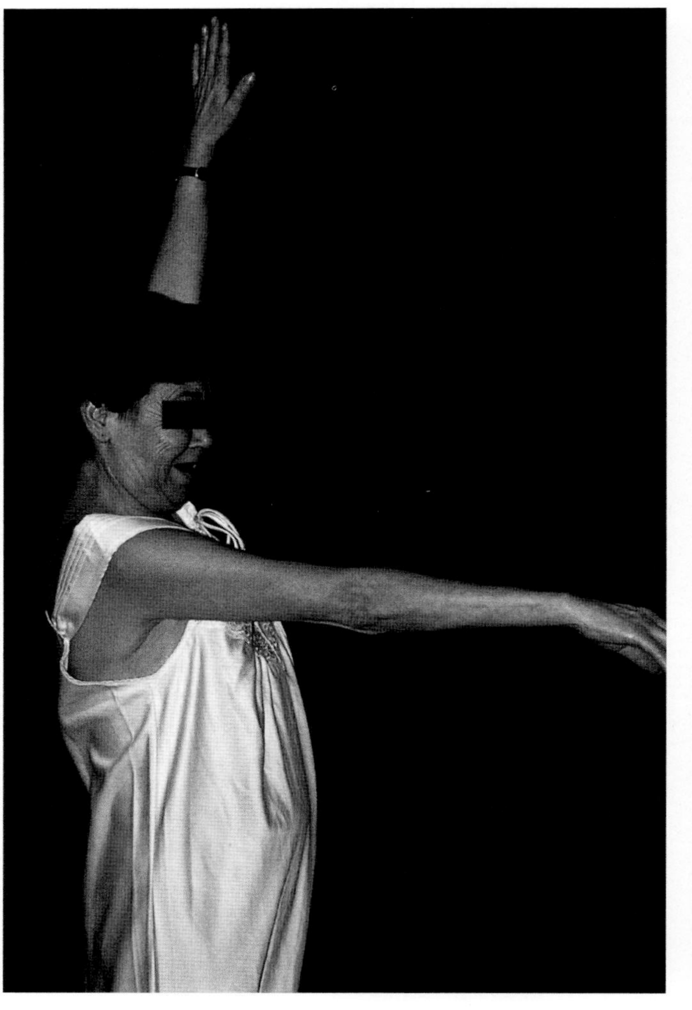
(A)

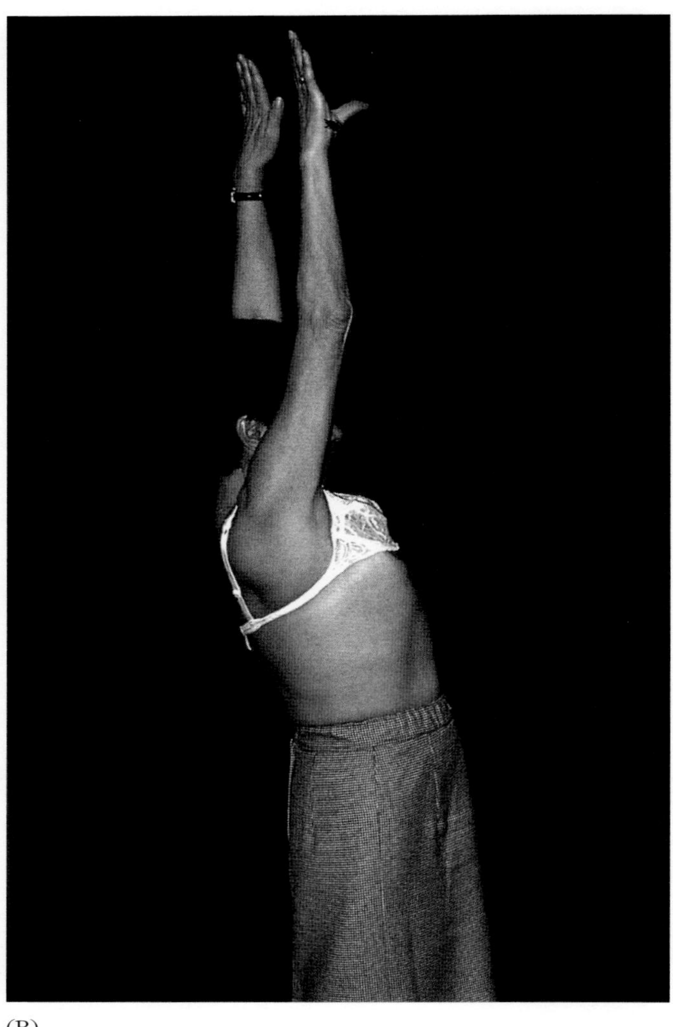
(B)

Figure 17.3
This patient has a complete trapezius paralysis after radical neck dissection, with reconstruction of trapezius function by the Eden–Lange procedure. (A) Preoperative; (B) postoperative.

Nonabsorbable sutures may be used, but we prefer to use either a screw or a Mitek anchor. The arm is immobilized at 90° abduction for 6 weeks. Passive range of motion is started after 6 weeks of immobilization. Active range of motion is started at 3 months postoperatively (Figure 17.3).

Narakas has performed two transfers using the entire latissimus dorsi (Narakas 1988). The muscle was completely dissected and then turned on itself like a page in a book. Its distal portion was fixed onto the spinous processes from T6 to T1, and its humeral tendon was transferred on the acromion. This was an aggressive procedure requiring extensive dissection of the back. As commonly occurs with the harvesting of the latissimus dorsi, a seroma developed and persisted for several months. The results were no better than those following Eden's procedure and we have since abandoned this procedure.

Long thoracic nerve (nerve to the serratus anterior)

Anatomy

The long thoracic nerve arises from C5–C6–C7. Contributions from C4 are frequent, whereas they are rare from C8. The branches from C5 and C6 roots emerge from the scalenus medius, the branch from C7 courses anterior to the muscle. They merge forming the long thoracic nerve at the level of the first intercostal space. The nerve then passes under a fascial band that is an extension of the insertion of the scalenus medius into the first digitations of the serratus antenor. The nerve may be compressed under this fascia (Hester et al 2000). The nerve then travels down along the chest wall 6–7 cm anterior to the scapula and innervates the serratus anterior muscle.

In flexion and/or abduction, the serratus anterior draws the scapula forward and outward. By the combined actions of the trapezius and serratus anterior, the scapula rotates upwards to allow full flexion and abduction. This function (scapular winging) is performed by the lower digitations of the serratus anterior that are innervated by C7.

Etiology

Scalenectomy or first rib resection through a transaxillary approach for thoracic outlet syndrome may be associated with iatrogenic injury to the long thoracic nerve. Following a cadaveric study, Salazar et al (1998) recommended a more anterior approach (7.5 cm anterior to the lower tip of the scapula) in order to avoid a long thoracic nerve lesion. After radical neck or axillary dissection, 30% of patients had a transient serratus anterior paralysis. Cervical or axillary radiotherapy may cause a serratus anterior paralysis. Serratus anterior paralysis has been described following general anesthesia.

Traumatic injury to the long thoracic nerve may occur following a stab or gunshot wound. The serratus anterior is also paralyzed following C5–C6–C7 root avulsion.

An entrapment neuropathy of the long thoracic nerve may result from compression by either the scalenus medius or on the second rib. Workers in occupations where heavy loads are carried on the shoulders are at greater risk because of the combined action of scalenus muscle contraction, bulging of the pleura, and lowering of the clavicle. The fascial band described by Hester et al (2000) may also compress the long thoracic nerve. Sports like swimming, golf, archery, basketball, or volleyball also pose a risk.

Parsonage–Turner syndrome or neuralgic shoulder amyotrophy is a rare disorder. It is characterized by acute onset of severe pain in one shoulder. After several days, the pain subsides and weakness of the shoulder girdle muscles appears. Usually, the serratus anterior is involved, but the spinatii, deltoid and trapezius muscles may also be affected. Amyotrophy is evident after several weeks. A sensory deficit along the outer aspect of the shoulder is present in 25% of cases. The etiology is not known. The course of Parsonage–Turner syndrome is usually benign. Three-quarters of the patients make a functional recovery within 2 years and 90% by 4 years (Wilbourn 1993). Finally, scapular winging due to serratus anterior paralysis may be the most visible sign of a C7 radiculopathy (Makin et al 1986).

Symptomatology

Subjective finding

Patients complain of shoulder pain, muscle spasm and weakness, and decreased shoulder flexion.

Objective findings

At rest, the levator scapulae, trapezius, and rhomboid muscles pull the scapula upwards. In abduction and flexion, the scapula translates towards the midline, its lower tip becoming more prominent (i.e. scapula alata) as it is pulled by the trapezius. Scapular winging increases when the patient is asked to lean forward against a wall in a push-up position. The scapulohumeral angle on the affected side is greater than that on the unaffected side. On X-ray examination, the glenoid fossa points downwards so that flexion and abduction are limited.

Treatment

Incorrect diagnosis and/or treatment are commonly seen in patients with long thoracic nerve palsy (Warner and Navarro 1998). Once the diagnosis is made, the treatment will depend on the etiology of the palsy. Following iatrogenic injury, permanent sequelae are common (Kauppila and Vastamaki 1996). Because of poor outcome, attempts should be made to repair the nerve surgically. Surgical repair is technically difficult and sometimes requires a double exposure, both supraclavicular and transaxillary. In entrapment neuropathy, neurolysis is recommended. In Parsonage–Turner syndrome, treatment is conservative. Reconstructive surgery is recommended when scapula alata has been present for 2–3 years (Wiater and Flatow 1999).

Reconstructive surgery

Two types of procedures exist for the reconstruction of serratus anterior paralysis: (1) static stabilization of the scapula or (2) dynamic muscle transfers.

Static stabilization

Static stabilization involves fixing the medial border of the scapula to the spinous processes or the lower angle of the scapula to the ribs by means of a strip of fascia. Unfortunately, this type of repair may loosen within 1 or 2 years. To avoid fascial sling loosening, Vukov et al (1996) use a synthetic ligament. This simple technique may be indicated in the elderly patient. As with trapezius paralysis, complete scapulothoracic fusion is not indicated because it severely limits shoulder function.

Dynamic muscle transfers

The rhomboids, levator scapulae, teres major, and latissimus dorsi have all been transferred in attempts to stabilize the medial border of the scapula. Currently, the most common dynamic transfers for serratus anterior paralysis

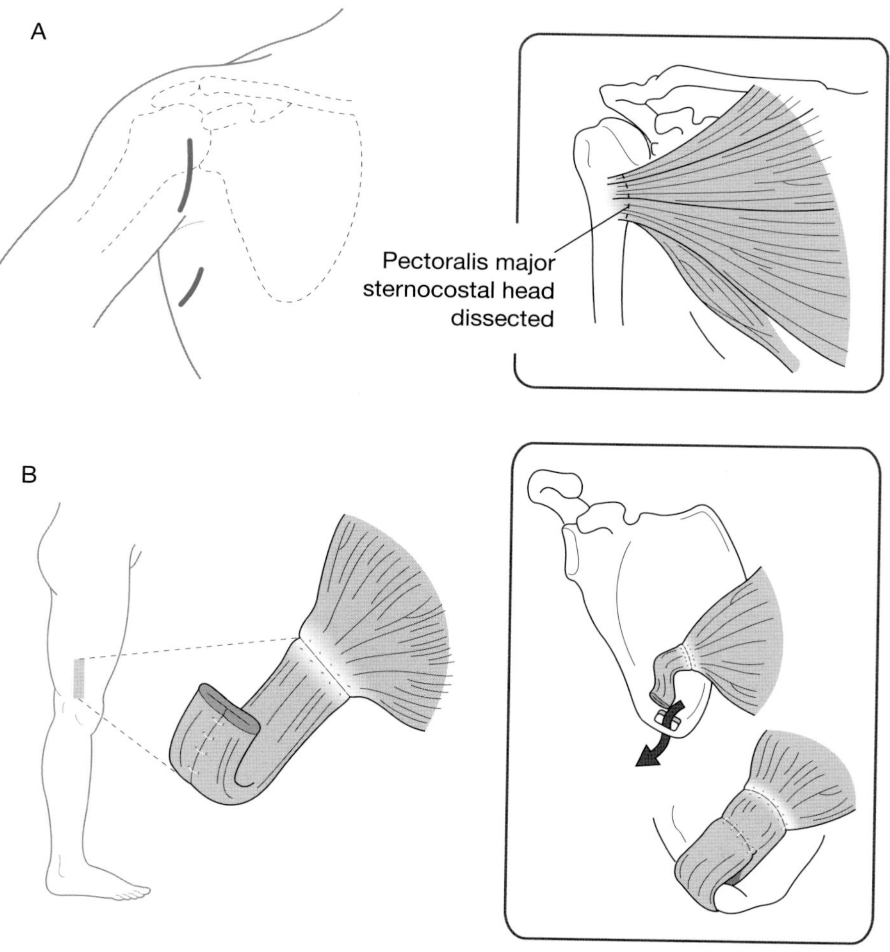

Figure 17.4

Transfer of the sternal head of pectoralis major. (A) Anterior approach for division of sternal head only. (B) Posterior view: the sternal head of pectoralis major is lengthened by a strip of fascia lata, passed through a hole in the scapula and sutured on itself with maximal tension.

use the pectoral muscles. In theory, transfer of the pectoralis minor offers the advantage of decreasing the downward traction on the coracoid process caused by this muscle (Chaves 1951). We have found this transfer to be weak and we now prefer to transfer the sternal head of the pectoralis major.

Transfer of the pectoralis major
Use of the sternal head of the pectoralis major is an excellent transfer, because both the pectoralis major and serratus anterior function together during shoulder flexion. Following the procedure, patients do not need to relearn how to use the transferred muscle. Tubby in 1904 used the sternal head of the pectoralis major tendon and fixed it to the paralyzed serratus anterior. Durman in 1945 modified the technique by lengthening the pectoralis major tendon with a strip of fascia lata. He passed the tendon across the axilla and fixed it to the scapula through a hole placed 5 cm from the lower angle and border of the scapula. The tension is set so as to pull the scapula forwards. Postoperatively, the arm is immobilized for 6 weeks. General use of the arm is limited for 6 months (Figures 17.4, 17.5).

Post in 1995 and later Perlmutter and Leffert in 1999 modified the technique by reinforcing the strip of fascia lata so as to avoid secondary loosening. In 1998, Warner and Navarro recommended using the semitendinous and gracilis tendons, as they may be stronger than fascia lata. Recently, Povacz suggested directly attaching the tendon to the scapula without an intermediate graft (Povacz and Resch 2000) and Perlmutter and Leffert (1999) recommended using the whole pectoralis major muscle in order to avoid a tenodesis effect, and fixing it to the medial border of the scapula. We do not see any advantage to this technique. We prefer to use a fascial strip passed through a hole in the scapula because it is the only technique that allows for precise tension setting.

Combined paralysis of the trapezius and the serratus anterior muscles

Trapezius and serratus anterior paralysis may spontaneously occur together. This may be a variant of Parsonage–Turner

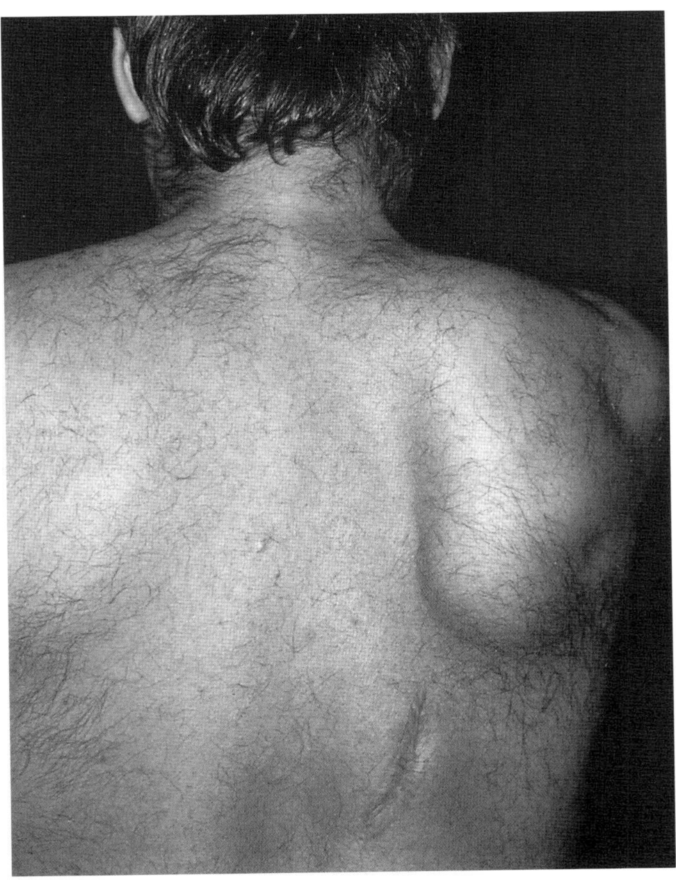
(A)

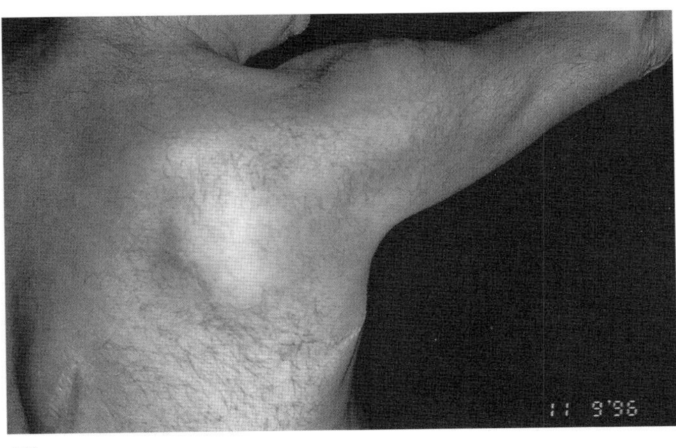

(B)

Figure 17.5
This patient suffers from a complete serratus anterior palsy caused by Parsonage–Turner syndrome.(A) The patient presented with a recurrence of scapular winging after a transfer of the pectoralis minor on the scapula. (B) Postoperative result after transfer of the sternal head of the pectoralis major.

syndrome. This combined paralysis also occurs in the facioscapulohumeral dystrophy. This disorder is with an estimated autosomally dominant prevalence of 1:20,000 (Kissel 1999). Patients present with a facial and scapular muscle weakness. The deltoid and spinatii are preserved.

With combined paralysis the scapula becomes completely unstable and patients have a major functional deficit and chronic pain due to permanent traction on the shoulder girdle. The functional deficit may be improved and chronic shoulder pain may be alleviated following scapulothoracic arthrodesis (Copeland et al 1999).

Suprascapular nerve

Anatomy

The suprascapular nerve arises from C5 and C6–C4 makes an inconsistent contribution in the prefixed plexus. The nerve leaves the upper trunk 3 cm above the clavicle and travels posterior and deep to the omohyoid muscle to the scapular notch. It passes under the superior transverse ligament while the vessels pass above it. The notch is rarely bridged by bone. In the supraspinatus fossa, the nerve gives off a short branch to the supraspinatus muscle and branches to acromioclavicular and glenohumeral joints. It may also innervate the skin over the acromioclavicular joint (Ajmani 1994). From the supraspinatus fossa, the nerve travels around the base of the spine of the scapula under the spinoglenoid ligament into the infraspinatus fossa. Here it ends in branches to the infraspinatus muscle.

Etiology

The suprascapular nerve must glide freely through the scapular notch during shoulder abduction and flexion. Sports or physical activities associated with excessive scapulothoracic gliding may cause local inflammation and later chronic compression of the suprascapular nerve at the notch (Witvrouw et al 2000). Sports like tennis, rowing, canoeing, shot-put, javelin, and volleyball may have a higher incidence of suprascapular nerve compression.

With trapezius paralysis, the chronic inferior position of the scapula may result in compression of the nerve at the scapular notch (Mizuno et al 1990). A ganglion originating from the acromioclavicular or glenohumeral joint may compress the nerve (Moore et al 1997). The notch itself may be too small because the ligament becomes too thick or ossified. Rarely, iatrogenic palsy may occur following excessive traction on the supraspinatus tendon during repair of an extensive rotator cuff lesion (Warner et al 1992, Zanotti et al 1997). The suprascapular nerve may be affected by neuralgic shoulder amyotrophy.

All scapular fractures through the notch or involving the base of the scapular spine may lead to direct nerve injury or to secondary nerve compression as callus forms. The suprascapular nerve is involved in 98% of brachial plexus lesions, either through a C5–C6 injury, or in more distal lesions between the upper trunk and the notch, or at the notch level. In one-third of axillary nerve lesions, there is an associated injury to the suprascapular nerve (Bonnard et al 1999). The lesion is situated at the notch level or distally. It is not uncommon that the branch to the supraspinatus is avulsed from the muscle while the longer branch to the infraspinatus muscle has been stretched or ruptured; the short length of the supraspinatus branch is believed to play a role in this pattern.

Symptomatology

Subjective symptoms

Chronic compression of the suprascapular nerve is associated with pain. The pain is constant and localized to the supraspinatus fossa. It may be triggered by pressure at the notch. The notch is clinically located just before the spine, at the junction between its medial two-thirds and its lateral third. Discomfort increases during the night, particularly when the patient lies on the involved side.

Objective findings

Shoulder flexion increases pain. The cross-body test is positive: pain occurs when, the patient having placed the hand of the affected side on the opposite shoulder, the examiner pushes the elbow forcefully to the normal side, causing full forward gliding of the scapula.

The strength of external rotation and abduction (especially between 60° and 90°) is decreased to one-half of normal. Movements are usually complete because of normal function of the deltoid and teres minor muscles. Later, atrophy becomes evident, especially in the infraspinatus fossa. The trapezius masks atrophy of the supraspinatus muscle.

Investigations

Routine investigations include standard X-rays of the shoulder and scapular notch. An MRI is ordered if a ganglion is suspected. EMG studies show decreased conduction at the notch level and signs of denervation or polyphasic action potentials in the spinatii.

Treatment

Entrapment neuropathy

Some authors (Martin et al 1997) recommend conservative management (i.e. discontinuation of all sports, local steroid injection, and physiotherapy). Surgical decompression is considered only when the pain persists. However, in our experience, when there is atrophy or when EMG studies show signs of denervation we proceed with nerve decompression.

Decompression of the suprascapular nerve

We use a trans-trapezial approach. A longitudinal skin incision is made between the free edge of the trapezius and the scapular spine down to the acromioclavicular joint. The fibers of the trapezius are split. The fat in the supraspinatus fossa is retracted together with the supraspinatus muscle. Deep to these structures, the notch is identified with the vessels above. They are retracted, the coracoid ligament is divided, and the nerve is released. The suprascapular nerve may have a pseudoneuroma in front of the notch, which confirms compression at this site. This approach may be extended posteriorly and vertically in order to assess the nerve beyond the base of the spine. The arm is held in abduction to facilitate dissection. The posterior deltoid is retracted upwards and the infraspinatus medially. The base of the spine along with the spinoglenoid ligament and the terminal branches of the nerve are easily explored.

In our experience, neurolysis of the suprascapular nerve is associated with pain relief in over 90% of cases. In contrast, amyotrophy showed improvement in only 9 out of 19 cases treated. Birch et al (1998) and Antoniadis et al (1996) have described a similar experience. When a ganglion is present, it may be resected arthroscopically (Iannotti and Ramsey 1996).

Traumatic lesions

Fracture dislocations of the scapula may injure the suprascapular nerve either at the notch or at the base of the spine. Occasionally, the short branch to the supraspinatus is avulsed from the muscle and should be repaired by neuromuscular neurotization. The long branch to the infraspinatus is often stretched at the base of the spine and may require grafting. Even if EMG studies confirm reinnervation, clinical recovery may be disappointing because of the association of orthopedic (e.g. dislocated scapula fracture) with neurologic lesions (e.g. suprascapular nerve paralysis). However, we continue to repair this nerve because we are convinced that nerve repair alleviates pain, and because in cases without orthopedic lesions, results may be excellent.

Reconstructive surgery

When the axillary nerve is intact, suprascapular nerve palsy does not usually require a muscle transfer because shoulder function is usually normal. Muscle transfers are not strong enough to dramatically improve strength. In rare cases where active shoulder function is limited, a muscle transfer may be indicated.

Axillary nerve

Anatomy

The axillary nerve arises from C5 and C6. Its fibers pass through the upper trunk and along the posterior cord. The nerve leaves the posterior cord at the coracoid process, travelling dorsally to leave the axilla through the quadrangular space, where it gives off branches to the glenohumeral joint and a small branch to the teres minor muscle. At the posterior aspect of the shoulder, the nerve divides into a sensory and motor branch. The sensory branch innervates skin over the deltoid muscle and the dorsal lateral aspect of the upper arm. The terminal motor branch travels around the neck of the humerus and innervates the three parts of the deltoid muscle in a posterior to anterior fashion. Throughout its course, the axillary nerve is in close contact with the glenohumeral joint and the neck of the humerus.

Etiology

The proximity of the axillary nerve to the glenohumeral joint accounts for the high frequency of nerve lesion following shoulder trauma: 9.3–37% of shoulder traumas present with an axillary nerve lesion (Gumina and Postacchini 1997, Visser et al 1999). Documentation of all clinical findings before closed reduction of a glenohumeral dislocation is important. Reduction of the glenohumeral joint can result in axillary nerve palsy. When axillary nerve injury is caused by a low-energy trauma, spontaneous recovery is common. Axillary nerve palsy due to a high-energy injury fails to recover spontaneously in 44% of cases (Narakas 1989).

The point of traumatic impact accounts for the level of axillary nerve lesion and the type of associated lesions (Bonnard et al 1999). An isolated axillary nerve lesion is caused by a direct trauma across the glenohumeral joint: the axillary nerve is injured in the quadrangular space and the nerve lesion is commonly associated with a rotator cuff injury. When the axillary nerve injury is associated with an infraclavicular plexus lesion(s), the trauma corresponds to the first stage of scapulothoracic dissociation. The axillary nerve is injured in front of the quadrangular space, the subclavian vessels are ruptured in one out of two cases, and fractures of the scapula and the clavicle are frequent. In this group, rotator cuff lesions are rare.

The proximity between the axillary nerve and the shoulder joint accounts for the risk of a iatrogenic nerve lesion in shoulder surgery (Boardman and Cofield 1999). The prognosis for these iatrogenic injuries is poor (McIlveen et al 1994).

Rarely, entrapment neuropathy of the axillary nerve may occur when it is compressed in the quadrangular space. We have seen four cases of suspected axillary nerve compression at the quadrangular space. Three cases were taken to the operating room, and in two of these, a sharp triceps tendon was found compressing the nerve.

Symptomatology

Subjective findings

Patients usually complain of fatigue and lack of strength in abduction, especially between 90° and 160°. Another difficulty described is placing the hand in a pocket; this combined movement of shoulder extension and abduction requires a normal posterior deltoid.

Objective findings

The deltoid and teres minor muscles are paralyzed. Atrophy is seen after a few months, at which time the humeral head and the acromion are prominent. Shoulder function is normal in 36% of cases (Bonnard 1997). A major functional deficit suggests an associated rotator cuff lesion of either orthopedic or neurological (i.e. suprascapular nerve lesion) origin. Sensory deficits vary in terms of area and location over the lateral aspect of the shoulder.

Nonspecific shoulder pain, tenderness over the quadrangular space, dysesthesia on the lateral aspect of the shoulder, and fatigue are the main complaints in entrapment neuropathy (Francel et al 1991). These symptoms start during or after repetitive activities above the horizontal plane (e.g. butterfly stroke, squash, or volleyball). These signs are often misinterpreted as thoracic outlet syndrome.

Investigations

EMG studies are performed at 3 weeks post-trauma. When shoulder function is near normal, only the axillary nerve and deltoid are assessed. If not, both suprascapular and axillary nerves are tested. In spontaneous recovery, the first signs of reinnervation should appear within 3 months. Initially, the posterior head of deltoid is reinnervated followed by the middle and anterior deltoid. X-rays of the shoulder are done routinely. An MRI or CT-arthrography are performed if a rotator cuff lesion is suspected (Bonnard et al 1999).

In entrapment neuropathy, EMG studies may reveal signs of denervation and reinnervation. Doppler studies or angiography help identify compression of the circumflex humeral artery. Compression becomes evident during shoulder abduction. An MRI may show selective atrophy of the teres minor (Linker et al 1993).

Treatment

In traumatic cases, surgical repair is recommended if at the end of 3 months following injury, the deltoid and teres minor paralysis persist with a sensory deficit on the lateral aspect of the shoulder. EMG studies must confirm a complete paralysis. In entrapment neuropathy, conservative treatment is recommended except when EMG studies and Doppler are positive, in which case neurolysis/decompression is performed.

Exposure of the axillary nerve

In isolated axillary nerve lesions, a double approach is required in 73% of cases. In lesions associated with infraclavicular plexus injuries, an anterior approach is sufficient in 71% of cases (Bonnard et al 1999). The anterior approach involves exposure of the infraclavicular plexus through the deltopectoral groove. The proximal stump of the axillary nerve is usually found in scar tissue in front of the quadrilateral space. The posterior incision is placed along the posterior border of the deltoid muscle. The cutaneous branch of the axillary nerve is identified and followed into the depths of the quadrilateral space. The distal stump of the axillary nerve is identified below the vessels. The tunnel is dissected and the nerve is prepared. Grafts are sutured to the distal stump, passed anteriorly, and then sutured to the proximal stump.

Results

Results after repair of an isolated lesion of the axillary nerve have been described as good in 50–84% of cases (Mikami et al 1997, Birch et al 1998, Alnot 1999, Bonnard et al 1999). We have shown that results are statistically better when patients have surgery within the 6 months following injury. Results after repair of a combined axillary and suprascapular nerve lesion disappointing – one-third of the patients recover shoulder abduction >160°, one-third recover shoulder abduction between 60° and 155°, and one-third recover little to no abduction (Bonnard et al 1999).

Reconstructive surgery

Muscle transfer, humeral osteotomy or glenohumeral arthrodesis are recommended when nerve repair has failed. These reconstructive procedures were initially described for the restoration of upper extremity function in infants with poliomyelitis or obstetrical palsy. Later they were recommended for use in adult patients with the long-term sequelae associated with brachial plexus lesions.

Muscle transfers

The prerequisite criteria for muscle transfers are as follows: (1) normal motor strength of the transferred muscle, (2) full passive range of motion of glenohumeral joint, (3) normal scapular control, and (4) the shoulder must not be flail. We have performed 30 muscle transfers for the restoration of abduction and/or external rotation in adults with brachial plexus lesions.

To improve abduction alone, we use the levator scapulae transfer or transfer the trapezius to the humerus with a mean gain in abduction of 22.5°. To improve external rotation alone, we transfer the teres major, latissimus dorsi, or both, to infraspinatus. This group of transfers has resulted in a mean gain in external rotation of 44.6° and an associated gain of 19.5° in abduction. The additional improvement in abduction seen with this group of transfers is caused by the more functional position of the humeral head during abduction (Figure 17.6).

The above transfers may be combined (i.e. double transfer) to improve abduction (+35°) and external rotation (+37.8°) (Figure 17.4). A triple transfer may be indicated in more severe cases. Narakas' triple transfer involved the transfer of (1) levator scapulae to supraspinatus to restore abduction, (2) teres major to infraspinatus to restore external rotation, and (3) latissimus dorsi to anterior deltoid to restore shoulder flexion. Results have been disappointing (abduction +17.5° and external rotation +27.5°), which may be explained by the severity of the nerve injury and extensive shoulder girdle paralysis.

Trapezius transfer may be performed in cases of flail shoulder. The gain in abduction described ranges from 30.3° to 42° (Aziz et al 1990, Kotwal et al 1998, Rühmann et al 1998). In addition, this transfer corrects subluxation of the humeral head.

Transfer of the levator scapulae to supraspinatus

The levator scapulae is dissected with a strip of periostium and completely freed from the scapula. A second longitudinal incision is placed over the humeral head. The deltoid is split and the subdeltoid bursa is opened. The insertion of the supraspinatus tendon is verified. The levator scapula is passed to the second incision through the subacromial space. There is usually enough space under the acromion because of supraspinatus atrophy. If

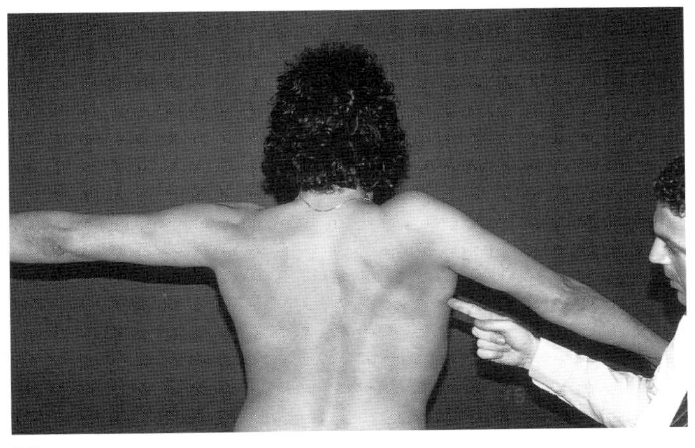

(A)

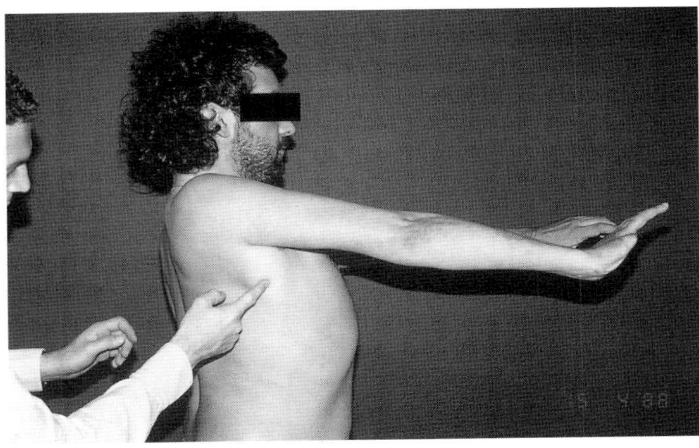

(B)

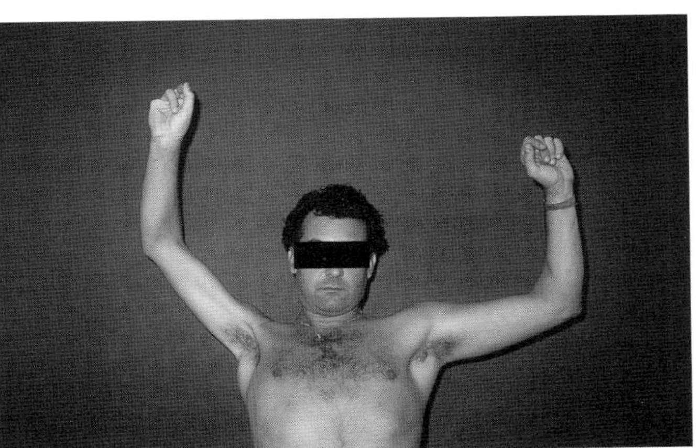

(C)

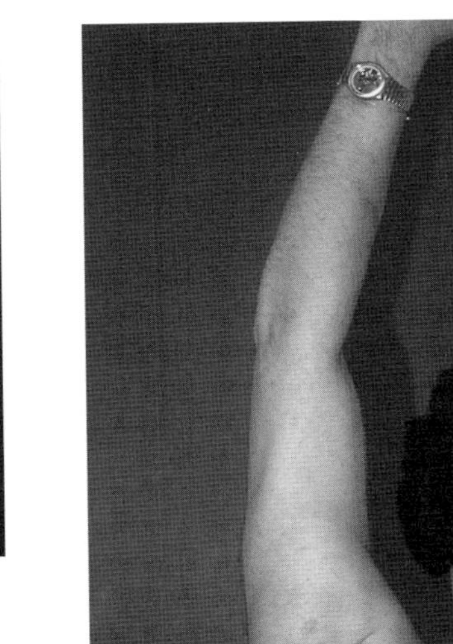

(D)

Figure 17.6

This patient had a C5 and C6 traction injury and a rupture of the musculocutaneous nerve (which recovered well after grafting). (A) and (B) Four years after the plexus reconstruction, he still has a deficit in external rotation and in abduction with an M4 deltoid and a normal serratus anterior (the finger shows the tip of the scapula which moves forward normally during abduction and flexion). (C) and (D) Improvement of external rotation and abduction after transfer of the latissimus dorsi and teres major to the rotator cuff and transfer of the levator scapulae onto the supraspinatus.

not, an acromioplasty is performed. The levator is attached to the trochanter with transosseous sutures or a Mitek anchor. Postoperatively, the extremity is immobilized in a spica cast for 6 weeks. Rehabilitation is similar to that described following rotator cuff repair (Saha 1967).

Transfer of the latissimus dorsi and teres major to infraspinatus

A zigzag skin incision is made on the posterior border of the axilla, and lengthened obliquely onto the chest over the anterior border of the latissimus dorsi. The latissimus dorsi and teres major are dissected to their insertion on the humerus from where their tendons are divided. The deltoid is elevated through the same incision. A second deltoid-splitting incision is made to expose the rotator cuff. The teres major and latissimus dorsi are passed over the teres minor and infraspinatus and under the deltoid. The two muscles are then brought out of the second incision and sutured to the posterior aspect of the rotator cuff (Narakas 1993b).

Trapezius transfer
The trapezius is harvested with a section of acromion that is freed from the scapular spine and the lateral third of the clavicle by oblique osteotomy. The proximal humerus is exposed and after holding the arm in 90° abduction, the acromion is fixed with two 4.5 mm screws below the greater tuberosity. Tension should be set as tightly as possible (Saha 1967).

Humeral osteotomy

Humeral osteotomy is an option for the restoration of external rotation. A humeral osteotomy is performed at the subcapital level. An osteotomy does not increase the overall shoulder range of motion but it does improve its orientation. We perform humeral osteotomy primarily in infants and rarely in adults (Alnot 1999).

Glenohumeral arthrodesis

Shoulder arthrodesis is indicated in two clinical situations. In the first situation, there is normal scapular control, poor glenohumeral function, adequate biceps function, and near normal hand function. Shoulder arthrodesis improves global arm control and elbow flexion strength. In the second situation, the shoulder is flail. Shoulder arthrodesis is recommended in order to decrease shoulder pain caused by excessive traction on the glenohumeral joint capsule.

The position of the arthrodesis must allow for a strong brachiothoracic grip and hand-to-mouth positioning. Chammas et al (1996) recommend the following position: 25° of abduction, 18° of flexion, and 22° of internal rotation. The gain in function and strength may be slightly better than following muscle transfers. Complications such as pseudarthrosis, secondary humeral fracture, and infection are frequent. Persistent discomfort following arthrodesis has been described (Rühmann et al 1999). Nevertheless, shoulder arthrodesis is recommended for patients requiring maximum function and strength in shoulder girdle and optimal use of elbow and hand.

Conclusions

Following trauma, the first step in the treatment of shoulder girdle paralysis is nerve repair, which should be performed within 6 months post-trauma. When sequelae persist, secondary reconstruction is recommended.

In cases of trapezius or serratus anterior definitive paralysis, dynamic muscle transfers are recommended; while in the combined permanent paralysis of the trapezius and serratus anterior, scapulo-thoracic arthrodesis improves motion and alleviates chronic shoulder pain.

In cases of spinatii and/or deltoid paralysis, a trapezius transfer or combined transfers using levator scapulae, teres major, and latissimus dorsi may improve abduction, external rotation, and flexion. The main advantage of dynamic muscle transfers is to keep the joint mobile while improving shoulder function and stability. Glenohumeral arthrodesis may be indicated when passive range of motion is limited or when the patient requests maximal function and strength. Significant complications are associated with glenohumeral arthrodesis. We continue to recommend muscle transfers in these cases.

References

Ajmani ML (1994) The cutaneous branch of the human suprascapular nerve, *J Anat* **185**: 439–42.

Alnot JY (1999) Paralytic shoulder secondary to post-traumatic peripheral nerve lesions in the adult, *Acta Orthop Belg* **65**: 10–17.

Alnot JY, Aboujaoude J, Oberlin C (1994) Traumatic lesions of the spinal accessory nerve, II: clinical study and results of a series of 25 cases, *Rev Chir Orthop Reparatrice Appar Mot* **80**: 297–304.

Antoniadis G, Richeter HP, Rath S et al (1996) Suprascapular nerve entrapment: experience with 28 cases, *J Neurosurg* **85**: 1020–5.

Aziz W, Singer RM, Wolff TW (1990) Transfer of the trapezius for flail shoulder after brachial plexus injury, *J Bone Joint Surg* **72**: 701–4.

Bigliani LU, Compito CA, Duralde XA, Wolfe IN (1996) Transfer of the levator scapulae, rhomboid major, and rhomboid minor for paralysis of the trapezius, *J Bone Joint Surg* **78A:** 1534–40.

Birch R, Bonney G, Wynn Parry CB (1998) *Surgical Disorders of the Peripheral Nerves* (Churchill Livingstone: Edinburgh).

Boardman ND 3nd, Cofield RH (1999) Neurologic complications of shoulder surgery, *Clin Orthop* **368**: 44–53.

Bonnard C (1997) Les lésions du nerf axillaire isolées ou associées au nerf scapulaire supérieur ou musculo-cutané. In: Alnot JY, ed., *Les Lésions Traumatiaues des Nerfs Périphérques* (Cahiers denseignement de la SOFCOT. Expansion Scientifique Française: Paris) 57–64.

Bonnard C, Anastakis DJ, Van Melle G et al (1999) Isolated and combined lesions of the axillary nerve. A review of 146 cases, *J Bone Joint Surg* **81B**: 212–17.

Chammas M, Meyer zu Reckendorf G, Allieu Y (1996) Arthrodesis of the shoulder for post-traumatic palsy of the brachial plexus. Analysis of a series of 18 cases, *Rev Chir Orthop Reparatrice Appar Mot* **82**: 386–95.

Chaves JP (1951) Pectoralis minor transplant for paralysis of the serratus anterior, *J Bone Joint Surg* **33B**: 228–30.

Coessens BC, Wood MB (1995) Levator scapulae transfer and fascia lata fasciodesis for chronic spinal accessory nerve palsy, *J Reconstr Microsurg* **11**: 277–80.

Copeland SA, Levy O, Warner GC, Dodenhoff RM (1999) The shoulder in patients with muscular dystrophy, *Clin Orthop* **36**: 80–91.

Dewar FP, Harris RY (1950) Restoration of function of the shoulder following paralysis of the trapezius by fascial sling fixation and transplantation of the levator scapulae, *Ann Surg* **132**: 1111–15.

Durman DC (1945) An operation for paralysis of the serratus anterior, *J Bone Joint Surg* **27**: 380–2.

Eden R (1924) Zur Behandlung der Trapeziuslähmung mittelst Muskelplastik, *Deutsche Zeitschrift Chirurgie* **184**: 387–97.

Francel TJ, Dellon AL, Campbell JN (1991) Quadrilateral space syndrome: diagnosis and operative decompression technique, *Plast Reconstr Surg* **87**: 911–16.

Gumina S, Postacchini F (1997) Anterior dislocation of the shoulder in elderly patients, *J Bone Joint Surg* **79B**: 540–3.

Hester P, Caborn DN, Nyland J (2000) Cause of long thoracic nerve palsy: a possible dynamic fascial sling cause, *J Shoulder Elbow Surg* **9**: 31–5.

Iannotti JP, Ramsey ML (1996) Arthroscopic decompression of a ganglion cyst causing suprascapular nerve compression, *Arthroscopy* **12**: 739–45.

Kauppila LI, Vastamaki M (1996) Iatrogenic serratus anterior paralysis. Long-term outcome in 26 patients, *Chest* **109**: 31–4.

Kissel JT (1999) Facioscapulohumeral dystrophy, *Semin Neurol* **19**: 35–43.

Kotwal PP. Mittal R, Malhotra R (1998) Trapezius transfer for deltoid paralysis, *J Bone Joint Surg* **80B**: 114–16.

Lange M (1951) Die Behandlung der irreparablen Trapeziusliihmung, *Archiv für Klinische Chirurgie* **270**: 437–9.

Linker CS, Helms CA, Fritz RC (1993) Quadrilateral space syndrome: findings at MR imaging, *Radiology* **188**: 675–6.

Mcllveen SJ, Duralde XA, D'Allesandro DF, Bigliani LU (1994) Isolated nerve injuries about the shoulder, *Clin Orthop* **30**: 54–63.

Makin GJ, Brown WF, Ebers GC (1986) C7 radiculopathy: importance of scapular winging in clinical diagnosis, *J Neurol Neurosurg Psychiatry* **49**: 640–4.

Martin SD, Warren RF, Martin TL et al (1997) Suprascapular neuropathy. Results of non-operative treatments, *J Bone Joint Surg* **79A**: 1159–65.

Matz PG, Barbaro NM (1996) Diagnosis and treatment of iatrogenic spinal accessory nerve injury, *Am Surg* **62**: 682–5.

Mikami Y, Nagano A, Ochiai N et al (1997) Results of nerve grafting for injuries of the axillary and suprascapular nerves, *J Bone Joint Surg* **79B**: 527–31.

Mizuno K, Muratsu H, Kurosaka M et al (1990) Compression neuropathy of the suprascapular nerve as a cause of pain in palsy of the accessory nerve, *J Bone Joint Surg* **72A**: 938–9.

Moore TP, Fritts HM, Quick DC, Buss DD (1997) Suprascapular nerve entrapment caused by supraglenoid cyst compression, *Shoulder Elbow Surg* **6**: 455–62.

Narakas AO (1988) Paralytic disorders of the shoulder girdle, *Hand Clin* **4**: 619–32.

Narakas AO (1989) Lésions du nerf axillaire et lésions associées du nerf supra-scapulaire, *Rev Med Suisse Romande* **109**: 545–56.

Narakas AO (1993a) Paralytic disorders of the shoulder girdle. In: Tubiana R, ed., *The Hand*, Vol IV (Masson: Paris) 112–25.

Narakas AO (1993b) Muscle transpositions in the shoulder and upper arm for sequelae of brachial plexus palsy, *Clin Neurol Neurosurg* **95** Suppl: S89–S91.

Newsom-Davis J, Thomas PK, Spalding JMK (1984) Diseases of the nineth, tenth, eleventh and twelfth cranial nerves. In: Dyck PJ, Thomas PK, eds, *Peripheral Neuropathy*, 3rd edn (WB Saunders: Philadelphia) 1337–47.

Perlmutter GS, Leffert RD (1999) Results of transfer of the pectoralis major tendon to treat paralysis of the serratus anterior muscle, *J Bone Joint Surg* **81A**: 377–84.

Post M (1995) Pectoralis major transfer for winging of the scapula, *J Shoulder Elbow Surg* **4**: 1–9.

Povacz P, Resch H (2000) Dynamic stabilization of winging scapula by direct split pectoralis major transfer: a technical note, *J Shoulder Elbow Surg* **9**: 76–8.

Rühmann O, Wirth CJ, Gosse F, Schmolke S (1998) Trapezius transfer after brachial plexus palsy. Indications, difficulties and complications, *J Bone Joint Surg* **80B**: 109–13.

Rühmann O, Gosse F, Wirth CJ, Schmolk S (1999) Reconstructive operations for the paralyzed shoulder in brachial plexus palsy: concept of treatment, *Injury* **30**: 609–18.

Saha AK (1967) Surgery of the paralyzed and flail shoulder, *Acta Orthop Scand* **97**: 5–90.

Salazar JD, Doty JR, Tseng EE et al (1998) Relationship of the long thoracic nerve to the scapular tip: an aid to prevention of proximal nerve iniury, *J Thorac Cardiovasc Surg* **116**: 960–4.

Spira E (1948) The treatment of the dropped shoulder. A new operative technique, *J Bone Joint Surg* **30A**: 229–33.

Tubby AH (1904) A case illustrating the operative treatment of paralysis of the serratus magnus by muscle grafting, *BMJ* **2**: 1159–60.

Visser CP, Coene LN, Brand R et al (1999) The incidence of nerve injury in anterior dislocation of the shoulder and its influence on functional recovery. A prospective clinical and EMG study, *J Bone Joint Surg* **81B**: 679–85.

Vukov B, Ukropina D, Bumbasirevic M et al (1996) Isolated serratus anterior paralysis: a simple surgical procedure to reestablish scapulo-humeral dynamics, *J Orthop Trauma* **10**: 341–7.

Warner JJ, Navarro RA (1998) Serratus anterior dysfunction. Recognition and treatment, *Clin Orthop* **349**: 139–48.

Warner JP, Krushell RJ, Masquelet A, Gerber C (1992) Anatomy and relationships of the suprascapular nerve: anatomical constraints to mobilization of the supraspinatus and infraspinatus muscles in the management of massive rotator-cuff tears, *J Bone Joint Surg* **74A**: 36–45.

Wiater JM, Bigliani LU (1999) Spinal accessory nerve injury, *Clin Orthop* **368**: 5–16.

Wiater JM, Flatow EL (1999) Long thoracic nerve injury, *Clin Orthop* **368**: 17–27.

Wilbourn AJ (1993) Brachial plexus disorders. In: Dyck PJ, Thomas PK, eds. *Peripheral Neuropathy*, 3rd edn (WB Saunders: Philadelphia) 911–50.

Witvrouw E, Cools A, Lysens R et al (2000) Suprascapular neuropathy in volleyball players, *Br J Sports Med* **34**: 174–80.

Zanotti R, Carpenter JE, Blasier RB et al (1997) The low incidence of suprascapular nerve injury after primary repair of massive rotator cuff tears, *J Shoulder Elbow Surg* **6**: 258–64.

18 Obstetrical paralysis

Alain Gilbert

Introduction

The term obstetrical palsy was used in 1867 by Duchenne de Boulogne (la paralysie obstetricale) in his book: *De l'Electrisation Localisée.* He recognized the traumatic origin of the lesion, although some controversy has existed until recently. Modern series in which operative explorations have been carried out have confirmed the pathology.

The aetiology is always a tearing force due to traction on the head or arm. There are two basic types of lesion:

1. Overweight babies (over 4 kg) with vertex presentation and shoulder dystocia who require excess force by traction, often with forceps or ventouse extraction for delivery. This results in upper plexus injury, most commonly to the C5 and C6 and occasionally the C7 roots, but never the lower roots (Figure 18.1).
2. Breech presentation, usually of small (under 3 kg) babies, requiring excessive extension of the head and often manipulation of the hand and arm in a manner that exerts traction on the upper roots as well as on the lower roots. This may cause rupture or avulsion of any or occasionally all of the roots (Figure 18.2).

Clinical presentation

The initial diagnosis is obvious at birth. After a difficult delivery of an obese baby by vertex presentation or a small baby by breech presentation the upper extremity is flail and dangling. A more detailed analysis of the paralysis patterns of the various muscles of the upper extremity is not necessary, as the picture will change rapidly. Examination of the other extremities is important to exclude neonatal quadriplegia or diplegia. Occasionally birth palsy may be bilateral. Forty-eight hours later a more accurate examination and muscle testing can be performed. At this stage it is usually possible to differentiate the two types of paresis:

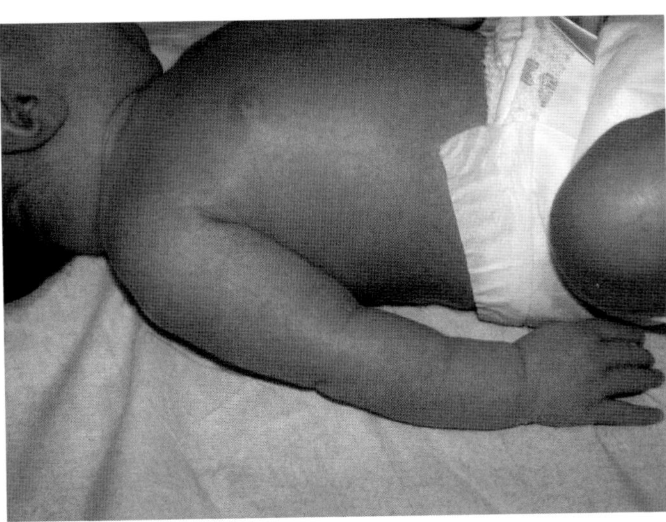

Figure 18.1
A typical C5, C6 paralysis.

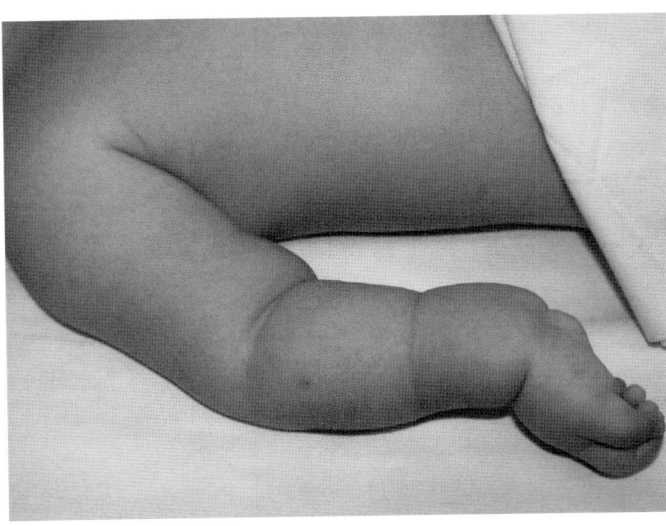

Figure 18.2
Complete paralysis.

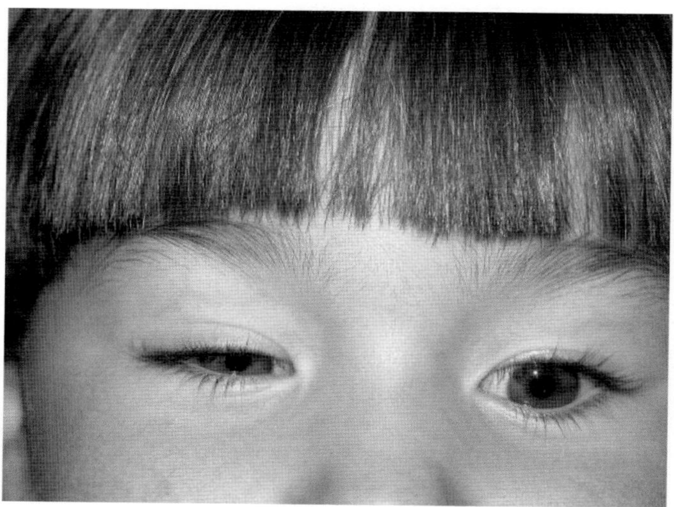

Figure 18.3
Horner's sign.

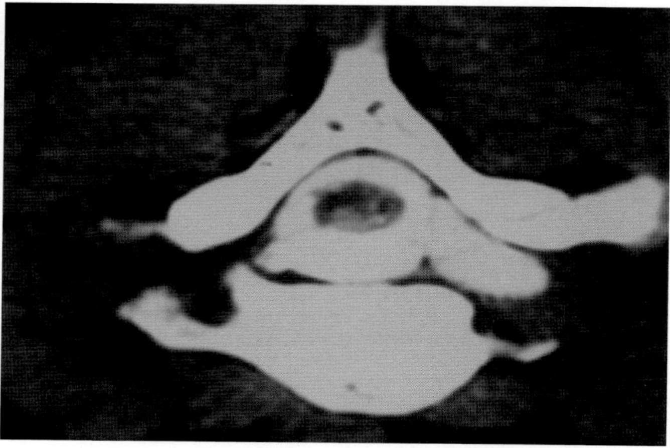

Figure 18.4
Myelo-scan showing a large meningocoele.

1. The Erb–Duchenne-type paralysis of the upper roots. The arm is held in internal rotation and pronation. There is no active abduction or elbow flexion (Figure 18.1). The elbow may be slightly flexed (lesion of C5–C7) or in complete extension (lesion of C5, C6). The thumb is in flexion and sometimes the fingers will not extend. As a rule the thumb flexor and the flexors of the fingers are functioning. The pectoralis major is usually active, giving an appearance of forward flexion of the shoulder. There are no vasomotor changes and there is no gross impairment of distal sensation.
2. Complete paralysis. The entire arm is flail and the hand clutched (Figure 18.2). Sensation is diminished and there is vasomotor impairment, giving a pale or even 'marbled' appearance to the extremity. Often a Horner's sign is present on the affected side (Figure 18.3).

A shoulder X-ray should be taken to eliminate fracture of the clavicle or the upper humerus (Babbitt and Cassidy 1968), which can occur in association with the paresis. Occasionally a phrenic nerve palsy can be detected by fluoroscopy.

The clinical development during the first month is variable and many pareses will recover during this stage (Bennet and Harrold 1976). However, Wickstrom et al (1971) reported that only 10% of total palsies recover to any useful extent. These patients should be carefully evaluated at the age of 3 months – clinically, electromyographically and by cervical myelography. Gentle physiotherapy should be used during this recovery period to minimize the development of contractures while awaiting spontaneous recovery. At this stage complete paralysis with Horner's sign will remain unchanged and early operation should be considered in these babies at 3 months.

Paralysis of the upper roots may show spontaneous recovery during the first 3 months. These babies should be treated with physiotherapy and assessed clinically and electromyographically by the age of 3 months.

Spontaneous recovery

The literature reports varying rates of spontaneous recovery, from 7% to 80%. Useful guidelines are given by Tassin (1984), who came to the following conclusions:

1. Complete recovery is seen in those infants showing some contraction of the biceps and the deltoid by the end of the first month and a normal contraction by the second month.
2. No infant in whom neither the deltoid nor the biceps contract by the third month can be expected to obtain a good result. Testing the deltoid can be difficult. As a result assessment of the biceps is the most reliable indicator for operative intervention. If there is no evidence of any recovery in the biceps by the end of the third month operation is indicated. Clinical assessment is more reliable than electrical testing. If surgery is not undertaken some recovery will continue to take place spontaneously, but it is likely to be less satisfactory than that following surgery.

Indications for operation

If recovery of the biceps has not begun by 3 months the prognosis is poor and surgical repair of the plexus is indicated. The following clinical situations pose particular problems:

1. Complete palsy with a flail arm after 1 month, particularly with Horner's syndrome, will not recover spontaneously and is a prime candidate for surgery. These babies are best treated by early operation at the age of 12 weeks. Absence of recovery of the hand is the most important factor, even with recovery of the shoulder or elbow.
2. Complete palsy of C5 and C6 occurring after breech delivery with no sign of recovery by the third month.
3. The commonest C5, C6 and sometimes C7 palsies almost always show some sign of recovery, which can be misleading, and has in the past encouraged a conservative approach. If, however, after careful examination the biceps function is completely absent at 3 months, surgery should be considered. Great difficulty arises when infants are seen late, i.e. towards the 6th to 8th month, and show minimal recovery of biceps function. The parents are often encouraged by the beginning of recovery and will not accept the idea of an unsatisfactory final result. Under these conditions it is difficult for the surgeon to advise surgery that cannot promise a definitive result. To avoid this situation it is important to try to make decisions by the third month. When the operation has been decided, the patient should be explored in depth to minimize any operative or anaesthetic risks and to predict as precisely as possible the lesions.

Preoperative explorations

Electromyography

Electromyography (EMG) is done at this stage. Although it rarely gives precise indications as to the extent of the lesion and the quality of recovery, it may be very useful in predicting avulsion injuries. The association with evoked potentials will give even more precision. The avulsion of an isolated root in the central or lower part of the plexus is not clearly shown by EMG. Association with Horner's syndrome will be almost pathognomonic of T1 avulsion (Al Qatan 2000).

However, in upper root avulsions, especially after breech delivery, the EMG is very clear, showing a total absence of muscle reinnervation. This absence, in conjunction with the obstetrical record, will almost certainly confirm the avulsion at exploration.

Some authors (Bisinella et al 2003) have developed methods of exploration that could give improved precision in the prognosis of the obstetrical lesions.

Radiology

Conventional radiology is necessary to assess the possibility of diaphragmatic paralysis, which can sometimes occur at birth concurrently with the plexus lesion. It is important to know the status both medically and legally before the operation.

We had a case of a 3-month-old baby, which had at birth a contralateral phrenic paralysis and a postoperative paralysis on the other side. This bilateral paralysis led to severe respiratory distress with a 3-week period of intubation and intensive care therapy.

Myelogram and CT myelography

For many years we used to perform myelograms on our patients (Neuenschwander et al 1980). The results were not entirely satisfactory, with a large number of false positives and false negatives. The advent of CT myelography has changed the situation and gives much precise information. However, the indications for CT myelography are rare, as it provides little information that will not be provided by direct observation during operation. Furthermore, this examination needs a general anaesthesic in a neonate. It can be useful mostly in upper root lesions suspected of avulsion. In these cases the roots are often in place and the operative diagnosis is difficult. The myelogram may be very useful in these cases (Figure 18.4).

Magnetic resonance imaging

Magnetic resonance imaging (MRI) has been used extensively for brachial plexus injuries (Miller et al 1993, Francel et al 1995, Chow et al 2000). Although it may give excellent results in adults, we feel that it is unreliable in children (Figure 18.5). With the improvement of the surface antennas, this will probably change but at the moment the necessity for general anaesthesia and the lack of information lead us to prefer, when necessary, the CT myelogram.

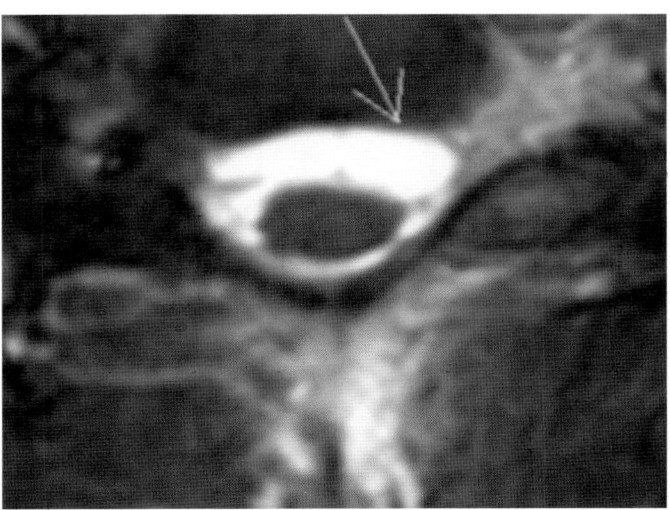

Figure 18.5
The MRI is more difficult to interpret.

Surgical approach

Anaesthesia

It has been well demonstrated (Cohen et al 1990) that after 1 month, the anaesthetic risks decrease. The respiratory system represents the main area of risk, represented essentially by central or occlusive apnoea (Borrero 2001). The main respiratory problem related to surgery is diaphragmatic paralysis, either pre-operative or postoperative; it has to be carefully assessed pre-operatively by fluoroscopy.

Temperature will be monitored throughout the operation. With good warming blankets or lamps and as soon as the infant is covered with drapes, there is no need to raise the room temperature as sometimes routinely proposed. The potential infectious consequences of a higher temperature overcome the advantages.

Large venous access is necessary and, in some instances, it is possible to place a large catheter intraoperatively in the subclavian vein.

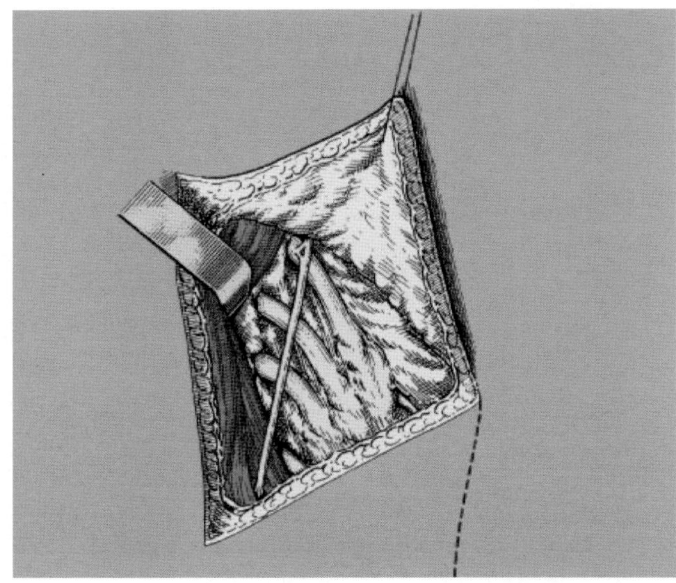

Figure 18.6
Opening the supraclavicular approach.

Position

The child is in a supine position, with a small towel rolled and placed under the superior spine and scapula, to allow a wide opening of the neck and thoraco-brachial area. The head is turned completely to the opposite side with the neck in slight hyperextension. The neck and upper thorax are prepped, as well as the entire upper extremity and both legs and knees. No tourniquet is used.

For several years, we have used preoperative evoked potentials (Laget et al 1967) but we have stopped this practice, as the results were quite unpredictable and the variations due to anaesthesia or temperature were too large.

The incision will vary according to the type of injury. For C5, C6, C7 lesions, we use only a supraclavicular triangular flap based on the posterior border of the sternocleidomastoid (SCM) muscle and the superior aspect of the clavicle.

In complete palsy, the incision extends distally over the delto-pectoral groove. The skin is infiltrated with a 1/1000 solution of adrenaline; this usually raises the heart rate by 15 or 20/min. In order to obtain a good efficiency and a bloodless field, it is best to wait for the rhythm to return to its pre-injection level.

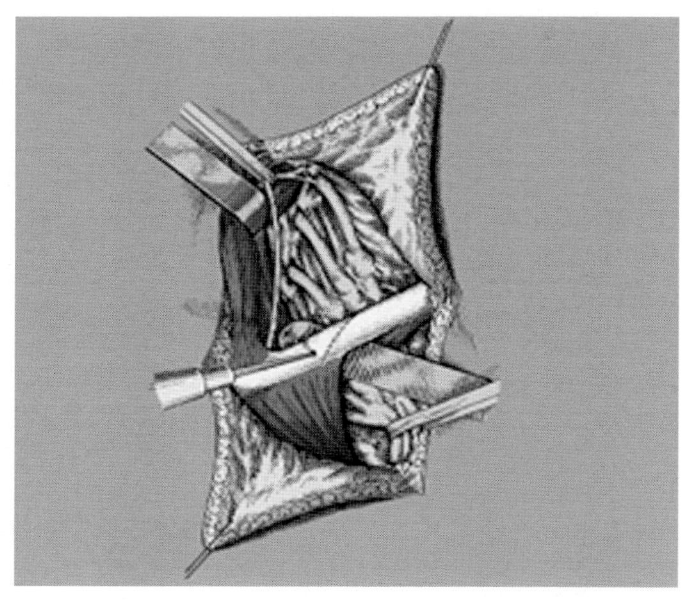

Figure 18.7
The infraclavicular approach is performed.

Approach

After supraclavicular incision, the skin and subcutaneous fat are lifted and held with a stay suture (Figure 18.6). If the SCM muscle insertion on the clavicle extends laterally, it may be necessary to detach its lateral part.

The plexus is covered with a thick layer of fat and multiple ganglions. This layer is lifted from its medial position, over the jugular vein and reflected laterally. The field is then stabilized with a self-retaining retractor.

To approach the plexus, it will be necessary to cut the omohyoid muscle and divide the transverse cervical vessels.

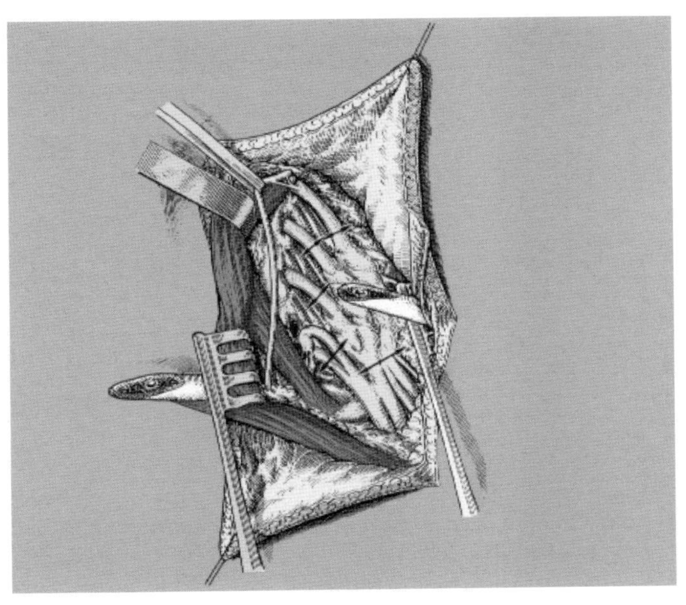

Figure 18.8
The clavicle is cut obliquely.

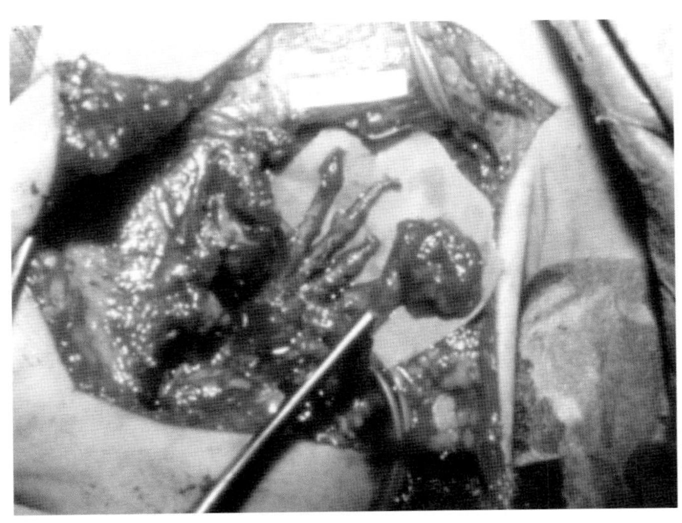

Figure 18.9
A complete lesion with rupture of two upper roots and avulsion of the others.

The plexus is then visible and the first move is to separate and protect the phrenic nerve. In following it upwards, C5 is found automatically as the nerve has a connection with the root in almost every case.

The anterior scalene is retracted gently and the roots can be seen and dissected free. As they are followed distally, the neuroma is obvious, hard, surrounded with scar, often reaching the superior part of the clavicle.

The suprascapular nerve is systematically dissected free as well as the long thoracic nerve and its branches when the neuroma is lifted.

Assessment of the extent of the lesion, the quality of the roots and the length of the defect can then be done.

When the infraclavicular approach is needed, the second flap is lifted and sutured to the skin of the thorax. The pectoralis major is detached from the inferior part of the clavicle and retracted. The retractor will also take the pectoralis minor, demonstrating the upper, middle and lower trunks and their branches (Figure 18.7).

A large periosteal flap is created on the clavicle with a lateral pedicle. It is elevated and the posterior periosteum is elevated. The clavicle is then cut obliquely, using an electric saw. Using a 12G K-wire, holes are drilled into the two opposite pieces of bone. Once they are elevated, the posterior periosteum is sectioned laterally, making another flap. It is also necessary at this stage to cut the subclavian muscle. The two parts of the clavicle are held with a self-retaining retractor and the whole plexus appears (Figure 18.8).

Every trunk is dissected and isolated. Care is exercised not to injure the subclavian artery and vein. The lower trunk has to be followed up to its division from C8 and T1 and the two nerves dissected up to the foramen. This may be dangerous due to the proximity of the vessels. However, it is absolutely necessary and no decision can be taken without appraisal of the roots at the level of the foramen (Figure 18.9).

Intraoperative stimulation may be of help, especially when there is a suspicion of avulsion (Horner, EMG) and the root is found in the foramen. In these cases, if there is no response to direct stimulation, the root will be considered as avulsed, cut at the foraminal level and grafted.

Early in our experience, we left several of these roots in place, with the hope of some recovery if there was no visible proof of avulsion. We always regretted it and these patients went on to have poor results in the hand. The situation is different in the upper roots, after breech delivery, as described later in the chapter.

Repair of the lesions

The neuromas are excised widely and systematically. There is no point in doing neurolysis if the clinical situation has led to a surgical exploration. Neurolysis does not provide improvement (Clarke et al 1996) and there are very few indications left.

When the roots are avulsed, the ganglion is often found with its small motor branch. This part should not be sacrificed, as sometimes only one or two roots are available for grafting. Directing the grafts on the small motor root will allow the grafting of all the plexus, which otherwise could not be repaired owing to the discrepancy between the donor roots and the large volume of

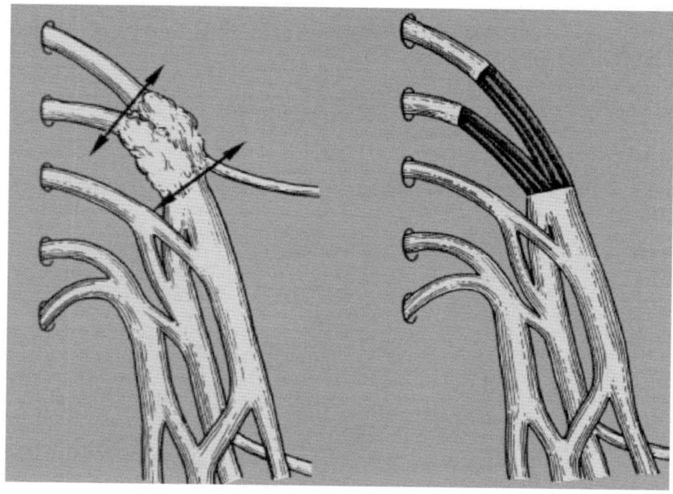

Figure 18.10

Repair of a simple upper root rupture.

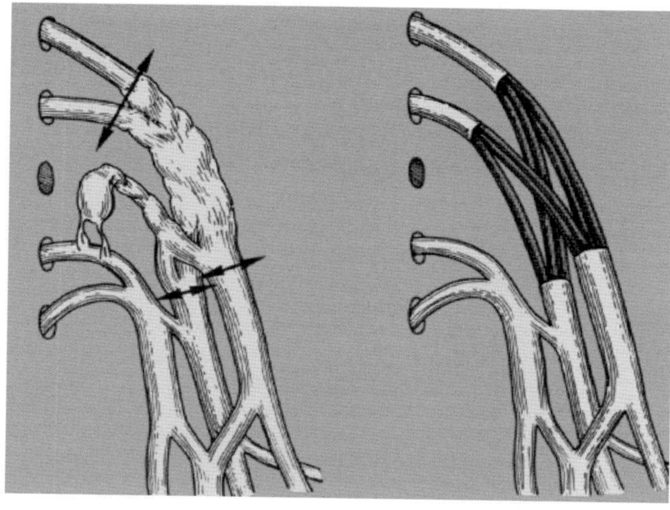

Figure 18.11

With one root avulsed, the repair is similar.

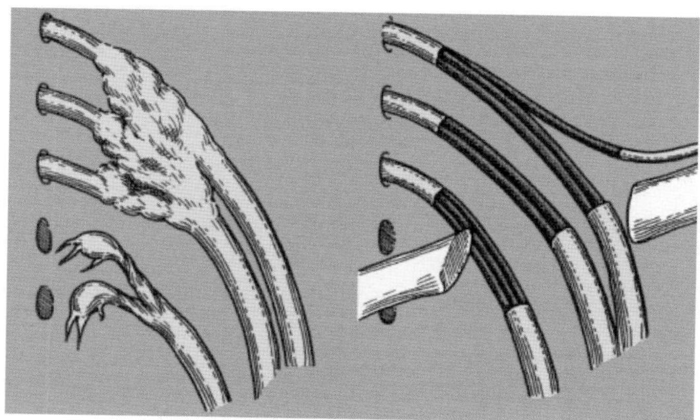

Figure 18.12

When the two lower roots are avulsed, the entire plexus can still be repaired.

the trunks to graft (Figure 18.10). When performed directly on the motor component these repairs have given some very satisfactory results.

Harvesting the nerve grafts

In babies we use only the sural nerve and on rare occasions the superficial cervical plexus. We feel that the use of trunk grafts, for example, the vascularized ulnar nerve, should never be done as it could sacrifice the chances of recovery in the hand.

The sural nerves are harvested by posterior zigzag incisions, after adrenaline injection. The nerve is too fine to be taken by separate incisions and its anatomy precludes the use of a stripper (Gilbert et al 1984).

Some authors (Hallock 1995, Kobayashi 1995) have proposed harvesting the sural nerve endoscopically. Capek et al (1996) have applied the technique to paediatric cases. It is appealing, as the scars in this area are usually visible. The drawbacks are the necessity to start the operation in a prone position and then turn the patient over and particularly the length of the procedure, which in some cases took several hours.

Preparing the nerve grafts

The sural nerve is Y-shaped in most cases (Gilbert 1984) and it is important to keep as much length as possible.

The defect between the two ends is measured at the plexus level and the grafts (usually both legs) are divided on the table, to produce a cable. We feel that the discussion about the direction of the grafts is not important; if one chooses to use the graft in an anterograde direction, there will be a loss of axons through the multiple branching; if it is used in a retrograde manner, the distal part will have many empty conduits. There has never been any proof that one way or another was better. The grafts are cut and placed on the table for their final organization. The end of each cable bundle is then glued so as to make a trunk and this trunk is sharply cut transversally. Then, in a bloodless field, the graft is placed immediately between the plexus extremities and simply glued in place.

We started glueing the nerves almost 20 years ago, immediately after Egloff and Narakas (1983). The fibrin glue has proven to be safe in our hands and has given better results than sutures. We use only glue without any sutures. It is also used with end-to-end and end-to-side anastomoses.

End-to-side anastomoses

Several authors (Viterbo et al 1995, Mennen 1999, Franciosi et al 1998) have shown the feasibility and effectiveness of end-to-side anastomoses in the experimental arena. To date, very few reports have described the results in the clinical arena.

There are cases where there is no simple solution to repair the plexus:

- In isolated avulsion of one or two roots. This may occur especially with breech delivery. The alternative may be a complicated extraplexual neurotization (Figures 18.11 and 18.12).
- In repair of extensive lesions, when there is a lack of donor area (rupture of a small C5 avulsion of C6, C7 with intact C8, T1). A relatively less important root (C7) may be sutured to C8 (Figures 18.13 and 18.14).
- In complete upper roots avulsion, the neurotization of a musculocutaneous nerve by the ulnar trunk (Oberlin et al 1994) may be done as end-to-side instead of sacrificing a bundle from the ulnar nerve. The recipient root is dissected and the perineurium is split longitudinally. No dissection is done inside the nerve. The end of the avulsed nerve is placed into the opening and simply glued. It should hold without tension and we do not use sutures even in this situation.

If it is proven that the results of end-to-side anastomosis equal those of neurotization, the simplicity of this approach will make it a valuable tool.

Neurotization

A large number of extraplexual neurotizations have been described in the literature, mainly for adults. We have used many of them in obstetrical palsy, but the development of multiple intraplexual repairs and end-to-side anastomoses have reduced their indications. We are reluctant to use the intercostal nerves, especially in complete paralysis, since we studied the ventilatory capacity in these children and showed that the extensive use of intercostal nerves would severely decrease this capacity (Gilbert et al 1980). This was confirmed recently (Gu 2002).

The occipital nerve (Romana 2000) is very small and too far from the plexus.

We still use the terminal part of the spinal accessory nerve. It can be found in the wound and its size allows repair or grafting of a suprascapular nerve or a musculocutaneous nerve. It should be taken after its division, so as not to affect the trapezius muscle.

We have used the medial nerve of pectoralis major many times. It is easy to find, of good size and can be sutured end-to-end with the musculocutaneous nerve. It is very useful in cases of upper roots avulsion. However, our results show that it is better to use it in pure C5, C6 lesions but that it is often too weak when C7 is injured. The results were not so good in these cases.

The contralateral C7 root has been used by some surgeons (Gu 1989, Gu et al 1991) and applied to obstetrical paralysis by others (Chuang et al 1993, Terzis et al 1999). The medico-legal situation as well as the length of grafts necessary have prevented us from using it. The possible advent of end-to-side anastomoses will reduce the indications for this procedure.

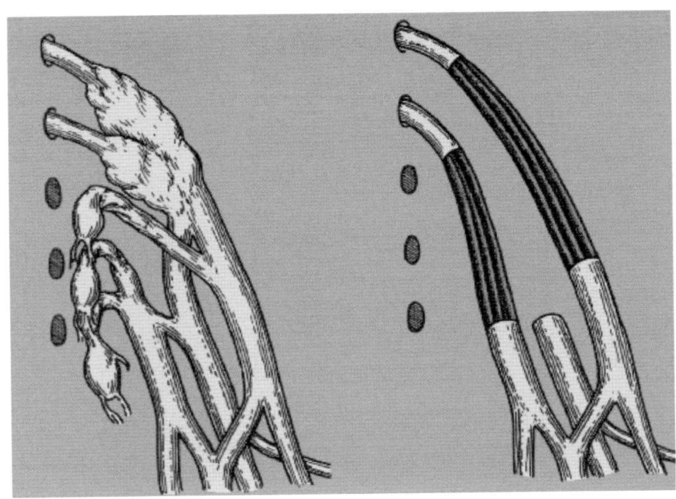

Figure 18.13
With three avulsed roots, it may be necessary to sacrifice some parts of the plexus.

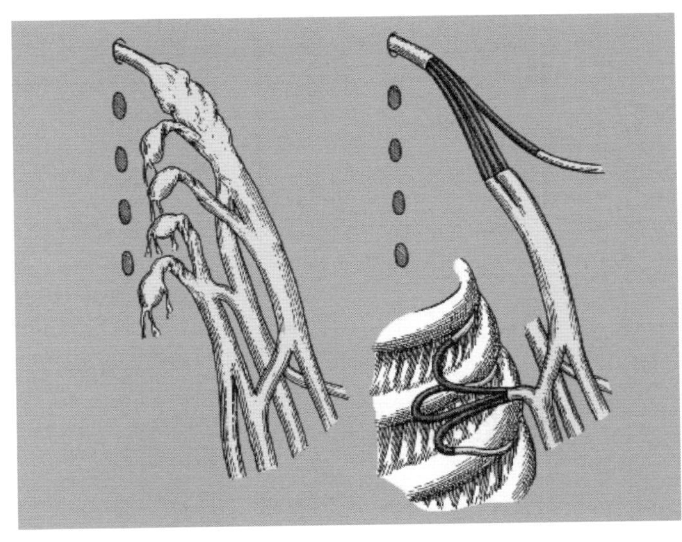

Figure 18.14
When one or no roots are left, extraplexual neurotization is necessary.

The lesions

Many types of lesions are encountered in obstetrical plexus paralysis. The most common is the neuroma in continuity. It is mostly found in the upper plexus; the level is usually at the junction of C5 and C6 but it can extend sometimes proximally, often distally to the clavicular area.

When confronted by this lesion, there has been a temptation for several authors (Janec et al 1968, Clarke et al 1996) to preserve the continuity and only perform a neurolysis. Some authors have been able to assess their patients and demonstrate the inefficiency of the procedure (Clarke et al 1996). We have always considered that, when the clinical decision to repair the plexus has been taken, the neuroma must be removed and grafted. Early in our experience (1979), a small series of 15 of these neuromas were excised and sent to pathology for serial studies. They showed the almost complete absence of fibres at the distal end of the neuroma. There are almost no indications for isolated neurolysis in this surgery. The intraoperative discovery that neurolysis may be the appropriate treatment generally comes from excess in the operative indication.

Rarely there is a complete rupture of the roots or trunks. The extremities may be difficult to find in a scarred area.

Avulsion injury is the most severe lesion. It may be suspected during the approach if there is an unusual amount of scar tissue, with difficult dissection of the roots. The spinal ganglion and the motor branch are usually found; it is important to preserve them, as it may be useful to repair the motor root directly.

No diagnosis of avulsion should be accepted until the root has been dissected up to the foramen. In several papers, authors determined the diagnosis of avulsion on clinical grounds, combined with EMG and myelography results. These examinations are very helpful, but only dissection can confirm the diagnosis.

This exploration of the lower roots C8, T1 can only be done safely with osteotomy of the clavicle.

There are difficult cases where the root is inside the foramen with all the signs of avulsion. This situation is found, in particular, in upper root lesions after breech delivery.

It is then necessary to make a decision. In upper root lesions, we know from experience (Geutjens et al 1996, Sloof et al 2001) that approximately 50% of these roots will recover, at least partially. We prefer to close the wound and wait 6 months. After this delay, those patients who have not recovered will be reoperated and these roots, considered as avulsed, will be neurotized. With lower roots, a decision has to be taken immediately as reoperation may become dangerous in this area. If there is an associated Horner syndrome and no response to electrical stimulation, the root is considered as avulsed, and cut at the foramen, to be neurotized.

Strategy of repair

When there are enough donor roots, repair by grafts is not a problem. The problems start when there are no donor roots (isolated avulsion) or only one or two roots with three or four avulsed roots. We then have to mix grafts, neurozations and end-to-side sutures. The technical aspects may vary with the lesion, its extent, the length of grafts, etc. The philosophy stays the same, we have priorities:

- The first priority is hand function and especially finger flexion and thumb movements. These movements are almost impossible to recover through secondary transfers.
- Wrist and finger extension are also a must if the hand is to be usable.
- The next most important movement will be elbow flexion, which can be used only with shoulder external rotation.
- Elbow extension and shoulder abduction will come later.

The choice of distal grafting will be determined by these priorities. According to the number of usable roots, the repair can be more or less ambitious. In using this strategy, one of the main questions was the function achievable after use of a single root to try to repair several movements, sometimes antagonists.

Our experience of very severe lesions (Gilbert 2001) has shown that in many cases, the child is able to control independently the movements he will recover, even from the same root.

In some instances, we have found co-contractions between biceps and triceps, which are difficult to treat (see later).

In terms of reliability, at that stage, we will use the grafts for the key movements; some neurotizations (spinal accessory, ulnar nerve, pectoralis major nerve) for the biceps and use end-to-side for the secondary aims or if nothing else is possible. The results in 436 cases operated on up until 1996 showed the following distribution of root lesions:

1. C5 and C6: 48%
2. C5 to C7: 29%
3. Complete involvement: 23%, of which almost all were avulsions.

Postoperative care

Stretching of the reconstructed area must be avoided in the first 3 weeks postoperatively. This can be achieved by the use of a plaster cast. Physical therapy is then resumed by gentle passive exercises and encouraging voluntary movement. Every effort should be made to counteract retraction and internal rotation of the shoulder and flexion of the elbow. Physiotherapy should be continued throughout the recovery period, usually for 2 years, but regular physiotherapy should then be discontinued. The recovery is slow. It can be seen 4–6 months after direct suture and at 6–10 months following graft reconstruction. It can continue in upper plexus lesions for more than 2 years and in complete lesions for more

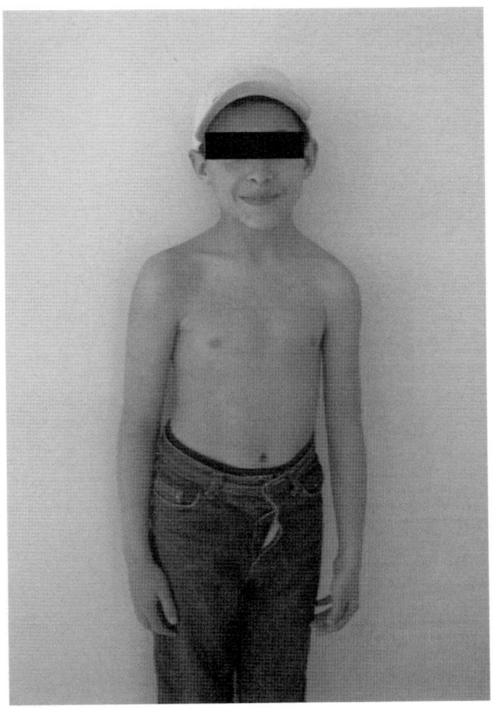
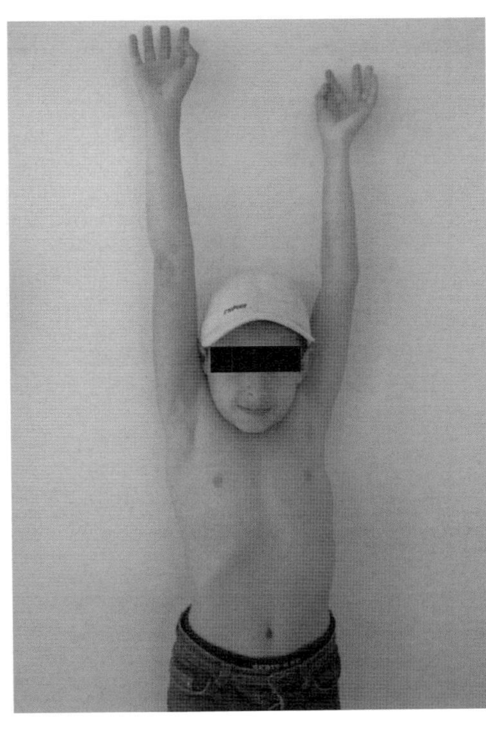

Figures 18.15 and 18.16
Results at 10 years after C5, C6 repair.

than 3 years (Gilbert 1997, Gilbert and Berger 1997, Gilbert et al 1988a, 1991).

Results

A total of 436 patients operated on between 1976 and 1995 have been reviewed, with more than 4 years' follow-up. The results in the shoulder using the Mallet scale (1972) were as follows. For C5, C6 lesions at 2 years, the results were > grade IV (good-excellent), 52%; grade III, 40% and grade II,. 8%. After 2 years one-third of the patients had secondary surgery: 13 subscapularis releases, 33 latissimus dorsi transfers and 6 trapezius transfers, and a new evaluation was done at 4 years. At 4 years (after tendon transfers) the results were as follows (Figures 18.15 and 18.16): > grade IV, 80%; grade III, 20% and grade II 0%.

For C5, C6, C7 lesions at 2 years the results were > grade IV, 36%; grade III, 46% and grade II, 18%. After 2 years, one-quarter of the patients had secondary surgery: 7 subscapularis releases, 24 latissimus dorsi transfers and 1 trapezius transfer, and the results were evaluated again at 4 years. At 4 years the results were > grade IV, 61%; grade III, 29% and grade II, 10%.

Complete paralysis

The shoulder results in complete paralysis are less satisfactory because part of the upper roots destined for the shoulder and elbow have to be sacrificed to obtain function in the hand. The shoulder results at 4 years are as follows: class IV, 22.5%; class III, 42%; class II, 35.5%.

Alternatively, the prognosis for the hand which is very poor following spontaneous recovery alone provides 83% of hands with some function and useful function in 75% of patients 8 years after a neurotization.

Complications

There have been no operative deaths. The overall complication rate in the present series was 1%, including phrenic nerve lesions, lesions of the thoracic duct, wound infections and vascular lesions, all of which have been managed satisfactorily without late sequelae.

Conclusions

Based on the results of the author's series, the following recommendations can be made:

1. Babies who do not recover biceps function by the age of 3 months should be considered for immediate operation.
2. Primary suture without tension is rarely possible. Nerve grafting is usually necessary for root or trunk ruptures.
3. In the presence of root avulsions an internal neurotization should be attempted between different roots,

particularly as children seem to have a far greater capacity to accommodate to differential neurotizations.
4. When it is not possible to perform an internal neurotization, an external neurotization can be performed using one or more of the following donor nerves in the following order of preference: the pectoral nerves, the intercostal nerves, the accessory nerve.
5. The reconstruction should be protected from excessive motion for the first 3 weeks.
6. Physiotherapy should be continued up to 2 years of age but then continued by the parents in the form of play and activities of daily living.
7. Secondary surgery can be considered when it is clear that recovery following reconstruction is unsatisfactory.

Sequelae

Immediately after the injury, the factors responsible for the late bone, joint and soft tissue sequelae are present: paralysis, imbalance of muscles, contractures.

Although it is possible to maintain the passive range of motion of the joints by active physiotherapy in the first few months, after 6–8 months some muscle contractures are present and may need treatment. The particular severity of the long-term complications is due to the sequence of paralysis, imbalance, contracture and joint deformities. At every stage the lesion may be reversible but will need continuous attention with physiotherapy, splinting and in some cases surgery.

The turning point is the appearance of a joint deformity. When the malpositions of the joint have been maintained for several months or years, growth will induce a joint anomaly, which may preclude any further surgery.

The existence of contractures and joint deformities as well as co-contraction will influence the treatment. All the evaluation systems that we designed can be used only when the contractures are treated. No tendon transfer can be done on a stiff joint.

Shoulder

The shoulder is the most complex joint of the upper limb. After upper root palsy, the external rotators are paralysed, as well as the deltoid. The subscapularis is either spared or recovers quickly, acting as a medial rotator. With no antagonist, the muscle may become hyperactive and contracted. Even very active physiotherapy may not allow the recovery of a good passive external rotation (Fairbank 1913).

The measurement of the range of rotation should be done with the arm in adduction. This passive external rotation can go up to 90° in a baby and decreases with age. The acceptable limit is 30°. Once this limit has been reached, there should be a very strict follow-up and if after 3 months of adequate mobilization the limitation does not improve or becomes worse, the patient should be operated.

If the child has recovered some abduction, the limitation will be responsible for a 'clarion sign'. When the child wants to put his hand to the mouth, he has to lift his elbow to compensate for the lack of rotation.

When surgical release has been decided upon, it is necessary to check the shape of the joint. It has been our experience that there is usually no risk of joint anomaly before 3 years old. In older children the glenohumeral joint can be studied by MRI or CT arthrogram and after 8–9 years old a simple CT scan can be performed.

Treatment of medial rotation contracture

This medial rotation contracture is treated continuously by physiotherapy. In the 1970s, the use of 'statue of liberty', splints was systematically recommended for babies in the recovery phase (Dubousset 1972). It was probably useful for the medial contracture but its consequences were often problematic. After a few months of splinting, a lateral rotation contracture was not unusual, with a spontaneous position in slight abduction and external rotation of the upper limb. Although the medial rotation contracture can be treated successfully, the lateral rotation contracture is extremely difficult to overcome. There is no real surgical treatment. For this reason, most authors have abandoned the abduction splint.

The cause of medial rotation deformity is the hyperactivity of the unopposed subscapularis muscle.

Although the pectoralis major is partly a medial rotator, it is mainly an adductor and its release is not necessary when treating the contracture.

The joint capsule is part of the poor position, but as a consequence of the medial rotation. It is not necessary to open the joint in younger children (under 8-9 years old).

Treatment is based on the release of the subscapularis. Sever (1927) proposed an anterior release with tenotomy of the subscapularis tendon and joint release. The consequence was an excellent external rotation but the loss of any internal rotation. However, it is still used by some authors (Strecker et al 1990, Covey et al 1992).

To avoid these consequences, Saloff-Coste (1965, 1966) proposed a lengthening of the subscapularis tendon. The principle is more functional but on a contracted muscle, a large lengthening of the tendon will lead to very limited excursion of the muscle. Based on the principles described by Scaglietti (1941), Carlioz and Brahimi (1971) and Rigault (1972); Pichon and Carlioz (1979) cited their preference for the subscapularis release. The muscle slide will allow free movements of the joint and respect its functionality (Figures 18.17 and 18.18).

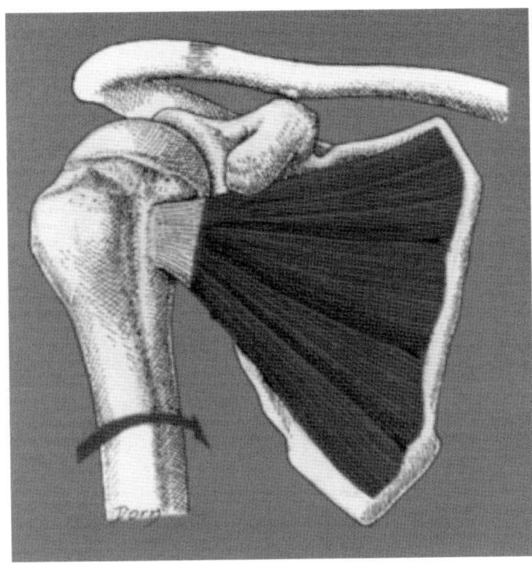

Figure 18.17
Tightness of the subscapularis is responsible for internal rotation contracture.

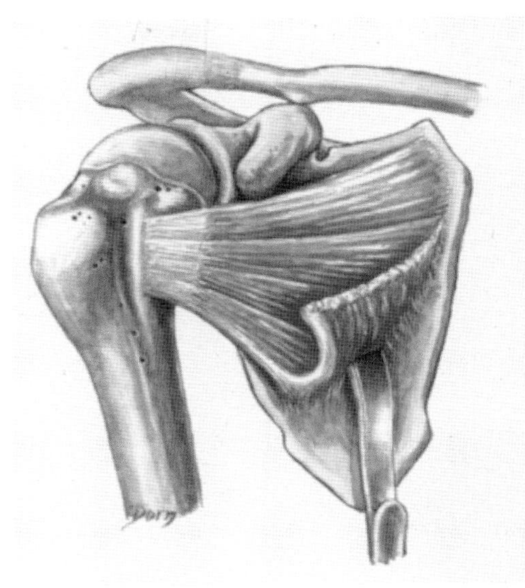

Figure 18.18
The subscapularis is detached from the scapula.

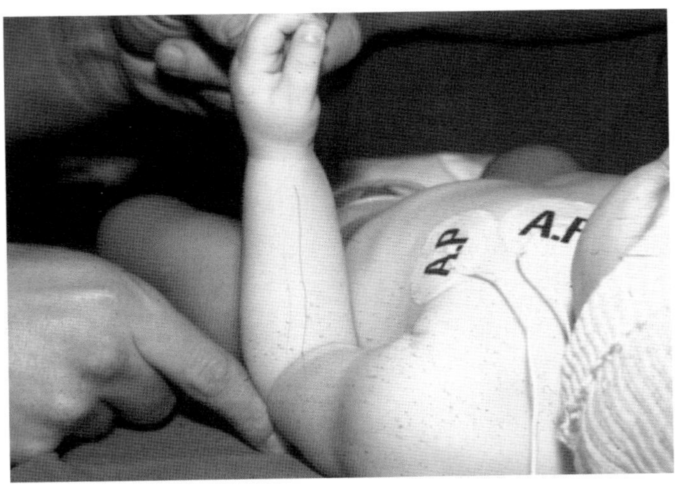

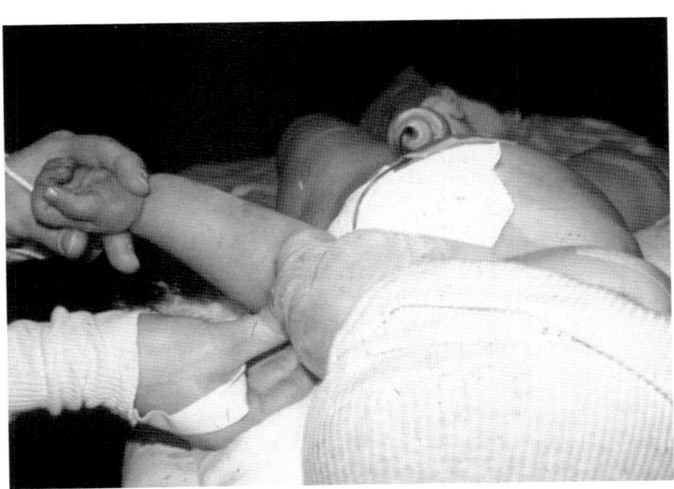

Figures 18.19 and 18.20
Subscapularis release: preoperative and postoperative.

The release of the contracture can always be overcome by the operation but the result can be maintained only if the external rotator muscles become active and if there are no sequelae from the long period of joint malposition.

We have reviewed a series of patients operated for medial shoulder contracture (Gilbert 2000, Gilbert et al 1988b) (Figures 18.19–18.24); it was necessary to do a secondary tendon transfer to the rotator cuff in 18% of the cases. Only 52% of the patients recovered spontaneously. The other patients either did not feel they needed transfer or refused the operation. These results show that after release of the contracture of the joint, many patients will recover sufficiently to avoid any transfer and that the systematic association of the release and a tendon transfer (l'Episcopo 1934, Hoffer et al 1978) is not always necessary.

We prefer to follow an intensive physiotherapy programme for 6 months. In many cases, the external rotators will recover progressively and maintain the passive rotation.

In some cases, after a few months, the external rotation regresses progressively despite a good physical programme. If, from 80° of passive external rotation the shoulder progresses in 3 months to 60°, then 40°, it is

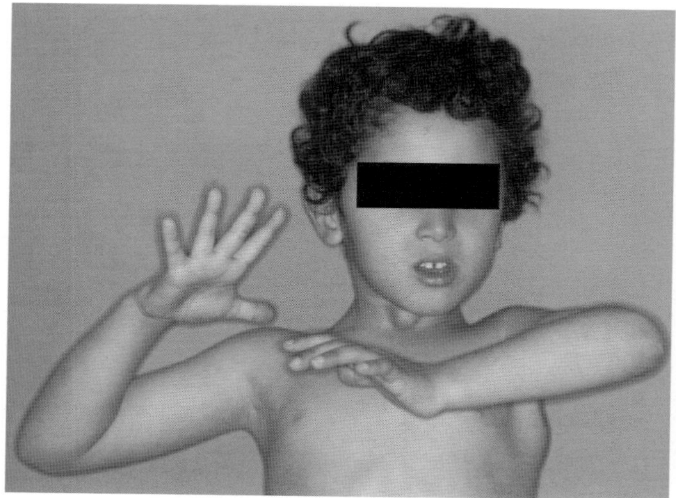

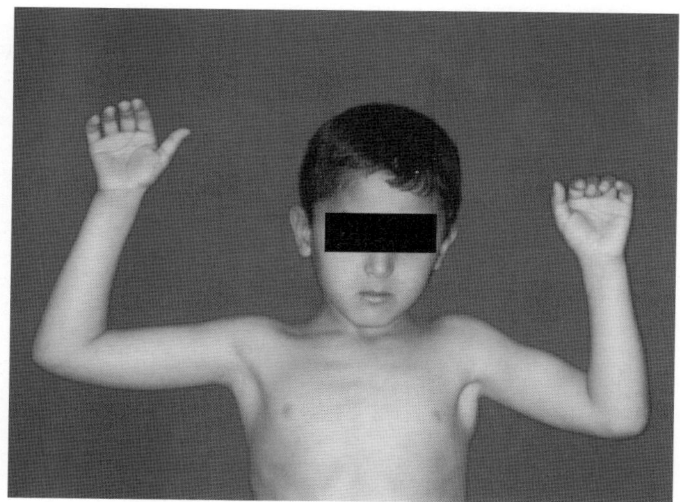

Figures 18.21 and 18.22
Pre and post release.

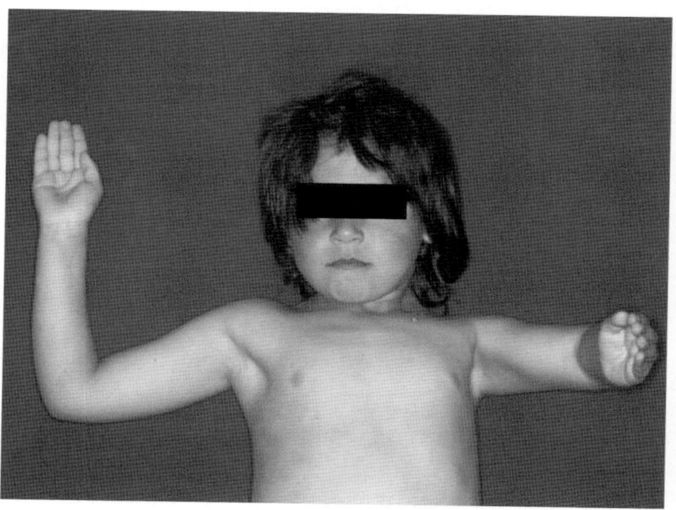

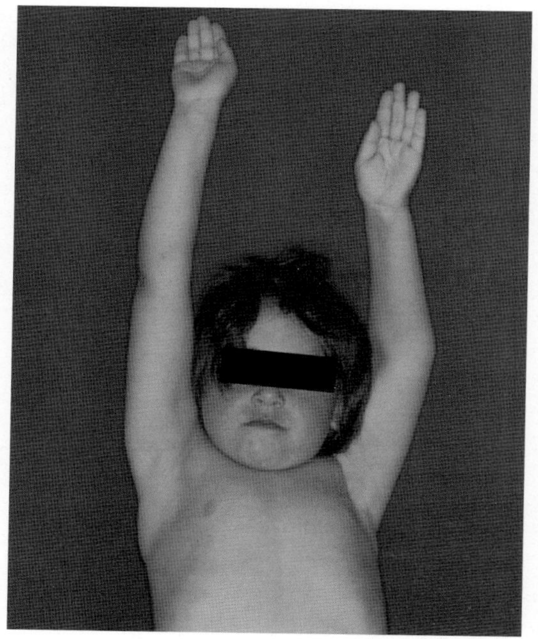

Figures 18.23 and 18.24
Abduction improved only by subscapularis release.

necessary to do a tendon transfer to avoid recurrence. If this rule is well followed, the final results will be very satisfactory and we found excellent stability of the result at 4 years follow-up:

However, there are some indications for combining the release and the tendon transfer: for example, patients who cannot be adequately followed, older children with no chance of recovery, patients who do not comply with the physiotherapy programme. In these cases, the risks of recurrence overcome the possibility of spontaneous recovery of external rotation. In older children, the problems become more complex as the joint deformities must be taken into account. After the age of 3 or 4 years, it has long been our belief that the joint anomalies preclude the use of subscapularis release. Recently, we have operated on a series of older children (8–12 years old) with interesting results, even if the shoulder joint was not perfectly congruent.

Treatment of paralytic shoulder

When the joint is free but paralytic, tendon transfers are possible. Several muscles have been used in the past, from the trapezius (Mayer 1927, Saha 1967a, 1967b) to the latissimus dorsi (Schulze-Berge 1917, Zachary 1947) either alone (Gilbert et al 1988b) or with teres major (L'Episcopo 1939, Price and Grossman 1995).

Other muscles – levator scapulae (Narakas 1993), teres major (Chuang et al 1998), pectoralis major and triceps – have been used, alone or in combination.

Immediately after removal of the plaster, intensive rehabilitation is started. The result is obtained rapidly, usually after 2 or 3 weeks. Itoh et al (1987) have proposed using the latissimus dorsi as an island, and moving it over the shoulder to replace a deltoid; this technique was used by Narakas (1993) a few times with some favourable results. The operation is very extensive, there are multiple scars and these may be too much for a hypothetical result.

The results of this operation are good in our hands: 203 children (male 110; female 93) underwent latissimus dorsi transfer between 1982 and 1999; 89 babies had had a C5,6 palsy, 73 a C5, 6, 7 palsy, 41 had a total brachial plexus palsy. In 20.2% (41) of the babies we performed a subscapularis release before the Hoffer procedure, at a mean age of 2.46 ± 2.07 years. Clinical evaluation has been performed up to 15 years. Using our shoulder classification, we divided the babies into three preoperative groups: group 0–1 (26), group 2–3 (121 babies) and group 4–5 (56 babies).

In C5,6 palsy, comparing the mean preoperative abduction value (105°) with the postoperative values at 1 (131°), 3 (136°) and 6 years (129°) we found a highly significant improvement ($P < 0.001$). On the other hand, abduction decreased progressively, reaching a value of 119° and 105° after 10 and 15 years respectively, and statistical differences from the preoperative values are no longer detectable ($P > 0.05$).

A statistically significant passive external rotation (RECC) improvement ($P < 0.01$) was detected only when comparing the preoperative value (56°) with the value recorded after 1 year (65°), while no significance was observed after 3, 6, 10 or 15 years ($P > 0.05$).

The active external rotation improvement was highly significant at each follow-up point ($P < 0.001$), increasing from 0.4 preoperatively to 1.5 after 1 year and also maintaining high values after 15 years (1.4).

In C5, C6, C7 palsy, the mean preoperative abduction value (82.5°) is lower than that recorded in C5, C6 palsies (105°). The postoperative improvement is significant after 1 (104°), 3 (104°), 6 (100°) and 10 years (98.4°), but no longer significant after 15 years (75°).

Compared with the preoperative values (58.68°), the improvement in the passive external rotation (RECC) was significant only at 1 (69.4°), 3 (68.77°) and 6 years (68°). A worsening with no significant differences from the preoperative data was observed at 10 (66.36°) and 15 years (62.5°).

The active external rotation improvement was highly significant at each follow-up, increasing from 0.5 preoperatively to 1.5 after 1 year and also maintaining high values after 6 (1.6), 10 (1.6) and 15 years (1.4).

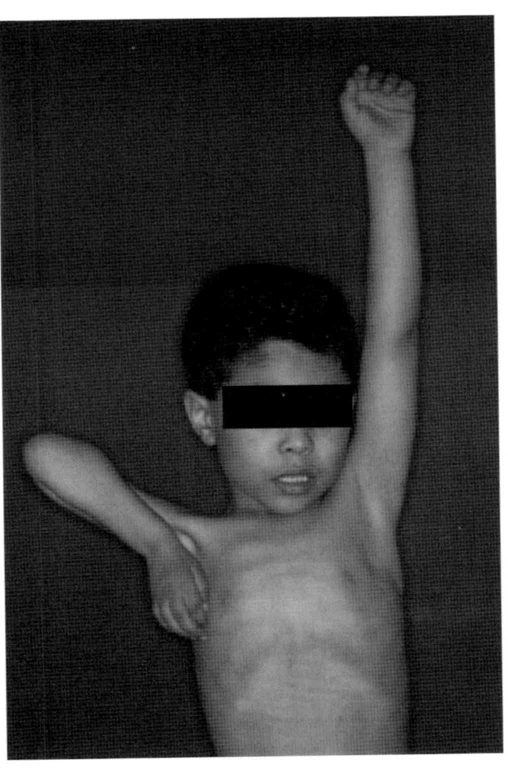

Figure 18.25
Lack of active external rotation.

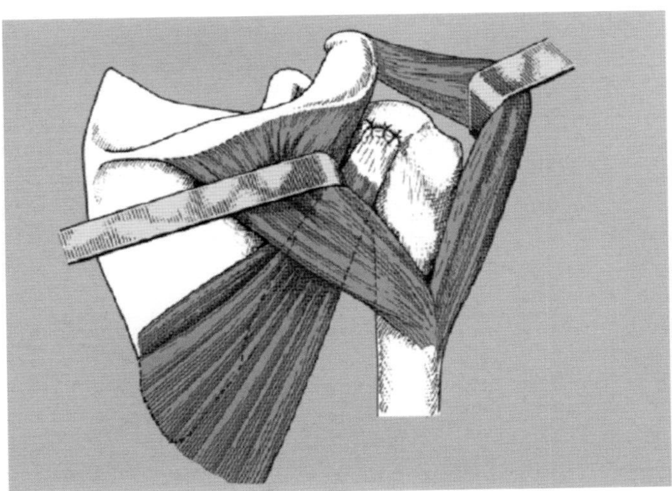

Figure 18.26
Transfer of the latissimus dorsi to the rotator cuff.

In complete brachial plexus palsy, the improvement in shoulder abduction was significant compared with preoperative data (76°) only after 1 (99°) and 3 years (98.5°), and a progressive worsening was observed after 6 (82.8°) and 10 years (68.4°).

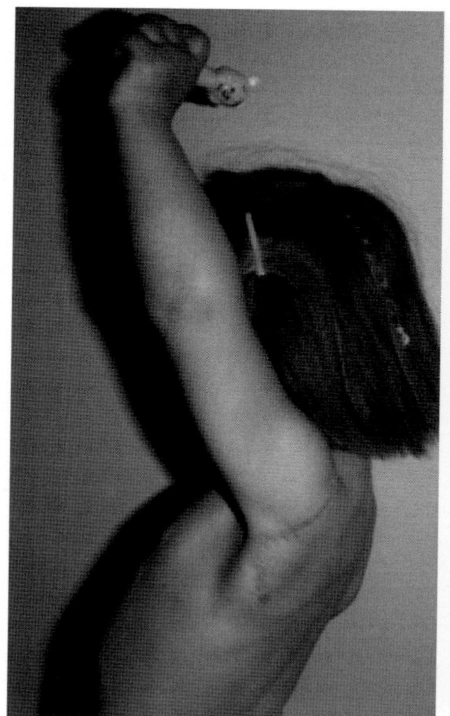

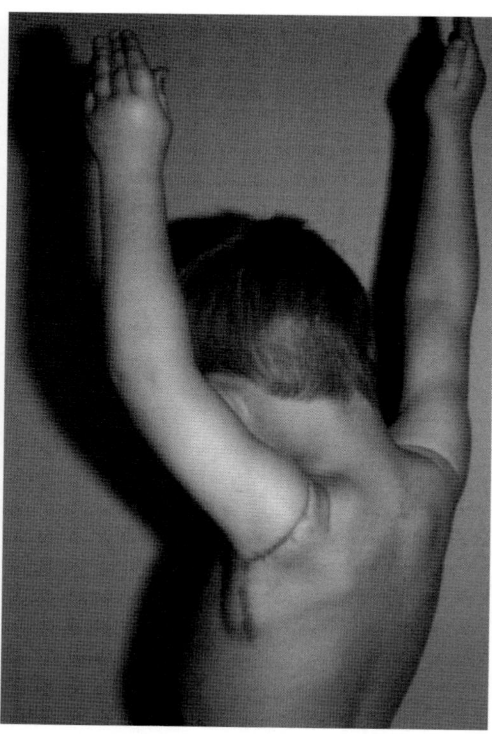

Figures 18.27 and 18.28
Results after latissimus transfer.

A statistically significant passive external rotation (RECC) improvement was detected only when comparing the preoperative value (49.7°) with the value recorded after 1 year (60.7°) and 3 years (62°), while no significance was observed after 6, 10 and 15 years (*P* >0.05).

The active external rotation improvement was highly significant at 1, 3, 6 and 10 years follow-up (*P* <0.001 or *P* <0.005), increasing from 0.2 preoperatively to 1.2 after 1 year and to 1.2 after 3 years. A weak external rotation was recorded after 6 (1.1) and 10 years (0.9).

The conclusions of this study are as follows:

- The latissimus transfer is effective in improving abduction for a few years after surgery (Figures 18.25–18.28).
- The long-term results on abduction decrease as the child approaches adolescence.
- These results are good in reconstructing active external rotation and, contrary to abduction, are maintained in the long term.

In the literature, there are few papers with a large number of patients (Chuang et al 1998, Edwards et al 2000) except the long-term experience of Phipps and Hoffer (1995). In the follow-up of 56 patients, they found an average improvement of 45° and a constant improvement of external rotation.

In other cases, either the latissimus dorsi is not usable or two muscles need to be combined and the trapezius is then also used. This muscle is always of good quality after a brachial plexus injury, as its innervation comes from higher roots; however, if the shoulder has been paralysed for several years, there is a tendency for a contracture of the trapezius. The muscle may become too short for a direct transfer and will need to be extended by a tendon graft or a piece of bone. Physiotherapy will be lengthy and difficult, it is best done lying down and in a pool as the trapezius is rarely strong enough to obtain a direct abduction rapidly.

The results of our trapezius transfers have been reviewed. In 17 patients, the average improvement has been 41° (Figures 18.29 and 18.30). These results are in accordance with the literature (Yadav 1978, Mir-Bullo and Hinarejos 1998, Ruhmann et al 1998, 1999, Aziz et al 1990).

Raimondi et al (2001) regularly uses the levator scapulae transfer. The use of this transfer is indicated in severely paralysed shoulders (grade 0) in which neither abduction nor external rotation are present. The rationale is to actively centre the humeral head into the glenoid fossa to improve the action of the transfer to deltoid. As the levator scapulae muscle is innervated by the cervical plexus it is always active even in severe obstetric paralysis and can be usefully transferred.

After the insertion of levator scapulae transfer to the humerus, the trapezius is transferred to substitute the paralysed deltoid (Egloff et al 1995).

Narakas (1993) likes to combine latissimus dorsi and teres major, as reported earlier by Sever (1939) and D'Aubigné and Deburge (1967). Gilbert et al (1988b) prefer to add the trapezius to the latissimus dorsi.

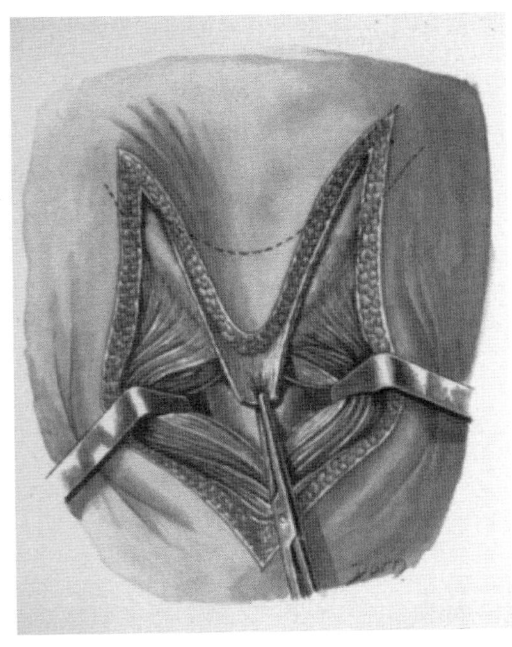

Figure 18.29
The trapezius is fixed on the posterior border of the bicipital groove.

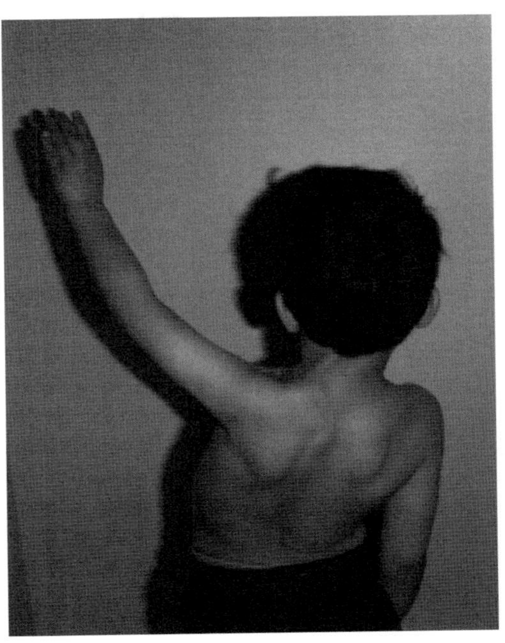

Figure 18.30
Result after trapezius transfer.

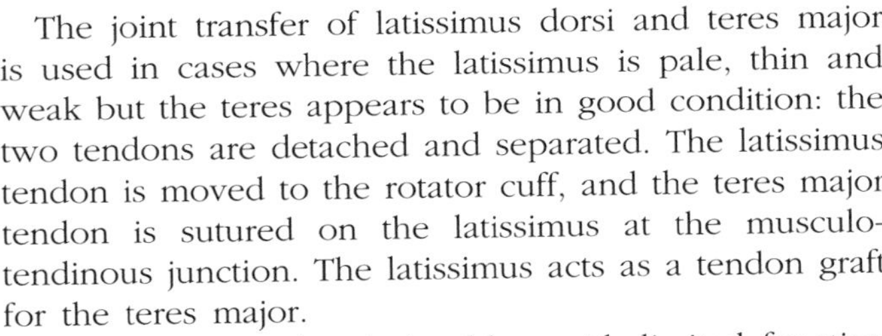

The joint transfer of latissimus dorsi and teres major is used in cases where the latissimus is pale, thin and weak but the teres appears to be in good condition: the two tendons are detached and separated. The latissimus tendon is moved to the rotator cuff, and the teres major tendon is sutured on the latissimus at the musculo-tendinous junction. The latissimus acts as a tendon graft for the teres major.

In severely paralysed shoulders with limited function (shoulder grade I) we like to combine trapezius with levator scapulae and latissimus dorsi or latissimus dorsi plus teres major (if they are usable). In 20 patients, this procedure has made it possible to obtain a shoulder grade III in 17 cases with a good scapulo-thoracic function and shoulder grade II in three patients when the scapulo-thoracic joint was unstable.

Indications

- Shoulder III–IV: isolated latissimus dorsi transfer.
- Shoulder II: trapezius transfer + latissimus dorsi or levator scapulae.
- Shoulder 0–I: trapezius (± levator scapulae).

Medial rotation contracture

Lack of active internal rotation is not rare but does not usually need treatment. In the past 25 years, we have had to treat this defect in only seven cases. In these cases, the pectoralis major is active, showing that it has no important role in medial rotation. The pectoralis can be used for reconstruction of internal rotation. This procedure gives some internal rotation but never a complete result.

Late shoulder deformity

In patients where the imbalance has not been treated or if the treatment has failed, the long-standing malposition will induce joint deformities, which will be more severe as time passes:

- Flattening and posterior subluxation of the humeral head with retroversion of the humeral neck. The glenoid does not develop normally, it is flat and retroverted (Figure 18.31).
- Later, the joint becomes non-congruent, with posterior dislocation and severe medial rotation. The coracoid is elongated and has a downward position. The acromion may be larger anteriorly and laterally (Pollock and Reed 1989). The glenoid is retroverted (Pearl and Edgerton 1998, Waters et al 1998, Beischer et al 1999).
- The child or adolescent is seen with a deformed shoulder, the head can be seen posteriorly. Abduction is limited; there is usually no external rotation.

The situation has to be studied radiologically: either by ultrasonography (Hunter et al 1998) or CT scan (Hernandez and Dias 1988) or MRI (Gudinchet et al 1995). We feel that the best and most accurate results can be obtained with a CT scan 3-D reconstruction, which shows the extent of the anomalies.

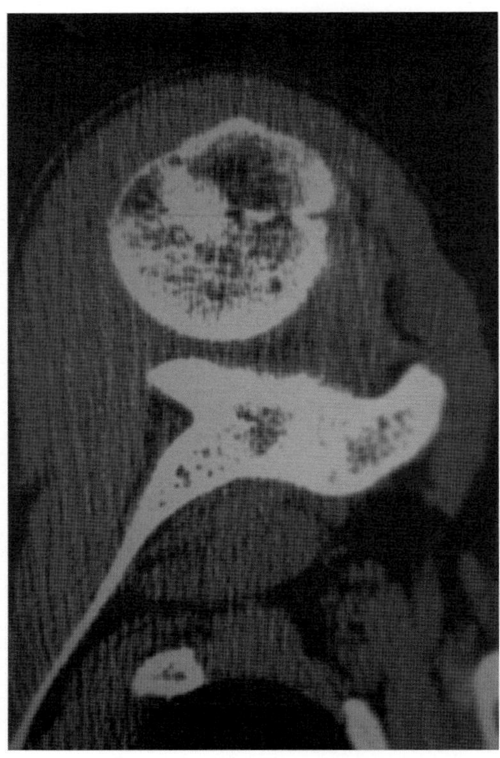

Figure 18.31
In late cases, the humeral head is subluxated and the glenoid is flattened.

There is sometimes slight pain, although very often the situation is painless but the patient seeks functional and cosmetic improvement.

The difficult questions for the surgeon are: Can we improve the situation? At what cost? Even if the functional improvement is limited, should we try to reintegrate the humeral head in order to prevent later arthritis and pain?

The answers to these questions are not easy and certainly differ. Several authors (Dunkerton 1989, Hoffer and Phipps 1998, Cullu 1999) advocate a surgical reduction, even in cases of posterior dislocation, using soft-tissue releases, often associated with tendon transfers and sometimes with rotation osteotomies.

Birch (1993) advocates, at least in the less severe cases, reintegrating the head and reconstructing the joint with a complex operation combining:

- Osteotomy of the coracoid.
- Lengthening of the subscapularis tendon.
- If necessary, medial rotation osteotomy to correct the retroversion, once normal external rotation is obtained.

This is certainly a very interesting suggestion but we still need to see the long-term functional results of these operations.

To date, we have tried in several cases to treat the medial rotation contracture in isolation by resection of the coracoid and resection of the coraco-humeral ligament. This can be done either in these older children or even after recurrence of subscapularis release and any case where the release is contraindicated because of some anomaly in the joint. The results of this simple operation are excellent and give a constant improvement – limited but enough to make the patient happy.

This does not solve the problem of the patient with posterior dislocation. In some cases, after coracoidectomy, the head reintegrates the glenoid in external rotation, but during medial rotation it comes out again.

The retroversion could be treated by a medial osteotomy like Birch et al (1988) but there is also a severe anomaly of the glenoid. In two cases we have tried to add a posterior approach with stabilization by a bone block, as the glenoid is too small for an osteotomy. The head has been stabilized but at the cost of more stiffness to the shoulder.

The treatment of late shoulder deformities is so unsatisfactory that anything should be done to avoid these anomalies. It is paramount to follow-up and treat any type of shoulder deformity in the young child immediately. Otherwise, if we consider that this shoulder dislocation cannot be treated and does not represent a particular risk for the future, osteotomy of the humerus can give excellent cosmetic and functional improvements (Goddard and Fixsen 1984, Al Zahrani 1993, 1997, Kirkos and Papadopoulos 1998).

The elbow

Recovery of elbow movements is usually very good in any type of paralysis. We saw that even in complete paralyses the recovery is excellent (close to 80%) after 2 years. The need for secondary surgery is rare. There are three main problems: paralysis of elbow flexion, paralysis of elbow extension and flexion contracture of the elbow.

Paralysis of elbow flexion

Absence of elbow flexion is not equivalent to absence of recovery. There are cases where even with proven recovery of the biceps with notable contraction, the elbow does not flex. This may be due to difficulties of brain control and the solution may only be achieved with physiotherapy and muscle stimulation. In other cases the presence of co-contraction with the triceps is the cause of absence of flexion. The treatment of these co-contractions will be described later in this chapter.

When the absence of biceps recovery is responsible for the elbow paralysis, several procedures can be used.

Several muscles can be transferred to replace the biceps; our favourite transfer is the latissimus dorsi, which can be used if it has not been used at the shoulder. This transfer was used by Hovnanian (1956) and modified by Zancolli (1973) to become bipolar. Several authors have used it with excellent results (Moneim and Omer 1986). Rehabilitation will need splinting and stimulation. The complete result may take a long time to achieve.

Even though the procedure is complex, and the postoperative care delicate, this operation gives good results. In 11 cases, we have found improvement in all patients, with the ability to perform hand to mouth movements in seven cases. This movement needs not only an elbow flexion superior to 110° but also an active external rotation of the shoulder.

When the latissimus dorsi is not available, it is possible to use other muscles. Pectoralis major can give some excellent results but the sacrifice of this muscle may be detrimental as it induces the loss of adduction. If the shoulder is flail, this loss is unacceptable. It also gives a poor cosmetic appearance but can give a strong flexion (Tubiana et al 1999).

Pectoralis minor can also be used for elbow flexion but it has two drawbacks: the muscle is situated behind pectoralis major and can only be assessed with great difficulty if pectoralis major is active; and it is a small and weak muscle and cannot pretend to replace a biceps.

In fact, the indication for using pectoralis minor is when a weak biceps has to be supplemented. The scars are extensive on the thorax, making it difficult to use in girls (Tubiana et al 1999). Another transfer can be very useful, i.e. the triceps. It is a simple operation (Tubiana et al 1999) but extremely effective. After discarding the immobilization, the result is obtained very rapidly. Unfortunately, the loss of elbow extension is a great disability. It can be compensated by gravity but only in certain positions.

In upper root palsy (C5, C6 or C7), the muscles of the shoulder girdle cannot be used and it is necessary to find another option. The best solution is the use of the Steindler procedure (Steindler 1923). The transfer of the flexor muscles from the medial epicondyle can give excellent flexion but the technique has to be very precise (Van Egmond et al 2001).

Rehabilitation after this operation is difficult. As the child has to learn to flex the elbow in contracting the flexors, the wrist extensors must be active. Only in this case can the procedure be done. In some rare cases it has been possible to add the transfer of the distal flexor carpi ulnaris (FCU) to the wrist extensors to the Steindler procedure. However, the transfer may flail and it is preferable to start by reconstructing the wrist extension first.

When starting the physiotherapy programme, it is necessary to use a wrist extension splint. It may take a few weeks for the child to control the wrist extension necessary to initiate elbow flexion.

In some cases there is a weak elbow flexion due to the brachioradialis, improperly called the 'Steindler effect'. In cases of pure C5 and C6 lesion, the biceps is paralysed and the brachioradialis may be spared. It is then possible to improve the moment of action of the brachioradialis by detaching the distal part of the humeral insertion. The muscle is lifted by a lateral incision, leaving its most proximal part inserted. Rehabilitation can be started early.

In cases where the whole arm is very weak and no transfers are possible, the only possibility will be a free muscle transfer. It is first necessary to find a good donor nerve. The plexus itself cannot be used and we have tried the spinal accessory nerve or the intercostal nerves but the best results have been obtained by using the contralateral pectoralis major nerve (Gilbert et al 1980). In the first stage a sural nerve is sutured on the healthy side to the superior pectoral nerve using an infraclavicular approach and passed subcutaneously to the paralysed upper arm. One year later a free gracilis muscle is raised with its neurovascular bundle and moved to the affected arm. The extremity of the sural nerve is examined, for the return of axonal growth. Then the vascular and nerve sutures are done and the muscle is fixed to the coracoid or the pectoralis major tendon proximally and distally to the biceps tendon. Reinnervation of the muscle will start after 6–8 months. We have carried out five cases of biceps reconstruction in obstetrical palsy. All of them were reinnervated and four obtained an active elbow function over M3.

All the above techniques will allow almost every patient to end their growing period with an active elbow flexion.

Paralysis of elbow extension

Although it is not often a source of complaints from patients, weak or absent elbow extension is not rare. It may even be an isolated feature of the C7 isolated avulsion syndrome (Brunelli and Brunelli 1991).

Lack of elbow extension can become a serious defect if the patient has excellent abduction, as they cannot reach out to anything.

Isolated neurotization is difficult as the branches to the triceps are multiple.

Reconstruction of extension can be done by several means.

- Latissimus dorsi transfer (Jones et al 1985), which can give excellent function. Unfortunately the muscle may have to be used for the shoulder or even for elbow flexion, which are priorities.
- Posterior deltoid, proposed for reconstruction of the tetraplegic upper extremity (Moberg 1975). The operation is easy and the transfer can be done directly on the triceps without a tendon graft.
- Teres major can be used and transferred directly on the tendon of the triceps at the level of the glenohumeral joint. The muscle is powerful but is active only in abduction of the shoulder, which answers only one of the concerns of the patients.

Flexion contracture of the elbow

This defect is very common but remains limited in many cases (Ballinger and Hoffer 1994). There is no clear explanation for this contracture. It happens even when the biceps is weak. The most conclusive explanation is that the retraction is due to a contracture of the biceps when it recovers. The two consequences of this contracture are lengthening and deviation of the coracoid proximally and elbow flexion.

The long-standing elbow flexion will provoke shortening and contracture of all the muscles around the elbow (brachialis, brachioradialis, FCU) and the joint capsule.

For many years there is no joint or bone deformity. This contracture may start at 2 years and continue until the age of 12. The maximum contracture occurs at around 8–10 years. As soon as the elbow contracture is diagnosed and is more than 10°, a night splint must be worn each night. By using this splint it is possible to control the contracture and, if not to reduce it, at least to stabilize it. In some cases, the contracture cannot be stopped or the splint is not worn regularly. The contracture progresses and may reach 45–60° or even 70°.

There is then no other option than surgical treatment. For many years, the only accepted possibility was to do an extension osteotomy of the distal humerus. The advantages include simplicity, the possibility of simultaneously performing a rotation osteotomy and no interference with the muscles. The drawbacks are the need to wait for the end of growth, the cosmetic aspect of the elbow and essentially the fact that we obtain a change in the arc of motion but not the range of motion. What is gained in extension will be lost in flexion. For a severe contracture, the recovery of a satisfactory extension will mean the loss of hand to mouth movements.

For these reasons we prefer to use an anterior soft tissue release which can be done at any age. We use a lateral approach which allows us to cut the anterior joint capsule. Although very tight, we never lengthen the biceps tendon, as this procedure may give a loss of elbow flexion. The physiotherapy focuses on the recovery of elbow flexion as the night splint, maintained for 2 or 3 months, will prevent any recurrence. This is a delicate operation and the two main complications are radial nerve paresis and weakness of elbow flexion.

The forearm

In upper root palsy the forearm is usually in pronation due to weakness of the supinator and the biceps. In contrast, complete paralysis provokes a supination contracture essentially due to the fact that for a long time, the only muscle active on the prosupination will be the biceps. There is no antagonist and the forearm stays in complete supination, with a hyperextended wrist.

We feel that the treatment of pronation deformity is not necessary: the functional position is acceptable and patients do not ask for treatment. Some series have demonstrated the possibility of these operations (Liggio et al 1999, Zancolli 2001), using the procedures designed for spastic contractures (lengthening of pronator teres, fascia release, flexor lengthening).

Often the patients' families complain about this excessive pronation, but most of these complaints are due to absence of external rotation of the shoulder. Usually when the shoulder is stabilized and the child has recovered external rotation, there are no more complaints.

On the contrary, supination contracture is a severe disability, as it makes prehension very difficult. The cosmetic aspect of the 'beggar's hand' is also a problem for the child and the family.

Supination contracture should be treated. It is important to differentiate between the pure paralytic cases that remain in supination most of the time and where the passive prosupination is free and the older cases.

After a few years, the contracture appears: passive pronation is impossible, the interosseous membrane is contracted and the bony anomalies may become obvious: bowing of the radius, dislocation of the radial head.

These two situations are totally different, as in the early case the treatment of imbalance of the muscles will be sufficient to re-establish function; in the later case, the treatment of contractures and bone procedures will be necessary. However, there is one absolute contraindication to the treatment of supination of the forearm and this is absence of wrist extension: if the forearm is put in pronation without wrist extension, the result will be disastrous. In the case of absence of wrist extension, it should be treated first and only after success of the transfer can the forearm be treated.

Often in these supination contractions the wrist extension is present but very weak, due to the prolonged hyperextended position. It can be improved by preoperative physiotherapy with the shoulder abducted.

In younger children (3–4 years) a contracture has not usually developed. The best proposition is biceps rerouting (Figure 18.32). This operation was proposed by Grilli (1959). The biceps is sectioned and refixed to the radial head in pronation. Zancolli (1967) made a modification, which gives a more functional result and is now used by most surgeons (Owings et al 1971, Dubousset 1972, Gualtieri et al 1976, Manske et al 1980, Manfrini and Valdiserri 1985). Other modifications have been proposed, such as moving the radial tuberosity (Eberard 1997).

The problem is different when the forearm is stiff or when the radial head is dislocated (Figure 18.33). Zancolli and Zancolli (1988) advocate the complete release of the interosseous membrane in cases of stiffness. To be effective this release must be extended, particularly at the two extremities. In our experience, this release can be useful when the stiffness is limited to the lack of 40° or 60°, but when the forearm is completely

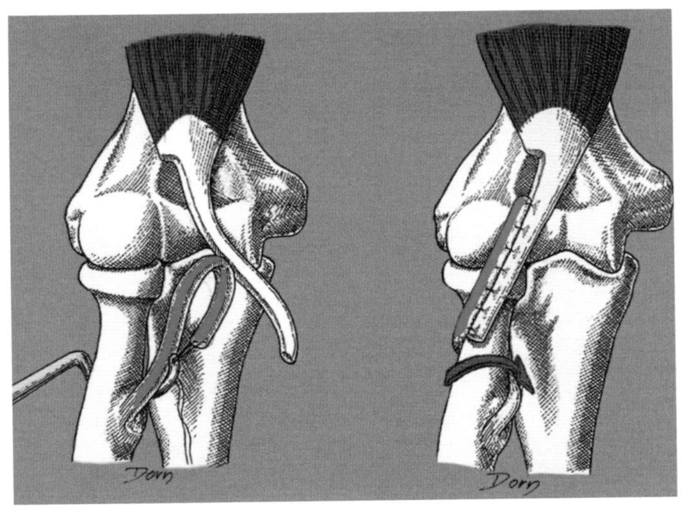

Figure 18.32
Rerouting of the biceps tendon according to Grilli–Zancolli.

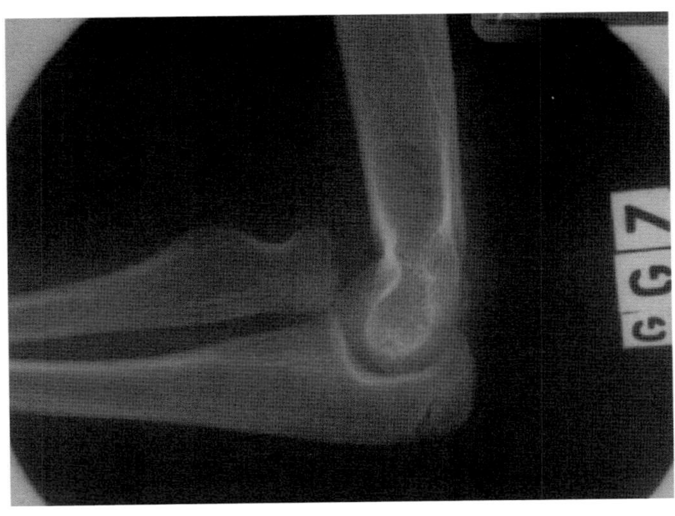

Figure 18.33
Dislocation of the radial head precludes the rerouting operation.

or almost completely stiff, the release is rarely effective as the bones are deformed.

Dislocation of the radial head precludes the use of the rerouting operation. We have tried several times to reduce the dislocation and fix the head (Zancolli 1967) but in all cases the dislocation recurred. The only way to keep the radial head reduced would be to detach the biceps tendon from the tuberosity and fix it again on the ulna.

In cases where tendon rerouting is not possible, the only possibility is a rotation osteotomy of the radius. This osteotomy can be done even at a very late stage and will be sufficient in most cases. In some late cases with hypersupination and bone deformities, it may be necessary to osteotomize both bones.

The results of the treatment of supination contracture are good. The osteotomy gives sufficient pronation intraoperatively, but there is a tendency to recurrence (9 recurrences out of 44 patients). However, soft tissue treatment (22 cases) had kept a good result even at long-term follow-up (Allende and Gilbert 2004) (Figures 18.34 and 18.35) .

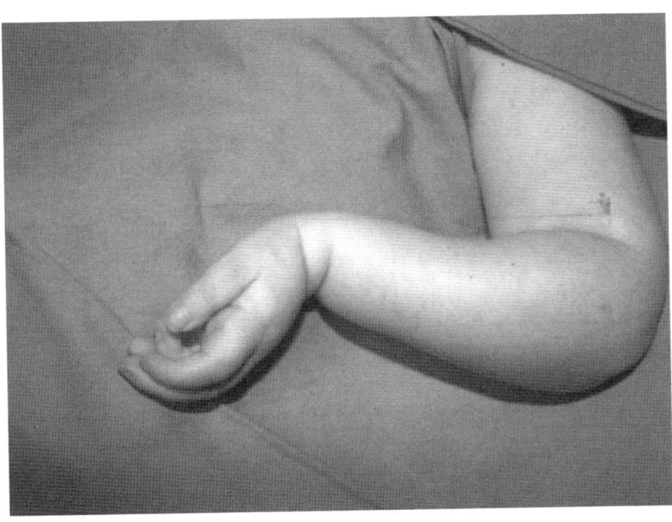

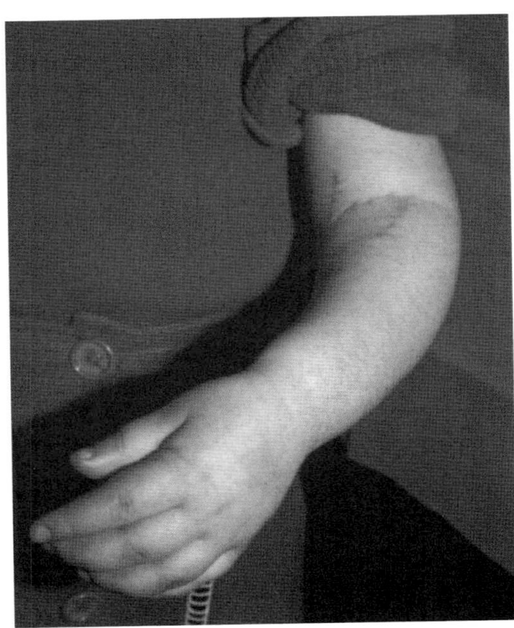

Figures 18.34 and 18.35
Before and after rerouting operation.

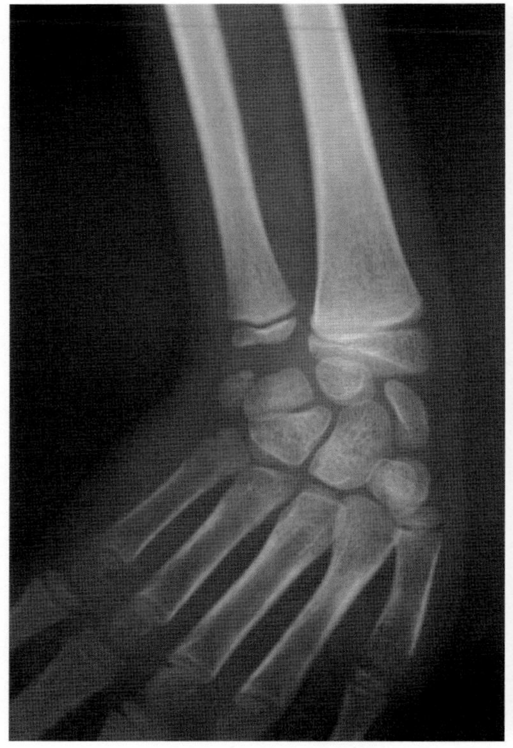

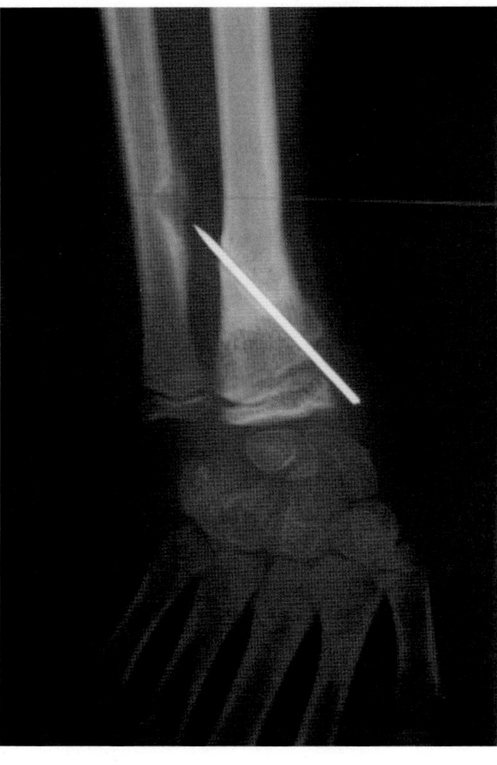

Figures 18.36 and 18.37

Ulnar deviation: before and after osteotomy.

The wrist and hand

Extension of the wrist is the key for hand function. It allows good use of finger flexors and improves pinch by the tenodesis effect. Unfortunately extension does not recover perfectly well and this recovery is late. The lack of extension is a severe disability and will need treatment.

Classically, wrist extension paralysis gives excellent results after treatment, especially after radial nerve palsy. After brachial plexus injury, the muscles have been either paralysed or weakened.

The most commonly used donor muscle will be the FCU. It is preserved in C5, C6, C7 lesions, and is one of the few muscles that regularly recovers after complete paralysis.

The FCU transfer has been the most commonly used (Duclos and Gilbert 1995). It can be transferred either on the ulnar border of the forearm or through the interosseous membrane. Although it seems logical to pass through the membrane with a direct pull and avoiding ulnar deviation, the results are inferior to when passing around the forearm. The relatively poor results after passing through the membrane are probably due to adhesions of the tendon.

When we expect that the muscle will be too weak, it is possible to do a double transfer of FCU and pronator teres (Duclos and Gilbert 1995, 1999). In cases where the FCU cannot be used, a flexor superficialis can be transferred.

In the long term, wrist extension usually increases but is balanced by the lack of wrist flexion. Progressively the wrist may become stiff on extension with dorsal capsule contracture. Attempts at surgical release of the joint are mainly unsuccessful.

Ulnar deviation of the wrist and hand

This is quite a common feature after complete paralysis. The extensor carpi radialis brevis (ECRB) and longus (ECRL) are weak and most extension is done by the extensor carpi ulnaris (ECU). The FCU is also often active. Progressive deviation occurs and after several years this deformity becomes fixed (Zancolli and Zancolli 1988).

At the beginning, when passive correction is possible, it is necessary to reinforce lateral forces by transferring ECU on ECRL. If the ECU is weak or if there is no active extension, the FCU can be transferred on the ECRL. Zancolli (2001) uses an original technique, passing the ECU volarly through the interosseous membrane and fixing it dorsally on the ECRB and ECRL.

When the child is seen late or if the deviation has not been treated, the deformity is fixed and the child asks for correction for cosmetic reasons. This can be done at the end of growth. A triangular piece of bone is resected, allowing correction of the deviation without disturbance of the distal radio-ulnar joint (Figures 18.36 and 18.37).

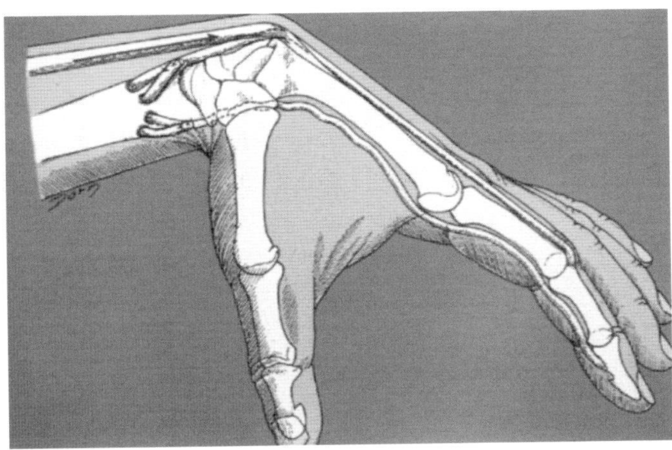

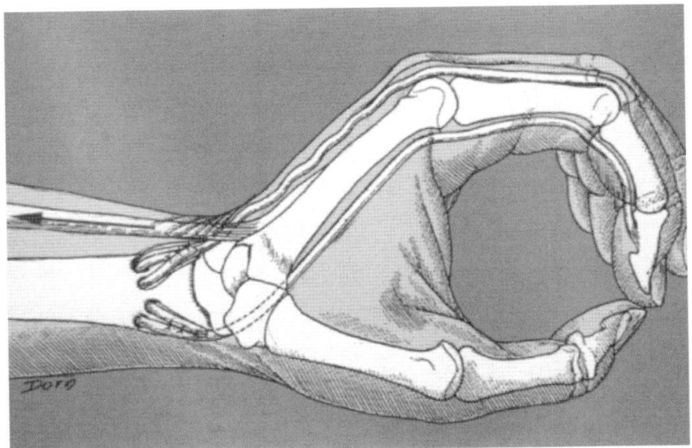

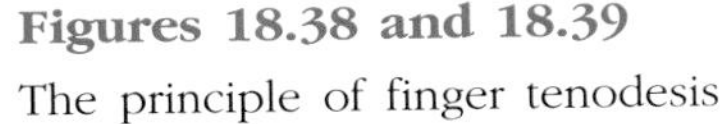

Figures 18.38 and 18.39
The principle of finger tenodesis.

The hand

In cases of severe paralysis of the lower roots the hand may stay very weak, even after repair of the roots. The hand has to be assessed carefully before any treatment is proposed. The deficits are multiple and some can be treated simply:

- Metacarpophalangeal (MP) joint stiffness can be treated by posterior release.
- Thenar muscle paralysis can be treated by flexor superficialis transfer.
- Finger extension defect can be treated by transfer of one or two flexor superficialis.
- Claw hand can be treated by capsulodesis or the lasso procedure.

When the paralysis is more extensive there may not be any tendon transfer possible. There is a need to use an extrinsic tendon. When there is some wrist extension, even with little or no finger flexors, it is possible to give the patient an automatic pinch by using different types of tenodeses.

- The flexor tendons are fixed on the radius through the bone.
- The extensor tendons are fixed dorsally in the same manner (Ochiai et al 1995).

These are the simplest tenodeses, but it is often necessary to add a better movement of the fingers (interosseous tenodesis) or to the thumb (antepulsion and opposition). These more sophisticated tenodeses can be done only if a few muscles are active. The results of this tenodesis may be spectacular, but in several cases it is not so satisfactory as:

- The precision of tension is paramount.
- There will be some lengthening of the tenodesis with time.

For several weeks, the thumb can be protected with strapping using an elastic bandage. This elastic tenodesis can also be used preoperatively to train the child before the surgical tenodesis (Figures 18.38–18.41).

In some cases, the patient has recovered enough finger flexion but cannot achieve a good grip because of interosseous muscle paralysis. It is then possible to use the Parkes technique (Parkes 1973), where the tendon grafts are sutured to the anterior carpal ligament and pass anteriorly to the intermetacarpal ligaments. Active flexion of the fingers will bring automatic flexion of the MP joints.

Another possibility is the Fowler technique in which the tendon grafts are sutured dorsally to the dorsal carpal ligament and passed through the intermetacarpal spaces, anteriorly to the metacarpal ligaments and fixed to the intrinsic tendons. In this case, wrist flexion provokes flexion of the MP joint.

Other tenodeses can be used. When there is no extension of the wrist but activity in the finger flexors, repositioning of the thumb can be done using the flexor pollicis longus.

There are even worse cases, when the hand is totally flail and there is no wrist extension. In selected cases, it may be possible to try improving these desperate situations.

If there is no wrist extension, either it may be possible to use some kind of extrinsic transfer, or it could be one of the very few indications for wrist fusion.

If we have a very limited number of muscles, reconstruction of extension is a priority. The ideal situation is when two transfers can reconstruct both wrist extension and finger extension. When we have only one transfer the best solution, although non-conventional, is to recon-

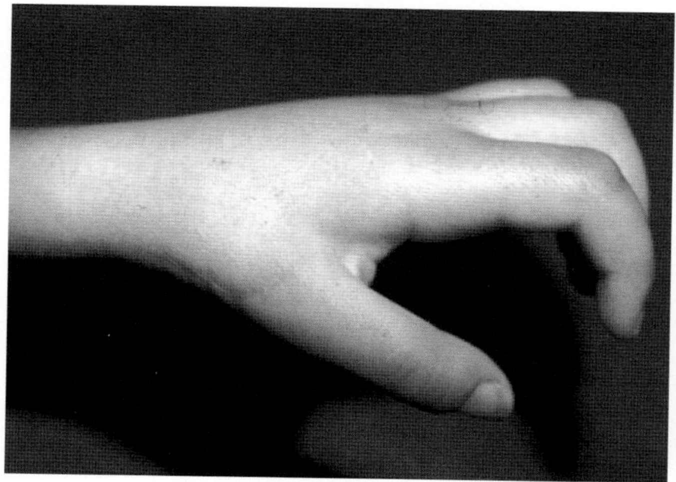

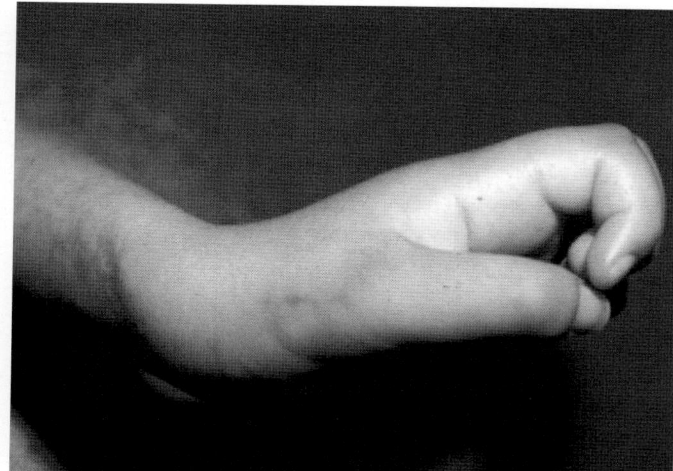

Figures 18.40 and 18.41
Results of flexors and thumb tenodesis.

struct only the fingers' extension, but with some technical modifications. The transfer must be very tight and the dorsal carpal ligament is opened, suppressing its pulley effect. We have used this technique in several adults and children with severe brachial palsy and obtained excellent results.

There are several extrinsic transfers that can be used in these completely paralysed hands.

- The transfer of the biceps tendon to the flexor profundus muscle is a simple operation. The distal tendon is detached from the radius and prolonged by a tendon graft, usually the paralysed FCU or brachioradialis. Rehabilitation is not easy and should be done with a splint, maintaining the elbow in extension. To use this transfer, the patient must have a triceps and unfortunately this is not a common situation.
- Another possibility is the transfer of an extended latissimus dorsi (Gousheh et al 2000). The latissimus is extended down to the gluteal fascia (Tubiana et al 1999). The muscle is now long enough to go to the hand (Figure 18.42). It may be used either to reconstruct extension or flexion of the fingers. On the dorsal aspect of the wrist, the bulk of the muscle needs a skin flap for coverage. Raising the flap with the muscle too distally may jeopardize its vitality. Rehabilitation is started at 6 weeks but in some cases it is possible to start immediately in the postoperative period.
- When no transfer is possible from the arm, there is still the option of a free muscle transfer. Several authors have used free muscle transfers (Akasaka et al 1990, Doi et al 1995, 2000) and proposed various donor muscles; however, most authors prefer to use the gracilis muscle, which is longer and has a well defined neurovascular pedicle.

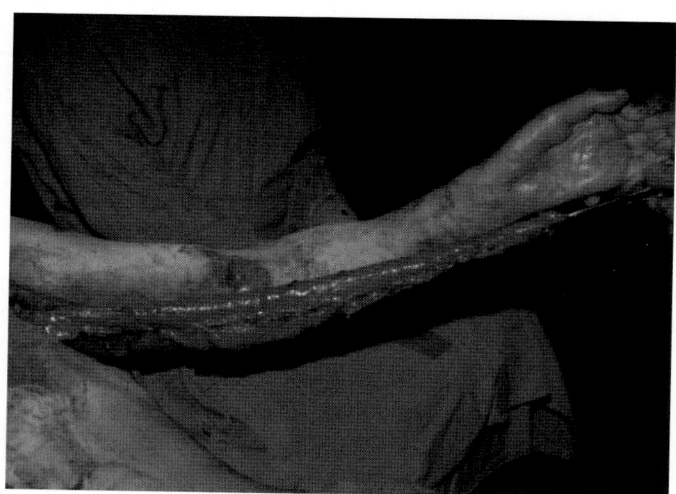

Figure 18.42
The latissimus can be extended to the fingers.

This technique is used in desperate cases and it is rare that a local nerve can be used. More often, the nerve has to be brought from far away. For 20 years our preferred donor nerve has been the pectoralis major nerve from the opposite side. The operation is done in two stages (see the section on the Elbow). In the first stage, a cross-thoracic nerve graft is sutured to the donor nerve of the contralateral side, and its free extremity is left in the upper arm for a year. After a year, the second stage is done. The muscle is harvested with its entire distal tendon, giving the possibility of reaching the wrist.

These complex secondary operations are done mostly for flexor reconstruction. In some cases it is possible to combine two of the techniques to recover flexion and extension.

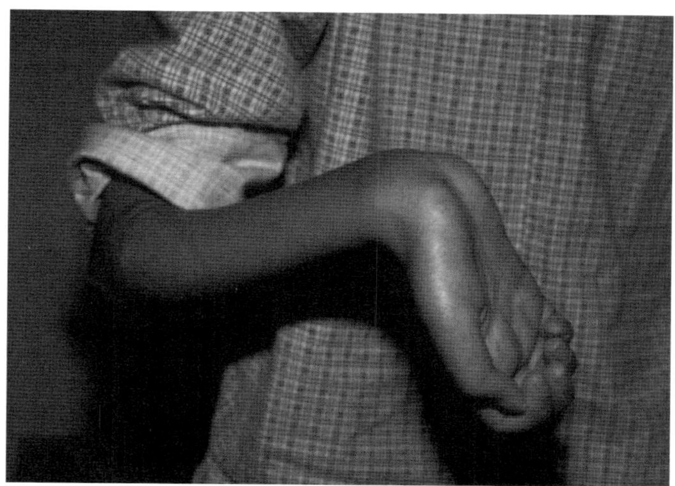

Figure 18.43
Severe hand paralysis.

The indications must be very well selected: the operations are complex, with long periods of immobilization, intensive physiotherapy and many unsatisfactory results. The family must understand that we are close to the borders of the impossible result. The function obtained will be of little use but may be psychologically very important for the child (Figures 18.43–18.45).

Co-contraction

The name is given to situations when several muscles contract when the patient tries to produce a precise movement. The co-contraction provokes simultaneous activity of antagonist muscles (i.e. biceps and triceps) resulting in complete dysfunction: each time the patient contracts the biceps, the triceps is activated and flexion is not possible.

Co-contractions may exist between different groups of muscle; the most classic is the co-contraction of the latissimus dorsi and teres major or more often the teres major alone, during abduction.

These co-contractions are more common with spontaneous recovery than after repair of the plexus. This difference is even one of the main advantages of surgical repair over spontaneous recovery.

The treatment of these co-contractions is very difficult: selective physiotherapy, electrical stimulation and splinting can help, but are mostly inefficient in treating the situation.

The aim of any treatment is to try to train the brain into controlling the groups of muscle selectively. One of the possibilities is to temporarily suppress the activity of one of the muscles and train the other during that time. By lengthening of the tendon, the muscle can be weakened. This technique can be used for the co-contraction of biceps-triceps. The triceps tendon is lengthened and weakened. It will recover its activity after 3–4 months.

In the shoulder, it may be necessary in some instances to simply tenotomize the teres major tendon. Recently, it has been proposed (Rollnik 2000) that botulin toxin injections are used to obtain the same result. After injection, the muscle is paralysed for 3–6 months. The injection can be done in the triceps, the subscapularis and other muscles. The early results (Rollnik 2000, Desiato and Risina 2001) and our own results are very encouraging but we have obtained better control of elbow flexion than abduction.

Age at operation

The age at operation is crucial, as we know that muscle imbalance can rapidly lead to joint deformities.

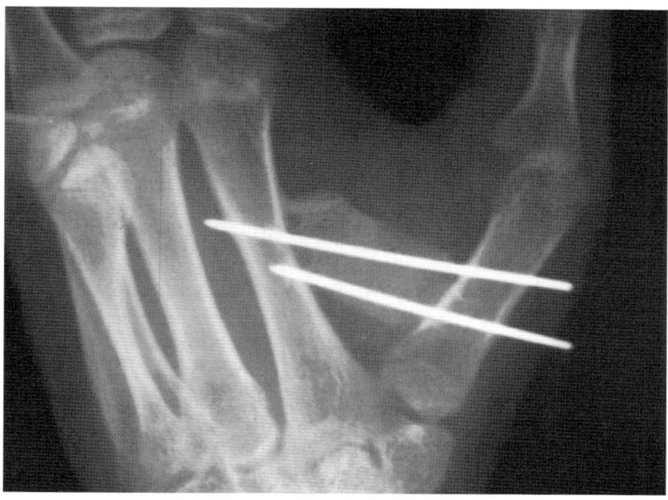

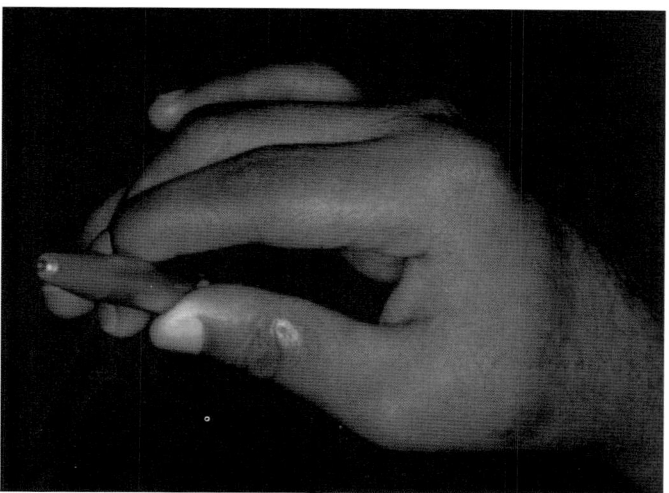

Figures 18.44 and 18.45
Can be improved cosmetically by wrist and thumb arthrodesis.

the muscles. According to Dellon (1981), progression of the clinical signs occurs as follows: first, distal sensory changes, then muscle weakness and finally motor paralysis. Distal sensory changes first affect perception of touch and vibration conducted by large nerve fibres. Perception of pain (conducted by small nerve fibres) is involved later. The tuning fork may be a useful clinical tool in the early diagnosis of compartment syndrome. Direct measurement shows that tissue pressures are more than 30 mmHg. The role of ischaemia is obvious in certain severe chronic compartment syndromes like Volkman syndrome of the forearm where late atrophy of median and/or ulnar nerve may be observed for a long distance in the middle of the compartment.

Experimental external nerve compression by inflatable cuff in man

Besides the ordinary mixed sensorimotor palsies, several clinical cases of purely motor paralysis have been published after localized compression or after nerve war injury (Erb 1876, quoted by Denny-Brown and Brenner 1944).

In human experimentation using a sphygmomanomter cuff at a pressure from 150 to 300 mmHg the paralysis commenced after about 25 minutes and had a centripetal onset and 'affected touch before pain and pain before motion' (Lewis et al 1931). With a pressure just sufficient to occlude the brachial artery, a block of nerve conduction was observed within 15–45 minutes (Lundborg 1970). The paralysis developed at the same rate if the pressure was increased from 150 mmHg to 300 mmHg. Latency between the onset of compression and conduction impairment, as well as length of recovery were extremely variable, but the shortening of the latency with repetition of compression was considered as characteristic of a mechanism of ischaemia.

In more recent experiments (Hurst et al 1981), conduction times could be measured in different zones: under the cuff, distal to the cuff (ischaemic zone) and at the two border zones at the distal and proximal edges of the cuff. Increased conduction time followed by conduction block occurred in the following sequence: 1) after 5–10 minutes across the proximal tourniquet zone; 2) later, at the level of the tourniquet and in the distal border zone; 3) after about 30 minutes of compression, in the segment distal to the tourniquet, in the 'ischaemic territory'. According to the results of this study, the direct, mechanical role of the hyper-pressure under the tourniquet zone can be considered as possible.

In conclusion the results of the pathological, clinical and experimental studies in man show that severity, duration and sequence in sensory and motor disorders are variable. In the early stage of compression and in reversible cases, ischaemia seems to offer a reasonable explanation for the nerve conduction disorders. Nevertheless, the direct mechanical role of the pressure cannot be excluded, especially when paralysis is purely motor.

Nerve compression in animals: observations of spontaneous nerve entrapment and animal experimentation

Animal pathological data

Animal pathological data were provided by guinea pigs, which develop carpal tunnel syndrome after 2 years of life (Fullerton and Gilliat 1967, Ochoa and Marotte 1973). Studies on single fibres showed that before the demyelinization stage there was asymmetry of the myelin sheath, which was thinned at one end of the intranodal segment and swollen at the other. The myelin was concentrated on each side away from the centre of the lesion. Completely demyelinated intranodal segments could be seen in the central part of the lesion. These morphological changes seemed to correspond to advanced stages of nerve entrapment (Figure 19.3).

Experimental models in animals

Experimental models in animals have made it possible to study not only compression of short duration (maximum several hours), as is possible in man, but also chronic compression (several weeks or months).

Short duration, experimental model in animals

As early as 1929, Gasser and Erlanger showed that nerve compression in animals produced early changes in the shape of the nerve electrical compound action potentials. Moreover, there was a difference in the relative susceptibility of the nerve fibres to pressure: the larger fibres were first affected when pressure increased. Short duration nerve compression was performed by Denny-Brown and Brenner (1944) by direct compression of an exposed nerve with a mercury pressure bag. The results were extremely variable according to the subject. The minimum time before the impairment of conduction was 20 seconds. The minimum time before the complete block of conduction was 120 seconds. The minimum pressure able to modify the conduction was about 16 cm of mercury. Note that this pressure was much higher than the tissue pressure recorded in experimental local hyper-pressure on the carpal tunnel in man (Lundborg et al 1982). After a short duration of compression, no histological lesion of the nerve was seen.

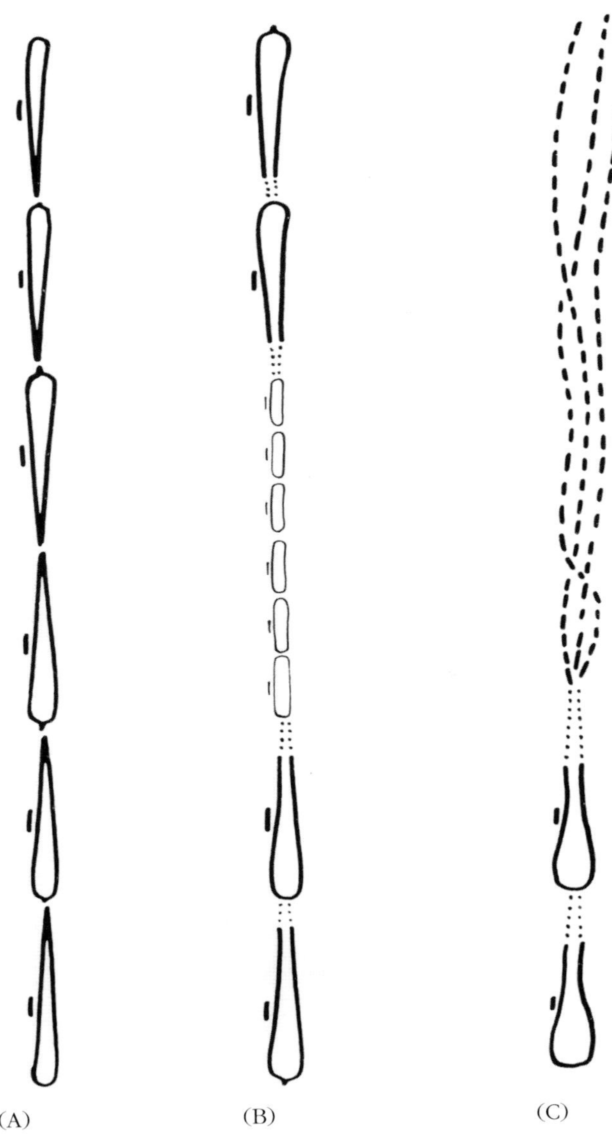

Figure 19.3

Diagrammatic representation of primary lesion of myelinated fibres underlying chronic entrapment and its progression. (A) Distorted myelin segment from median nerve of young guinea pig. Polarity is reversed at wrist, represented at the centre of the figure. (B) Increased deformity of myelin segments with partial exposure of axon toward tapered ends of internodes. Thinly remyelinated segments repair extensive local demyelinization at wrist. (C) Grotesque bulbous ends of distorted internodes and signs of wallerian degeneration at wrist. (From Ochoa J (1980) Histopathology of common mononeuropathies. In: Jewett DL, McCarroll HR, eds, *Nerve Repair and Regeneration* (Mosby: St Louis).)

Intermediate duration, experimental model in animals

Application of a rubber or a string tourniquet in cats for 45–120 minutes at a pressure varying from 30 to 20 cm of mercury was followed by a complete paralysis or a 'weakness' in 17 of 24 cases (Denny-Brown and Brenner 1944). Motor block was observed in 14 cases and sensitive block in only one case. Histological lesions were observed in 19 of 24 cases. In 6 of 19 cases, these lesions were considered as to be 'slight'. In 2 of 19 cases the lesion was a wallerian degeneration. In all cases in which the animal was killed on the same day as the experiment, no histological change was observed. Lesions that were presumably due to ischaemic pressure appeared within 24–48 hours and progressed to about the tenth day. In the typical cases of these purely or almost purely motor blocks, lesions were localized within 10–20 mm and could be described as follows:

- Between the second and the fifth day: localized oedema, thickening and vacuolation of the axons, vacuolation of the myelin, neurofibrillar condensation at the nodes of Ranvier.
- At the seventh day, demyelinization appeared at the nodes of Ranvier, whereas the axons became thin at the level of the nodes and distal to them.
- After 2 weeks, lesions were predominant at the nodes with alternating thinning, thickening or absence of staining of the axons.
- Reappearance of myelin and normalization of the axons was then observed more or less early according to the severity of the lesion.

Finally, a staging of four degrees of nerve pressure lesions was proposed by Denny-Brown and Brenner (1944):

1) Nil.
2) Paralysis with rapid recovery on release of pressure.
3 Paralysis with delayed recovery with preservation of gross sensation without degeneration (intermediate pressure lesion).
4 Complete anatomic lesion with degeneration.

A model of direct compression of rabbit tibial nerve by a miniature transparent cuff was developed by Rydevik et al (1981). The model made possible direct observation of neural vessels during and after the compression phase. Permeability of the intraneural vessels was studied by infusion of Evans' blue (Rydevik and Lundborg 1977). Direct measurement of endoneural fluid pressure (EFP) (Lundborg et al 1983) and assessment of axonal transport (fast and slow, anterograde and retrograde) were also performed (Rydevik et al 1980, Dahlin and McLean, 1986). Extraneural pressure of 20 mmHg reduced epineural venous flow (Rydevik et al 1981). The threshold of 30–50 mmHg for two hours was the critical pressure beyond which abnormalities such as epineural oedema and partial or complete block of axonal transport appeared (Dahlin and McLean 1986). Oedema was initially epineural and then became subepineural, then endoneural. The perineural barrier is broken, thus allowing the macromolecules to pass into the endoneurial space. The EFP increases to up to three or four times the normal level and may remain abnormally high after releasing the compression, as in a 'mini compartment syndrome' (Lundborg and Dahlin 1992). Block of axonal transport becomes reversible only after several days; slow and retrograde axonal transports are affected as well as the nerve cell bodies, which undergo marked morphological changes similar to those seen after division of the axons (Dahlin and Lundborg 1990, MacKinnon et al 1985).

Beside these ischaemic consequences, structural changes were also observed after an intermediate duration nerve compression by cuff (Dyck et al 1990). A special method of fixation was used after a few minutes of compression, allowing observation of pressure- and time-related early structural changes. These changes were different under the cuff and at the edge of the cuff. Under the cuff, they observed decreased fascicular area, compression and expression of axoplasm, sometimes to the point of fibre transection, lengthening of internodes and obscuration of nodes of Ranvier due to cleavage and displacement of myelin and overlapping of nodes by displaced loop of myelin. At the edge of the cuff they observed an increase of the fascicular area, a widening of the nodal gap, and a disordered structure of the axoplasm.

Long duration, experimental compression in animal

The histopathological changes observed after experimental compression in rats and primates appear to be consistent with the histopathological data harvested in specimens of chronic nerve compression from humans and guinea pigs. A breakdown in the blood–nerve barrier may be observed with a very slight compression after 2 months (MacKinnon and Dellon 1986). Further modifications include increased vascularity and increased number of microvessels, thickening of the perineurium and the external and internal epineurium, and a fall-out of the large myelinated fibre group at the periphery of the fascicles. As a consequence, the percentage of myelin may fall from 63% (normal) to 34% after 12 months. An increased number of small unmyelinated fibres is observed at the site of the compression. This phenomenon may be interpreted as an attempted regeneration (MacKinnon and Dellon 1986). The last stage is characterized by wallerian degeneration distal to the nerve compression. It has been stressed that there is an intraneural variation in the severity of the lesion. The peripheral fascicles are more severely damaged than the deep ones (MacKinnon and Dellon 1986). The peripheral nerve fibres and the large myelinated fibres are more severely damaged than the deep and/or small fibres. The consequence of the uneven distribution of the damage is that 'the pathologic changes in the worst fascicles represent the patient's most severe symptoms, the normal large myelinated fibres in the best fascicles provide the basis for normal nerve conduction studies' (MacKinnon and Dellon 1986).

Discussion

When dealing with nerve compression, the large variety of possible aetiological factors, often combined, must be borne in mind.

The severity of nerve compression lesions is extremely variable, depending on the intensity and duration of the pressure. The distribution of the pressure along the nerve, the surface bearing the pressure and the possible displacement of the nerve are also important factors. Nerve compression frequently involves other types of mechanisms such as traction or shearing forces.

Several classifications of nerve compression injuries have been proposed. Table 19.2 summarizes the two types (A and B) of 'metabolic disorders' described by Lundborg (1988) and Sunderland's classification in five stages from neurapraxia to neurotmesis.

Sunderland's classification (Sunderland 1978) supposes that the anatomical structures are damaged from the deep part to the surface of the nerve according to the following sequence: myelin (type 1), axon (type 2), endoneurium (type 3), perineurium (type 4), epineurium (type 5). The Sunderland classification for nerve compression injuries may be debatable, as the compression seems to affect the epineural compartment first, and then the perineurial compartment.

Comparison with the classical classification of Denny-Brown and Brenner (1944) is also difficult: the stage of immediately reversible disorders described by Denny-Brown and Brenner corresponds to the 'local metabolic disorder' of Lundborg (1988). The 'intermediate pressure lesion' (Denny-Brown and Brenner) corresponds to neurapraxia (Seddon 1943). The 'complete anatomic lesion' of Denny-Brown and Brenner corresponds to the 'axonotmesis' described by Seddon.

We need further information about the stage at which lesions of the perineurium and epineurium arise, with their consequences for intraneural disorganization. There is no general agreement about the sequence of nerve compression disorders. In the 'intermediate' stage of Denny-Brown and Brenner, the paralysis is first motor, corresponding to the 'purely motor paralysis' which was first described by Erb in 1876 (quoted by Denny-Brown and Brenner 1944). However, according to other authors, touch and pain are affected before motion (Lewis et al 1931, Dellon 1981).

Several degrees of lesion are frequently associated in a compression-damaged nerve depending on the site, more or less superficial, of the fascicle into the nerve or of the fibre into the fascicle. The large myelinated fibres are more subject to compression lesions than the small ones (Gasser and Erlanger 1929). The efferent fibres to the muscles, the fibres of touch receptors and the fibres of nociceptors have a mean diameter of 13, 9 and 4 microns respectively (Boyd and Davey 1968). This could account for the sequence of the nerve compressive lesions which, according to certain authors, involve the motor fibres first.

Finally, the mechanism by which the pressure leads to nerve tissue damage remains unclear: ischaemia explains the relationship betwen the blood pressure threshold and the sensory block of conduction (Szabo et al 1983, Lundborg 1988). The delay of the conduction block is similar to the delay of inexcitability of the nerve after limb amputation (Gignoux et al 1970). Nevertheless, recent experiments in animals (Dyck et al 1990) have shown that structural nerve lesions, different from ischaemic lesions, could be observed immediately during compression. More complex biochemical disorders may also arise, such as adhesion mechanisms mediated by cytokines (Germann et al 1997).

References

Amadio PC (1987) Carpal tunnel syndrome, pyridoxine and work place, *J Hand Surg* **12A**: 875–9.

Boyd IA, Davey M (1968) *Composition of Peripheral Nerves* (Livingstone: Edinburgh) 41.

Chaise F, Witvoet J (1984) Mesures des pressions intracanalaires dans le syndrome du canal carpien idiopathique non déficitaire, *Rev Chir Orthop* **70**: 75–8.

Dahlin LB, McLean WG (1986) Effect of graded experimental compression on slow and fast axonal transport in rabbit vagus nerve, *J Neurosci* **72**: 19–30.

Dahlin LB, Lundborg G (1990) The neuron and its response to peripheral nerve compression, *J Hand Surg* **15B**: 5–10.

Davis TRC (2001) Miners' nystagmus, *J Hand Surg* **26B**: 399.

Dell PC, Guzewicz RM (1992) Atypical peripheral neuropathies, *Hand Clin* **8**: 275–83.

Dellon AL (1981) *Evaluation of Sensibility and Reeducation of Sensation in the Hand* (William & Wilkins: Baltimore).

Denny-Brown D, Brenner C (1944) Paralysis of nerve induced by direct pressure and by tourniquet, *Arch Neurol Psychiatry* **51**: 1–26.

Dyck PJ, Lais AC, Giannini C, Engelstad JN (1990) Structural alteration of nerve during cuff compression, *Proc Natl Acad Sci USA* **87**: 9828–32.

Friden F (2001) Vibration damage to the hand: clinical presentation, prognosis and length and severity of vibration required, *J Hand Surg* **26B**: 471–4.

Fuchs PC, Nathan PR, Myers LD (1991) Synovial histology and carpal tunnel syndrome, *J Hand Surg* **16A**: 753–8.

Fullerton PM, Gilliat RW (1967) Pressure neuropathy in the hindfoot of the guinea pig, *J Neurol Neurosci Psychiat* **30**: 18–25.

Gasser HS, Erlanger J (1929) The role of fiber size in the establishment of a nerve block by pressure or cocaine, *Am J Physiol* **88**: 581–91.

Gelberman RH, Hergenroeder PT, Hargens AR, Lundborg GN, Wayne HA (1981) The carpal tunnel syndrome: a study of carpal tunnel pressures, *J Bone Joint Surg* **63A**: 380–3.

Gelberman RH, Yamaguchi K, Hollstien SB et al (1998) Changes in interstitial pressure and cross-sectional area of the cubital tunnel and the ulnar nerve with flexion of the elbow: an experimental study in human cadavera, *J Bone Joint Surg* **80A**: 492–501.

Germann G, Drücke D, Steinau HU (1997) Adhesion receptors and cytokine profile in controlled tourniquet ischemia in the upper extremity, *J Hand Surg* **22B**: 778–82.

Gignoux M, Firica A, Ray A (1970) Effet de l'ischémie et de l'oxygène hyperbare sur l'exitabilité neuro-musculaire de la patte du chien, *Lyon Chir* **66**: 126–8.

Greening J, Lynn B, Leary R, Warren L, O'Higgins P, Hall-Craggs M (2001) The use of ultrasound imaging to demonstrate reduced movement of the median nerve during flexion in patients with non-specific arm pain, *J Hand Surg* **26B**: 401–6.

Guillain G, Courtellemont (1905) L'action du muscle court supinateur dans la paralysie du nerf radial, *Presse Med* **18**: 50–2.

Hurst LN, Weiglein O, Brown WF, Campbell GJ (1981) The pneumatic tourniquet: a biomechanical and electrophysiological study, *Plast Reconstr Surg* **67**: 648–52.

Lewis T, Pickering GW, Rothschild P (1931) Centripetal paralysis arising out of arrested bloodflow to the limb, including notes on a form of tingling, *Heart* **16**: 1–32.

Lundborg G (1970) Ischemic nerve injury. Experimental studies on intraneural microvascular physiopathology and nerve function in a limb subjected to temporary circulatory arrest, *Scand J Plast Reconstr Surg Suppl* **6**: 3–113.

Lundborg G (1988) *Nerve Injury and Repair* (Churchill Livingstone: Edinburgh).

Lundborg G, Dahlin LB (1992) The pathophysiology of nerve compression, *Hand Clin* **8**: 215–27.

Lundborg G, Gelberman RH, Minteer-Convery M, Lee YE, Hargens AR (1982) Median nerve compression in the carpal tunnel: functional response to experimentally induced controlled pressure, *J Hand Surg* **7**: 252–9.

Lundborg G, Myers R, Powell H (1983) Nerve compression injury and increased endoneurial fluid pressure: "miniature compartment syndrome", *J Neurol Neurosurg Psychiatr* **46**: 1119–24.

Mackinnon SE (1999) Peripheral nerve injuries. In: Light TR, ed, *Hand Surgery Update II* (American Academy of Orthopedic Surgery: Rosemont) 199–210.

MacKinnon SE, Dellon AL (1986) Experimental study of chronic nerve compression, *Hand Clin* **2**: 639–50.

MacKinnon SE, Dellon AL, Hudson AR, Hunter DA (1985) A primate model for chronic nerve compression, *J Reconstr Microsurg* **1**: 185–94.

MacQuarrie IG (1973) The effect of the conditioning lesion on the regeneration of motor axons, *Brain Res* **152**: 597–602.

Marie P, Foix C (1913) Atrophie isolée de l'éminence thénar d'origine névritique. Rôle du ligament annulaire antérieur du carpe dans la pathogénie de la lésion, *Rev Neurol* **26**: 647–9.

Millesi H, Zöch G, Rath Th (1990) The gliding apparatus of peripheral nerve, *Ann Hand Surg* **9**: 87–98.

Nakamichi K, Tachibana S (1995) Restricted motion of the median nerve in carpal tunnel syndrome, *J Hand Surg* **20B**: 460–4.

Neary D, Ochoa J, Gilliat RW (1975) Subclinical entrapment neuropathy in man, *J Neurosci* **24**: 283–98.

Ochoa J (1980) Histology of common neuropathies. In: Jewett DL, MacCaroll HL, eds, *Nerve Repair and Regeneration* (Mosby: St Louis) 36–52.

Ochoa J, Marotte L (1973) Nature of the nerve lesion underlying chronic entrapment, *J Neurosci* **19**: 491–9.

Rempel D, Dahlin L, Lundborg G (1999) Pathophysiology of nerve compression syndromes: response of peripheral nerves to loading, *J Bone Joint Surg* **81A**: 1600–10.

Rydevik B, Lundborg G (1977) Permeability of intraneural microvessels in perineurium following acute graded experimental compression, *Scand J Plast Reconstr Surg* 11: 179–87.

Rydevik B, McLean WG, Sjöstrand J, Lundborg G (1980) Blockage of axonal transport by acute graded compression of the rabbit vagus nerve, *J Neurol Neurosurg Psychiatry* **43**: 690–8.

Rydevik B, Lundborg G, Bagge U (1981) Effect of graded compression on intraneural blood flow. An in vitro study on rabbit tibial nerve, *J Hand Surg* **6**: 3–12.

Seddon H (1943) Three types of nerve injuries, *Brain* **66**: 237–88.

Sunderland S (1978) *Nerve and Nerve Injuries*, 2nd edn (Churchill Livingstone: Edinburgh) 32.

Szabo RM (1999) Nerve compression syndromes. In: Light TR, ed,

Hand Surgery Update II (American Academy of Orthopedic Surgery: Rosemont) 183.

Szabo R, Gelberman R, Williamson RV, Hargens A (1983) Effect of increased systemic blood pressure on the tissue fluid pressure. Threshold of peripheral nerve, *J Orthop Res* **1**: 172–8.

Szabo R, Gelberman RH, Williamson RV, Dellon AL, Yaru NC, Dimick MP (1984) Vibratory sensory testing in acute peripheral nerve compression, *J Hand Surg* **9A**: 104–9.

Thomas PK, Fullerton PM (1963) Nerve fiber size in the carpal tunnel syndrome, *J Neurol Neurosurg Psychiatry* **26**: 520–7.

Upton AR, McComas AJ (1973) The double crush in nerve entrapment syndromes, *Lancet* **2**: 359–62.

Zimmerman NB, Zimmerman SI, Clark GL (1992) Neuropathy in the workplace, *Hand Clin* **8**: 255–62.

20 Anatomical bases for brachial plexus and subclavian artery compression

Luciano A Poitevin

Introduction

The neurovascular bundle to the upper limb proceeds through several confined spaces. The subclavian artery and brachial plexus go together while the vein follows a different route. The brachial plexus arises mostly from the cervical spine. At the same time, the subclavian artery leaves the adjacent mediastinum, while its accompanying vein enters. These neurovascular elements run through narrow passages located at the root of the neck, the thoracic outlet and the axilla.

Owing to the extent of these spaces, which belong to different topographic regions, we feel that the term 'thoracic outlet' is misleading. Therefore, we propose the term 'upper limb inlet' (ULI), which includes complete and incomplete tunnel-like spaces spanning from the axial skeleton of the thorax and cervical spine to the lower border of pectoralis major muscle.

These narrow spaces are as follows:

1. Spaces of the suprapleural membrane
2. Interscalene spaces
3. Costo-clavicular space
4. Clavi-pectoral region
5. Retro-pectoralis minor space
6. Prehumeral head passage
7. Median nerve compass
8. Prescalene space.

Some of these spaces are permanent, others develop when the upper limb is placed in a forced extreme position of abduction and/or retraction.

In fact, the term upper limb inlet (ULI) stresses two important facts:

1. That narrow passages and therefore possible neurovascular compressions are not restricted to the thoracic exit, but rather extend to the neck and axilla.
2. That symptoms due to compression are referred to the arm and not to the thorax.

This chapter describes the results of part of our research work on several non-embalmed specimens, which includes intra-arterial injections, dynamic radiographs, dissections, pressure recordings and linear measurements. Clinical correlations will also be made. The description will be limited to the suprapleural membrane (SPM) and interscalene (IS) spaces, the most proximal and common entrapment sites.

Anatomical description

Spaces of the suprapleural membrane (pleura suspensory apparatus)

Suprapleural membrane (Figures 20.1, 20.2)

The subclavian vessels – mainly the artery – describe an arch over the lung summit. In fact, the lung summit is covered, from bottom to top, by two contiguous layers of tissue: a serous membrane, i.e. the apical pleura; and a fibrous membrane, which is on top, i.e. the suprapleural membrane or septum, also called Sibson's membrane or Truffert's fascia.

This membrane attaches laterally to the inner border of the first rib and its inferior aspect; and dorsally to the neck of the first rib and the anterior tubercle of the transverse processes of C6 and C7 vertebrae.

The membrane is easily detachable from the apical pleura. It is composed of an inferior fibrous layer and a superior areolar layer blending with the subclavian artery. It is reinforced by fibres coming from the scalene muscles, and held back to the cervical spine by fibrous bundles. It is in continuity with the intrathoracic fascia. Its lateral aspect is thicker than the medial.

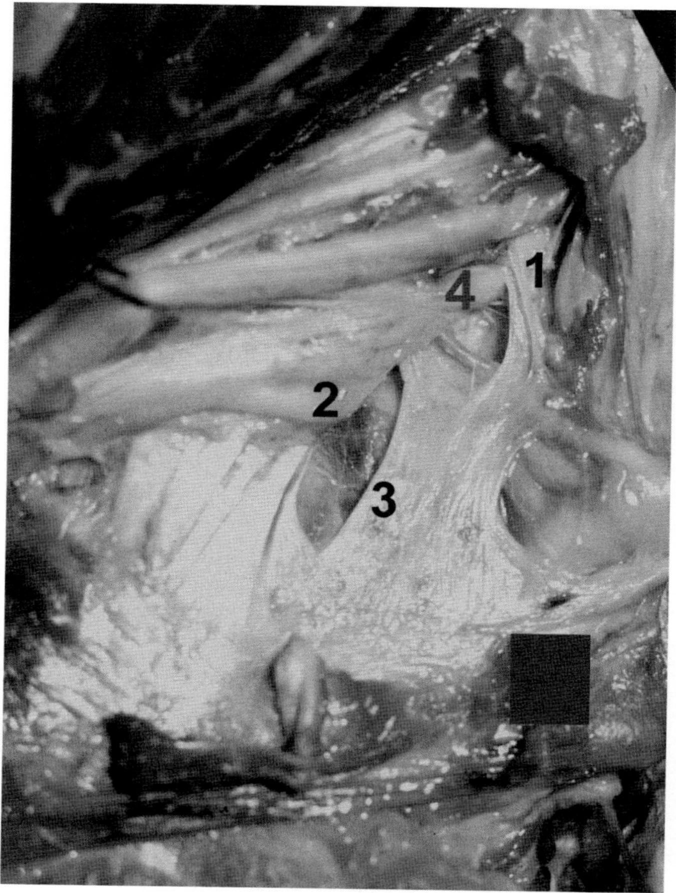

Figure 20.1
The suprapleural membrane
1 Transverse-septo-costal ligament
2 T1 root
3 Costo-septo-costal ligament and suprapleural membrane
4 C8 root

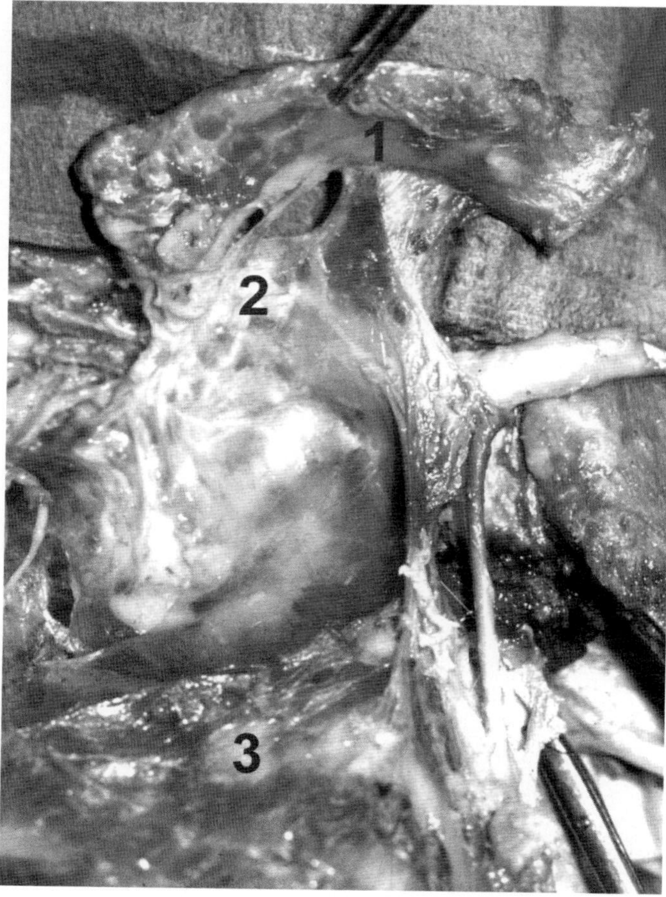

Figure 20.2
The suprapleural membrane
1 1st rib lifted
2 Suprapleural membrane
3 Apical pleura

Septal ligaments (Figures 20.1, 20.3, 20.4)

These ligaments are also called 'pleura suspensory ligaments' (Sebileau). They bind the suprapleural membrane to the lower cervical spine and the neck of the first rib. Various ligaments can be distinguished:

- Vertebro-septal ligament. Origin: body of C7 vertebra. Insertion: suprapleural membrane.
- Transverse-septo-costal ligament (Figures 20.1 and 20.3). Origin: anterior tubercle of the transverse process of C7 vertebra. Insertion: suprapleural membrane, often reaching the attachment of the anterior scalene muscle. In 50% of cases, this ligament is replaced by a muscle belly: the scalene minimus muscle (Figure 20.6).
- Costo-septo-costal ligament (Figures 20.1, 20.4). Origin: neck of first rib. Insertion: suprapleural membrane, medial border of the first rib and scalene tubercle.

Septal spaces

The septal ligaments, along with the first rib, bound three spaces:

- Supra-retro-pleural fossa (Figure 20.6), inbetween the vertebro-septal and transverse-septo-costal ligamnts. It contains the stellate or inferior cervical ganglion.
- Suprapleural biceps (Sebileau) (Figures 20.1 and 20.4), inbetween the transverse-septo-costal ligament (or scalene minimus muscle) and costo-septo-costal ligament. It gives way to the C8 nerve.

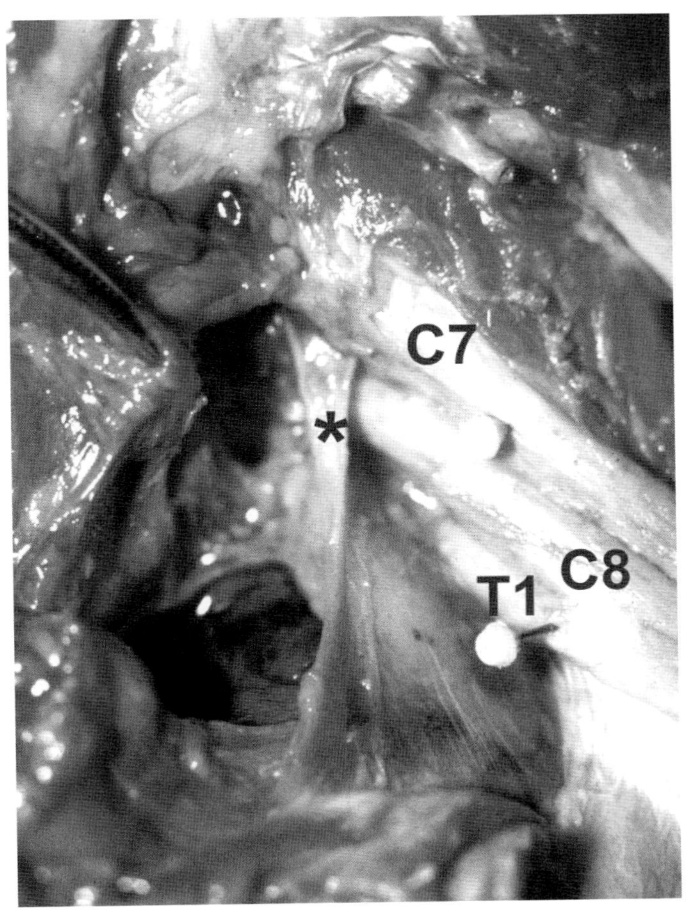

Figure 20.3
Transverse-septo-costal ligament
C7–C8–T1: roots of the braichial plexus
*: Transverse-septo-costal ligament

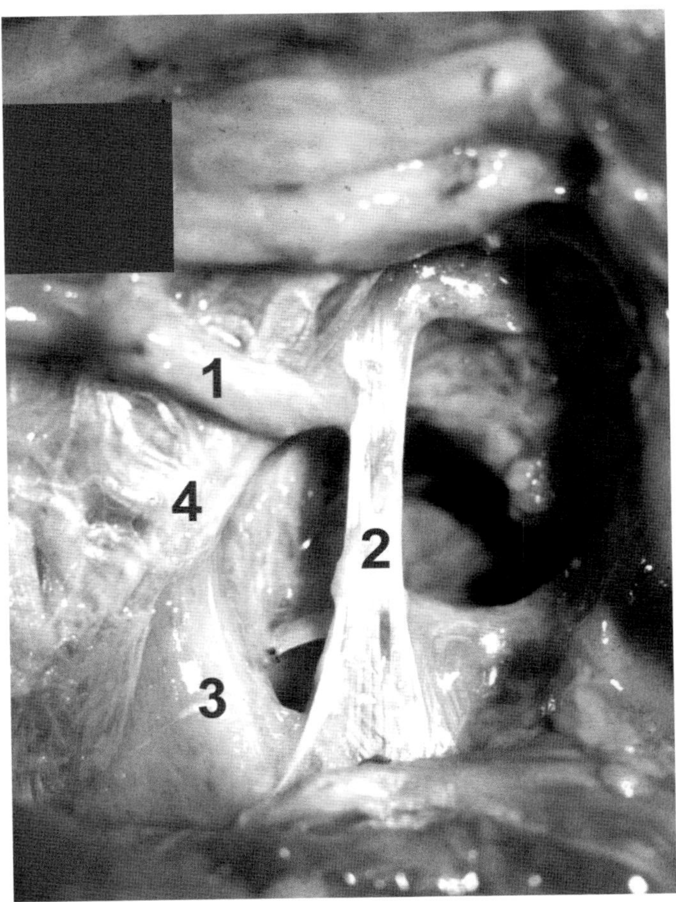

Figure 20.4
Costo-septo-costal ligament
1 T1 root
2 Costo-septo-costal ligament
3 1st rib
4 Middle scalene muscle

- T1 buttonhole (Figure 20.3), limited medially by the costo-septo-costal ligament and laterally by the inner border of the first rib. It allows the passage of T1 nerve.

In fact, the anterior branch of the first thoracic nerve describes a double, S-shaped curve around the first rib, as it comes not only from inside but also from below and behind, due to its origin at the beginning of the thoracic kyphosis. Any increase in this arrangement can produce an elongation and consequent damage to the nerve, as described later.

Besides the spaces just described, the transverse-septo-costal ligament (or the scalene minimus muscle) splits the interscalene space into two parts, as discussed below (Figures 20.7 and 20.8).

Interscalene spaces

The scalene complex

According to classical descriptions, there are three scalene muscles, joining the cervical spine to the first and second ribs. The anterior scalene muscle originates from the anterior tubercles of transverse processes of vertebrae C3–C6, and ends in the scalene tubercle of the first rib. The middle scalene muscle arises from the anterior tubercles of transverse processes of vertebrae C2–C7, and attaches to the superior aspect of the first rib, behind the anterior scalene muscle and leaving a groove inbetween where the subclavian artery lies. The posterior scalene muscle joins the posterior tubercles of transverse processes of vertebrae C4–C6 to the first and second ribs. The

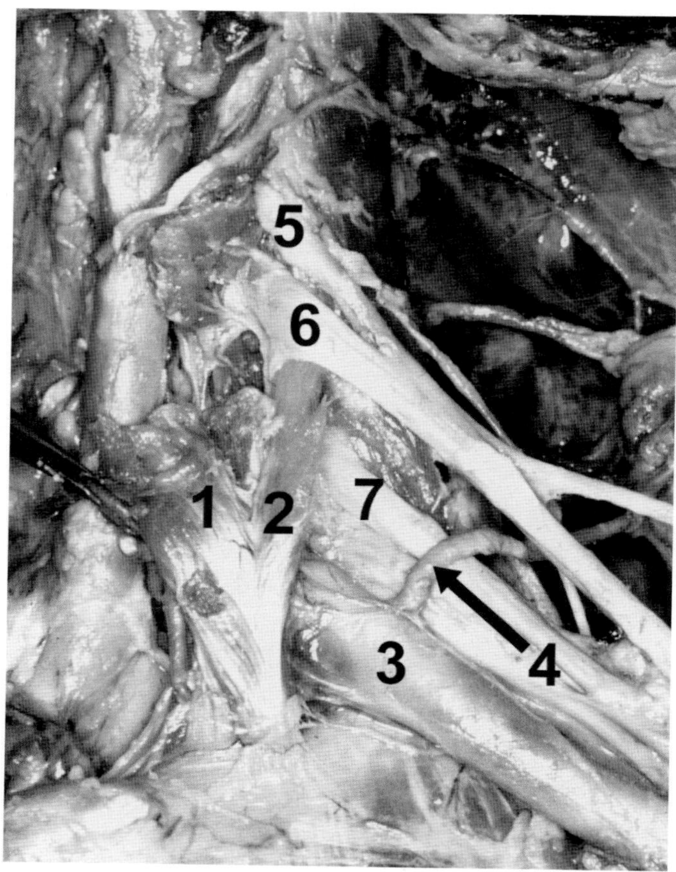

Figure 20.5
Upper interpedicle scalene
1 Anterior sccalene
2 Upper interpedicle scalene
3 Subclavian artery
4 Posterior scapular artery
5 C5 root
6 C6 root
7 C7 root

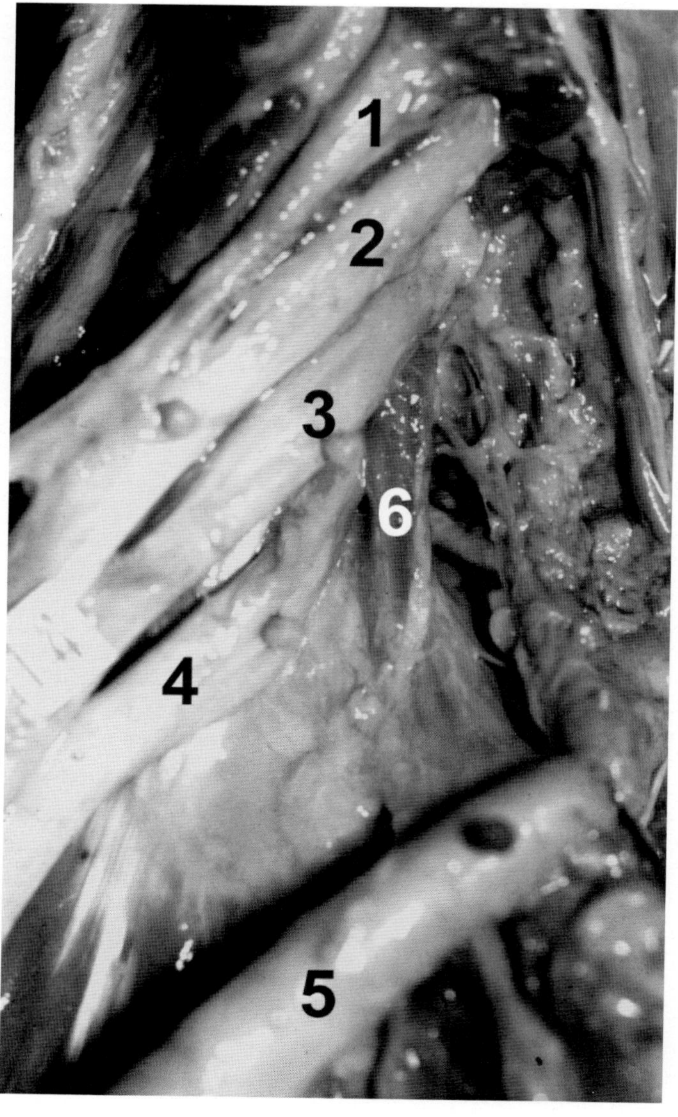

Figure 20.6
Lower interpedicle scalene
1 C5
2 C6
3 C7
4 C8
5 Subclavian artery
6 Lower interpedicle scalene (scalene minimus)

subclavian artery and the brachial plexus pass inbetween the anterior scalene muscle (in front) and the middle and posterior scalene muscles (behind). The subclavian vein passes in front of the anterior scalene muscle.

However, the scalene muscles should be considered as a single mass which has become fragmented in a variable way during embryological development, due to the growth and transverse passage of the neurovascular (NV) structures to the upper limb. Thus – with the exception of the subclavian vein, which is always in front of the scalene mass – the vessels and nerves will separate an anterior part (prepedicle), which will become the so-called anterior scalene muscle, and a posterior part (retropedicle), which will originate the middle and posterior scalene muscles.

Remnants of the original single mass are very often present, joining the middle to the anterior scalene muscles and passing inbetween the elements of the NV bundle; they are the interpedicle muscles (Figures 20.5–20.8).

These muscles can either: (a) form bridges passing inbetween C6 and C7 nerves and then in front of the subclavian artery (upper interpedicle muscle; Figures 20.5, 20.7 and 20.8), or (b) originate from C7 anterior

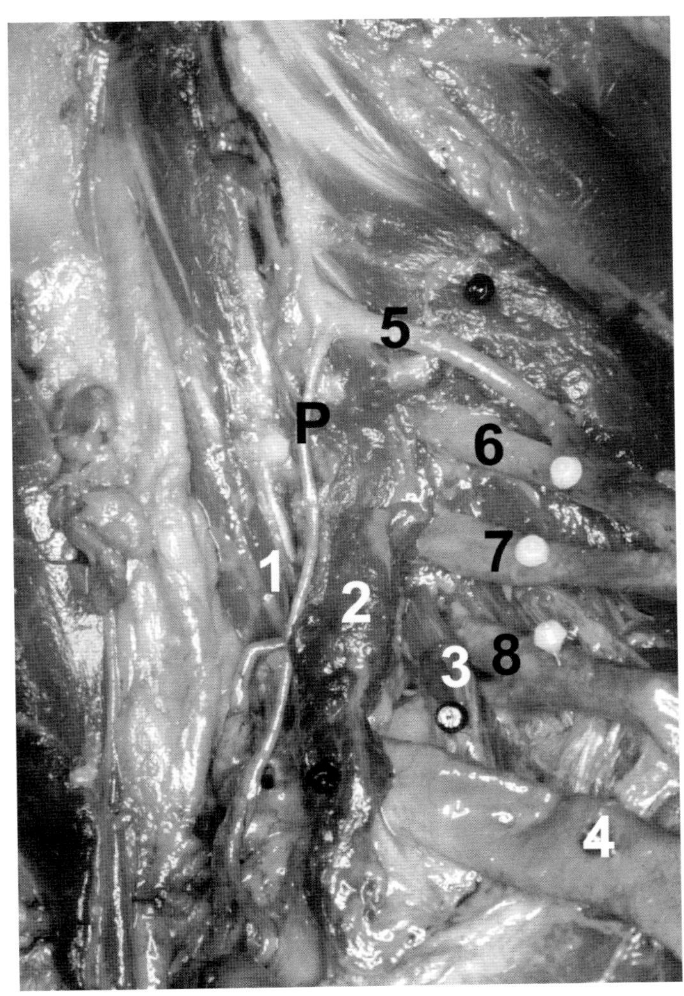

Figure 20.7

Interscalene passages

1 Anterior scalene muscle
2 Upper interpedicle scalene
3 Lower intermediate sccalene
4 Subclavian artery
5 C5
6 C6
7 C7
8 C8
P: Phrenic nerve

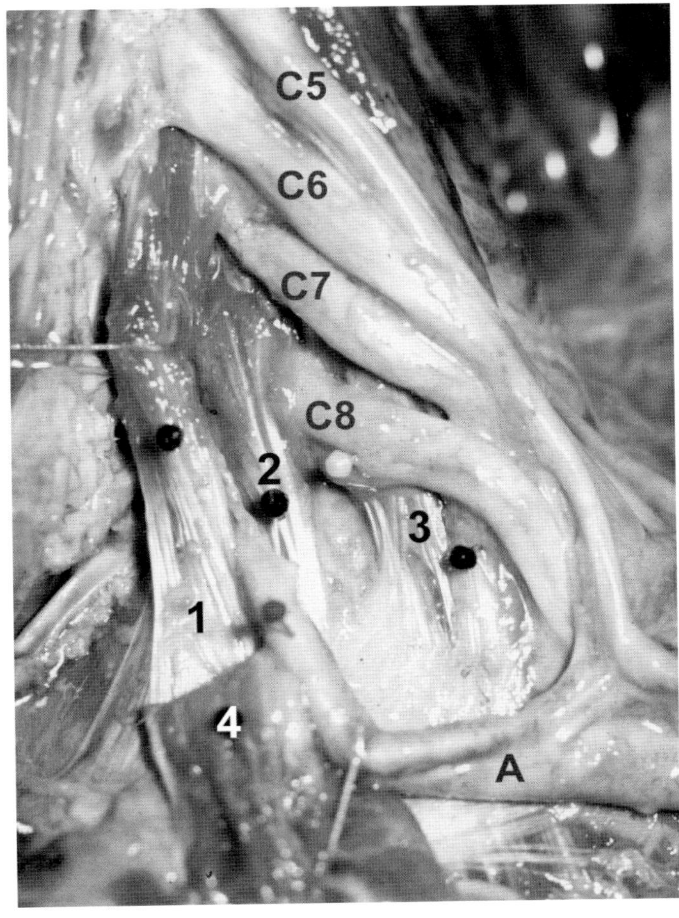

Figure 20.8

Interscalene passages

1 Upper interpedicle scalene
2 Lower interpedicle scalene
3 Middle scalene
4 Anterior scalene
C5–C6–C7–C8: roots of the brachial plexus
A: Subclavian artery

tubercle, passing in front of C8 and T1 and behind the subclavian artery – lower interpedicle muscle – which constitutes the scalene minimus muscle (Figures 20.6–20.8).

Sometimes, there will be no muscle left in front of the uppermost roots of the brachial plexus, C5 thus becoming superficial and uncovered.

In summary, there is a scalene complex which can be broken up as follows:

1. Prepedicle muscle = antenior scalene muscle.
2. Retropedicle muscles = middle and posterior scalene muscles.
3. Interpedicle muscles:
   – Upper = muscular bridges inbetween C6 and C7 nerves (14% of cases)
   – Lower = Scalene minimus muscle (present in 50% of cases, often replaced by a fibrous band, the transverse-septo-costal ligament), passing inbetween the artery and nerves C8 and T1. Besides the osseous insertion, the scalene complex also attaches to the suprapleural membrane, blending with its fibres.

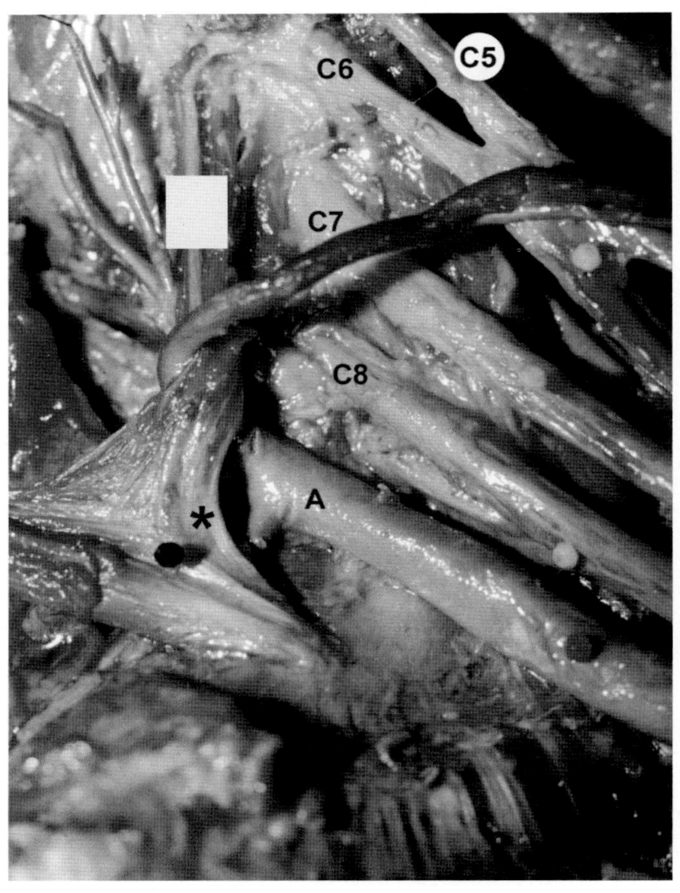

Figure 20.9A

Anterior scalene. Sharp edge

C5–C6: Roots of the brachial plexus
C7–C8: roots of the brachial plexus
A: Subclavian artery
*: Sharp edge of anterior scalene

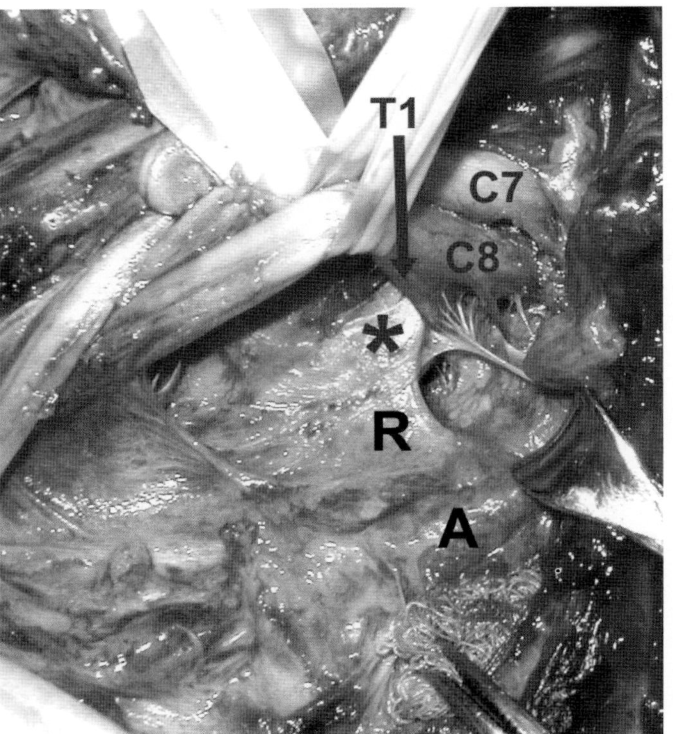

Figure 20.9B

Middle scalene. Sharp edge

C7–C8–T1: Roots of the brachial plexus
R: 1st rib
A: Subclavian artery
*: Sharp edge of middle scalene

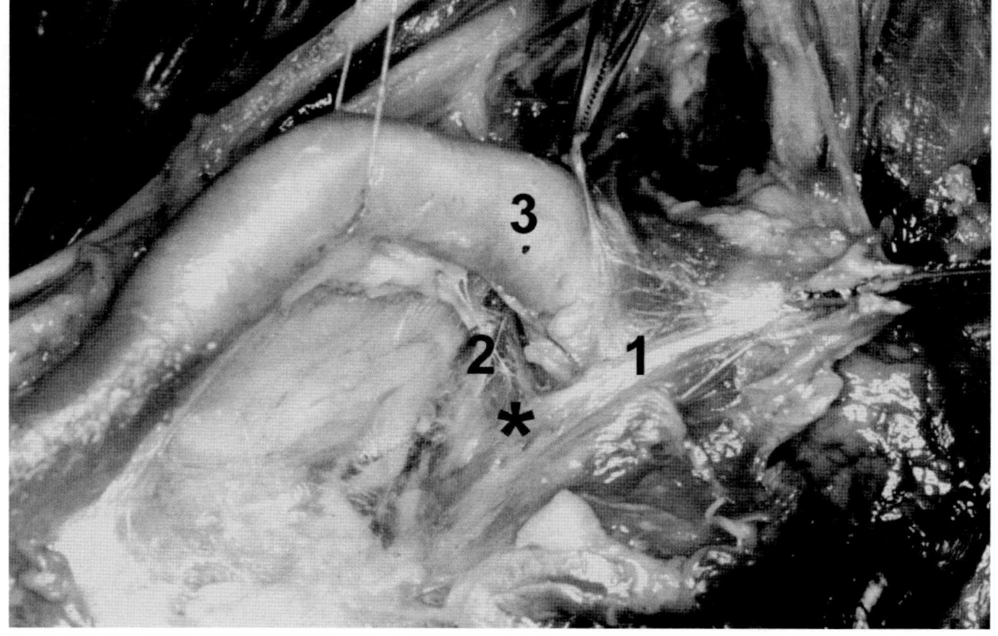

Figure 20.9C

Overlapping of scalene insertions

1 Anterior scalene muscle
2 Middle scalene muscle
3 Subclavian artery
*: Overlapping of both scalenes

Interscalene spaces (Figures 20.7, 20.8)

Reality differs from classic description, due to the presence of interpedicle muscles. Therefore, the following can be distinguished.

The anterosuperior interscalene space (ASI) is a neurovascular space (Figures 20.7 and 20.8).

- Anterior wall: anterior scalene muscle.
- Posterior wall: from top to bottom – middle scalene and scalene minimus.

This space contains several neurovascular elements, arranged as follows:

- In a posterior plane: C5, C6 and C7 nerves.
- In an anterior and lower level: the subclavian artery, right inbetween the convergent anterior and minimus scalene muscles.

In some cases, when there is an upper interpedicle muscle, this ASI space is further subdivided into an upper compartment containing C5 and C6 nerves, and a lower one, containing C7 nerve and the subclavian artery.

The postero-inferior interscalene space (PII) is a neural space (Figures 20.7 and 20.8).

- Anterior wall: scalene minimus muscle.
- Posterior wall: middle scalene muscle.

This space contains two nerves: C8 and T1, separated from each other by means of the costo-septo-costal ligament.

Variations in scalene muscles

Variations in the insertions and in the extent of IS space (Figure 20.9A)
Insertions of scalene muscles on the first rib can vary in extent, determining variations in the IS space wtdth, when measured over the first rib. The distance varies between 0 and 2.08 cm, with a mean of 1.04. The smaller the interscalene space, the higher the position of the subclavian artery over the first rib (mean 0.72 cm, between 0 and 1.60 cm). Furthermore, the scalene minimus muscle also lifts the artery, separating it from the first rib.

When the scalene minimus muscle is short and attaches close to the middle scalene muscle, it can impinge against the C8 nerve and the lower trunk.

Variations in shape (Figure 20.9)

- The anterior scalene, in 12% of cases, presents a sharp posterior edge, impinging on the subclavian artery (Figure 20.9A).
- The membranous insertion of the middle scalene muscle can form a sharp edge, impinging from behind on the lower trunk of the brachial plexus (Figure 20.9B).
- Insertions of the scalene muscles may overlap, forming a girth under the artery and the lower trunk (Figure 20.9C)

Variations in number
The scalene minimus and the upper interpedicle muscles are described above.

Compressions

The brachial plexus and the subclavian artery, while passing through these narrow spaces, can suffer mechanical damage due to elongation, bending, compression and combined mechanisms. Sustained extreme positions of the upper limb can further reduce these passages. Muscle variations, as well as the presence of a cervical rib, will also decrease the available space for the NV structures.

The causes of compression can be classified into morphological and functional; these mechanisms can be present in combination.

Morphological compressions

These may be due to various factors.

Cervical rib

The presence of a cervical rib (0.5–1%) reduces the IS spaces and lifts the artery and the lower trunk of the brachial plexus, elongating them and increasing their loop. The rib can be complete, articulating with the sternum, or incomplete, and may or may not reach the first rib. In the latter case, it is usually prolonged by an anterior fibrous band, which must be severed during the operation.

Variations in scalene muscles

The presence of an overdeveloped interpedicle muscle, a sharp edge of a scalene muscle, or an abnormal extension of scalene insertions on the first rib, can act on the plexus and artery.

Shoulder girdle descent

Related to man's standing position, there is a progressive drop of the shoulder girdle in relationship to the thorax, throughout the whole of life. This fact is exaggerated by a hypotonus of the girdle elevators or the carrying of heavy weights, the arm beside the body. This circumstance will increase the T1 loop around the first rib, elongating the nerve.

Functional compressions

- Downward pull, as in carrying heavy weights, will produce an elongation mainly of T1, as well as a costoseptal entrapment of this nerve.
- 90° abduction + retraction: T1 nerve may become pinched at the posterior angle of T1 buttonhole (inbetween the first rib and the costo-septo-costal ligament).
- 180° hyperabduction brings the clavicle against C5–C6–C7 nerves at their exit from the IS space.

Conclusions

- The brachial plexus and the subclavian artery are prone to mechanical damage while passing through confined spaces at the cervico-thoracic junction.
- These narrow passages are related to the suprapleural complex ('pleura suspensory apparatus') and the scalene muscle complex.
- The suprapleural complex includes a membrane and three ligaments: vertebro-septal, transverse-septo-costal and costo-septo-costal.
- Suprapleural ligaments bound spaces for the passages of C8 and T1 nerves.
- The scalene complex is a common mass running from the cervical vertebrae and reaching the first and second ribs. During development, this mass is fragmented in a variable fashion.
- As a result of this fragmentation, muscular bridges remain joining anterior and middle scalene muscles, passing inbetween the neurovascular structures.
- These bridges pass either inbetween C6 and C7 nerves (upper interpedicle muscles), or inbetween the subclavian artery and nerves C8 and T1 (lower interpedicle scalene minimus muscle).
- Bridges subdivide and reduce the IS space.
- Variations in the shape, number and extension of insertions of scalene muscle can also reduce the IS space.
- A cervical rib will also reduce the IS space and kink the subclavian artery and the lower trunk.
- Shoulder drop elongates T1 nerve, increasing its loop around the first rib.
- Forced abduction and other functional positions can produce compression.
- Structural and dynamic factors can combine to cause mechanical damage.

21 Thoracic outlet syndrome, scalene complex and interscalene passages: new concepts

Luciano A Poitevin

Introduction

Thoracic outlet syndrome (TOS) is a proximal entrapment neuropathy of the upper limb. Sometimes an X-ray will demonstrate a cervical rib, but in less straightforward situations there is no cervical rib and yet neurovascular signs and symptoms are found. Several authors have identified anatomical variations at the cervico-brachial junction (Shore 1926, Adson and Coffey 1927, Gage and Parnell 1947, Leblanc 1937, Delmas 1938, Kirgis and Reed 1947, Fernández 1957, Naffziger and Grant 1938, Rosati and Lord 1961, Sunderland 1978, Poitevin 1982, 1986, 1988a, 1988b, 1988c, 1988d, 1991, 1993, Narakas et al 1986). Roos (1976, 1979, 1982) has described nine different types of bands (Wood et al 1988); however, interpretation of these bands is not always clear. This chapter describes studies that aimed to determine the anatomic and functional variations in the arrangement of the scalene muscles, their importance in causing thoracic outlet syndrome and whether the 'abnormal' muscles and fibrous bands are anatomical variations.

Materials and methods

In all, 42 non-embalmed specimens were injected with latex and lead compounds via the thoracic aorta. Thoracic outlet passages were identified and measured. Pressures within these spaces were recorded in normal position, hyperabduction (Figure 21.1) and downward pull (Figure 21.2). Radiographs were also taken in these positions of the shoulder, recording the shape and calibre of the subclavian-axillary artery (Figure 21.3). Dial calipers and a balloon connected to a water manometer (Figure 21.4) were employed as measuring instruments. Anatomical, metric and radiological data were correlated.

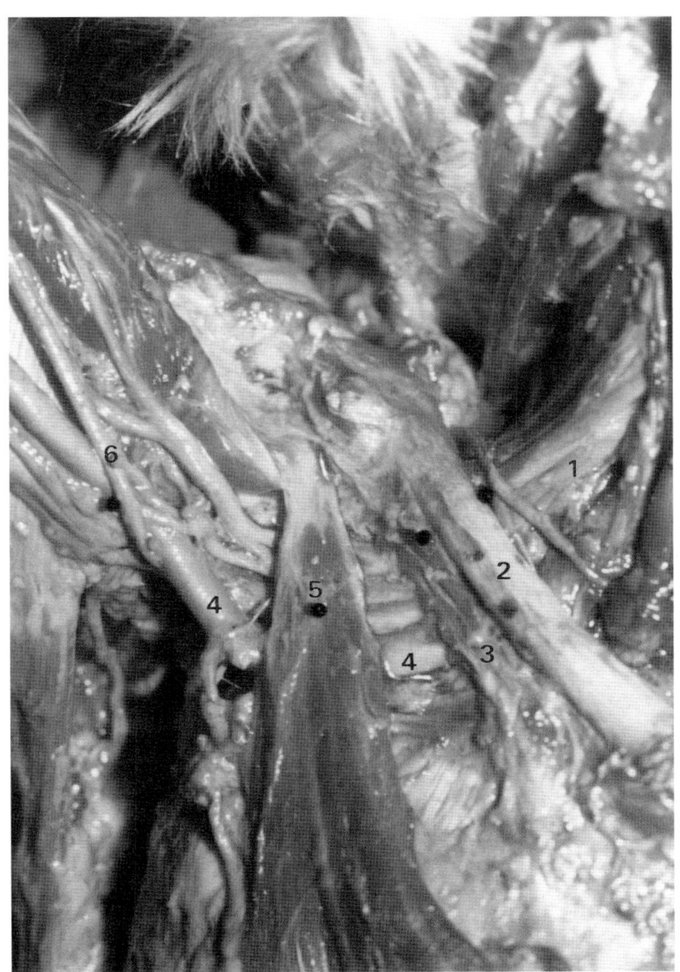

Figure 21.1

Hyperabduction – right side 1, brachial plexus; 2, clavicle; 3, subbclavius muscle; 4, axillary artery; 5, pectoralis minor; 6, median nerve.

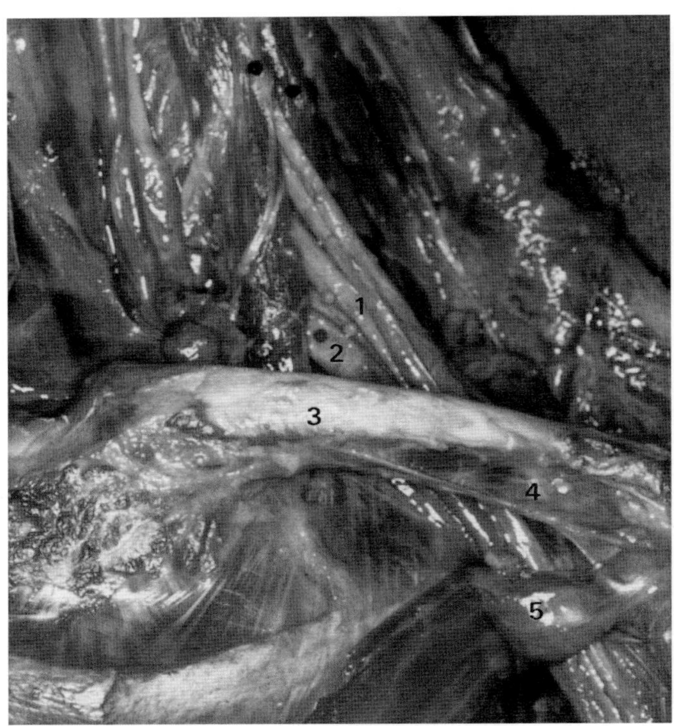

Figure 21.2
Downward pull – left side. 1, brachial plexus; 2, subclavian artery; 3, clavicle; 4, subclavius muscle and fascia; 5, pectoralis minor.

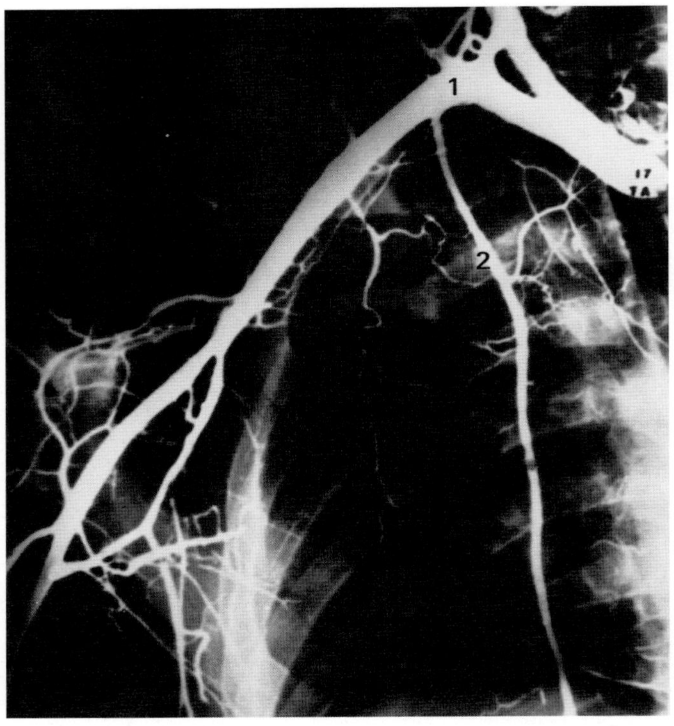

Figure 21.3
Subclavian-axillary arteriography – right side. 1, subclavian artery; 2, internal mammary.

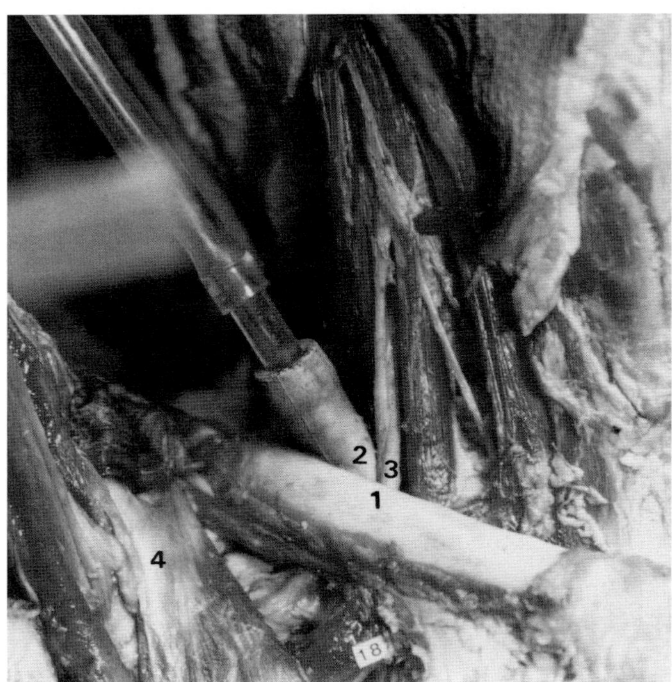

Figure 21.4
Recording pressures – right side, hyperabduction. The rubber balloon is inbetween the clavicle and the NV bundle. 1, clavicle; 2, pressure gauge behind the clavicle; 3, brachial plexus; 4, pectoralis minor.

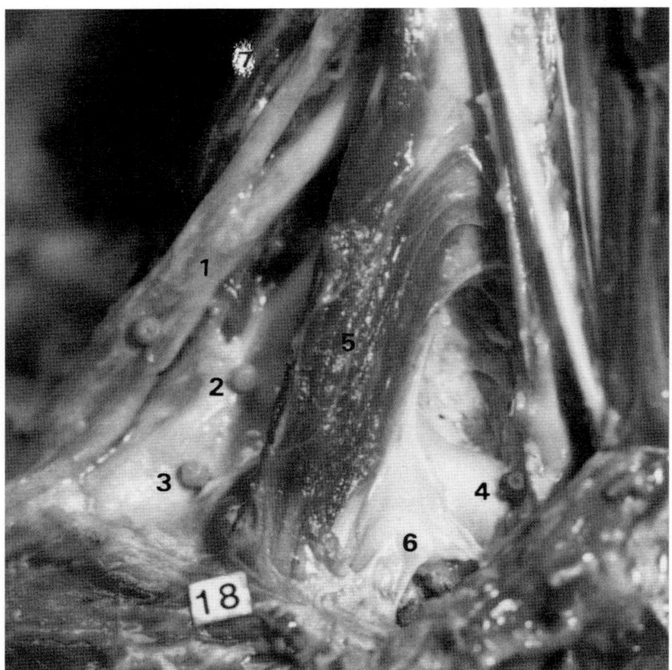

Figure 21.5
The scalene complex. 1, upper trunk; 2, middle trunk, 3, lower trunk, 4, subclavian artery; 5, anterior scalene; 6, suprapleural membrane (septum) and septal insertions of anterior scalene; 7, middle scalene.

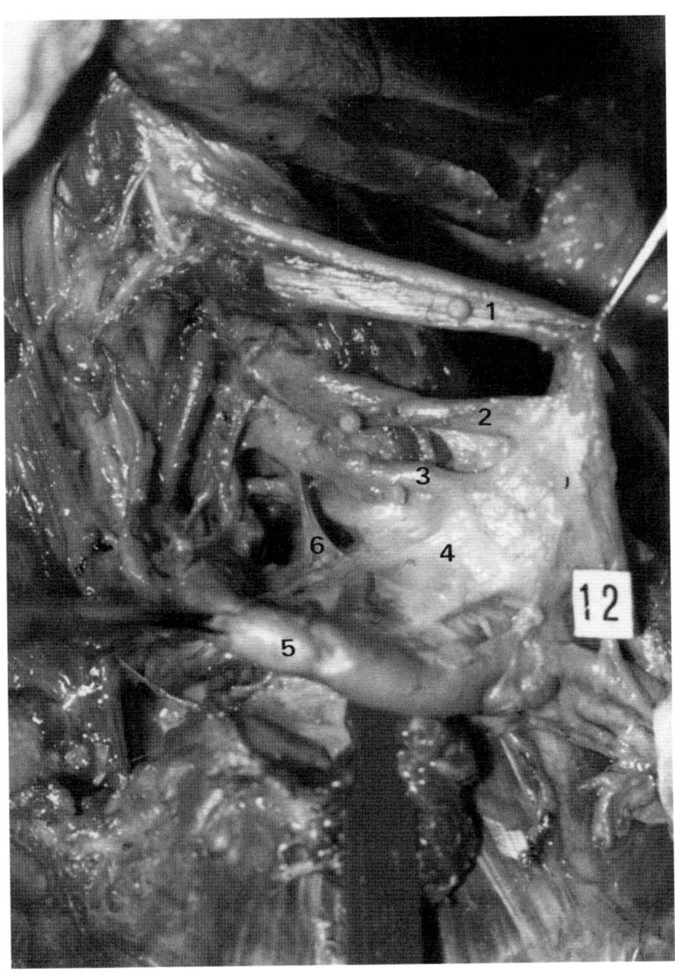

Figure 21.6

The suprapleural membrane – left side. 1, upper trunk; 2, middle trunk; 3, lower trunk; 4, suprapleural membrane and subclavian artery fascia; 5, subclavian artery; 6, costo-septo-costal ligament.

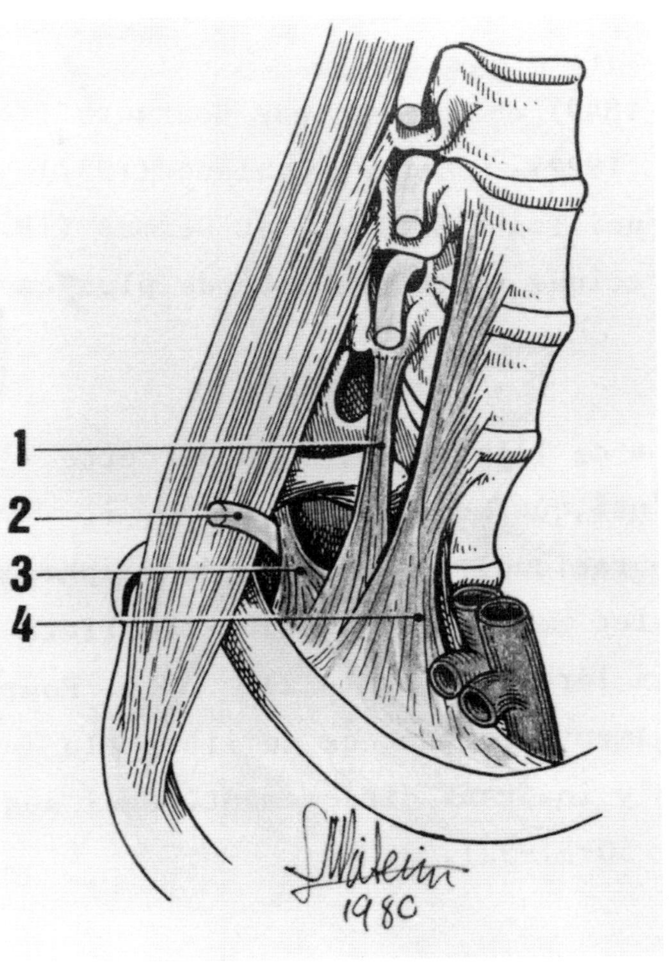

Figure 21.7

The suprapleural suspending apparatus – right side. 1, Transverse-septo-costal ligament; 2, T1 nerve; 3, costo-septo-costal ligament; 4, vertebro-septal ligament.

Results and discussion

Scalene complex

The scalene muscles are a common mass which originates from the transverse processes of the cervical vertebrae and fans downward to insert into the suprapleural membrane (membranous or septal insertions) and the first and second ribs (bony insertions) (Figure 21.5).

The suprapleural membrane (also called septum) (Figure 21.6) is a fibrous sheath over the apical pleura and the lung apex, dependent on the fascia of the subclavian artery (Truffert 1922, Leblanc 1937, Cordier-Devos 1938, Delmas 1938, Sunderland 1978, Poitevin 1980, 1982, 1986, 1988a, 1988b, 1988c, 1988d, 1991, 1993). It attaches to the inner border of the first rib and blends with the endothoracic fascia. It is held back to the cervical spine by three ligaments which form the suprapleural suspending apparatus (Figure 21.7) and by the septal insertions of the scalene muscles (Figure 21.5).

The common musclar mass or scalene complex is divided into an anterior segment (the anterior scalene muscle), a posterior segment (the middle and posterior scalenes) and an intermediate segment.

Intermediate segment

Two different muscles were found in this section: the upper intermediate scalene and the lower intermediate scalene. The upper intermediate scalene (14%) (Figures 21.8A and B and Figure 21.9) comes from behind,

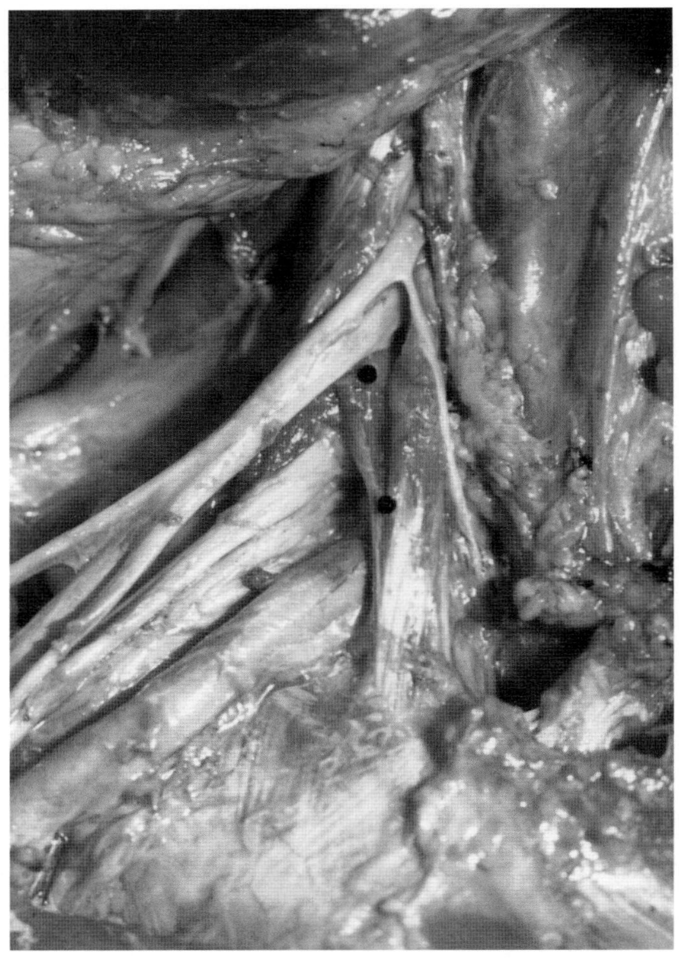

(A)

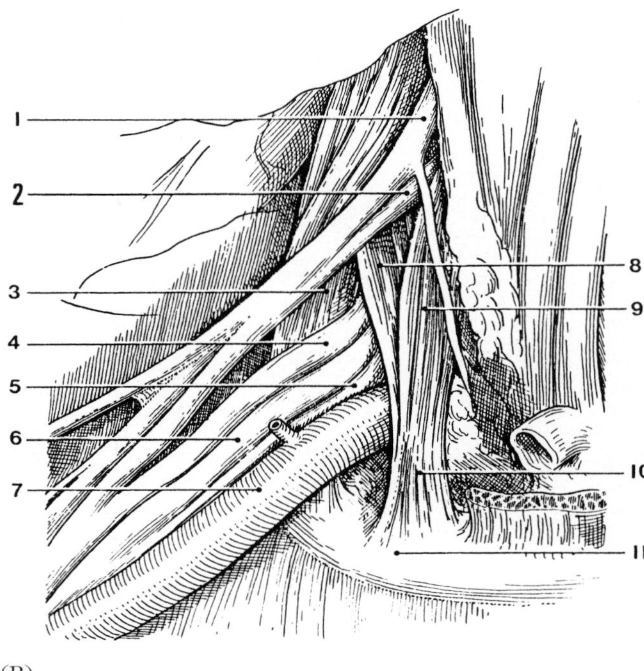

(B)

Figure 21.8

(A) The upper intermediate scalene – right side. (B) Diagrammatic illustration of (A). 1, C5 nerve; 2, C6; 3, middle scalene; 4, C7; 5, T1; 6, C8; 7, subclavian artery; 8, upper intermediate scalene; 9, anterior scalene 10, anterior scalene tendon; 11, first rib.

detaching from the middle scalene, passes between C6 and C7 nerves and then in front of the artery, to join the insertion of the anterior scalene into the first rib. This muscle can compress the middle trunk of the brachial plexus and mimic a carpal tunnel syndrome.

The lower intermediate scalene (50%) (Figures 21.10–21.14) is the scalene minimus (Fawcett 1896, Shore 1926, Leblanc 1937, Delmas 1938, Kirgis and Reed 1948, Lazorthes 1952, Rosati and Lord 1961, Lord and Rosati 1971, Roos 1976, 1979, 1982, Sunderland 1978, Poitevin 1980, 1982, 1986, 1988a, 1988b, 1988c, 1988d, 1991, 1993). It arises from the anterior tubercle of the transverse process of C7 vertebra. It proceeds downward and anteriorly, passing between the subclavian artery (which is in front) and C8 and T1 nerves (which lie behind). It ends by attaching to the suprapleural membrane in a fan-like fashion (short variety). It frequently reaches the scalene tubercle of the first rib, fusing with the anterior scalene (long variety).

Quite frequently, the muscle is replaced by a fibrous band: the transverse-septo-costal ligament (Figure 21.15). Its origin is on the anteribr tubercle of the transverse process of C7 vertebra. The insertion is into the suprapleural membrane and the scalene tubercle of the first rib.

This muscle (or the transverse-septo-costal ligament) can compress the subclavian artery (long variety) and/or the lower trunk of the brachial plexus (short variety), producing the classic symptoms of TOS.

According to classical descriptions, there are three scalene muscles: anterior, middle and posterior. The subclavian artery and the brachial plexus pass through the space inbetween the anterior scalene muscle (in front), and the middle and posterior scalene muscles (behind). The subclavian vein passes in front of the anterior scalene muscle.

However, very often we have found four and even five scalenes, some of them passing between the elements of the neurovascular (NV) bundle. These findings confirm that scalene muscles originally consist of a single muscular mass (Orts-Llorca 1970), extending from the transverse processes of the cervical vertebrae

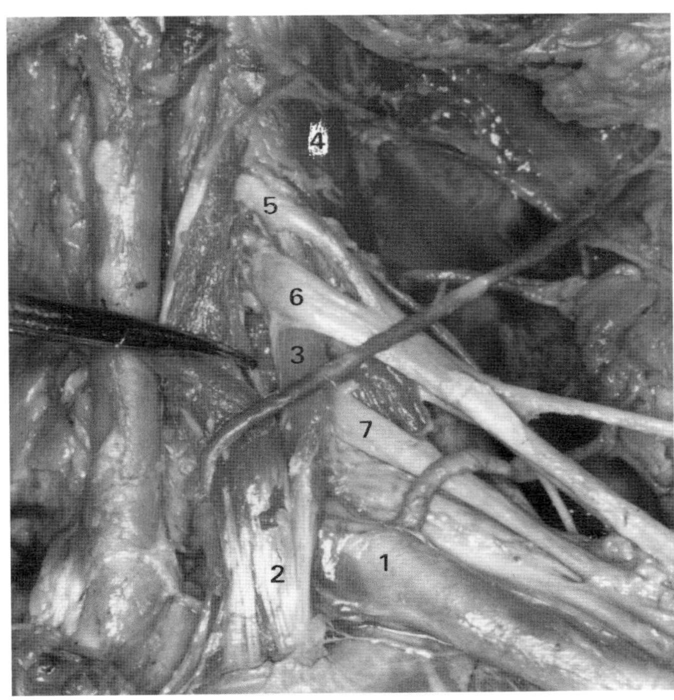

Figure 21.9

The upper intermediate scalene – left side. 1, subclavian artery; 2, anterior scalene tendon; 3, upper intermediate scalene; 4, middle scalene; 5, C5 nerve; 6, C6; 7, C7.

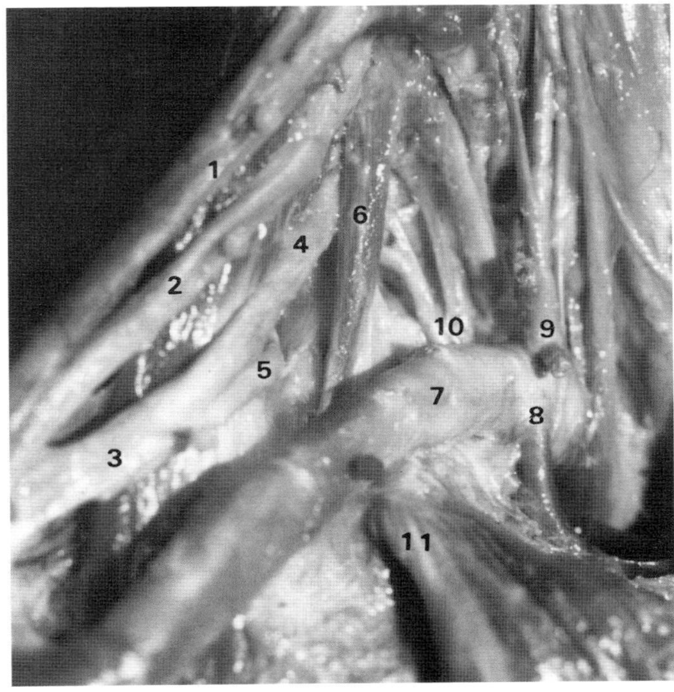

Figure 21.10

The lower intermediate scalene – right side. 1, upper trunk; 2, middle trunk; 3, lower trunk; 4, C8 nerve; 5, T1 nerve; 6, lower intermediate scalene (scalene minimus); 7, subclavian artery 8, internal mammary; 9, thyro-cervical trunk; 10, superior intercostal artery; 11, anterior scalene severed and retracted.

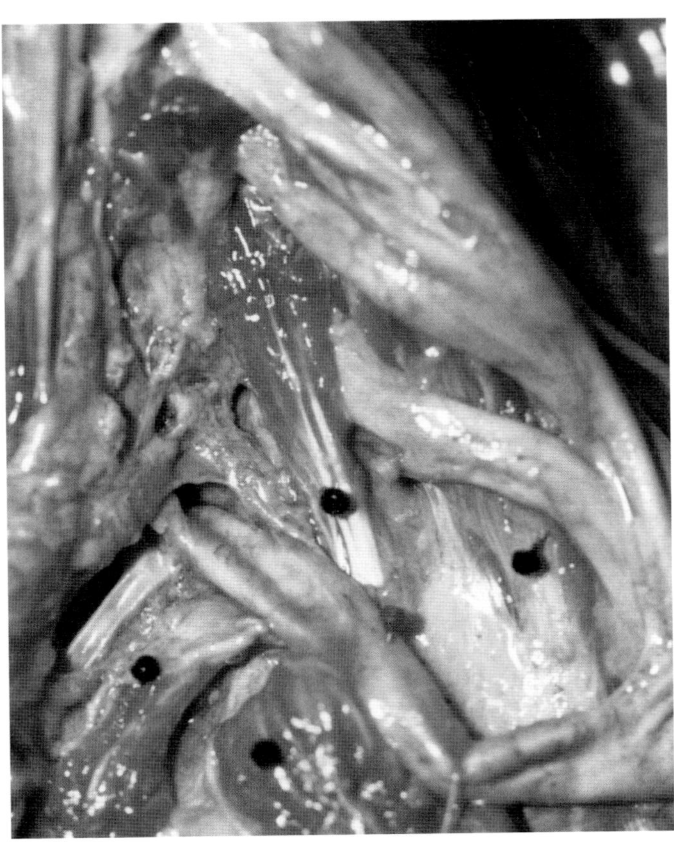

(A)

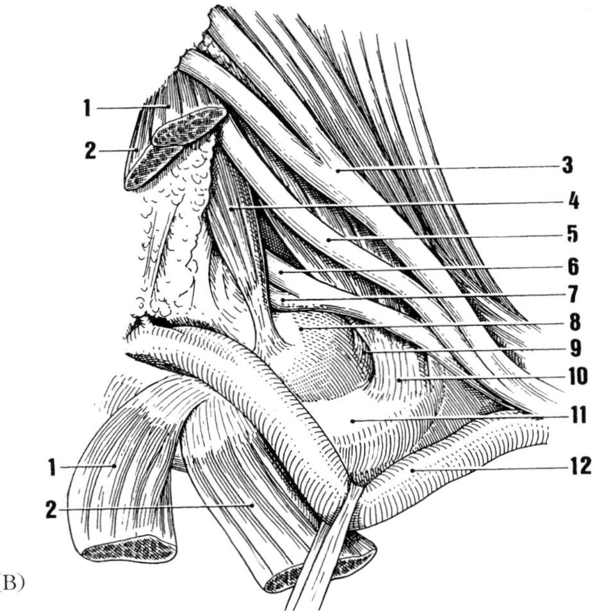

(B)

Figure 21.11

(A) The lower intermediate scalene – left side. (B) Diagrammatic illustration of (A). 1, anterior scalene, superficial part; 2, anterior scalene, deep part; 3, upper trunk; 4, lower intermediate scalene (scalene minimus); 5, middle trunk; 6, C8; 7, T1; 8, suprapleural membrane (septum); 9, septal insertions of middle scalene; 10, middle scalene tendon; 11, first rib; 12, subclavian artery.

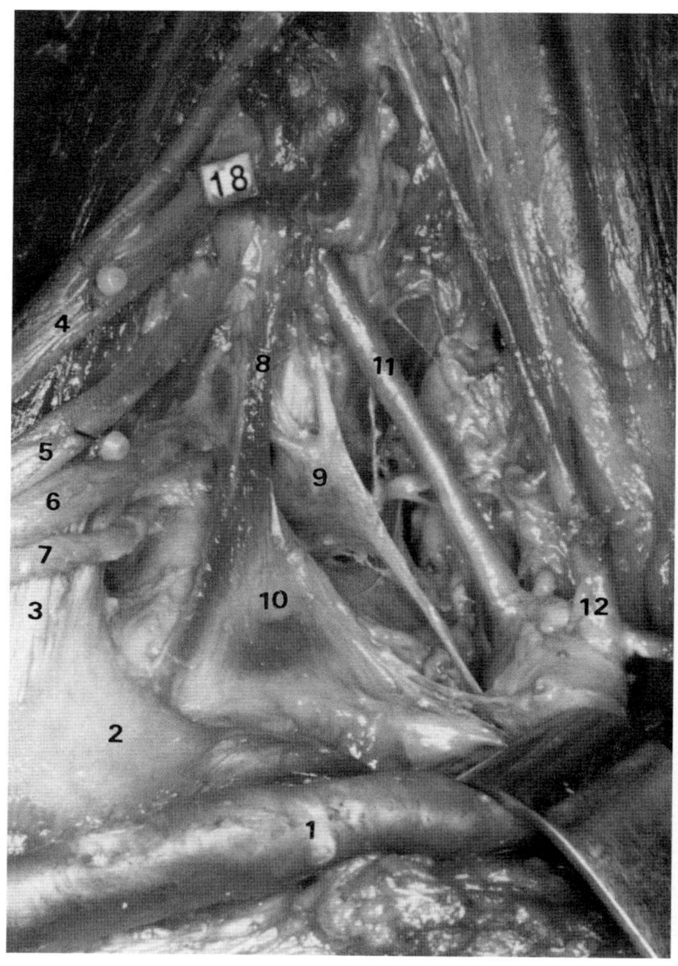

Figure 21.12

The lower intermediate scalene – right side. 1, subclavian artery; 2, first rib; 3, middle scalene tendon; 4, upper trunk; 5, C7 trunk; 6, C8; 7, T1; 8, lower intermediate scalene (scalene minimus); 9, stellate ganglion; 10, suprapleural membrane (septum); 11, vertebral artery; 12, subclavian artery.

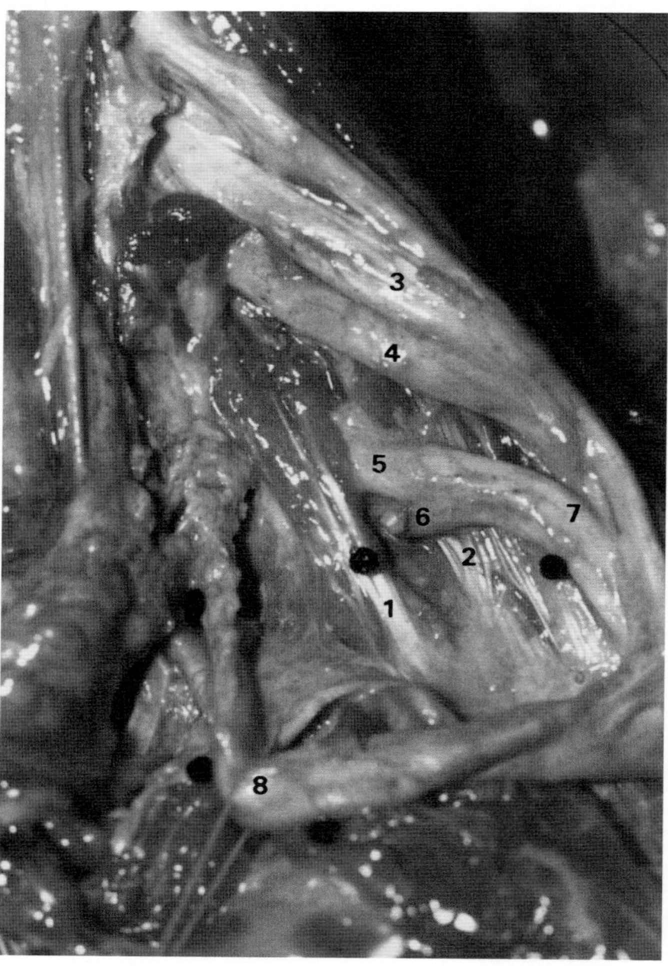

Figure 21.13

The lower intermediate scalene – left side. 1, lower intermediate scalene; 2, middle scalene; 3, C6 nerve; 4, C7; 5, C8; 6, T1; 7, inferior trunk; 8, subclavian artery retracted medially.

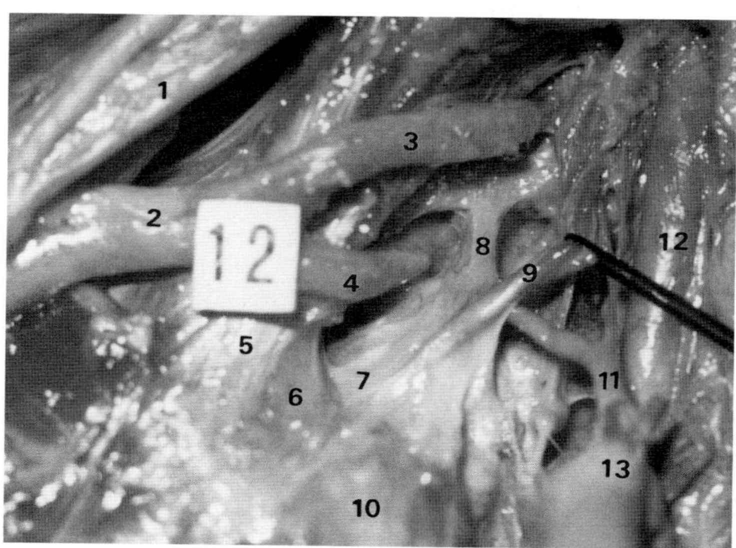

Figure 21.14

The lower intermediate scalene – right side. 1, middle trunk; 2, lower trunk; 3, C8 nerve; 4, T1; 5, middle scalene; 6, first rib; 7, suprapleural membrane; 8, costo-septo-costal ligament; 9, lower intermediate muscle (scalene minimus); 10, anterior scalene insertion; 11, superior intercostal artery; 12, vertebral artery; 13, subclavian artery retracted.

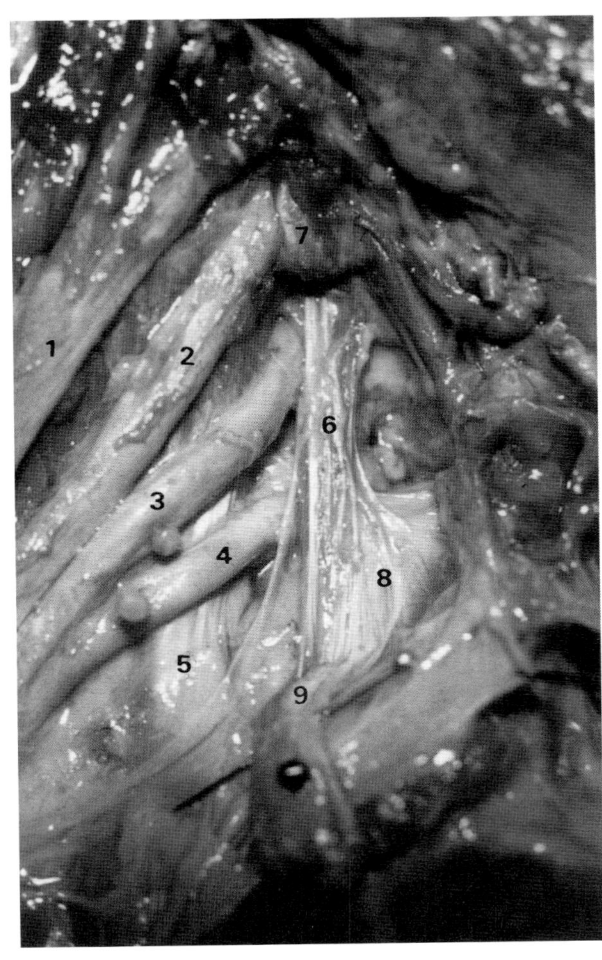

Figure 21.15

The transverse-costo-septal ligament – right side. 1, upper trunk; 2, middle trunk; 3, C8 nerve; 4, T1; 5, middle scalene; 6, transverse-septo-costal ligament; 7, proximal end of severed lower intermediate scalene; 8, suprapleural membrane or septum; 9, distal end of severed lower intermediate scalene.

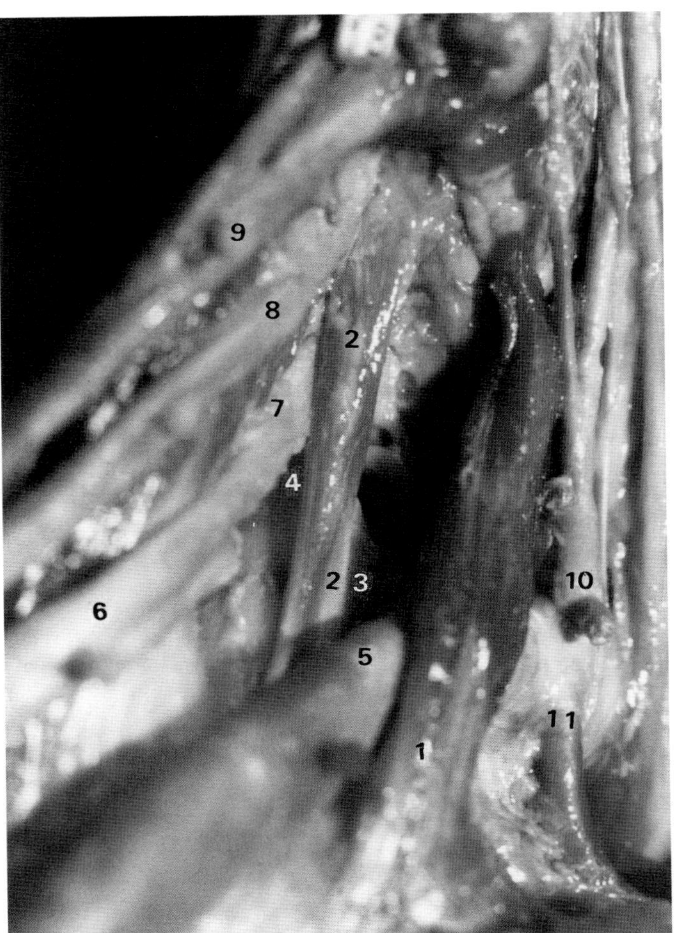

Figure 21.16

The interscalene passages – right side. 1, anterior scalene; 2, lower intermediate scalene (scalene minimus); 3, anterosuperior innterscalene passage; 4, postero-inferior interscalene passage; 5, subclavian artery; 6, lower trunk; 7, C8 nerve; 8, middle trunk; 9, upper trunk; 10, thyro-bicervical arterial trunk; 11, internal mammary artery.

to the first and second ribs and the suprapleural membrane. This common mass – the scalene complex – becomes fragmented in a variable fashion during embryological development, due to the growth and transverse passage of vessels and nerves to the upper limb. The subclavian vein remains anterior to the scalene complex. The artery and brachial plexus will split the scalene mass into an anterior segment (which will become the anterior scalene muscle) and a posterior segment (the future middle and posterior muscles). Very often, remnants of the original common mass can be noticed as muscle bridges which connect the posterior and the anterior segment passing between the artery and the trunks of the achial plexus. This is the intermediate segment.

Roos described nine different clinical types of bands. We were not able to find types 5, 7 and 8. Type 3 is a normal structure, the costo-septo-costal ligament (Figures 21.6, 21.7 and 21.14). Type 1 is a very frequent anatomic variation of the scalene complex: the transverse-septo-costal ligament (Figures 21.7 and 21.15). Types 4–6 are other variations of the scalene complex. The scalene minimus (Roos types 5 and 6) was present in 50% of the specimens (Figures 21.10–21.18).

The frequent presence of these bands as normal variations means that they are not enough to produce symptoms by themselves. We believe like Fernández (1957) that additional factors are necessary, such as an overdevelopment of the muscle or band and/or a sustained extreme position of the upper limb.

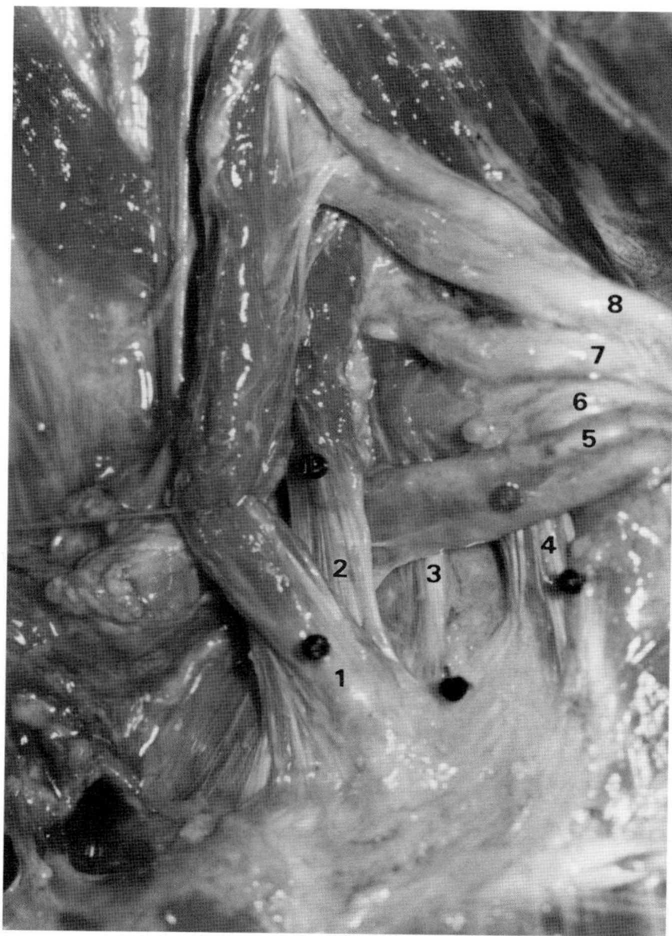

Figure 21.17
The interscalene passages – left side. 1, anterior scalene; 2, upper intermediate scalene; 3, lower intermediate scalene (scalene minimus); 4, posterior scalene; 5, subclavian artery; 6, lower trunk; 7, middle trrunk; 8, upper trunk.

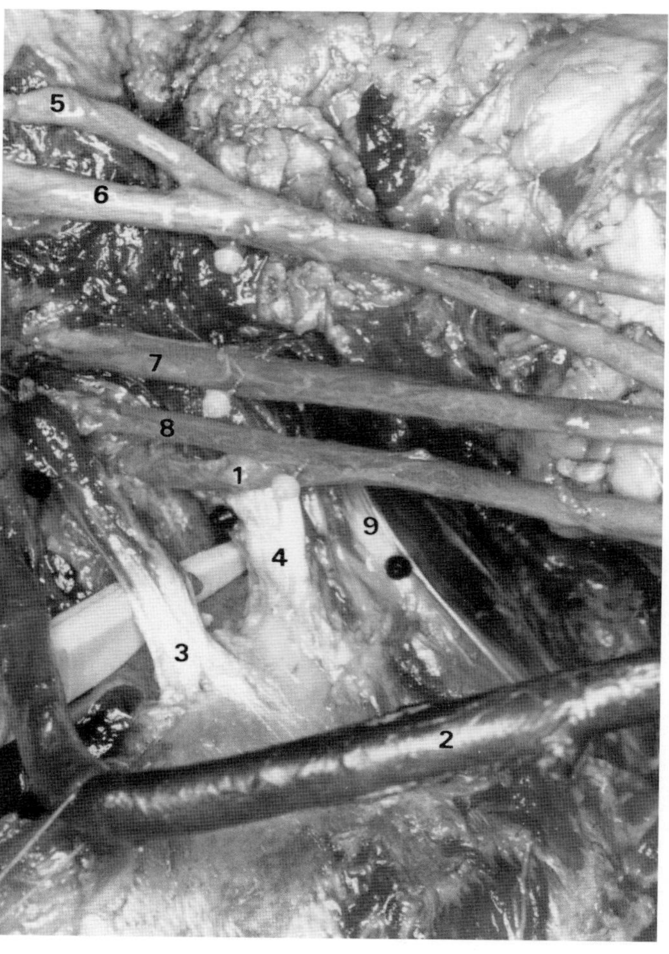

Figure 21.18
The interscalene passages – left side. 1, T1 nerve; 2, subclavian artery; 3, lower intermediate scalene; 4, middle scalene; 5, C5; 6, C6; 7, C7; 8, C8; 9, posterior scalene.

Interscalene passages

The presence of three segments in the scalene complex makes up several interscalene passages, instead of a single one (Figures 21.16–21.18).

Antero-superior interscalene passage (Figure 21.16)

This is a neurovascular space, bounded in front by the anterior scalene muscle and behind by the middle scalene (above) and the scalene minimus (below). It is the largest space. It contains, in a posterior plane, the nerves C5, C6 and C7. In the anterior and inferior aspect, the subclavian artery can be seen. It lies on the apex of the angle formed by the anterior and the scalene minimus muscles.

When there is an upper intermediate scalene (Figures 21.8, 21.9 and 21.17), this space is further divided into an upper stage, occupied by C5 and C6 nerves; and a lower stage, occupied by C7 and the subclavian artery.

Postero-inferior interscalene passage (Figures 21.10, 21.16 and 21.18)

This is a neural space, bounded in front by the scalene minimus and behind by the middle scalene. It gives way to the nerves C8 and T1.

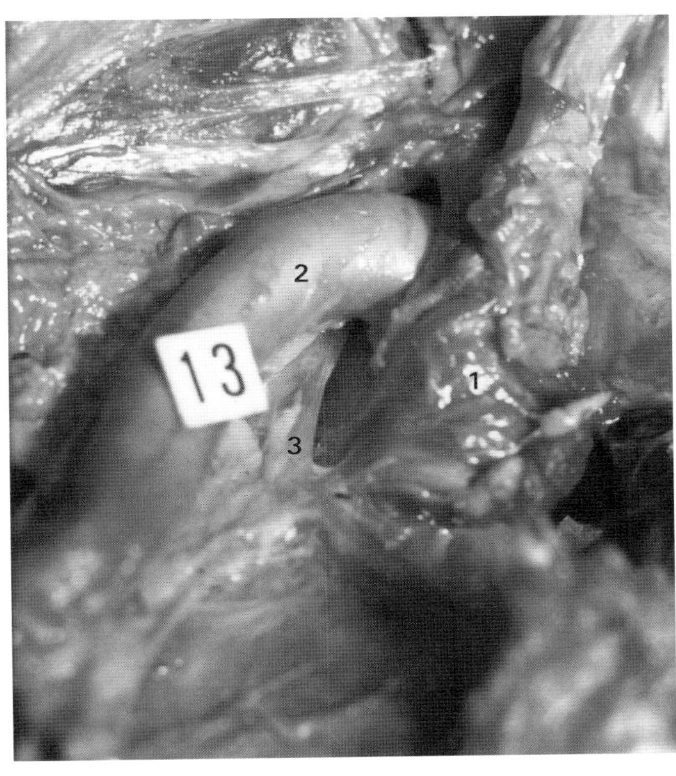

Figure 21.19

Overlapping of the insertions of the scalenes – right side. 1, anterior scalene advancing posteriorly and lifting the subclavian artery; 2, subclavian artery; 3, middle scalene and its septal insertions.

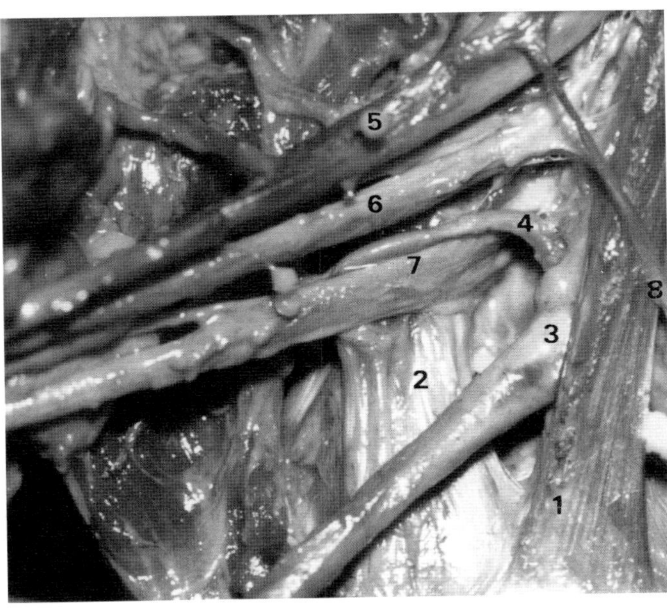

Figure 21.20

Falciform middle scalene, interscalene passages – right side. 1, anterior scalene; 2, middle scalene; 3, subclavian artery; 4, posterior scapular artery; 5, upper trunk; 6, middle trunk; 7, lower trunk; 8, phrenic nerve.

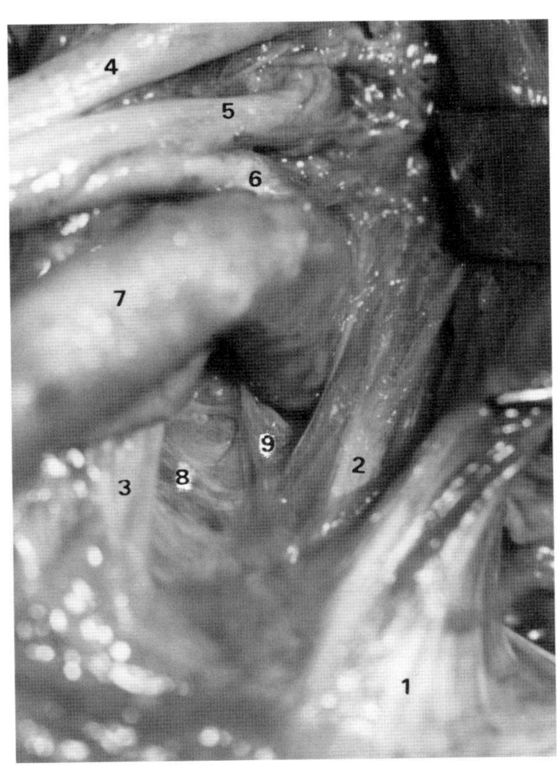

Figure 21.21

Sharp edges of scalene muscles – right side. 1, anterior scalene, superficial part; 2, anterior scalene, deep part with a sharp edge impinging on the artery; 3, middle scalene, anterior sharp edge; 4, C5 nerve; 5, C6; 6, C7; 7, subclavian artery; 8, septal insertions of the middle scalene; 9, costo-septo-costal ligament.

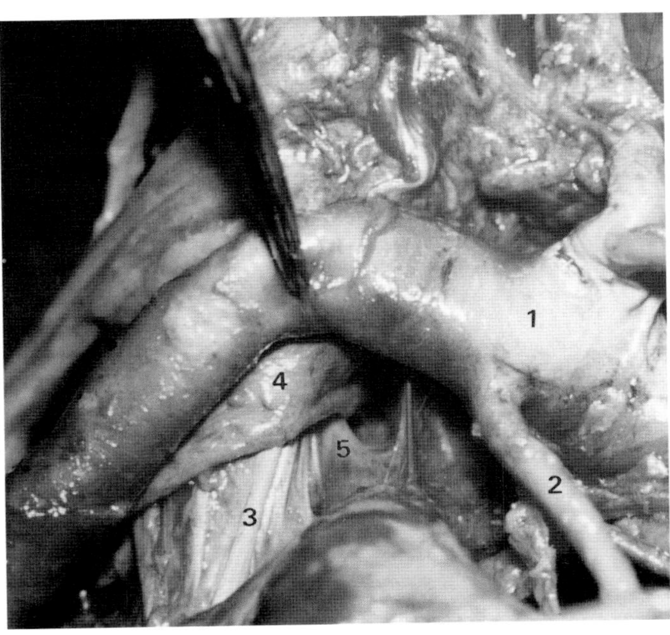

Figure 21.22

Sharp edge of middle scalene – right side. 1, subclavian artery; 2, internal mammary; 3, middle scalene tendons; 4, lower trunk; 5, septal insertions of the middle scalene.

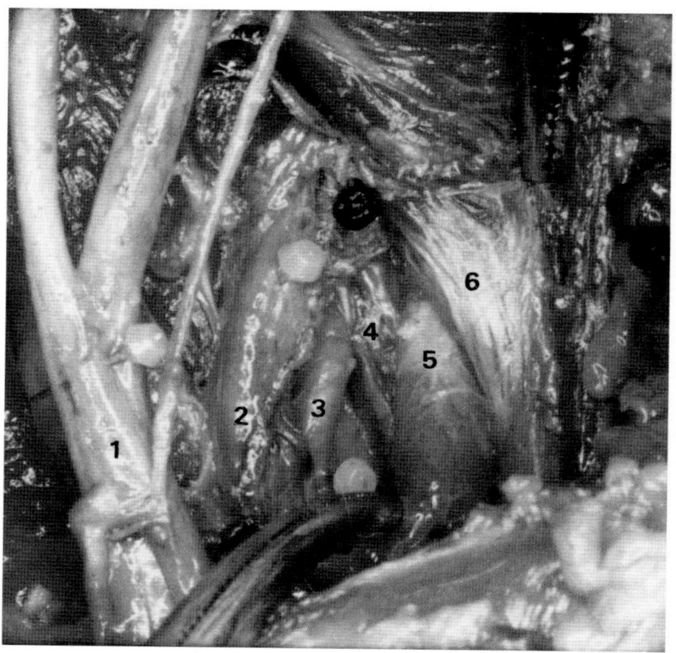

Figure 21.23

Sharp edge of anterior scalene – right side. 1, upper trunk; 2, middle trunk; 3, lower trunk; 4, lower intermediate scalene; 5, subclavian artery; 6, anterior scalene with a posterior edge.

These narrow passages can be further reduced by an overdevelopment of any of the muscles and/or an extreme position of the upper limb.

Extent of the insertions into the first rib

The mean distance between the insertions of the anterior and posterior scalene segment into the first rib is 1.04 cm. This width will allow the uneventful passage of the subclavian artery and the lower trunk of the brachial plexus. However, in 28% of cases, the distance is lesser than the diameter of the artery (Figure 21.19). In this situation, there is not enough room for the lower trunk and the artery, which are lifted and bent. Pressure recordings in extreme positions are higher in these specimens.

Variations in shape

The insertions of the anterior or middle scalene may present sharp edges (12%). They can be fibrous or muscular. The insertions of the middle scalene into the suprapleural membrane (Delmas 1938, Poitevin 1980, 1986) (Figures 21.20–21.22) and less frequently into the first rib (Telford and Mottershead 1948, Williams 1952, Fernández 1957, Sunderland 1978) can form an anterior sickle which will impinge on the lower trunk of the brachial plexus. This is a common cause of isolated neurological compressions.

This sickle-like arrangement can also be seen in the tendon of the anterior scalene (Poitevin 1980, 1982, 1986, 1988a, 1988b, 1988c, 1988d) (Figures 21.21, 21.23 and 21.24). It points dorsally and may compress the subcla-

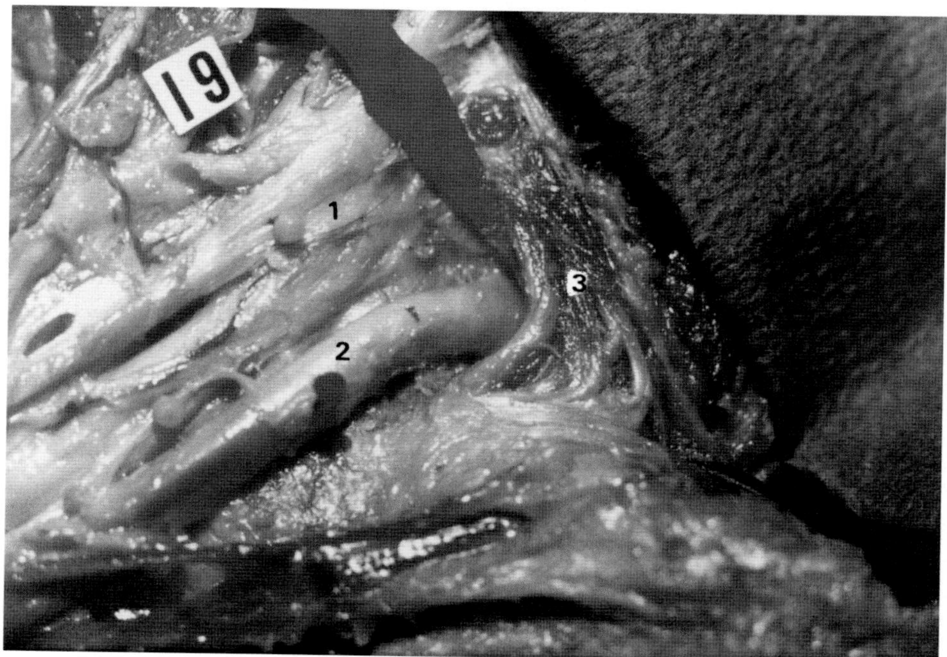

Figure 21.24

Falciform anterior scalene (muscular) – right side. 1, brachial plexus; 2, subclavian artery; 3, anterior scalene muscle.

vian artery and lower trunk; for instance in workers who hold their arms further forward than normal (Leffert 1993). The septal insertions of the anterior scalene (Delmas 1938, Poitevin 1980, 1986) may also impinge on the NV bundle.

Conclusions

1. Variations in number and arrangement. Abnormal muscles and bands are just anatomical variations of the scalene complex, formed by up to five scalenes (anterior upper intermediate (14%), lower intermediate (48%), middle and posterior) and one fibrous band (the transverse-septo-costal ligament). The scalene muscles should be considered as a scalene complex.
2. These variations in arrangement lead to the appearance of several interscalene passages, which can be further reduced by an overdevelopment of any of the muscles.
3. Extent of the insertions into the first rib. This is variable, and in 28% there is not enough room for the lower trunk and the artery. Pressure recordings in extreme positions are higher in these specimens.
4. Variations in shape. The insertions of the anterior or middle scalene may present sharp edges which can produce an impingement on the NV bundle in hyperabduction or shoulder girdle descent.
5. These findings explain clinical situations of TOS in the absence of a cervical rib.

References

Adson AW, Coffey JR (1927) Cervical rib – a method of anterior approach for relief of symptoms by division of the scalenus anticus, *Ann Surg* **5**: 839.

Cordier-Devos A (1938) Le dôme plévral. Aspect endothoracique, *Ann Anat Pathol* **15**: 465.

Delmas A (1938) *L'orifice Supérieur du Thorax.* Etude morphogénetique de ses éléments constitutits osseux et fibreux. Thesis Médecine, Montpellier.

Fawcett E (1896) What is Sibson's muscle (scalenus pleuralis)? *J Anat Physiol* **30**: 433.

Fernández LL (1957) Compresiones vásculo-nerviosas supraclaviculares. Ténica de la exploración quirúrgica, *Pr Méd Arg* **44**: 871.

Gage M, Parnell H (1948) Scalenus anticus syndrome, *Am J Surg* **73**: 252.

Kirgis AD, Reed AF (1948) Significant anatomic relations in the syndrome of the scalene muscles, *Ann Surg* **127**: 1182.

Lazorthes C (1952) La boutonnère scalénique, *CR Assoc Anat* 312.

Leblanc E (1937) L'appareil musculo-fibreux du septum cervico-thoracique et le petit scalène, *Ann Anat Pathol* **14**: 809.

Leffert RD (1993) Thoracic outlet syndrome. In: Tubiana R, ed., *The Hand*, Vol. IV (WB Saunders: Philadelphia) 343.

Lord JW, Rosati LM (1971) Thoracic outlet syndromes, *Clin Symp Ciba* **23**: 1.

Naffziger HC, Grant WI (1938) Neuritis of the brachial plexus mechanical in origin, *Surg Gynecol Obstet* **67**: 722.

Narakas A, Bonnard C, Egloff DV (1986) The cervico-thoracic outlet compression syndrome. Analysis of surgical treatment, *Ann Chir Main* **5**: 195.

Orts-Llorca F (1970) *Anatomia Humana* (Ed Cientifico Médica: Barcelona).

Poitevin LA (1980) Les Défilés Thoraco-cervico-brachiaux, *Mém Lab Anat, Paris* **42**.

Poitevin LA (1982) Données antrhopométriques du carrefour cervico-brachial, *Cah Antropol* **1**: 1.

Poitevin LA (1986) *Los Desfiladeros Tóraco-cervico-braquiales. Investigaciones anatómicas, dinámicas y radiológicas.* Thesis, University of Buenos Aires Medical School, Argentina.

Poitevin LA (1988a) Bases anatómicas de las compresiones cérvico-braquiales. Parte I: Factores estáticos, *Rev Asoc Arg Ortop y Traumatol* **53**: 175.

Poitevin LA (1988b) Bases anatómicas de las compresiones cérvico-braquiales. Parte II: Factores dinámicos. Patogencia de las compresiones, *Rev Asoc Arg Ortop y Traumatolog* **53**: 199.

Poitevin LA (1988c) Proximal compressions of the upper limb neurovascular bundle. An anatomic research study, *Hand Clin* **4**: 575.

Poitevin LA (1988d) Thoraco-cervico-brachial confined spaces. An anatomic study, *Ann Chir Main* **7**: 5.

Poitevin LA (1991) Compressions de la confluence cervicobrachiale. In: Tubiana R, ed., *Traité de Chirurgie de la Main* (Masson: Paris) 362.

Poitevin LA (1993) Proximal compressions of the upper limb neurovascular bundle. In: Tubiana R, ed., *The Hand*, Vol. IV (WB Saunders: Philadelphia) 433.

Roos DB (1976) Congenital anomalies associated with thoracic outlet syndrome. Anatomy, symptoms, diagnosis and treatment, *Am J Surg* **132**: 771.

Roos DB (1979) New concepts of thoracic outlet syndrome that explain etiology, symptoms, diagnosis, and treatments, *Vasc Surg* **13**: 313.

Roos DB (1982) The place for scalenectomy and first-rib resection in thoracic outlet syndromes, *Surgery* **92**: 1077.

Rosati LM, Lord JW (1961) *Neurovascular Compression Syndromes of the Shoulder Girdle* (Grune & Stratton: New York).

Shore LR (1926) An example of the muscle scalenus minimus, *J Anat* **60**: 418.

Sunderland S (1978) *Nerves and Nerve Injuries* (Churchill Livingstone: Edinburgh).

Telford ED, Mottershead S (1948) Pressure at the cervicobrachial junction, *J Bone Joint Surg* **30B**: 249.

Truffert P (1922) *Le Cou. Anatomie Topographique. Les Aponévroses. Les Loges* (Arnette: Paris).

Williams AF (1952) The role of the first rib in the scalenus syndrome, *J Bone Joint Surg* **34B**: 200.

Wood VE, Twito R, Verska JM (1988) Thoracic outlet syndrome. The results of first rib resection in 100 patients, *Orthop Clin North Am* **19**: 131.

22 Thoracic outlet syndrome

Michel Merle, Jacques Borrelly and Stuart W Wilson

Introduction

The large number of names given to compression syndromes of the brachial plexus and the subclavian vessels during the last century bears testimony to the difficulty in teaching this condition, with its difficult diagnostic reputation and even more controversial treatment. Narakas (1991) has described more than 18 different types of compression syndromes arising between the cervical spine and the lateral border of the pectoralis major. From our point of view, these can, without oversimplifying, be named under the general term (in French) *syndrome de la traversée cervico-thoraco-brachiale* (STCTB). A review of the last 250 references in the literature which deal with STCTB in general, and which in the English literature come under the term 'thoracic outlet syndrome' (TOS), reveals a wide variation in the aetiological, diagnostic and therapeutic approach. This condition is managed by vascular-trained surgeons, as well as upper limb surgeons trained in brachial plexus and peripheral nerve surgery. Each speciality tends to prefer its own pathological description, on one hand stressing the importance of vascular syndromes, on the other stressing the frequency of neurological syndromes and combined neurovascular syndromes. To simplify the approach of these two specialties, the treatment options can be described in the following way.

Vascular surgeons believe that resection of the first rib, usually via the axillary route, deals with vascular compressive problems just as well as neurological ones, while brachial plexus surgeons argue that the majority of neurological syndromes can be addressed by a straightforward cervical approach, and rarely by a combined cervical and axillary approach when the pathology is neurovascular in origin. Over the past 20 years we have combined our experience of brachial plexus surgery (M.M.) and thoracic surgery (J.B.) (Borrelly et al 1984, Merle 1995, Merle and Borrelly 1987, 2002). While we have carried out both cervical and axillary approaches in the last 15 years, we have preferred the supra- and infra-clavicular route when we have had to treat vascular or neurovascular forms of compression; the cervical route being reserved exclusively for purely neurological compression and removal of the first rib alone, when this is the sole cause of the clinical findings.

As we can see from the most recent anatomical studies, compression of the plexus and the subclavian vessels can take place at six distinct levels (Table 22.1). This means that the examining doctor must have a good knowledge of the anatomy of the thoracic outlet, as well as a wide knowledge of other possible pathologies in this anatomical region. Despite progress in electromyographic and imaging techniques, clinical examination remains the most important aspect in diagnosis and directing treatment, whether this be conservative or surgical. The selection of a specific surgical technique will depend on the determination of the cause of the pathology of the brachial plexus and subclavian vessels. Within one century, the difficulty encountered by surgeons has, despite everything, led to the development of pathways for treatment which are becoming ever clearer as we become more familiar with the anatomy,

Table 22.1 *The spaces traversed by the brachial plexus and the subclavian and axillary vessels*

	Space	
Brachial plexus →	1 – Region of the suspensory apparatus of the pleura	
Brachial plexus	2 – Interscalene space ←	Subclavian and axillary artery
Brachial plexus	3 – Costoclavicular space ←	Axillary and subclavian vein
Brachial plexus	4 – Clavipectoral region	
Brachial plexus	5 – Region posterior to pectoralis minor	
Brachial plexus →	6 – Region anterior to the head of the humerus ←	Subclavian and axillary artery; Axillary and subclavian vein

and the limitations of each type of surgical treatment. During the last decade, it appears that this condition has become increasingly commonplace and there has been an increase in the number of surgical procedures to resect the first rib, particularly in well-developed countries; this seems excessive to us. The morbidity of the transaxillary approach of Roos is far from negligible, and Dale demonstrated in 1982 that surgery for TOS was the commonest cause of litigation against thoracic surgeons in the USA. More recently, Roos (1990), who published a series of more than 1500 cases of resection of the first rib with a very low complication rate, remains convinced that the diagnosis of TOS is under-estimated, while Wilbourn (1990) believes that this is a syndrome which is too frequently diagnosed incorrectly. In our experience we have had to take on several surgical revisions following first rib resections by the Roos technique (usually partial rib resections). This surgery should not be under-estimated, as the anatomical variations and technical pitfalls can be formidable.

Historical background

The reader who wishes to explore the history of TOS in more depth should not miss the accounts of Narakas (1989, 1991) who, in his own erudite way, relates a memorable historical account which we are pleased to summarize. In 1627 William Harvey described a subclavian artery aneurysm which manifested as TOS. Sir Astley Cooper identified a clinical case in 1821, but it was not until a publication by Mayo in 1835 that there was a description of the symptoms created by the presence of a subclavian artery aneurysm. Willshire described the syndrome of the cervical rib in 1860. In 1906, Murphy, in the USA, described the role played by the scalenus anterior muscle in brachial plexus palsies caused by the presence of an accessory rib. Another Murphy, in Australia, in 1910, successfully resected the first rib, which was recognized as the principal cause of compression, as had been reported by Bramwell in 1903. However, at the start of the twentieth century, resection of the first rib remained a dangerous surgical treatment and the suggested procedure of scalenotomy put forward by Adson and Coffee in 1927 simplified the therapeutic approach. Around the same time, several workers stressed the importance of the scalene space as a cause of these brachial plexus palsies, and the anatomical concept of the interscalene trigone is attributed to Puusepp in particular (Puusepp 1931). Other authors, such as Gaupp in 1894 and Clerck et al in 1917, stressed the role of the scalenus medius in compression of the lower roots of the brachial plexus, an idea which was re-visited by Nichols in 1986 and by Allieu et al in 1991. The interscalene space was considered the principal cause of plexopathies causing chronic arm pain for several decades, and in 1938 Naffziger and Grant, relying on a clear clinical study, defended scalenotomy, which was practised up until the 1960s, despite a high failure rate. The widespread use of this technique somewhat obscured an important work carried out by Brickner in 1927, who stressed the importance of the role played by the first rib in subclavian artery compression; observations that were reported later by Leriche in 1941, and Falconer and Weddell in 1943. However, the clinical picture was not due entirely to compression of the subclavian artery; thrombosis of the subclavian vein was also described as a cause, under the name 'Paget-Schrötter syndrome' (Paget 1875, Schrötter 1884). In 1945, Wright stressed the importance of nerve root compression caused by hyperabduction of the arm, which produced a compression of the root deep to the coracoid and the pectoralis minor. The 1960s saw more and more adventurous surgical treatments proposed, from resection of the clavicle to abolish the effect of costoclavicular compression, to the re-appearance of first rib resection, carried out first by a posterior approach and then by an anterior approach. These approaches to the first rib were nothing new to thoracic surgeons. Noteworthy during this era was the experience of one of them, Mark Iselin, who subsequently became one of the pioneers of hand surgery.

In 1956, workers at the Mayo Clinic, led by Peet et al, suggested rehabilitation protocols which avoided surgical intervention in more than half of the patients. This interesting conservative approach did not enjoy the same success in the hands of other teams of therapists. An important turning point in treatment was the proposition of Roos in 1966, who carried out first rib removal by a transaxillary approach. This surgical treatment was undoubtedly a great success, as it had the attraction of an unobtrusive surgical approach, which avoided aesthetic sequelae, but above all it allowed visualization of all the planes up to the C8-T1 roots. The first rib resection, which of necessity led to disinsertion of the scalenus anterior, allowed the interscalene space to be opened up and to free up extensively the subclavian vessels. Certain accomplished surgeons even suggested resection of cervical ribs by this approach. The enthusiasm for this technique was confirmed by the first statistics published by Roos in 1966, concerning 106 costal resections, which resulted in cure of neurological symptoms in 88% and improved symptoms in 12%; and recovery of vascular symptoms in 42% and deterioration in 53%. The quality of these results is probably explained by Roos' rigorous technique, because at this time the anatomical variations at the level of the interscalene trigone and at the suspensory apparatus of the pleura had not yet been clarified by the anatomical studies of Poitevin (1980a, 1980b). This would explain certain failures of treatment reported in the literature between the 1970s and 1980s, which led to a successful return to the cervical approach for TOS.

Between 1980 and 1990, a number of publications criticized treatment by the transaxillary approach, in favour of the supraclavicular approach. Dale's publication in 1982, quoting complications produced by first rib resection via the transaxillary route, reduced the indications for this approach. The anatomical studies on the scalenus anterior, reported by Machleder et al in 1986, restored interest in muscle sectioning, specifically resection of scalenus anterior, justified on the grounds of the presence of the more important type 1 muscle fibres, which predisposed to permanent contracture of this muscle. A review of different series confirms that in cases when neurological origin is predominant or pure, quite often the cervical approach allows access to and excision of all the pathological structures causing the compression, or producing a 'saddle' effect at the level of the roots and the trunks of the brachial plexus. On the other hand, this approach seems inadequate in situations caused by purely neurovascular or vascular causes, in which, without doubt, first rib resection is fully justified. It is interesting to note that Narakas (1991), known for his careful studies of the aetiology and pathology of nerve palsy, predicted a double approach using the transaxillary and cervical route in a situation where a single underlying cause was not evident. Experience from leading units in brachial plexus surgery completely justified the sound basis of this approach, taking into account the complexity of the anatomical structures and anatomical variation at the supraclavicular level. The treatment approach that we have followed is close to that of Narakas, but in order to avoid two operative fields, we have preferred the supra- and infra-clavicular approach, which allows precise control of the subclavian vessels and the brachial plexus.

Clinical examination and electromyography (EMG) tends to favour, probably incorrectly, a proximal compression of the brachial plexus, obscuring compression of the median nerve in the carpal tunnel, or compression of the ulnar nerve at the elbow. According to Narakas (1991) these multi-level compressions occur in 30% of cases. Most often, after release of the obstruction at the level of the thoracic outlet, the patient considers himself cured, or at least greatly improved, and avoids returning to the clinic for further consultations for several months, even several years. After this time, the patient returns with complaints which could suggest recurrence of the TOS. In fact, the compression syndrome appears clear-cut both clinically and electromyographically, in the case of the carpal tunnel as well as the cubital tunnel.

It should be understood that, despite the protocols of Peet et al, which were widely circulated in 1956, but probably poorly understood, the results of conservative treatment could not be retained as the treatment of choice in proven TOS. Few workers were able to establish which patients were significantly improved by prolonged periods of rehabilitation in adults. It is interesting to note that Sallstrom and Celegin (1983) believed that such protocols could lead to worsening of symptoms in 10–20% of cases and thereby precipitate the decision to operate.

Anatomical and anatomico-pathological basis of TOS

Levels of compression of the brachial plexus and surrounding vessels

Poitevin (1980a, 1991), quoting an extremely important anatomical study, defined six levels of compression of the brachial plexus:

1. The region known as the suspensory apparatus of the pleura
2. The interscalene space
3. The costoclavicular space
4. The clavipectoral region
5. The region posterior to pectoralis minor
6. The region anterior to the head of the humerus.

Region of the suspensory ligament of the pleura (Figure 2)

Sebileau (1892) described three structures emerging from the seventh cervical vertebra and from the first rib which

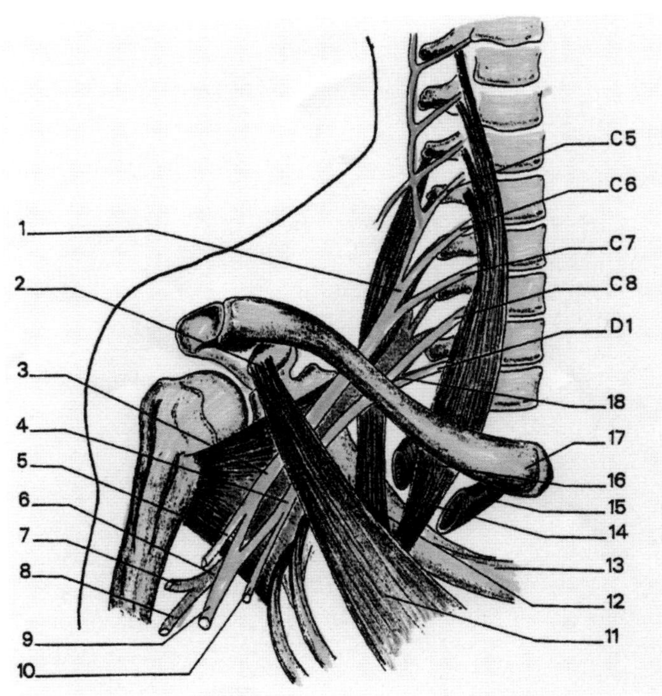

Figure 22.1

Anatomy of the brachial plexus. 1, Upper trunk; 2, coracoid process; 3, lateral cord; 4, medial cord; 5, musculocutaneous nerve; 6, posterior cord; 7, axillary nerve; 8, radial nerve; 9, median nerve; 10, ulnar nerve; 11, pectoralis minor; 12, scalenus medius; 13, first rib; 14, scalenus anterior; 15, subclavian vein; 16, subclavian artery; 17, clavicle; 18, lower trunk.

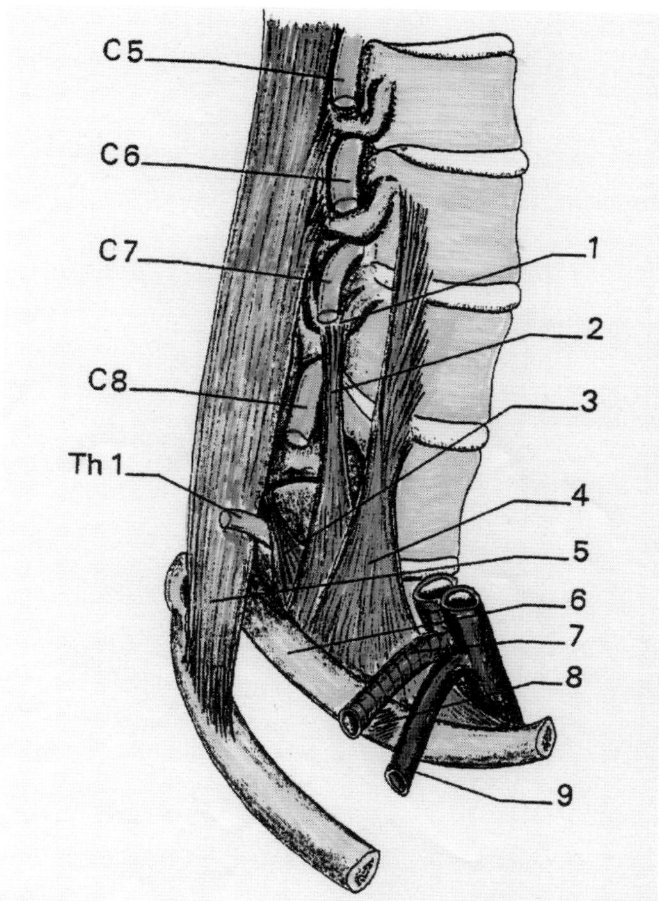

Figure 22.2
Region of the suspensory ligament of the pleura.
1, Transverse process of C7; 2, transversoseptocostal ligament; 3, costoseptocostal ligament; 4, scalenus minimus (equivalent: scalenus minor); 5, scalenus posterior; 6, first rib; 7, subclavian artery; 8, insertion of scalenus anterior; 9, subclavian vein.

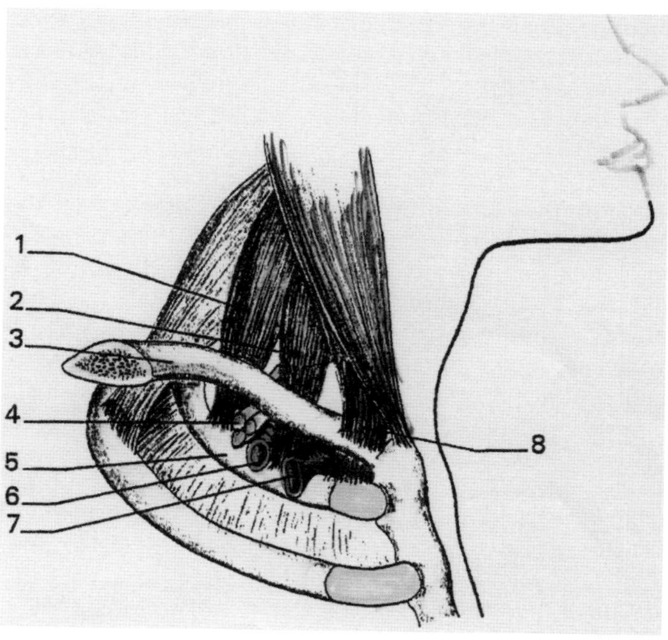

Figure 22.3
The interscalene space. 1, Scalenus medius; 2, scalenus anterior; 3, clavicle; 4, brachial plexus; 5, first rib; 6, subclavian artery; 7, subclavian vein; 8, sternocleidomastoid.

insert onto the supra-pleural membrane. The transversoseptocostal ligament inserts onto the anterior tubercle of the transverse process of C7 and has an attachment in the region of the scalenus anterior muscle. The costoseptocostal ligament attaches posteriorly into the neck of the first rib and reaches the posterior border of the first rib, creating a true buttonhole, through which the root of T1 can pass, and where it can be seriously injured during resection of the first rib by the transaxillary approach. The transversoseptocostal ligament, or its equivalent the scalenus minimus, which emerges from the interscalene space, abuts the artery anteriorly, while impinging on the lower trunk posteriorly.

The interscalene space (Figure 3)

The subclavian artery and the brachial plexus are surrounded by the scalenus anterior muscle in front and the scalenus medius and scalenus posterior behind, and the subclavian vein is situated anterior to the scalenus anterior. Within the interscalene space, the presence of a scalenus minor or its equivalent, the transversoseptocostal ligament, creates an anterior space in which the artery runs, and a posterior space where the roots of the brachial plexus can be found. The scalenus medius muscle may be one of the causes of direct compression of the lower trunk and the subclavian artery in their passage inferiorly. During abduction and extension movements, the interscalene space participates directly in compression of neurovascular structures.

Costoclavicular space

This space, bounded by the clavicle superiorly and the first rib inferiorly, is more or less open during contraction of the subclavian muscles and in the majority of arm positions. The costoclavicular space is obliterated by retropulsion of the shoulder and also by progressive muscular atrophy, which leads to the descent of the shoulder girdle. This progressive alteration of the normal anatomical relationship leads at the same time to stretching of the inferior trunk and the subclavian artery, and causes these structures to be bent around the first rib.

Clavipectoral region

The medial coracoclavicular ligament is in direct contact with the subclavian vein and can be directly involved in its compression.

Region posterior to pectoralis minor

Bound anteriorly by the pectoralis minor and posteriorly by the posterior wall of the axilla. Structures can be trapped here during hyperabduction movements of the arm.

Region anterior to the head of the humerus

When the arm is abducted and extended, the axillary artery and the terminal branches of the brachial plexus are in direct contact with the humeral head, which can compress them anteriorly. The 'M' of the median nerve is the most at risk of stretching. It should be noted here that there may be a Langer's muscle, which creates a tight sling anteriorly around the neurovascular structures, between the latissimus dorsi and pectoralis major.

Anatomical variations of the cervical rib and its incidence in TOS

A cervical rib is found in between 0.004% and 1% of the population. In 9 cases out of 10 this is asymptomatic. It is found three times more commonly in females than males and is present bilaterally in one case out of two. Gruber (1869) suggested a classification into four types:

- Type 1: short cervical rib measuring < 2.5 cm.
- Type 2: cervical rib of > 2.5 cm with a tapered end which continues as fibrous bands or muscle (Figure 22.4).
- Type 3: attaches to the first rib (Figure 22.5).
- Type 4: a complete rib which articulates with the first rib or the sternum.

Type 3 is most commonly encountered in cases of TOS. The cervical rib is situated below the root of C7 and above that of C8. The fibrous bands related to a type 3 cervical rib can produce a 'saddle' effect in the region of the lower trunk and the subclavian artery.

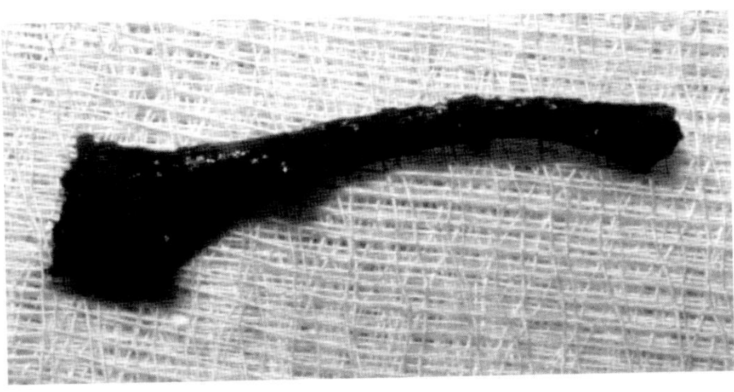

Figure 22.4
Cervical rib with tapered end (type 3).

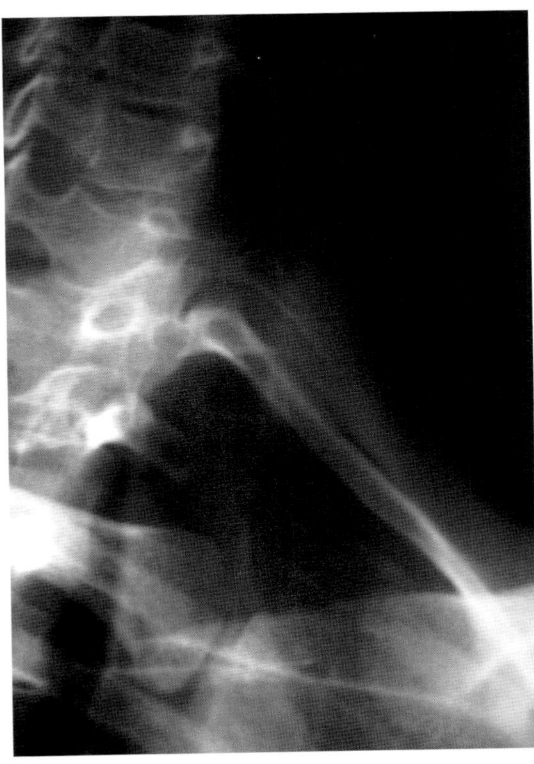

Figure 22.5
Resection of a type 3 cervical rib, the end of which is attached to the first rib.

Pathophysiology of compression

The diagnostic difficulty associated with TOS arises from the variety of symptoms produced by compression of the brachial plexus, together with possible symptoms of occlusion of the subclavian artery and vein. With the exception of the suspensory ligament of the pleura, the subclavian artery and axillary artery cross the same spaces as the brachial plexus. In contrast, the axillary vein and subclavian vein have a less exposed course, as they run successively in front of the humeral head, in the retropectoral space, the clavipectoral space and the costoclavicular space (Figure 1). A sound knowledge of the anatomy of the thoracic outlet, together with an understanding of the neurology of the upper limb, is absolutely essential in reaching a diagnosis of the cause of TOS. Proximal types of TOS involving roots C5, C6, C7, upper and middle trunks are the exception; the description of Swank and Simeone (1944) reported functional problems in extension of the wrist and the fingers accompanied by paraesthesiae in the territory of the median and cutaneous nerves. The cause could be the presence of a fibrous band behind the scalenus anterior associated with a contracture of the scalene muscles.

Table 22.2 *Symptoms of upper (C5-C6-C7) and lower (C8-T1) TOS*

	Upper TOS C5-C6-C7	*Lower TOS C8-T1*
Pain	Lateral cervical	Posterior
Radiation	Lateral border of upper limb	Posterior surface of shoulder – root of axilla Medial border of upper limb
Hypoaesthesia	Radial nerve territory	Ulnar nerve territory
Paraesthesia	Rarely in the hand (musculocutaneous ± median)	Hand: fourth and fifth rays
Loss of endurance	At the elbow, wrist and hand (weakness of extension)	Hand: weakness of interossei
Tinel sign	Supraclavicular	Supra- and infra-clavicular

Table 22.3 *Anatomical and functional causes of TOS*

Anatomical and functional causes		*Consequences*
Complete cervical rib or cervical rib with fibrous band		Elevation of the lower trunk and/or subclavian artery
Static compression	Depression of shoulder girdle by muscular weakness	Lower trunk and subclavian artery subjected to stretching over first rib
	Extensive posterior insertion of scalenus anterior	Narrowing of interscalene space
	Falciform configuration of scalenus medius	Elevation of lower trunk and subclavian artery
	Scalenus minor muscle or transversoseptocostal ligament	Narrowing of interscalene space Lower trunk compressed posteriorly Subclavian artery forced anteriorly
	Fibrous connections between scalenus medius and scalenus anterior	Separates the upper roots from the lower roots of the plexus
	Langer's muscle (fibres between pectoralis major and latissimus dorsi)	Compresses the neurovascular pedicle
Dynamic compression	By abduction and extension of the arm	Closes the interscalene space
	Axial traction	Compression of vessels and nerves on first rib
	By hyperabduction	Closes the costoclavicular space Compression of the subclavian vein and the medial cord by the coracoclavicular ligament
	By abduction and retroposition	Compression of median nerve at the level of the humeral head

TOS cases involving the lower plexus are, on the other hand, more frequent and involve the roots from C7 to T1: the middle trunk, the lower trunk and the medial cord, and may or may not be associated with compression of the artery and/or the subclavian and axillary veins. Table 2 summarizes the symptoms of upper and lower plexus TOS, and Table 3 illustrates the anatomical and functional causes that can aid in diagnosis.

Diagnosis

Clinical study and complementary examination

The approach must be meticulous, and a search must be made for unusual anatomical structures: cervical rib, axillary muscle of Langer. The examination of the anatomical make-up of the patient who presents with a dropped shoulder due to muscle atrophy; the funnel chest; as well as the search for a traumatic origin – particularly for proximal TOS involving C5-C6-C7; patients carrying heavy weights on the point of the shoulder, typical carrying position of a backpack, etc., are all points that lead to the diagnosis.

As far as symptoms are concerned, it is convenient to differentiate cases of TOS of the upper plexus involving roots C5-C6-C7-C8 (Table 2). Those types involving the upper plexus present with lateral cervical pain radiating to the lateral border of the upper limb. The area of paraesthesia involves the musculocutaneous nerve territory and occasionally encroaches on that of the median nerve. The patient complains of lack of endurance in extension movements of the elbow, wrist and digits, but it is unusual for this clinical picture to present with acute

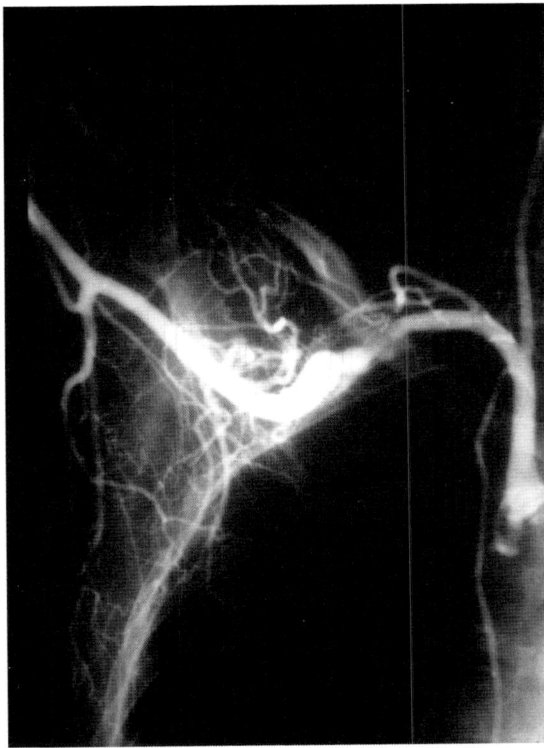

Figure 22.6
Post-stenotic aneurysm of the subclavian artery.

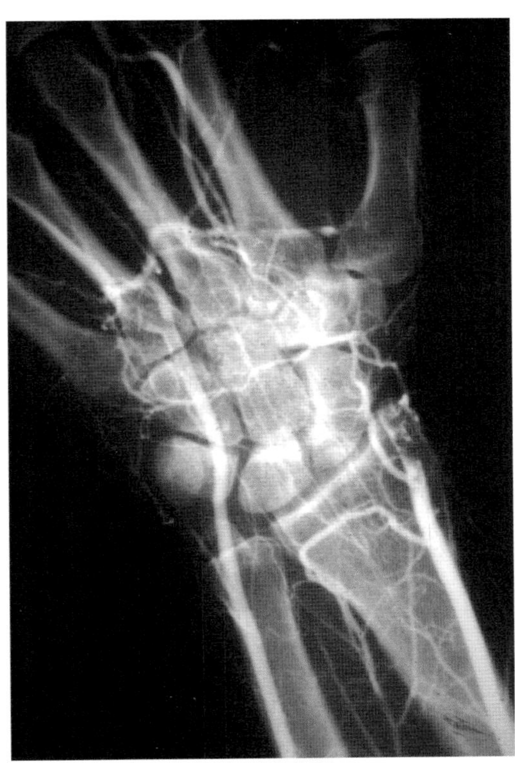

Figure 22.7
Thrombosis of the radial artery.

motor weakness. There is a positive Tinel's sign in the supraclavicular fossa.

- The lower forms (C8-T1 or C7-C8-T1) are found in the presence of dorsal pain which radiates to the posterior surface of the shoulder, reaching the apex of the axilla and the medial surface of the upper limb. The paraesthesia is found essentially in the territory of the ulnar nerve. However, this clinical picture, if present for several years, can present with a serious loss of strength in the hand due to marked wasting of the interossei.
- Association with vascular types of compression is frequent and, in addition to direct nerve compression, there are signs of nerve ischaemia due to intermittent compression of the main vessels. Cold sensitivity is sometimes seen here, and a diagnosis of Raynaud's syndrome made.
- Long-standing arterial lesions are less common and can lead to a clinical picture of ischaemia due to partial thrombosis of the artery and to the development of a post-stenotic aneurysm (Figures 6 and 7). Rarer still is the venous thrombosis, an extension of which can be dramatic when complicated by emboli (Aziz et al 1986) (Figure 8).

Auscultation of the vessels with the arm held in different positions, searching for a bruit or signs of obstruction, must be meticulous.

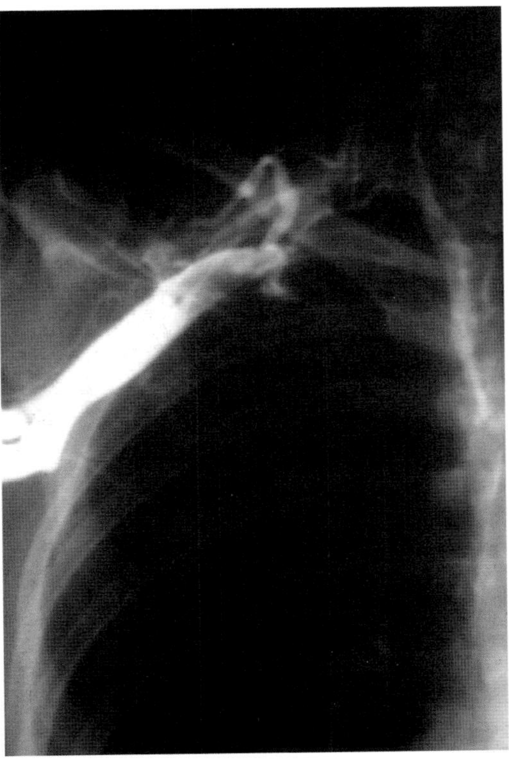

Figure 22.8
Thrombosis of the subclavian vein.

Table 22.4 *Clinical tests to diagnose TOS of neurological, vascular or mixed origin*

Neurological TOS	*Neurovascular TOS*	*Vascular TOS*
Morley's sign ⇓ Compression of transverse process of C7 Modified Adson #2 test Turn the head to opposite side Chin elevated Deep inspiration Posterior projection of shoulders, hands on thighs	Greenstone's sign ⇓ Compression of scalenus anterior Falconer and Weddel's test or 'at attention' Closes the costoclavicular pincer by raising the chin and lowering the shoulders Compresses the artery and produces paraesthesia	Allen's sign ⇓ Arm elevated to 90° Elbow flexed External rotation Head turned to opposite side Check pulse Followed by:
	Adson #1 test Head turned to injured side Demonstrates interscalene neurovascular compression Vascular form if the arm is positioned posteriorly	Roos' sign Opening/closing of hand 20–40 times Onset of paraesthesia
	Progressive abduction to 90° Diminution of the pulse Appearance of paraesthesia in C8-T1	Chandelier test For 1–3 minutes (static test) Sign of Wright or 'Lord and Rosati' Hyperabduction test Diminution of pulse (in 50% of asymptomatic subjects)

Clinical tests

The large number of clinical tests that have been proposed just goes to show their lack of complete reliability. It is possible, however, to distinguish those tests that point more to a neurological cause, from those that signal a vascular occlusion. It should be remembered that a vascular occlusion from ischaemia or stasis induces nerve ischaemia which leads rapidly to a clinical picture of nerve compression. Table 4 categorizes those clinical tests that allow TOS to be ascribed to a neurological, a vascular or mixed origin. We should remember the sign described by Morley (1913), which consists of compression of the transverse process of C7, and which reproduces the neurological symptoms of TOS, and has a reputation for reliability. The modified Adson test (Adson and Coffey 1927) reproduces the same symptoms that may be superimposed: the head is turned to the opposite side, the chin raised, the patient seated, holds his breath in full inspiration, thrusts the shoulders back and places the hands on the thighs. The Allen test has the same value in arterial forms of compression; the arm, with the elbow flexed, is elevated to 90°, is rotated externally, while the head is turned to the opposite side. In this position the absence of the radial pulse is confirmed. This test can be prolonged in this position, to look for Roos' sign (Roos 1979) in which the hand is opened and closed 20–40 times, until the onset of paraesthesia. The same clinical findings are often produced by the so-called 'chandelier test' in which the arm is placed as high as possible for 1–3 minutes.

The various neurovascular tests can bring on symptoms, in particular the Greenstone test (Narakas 1991), which involves compression of the scalenus anterior muscle on its costal insertion for 30 seconds. Closure of the costoclavicular space can be produced by the 'sentry' position, as in the tests suggested by Falconer and Weddel (1943). The Adson test consists of turning the head to the injured side thereby closing the interscalene space, producing compression of the neurovascular structures.

Placing the arm in progressive abduction to 90°, until a reduction or cessation of the radial pulse and the onset of paraesthesia in the C8-T1 territory is, according to Narakas (1991), a very reliable test for diagnosis of lower TOS.

The clinical neurological assessment must include a search for median nerve compression in the carpal tunnel or deep to the pronator teres; for ulnar nerve compression at the elbow and in Guyon's canal; and also for radial nerve compression at the level of supinator. Wood et al (1990) and Narakas (1990) have reported, respectively:

- 19% and 31% of cases of TOS with associated compression of the median nerve in the carpal tunnel,
- 2% and 15% with compression of the radial nerve at the supinator,
- 7% and 9% with ulnar nerve compression at the elbow. In total Wood and colleagues (1990) have found 44% of patients with segmental nerve compressions, and Narakas (1990) found 32.5%.

This association of nerve lesions can confuse the clinical picture and lead to misdiagnosis. It is here that EMG studies can most often contribute by helping to organize the surgical plan into a hierarchy.

Supplementary examinations

Radiological assessment

Frontal and lateral X-rays of the cervical spine are arranged routinely. It should be possible to assess this with depression of the shoulders, which allows the visualization of all seven cervical bodies in lateral view. It is important to establish the presence of a cervical rib, and this may be unilateral or bilateral (in 50% of cases). Assessment of the configuration and associated anomalies of the first rib is equally systematic. Rarely, there is evidence of malunion of the clavicle leading to neurovascular compression. Hypertrophy of the coracoid process or in exceedingly rare cases pseudoarthrosis of the first rib (Borelly et al 1984) can be the cause of TOS.

CT scans

Any indication is limited to a search for bony lesions or tumours.

Magnetic resonance imaging

The contribution of magnetic resonance imaging (MRI) appears much more promising insofar as this allows visualization of the brachial plexus, muscle tissue and fibrous bands attached to the origin of C7. These scans can be used to delineate an anomalous course of the brachial plexus and adjacent vessels. Interpretation of MRI scans is still difficult but in the future improvement in image quality should allow much greater precision in assessing which anatomical structures are effectively the cause of the vascular or neurological compression.

Arterial and venous Doppler studies

In a systematic evaluation, the goal of this approach is to search for a vascular complication in the form of a stenosis, a post-stenotic aneurysm or a partial thrombosis. In cases of vascular anomaly found by Doppler, it is appropriate to arrange arteriography.

Arteriography

Arteriography is as much indicated following identification of lesions by Doppler, as when the patient is found to have bony abnormalities, particularly a cervical rib (Figures 4 and 5). While the majority of authors acknowledge that the general views obtained during the course of arteriography are of little interest, on the other hand angiography itself allows clarification of the degree of compression of the subclavian artery by the first rib and by the scalenus anterior muscle in front. The finding of stenosis of the subclavian artery is most often accompanied by a post-stenotic dilatation (Figures 6 and 7). These lesions usually settle after removal of the compressing structure. In contrast, the presence of intrinsic abnormalities of the vessel wall will lead to intimal ulceration and produce an aneurysm, together with an array of possible associated complications such as thrombosis and thrombo-embolism. At this stage treatment of the compression alone does not suffice, and it is necessary to reconstruct the artery, usually preceded by embolectomy.

Venography

This is only justified in the presence of oedema of the hand or upper limb together with cyanosis and dilatation of the superficial venous system. The appearance of cramps, paraesthesia and heaviness of the upper limb should lead to the request for a Doppler study, which can confirm intermittent occlusion of the vein in various positions of the arm. This investigation should be complimented with venography, to assess the tributaries of the subclavian venous system. Venography and Doppler assessment are essential when there has been an acute venous thrombosis (Figure 8).

EMG with nerve conduction studies

This approach is chosen to distinguish the neurological forms of TOS. This must be carried out by an electromyographer trained in assessing nerve conduction velocity on either side of the clavicle, over short distances. There is undoubtedly a technical know-how which renders this examination more reliable. In those clinical cases that are not clear-cut, this examination allows a differentiation between neurological syndromes originating from C5-C6-C7, and those originating in C8-T1.

In long-standing cases of C8-T1 compression, EMG assessment can focus on the intrinsic muscles of the hand, denervation of which is a sign of prolonged compression of the plexus, and suggests a poor prognosis. Our experience has shown that, on those occasions in which diagnosis was made on EMG grounds, patients obtained good or excellent results following surgical decompression. On the other hand, when the diagnosis could not be clearly established using EMG techniques, but the clinical signs did however point towards a diagnosis of TOS, we have not been able to obtain such good results after surgery.

This examination should not be limited solely to the assessment of brachial plexus lesions; it should also be carried out routinely to assess the median nerve in its passage through the carpal tunnel and deep to the pronator teres, the ulnar nerve at the elbow and in Guyon's canal and, less frequently, for the radial nerve within the supinator. It should be borne in mind that a double level compression can be revealed in 30–40% of cases.

Sensory-evoked potentials

One criticism of EMG is the difficulty of stimulation of Erb's point in order to calculate conduction velocity. To get round this problem, one suggestion has been to carry out sensory-evoked potentials. Although this technique may be very precise, it should be recognized that the findings are not guaranteed to establish with any certainty compression of the brachial plexus and its branches as they pass through the thoracic outlet (Brudon 1989).

All in all, it is advisable to be rigorous when requesting complimentary investigations in TOS. When dealing with a predominantly vascular syndrome, the first investigation to request is the Doppler, which allows an assessment of flow within the arteries and veins or reductions in flow, or vascular occlusion with different positions of the upper limb. This examination should be supplemented by arteriography and venography in cases of confirmed anomalies. In contrast, in cases of TOS with a neurological origin, EMG studies carried out by a trained neurophysiologist are of most value in diagnosing either an upper lesion (C5-C6-C7) or a lower lesion (C8-T1). Studies using echography can be used to investigate vascular lesions that may be associated with a neurological syndrome. The use of sensory-evoked potentials produces uncertain results and should not be a first-line investigation.

In contrast, MRI is likely to be the investigation of the future, as this will allow delineation of the majority of anatomical anomalies in the supraclavicular region.

Differential diagnosis

Clinical examination of the cervical spine, the supraclavicular and axillary areas, the shoulder and the thoracic outlet region has to be thorough, as a large number of pathologies from these regions present with upper limb pain; TOS represents only 5% of such upper limb pain. It should be remembered that C5-C6 root pain is common and can result from cervical spondylosis, a herniated disc, following fractures, etc., and less frequently from a tumour. The symptoms and signs of rotator cuff compression usually allow a specific diagnosis which can be distinguished from that caused by a compression of the suprascapular nerve in the coracoid notch. The careful examiner may have difficulty distinguishing TOS from an algodystrophy syndrome of the upper limb with its collection of inflammatory signs and articular stiffness. The various peripheral nerve compression syndromes must be distinguished clinically from TOS, bearing in mind that these are frequently associated, and need to be taken into account in treatment. Finally, when neurological symptoms dominate the clinical picture, the possibility of other diagnoses, such as amyotrophic lateral sclerosis, multiple sclerosis, syringomyelia, scleroderma and Von Recklinghausen's disease among others, should be considered.

Treatment

Conservative treatment

An improved understanding of the various levels of lesions in TOS has led to the creation of logical rehabilitation protocols that aim to improve the posture of the spine, to open up the anatomical planes and to enhance abdomino-diaphragmatic respiration. The protocols put forward at the Mayo Clinic by Peet et al in 1956, then by Smith in 1979, Sallstrom and Celegin in 1983, Aligne and Barral in 1992 and Novak in 1992 have undoubtedly improved symptoms in young patients tackled early, presenting with a predominantly neurological clinical picture, and without bony anomalies of the cervical spine. Together these authors have reported improvements, even disappearance of symptoms, in 66–87.5% of cases, with a follow-up of > 4 years. In 10–20% of cases, the rehabilitation programme exacerbates the neurological and/or vascular symptoms, and precipitates a need for operative intervention, most often decompression in the interscalene space.

The protocol suggested by Aligne and Barral (1992) is logical. Repeated from the start, three times weekly, and accompanied by daily exercises, supervised by the same observer, this consists of seven types of exercise:

- Spinal posture re-education which aims to correct imbalances of the cervical spine.
- Respiratory kinestherapy to reinforce the abdominal muscles and the diaphragm.
- Massage techniques designed to decrease the contractions around the muscles of the neck and the scapular region.
- Movements designed to relax the muscles around the scapula using the weight of the upper limb.
- Active re-enforcement of the suspensory muscles of the scapular region.
- Global exercises to reinforce the musculature contributing to elevation and extension of the shoulder joint.
- Specific exercises aimed at the sternocleidomastoid muscle, the serratus anterior, the upper fibres of the trapezius and around the levator scapulae.

Together these exercises, followed for a period of 6–8 weeks, aim to reinforce the action of 'opening' muscles – namely the upper and middle fibres of trapezius, the muscles around the angle of the scapula, and sternocleidomastoid; and to relax the 'closing' muscles – which include the scalenus anterior and medius, subclavius, and pectoralis major and pectoralis minor muscles. It must be recognized that surgeons tend to be sceptical about this type of conservative treatment, as they tend only to see treatment failures in the clinic. It is equally likely that teams of therapists sufficiently familiar with these protocols and who have a good anatomical and pathophysiological knowledge of TOS are insufficient in number.

We have spoken to several teams of rehabilitation physicians about the success of these techniques, and they do not have the same enthusiasm for these as do the protagonists of rehabilitation protocols. Many treatment failures arise from a heterogeneous population of patients with uncertain diagnoses of TOS, and in whom motivation is not great. Better education of these teams and rigorous patient selection should, in the future, restore the place of conservative treatment.

Surgical treatment

The choice of surgical approach remains controversial. While Roos' transaxillary approach is used most frequently for ablation of the first rib, one should not underestimate the cervical approach, which is irreplaceable when carrying out resection of a cervical rib, and/or correction of ligamentous and muscular anomalies. Other surgical techniques, such as claviculectomy, infraclavicular, posterior, extra-plural, anterolateral, and trans-plural approaches, for carrying out resection of the first rib, have all become obsolete and have given way to approaches using the axillary, cervical, supra- and infraclavicular routes.

The cervical approach

The patient is placed supine with a support beneath the ipsilateral shoulder, the head is turned towards the contralateral side, and the operating table is adjusted so that the patient is inclined 30°. The upper limb is left completely free within the operative field so as to allow it to be placed in all the possible positions causing compression. A 5–6 cm transverse skin incision placed within a neck crease and located 2 cm from the clavicle begins at the lateral border of the sternocleidomastoid muscle, which is found by palpation. The platysma muscle is elevated with the skin flap and the external jugular vein is preserved. After dissection and preservation of the subcutaneous tissues, the lateral border of the sternocleidomastoid is freed up and retracted medially. The omohyoid is encountered next within the operative field, and is freed up and retracted with slings to allow access to the upper and middle trunks and the suprascapular nerve. The scalenus anterior muscle is isolated as far as its attachment to the first rib. The subclavian artery is easily identified and controlled with slings. The subclavian artery is easily identified and a vessel loop is placed around this. Before proceeding to scalenotomy or scalenectomy, it is important to visualize the phrenic nerve; usually this is found running along the medial border of the scalenus anterior, and does not interfere with the operative field. However, when a scalenectomy is required and the nerve is adherent to the anterior surface of the scalene muscle, it is necessary to dissect the nerve and retract it with slings. It is helpful to separate the inferior portion of the scalenus anterior with a dissector. Its detachment can be carried out quite safely without risk of damaging the subclavian artery. Upward retraction of the scalenus anterior allows a good view of the roots, and the upper and middle trunks of the brachial plexus. Dissecting the subclavian artery over several centimetres allows the artery to be retracted, and gives access to the C8-T1 roots. At this point in the procedure the anatomical structures in the supraclavicular region that are liable to compress the plexus and the vessels are displayed by placing the upper limb in various positions. Several options are available to the surgeon, as outlined below.

- Anterior scalenectomy is justified if the muscle mass is compressing or separating the roots of the plexus in the vicinity of the transverse processes, and also to avoid fibrous contracture, which can lead subsequently to intractable neurological symptoms.
- Division or resection of the scalenus medius is a further important procedure designed to free the inferior roots and the subclavian artery in their passage around this muscle. However, this manoeuvre does require complete visualization of the long thoracic nerve, whose passage is in part intramuscular. Identification of this 1-mm diameter nerve is not always straightforward, and we advise the use of a nerve stimulator set at 1 mA (Variostim) to help locate the nerve.

  Supernumerary fibres and muscular structures such as the scalenus minimus are most easily accessed once the scalenus anterior and scalenus medius are detached or resected. In this way it is possible to carry out excision of the transversoseptocostal ligament or its equivalent, the scalenus minimus, which can be found between the subclavian artery and the plexus. In the region of the first rib, the costoseptocostal ligament, which forms a true buttonhole around the T1 root, can be found with the finger.
- Exploration of the subclavian space is more difficult. It is possible, however, to proceed with excision of the subclavius muscle, but greater difficulty and greater danger are encountered with division of the medial coracoclavicular ligament, bearing in mind the poor visualization of the subclavian vein.
- Resection of a cervical rib is necessary irrespective of the anatomical type (four types of Gruber)

(Gruber 1869). It is recommended that the rib is disarticulated posteriorly and detached from the synostosis or synchondrosis with the first rib (Gruber type 3, which is the commonest), or to resect the fibrous or muscular bands which are attached in the incomplete type (type 2).

- Resection of the first rib: this is technically feasible, but can be difficult to carry out for several reasons. The approach to the posterior arc of the first rib, which allows its disarticulation, requires an extensive dissection of the brachial plexus to free it up medially. It is then preferable to choose an incision along the line of the sternocleidomastoid, as the disarticulation of the first rib without putting the brachial plexus at risk involves dissection of the upper trunk of the plexus and the C5-C6 roots. Frequently the surgeon struggling with the transverse cervical approach leaves behind a segment of > 1 cm of the posterior part of the rib, and this can produce a chronic neuralgia of the brachial plexus. On the other hand, the approach to the anterior part of the first rib is not easy because the narrow anatomical space does not allow control of the subclavian vein.

  In our experience we have only been able to carry out this type of first rib resection in tall thin patients who have good movement at the sternoclavicular joint. This type of manoeuvre carried out in heavier patients with a short neck can be hazardous for the vessels and the brachial plexus. For these reasons we would advise against this approach.
- Microsurgical neurolysis, usually involving roots C7-C8-T1, and limited to simple epineurotomy to decompress the fascicular groups which are encroached on by the epineural reaction.
- At the end of the procedure, it is advisable to confirm that haemostasis has been achieved, and this is done purely with bipolar coagulation. Each haematoma is a formidable complication for the brachial plexus, especially if intraneural neurolysis proves necessary. It is wise to place a suction drain beneath the skin of the neck for 3 days. In addition, the risk of breaching the pleura is significant; this can be confirmed by carrying out positive pressure ventilation after the subclavian space has been filled with Ringer's lactate solution. Usually this consists of several tears in the pleura which can be repaired with a simple suture, or sealed off with Tissucol®. In this situation no chest drain is used. Strict postoperative immobilization is not enforced. A sling is used to elevate the upper limb for 3 weeks. Working and sporting activities can be resumed between 3 and 4 weeks postoperatively.

The axillary approach (Figure 9)

The anatomical study of the Roos transaxillary approach (Merle and Borrelly 1987) demonstrated the feasibility of dissecting the medial cord of the plexus as far as the C8-T1 roots. To be able to do this requires careful positioning of the patient, who is placed in lateral decubitus, tilted to 60° with sandbags, and raised to 30°. This places the root of the axilla on a horizontal plane, the surgeon stands behind the patient, and requires two assistants – the first by the surgeon's side, to direct the lighting, the other opposite, who can lift the arm vertically, which allows distraction of the contents of the root of the axilla and its enclosed neurovascular structures. The skin incision is curved, running from the latissimus dorsi to the pectoralis major. The dissection is carried out along the whole length of the intercostal muscle, which is covered by the serratus anterior, all the while preserving both the thoraco-brachial nerve anastomosis emerging from the second intercostal nerve (damage to which can produce intolerable pain), as well as the long thoracic nerve. Theoretically it is better to carry out extra-periosteal resection of the first rib, to prevent new bone formation and possible recurrence of the compression. In reality the surgeon is concerned with detaching and separating the scalenus anterior and scalenus medius, and freeing all the ligamentous and muscular attachments from the first rib, which usually results in a subperiosteal resection. Narakas (1991) feels that subperiosteal rib resection does not represent any risk, as long as the surgeon is careful to divide the suspensory ligaments of the pleura, which allows the pleural dome to be lowered by several centimetres. Initially the rib is detached in a single manoeuvre at the level of its convexity, and then the scalenus anterior and medius are divided, taking great care to separate these from the fibrous arch which can unite them. Failure to carry out this manoeuvre leads to traction on the upper part of the plexus and the artery from the scalenus anterior and medius joined by this fibrous sling; this creates a

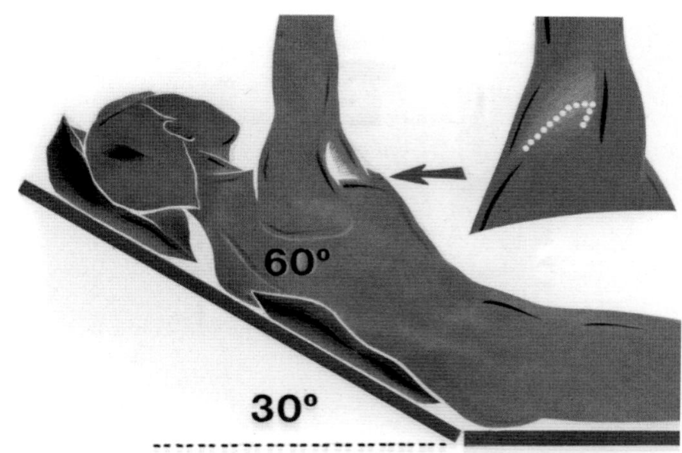

Figure 22.9

Patient position for the Roos approach.

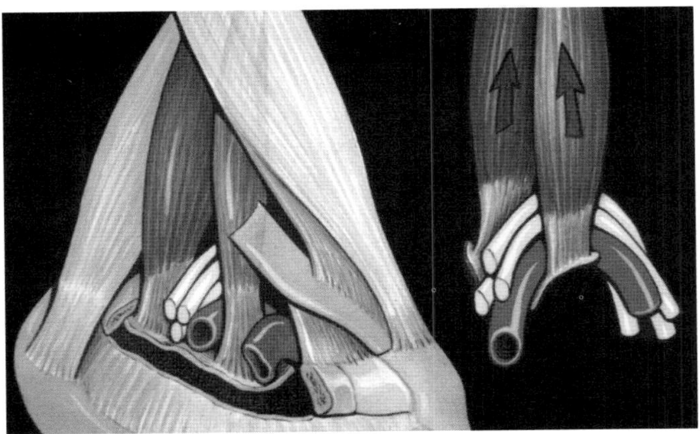

Figure 22.10

'Hammock' effect produced by a false aponeurosis between the scalenus anterior and medius. Postoperative exacerbation of symptoms is explained by traction created by the scalene muscles.

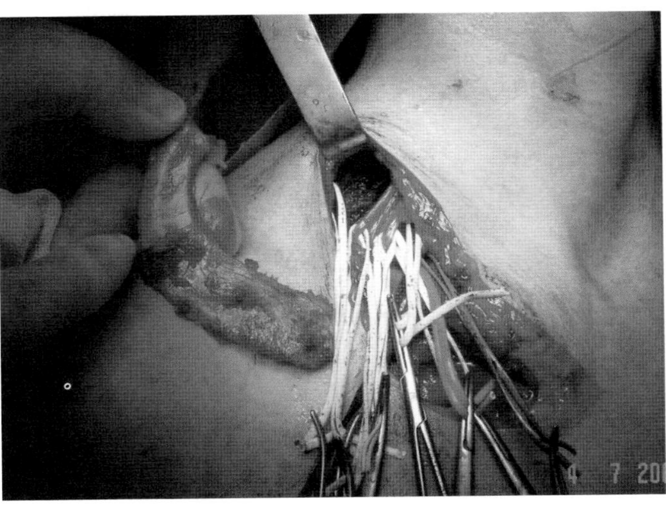

Figure 22.11

Resection of the first rib using the supra- and infra-clavicular approach of Cormier.

hammock effect, and the patient will experience an aggravation of symptoms in the postoperative period (Figure 10). Next, the concavity of the first rib is elevated and the costoseptocostal ligament (which produces a buttonhole effect, through which the T1 root may pass) is divided. Failure to carry out this manoeuvre may lead to avulsion of the root at the time of removal of the first rib. Usually division of the first rib can be carried out in two segments, and posterior disarticulation is achieved; however, when this approach is difficult, division of the rib can be carried out with a costotome, leaving a 1-cm fragment of rib, which can be rounded off or removed with the rongeur. Anterior division must be carried out painstakingly, as this takes place in the vicinity of the subclavian vein. Having completed resection of the rib, it is advisable to ensure that there are no remaining bony fragments which might damage the vein, the subclavian artery, or brachial plexus. The standard costotome leaves an oblique sharp bony stump in place. If any remaining fibres of the scalenus anterior remain attached to the stump, this can lead to compression of the subclavian vein. It is important to check for this possibility and to complete resection of the rib using a rongeur and a long narrow lighted retractor, which also helps to retract the subclavian vein. Neurolysis of C8-T1 is carried out at this point with the help of loupe magnification, as introduction of the microscope is not feasible. This manoeuvre is usually restricted to a decompression epineurotomy at the level of the epineural sheath. To carry this out we use titanium microsurgical forceps with long rounded stems and micro-claws (Fontax).

This axillary approach allows division of the following: the muscle of Langer, the coracoid attachment of the pectoralis minor and the medial coracoclavicular ligament. Although technically feasible, resection of a cervical rib by the axillary approach is not satisfactory insofar as this does not allow control of the supraclavicular musculo-ligamentous system, which may be involved in compression of neurovascular structures. Just as likely is the possibility that the axillary approach does not allow the surgeon to perform a scalenectomy. At the end of the procedure the operative field is irrigated with Ringer's lactate, which allows nerve stimulation of the brachial plexus and its various branches, to clear away any tissue debris from the operative field, and to confirm air-tightness of the pleura. Skin closure is carried out over a suction drain or a size 20 or 24 chest drain, if a pneumothorax has been noted.

Work and exercise are resumed at the end of the fourth postoperative week.

The supra- and infra-clavicular approach of Cormier (Figure 11)

This is the surgical approach (Ward and Cormier 1986, Cormier et al 1994) that we favour for treating vascular and neurovascular types of compression that demand resection of the first rib and decompression of the brachial plexus. We have modified the incision on aesthetic grounds. The incision begins three fingerbreadths from the mastoid process and runs along the lateral border of the sternocleidomastoid muscle as far as the superior border of the clavicle, which the incision follows as far as its middle third, and then forms a lazy 'S' and reaches the first intercostal space as far as the sternocostal junction.

The infraclavicular approach begins with the detachment of the most medial fibres of the pectoralis major by electrodissection, taking care to preserve the neurovascular pedicle of the muscle. The pectoralis minor does not necessarily obstruct the access, and this can be held with a Farabeuf retractor. The superior border of the anterior arch of the first rib is freed up using an elevator, as is the lateral border, which gives better access to the sternocostal joint. During this approach, which should be meticulous as the subclavian vein has not yet been brought under control, it is advisable to ask the assistant to elevate the shoulder to enhance the visibility of the costoclavicular space and to detach the most medial insertions of the scalenus anterior muscle.

When the subclavian vein is compressed by the pincer action of the costoclavicular junction, the vein can enlarge with a diameter up to 15 mm. Upward traction of the clavicle can lead to rapid emptying of the vein, and facilitates its dissection. Next the intercostal muscles are detached and the pleura, which is often adherent to the inferior border of the first rib, is lifted off, using pledgets or else just with the finger. It is at this point that the pleura can be torn, and this is not strictly a complication, but in fact a useful method of draining the operative field, as we shall demonstrate later. A tissue forceps is placed around the clavicle, avoiding breaching the periosteum to avoid damage to the bone, and this will help to elevate the clavicle in order to clear the costoclavicular space. The muscle and ligament detachments are carried out from the inferior border of the first rib towards its middle segment.

This is also a good approach for assessing the superior border of the first rib in the search for the presence of a possible costoseptocostal ligament, scalene attachments and vertebrocostal ligaments. At this point the first rib can be divided at the level of the sternocostal articulation using a rongeur; the mobility thus produced allows detachment of the musculotendinous structures further back on the middle segment of the rib, opening up the supraclavicular space.

For the supraclavicular approach the skin is elevated, paying attention to the sensory cervical nerve branches and also the emergence of the spinal accessory nerve at the posterior border of the sternocleidomastoid muscle, three finger-breadths from the mastoid process. The omohyoid muscle is easily located, dissected and retracted. This is a good anatomical landmark, because immediately behind the muscle the upper trunk of the brachial plexus can be found and 1 cm inferior on its lateral border is the emergence of the suprascapular nerve, which has a diameter varying from 1.5 mm to 2 mm. Access to the trunks of the brachial plexus is often hindered by an abundance of fatty connective tissue. This should be preserved and retracted laterally, as this tissue will help with recovery of the neurolysed brachial plexus. Having retracted the upper and middle trunks of the plexus as well as the suprascapular nerve, the dissection returns to the scalenus anterior muscle, which is still attached to the first rib by several of its fibres. The subclavian artery is now clearly visible, it is dissected over 2 cm to 3 cm and retracted, and the same procedure is carried out for the lower trunk, which lies side by side posterior to the artery. Division of a fibrous attachment to the first rib between the scalenus anterior and the scalenus medius is essential, to avoid the creation of a sling which could produce upward traction on the subclavian artery and the brachial plexus. Early in our experience we limited this to scalenotomy alone, taking great care to separate the scalenus anterior and scalenus medius, but we found that some of our patients developed fibrous contractures which resulted in intractable nerve pain. We have subsequently progressed to a total removal of the anterior scalene and partial resection of the scalenus medius. These two important manoeuvres require preliminary identification of the phrenic nerve and the long thoracic nerve.

The phrenic nerve is sometimes difficult to locate at the distal end of the scalenus anterior, in which case it is wise to look for it as it emerges from the C4-C5 roots and to retract it to allow anterior scalenectomy. Likewise the identification of the long thoracic nerve can be achieved by retracting the upper and middle trunks of the plexus medially, to allow visualization of the scalenus medius. If the nerve, which is < 1 mm in diameter, runs on the anterolateral part of the muscle, it is easily identified and dissected; however, if its course is intramuscular it is advisable to search for the nerve using a nerve stimulator (Variostim) calibrated to 1 mA.

At this stage all the neurovascular structures are under control and the approach to the middle and posterior segments of the first rib can continue. The entire brachial plexus is retracted medially and the freeing up which has been achieved as far as the upper roots C5-C6 facilitates access to the transversocostal junction.

The first rib has been freed of all its muscular and ligamentous attachments, particularly along the superior border, which can trap the T1 root when a costoseptal-costal ligament is present. Using a rongeur the posterior segment of the rib is divided immediately adjacent to the transversocostal articulation. In all cases the residual stump should not be greater than 1 cm and should be smoothed off with a nibbler to prevent later impingement on the trunks of the brachial plexus. Removal of the first rib is routinely carried out from a superior to inferior direction by the infraclavicular route.

Microsurgical neurolysis is carried out with the aid of loupe magnification and is usually limited to epineurotomy to avoid impairing the vascularity. Epineurotomy of the C7 root is often required, as the epineural thickening may be considerable. Likewise the C8-T1 roots are often arranged side by side with dense epineural covering, and neurolysis is often necessary. Lavage of the operative field with Ringer's lactate solution allows removal of all tissue debris while retaining the capacity for electrostimulation of the plexus. In the presence of a pneumothorax, a chest drain is placed in the anterior part of the second intercostal space and left for 2–3 days. This drainage is certainly essential for inflating the lung, but we have also found that this is equally good for draining the supra- and infra-clavicular spaces. Such

Table 22.5 *Results of surgical treatment of TOS by technique and author**

Authors	*Supraclavicular approach*									*Axillary approach of Roos*			*Axillary and cervical approach*		
	Cervical rib + scalenus			*First rib*			*Scalenectomy*								
	Excellent	*Good*	*Poor*	*Excellent*	*Good*	*Poor*	*Excellent*	*Good*	*Poor*	*Excellent*	*Good*	*Poor*	*Excellent*	*Good*	*Poor*
Adson (1947)	79	11.5	3.8				81	6	12						
Narakas (1989)	66.7	19	14.3	50	50	0	53.8	30.8	15.4	76.6	8.3	15	66.6	33.3	
Merle (1995)								54	30	16					
Cormier-Kieffer (1982)				56	31	13									
Sanders (1979)				72						86	4	10			
Roos (1982)										92.2	5.6	2.2			
Qvafordt et al (1984)													94.7	4.3	1

* Values are given as percentages.

patients develop less postoperative scarring in contrast to those we have seen treated with simple suction drains.

Closure of the supraclavicular approach is carried out by placing the fatty connective tissue over the neurolysed brachial plexus and suturing in two planes. In the infraclavicular approach, the pectoralis major is attached to the clavicle or surrounding tissues. The elbow is immobilized against the trunk for 3 weeks.

Complications and technical limitations of surgery

Experience with 125 patients between 1985 and 2001 has enabled us to carry out 192 surgical procedures, of which 115 used the cervical approach, 38 were transaxillary approaches and 40 used the supra- and infraclavicular approach of Cormier.

Table 5 summarizes the complications and technical difficulties encountered according to the approach used. Undoubtedly the axillary approach of Roos results in the majority of problems reported here; 30% of the Cormier approaches carried out by ourselves were revisions which we undertook following a failure of surgery by the axillary route.

Cervical approach

Peroperative complications

We have only encountered one palsy of the long thoracic nerve in which the nerve had an intramuscular course within the scalenus medius. Following this complication we routinely use a nerve stimulator to identify the long thoracic nerve before carrying out a scalenectomy. One chylothorax was successfully treated by thoracic drainage and low fat diet for 15 days.

Technical difficulties

In our series of 115 cervicotomies we have had to reoperate eight times to carry out first rib resection. Initially these eight patients had undergone surgery for an interscalene syndrome, without removal of the first rib, most commonly anterior scalenectomy. Narakas (1989) showed how this interscalene syndrome evolves into a costoclavicular syndrome. When the oblique plane of the first rib is further inclined, because it is no longer held by the scalenus anterior attachment, the neurovascular structures tend to move medially and to become blocked in the depth of the acute angle which makes up the costoclavicular 'pincer.' Sunderland also reported this complication and we have encountered a small series keeping the most medial costal attachments of the scalenus anterior while at the same time detaching the scalenus medius to allow the neurovascular pedicle to move backwards freely during abduction of the arm (Allieu et al 1991). Unfortunately this mechanistic approach has not allowed us to abolish all symptoms, particularly neurological symptoms, and we have returned to using as complete a scalenectomy as possible in the purely neurological types of compression. In contrast, in those nine cases in which we have had to re-operate, we have used the supra- and infra-clavicular approach of Cormier to achieve first rib resection safely.

Axillary approach of Roos

In our series (Merle and Borrelly 2002) the transaxillary approach of Roos resulted in a high level of complications or technical difficulties (28 of 38 cases, 73.6%), of which 13 revisions were in patients operated on by other surgeons. We have not counted a pneumothorax as a complication, as we feel that thoracic drainage allows better re-attachment of the pleural dome than extrapleural drainage.

Injury to the subclavian artery was complicated by aneurysm formation, leading to embolism of the radial artery. The aneurysm was treated with venous grafting, followed later by grafting of the radial artery, but without success. It is recommended that aneurysms are treated effectively. Melliere et al (1985) reported a case of corrective surgery to treat a double subclavian aneurysm caused by cervical rib, which culminated in amputation of the forearm. Peroperative injury to the subclavian vein is equally difficult to treat, and is often subject to a difficult repair owing to the restricted and deep surgical field, resulting in stenosis and occasionally a thrombosis.

The **phrenic palsy** which we report probably arose from a detachment of the scalenus anterior which was carried out without direct vision. With the cervical approach, the phrenic nerve is easily identifiable on the anterior surface of the scalenus anterior, on its upper part. It is not always visible, as the muscle runs medially lower down, and one can see how the nerve may not be seen directly in the transaxillary approach.

Narakas reported 1 case out of 102 operations, Batt et al (1983) reported 1 case out of 112 cases. The majority of authors report 0.5–6% (Sharp et al 2001) of phrenic palsy using the transaxillary approach.

Root avulsion of T1 is better understood following the anatomical studies of Poitevin. The lower trunk and the T1 root is on one hand adherent to the first rib and on the other hand can be trapped by a costoseptocostal ligament. En bloc removal of the first rib can result quite literally in intramedullary avulsion of the root. The surgeon's finger should examine the superior border of the first rib to confirm the absence of any remaining fibrous or ligamentous structures. Such a root injury is irreparable and leaves sensory and motor sequelae in the hand which often lead to medicolegal claims.

Paralysis of the long thoracic nerve results in a winged scapula, which is often poorly tolerated by the patient. The number of injured nerves in the transaxillary approach varies according to author, Wood et al (1988) reported 14 such cases in a series of 100, Sharp et al (2001) reported 1 out of 36, Batt et al (1983) 1 out of 112. The nerve, which has a tiny diameter (1 mm), can be completely concealed when its course is entirely intramuscular within the scalenus medius. A partial or total scalenectomy of the scalenus medius via the transaxillary route risks the continuity of the nerve. It is advisable to avoid this complication by using a nerve stimulator, which will identify its course without difficulty. For correction of this complication we have given up procedures which involve fixation with fascia lata, preferring instead the transfer of teres major onto the medial border of the scapula.

Causalgia syndrome with transient palsy of the brachial plexus is caused by excessive upward traction of the patient's arm by the assistant. It has to be admitted that the assistant's role is particularly thankless and uncomfortable, as the arm has to be placed under traction throughout the procedure to expose the superior border of the first rib and to open up the costoclavicular 'pincer' without having the slightest view of the operative field.

Overweight or very muscular patients require considerable traction, which may be the cause of neuropraxia, axonotmesis or avulsion of the C8-T1 roots of the brachial plexus. Horowitz (1985) reported four cases of causalgia syndromes following ablation of the first rib by the transaxillary approach. The symptoms encountered were suggestive of partial or total avulsion of the C8, T1 roots in three of the four published cases. The clinical picture is severe, with a causalgia syndrome leading to depression, a need for strong analgesics, accompanied by a sensorimotor deficit in the median and ulnar nerve territories. Throughout the operative procedure it is important to check the surgical assistant and to allow them to relax the upper limb so as to avoid not just severe and prolonged traction of the brachial plexus, but also ischaemia. The two cases we have encountered presented with a neurological deficit which resolved over a period of 1 year, suggesting a mixed neuropractic and axonotmetic lesion. These two well-built patients required treatment based on strong analgesics and antidepressants.

Partial or total lesions of the intercostobrachial nerve produce paraesthesiae or poorly tolerated anaesthesia along the medial and posterior border of the arm. The passage of time and local treatments such as massage, physiotherapy, infiltration of anaesthetic and steroids hardly ever help the situation. In our two cases we opted for extensive dissection of the neuroma and the surrounding tissue within the intercostal muscle. To avoid this complication we decided early on to use a curved incision, with superior convexity in the root of the axilla, so as to avoid this nerve crossing the operative field.

The 'hammock' syndrome (Borrelly et al 1984) (Figure 10) is formidable, and is produced by a failure of separation of the scalenus anterior and scalenus medius, which are joined together on the superior border or the first rib by pseudo-aponeurosis. Released by rouginage of the costal periosteum, this aponeurosis produces superior displacement of the subclavian artery and the lower trunk of the plexus, even the middle trunk (C7). On waking up, the patient develops a clinical picture of hyperalgesia, even partial ischaemia of the upper limb. These patients are wrongly labelled delicate, emotionally sensitive or depressives. The surgeon has the impression of a problem-free procedure, as he or she has carried out ablation of the first rib. This explains late revisions carried out by a different surgical team.

In those revisions carried out using a cervical approach, the dissection is always difficult, particularly with respect to the subclavian artery, which is literally crushed and stretched upwards by the hammock created by the scalenus anterior and medius. Once the scalenes are separated and resected, neurolysis of brachial plexus is made easier, the epineural reaction is always considerable and requires a decompressive epineurotomy.

Inadequate resection of fibrous or muscular structures. The suspensory ligament of the pleura (transversoseptocostal ligament, vertebroseptocostal ligament, costoseptocostal ligament, scalenus minimus) can lead to a chronic neuralgia involving the roots C7, C8, T1 and the lower trunk of the plexus. These structures are not readily accessible by the transaxillary approach and their 'en bloc' detachment explains the patient's residual pain. In our experience we have had to re-operate each time, using the supraclavicular approach to carry out resection of these residual ligamentous structures and also with the addition of neurolysis with epineurotomies.

Inadequate resection of the scalenus anterior and scalenus medius

Detachment of the scalenes in isolation is insufficient to guarantee a complete result that is long-lasting. Subperiosteal resection of the first rib can lead to regrowth of the first rib as described by Narakas (1991). The fibrous tissue developing from the scalenus anterior and scalenus medius once again creates a real constriction of the brachial plexus, which requires subsequent neurolysis via the supraclavicular approach. The transaxillary approach of Roos undoubtedly hinders the execution of scalenectomy without endangering the phrenic nerve and the long thoracic nerve. Many of the intermediate or poor results quoted in previous series can probably be explained by such technical difficulties.

Inadequate resection of the anterior segment of the first rib

This is a technical shortcoming which is largely neglected in the literature, in contrast to the majority of series which stress inadequacy of resection of the posterior segment of the rib (Urshel and Razzuk 1986). We were surprised by the five cases in which we undertook revision for clinical findings of oedema (two cases) and pain (five cases) requiring continued opiate treatment. It has to be admitted that it is only by increasing the number of radiographic examinations in the region of the first rib that the importance of the residual anterior segment of the rib has been demonstrated.

While the majority of authors make no mention of the residual anterior segment, this is because they have the operative impression that section of the rib has been carried out as close to the chondrosternal cartilage as possible. The anterior segments that we have excised as a secondary procedure all had a sharp oblique cut conforming to that of the costotome used. This bony prominence came into direct contact with the brachial plexus. By contrast, compression of the subclavian artery and vein is due to superior movement of the residual anterior segment of the rib under the influence of the scalene muscles that had not been fully resected. The two patients in whom subsequent resection of the anterior segment was carried out after several years noticed a resolution of their upper limb oedema several hours after the surgical procedure. While the costotome is invaluable in carrying out division of the first rib, it is also necessary to complete the resection at the level of the chondrosternal and costotransversal articulation using a rongeur. For carrying out these surgical revisions on the anterior segment of the first rib, we have made use of the supra- and infra-clavicular approach of Cormier, which allowed control of the subclavian vein by the infraclavicular route and of the entire brachial plexus and the subclavian artery by the supraclavicular route.

Chronic neuritis produced by widespread scarring

In three cases, we have had to re-operate for chronic neuritis associated with widespread scarring in the absence of scalene or ligamentous components in contact with the lower roots of the brachial plexus. These fibrous reactions have probably been caused by 'laborious' surgery, a poorly drained haematoma and premature rehabilitation. Our series demonstrates that it is just as easy to drain a haematoma with a chest drain placed following disruption of the pleura as by a drain placed in the region of the pleural dome. We feel that the residual scarring produced by the haematoma is subsequently less important. Furthermore, in the supraclavicular approach we preserve the fatty and connective tissue, which can be used to cover the brachial plexus at the close of the procedure, aiding recovery.

Finally, when considering the space left by ablation of the first rib, it is better for the patient to keep the elbow immobilized against the trunk for 3 weeks before undertaking overall rehabilitation of the upper limb.

This series of complications has led Roos to revise his technical criteria for prevention of recurrence:

1. Extraperiosteal resection of the first rib.
2. Costal stump as short as possible.
3. Resection of all abnormal musculo-aponeurotic structures.
4. Perfect haemostasis.
5. Repeated washing of the wound before closure.
6. Limited movement of the shoulder and the arm for 3 months.

Supra- and infra-clavicular approach according to Cormier

None of the complications described above with the axillary and cervical approaches has been encountered in this approach, with the exception of a dissection of the subclavian artery which became apparent immediately postoperatively, probably after a difficult dissection of the artery which had been very adherent to the remnants of the scalenus anterior. This had previously been the subject of a partial scalenotomy via a transverse cervicotomy, and ligature of a collateral artery situated very close to the subclavian artery. Placement of a stent allowed the immediate return of the radial pulse.

The aesthetic aspect of the cutaneous scar is open to criticism, as well as the localized atrophy of the pectoral muscle, which is inserted into the anteromedial border of the clavicle – although we have reduced these problems by modifying the incision. This modification using a lazy 'S' begins above the clavicle and runs along the sternocleidomastoid, turns horizontally 5 cm above the superior border of the clavicle, and then obliquely medial reaches the first intercostal space, ending in the vicinity of the chondrosternal junction. This approach reduces the risk of retractile scarring and hypertrophic scar, moreover this allows us to limit the detachment of the most medial fibres of the pectoralis major, and also allows comfortable access to the brachial plexus and extensive dissection of this as far as the C5-C6 roots, which will be required in surgical revisions when identifying the phrenic nerve and the long thoracic nerve, and providing access to the residual stump of the posterior segment of the first rib.

Surgical indications

Segmental compressions

Before deciding on decompression of neurovascular structures by the cervical, axillary or supra/infraclavicular approach, it is better to treat peripheral compression syndromes, which are seen in 30–40% of patients who present with TOS (carpal tunnel at the wrist, pronator syndrome, ulnar nerve at the elbow, radial nerve within supinator). We avoid combining plexus surgery and peripheral nerve surgery in the same operation. Resolution of the symptoms associated with peripheral nerve compression syndromes allows us to better define the clinical picture arising from TOS alone.

Moreover, like Narakas, each of us has been surprised to observe that patients suffering with TOS who showed no clinical or EMG signs of peripheral nerve compression syndrome, and who had been considered cured after release of the brachial plexus and the subclavian vessels, presented 8–12 months later with symptoms suggestive of ulnar nerve compression at the elbow. Is this a neurological syndrome associated with C8-T1 regeneration which reaches the level of the elbow, on a background of tissue atrophy? These patients are concerned about recurrence of their TOS, but simple neurolysis of the ulnar nerve at the elbow amends their symptoms. As for peripheral nerve compression syndromes produced by retraction of fibrous and aponeurotic structures, related to disuse of the upper limb, we remain convinced also by the fact that the nerve trunks are subject to significant volumetric variations during periods of denervation and reinnervation.

Cervical approach

This remains the current technique for carrying out ablation of cervical ribs and freeing the plexus from compressive structures – suspensory ligaments of the pleura, scalenus anterior, scalenus medius and scalenus minimus, subclavian tendon and muscle. This surgical approach is particularly indicated in traumatic cases. Only in particularly long-limbed and thin patients should this route be used for ablation of the first rib, remembering that the sternochondral disarticulation in the vicinity of the subclavian vein is a difficult technical manoeuvre.

Axillary approach

This is undoubtedly an elegant approach for carrying out ablation of the first rib. This requires a good assistant who must fully retract the arm without overdoing this, to avoid axonotmetic damage which can produce a causalgia syndrome. The view is often satisfactory if the surgeon makes use of a lighted retractor.

Access to the C8-T1 roots as they emerge from the foramina is usual, and allows neurolysis under loupe magnification. No important structures are divided, while straightforward division of pectoralis minor or a muscle of Langer is possible if these structures are the cause of compression. The subclavian vein is sufficiently well exposed, freed-up and protected. However, this approach does not always allow complete resection of the anterior segment of the first rib. Finally, the transaxillary approach does not allow anterior scalenectomy, only allowing scalenotomy with the risk of developing a fibrous contracture at the level of the trunks of the brachial plexus. This surgical approach is applicable above all to vascular and neurovascular types of compression.

The supra- and infra-clavicular approach

This surgical approach is one of great safety, as it allows control of all the neurovascular structures. It seems to us that it is essential to have perfect control over the subclavian vein in cases of surgical revision, particularly when there is oedema of the upper limb, as the dilated vein takes up a considerable volume in the infraclavicular space and is therefore exceedingly vulnerable. This is an approach which we use for treating neurological and neurovascular forms and for carrying out surgical revisions to complete the resection of the first rib, the scalenus anterior, the suspensory ligament of the pleura, and finally for carrying out neurolysis of the brachial plexus when scarring is producing ongoing pain.

Results

Roos (1989), who has operated on more than 1500 cases of TOS, providing him with a unique world experience, reports 90–94% recovery or significant improvements after surgical treatment. It is difficult to compare results from different surgeons by technique because of the influence of the surgical specialty of each surgeon, be it predominantly vascular or predominantly neurological. Table 5 shows the results of different surgical units according to the technique used. It is noted that the supraclavicular approach results in 86–90% good or excellent results in the case of cervical rib with scalenotomy. Ablation of the first rib by the cervical approach in predominantly neurological forms of compression bears comparison with the transaxillary approach of Roos. We share the conclusions of Maxwell-Armstrong et al (2001) who, in a series of 126 procedures, carried out ablation of the first rib solely via the supraclavicular approach. They observed 86.5% improvement or resolution of symptoms. It is interesting to note the similarity of our own results with those of Narakas with respect to scalenectomy and resection of associated fibrous bands, without ablation of the first rib. The series of patients operated here is homogeneous in that they suffered predominantly neurological forms of compression. The transaxillary approach of Roos is a reliable technique for vascular or neurovascular forms in trained hands, and it is interesting to note the consistency of results published in the series of Narakas (1991) and Qvafordt et al (1984) when accompanied by a supraclavicular approach. To avoid this double surgical approach we have preferred the supra- and infra-clavicular approach of Cormier. Validation of the surgical approach to the first rib and the brachial plexus using the supra- and infra-clavicular approach in a continuous series of 40 procedures is confirmed by the absence of complications.

However, the evolution of our surgical approach shows that the diagnosis of a purely neurological form of compression is never certain, because in nine operative procedures using cervicotomy we have converted a scalene syndrome into a costoclavicular syndrome and we have demonstrated a tendency, without being able to predict this, for over-zealous removal of the first rib. The resolution of symptoms obtained in this series of 40 cases leads us to follow this therapeutic approach to avoid the risk of surgical revision, but which does not always prevent the patient developing chronic residual neuritis.

Conclusions

TOS syndromes are difficult diagnoses, bearing in mind the intricacies of the vascular and neurological symptoms. A sound anatomical knowledge is mandatory so as to clarify the mechanisms and the location of the lesions. Supplementary examinations may be limited to Doppler and EMG studies while awaiting further improvement in MRI techniques. Before undertaking surgery, it is recommended that all other causes of upper limb pain, as well as peripheral nerve compression syndromes that can coexist with TOS, are excluded. Rehabilitation protocols have been judged disappointing, probably as a result of a lack of education of therapists and patients. Surgery of the thoracic outlet can only benefit from an accumulation of knowledge in vascular surgery, thoracic surgery and microsurgery of the brachial plexus, to provide a better understanding of compression of the brachial plexus and the subclavian vessels. The increasing number of published series has led us to establish that the transaxillary approach of Roos does not prevent a significant number of complications or technical inadequacies (10–20%) and we fall short of the 92.2% excellent results claimed by Roos in his personal series (Roos 1987). Increasing use of the supraclavicular approach is justified in neurological forms when this can be confirmed, and does not require ablation of the first rib. It is then recommended to carry out an anterior scalenectomy and a partial or complete scalenectomy of the scalenus medius to allow the subclavian artery to move posteriorly during abduction manoeuvres of the arm. When complete ablation of the first rib is required, particularly in the case of surgical revision, we have adopted the supra- and infra-clavicular approach of Cormier, which allows a comfortable and safe operative procedure and shields the patient from some of the complications seen with the axillary approach.

References

Adson AW, Coffey JR (1927) Cervical rib. A method of anterior approach for relief of symptoms by division of the scalenus anticus, *Ann Surg* **85**: 839–57.

Adson AW (1947) Surgical treatment for symptoms produced by cervical rib and the scalenus anticus muscle, *Surg Gynecol Obstet* **85**: 687–700.

Aligne C, Barral X (1992) La rééducation des syndromes de la traversée thoracobrachiale, *Ann Chir Vasc* **64**: 381–9.

Allieu Y, Benichou M, Touchais S, Desbonnet P, Lussiez B (1991) Les formes neurologiques du syndrome du hile du membre supérieur: le rôle du scalène moyen, *Ann Chir Main Memb Super* **10**: 308–12.

Aziz S, Straehley CJ, Whelan JT (1986) Effort-related axillosubclavian vein thrombosis. A new theory of pathogenesis and a plea for direct surgical intervention, *Am J Surg* **152**: 57–61.

Batt M, Griffet J, Scotti L, Le Bas P (1983) Le syndrome de la traversée cervico-brachiale. A propos de 112 cas: vers une attitude tactique plus nuancée, *J Chir* **120**: 687–91.

Borrelly J, Merle M, Hubert J, Grosdidier G, Wack B (1984) Compression du plexus brachial par pseudarthrose de la première côte, *Ann Chir Main* **3**: 266–8.

Bramwell E (1903) Lesions of the first dorsal nerve root, *Rev Neurol Neurosurg Psychiatry* **1**: 236.

Brudon JR, Brudon F, Bady B, Descotes J (1989) Intérêt des potentiels évoqués somesthésiques dans les syndromes de la traversée thoracobrachiale, *J Mal Vasc* **14**: 303–6.

Clerc A, Didier R, Robbie J (1917) Anomalie de la première côte gauche, *Bull Acad* [Paris] 3e série, Vol LXXVII.

Cooper A (1821) On exostosis. In: Cooper A, Cooper B, Travers B, eds, *Surgical Essays*, 2nd Am. edn. (James Webster: Philadelphia).

Cormier F, Brun JP, Marzelle J, Fichele JM, Cormier JM (1994) Syndrome du défilé thoraco-brachial, *Actualités d'Angéiologie* **19**: 62–9.

Dale WA (1982) Thoracic outlet compression syndrome, *Arch Surg* **117**: 1437–45.

Falconer MA, Weddell G (1943) Costoclavicular compression of the subclavian artery and vein, *Lancet* **30**: 539–43.

Gaupp E (1894) Über die Bewegungen des menschlichen schulterguertels und die atiologie der sogenannten narkosenlaehmungen, *Zentr F Chir* **21**: 793–5.

Gruber W (1869) Ueber die Halsrippen des Menschen mit vergleichenden anatomischen Bemerkungen *Mem Acad Imper Sciences Saint-Petersbourg* 12.

Harvey W (1970) Exercitatio anatomica de motu cordis et sanguinis in animalibus (1627) Translated into English by CD Leake, 5th edn (C Thomas: Springfield) 36.

Horovitz SH (1985) Brachial plexus injuries with causalgia resulting from transaxillary rib resection, *Arch Surg* **120**: 1189–91.

Leriche R (1941) Les syndromes du défilé costo-claviculaire, l'insomnie par douleur du bras dans l'horizontale, *Presse Med* **64**: 825–6.

Machleder HI, Moll F, Verity MA (1986) The anterior scalene muscle in thoracic outlet compression syndrome, *Arch Surg* **121**: 1141–4.

Martinez NS (1979) Posterior first rib resection for total thoracic outlet decompression syndrome, *Contemp Surg* **15**: 13–21.

Maxwell-Armstrong CA, Noorpuri BS, Haque SA, Baker DM, Lamerton AJ (2001) Long term results of surgical decompression of thoracic outlet compression syndrome, *J R Coll Surg Edinb* **46**: 35–8.

Mayo H (1835) Exostosis of the first rib with strong pulsations of the subclavian artery, *London Med Phys J* **11**: 40.

Melliere D, Becquemin JP, Etienne G (1985) Les complications de la chirurgie des défilés thoraco-cervico-braciaiux, *J Chir* **122**: 151–7.

Merle M, Borrelly J (1987) Le traitement des formes neurologiques du syndrome du défilé cervico-axillaire par voie de Roos, *Chirurgie* **113**: 188–94.

Merle M (1995) Les syndromes de la traversée cervico-thoraco-brachiale. In: *Cahier d'Enseignement de la Société Française de Chirurgie de la Main* (Expansion Scientifique Française: Paris) 29–47.

Merle M, Borrelly J (2002) Complications de la chirurgie du défilé cervico-thoraco-axillaire, *Chirurgie* **3**: 23–8.

Morley J (1913) Brachial pressure neuritis due to a normal first thoracic rib: its diagnosis and treatment by excision of rib, *Clin J* **13**: 461–3.

Murphy JB (1906) The clinical significance of cervical ribs, *Surg Gynecol Obstet* **3**: 514–20.

Murphy T (1910) Brachial neuritis from pressure of the first rib, *Aust Med J* **15**: 582–4.

Naffziger HL, Grant WT (1938) Neuritis of the brachial plexus mechanical in origin. The scalenus syndrome, *Surg Gynecol Obstet* **67**: 722–30.

Narakas AO (1989) Revue critique du traitement conservateur et chirurgical du syndrome de la traversée thoraco-cervico-brachiale, *Rev Med Suisse Romande* **109**: 557–71.

Narakas AO (1990) The role of thoracic outlet syndrome in the double crush syndrome, *Ann Chir Memb Super.* **9**: 331–40.

Narakas AO (1991) Syndrome de la traversée thoraco-cervico-brachiale. In: Tubiano R, ed, *Traité de Chirurgie de la Main,* vol 4 (Masson: Paris) 378–418.

Nichols HM (1986) Anatomical structures of the thoracic outlet, *Clin Orthop* **207**: 13–20.

Novak CB (1992) Physical therapy management of musicians with thoracic outlet syndrome, *J Hand Therapy* **5**: 73–9.

Paget J (1875) *Clinical Lectures and Essays* (Longman, Green and Co.: London and New York).

Peet RM, Henriksen JD, Anderson PT, Martin GM (1956) Thoracic outlet syndrome: evaluation of a therapeutic exercice program, *Mayo Clin Proc* **31**: 281–7.

Poitevin LA (1980a) Etude des défilés thoraco-cervico-brachiaux: etude anatomique, dynamique et radiologique. Dissertation, Paris.

Poitevin LA (1980b) Les défilés thoraco-cervico-brachiaux. *Mem Lab Anat Paris* **42**: 1–207.

Poitevin LA (1991) Compressions à la confluence cervico-brachiale. In: Tubiana R, ed, *Traité de Chirurgie de la Main,* vol 4 (Masson: Paris) 362–78.

Puusepp L (1931) Kompression des plexus brachialis durch di normale 1. Brustrippe. *Folia Neuropath Eston* **II**: 93–5.

Qvarfordt PG, Ehrenfeld WK, Stoney RJ (1984) Supraclavicular radical scalenectomy and transaxillary first rib resection for the thoracic outlet syndrome, *Am J Surg* **148**: 111–15.

Roos DB (1966) Trans axillary approach for first rib resection to relieve thoracic outlet syndrome, *Ann Surg* **163**: 354–8.

Roos DB (1979) New concepts of thoracic outlet syndrome which explain etiology, symptoms, diagnosis and treatment, *Vasc Surg* **13**: 313–21.

Roos DB (1982) The place of scalenectomy and first rib resection in thoracic outlet syndrome, *Surgery* **92**: 1077–83.

Roos DB (1987) Thoracic outlet syndromes: update 1987, *Am J Surg* **154**: 568–73.

Roos DB (1990) The thoracic outlet syndrome is underrated, *Arch Neurol* **47**: 327–8.

Roos DB (1989) Récidives post-opératoires des syndromes de la traversée thoraco-brachiale. In: Kieffer E, ed, *Les Syndromes de la Traversée Thoraco-brachiale* (AERCV: Paris) 317–28.

Sällström J, Celegin Z (1983) Physiotherapy in patients with thoracic outlet syndrome, *Vasa* **12**: 257–61.

Sanders RJ (1979) Scalenectomy versus first rib resection for thoracic outlet syndrome, *Surgery* **85**: 109–21.

Schrötter L von (1884) Erkrankungen der Gefäse. In: *Nothnagel's Handbuch der Pathologie und Therapie* (Holder: Vienna).

Sebileau P (1892) *Démonstrations d'Anatomie* (G Steinheil: Paris).

Sharp WJ, Nowak LR, Zamani T et al (2001) Long-term follow-up and patient satisfaction after surgery for thoracic outlet syndrome, *Ann Vasc Surg* **15**: 32–6.

Smith KF (1979) The thoracic outlet syndrome: a protocol of treatment. *J Orthop Sports Phys Ther* **1**: 89–99.

Swank RL, Simeone EA (1944) The scalenus anticus syndrome, *Arch Neurol Psychiatry* **51**: 432–45.

Urshel HC, Razzuk MA (1986) The failed operation for thoracic outlet syndrome: the difficulty of diagnosis and management, *Ann Thorac Surg* **42**: 523–8.

Ward AS Cormier JM (1986) Thoracic outlet syndrome and upper limb revascularisation In: *Operative Techniques in Arterial Surgery* (MTP Press: Lancaster) 283–303.

Wilbourn AJ. The thoracic outlet syndrome is overdiagnosed, *Arch Neurol* **47**: 328–30.

Willshire WH (1860) Supernumerary first rib, *Lancet* 633–4.

Wright IS (1945) The neurovascular syndrome produced by hyperabduction of the arms, *Am Heart J* **29**: 1–19.

Wood VE, Tvito R, Verska JM (1988) Thoracic outlet syndrome. The results on first rib resection in 100 patients, *Orthop Clin North Am* **19**: 131–46.

Wood VE, Biondi J, Linda L (1990) Double crush nerve compression in thoracic outlet syndrome, *J Bone Joint Surg* **72A**: 85–7.

23 Radial nerve compression

Guy Raimbeau

Introduction

Compression neuropathy of the radial nerve is the least common of the nerve compression syndromes of the upper extremity. Neurologic signs and symptoms may be localized to the arm, the elbow, or the wrist, and may be manifested as pain, hypesthesia or dysesthesia, or weakness.

Disturbances of sensibility are most often related to a compression of the superficial branch to the wrist, occasionally at the level of the elbow. Pain is most often due to compression of the radial nerve at the level of the elbow, but may sometimes be due to compression of the terminal branches at the level of the wrist. Muscle weakness is due either to compression proximal to the elbow, in which case it often results in profound or even complete paralysis; or at the level of the elbow, in which case the paralysis is often incomplete.

Disturbances of sensibility

Compression of the superficial branch to the wrist

The first description of this syndrome was by Stopford in 1922 (Braidwood 1975), but it is better known by the name of 'Cheiralgia paresthetica', given to it in 1932 by Wartenberg (Ehrlich et al 1986).

The first symptoms are usually those of paresthesias, rapidly becoming mixed with disagreeable sensations, then becoming frankly painful. The symptoms of hypesthesia or anesthesia in the dorsal aspect of the first web space cause little functional impairment, but may cause significant annoyance to the patient. Patients are not awakened at night by the symptoms, and neither movement of the elbow nor elevation of the arm will modify the symptoms. Repetitive motions of supination, and especially pronation, or a history of twisting injury to the wrist are often reported. Descriptions of symptoms are often variable; burning pain, a feeling of thickness, or a sensation as if ants are crawling on the skin (formication) are often described. These sensations are usually felt in the first web space with radiation into the thumb and index and middle fingers. Symptoms are triggered or aggravated by wrist motion.

The regional character of these signs and symptoms makes their analysis difficult. The clinician must look for local signs of irritation along the course of the nerve, particularly in the proximal part of the distal third of the forearm, where the nerve emerges dorso-laterally. Flexion and ulnar deviation of the wrist triggers or aggravates the symptoms. This maneuver is similar to Finkelstein's test, but does not include simultaneous flexion of the thumb (Dellon and Mackinnon 1986). The differential diagnosis between radial nerve compression and De Quervain's tenosynovitis is often difficult, especially in view of the fact that these entities are often associated (Figure 23.1). It has been estimated that 10% of cases of tenosynovitis will have an associated neurologic syndrome (Foucher et al 1991).

Careful preoperative evaluation will reduce the chance of a disappointing outcome. Arthrosis of the trapezometacarpal joint can usually be detected by testing the range of motion of this joint and by the 'grind' test. Radiographs including specific views are often helpful in confirming this diagnosis. In theory, the test described above, similar to Finkelstein's test, should be negative in cases of De Quervain's tenosynovitis because the thumb ray is left free, but Dellon found this test be positive in 96% of Wartenberg's cases (Dellon and Mackinnon 1986). Dellon proposes a provocative maneuver in which the elbow is extended and the forearm is pronated (Figure 23.2). If the test is positive, paresthesias appear in 30–60 seconds, and can be augmented by ulnar deviation of the wrist and flexion of the fingers. The accuracy of this test can be influenced by the presence of carpal tunnel syndrome. In fact, according to Dellon, only nerve blocks with a local anesthetic can define the anatomical lesion with precision, given the frequent overlap of the territory of cutaneous nerve innervation. The overlap of the areas innervated by the radial nerve and the lateral antebrachial cutaneous nerves is of the order of 75% (Mackinnon and Dellon 1985). To carry out the selective blocks, the lateral antebrachial cutaneous nerve is first

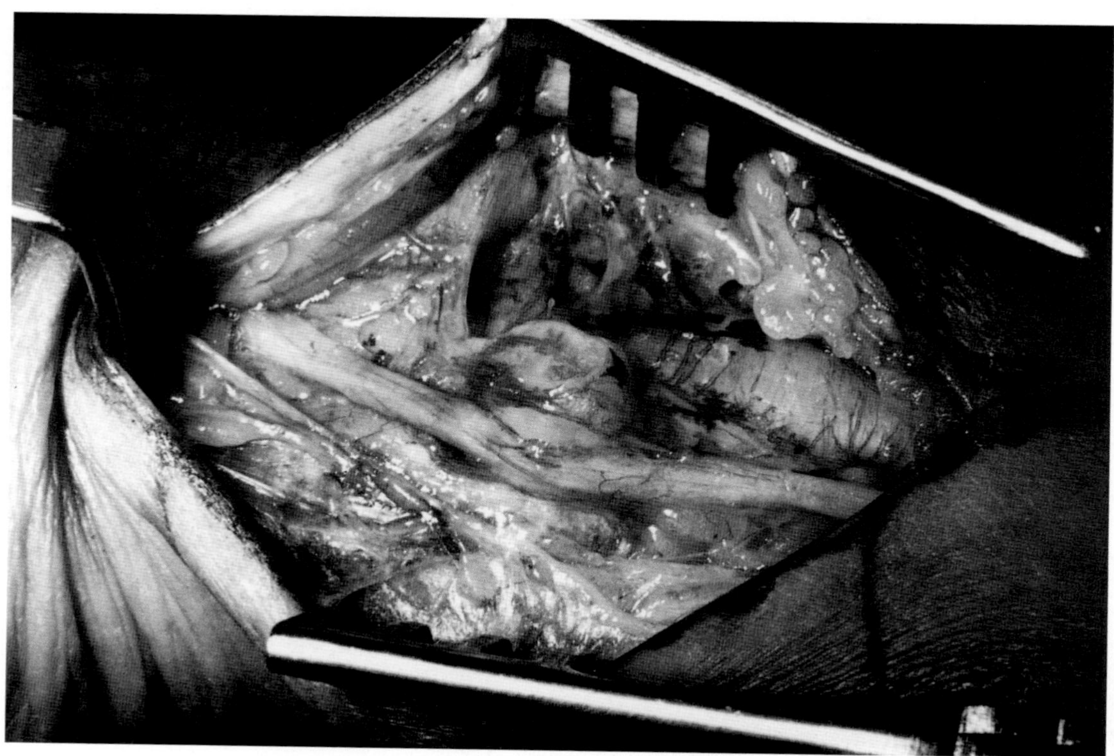

Figure 23.1
Intraoperative view – right wrist. Radial nerve compression associated with De Quervain's tenosynovitis.

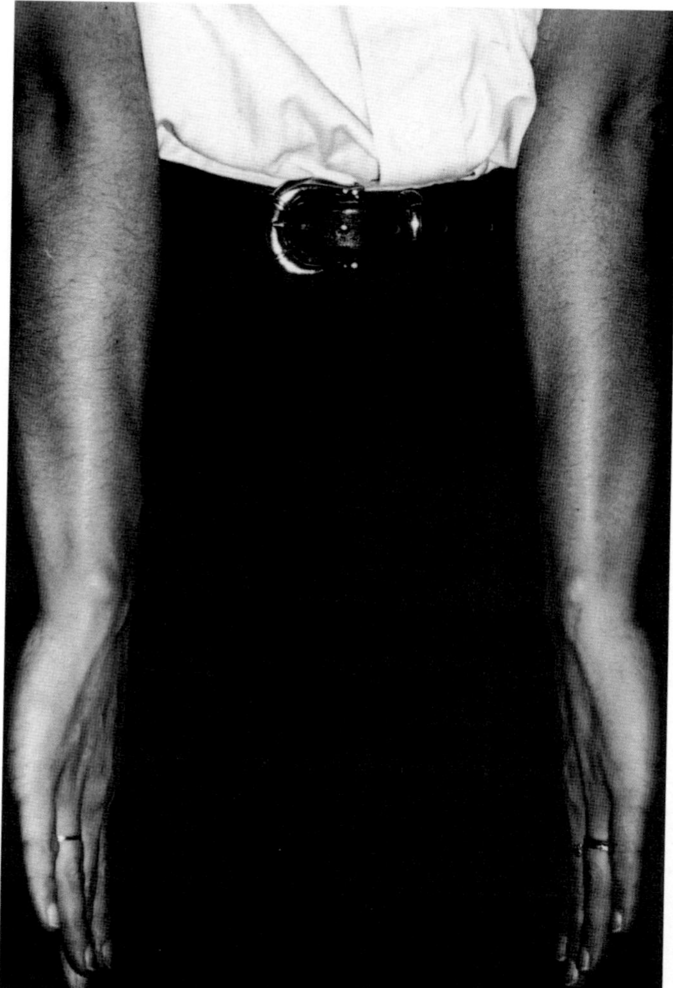

Figure 23.2
The provocative maneuver: paresthesias appear in 30–60 seconds when an entrapment of the superficial branch of the radial nerve exists.

blocked in the proximal part of the forearm, at the cephalic vein; then 10 or 20 minutes later the superficial branch of the radial nerve is blocked at the musculotendinous junction of the brachioradialis.

The electrodiagnostic tests are easily done, but are of significance only if they are abnormal. In fact, these tests are useful mainly to rule out polyneuropathies. The testing of the previously mentioned nerves must be carried out while keeping in mind the frequent overlap of their territories of innervation. Electromyography (EMG) may allow an anatomical diagnosis to be verified by demonstrating cervical root lesions, or occasionally by revealing an isolated lesion of the superficial branch in the forearm.

In practice, in the context of subjective sensory disturbances, the diagnosis is often evident. Apart from late sequelae of wounds or crushing injuries, the syndrome is often associated with wearing a constricting watchband or bracelet, or with a cast or dressing causing external compression (Rask 1979), or with repetitive motions causing compression from within. The treatment for the first 4–6 months is medical, with use of a splint and avoidance of activities that tend to increase symptoms. Injection of corticosteroids at the wrist is not recommended because of the risk of cutaneous atrophy. Continued irritation of the nerve is an indication for surgical intervention. All local problems, including nerve and tendon compression, may be surgically treated at the same operation. It is necessary to eliminate the scissors-like effect of the brachioradialis and extensor carpi radialis longus tendons, which close in pronation and open in supination. Care must be taken to ensure that the incision is placed so that it does not result in scarring about the nerve, causing recurrent neuritis (Mackinnon 1999).

Dellon's results were mixed (Dellon and Mackinnon 1986). He reported 86% good results, but only 43% of those operated on returned to their former work activities. The long history of pain and the high percentage of compensatable injuries (71%) in his patients were poor prognostic signs.

Lluch and Beasley (1989) proposed a release of the posterior interosseous nerve in all cases operated on for compression of the superficial sensory branch of the radial nerve. This treatment is based on the the observation that dysesthesias are often absent in cases of compression of the nerve proximal to its division into sensory and motor branches at the elbow. These authors expressed the opinion that the uninvolved branch permitted cerebral reception of stimuli which had their origin in the traumatized fibers of the other branch. Surgery for recurrence of symptoms in this region may include enveloping the nerve in a vein graft to diminish the incidence of adhesions.

Finally, in the syndromes of altered sensibility, the clinician must always consider the possibility of a tumor causing intrinsic or extrinsic nerve compromise. Schwannomas must be especially looked for (Figure 23.3). Appropriate imaging tests are indispensable in making the diagnosis of soft tissue tumor.

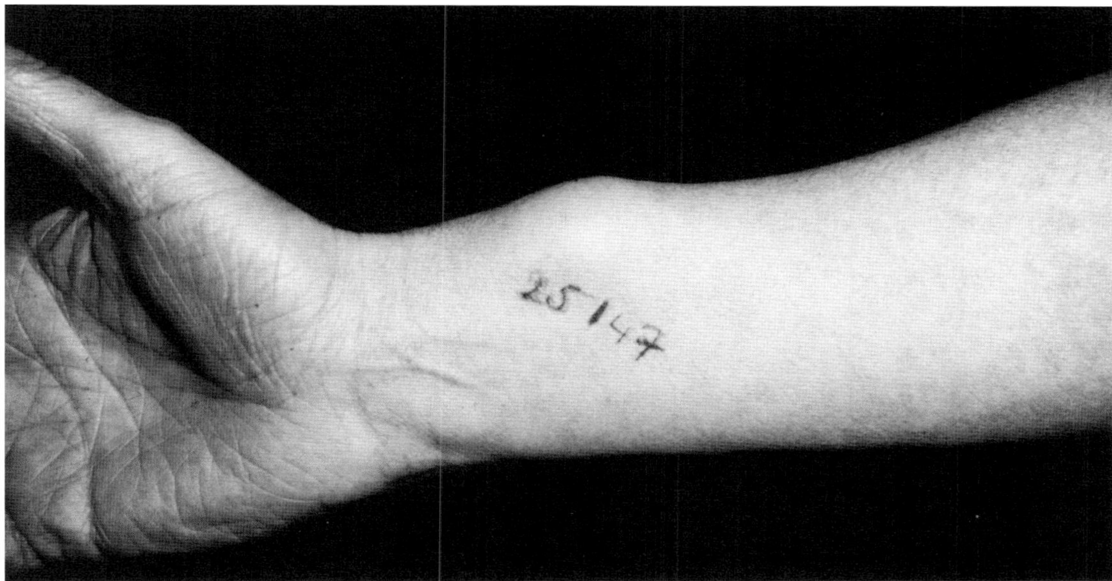

(A)

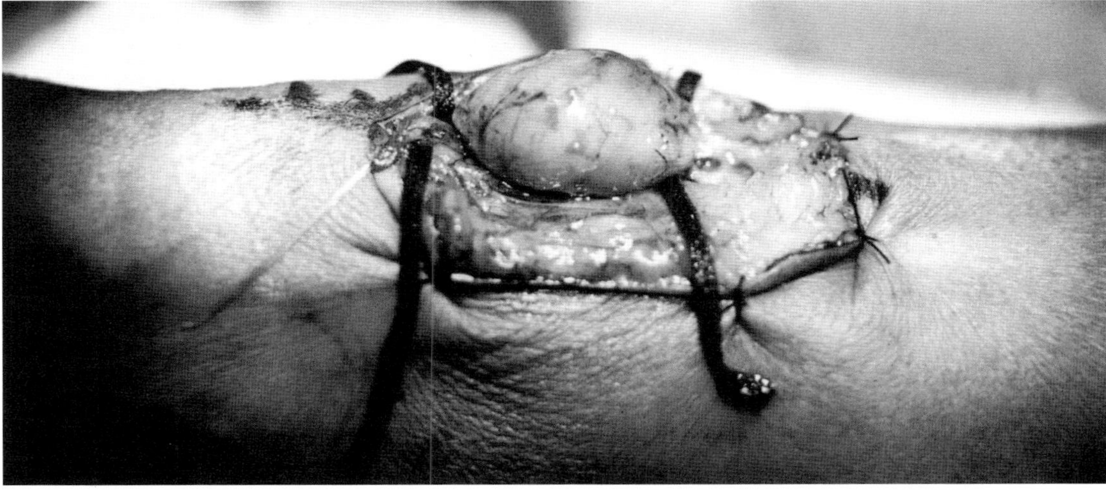

(B)

Figure 23.3
(A) Preoperative view. (B) Intraoperative view: schwannoma of the superficial sensory branch of the radial nerve.

At a distance from the wrist

The superficial branch of the radial nerve may be compressed proximal to the wrist. Since compression at this level may accompany a compression at the level of the brachial plexus or nerve trunk, it is important to analyse the neurologic symptomatology carefully. The atypical forms of this syndrome with disturbances of sensibility caused by compression in the radial tunnel will be discussed.

Painful syndromes

Painful syndrome of the posterior interosseous nerve at the wrist

This syndrome is manifested by dull dorsal pain, aggravated by pressure of the fourth compartment and by passive mobilization, either in maximum flexion or maximum extension of the wrist. Pseudo-bulbous termination at the capsule of the radio-carpal joint predisposes to the development of this syndrome (Carr and Davis 1985). After ruling out other causes of dorsal wrist pain, a therapeutic test comprising local nerve block of the posterior interosseous nerve can eliminate the possibility of anomalous innervation and confirm the diagnosis (Dumitru and Walsh 1988).

Initial treatment consists of wearing a splint for 1–3 months and restriction of those activities that tend to aggravate symptoms. If conservative treatment fails, resection of the terminal branches of the nerve back several centimeters is indicated (Dellon 1985).

Radial tunnel syndrome

The painful syndrome described by Roles and Maudsley (1972) is caused by compression of the deep branch of the radial nerve at the elbow. It is often put in the same category as epicondylitis, and is still sometimes called 'resistant tennis elbow'. Hagert et al (1977), then Werner (1979), published large studies. Since then, other authors have published smaller series, including several in French (Narakas 1974, Comtet et al 1976, Raimbeau et al 1990).

This compression syndrome must be differentiated from the paralytic syndrome of the posterior interosseous nerve. The confusion between these two syndromes is caused by the fact that the same structures are involved in the same location in both syndromes.

This compression syndrome is related to the anatomy of the elbow, which permits flexion-extension and pronation-supination at the same time. The study by Roquelaure et al (2000) demonstrated a statistical relationship between repetitive manual work and the development of the compression syndrome. From the anatomical point of view, conditions are set for restriction of movement of the deep branch of the radial nerve, which should follow the movements of pronation and supination of the forearm. The arc of motion of the radius is imposed on the deep branch of the radial nerve, which is confined between the two muscular layers of the supinator. In addition to the elasticity which all peripheral nerves possess (Grewal et al 1996), the radial nerve has a reserve connective structure in axial torsion. The sensory branch is not subject to such stresses in the proximal third of the forearm, since it follows the course of the brachioradialis.

In the radial tunnel, three possible sources of compression were described by Roles and Maudsley (1972) in their first description, and Lister et al (1979) added a fourth. These four elements have become classic: fibrous bands in front of the humero-radial capsule; the leash of vessels from a branch of the anterior recurrent radial artery; the tendinous proximal edge of the extensor carpi radialis brevis (ECRB); and the proximal margin of the supinator. A fifth source, rarely a problem, is the distal edge of the supinator. Compression at this point was described by Sponseller and Engber (1983).

Diagnostic criteria

The signs and symptoms of the radial tunnel syndrome may be spontaneous or provoked. This pain is easily recognized by those who have experience with the syndrome. The spontaneous pain is located distal to the epicondyle, on the lateral side of the forearm, radiating down the course of the radial nerve, most often descending toward the dorsum of the wrist without ever going beyond the MP joints of the central digits. Spontaneous ascending pain may also occur, especially at night. The usual nocturnal pattern is typical of the compression neuropathies, but the nocturnal pain may be inconstant and transient at first, becoming more cyclical in the chronic stages. The pain is usually relieved by shaking the hand or moving the elbow. Repetitive movements, especially those related to work, exacerbate the pain, which may persist and may occur with activities of daily living such as pouring water or shaking hands. There is often a feeling of weakness associated with the syndrome.

Palpation along the course of the nerve or putting the nerve under tension in the radial tunnel by different maneuvers can elicit pain which reproduces and exacerbates the spontaneous pain. At the radial point, 3–5 cm distal to the lateral epicondyle, pressure should be carefully applied by the examiner's finger and the degree of tenderness should be compared to the opposite side (Figure 23.4). We prefer to do this provocative test towards the end of the examination. This sign is relatively sensitive and should be combined with palpation of the nerve along its course from the lower third

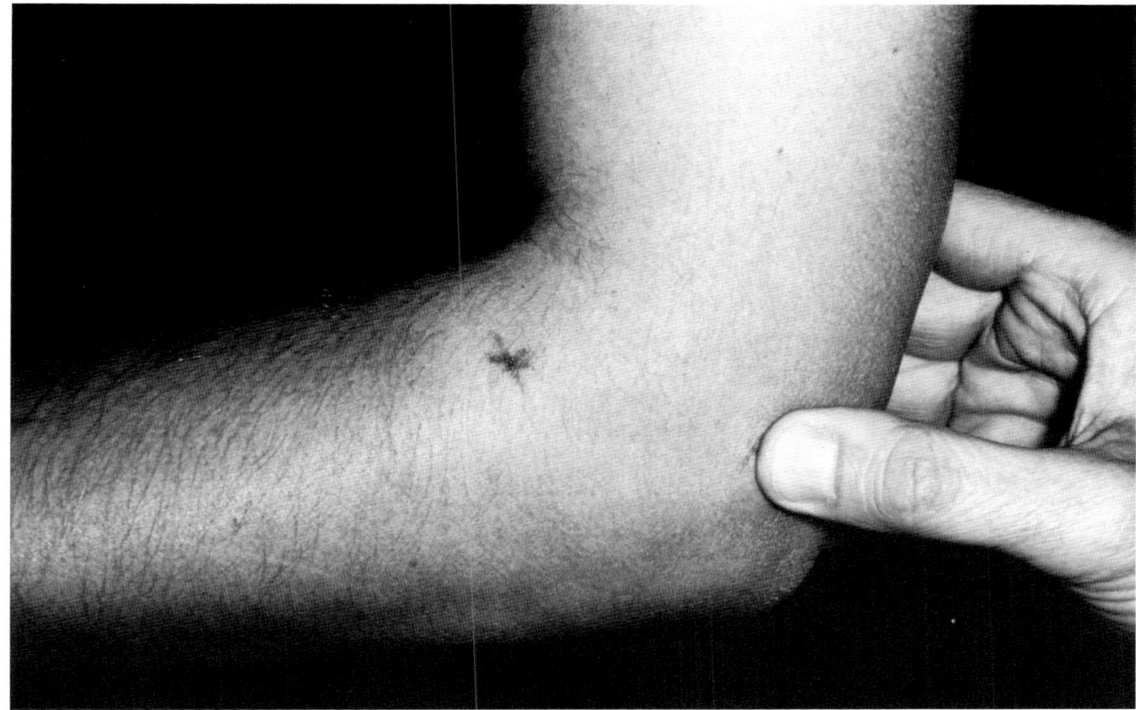

(A)

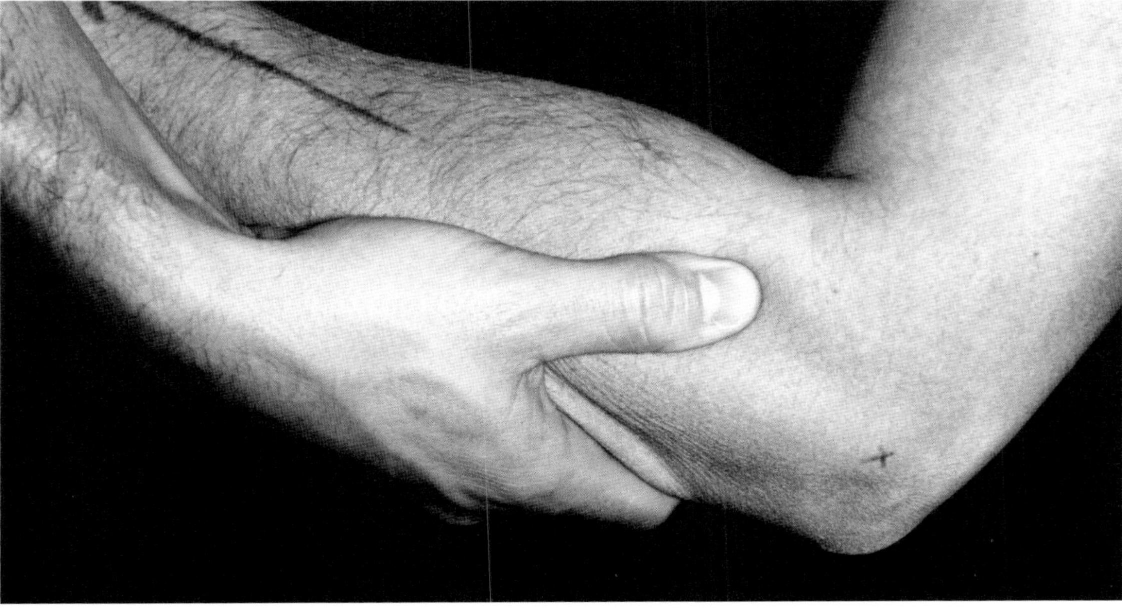

(B)

Figure 23.4
Left elbow; (A) Lateral epicondyle point. (B) A gentle pressure at the radial point exacerbates the spontaneous pain radiating down the course of the radial nerve.

of the arm to the lower third of the forearm. The study of resisted active motions is important; above all it is resisted active supination which brings out the pain. We carry out this test in two stages. First, with the flexed elbow supported on the table, the patient attempts to supinate from a position of full pronation, while the examiner holds the forearm to prevent this motion. This test is then repeated with the elbow in complete extension so that the nerve is under more tension. Finally, the examiner puts the supinator under tension by passively extending the elbow while passively pronating the forearm and flexing the wrist. These maneuvers, one passive with maximum tension on the nerve, the other active, are designed to flatten the arcade of the supinator on the radial nerve. In contrast, the pain on resisted extension of the middle finger while the elbow and wrist

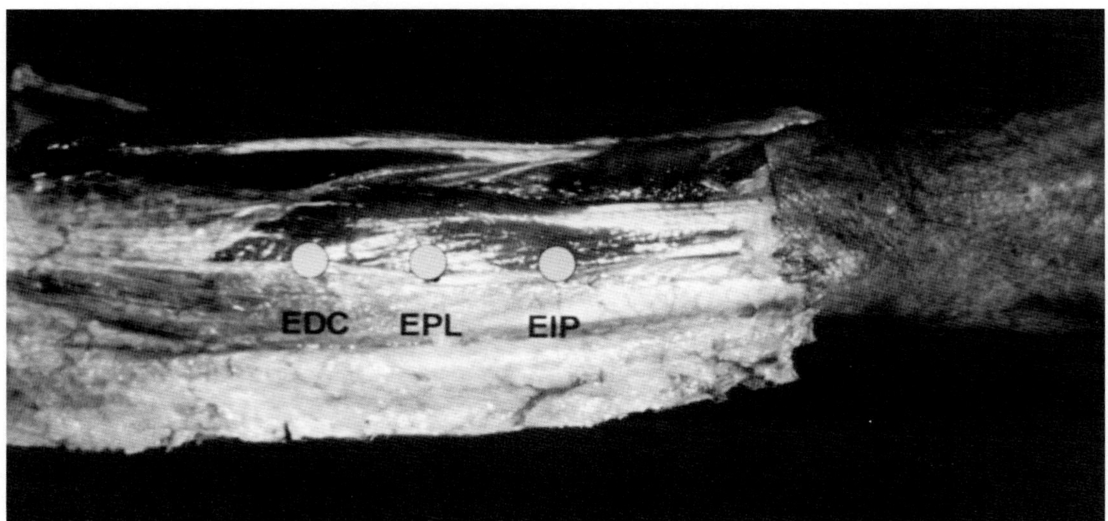

Figure 23.5

Specimen view – right forearm. The needles at 13, 16 and 20 cm from the lateral side of the flexor crease of the elbow are localized in the EDC, EPL, and EIP, respectively.

are extended, or Roles' sign (Roles and Maudsley 1972), does not seem to us to be specific for the radial tunnel syndrome, since it is frequently positive in cases of lateral epicondylitis. Some authors (Ritts et al 1987, Sotereanos et al 1999) have recommended the use of local anesthetics to block the radial nerve at the elbow. Motor weakness of the extensors, which might in principle be expected, is absent in the pure form of radial tunnel syndrome.

Electrodiagnostic studies

The value of EMG studies in radial tunnel syndrome is controversial (Van Rossum et al 1978, Comtet et al 1985, Ritts et al 1987, Jalovaara and Lindholm 1989, Verhaar and Spaans 1991, Younge and Moise 1994), and most authors believe that this test contributes little, because it is unreliable and is often normal. Since we are dealing with a painful syndrome without any consistent objective physical signs, we firmly believe that a decision to operate should not be made without objective evidence to confirm the diagnosis. With this requirement in mind, we have developed a protocol with Dr M-C Pelier-Cady (Raimbeau 2001).

The examination is long and difficult, often lasting as long as an hour, and it requires an experienced examiner. The examination may be normal in the early stages of the evolution of the syndrome, and it may be necessary to repeat the examination in 4–6 months if there is doubt. The examination should be done in a room at 23°C (82°F). The patient lies down with the forearm pronated.

Components of the examination
The examination includes:

- EMG.
- Determination of motor conduction velocities and distal latencies.
- Determination of sensory latencies of the anterior branch of the radial nerve (which are usually normal).
- Study of other nerves as indicated by associated symptomology, such as the median nerve at the wrist and ulnar nerve at the elbow, so as to detect a generalized sensitivity to compression.

EMG is indispensable because compression of the radial nerve at the elbow is often of the axonal type. The test is done using a needle electrode. At least three muscles are examined: the extensor digitorum (ED), the extensor pollicis longus (EPL), and the extensor indicis proprius (EIP). These three muscles are relatively easy to hit reliably, and they have been found on anatomical studies to have distances of 13, 16, and 20 cm from the lateral side of the flexor crease of the elbow (Figure 23.5). The extensor digitorum is a superficial muscle which is easy to explore (as cited in the majority of studies). On the other hand, we have noted that neurological abnormalities are more common in more distal muscles in the area where the deep branch of the radial nerve arborizes into its distal branches (EPL and EIP). To eliminate an area of compression more proximally, we conclude the study with an examination of the extensor carpi radialis longus (ECRL) and the brachioradialis. A semi-quantitative scale was used to classify the EMG signal.

Study of the motor conduction of the deep branch
This examination is composed of two parts:

1. **Distal latencies**. This study is carried out by stimulating the nerve at the level of the lateral brachial sulcus and reading the responses by means of a needle electrode in the three muscles ED, EPL, and EIP, at fixed distances of 13 cm, 16 cm, and 20 cm, according to our anatomical studies. The values in

milliseconds are: ED 3.12 ± 0.32; EPL 4.04 ± 0.22; and EIP 5.06 ± 0.26.

2. **Motor conduction velocities of the radial nerve**. The reading is made by surface electrode on the EIP muscle. The nerve is stimulated by a surface electrode applied at the level of the lateral humeral gutter, then at the lateral side of the flexor crease of the elbow, then in the forearm halfway between the epicondyle and the wrist, where the nerve is stimulated more easily. The normal value is 61.4 m/s ± 5.4 at the elbow. A velocity of <50 m/s is definitely pathological; between 50 m/s and 60 m/s is borderline. It may be necessary to use the opposite arm as a control. A difference of >5 m/s between the two sides may indicate an abnormality of conduction velocity.

Sensory conduction velocity
This velocity is calculated either by the classical orthodromic method, from the first web space to the distal third of the forearm, or by Schirali and Sanders' antidromic method, stimulating the nerve in the distal third of the arm and recording in the distal third of the forearm.

Positive electrodiagnostic test
We consider an electrodiagnostic test to be positive for radial nerve dysfunction when the following signs are present: anomalies on EMG in the three muscles mentioned above, while all other muscles are normal, or significant slowing of motor nerve conduction, or an association of several abnormalities.

It is important to study the C7 nerve root in a systematic manner.

Instead of using dynamic testing, which can be difficult to carry out because of technical problems and the incresased discomfort that the patient must tolerate, we prefer to do the EMG studies at the end of a working day. If necessary, this protocol may be repeated in 4–6 months.

Electrodiagnostic study of the radial nerve at the elbow does not consist only of an EMG study of the ED and a motor conduction velocity. An EMG study of several muscles innervated by the deep branch, and a study of sensory and motor conduction velocities of the nerve are needed before firm conclusions can be drawn.

Treatment

We recommend conservative treatment for 3–6 months, with limitation of those activities that exacerbate the pain, especially frequent and forceful pronation and supination. We do not recommend steroid injections. In addition to medical treatment with systemic anti-inflammatory medications, we recommend a rehabilitation program to aid the patient in achieving a balance between the flexor and extensor forces exerted during certain actions, especially those requiring forceful grip. We find that it is common for patients with these syndromes to exert much more gripping force than is necessary to carry out the intended task. If medical treatment is insufficient, the EMG study is repeated after 4–6 months, especially if the initial EMG is normal.

Surgical treatment

The operative treatment must be carried out carefully. The operation should be done in a facility that is equipped to treat peripheral nerve injuries, including magnifying loupes or an operating microscope. The operation should be done under general or regional anesthesia. We recommend that the pneumatic tourniquet is inflated to 20–25 mmHg above the systolic blood pressure, and that the arm is not fully exsanguinated, so engorged blood vessels that may contribute to nerve compression can be identified more easily.

Our preference is for the dorso-lateral longitudinal approach, as described by Hagert et al (1977), which permits an excellent view of the radial tunnel, and does not leave an unsightly scar. It is not necessary to use the long incision described by Mayer (in Hashizume et al 1996). The incision is made on a line drawn from the lateral epicondyle to the radial styloid process while the elbow is in 80° flexion and the forearm is in slight pronation. The usual incision is about 6–10 cm long, depending on the size of the patient and the experience of the surgeon. In the distal part of the incision, especially if it is rather long, a cutaneous sensory branch that is a branch of the posterior antebrachial cutaneous nerve must be identified and preserved. In the distal part of the incision, the ribbon-like aspect of the tendon of the ECRL, which is the key point to enter the inter-muscular space between the two radial extensors of the wrist, must be identified. Developing this intermuscular space proximally, the surgeon opens up the area of the radial tunnel and encounters fatty perineural tissue and an arteriovenous leash across the deep branch of the radial nerve. It is sometimes difficult to find the correct space. Often searches are made too far posterior, and in some cases there is some degree of fusion between the muscle bellies of the ECRB and the ECRL. In this case, it may be necessary to work from proximal to distal in developing this interval, beginning near the epicondyle and exposing the tendinous portion of the ECRB by dividing muscle fibers and ligating vessels as needed. Decompression of the nerve is accomplished by leaving it in its bed and incising, or sometimes excising, a portion of the proximal part of the superficial head of the supinator for several centimeters. In the absence of signs of compression of the nerve, the neurolysis should be continued as far as the distal part of the supinator. The medial border of the tendon of the ECRB is excised as needed if it represents an obstacle. Rarely, a fibrous band is encountered between the ECRL and the arcade

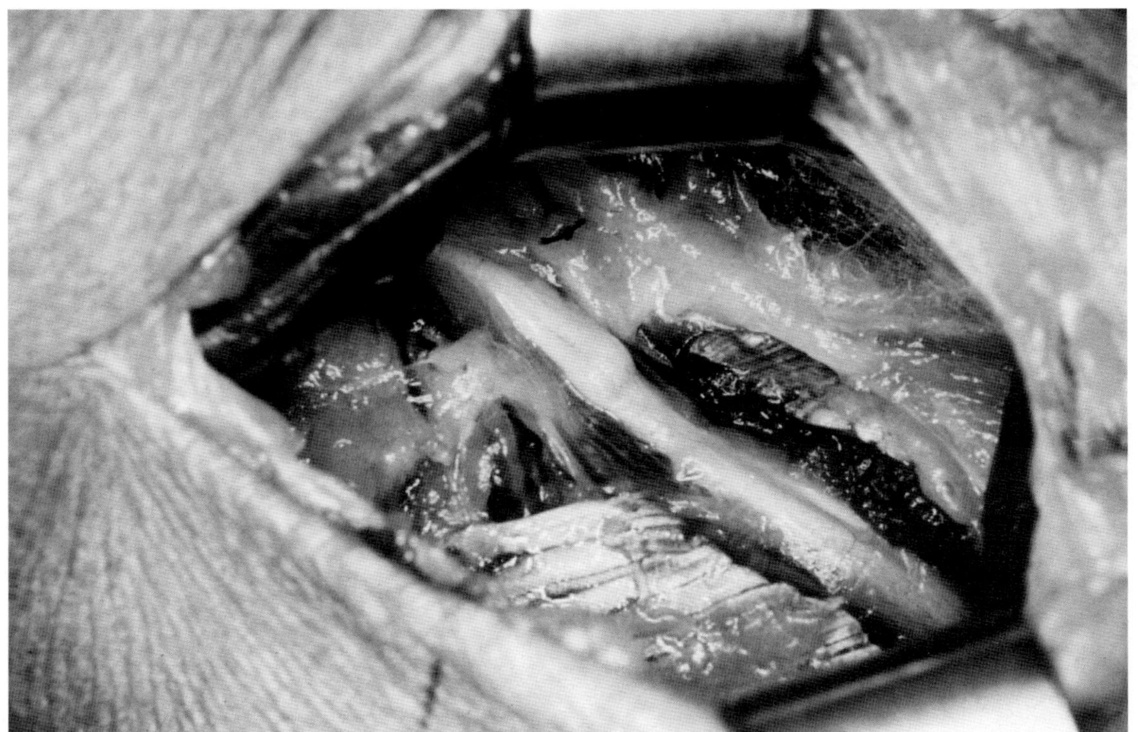

Figure 23.6

Intraoperative view – right elbow. Imprint at the proximal edge of the supinator muscle. The muscle is cut straight above the nerve. A loop of vessel proximal to the supinator had been excised.

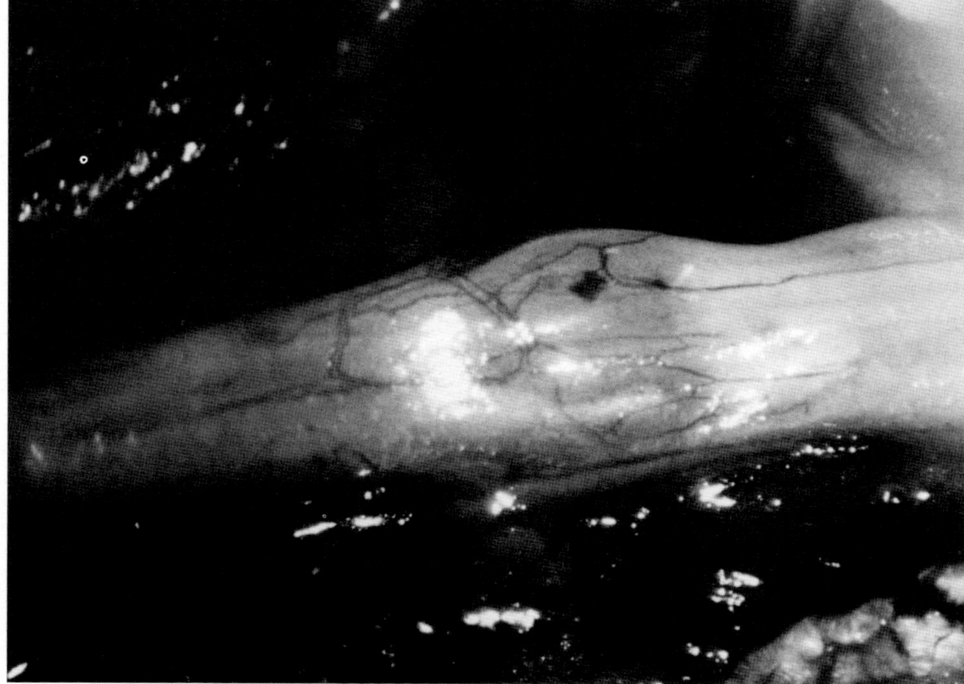

Figure 23.7

View through operating microscope – right elbow. After excision of the supinator muscle, the nerve deformation with post-stenotic dilatation is clear.

of the flexor digitorum superficialis. If found, this band should be resected. We do not consider an arcade of Frohse to be present unless the proximal edge of the supinator is fibrous for several millimeters. The exploration of the deep branch of the radial nerve should be methodical and systematic, not only at the proximal edge of the supinator, but also anterior to the radio-humeral joint, where fibrous bands may sometimes be found. Flexion of the elbow permits sufficient proximal exposure. It is important to ensure that the deep branch of the radial nerve is completely free during both flexion-extension and pronation-supination motions of the elbow. The anatomic lesions of the nerve will be even more visible if magnification is used (Figures 23.6 and 23.7). In this way, the surgeon can note whether there is simply a change in color of the nerve due to impaired microcirculation, or a loss of the transverse striations (Werner 1979), or a post-strictural dilation or even a neuroma in continuity in chronic cases (Hagert et al 1977, Raimbeau et al 1990).

We have noted the nerve to be attached by fibrous bands to the floor of the radial tunnel (due to post-inflammatory thickening), or constricted by a loop of vessels proximal to the supinator, or compressed by the proximal edge of the supinator, with or without an arcade of Frohse, or by the medial edge of the ECRB, or by a fibrous arcade at the distal margin of the supinator. Sometimes, the syndrome is purely dynamic in nature, because of increased intramuscular pressure. Werner (1979) has shown very high pressures (on the order of five times normal) during tetanic contractions of the supinator. A number of forces act on the nerve as it traverses the supinator, and a histologic study (Rath et al 1993) has shown a significant increase in fibrous tissue in the epineurium and interstitial connective tissue in this segment of the nerve. The edge of the ECRB can cause compression, either directly only in pronation (Spinner 1968) as it crosses over the nerve (Laulan et al 1994), or indirectly by putting pressure on the supinator, which in turn exerts pressure on the nerve.

If pathological conditions of the elbow joint or of a tendon are found in addition to a neuropathy, surgical measures to address these problems are carried out at the same operation, but the postoperative care may be different, with a period of immobilization of about 2 weeks after any operation on a tendon. When only neurolysis is done, mobilization is begun immediately.

Other approaches

Henry's classic approach is anterior, between the brachioradialis and the brachialis, but Roles and Maudsley (1972) and Lister et al (1979) recommend separation of the brachioradialis muscle. This approach has the disadvantage of leaving a scar which is sometimes cosmetically displeasing, even if the 'lazy S' advocated by Lister is used. To avoid this problem, Crawford (1984) has proposed using Henry's approach, but using a transverse skin incision. Posterior approaches give results that are more cosmetically pleasing. Capener (1966) goes between the ECRB and the EDC (Wigoda and Coleman 1999). We believe that this approach limits the exposure of the superficial branch of the radial nerve distal to the elbow. Mackinnnon (1999) goes between the brachioradialis and the ECRL. Hybrid approaches do not appear to us to be useful, since the posterior lateral approach that we use allows us to deal with all of the regional pathology (Hagert et al 1977, Werner 1979, Raimbeau et al 1990).

The published results of surgical treatment are variable (Atroshi et al 1995). Roles and Maudsley (1972) reported 92% good and excellent results, while Ritts et al (1987) reported only 51% of their results to be this good. The criteria of Roles and Maudsley are strict and should serve as a reference. We published a series of 35 cases in 1990, with 71% good or excellent results (Raimbeau et al 1990). The worst results were found in patients who had a long history of epicondylitis, especially in the context of a work-related condition (Sotereanos et al 1999). Nevertheless, Lawrence et al (1995) recommended surgical treatment, since they found 66% good results of surgical treatment for patients in this category.

Radial tunnel syndrome in cases of epicondylitis

Pain on the lateral side of the elbow may be caused by referred or radicular pain of cervical origin, by early arthritis of the radio-humeral joint, by inflammation or micro ruptures of the common extensor origins, or by radial tunnel syndrome. These last two conditions are frequently difficult to differentiate preoperatively, but it is at this stage that an attempt must be made to separate the two diagnoses. Epicondylitis is more common in athletes or those who do heavy manual work. In this condition, the pain is behind or on the epicondyle, and medical treatment (particularly local injections) gives temporary relief of symptoms. In the radial tunnel syndrome, it is a matter of dynamic pathology. The pain is worse in the muscular mass of the muscles which take origin on the epicondyle, and along the course of the radial nerve. Pain at rest is much more common in the radial tunnel syndrome than it is in epicondylitis. Other areas of nerve symptoms are not rare. After a long history of discomfort, the distinction between the signs and symptoms of these two syndromes becomes less marked, and we must look elsewhere for clues to enable us to distinguish between them. The best complimentary examination is, at present, the performance of the 'block test' with a local anesthetic (Ritts et al 1987, Sotereanos et al 1999, Wigoda and Coleman 1999). We believe that an inflammatory reaction in the area of the epicondyle that persists for several months can bring about a secondary reaction of the radial nerve by modifying the epineural environment of the nerve. Less than 10% of cases of epicondylitis cause irritation of the radial nerve; Werner (1979) found 5%. If lengthening of the conjoined tendon can relieve pressure on the supinator muscle, the effect on the nerve is far from being constant. Of Werner's cases, 12 had previous surgery for epicondylitis. On the other hand, neurolysis alone will not relieve the symptoms of epicondylitis (10% reoperation rate in Werner's series), except in rare cases by relief of proximal tension on the tendon of the supinator. Heyse-Moore (1984) concluded that epicondylitis might be treated either by lengthening of the ECRB or by opening up the arcade of the supinator. We believe, like van

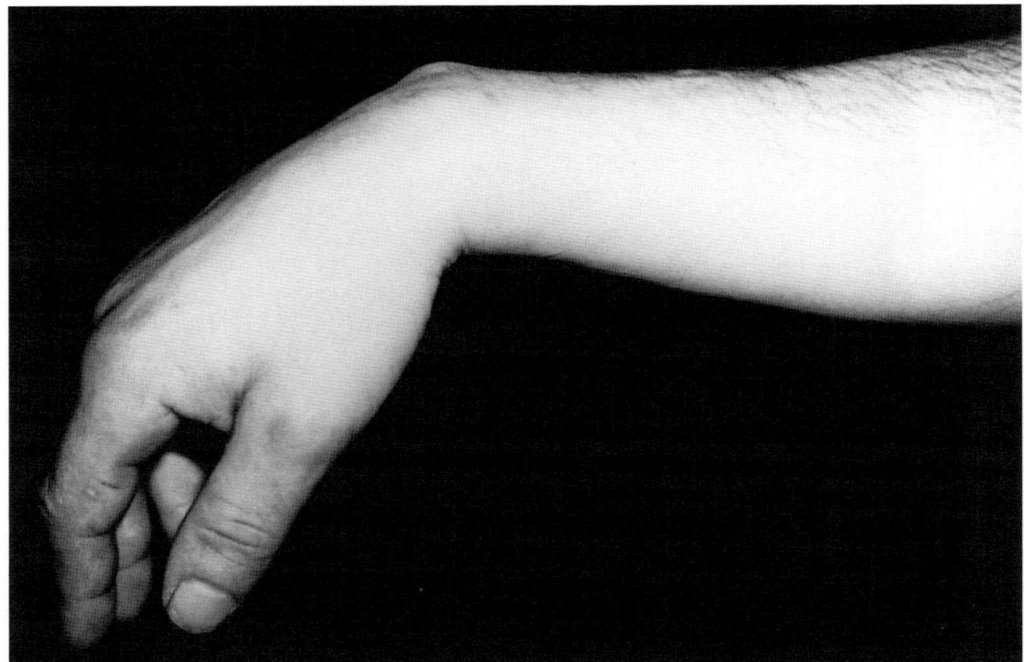

Figure 23.8

Right hand. High radial palsy: no extension of the wrist, no extension of the fingers.

Rossum et al (1978), that the radial tunnel syndrome does not cause epicondylitis, and we agree with Hagert et al (1977) and Crawford (1984) that the two conditions may coexist, especially in those who carry out forceful repetitive motions.

Compression of the superficial branch at the elbow

As to localization of the compression in the radial tunnel, there can be a component of irritation of the superficial branch. In this form of the syndrome, the pain radiates distally, and may extend all the way to the first web space and even to the thumb and index finger. Palpation of this branch is painful well proximal to the localization of Wartenberg's syndrome. This compression of the superficial branch at the elbow is relatively rare, but it was noted by Moss and Switser (1983), who reported this finding in four patients in their series of 15 cases of radial tunnel syndrome. These four patients were relieved of their symptoms by neurolysis of the two branches of the radial nerve. In one of these four cases, the tendon of the ECRB was the source of compression. In our experience, this lesion is very rare.

Paralytic form

High radial palsy

High radial palsy refers to compression of the nerve above its division into deep motor branch and superficial sensory branch. It is therefore a matter of localization proximal to the flexor crease of the elbow. Most often, it is in the context of a traumatic lesion or external compression syndrome (Lover's palsy or Saturday night palsy). All muscles are involved (Figure 23.8) except the triceps, the innervation of which is mainly from branches taking origin in the axilla. Weakness of the brachioradialis and the wrist extensors with wrist drop indicates a high radial palsy. In a high radial palsy, there may be hypesthesia in the dorsal aspect of the first web space. Wilhem (1991) emphasizes the impairment of sensibility on the postero-lateral aspect of the forearm, the spontaneous pain on the posterior part of the epicondyle, and the pain at the point of compression. High radial palsies of non-traumatic orgin are exceedingly rare. They are most often related to sustained muscular effort (Mitsunaga and Nakano 1988). The fibers of the triceps 'massage' the nerve behind the humerus with every active movement of the elbow, and the fibers of the lateral head of the triceps compress the radial nerve in its passage around the humerus in the lower part of the radial groove. This was described by Lotem et al (1971). Although their patients were not operated on, they consider that the lesion is related to the passage of the nerve under the fibrous arcade at the insertion of the lateral head of the triceps. This phenomenon was demonstrated by Nakamichi and Tachibana (1991) with a case of pseudo-neuroma. Elsewhere, a hereditary form has been reported (Lubahn and Lister 1983). On the other hand, Manske (1977) performed a late exploration, but did not find a fibrous arcade. Other reports describe muscular compression at the level of the change in direction of the trunk of the radial nerve. Wilhem (1991)

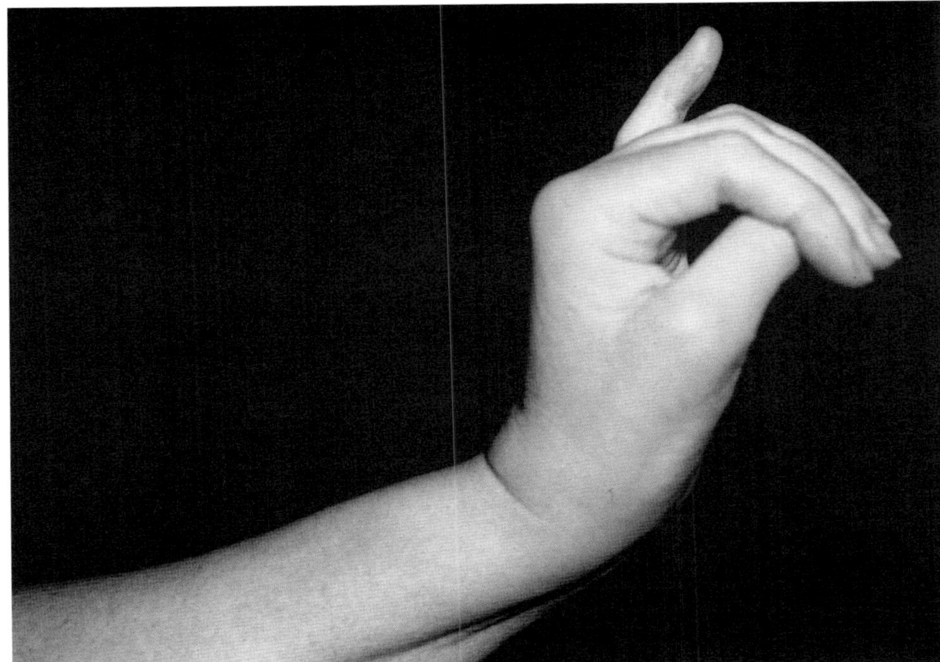

Figure 23.9
Left hand. Low radial palsy; note the extension of the wrist. Incomplete palsy is frequently like this case with the conservation of the extension of the fifth finger.

reported 19 non-traumatic cases. Lussiez et al (1993) effectively demonstrated the constraints on torsion of the nerve caused by flexion-extension movements of the elbow, with hourglass narrowing of the nerve, the fibrous arcade serving only to aggravate the dynamic phenomenon.

There are also cases of overuse syndromes of the upper extremity, without a history of recent excessive effort. Although these syndromes may exist without any anatomic constrictive element, true strictures of the nerve may be found, almost as if it had been ligated. The observations of Burns and Lister (1984) (three cases), of Palazzi et al (1983) (four cases, of which two were in the proximal third and two in the distal third of the arm) are documented. One case occurred in conjunction with periarteritis nodosa, but the others were not related to any evident disease.

We propose the hypothesis of an intraneural irreversible compartment syndrome (Lundborg et al 1983) which would leave intraneural scarrring (Rydevik et al 1981) that would be an obstacle to axial torsion of the nerve. To be complete, we must mention congenital compression, with or without amniotic grooves, as reported by Richardson and Humphrey (1989).

In all cases of high radial nerve palsies, the EMG can confirm the localization of the compression and differentiate it from a brachial plexus lesion, denervation involving all muscles except the triceps. In all non-traumatic etiologies, a period of observation of 3–4 months is indicated, with a repeat EMG during the third month. The absence of improvement during this period is indication of the need for neurolysis to obtain a good result.

Low radial palsy

Except for traumatic lesions of the nerve (laceration of the nerve or compression caused by fracture-dislocation of the elbow), radial nerve palsy at the elbow is often incomplete (Figure 23.9). A low radial palsy differs from a high radial palsy in that it spares the radial wrist extensors and the supinator. It is often called posterior interosseous nerve syndrome. Deficits of motor function are variable, and can at first be confused with tendon ruptures, particularly at the wrist. The onset of symptoms in the low radial nerve palsy may be abrupt or slow, but most importantly it is painless, except for the first few days. Weakness of the extensor carpi ulnaris results in radial deviation of the wrist during extension. Weakness of the extensor digitorum results in a deficit of metacarpal phalangeal extension, although extension of the interphalangeal joints – including that of the thumb – remains possible by action of the median and ulnar innervated lumbricals and interossei. Comtet and Chambaud (1975) emphasized that to detect weakness of the extensor digitorum, the wrist must be maintained in extension to eliminate the tenodesis effect of wrist flexion.

Extrinsic compression is the most important etiology, particularly that caused by a lipoma. The first description of this occurrence was in 1953 by Richmond (in Bieber et al 1986). A review of 48 tumors reported 35 lipomas (Werner 1991). A painless, sometimes palpable, mass develops on the dorso-lateral aspect of the elbow. An ultrasound or magnetic resonance image, or both, may be necessary to visualize the extent of the tumor mass. A lipoma may attain a size of 6–8 cm in diameter, and may be multilobulated. Excision of the mass and decompression of the radial nerve usually result in complete recovery of function in a few months (Capener 1966, Bieber et al 1986, Durandeau and Geneste 1988, Werner 1991).

Synovial cysts (Bowen and Stone 1966, Steiger and Vögelin 1998) present a more difficult problem, as do bursae of the bicipital tuberosity. In spite of the frequency of rheumatoid arthritis, development of synovial cysts causing compression of the radial nerve are relatively rare (Millender et al 1973).

Idiopathic paralysis, which occurs in the absence of intrinsic or extrinsic compression, is often preceded by a short period of pain, while the paralysis persists and worsens. It is often related to forceful repetitive motion, with constriction of the nerve at the proximal edge of the supinator. In this case, it often is a matter of a true arcade of Frohse. The first description of this anatomical structure was given in 1905 by Guillemain and Courtellemont (see Comtet and Chambaud 1975). The case was that of an orchestra conductor, but this syndrome can also be found in violinists, pianists, corsetieres, or other occupations that involve forceful repetitive work in pronation and supination coupled with flexion and extension of the elbow. Sharrard (1966) thought that capsular lesions might cause problems in full extension because he had found adhesions around the nerve. One case of dynamic paralysis in pronation due to a fibrous band just proximal to the supinator has been reported (Derkash and Niebauer 1981). The first surgical excision of the arcade was done by Capener (1966) for the relief of pain, but it was Sharrard who made the first observations of paralysis not due to tumor in 1966.

Comtet and Chambeaud (1975) discovered a double constriction of the nerve before it entered the supinator, as if two ligatures had been put around the nerve at 1-cm intervals. Kotani et al (1995) reported four cases. The constrictions found, with or without arcade of Frohse (Hashizume et al 1996, Inoue and Shionoya 1996), show that the nerve moves and that any anatomic anomaly in the radial tunnel can cause single or double constriction.

Electrodiagnostic studies nearly always show abnormalities that correlate well with the clinical findings. There is prolongation of the distal motor latency on conduction studies, and evidence of denervation of the extensor digitorum, extensor indicis proprius, and extensor digiti minimi, on EMG studies, while the muscles that are more proximally innervated are spared, and the superficial branch remains normal.

The treatment is surgical for all the compression syndromes caused by an expansile lesion, but in the absence of a mass, surgery should be deferred for 2 or 3 months to allow for spontaneous recovery. However, it is early decompression that brings about complete muscular recovery (Nielsen 1976). The surgical approach is, for us, dorso-lateral unless there is an anterior lesion.

Differential diagnosis

As with any non-traumatic peripheral neuropathy, metabolic, vascular, inflammatory, or degenerative causes must be ruled out. In asymmetrical neuropathies, diabetic mononeuropathy of the radial nerve is rare. In chronic lead poisoning, it is the classic description. Demyelinating diseases are usually easy to differentiate because they are multifocal and often symmetrical.

One of the diagnostic difficulties in cases of complete low radial palsy is the localization of the 'hérédopathie tomaculaire' which is a heritable neuropathy characterized by hypersensitivity to compression. It is most often manifested by painless motor and sensory loss, with remissions and exacerbations. More research needs to be done on this autosomal dominant heritable disorder. Radial nerve palsy in the Parsonage-Turner syndrome is quite rare. The diagnosis may be facilitated by signs of nerve deficit proximal to the shoulder. Hashizume et al (1996) insist on the notion of severe pain before the paralytic syndrome and the notion of an episode of a viral type which precedes the muscle atrophy. According to these authors, the paralysis is variable and changeable, whereas in compression syndromes, the paralysis would be progressive before becoming complete. The chronic compartment syndrome is usually seen in athletes or workers who carry out repetitive motions. The diagnosis can only be made by measuring intramuscular pressures and comparing them with those on the opposite side. It is probable that certain patients are relieved of symptoms by simple opening of the aponeurosis, through a radial nerve approach. Since the descriptions of Upton and MacComas in 1973 (in Wood et al 1990), double compressions should be considered. A C7 radiculopathy is relatively common in cases of non-traumatic neuropathy of the radial nerve. By contrast, association with nerve compression in the cervico-thoraco-brachial course is rare. Compression of the brachial plexus may be due to tumor, but it is more often due to anatomic anomalies, particularly of the scalenus anticus. Symptoms are usually proximal with lateral cervical pain which radiates distally to the lateral aspect of the upper extremity and especially with hypesthesias in the area innervated by the radial nerve. Muscular involvement is partial and mixed. The syndrome seems to be uncommon, since in their series, Wood et al (1990) and Narakas (1990) reported respectively 2% and 15% of compression associated with the radial nerve at the elbow, but 19% and 31% compression of the median nerve in the carpal tunnel.

Radiculopathy is the most common differential diagnosis, and it is the C6–C7–C8 lesions that interest us the most, with C7 lesions frequently manifested as paresthesias and pain referred to the the forearm and the dorsum of the hand. They can be aggravated by coughing. As with all double compressions (double crush syndromes), distal neurolysis improves the clinical situation, without bringing about a complete cure. Sometimes specific treatment of the cervical lesion is necessary.

Conclusion

Non-traumatic neuropathy of the radial nerve is better known in the context of a paralytic syndrome. However, we have seen the richness of other manifestations, particularly pain syndromes or disturbances of sensibility. In order to validate the clinical diagnosis of radial tunnel syndrome, and therefore to separate out the different etiologies of epicondylalgias, we insist on the mastery of a long and precise protocol for the performance of the EMG study. The pathophysiology of the nerve compression syndromes is not yet clear. We still do not understand why two manifestations that are so different (paralytic or pain syndromes) can result from the same anatomical abnormalities, and respond to the same mechanical solutions. At present, it seems that slow but continued compression is more likely to result in a paralytic syndrome, whereas intermittent compression is more likely to cause a pain syndrome. Future studies in neurophysiology may clarify this point.

Acknowledgement

Thanks are due to Dr FE Jones (Nashville, TN, USA) for his help with the translation of this manuscript from French to English.

References

Atroshi I, Johnsson R, Ornstein E (1995) Radial tunnel release, *Acta Orthop Scand* **66**: 255–7.

Bieber EJ, Russel Morre J, Weiland AJ (1986) Lipomas compressing the radial nerve at the elbow, *J Hand Surg* **11A**: 533–5.

Bowen TL, Stone KH (1966) Posterior interosseous nerve paralysis caused by a ganglion at the elbow, *J Bone Joint Surg* **48B**: 774–6.

Braidwood AS (1975) Superficial radial neuropathy, *J Bone Joint Surg* **57**: 380–3.

Burns J, Lister GD (1984) Localized constrictive radial neuropathy in the absence of extrinsic compression: three cases, *J Hand Surg* **9A**: 99–103.

Capener N (1966) The vulnerability of the posterior interosseous nerve of the forearm. A case report and an anatomical study, *J Bone Joint Surg* **48B**: 770–3.

Carr D, Davis P (1985) Distal posterior interosseous nerve syndrome, *J Hand Surg* **10A**: 873–8.

Comtet JJ, Chambaud D (1975) Paralysie "spontanée" du nerf interosseux postérieur par lésion inhabituelle, *Rev Chir Orthop* **61**: 533–41.

Comtet JJ, Chambaud D, Genety J (1976) La compression de la branche postérieure du nerf radial, *Nouv Presse Med* **5**: 1111–14.

Comtet JJ, Lalain JJ, Moyen B, Genety J, Brunet-Guedj E, Lazo-Henriquez R (1985) Les épicondylalgies avec compression de la branche postérieure du nerf radial, *Rev Chir Orthop* **71** (Suppl. II): 89–93.

Crawford GP (1984) Radial tunnel syndrome (letter), *J Hand Surg* **9**: 451–2.

Dellon AL (1985) Partial dorsal wrist denervation: resection of the distal posterior interosseous nerve, *J Hand Surg* **10A**: 527–33.

Dellon AL, Mackinnon SE (1986) Radial sensory nerve entrapment in the forearm, *J Hand Surg* **11A**: 199–205.

Derkash RS, Niebauer JJ (1981) Entrapment of the posterior interosseous nerve by a fibrous band in the dorsal edge of the supinator muscle and erosion of a groove in the proximal radius, *J Hand Surg* **6A**: 524–6.

Dumitru D, Walsh N (1988) Congenital hemihypertrophy associated with posterior interosseous nerve entrapment, *Arch Phys Med Rehabil* **69**: 696–8.

Durandeau A, Geneste R (1988) Un syndrome canalaire rare: la paralysie du nerf interosseux postérieur, *Rev Chir Orthop* **74** (Suppl II): 156–8.

Ehrlich W, Dellon AL, Mackinnon SE (1986) Cheiralgia paresthetica (entrapment of the radial sensory nerve), *J Hand Surg* **11A**: 196–9.

Foucher G, Greant Ph, Sammut D, Buch N (1991) Névrites et névromes des branches sensitives du nerf radial. A propos de quarante-quatre cas, *Ann Chir Main* **10**: 108–12.

Grewal R, Xu J, Sotereanos DG, Woo L-YS (1996) Biomechanical properties of peripheral nerves, *Hand Clin* **12**: 195–204.

Hagert CG, Lundborg G, Hansen T (1977) Entrapment of the posterior interosseous nerve, *Scand J Plast Reconstr Surg* **11**: 205–12.

Hashizume H, Nishida K, Nanba Y, Shigeyama Y, Inoue H, Morito Y (1996) Non-traumatic paralysis of the posterior interosseous nerve, *J Bone Joint Surg [Br]* **78B**: 771–6.

Heyse-Moore GH (1984) Resistant tennis elbow, *J Hand Surg* **9B**: 64–6.

Inoue G, Shionoya K (1996) Constrictive paralysis of the posterior interosseous nerve without external compression, *J Hand Surg* **21B**: 164–8.

Jalovaara P, Lindholm RV (1989) Decompression of the posterior interosseous nerve for tennis elbow, *Arch Orthop Trauma Surg* **108**: 243–5.

Kotani H, Miki T, Senzoku F, Nakagawa Y, Ueo T (1995) Posterior interosseous nerve paralysis with multiple constrictions, *J Hand Surg* **20A**: 15–17.

Laulan J, Daaboul J, Fassio E, Favard L (1994) Les rapports du muscle court extenseur radial du carpe avec la branche de division profonde du nerf radial. Intérêt dans la physiopathologie des épicondylalgies, *Ann Chir Main* **13**: 366–72.

Lawrence T, Mobbs P, Fortems Y, Stanley JK (1995) Radial tunnel syndrome. A retrospective review of 30 decompressions of the radial nerve, *J Hand Surg* **20B**: 454–9.

Lister GD, Belsole RB, Kleinert HE (1979) The radial tunnel syndrome, *J Hand Surg* **4**: 52–9.

Lluch L, Beasley RW (1989) Treatment of dysesthesia of the sensory branch of the radial nerve by distal posterior interosseous neurectomy, *J Hand Surg* **14A**: 121–4.

Lotem M, Fried A, Levy M (1971) Radial palsy following muscular effort, *J Bone Joint Surg* **53B**: 500–6.

Lubahn JD, Lister GD (1983) Familial radial nerve entrapment syndrome: a case report and literature review, *J Hand Surg* **8**: 297–300.

Lundborg G, Myers G, Powell H (1983) Nerve compression injury and increase in endoneurial fluid pressure: a miniature compartment syndrome, *J Neurol Neurosurg Psychiatry* **46**: 1119–24.

Lussiez B, Courbier R, Toussaint B, Benichou M, Gomis R, Allieu Y (1993) Paralysie radiale au bras après effort musculaire. A propos de quatre cas, *Ann Chir Main* **12**: 130–5.

Mackinnon SE, Dellon AL (1985) The overlap pattern of the lateral antebrachial cutaneous nerve and the superficial radial nerve, *J Hand Surg* **10A**: 522–6.

Mackinnon SE (1999) Surgical approach to the radial nerve, *Techniques in Hand and Upper Extremity Surgery* **3**: 87–98.

Manske PR (1977) Compression of the radial nerve by the triceps muscle, *J Bone Joint Surg* **59A**: 835–6.

Millender LH, Nalebuff EA, Holdsworth DE (1973) Posterior interosseous nerve syndrome secondary to rheumatoid synovitis, *J Bone Joint Surg* **55A**: 375–7.

Mitsunaga MM, Nakano K (1988) High radial nerve palsy following strenuous muscular activity, *Clin Orthop* **234**: 39–42.

Moss SH, Switzer HE (1983) Radial tunnel syndrome: a spectrum of clinical presentations, *J Hand Surg* **8A**: 441–20.

Nakamichi K, Tachibana S (1991) Radial nerve entrapment by the lateral head of the triceps, *J Hand Surg* **16A**: 748–50.

Narakas A (1974) Epicondylite et syndrome compressif du nerf radial, *Med Hyg* **32**: 2067–70.

Narakas A (1990) The role of thoracic outlet syndrome in the double crush syndrome, *Ann Hand Upper Limb Surg* **9**: 331–40.

Nielsen HO (1976) Posterior interosseous nerve paralysis caused by fibrous band compression at the supinator muscle – a report of four cases, *Acta Orthop Scand* **47**: 304–7.

Palazzi S, Palazzi C, Raimondi P, Aramburo F (1983) Syndromes compressifs du nerf radial. In: Souquet R, ed, *Syndromes Canalaires du Membre Supérieur* (Monogr GEM, Expansion Scientifique: Paris) 41–54.

Raimbeau G, Saint-Cast Y, Pelier-Cady MC (1990) Radial tunnel syndrome. Study of a continuous and homogenous series of 35 cases, *Rev Chir Orthop* **76**: 177–84.

Raimbeau G (2001) Radial nerve compression at the elbow. In: Allieu Y, Mackinnon SE, eds, *Nerve Compression Syndromes in the Upper Limb* (Martin Dunitz: London).

Rask R (1979) Watchband superficial radial neurapraxia (letter), *JAMA* **241**: 2702.

Rath AM, Perez M, Mainguene C, Masquelet AC, Chevrel JP (1993) Anatomic basis of the physiopathology of the epicondylagias: a study of the deep branch of the radial nerve, *Surg Radiol Anat* **15**: 15–19.

Richardson GA, Humphrey MS (1989) Congenital compression of the radial nerve, *J Hand Surg* **14A**: 901–3.

Ritts GD, Wood MB, Linscheid RL (1987) Radial tunnel syndrome – a ten-year surgical experience, *Clin Orthop* **219**: 201–5.

Roles NC, Maudsley R (1972) Radial tunnel syndrome: resistant tennis elbow as a nerve entrapment, *J Bone Joint Surg* **54B**: 499–508.

Roquelaure Y, Raimbeau G, Dano C et al (2000) Occupational risk factors for radial tunnel syndrome in industrial workers, *Scand J Work Environ Health* **26**: 507–13

Rydevik B, Lundborg G, Bagge U (1981) Effects of graded compression on intraneural blood flow, *J Hand Surg* **6A**: 3–11.

Sharrard WJ (1966) Posterior interosseous neuritis, *J Bone Joint Surg* **48B**: 777–80.

Sotereanos DG, Varitimidis SE, Giannakopoulos PN, Westkaemper JG (1999) Results of surgical treatment for radial tunnel syndrome, *J Hand Surg* **24A**: 566–70.

Spinner M (1968) The arcade of Frohse and its relationship to posterior interosseous nerve paralysis, *J Bone Joint Surg* **50B**: 809–12.

Sponseller PD, Engber WD (1983) Double-entrapment radial tunnel syndrome, *J Hand Surg* **8A**: 420–3.

Steiger R, Vögelin E (1998) Compression of the radial nerve caused by an occult ganglion, *J Hand Surg* **23B**: 420–1.

Van Rossum J, Buruma OJS, Kamphuisen HAC, Onvlee GJ (1978) Tennis elbow – a radial tunnel syndrome?, *J Bone Joint Surg* **60B**: 197–9.

Verhaar J, Spaans F (1991) Radial tunnel syndrome. An investigation of compression neuropathy as a possible cause, *J Bone Joint Surg* **73A**: 539–44.

Werner CO (1979) Lateral elbow pain and posterior interosseous nerve entrapment, *Acta Orthop Scand Suppl* **174**: 1–62.

Werner CO (1991) Radial nerve paralysis and tumor, *Clin Orthop* **268**: 223–5.

Wigoda P, Coleman DA (1999) A simple technique for decompression of the posterior interosseous nerve, *Techniques in Hand and Upper Extremity Surgery* **3**: 237–41.

Wilhelm A (1991) Compression proximale du nerf radial. In: Tubiana R, ed, *Chirurgie de la Main,* vol 4 (Masson Ed: Paris) 455–65.

Wood VE, Biondi J, Linda L (1990) Double crush nerve compression in thoracic outlet syndrome, *J Bone Joint Surg* **72A**: 85–7.

Younge DH, Moise P (1994) The radial tunnel syndrome, *Int Orthop* **18**: 368–370.

24 Median nerve compression

Michael Davidsen and Alain Gilbert

Introduction

The median nerve has attracted the attention of orthopaedic surgeons and hand surgeons for the last century like no other peripheral nerve. The disability and pain due to compression syndromes can dominate and invalidate the patient's well-being. For obvious reasons, carpal tunnel syndrome is most predominant in this group of patients, but the other entrapment syndromes of the median nerve should to be kept in mind when evaluating a differential diagnosis.

The median nerve is formed by the conjunction of the lateral and medial cord of the brachial plexus. It is composed of fibres from the C6, C7, C8 and T1 roots.

This chapter focuses on non-traumatic compression syndromes. Of course, any anatomical part of the median nerve can be damaged by blunt or sharp trauma or fractures of the upper extremity (Pritchard et al 1973, Rana et al 1974). Rare anatomical variations, such as aberrant muscles or vascular malformations, may cause compression syndromes of the nerve and knowledge of these variations is mandatory for the examining physician. There are five well described entrapment syndromes:

- The supracondylar spur, ligament of Struthers.
- Pronator syndrome.
- Entrapment of the anterior interosseus nerve.
- Carpal tunnel syndrome.
- Bowler's thumb.

The supracondylar spur, ligament of struthers

Not all entrapment syndromes of the upper arm present as purely neurological diseases, sometimes vascular symptoms and findings are involved. Median nerve symptoms are not always distinguishable from ulnar nerve symptoms. When this mixed picture presents itself to the hand surgeon, a proximal entrapment such as the combined supracondylar spur and ligament of Struthers should be considered (Gessini et al 1983, Kessel and Rang 1966, al Naib 1994).

Anatomy

A supracondylar foramen, containing the median nerve and brachial artery, can be seen in lions. In humans this 'bridge' is not common, but sometimes a spur is visible on plain X-rays (Figure 24.1). From this spur, the

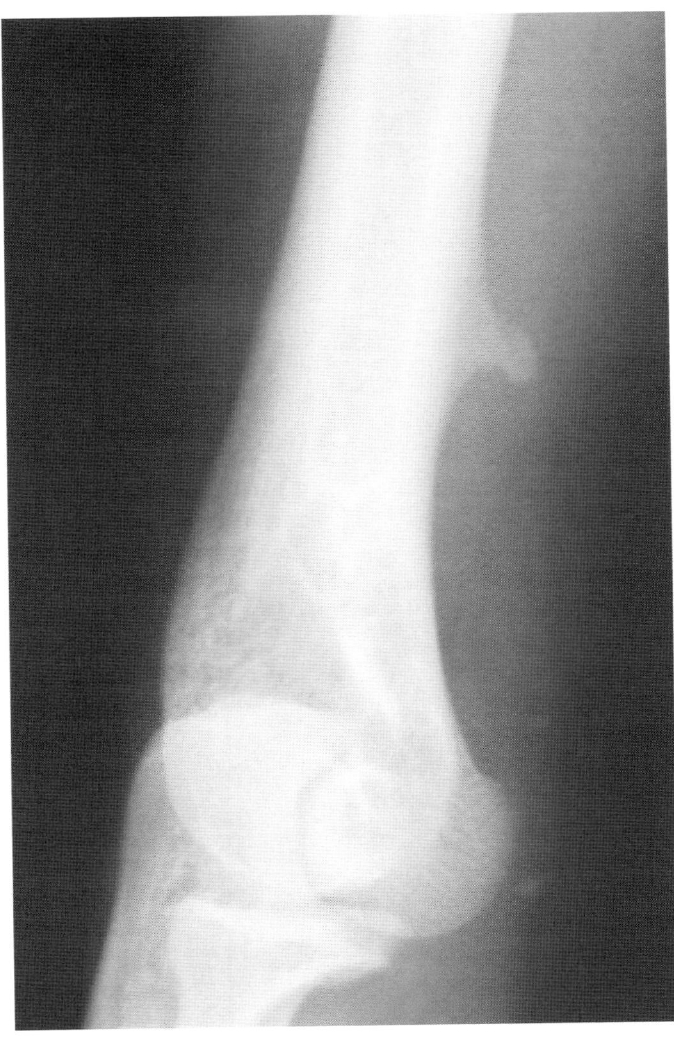

Figure 24.1

A supracondylar spur of the humerus is seen on the X-ray.

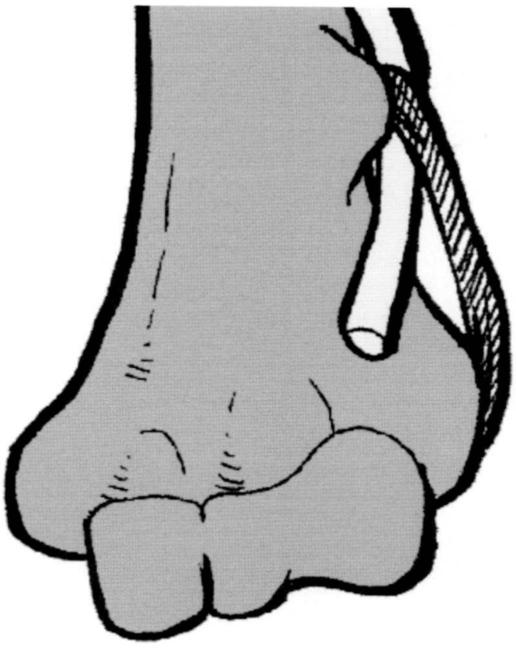

Figure 24.2
The ligament of Struthers with the median nerve passing under it.

ligament of Struthers extends downward to the humerus, thus forming a supracondylar foramen. The spur and ligament originate from the antero-lateral, distal part of the humerus and continue as a ligament onto the medial epicondyle. The median nerve and brachial artery will pass under this structure (Figure 24.2), but the ulnar nerve and ulnar artery can also be involved. The median nerve takes a slightly curved course to the anterior part of the arm.

Clinical features

History

When no spur or ligament of Struthers is present, the movement of the nerve is free, but when the nerve is fixed by these structures, stretching of the nerve causes pain. Thus, pain will be caused by:

- supination, especially on the stretched elbow
- extension of the elbow
- stretching of fingers and hand.

Patients can complain about coldness or numbness in the fourth and fifth fingers and the hypothenar region, when working with the arm in supination combined with elbow extension (al Naib 1994).

Clinical findings

Tinel's sign can be positive at the site. Sensibility and motor skills will be affected in the whole median nerve area. Ulnar nerve neurological findings can also be present when there is an involvement of the ulnar nerve. Sensory disturbances will often vary with the position of the antebrachium (see above). Vascular involvement is difficult to demonstrate clinically and peripheral pallor on physical exercise may be present. Electromyography (EMG) might help to locate the site of entrapment. The process (spur) might be palpable (al Naib 1994).

Diagnosis

A conventional X-ray is mandatory. The mixed clinical picture and the finding of a spur at the medial, distal humerus should point in the right direction.

Differential diagnosis

Myositis ossificans, myositis fibrosa generalisata, supracondylar fracture, other entrapment syndromes.

Operative treatment

If the spur is palpable, it should be marked on the skin. If it is not palpable, the image intensifier can be used to locate it. The arm is positioned on a radiolucent arm table. Often a sterile tourniquet has to be used, due to the limited space. An incision from the elbow crease along the medial border of the biceps tendon is made. The incision is centred over the spur. The brachial artery and median nerve are found distally and followed proximally. The ligament of Struthers and the supracondylar

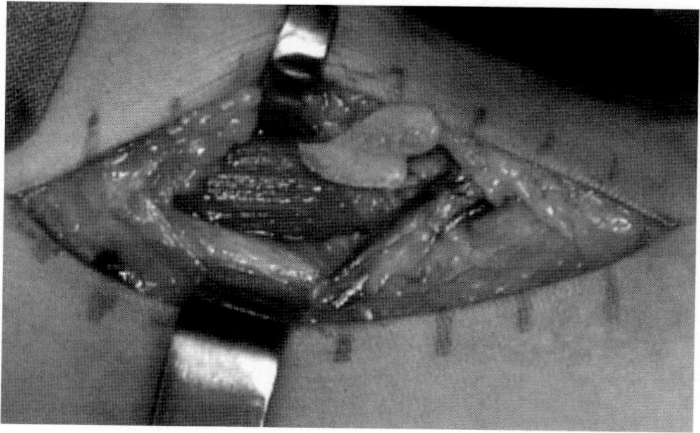

Figure 24.3
The supracondylar spur is resected.

spur are located and freed from surrounding tissue. The spur is resected close to the bone (Figure 24.3), and the ligament is excised and not transected. The bone surface is waxed. Failure to excise the ligament-like structure greatly increases the risk of recurrence of a constrictive band. If needed, the incision can be continued distally to explore the trunk of the median nerve. Postoperatively, a soft dressing is applied and, after a few days, exercises can start.

The pronator syndrome

Entrapment of the median nerve where it enters the forearm is called the pronator syndrome. This entrapment is not as common as carpal tunnel syndrome, but patients are often much younger. This syndrome is seen especially in sports where pronation of the forearm is performed repeatedly. Also, ballgames involving repeated catching might cause a pronator syndrome, as well as blunt trauma to the forearm by production of local oedema and sometimes haemorrhage. Conservative treatment might be effective (Asami et al 1999, Gessini et al 1987, Berlit 1989, Gainor 1990, Rehak 2001).

Anatomy

When the median nerve enters the antebrachium, and passes between the two heads of pronator teres, under the lacertus fibrosus, it may be compressed. The possible presence of a tumour should be considered.

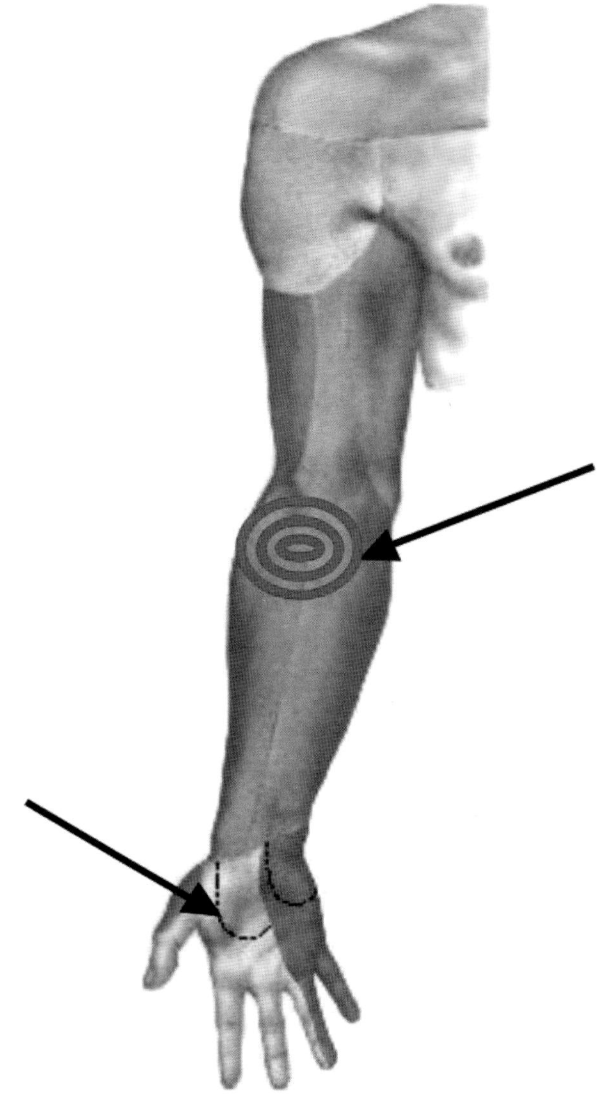

Figure 24.4
The red circle marks the site of pain in pronator syndrome.

Clinical features

Normally the disease evolves gradually with pain at the anterior surface of the forearm. Both strength and sensation will be reduced in the three radial fingers, but especially in the thumb and index finger. The intensity of the pain increases with workload and vice versa. There will normally be no disturbance of sleep by night pain.

Tinel's sign will be positive at the proximal anterior part of the forearm. There will be no findings at the carpal tunnel, Phalen's test is negative. Flexion of the distal phalanges of the three radial fingers will be decreased and the small muscles of the thenar eminence may be affected. Sensibility of the radial fingers can be decreased. The following might give a hint as to the more specific site of entrapment (Figure 24.4):

- When flexion (against resistance) of the elbow in a supine position causes pain, the lacertus fibrosus (the aponeurosis of the biceps tendon) may be the cause of compression.
- When pronation (against resistance) of the supinated, stretched elbow causes pain, the pronator teres may be causing compression. This test must be done with the elbow nearly extended owing to the relaxation of the humeral head of the pronator teres when the elbow is flexed.
- When flexion (against resistance) of the third finger's proximal interphalongeal (PIP) joint, with hyperextension of the second, fourth and fifth fingers (use of the third flexor digitorum superficialis), causes pain, the ligamentum arcuatum, tendinous origin of the flexor digitorum superficialis, may be the cause of entrapment (Gessini et al 1987, Gainor 1990, Rehak 2001).

Diagnosis

The absence of night symptoms, the lack of findings at the carpal tunnel and the presence of pain, tenderness and a positive Tinel's sign at the volar aspect of the proximal forearm will help the examiner. Decreased sensibility of the radial fingers will distinguish the pronator syndrome from other diseases: entrapment of the anterior interosseus nerve, carpal tunnel syndrome, and rupture of flexor pollicis longus or flexor digitorum to index or third finger.

Conservative treatment

Splinting and non-steroidal anti-inflammatory drugs (NSAIDs) may be tried for a couple of months. The splint should keep the elbow flexed in 45°, in pronation to release the tension of the humeral head of the pronator teres. The wrist should be in neutral position. Rather than immobilizing the arm, the splint should keep the patient from overexertion during activities.

Operative treatment

If conservative treatment has no effect, surgical release of the nerve should be carried out. The operation is done in a bloodless field, using a tourniquet. In the anterior surface of the cubital region a 5 cm incision is made along the medial border of the biceps tendon. Distally this incision is continued in a Z-fashion in the forearm. The length of the incision in the forearm must cover the proximal two-thirds thirds of the forearm. Subcutaneous veins are ligated. The fascia is incised and the nervus cutaneus antebrachii lateralis is located and isolated, between the biceps tendon and the medial border of the brachioradialis muscle. The median nerve (Figure 24.5) and the brachial artery are found lying on the lateral aspect of the nerve. The lacertus fibrosus, the aponeurosis of the biceps tendon, is divided with great care, respecting the radial artery which originates from the brachial artery just underneath the aponeurosis. The median nerve is dissected distally and the origin of the anterior interosseus nerve is located just before they pass between the humeral and ulnar heads of the pronator teres muscle. A Z-incision in the distal part of the humeral head of the pronator teres muscle is made close to its insertion on the radius. Reconstruction of this normally very tense muscle is facilitated by the lengthening Z-reconstruction. Then the origin of the branch to the flexor pollicis longus muscle is found. All nerves pass beneath the origin of the flexor digitorum superficialis muscle which forms a ligament, the arcuate ligament. This is the most common site of entrapment. Look for a persisting median artery or other pathology. Good haemostasis is secured with a bipolar coagulator. Only the skin is sutured and a soft dressing is applied. Postoperatively, the arm is immobilized for 6 weeks with a hard bandage from the upper arm to the metacarpophalangeal (MP) joints. The position of the arm should be 90° at the elbow with the forearm in 45° pronation to release the tension on the sutured pronator teres (Gessini et al 1987, Idler et al 1991, Rehak 2001).

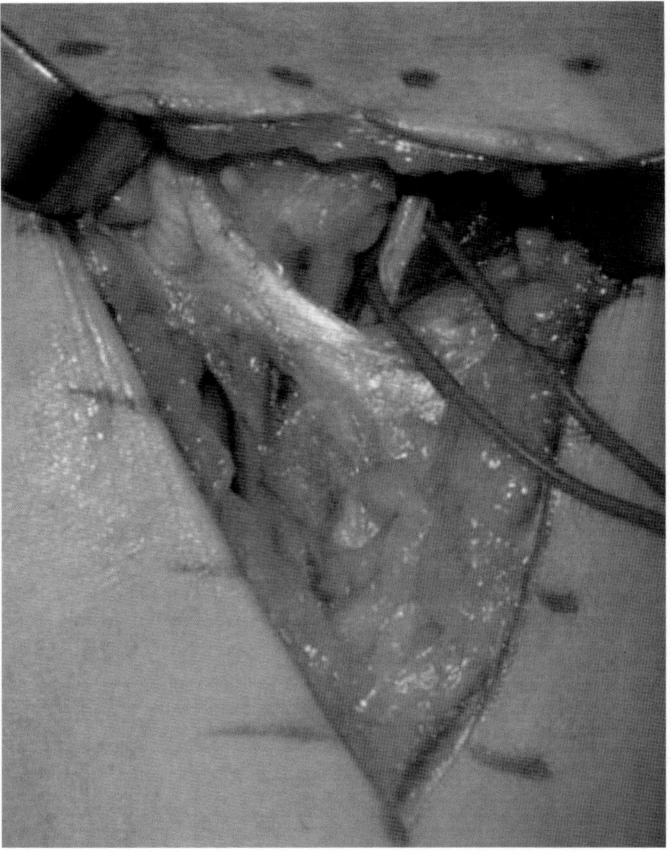

Figure 24.5
The median nerve is located (and marked with the band) just when it passes under the lacertus fibrosus (also seen).

Entrapment of the anterior interosseus nerve

Sudden decrease of flexion force of the thumb and index finger can be a sign of entrapment of the anterior interosseus nerve. Patients complain about difficulties with fine motor skills, such as picking up small objects and using the pinch grip. Pain at the anterior surface of the arm is often present. This entity is sometimes misdiagnosed as a carpal tunnel syndrome or even as reflex dystrophy. Patients will often go 'doctor shopping' or

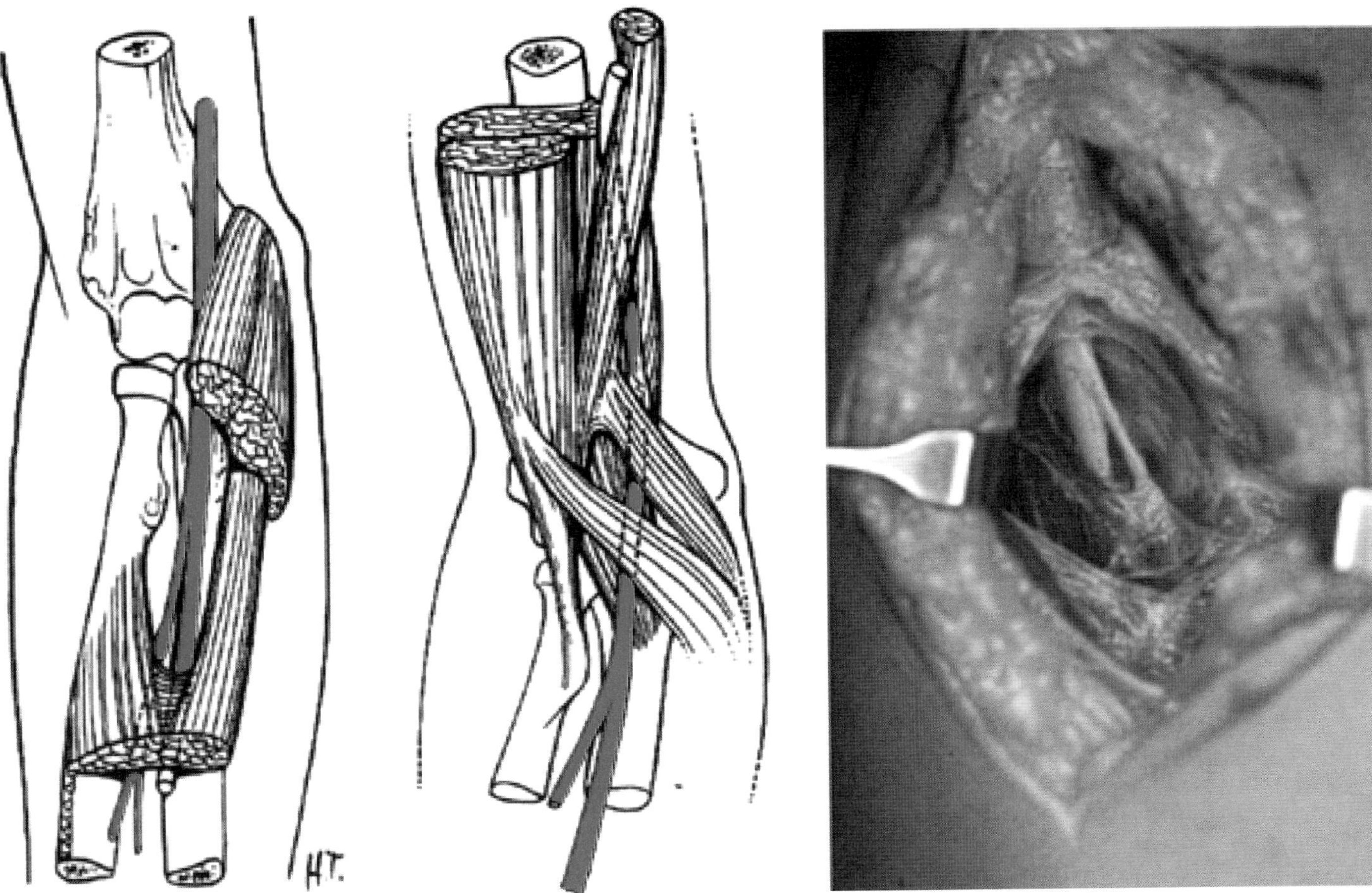

Figure 24.6
The location of the anterior interosseus nerve and its origin.

even try alternative treatments before a correct diagnosis is made (Gessini et al 1988, Creighton et al 1991, Carmant and Veilleux 1993, Axmann and Mailander 1995, Ashworth et al 1997, Haug and Bertheussen 1998). Hyperextension of the elbow, especially combined with supination or traction injuries, are common causes of this disease, as may occur in waterskiing or gymnastics. Other causes are blunt trauma or fractures of the forearm. In mild cases or slowly evolving cases, a neuropraxia is present and full recovery should be expected. More severe cases following blunt trauma or fracture of the forearm can lead to axonotmesis with a slow and long restitution. Successful treatment should be expected to be followed by a recovery period of up to 6 months. Different authors disagree on whether to treat this entrapment conservatively or to decompress the nerve.

Anatomy

The anterior interosseus nerve is a motor branch from the median nerve (Figure 24.6). It innervates the flexor pollicis longus, the deep flexor to the index finger and the pronator quadratus muscle. This nerve also provides the central nervous system with proprioceptive information from the joint capsule and ligaments but it does not contain any sensory information from the skin. At the level of the radial neck, the nerve originates from the median nerve and passes together with the median nerve between the humeral and ulnar head of the pronator teres muscle. The first motor branch to the flexor pollicis longus muscle originates about 4 cm from the origin of the anterior interosseus nerve. All these median nerves pass under the tendinous origin of the flexor digitorum superficialis muscle, the ligamentum arcuatum. En route to the pronator quadratus muscle the nerve is joined by the interosseus artery lying between the flexor pollicis longus and the flexor digitorum profundus muscle, on the interosseus membrane.

Exploration of the nerve often shows entrapment under the arcuate ligament. The nerve can be swollen in an 'hourglass'-like fashion. Fibrosis can be seen if the problem has been present for a longer period.

Clinical features

This entrapment evolves gradually, but can also occur as an acute problem, after trauma when lifting heavy objects.

Patients will complain of:

- Weak pinch grip because of decreased strength in the flexor pollicis longus muscle and flexor digitorum profundus muscle to the index finger. Fingers feel 'clumsy' and small objects like coins or needles are picked up with great difficulty.
- Pronation of the forearm is weak, producing difficulty in turning a key in the lock, or unscrewing a screw with a screwdriver.
- Pain at the elbow crease which worsens during work and is relieved at rest.

There will be no complaints about loss of sensation.

Objective findings

- Abnormal position of the distal phalanx of the thumb and index finger when performing the pinch grip due to weak flexor pollicis longus and weak flexor digitorum profundus to the index finger. This is often referred to as the 'O'-sign, which is rather misleading as a normal grip should present an 'O', whereas these patients do not (Figure 24.7)!
- Decreased power of the flexor pollicis longus and the flexor digitorum profundus to the index finger.
- Decreased force of pronation due to a weak pronator quadratus muscle. This test is done with the elbow in maximal flexion, to eliminate the action of the humeral head of the pronator teres muscle.

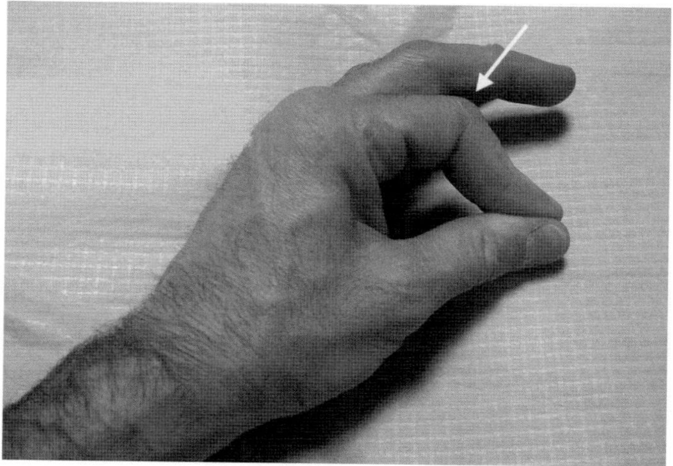

Figure 24.7
The lack of 'O' sign, due to the weak flexor pollicis longus.

- Normal sensation in the area innervated by the median nerve, with a positive Tinel's sign at the ligamentum arcuatum.

Pitfalls:

- The anterior interosseus nerve may act on the deep flexor to all digits, and thus all distal interphalangeal (DIP) joints may be affected.
- The anterior interosseus nerve may act on the superficial flexor muscles to digits, thus affecting the flexion force of the PIP joints.
- In 15% of normal individuals, the anastomosis of Martin Gruber is present, a shortcut to the motor branch of the ulnar nerve to the small hand muscles, and these muscles may be weakened.

Differential diagnoses

- Rupture of the flexor pollicis longus tendon. In this case there will be normal flexion force of the DIP joint of the index finger and normal pronation force.
- Pronator syndrome paraesthesias will be present. There will be loss of sensation in the area innervated by the median nerve.
- Carpal tunnel syndrome. Paraesthesias in radial fingers. Good pronation force with the elbow flexed. Weakness of thenar eminence muscles.

Conservative treatment

Splinting and NSAIDs can be tried. Two authors have recommended electrical stimulation of affected muscle until recovery (Vichare 1968, Turek 1977).

Operative treatment

The operation is done in a bloodless field, using a tourniquet. The patient is positioned supine and the arm rests in supination on an arm table. A 5-cm incision is made along the medial border of the biceps tendon in the anterior surface of the cubital region (Figure 24.8). Distally this incision is continued as a lazy Z-incision in the central part of the forearm. The length of the incision in the forearm must cover the proximal two-thirds of the forearm. The fascia is incised and the nervus cutaneus antebrachii lateralis is located and isolated, between the biceps tendon and the medial border of the brachioradialis muscle. The median nerve and the brachial artery, lying lateral to the nerve, are located. The lacertus fibrosus, the aponeurosis of the biceps tendon, is divided with great care, respecting the radial artery, which originates from the brachial

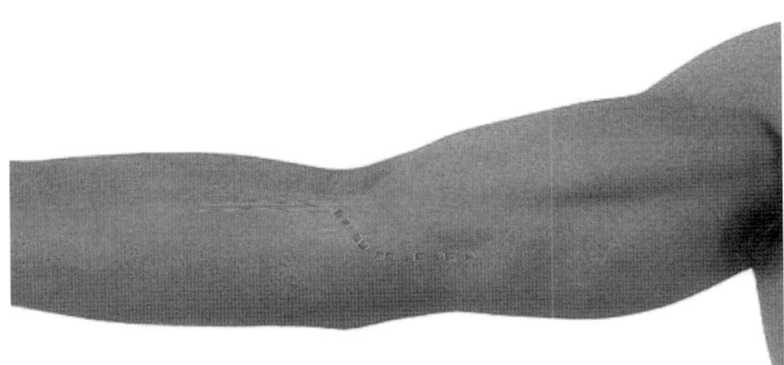

Figure 24.8
The incision for exploring the anterior interosseus nerve.

artery just underneath the aponeurosis. The median nerve is dissected distally and the origin of the anterior interosseus nerve is located just before both nerves pass between the humeral and ulnar head of the pronator teres. A Z-incision in the distal part of the humeral head of the muscle is made close to its insertion on the radius. Reconstruction of this normally very tense muscle is facilitated by the lengthening Z-reconstruction. Shortly after, the origin of the branch to the flexor pollicis longus muscle is found. All nerves pass beneath the origin of the flexor digitorum superficialis muscle, which forms a ligament, the arcuate ligament. This is the most common site of entrapment. Look for a persisting median artery or other pathology. The Z-incision in the humeral head of pronator teres muscle is sutured, elongating it 2 cm. Good haemostasis is secured with a bipolar coagulator. Only the skin is sutured and a soft dressing is applied. Postoperatively the arm is immobilized for 4 weeks with a hard bandage for the upper arm to the MP joints. The position of the arm should be 90° at the elbow with 45° pronation of the forearm, to release the tension of the sutured pronator teres.

Carpal tunnel syndrome

Carpal tunnel syndrome (CTS) is by far the most common nerve entrapment in the upper extremity (Tubiana 1990), probably in the whole body. No other entity has so prompted attempts to understand the mechanism and pathophysiological changes of entrapment neuropathies. It is seen two-to-three times more often in women than in men, and most often affects middle-aged women (Tubiana 1990, Boeckstyns and Sorensen 1999). Conditions that alter the volume of the subcutaneous and connective tissues can often produce CTS, including pregnancy, diabetes mellitus, rheumatoid arthritis or renal insufficiency. In patients on haemodialysis with a fistula in the affected arm, amyloidal substances may reduce the space in the carpal tunnel. In approximately 25% of patients, the disease is bilateral (Bodofsky et al 2001).

If the history is short, especially in diabetes, conservative treatment might have an effect. Operation quickly relieves the patient of night pain, whereas decrease of sensibility takes a little longer to improve. If the history has lasted for several years, and there is muscle atrophy at the thenar eminence, complete recovery is rare and loss of muscle mass is often permanent (Michelsen and Posner 2002). Around 80–95% of patients will have complete recovery (Gerritsen et al 2002, Okada et al 2000, Braun et al 2002, Chow and Hantes 2002).

Aetiology

CTS is caused by elevated pressure on the contents of the carpal tunnel.

1. Swollen tendon sheaths. Thus is one of the most common causes, as seen in diabetes; 15% of patients with CTS have diabetes. Pregnant women who develop CTS will have symptoms in the sixth to ninth month of pregnancy and often with bilateral affection. Rheumatoid arthritis is found in up to 12% of patients with CTS.
2. Colles' or Schmidt's fracture. In Colles' fracture, the distal fragment is displaced dorsally and the fracture is reduced by deviating the hand and immobilized in a volar and ulnar manner, thus reducing the volume of the carpal tunnel. Bleeding may also decrease the volume of the tunnel. Symptoms will often disappear after neutralizing the hand. If the fracture cannot be stabilized in this neutral position, internal fixation should be performed. The frequency of CTS following Colles' fracture can be as high as 17% and often requires surgical treatment.
3. Expanding processes. A ganglion from a tendon sheath is seen in 2% of cases. Lipomas have been described, but have never been seen by these authors.
4. Anatomical variations. Anomalies of the flexor digitorum superficialis muscle, reverse palmaris longus muscle, long small muscles in the hand or other abnormal structures are all rare.
5. Double crush. When a proximal entrapment is present, e.g. pronator syndrome, the distal part of the nerve is more sensitive to compression.

Anatomy

The carpal tunnel is a well defined space, surrounded by hard surfaces. Radially the tuberosity of the scaphoid and the trapezoid bone limit the tunnel. On the ulnar side, it is bordered by the hook of hamate and the pisiform bones. The floor is made of the carpal bones and ligaments, and the roof is formed by the thick transverse carpal ligament. Through the tunnel pass:

- The flexor pollicis longus tendon, in its own tendon sheath.
- The deep and superficial flexor tendons in a common tendon sheath.
- The median nerve.

Many anatomical variations are seen, such as:

- Branching of the median nerve, proximal to the tunnel.
- Aberrant muscles.
- Motor branch to the thenar arising proximally to the tunnel or even from the ulnar side of the median nerve.
- Sensory branch to the thenar skin arising anywhere on the distal median nerve, even penetrating the ligament.

The last mentioned sensory branch is often neglected and may be cut, especially in trauma surgery, where the surgeon wants to put a volar T-plate on the distal radius to stabilize a Schmidt's fracture. Having put the plate in place, the inexperienced surgeon, who also wants to decompress the carpal tunnel, continues the incision distally, thereby cutting the sensory branch to the the thenar. Patients will complain about loss of sensibility and numbness in the thenar region for several years.

Clinical features

The patient will complain about a variety of symptoms. The duration of symptoms will vary. Some patients have symptoms for a few weeks only and experience slight paraesthesia in the fingertips. Others will have had symptoms for several years with total loss of thenar muscle mass.

1. Paraesthesias. The first, second, third and the radial half of the fourth finger feel numb at night. Often this symptom is most severe in the third finger. In the beginning these sensations are intermittent and work-related. Characteristic are the nightly symptoms after a few hours of sleep. The patient wakes up and has to shake the hand, hold it downwards or even put it in cold/hot water to make it 'come alive'. Some patients will sleep with the hand in a distinct position.
2. Pain. Pain can be felt in the whole area of the median nerve distribution, in the hand and wrist, sometimes going up to the shoulder.
3. Reduced fine motor skills. There is reduced ability to pick up small objects, like needles, small coins or paper clips.
4. Reduction of thenar force. The abductor pollicis brevis and opponens pollicis muscles are weakened, and the pinch grip is reduced. This can be measured by a special instrument.

Objective findings

1. Sensation. Sensibility to both sharp and blunt objects will be reduced. Two-point discrimination can be affected, although this is not always the case. The area of reduced sensation is the classical median nerve area covering the first, second, third and the radial half of the fourth finger, but does not necessarily involve the whole area. Reduced sweat production, as shown with the ball-pen traction test, or even a ninhydrin test, is only seen in the most severe cases. If the whole thenar area is involved (also the proximal part) one must suspect that the palmar sensitive branch of the thenar arises beneath the ligament.
2. Muscle strength. M. abductor pollicis brevis may be affected. This can be demonstrated by:
   - Test A, with the hand lying on the back, the patient is asked to abduct the thumb against the examiner's own finger. If unilateral involvement of the nerve is present, the hand is compared with the contralateral hand. A reduced force is quite easy to recognize.
   - Test B, holding the hands with the palms facing each other at a distance of 10 cm apart, the patient is asked to press the thumbs against each other, or hold a piece of paper that the examiner tries to pull on. This of course works best in a unilateral case.
3. Atrophy of the thenar muscles is seen in more severe cases.
4. Phalen's test (Figure 24.9). The hand is flexed which reduces the volume of the carpal tunnel. After seconds or minutes paraesthesias will occur. This test can also be done as the reversed Phalen in extension. The test is reliable.
5. Tinel's sign. Tapping the tunnel with a finger or reflex hammer will produce paraesthesias. This test

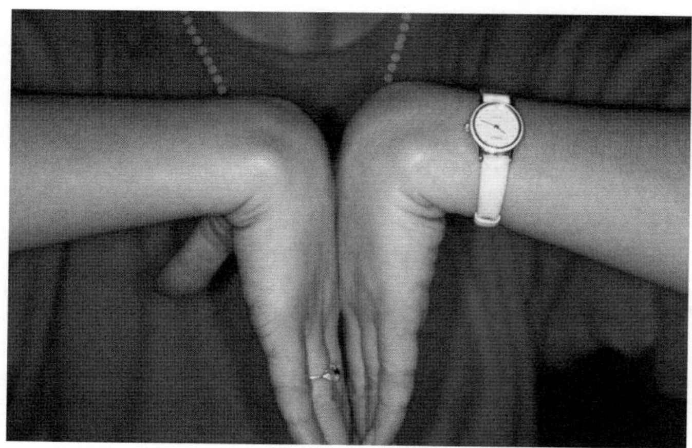

Figure 24.9
The Phalen test.

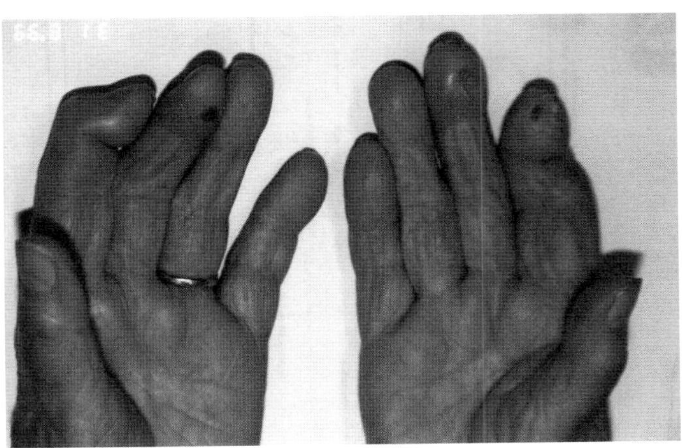

Figure 24.10
Acronecrosis in severe carpal tunnel syndrome.

is good for localizing the site of entrapment. The test is highly specific.

6. Durkan's sign. Compression of the carpal tunnel will produce paraesthesias after seconds or minutes. Not a reliable test.
7. Gilliat's sign. A tourniquet is applied to the suspected arm. Paraesthesias are produced after seconds to minutes. Difficult to interpret because of vascular signs produced by the test.
8. Raised arm test. Raising both arms will produce paraesthesias. A quick and easily done test.
9. Acronecrosis (Figure 24.10). Ulceration on the fingertips may be seen in more severe cases.

EMG

The question as to whether EMG will elucidate CTS further in diagnosis is not yet fully resolved; it seems that this discussion is more of a debate between neurophysiologists and surgeons. On a broad basis, around 90% of patients who will benefit from an operation will have reduced sensory nerve conduction, and 65–90% will have reduced motor nerve conduction. Thus a normal EMG will sometimes be false negative. Tests on the normal population also show some degree of false positive EMG results (Cho and Cho 1989, Anastosopoulos and Chroni 1997, Wiederien et al 2002). Having said that, one should not neglect the usage of EMG, which is very helpful when:

- Symptoms and findings are not specific, making the diagnosis uncertain.
- Monitoring of the evolution of the disease is needed.
- Symptoms have been present for a long time. Symptoms will not disappear as quickly as when symptoms have been present for a short time. The lack of relief will make a hand surgeon suspect an incomplete decompression, but EMG will often show improvement before the patient senses it.

Diagnosis

In simple straightforward cases where symptoms and signs are clear, the diagnosis should be easy, but if in doubt, do not hesitate to perform an EMG. Remember to check for diabetes. If EMG is normal an injection of steroid could be tried as a test.

Thoracic outlet syndrome can be either a differential diagnosis or an associated one.

Conservative treatment

Conservative treatment can be tried out in pregnant women, or where the duration of symptoms is short. An immobilizing cast is made with the hand in a neutral position. NSAIDs can help to reduce inflammation. Some authors recommend injection of steroid in the carpal tunnel, but there is a risk of injecting into the nerve and thereby damaging the nerve.

Conservative treatment should not be tried when there are hyperaesthesias or there is atrophy of the thenar muscles (Ebskov et al 1997, Bodofsky 2002, Osterman et al 2002).

Operative treatment

Several methods exist. The range goes from one-hole endoscopic techniques, to minimal incision techniques to fully open decompression and internal neurolysis using a microscope. The choice of operation is often affected by the skills of the surgeon and the traditions of the hospital. Generally speaking the surgeon should choose the method that works best in his hands, but he should also be aware of possibilities of improvements, even if it takes a completely new technique, like endoscopic release, to maximize the success of the operation. A good result of an operation is not just a well executed decompression, but also sends the patient back to work quickly, saves him from tenderness of the palm when supporting his weight on it, relieves him of symptoms, does no further damage, and prevents return of symptoms. Endoscopic decompression with its clear advantages should be reserved for straightforward cases. If there is any doubt as to whether anatomical variations are present, or after a wrist fracture, or when there is a synovitis that needs synovectomy, an open approach should be chosen.

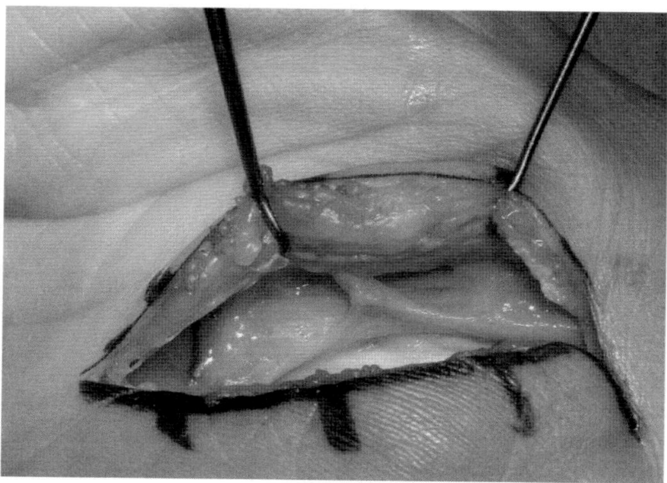

Figure 24.11
An open visualization of the carpal tunnel.

Open method (Figure 24.11)

The patient is positioned supine with the arm on an arm table. A tourniquet is applied. The whole hand and forearm must be free. Distally the incision should commence at a point on a transverse line through the bottom of the first webspace. A curved incision is made along the thenar crease to the distal flexion crease of the wrist. From there the incision continues obliquely towards the ulnar edge for 3–4 cm. Proximally at the ulnar side of the palmaris longus tendon, the median nerve is found. Look for a longitudinal grey structure that is not smooth surfaced, rather than a blank white shiny structure. The presence of vasa nervorum will indicate that a nerve has been found. Once the nerve has been found it is followed distally while keeping in the ulnar side of the tunnel so as not to damage the motor branch of the thenar. The ligament is completely divided. Care must be taken at the distal part where the nerve to the third and fourth fingers curves ulnarly. Take care not to damage the arterial arcade. There is no need to dissect the epineurium and there is also no need to dissect the motor thenar; the risk of damaging rather than benefiting the patient is too great. A good haemostasis is secured and only the skin is sutured. Postoperatively, a soft dressing is applied and the wound is inspected after 1 week. After open decompression one should wait for 2 weeks before removing stitches. Some tenderness of the palm can be expected, especially after open treatment. This can take up to 5 months to disappear.

- Night pain will be the first to disappear. Often patients will report that the night after the operation was the first night for a long time that they were not woken up by pain.
- Loss of sensation may take several weeks or months to improve.
- The fine motor skills will take months to recover.
- Muscle atrophy will often never disappear.

Endoscopic method (Figure 24.12 and 24.13)

In the two-portal technique a small, 5-mm transverse incision is made at the proximal flexion crease of the wrist. The skin is lifted with a hook, and dissection to the carpal tunnel is carried out. A blunt instrument such as Mayo scissors is introduced into the tunnel, following the ulnar border of the tunnel, and the transverse carpal ligament can be palpated. A space is created under the ligament. The tip of the introducer is protruded and palpated in the palm of the hand, and the second opening is made right over the tip of the introducer. In

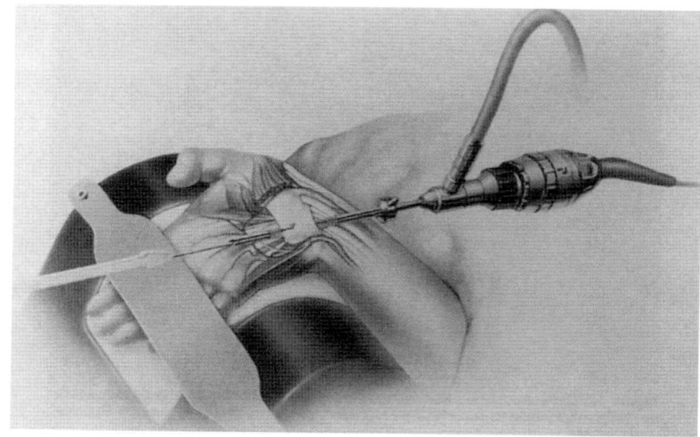

Figure 24.12
Two-portal endoscopic technique.

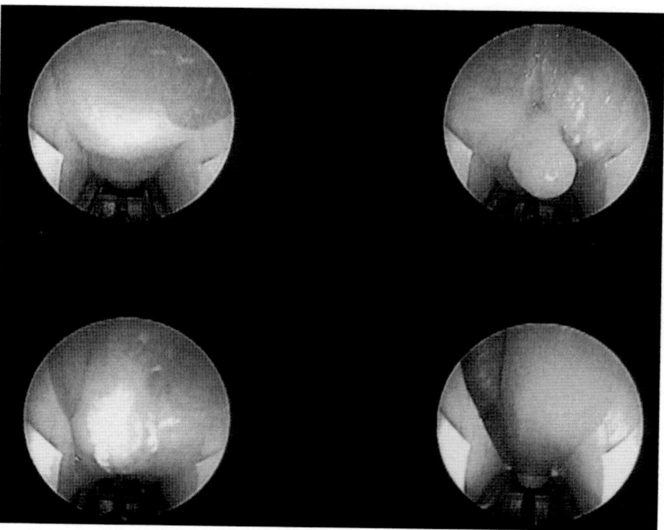

Figure 24.13
Four views through the endoscope showing the 'roof' of the carpal tunnel, the fat pad bulging down when cutting the ligament, and the completed procedure.

this way, a canal is produced. The endoscope is then introduced. The ligament is visualized and cut under vision. Skin is sutured and a soft dressing is applied.

Results after treatment of CTS

Results after open decompression

In many centres, open decompression is considered the 'gold standard'. The complete visualization of all the structures and abnormalities in the carpal tunnel satisfies many surgeons, but what about the patient's own opinion? In an article by Boeckstyns et al (1999) no difference was found in the complication rate between the two methods, and return to work was quicker after endoscopic treatment. In another article, the focus on scar tenderness and risk of reflex sympathetic dystrophy, did not favour the open treatment (Braun et al 2002).

Results after endoscopic decompression

Endoscopic decompression has been performed in our centre for more than 10 years. Table 24.1 provides an analysis of 14,666 cases. The average age of these patients was 54.1 years (range 19–96). In 1.2% of cases the procedure had to be converted to open surgery. In a paper from Elmaraghy and Hurst (1996) the rate of infection was 1.5%. Another paper by Agee et al (1992) showed nerve injuries in 0.6% of cases and tendon injuries in 0.08%. The recurrence rate was 1.2%.

Table 24.1 *Results after endoscopic decompression*

Result	*Number*	*%*
Tendon injuries	0	0
Bleeding/haematoma	0	0
Infection	10	0.07
Tender scar	35	0.2
Recurrence/persistent symptoms	52	0.4
Pillar pain	210	1.4

Thus our series provides sufficient arguments to justify the method, with very low complication rates. In our hands this treatment is considered safe and is recommended, and several articles on this subject support view (Ebskov et al 1997, Boeckstyns and Sorensen 1999, Okada et al 2000, Braun et al 2002, Nagle 2002).

Bowler's thumb

Bowler's thumb is caused by constant pressure on the ulnar digital nerve of the thumb. The entity is seen in bowlers when grip of the bowling ball squeezes the nerve. In countries like the USA where bowling is very popular, this sport is the predomir cause of the disease. The disease can also be work-related, especially in people changing to manual work and gripping a tool with a sharp edge. Fibrosis of the epineurium eventually occurs and often a true neuroma is found when the nerve is exposed (Rayan 1990). The bowling syndrome produces a spindle neuroma (Herndon et al 1976), justifying conservative treatment.

Clinical features

The patient will report pain, especially when participating in their sport or work. Later paraesthesias will appear. There is no pain during sleep.

Tenderness of the ulnar sesamoid bone is found as the first sign. Later Tinel's sign may be positive. Sensibility in the area of the affected nerves is decreased, often with increased two-point discrimination. Occasionally, hyperaesthesia with pain on the slightest touch is seen, this is present in the whole innervation area of the nerve. Flexion of the thumb, especially at the MP joint, may be decreased.

Conservative treatment

Splinting of the thumb and hand may be helpful. Sport or work activities should be modified. The patient can try placing the thumb only halfway down the hole in the ball. Another placement of the holes in the ball may also help to move the pressure to another region.

Operative treatment

If conservative treatment fails, a neurolysis or even resection can be done. Resection is only done in the most severe cases and after obtaining the acceptance of the patient (it is most often done secondarily, after trying neurolysis). The sesamoid bone should not be removed. Postoperatively, a soft dressing is applied. The wound is inspected after 4 days, and exercises are begun after removal of the stitches. Care should be taken to alter the sport or work, to avoid recurrence of the symptoms.

Conclusion

Treatment of median nerve compression syndromes is a challenge to many surgeons worldwide. Knowledge of the anatomy with its variations, as well as the variability in symptoms, is absolutely essential. Diagnosis may sometimes be very difficult due to the common associations. Electrodiagnostic techniques may be of great help, but the physician needs a detailed knowledge of anatomy.

References

Agee JM, McCarroll HR Jr, Tortosa RD, Berry DA, Szabo RM, Peimer CA (1992) Endoscopic release of the carpal tunnel: a randomized prospective multicenter study, *J Hand Surg [Am]* **17**: 987–95.

al Naib I (1994) Humeral supracondylar spur and Struthers' ligament. A rare cause of neurovascular entrapment in the upper limb, *Int Orthop* **18**: 393–4.

Anastasopoulos D, Chroni E (1997) Effect of carpal tunnel syndrome on median nerve proximal conduction estimated by F-waves, *J Clin Neurophysiol* **14**: 63–7.

Asami A, Takayama G, Hotokebuchi T (1999) Pronator teres syndrome associated with mononeuritis multiplex in polyarteritis nodosa, *Hand Surg* **4**: 189–92.

Ashworth NL, Marshall SC, Classen DA (1997) Anterior interosseous nerve syndrome presenting with pronator teres weakness: a case report, *Muscle Nerve* **20**: 1591–4.

Axmann HD, Mailander P (1995) [Anterior interosseus syndrome from the surgical viewpoint], *Nervenarzt* **66**: 610–13.

Berlit P (1989) [Pronator teres syndrome caused by neurinoma of the median nerve], *Nervenarzt* **60**: 184–6.

Bodofsky E (2002) Treating carpal tunnel syndrome with lasers and TENS, *Arch Phys Med Rehabil* **83**: 1806–7.

Bodofsky EB, Greenberg WM, Wu KD (2001) Median nerve compression at the wrist: is it ever unilateral? *Electromyogr Clin Neurophysiol* **41**: 451–6.

Boeckstyns ME, Sorensen AI (1999) Does endoscopic carpal tunnel release have a higher rate of complications than open carpal tunnel release? An analysis of published series, *J Hand Surg [Br]* **24**: 9–15.

Braun RM, Rechnic M, Fowler E (2002) Complications related to carpal tunnel release, *Hand Clin* **18**: 347–57.

Carmant L, Veilleux M (1993) Anterior interosseous neuropathy in the postpartum period, *Can J Neurol Sci* **20**: 56–8.

Cho DS, Cho MJ (1989) The electrodiagnosis of the carpal tunnel syndrome, *S D J Med* **42**: 5–8.

Chow JC, Hantes ME (2002) Endoscopic carpal tunnel release: thirteen years' experience with the Chow technique, *J Hand Surg [Am]* **27**: 1011–18.

Creighton JJ Jr, Strickland JW, Idler RS (1991) Anterior interosseous nerve palsy, *Indiana Med* **84**: 192–4.

Ebskov LB, Boeckstyns ME, Sorensen AI (1997) Operative treatment of carpal tunnel syndrome in Denmark. Results of a questionnaire, *J Hand Surg [Br]* **22**: 761–3.

Elmaraghy MW, Hurst LN (1996) Single-portal endoscopic carpal tunnel release: agee carpal tunnel release system, *Ann Plast Surg* **36**: 286–91.

Gainor BJ (1990) The pronator compression test revisited. A forgotten physical sign, *Orthop Rev* **19**: 888–92.

Gerritsen AA, de Vet HC, Scholten RJ (2002) Splinting vs surgery in the treatment of carpal tunnel syndrome: a randomized controlled trial, *JAMA* **288**: 1245–51.

Gessini L, Jandolo B, Pietrangeli A (1983) Entrapment neuropathies of the median nerve at and above the elbow, *Surg Neurol* **19**: 112–16.

Gessini L, Jandolo B, Pietrangeli A (1987) The pronator teres syndrome. Clinical and electrophysiological features in six surgically verified cases, *J Neurosurg Sci* **31**: 1–5.

Gessini L, Jandolo B, Landucci C, Pietrangeli A (1988) Anterior interosseous nerve syndrome, *Ital J Neurol Sci* **9**: 41–5.

Haug M, Bertheussen K (1998) [Anterior interosseus nerve syndrome], *Ugeskr Laeger* **160**: 5192–3.

Herndon JH, Eaton RG, Littler JW (1976) Management of painful neuromas in the hand, *J Bone Joint Surg [Am]* **58**: 369–73.

Idler RS, Strickland JW, Creighton JJ Jr (1991) Pronator syndrome, *Indiana Med* **84**: 124–7.

Kessel L, Rang M (1966) Supracondylar spur of the humerus, *J Bone Joint Surg [Br]* **48**: 765–9.

Michelsen H, Posner MA (2002) Medical history of carpal tunnel syndrome, *Hand Clin* **18**: 257–68.

Nagle DJ (2002) Endoscopic carpal tunnel release, *Hand Clin* **18**: 307–13.

Okada M, Tsubata O, Yasumoto S, Toda N, Matsumoto T (2000) Clinical study of surgical treatment of carpal tunnel syndrome: open versus endoscopic technique, *J Orthop Surg [Hong Kong]* **8**: 19–25.

Okada M, Tsubata O, Yasumoto S, Toda N, Matsumoto T (••••) Open versus endoscopic technique,

Osterman AL, Whitman M, Porta LD (2002) Nonoperative carpal tunnel syndrome treatment, *Hand Clin* **18**: 279–89.

Pritchard DJ, Linscheid RL, Svien HJ (1973) Intra-articular median nerve entrapment with dislocation of the elbow, *Clin Orthop* **90**: 100–3.

Rana NA, Kenwright J, Taylor RG, Rushworth G (1974) Complete lesion of the median nerve associated with dislocation of the elbow joint, *Acta Orthop Scand* **45**: 365–9.

Rayan GM (1990) Stenosing tenosynovitis in bowlers, *Am J Sports Med* **18**: 214–15.

Rehak DC (2001) Pronator syndrome, *Clin Sports Med* **20**: 531–40.

Tubiana R (1990) Carpal tunnel syndrome: some views on its management, *Ann Chir Main Memb Super* **9**: 325–30.

Turek SL (1977) *Orthopaedics. Principles and their Applications* (Lippincott: Philadelphia) 907–9.

Vichare NA (1968) Spontaneous paralysis of the anterior interosseous nerve, *J Bone Joint Surg [Br]* **50**: 806–8.

Wiederien RC, Feldman TD, Heusel LD et al (2002) The effect of the median nerve compression test on median nerve conduction across the carpal tunnel, *Electromyogr Clin Neurophysiol* **42**: 413–21.

25 Other nerve compression lesions in the upper extremity

Robert J Spinner and Peter C Amadio

Introduction

While the most common peripheral nerve lesions of the upper limb involve the median nerve at the wrist, the ulnar nerve at the elbow and the wrist, and the radial nerve in the arm, physicians dealing with upper extremity or peripheral nerve problems will see patients from time to time with other rare compressive lesions. These may involve the proximal median nerve (anterior interosseous nerve and pronator syndrome), posterior interosseous nerve, superficial radial nerve, and the digital nerves. These compression syndromes have an anatomical basis and a classic clinical presentation. Knowledge of these nerve compression syndromes is important both in establishing the correct diagnosis and also in excluding the other more common syndromes which frequently have similar presentations.

Ligament of Struthers complex/median nerve entrapment

Median nerve entrapment can rarely occur above the elbow due to compression by the ligament of Struthers. This variant ligament typically connects a humeral supracondylar process with the medial epicondyle. The spur and the ligament of Struthers form the fibro-osseous roof of a small tunnel, through which the median nerve and the brachial (or ulnar) vessels traverse. The supracondylar spur, which is present in approximately 1% of the normal population, may be rudimentary or even absent. Other associated anatomic variants may include: high origin of the pronator teres, high division of the brachial artery, high origin of the anterior interosseous nerve branch, or variant position of the ulnar nerve.

Compression of the median nerve at this site is relatively uncommon, even in patients with the bony spur. Patients may present with signs and symptoms of neurovascular compression syndromes. The ligament of Struthers' complex should be considered in the differential diagnosis as a localizing site in every patient with high median nerve, ulnar nerve, or brachial artery pathology. Physicians should palpate the elbow region for a bony spur on the anteromedial surface of the humerus (about 5 cm above the medial epicondyle), and should examine this site for percussion tenderness. Surgical decompression with release of the ligament is usually helpful in the rare patient with this entrapment lesion.

Anterior interosseous nerve

Anterior interosseous nerve syndrome or Kiloh-Nevin syndrome (Kiloh and Nevin 1952) is caused by compression of the anterior interosseous branch, the major motor branch of the median nerve. The anterior interosseous nerve is most commonly compressed by fibrous bands related to the deep head of the pronator teres, but it may also be compressed by tendinous bands of the superficial head of the pronator teres, the flexor digitorum superficialis arch or, rarely, other accessory muscles. Compression may occur spontaneously or may be directly related to repetitive forearm activities or prolonged pressure on the forearm. Other lesions of the anterior interosseous nerve may be related to traumatic events (e.g. pediatric supracondylar fractures, both-bone forearm fractures, elbow dislocations), iatrogenic injury (e.g. plating a radius fracture or performing the flexor-pronator slide procedure), or in association with masses.

Anterior interosseous nerve syndrome is a pure motor neuropathy, as cutaneous sensation is unaffected. Patients with lesions of the anterior interosseous nerve present with vague forearm pain followed by weakness in the thumb, index and middle finger flexion (Sharrard 1968). Weakness may arise acutely or gradually. The anterior interosseous nerve innervates the flexor pollicis longus, flexor digitorum profundus to the index (and in 50% of cases, the middle finger), as well as the pronator quadratus. Patients may note difficulty in writing. Examination characteristically reveals the patient's inability to make the 'okay' sign (Figure 25.1A), to clench their fist (Figure 25.1B), or to oppose the flexed thumb

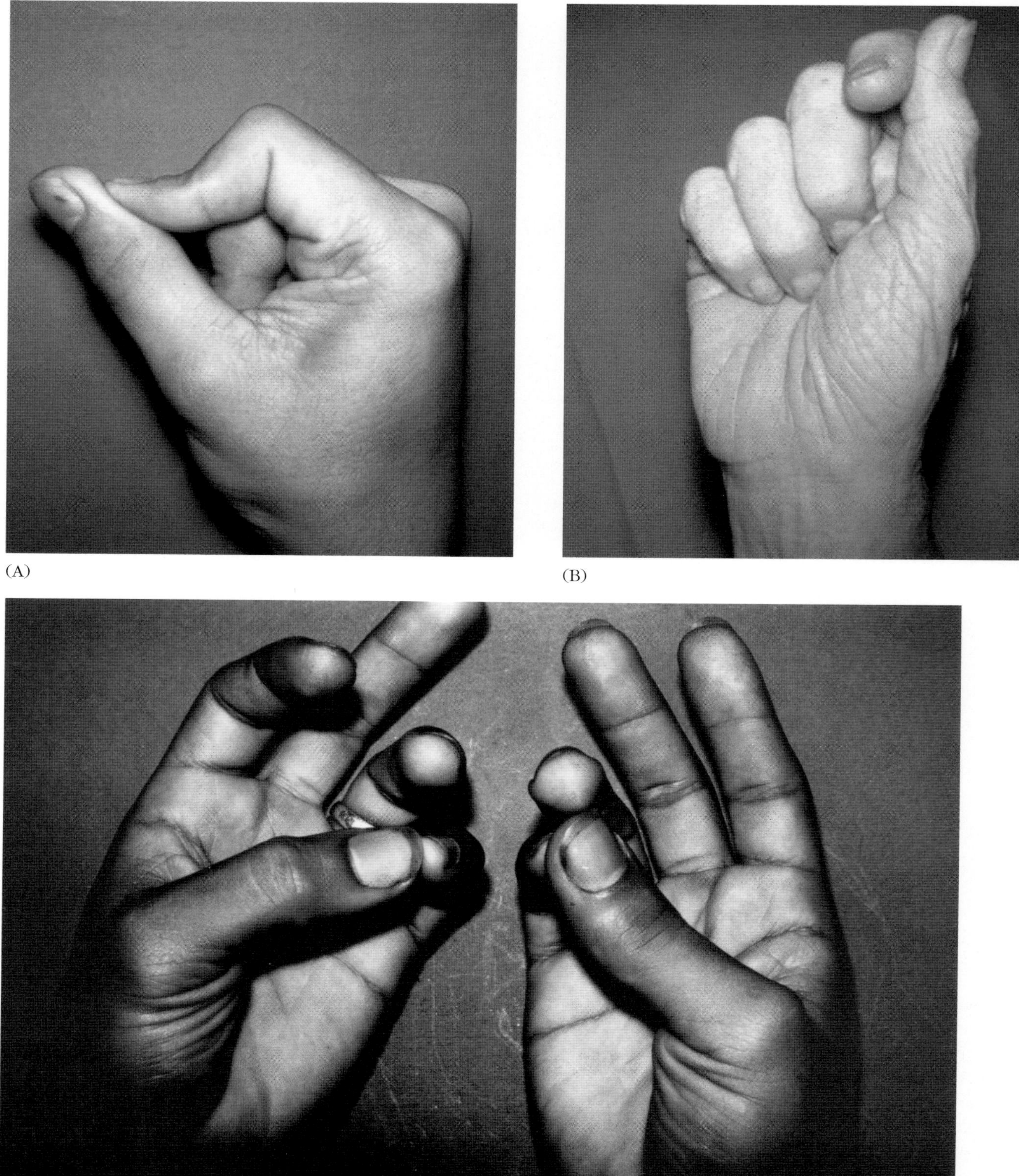

(A)

(B)

(C)

Figure 25.1

Hand attitudes of patients with anterior interosseous nerve palsy. (A) The patient has a square pinch due to inability to flex the terminal phalanges of the thumb and the index finger. (B) The patient is unable to clench his fist with his thumb and index finger. (C) With opposition, there is no flexion of the interphalangeal joint of the thumb in the affected right limb.

(Figure 25.1C). Weakness of the pronator quadratus is tested with the elbow flexed. Sensation is unaffected. Incomplete anterior interosseous nerve palsy also exists when only the thumb or index finger is affected (Hill et al 1985). Anatomic variations may lead to atypical presentations (Spinner 1970); patients may have some hand intrinsic muscle paralysis from a Martin-Gruber anastomosis when ulnar nerve input occurs via the anterior interosseous nerve. In addition, the anterior interosseous nerve may supply the ring finger of the flexor digitorum profundus or the flexor digitorum superficialis.

Patients should be treated non-operatively for a period of 6 months because of the frequent spontaneous improvement of the weakness either from a nerve compression etiology or from Parsonage-Turner syndrome (idiopathic brachial neuritis) (Parsonage and Turner 1948). Electrodiagnostic studies are quite helpful in delineating the extent of the denervation (especially in the pronator quadratus and the flexor pollicus longus) and the presence of reinnervation. Anterior interosseous nerve syndrome must be differentiated from Parsonage-Turner syndrome, which is typically characterized by shoulder pain followed by patchy neurologic loss affecting several peripheral nerves. Occasionally isolated nerves, particularly the anterior interosseous nerve (England and Summer 1987), can be affected, making this differential diagnosis more difficult. The differential diagnosis of anterior interosseous nerve compression also includes tendon rupture, more proximal anterior interosseous nerve involvement (pseudo-anterior interosseous nerve), or other more proximal median nerve lesions, and congenital absence of the flexor pollicis longus.

Surgery can be performed using an internervous plane. The median and anterior interosseous nerves can be explored through an incision spanning from the distal third of the arm to the mid-forearm. The median nerve can be identified proximal to the lacertus fibrosus and traced distally. The lacertus fibrosus is divided, the superficial head of the pronator teres is mobilized and the sublimis bridge is released. Rarely, when no extrinsic site of compression is identified, intratruncal fascicular dissection within the median nerve will demonstrate pathology localized to the anterior interosseous nerve fascicle(s).

The anterior interosseous nerve is given off from the median nerve approximately 6 cm distal to the medial epicondyle. Individual anterior interosseous nerve fascicles can be identified several centimeters proximal to its branching point within the median nerve. In 80% of cases, the median nerve courses between the two heads of the pronator teres; in rare cases, the deep head is absent, or it may pass deep to both heads or through the superficial head. The anterior interosseous nerve branch usually arises as a discrete branch near the distal edge of the pronator teres. Near the tendinous origin of the flexor digitorum superficialis, the anterior interosseous nerve gives off major branches to the flexor pollicus longus and flexor digitorum profundus.

Overall, satisfactory surgical results have been obtained in about 70% of patients. Tendon transfers can restore function in those patients not significantly improved by neurolysis.

Pronator syndrome

The pronator syndrome is a more controversial syndrome, thought to be due to compression of small median nerve pain fibers by the pronator teres, the flexor digitorum superficialis, and the lacertus fibrosus (Johnson et al 1979). It is characterized by diffuse chronic pain in the proximal forearm that is worse with resisted forearm pronation (Kopell and Thompson 1958, Hartz et al 1981). Vague sensory symptoms may be felt in the median nerve distribution of the hand. Symptoms may begin insidiously, follow episodes of sudden lifting or pushing heavy objects, or be associated with repetitive forearm pronation/supination. Typically symptoms occur during the day and are relieved at night with rest.

Percussion or pressure over the median nerve may help to determine the specific site of neural pathology. Certain provocative tests may produce pain or paresthesias and also help to localize the level of the nerve lesion. These maneuvers are thought to reproduce a dynamic mechanical compression of the median nerve by overlying soft tissue structures. These include extending the flexed, pronated limb (pronator teres); resisted flexion of the middle finger (flexor digitorum superficialis); resisted elbow flexion and supination of the forearm (lacertus fibrosus). Electromyography is often normal, and the diagnosis often remains a clinical one. The prevalence of carpal tunnel syndrome is significantly higher than that of pronator syndrome, although occasionally median nerve compression at the wrist may coexist with pronator syndrome. The diagnosis of carpal tunnel syndrome must therefore be carefully excluded. Sensory disturbance in the palm and/or median-innervated weakness of wrist or finger flexors bespeaks a lesion proximal to the carpal canal, whereas percussion tenderness over the carpal canal and a positive Phalen's test are indicative or carpal tunnel syndrome.

Conservative management consists of avoidance of exacerbating activities or positions, splinting, and the judicious use of non-steroidal agents and local steroid injections. A trial of these modalities is often effective, especially in those with mild or intermittent symptoms. Surgery is performed after non-operative measures are exhausted. The same surgical approach as for exposure of the anterior interosseous nerve is performed and the sites of potential compression are released. At surgery, fibrous bands, anomalous origins of the pronator teres, and hypertrophied muscles have been described. The most common finding is a variably sized band in the interval between the pronator teres and the flexor carpi radialis. Several series have produced excellent results in over 80% of patients (Johnson et al 1979, Hartz et al 1981).

Posterior interosseous nerve compression/radial tunnel syndrome

The posterior interosseous nerve is most susceptible to compression at the level of the arcade of Frohse (proximal edge of the supinator) (Spinner 1968), but it may also result from fibrous bands at the radiocapitellar joint, the recurrent leash of Henry, the extensor carpi radialis brevis, or within the middle or distal edge of the supinator. Patients may develop compression spontaneously (Capener 1964). In these cases, variations such as a fibrous edge of the supinator or the extensor carpi radialis brevis might result from repetitive forearm rotation and predispose patients to the development of symptoms from irritation or dynamic compression of the posterior interosseous nerve (Spinner 1968, Roles and Maudsley 1972). Posterior interosseous nerve lesions may be due to elbow trauma (e.g. radial head fractures, Monteggia fracture-dislocations), iatrogenic injury (e.g. radial head resection, arthroscopy) (Strachan and Ellis 1971, Capener 1996) or masses (most commonly lipomas or ganglia) or inflammation (e.g. synovitis).

Patients present with forearm pain which is normally followed by thumb and finger drop. Strength in wrist dorsiflexion is preserved as the extensor carpi radialis longus and extensor carpi radialis brevis are innervated proximally to the posterior interosseous nerve; wrist dorsiflexion is performed in the radial direction (owing to loss of the extensor carpi ulnaris). Patients may have a complete or a partial posterior interosseous nerve lesion (Figure 25.2A). Some partial lesions may become complete over time. There is no sensory abnormality. Electrodiagnostic studies help to localize the lesion, and imaging can help to rule out an underlying mass lesion (Figure 25.2B). The differential diagnosis includes radial nerve compression, Parsonage-Turner syndrome, extensor tendon rupture, and metacarpophalangeal joint dysfunction.

Surgery is indicated in cases where spontaneous clinical or electrical improvement has not occurred within 3–6 months. We favor the anterior (Henry) approach when the pathology is centered at the proximal supinator (Figure 25.2C and D). This approach uses the internervous plane between the brachioradialis and the brachialis proximally, and the brachioradialis and the pronator teres more distally. We perform the posterior (Thompson) approach for exposure of the distal supinator; this approach uses the plane between the extensor carpi radialis brevis and extensor digitorum communis. The posterior interosseous nerve branches from the radial nerve near the elbow joint. Approximately 1 cm distal to exiting the supinator, the posterior interosseous nerve arborizes into its terminal branches (Elgafy et al 2000).

Radial tunnel syndrome

It is thought that compression of the posterior interosseous nerve by the same anatomic structures can also produce a pain syndrome: radial tunnel syndrome or refractory tennis elbow (Roles and Maudsley 1972, Lister et al 1979, Werner 1979). Patients typically have proximal forearm pain localized to the region of the supinator rather than the lateral epicondyle in tennis elbow; however, radial tunnel syndrome may overlap with lateral epicondylitis. Neurologic examination in this syndrome is normal. Pain may be provoked by resisted middle finger extension with the elbow extended or resisted forearm supination with the elbow flexed. Unlike in posterior interosseous nerve compression, electrodiagnostic studies in radial tunnel syndrome are usually normal. Local injection may be diagnostic and therapeutic. Splinting may also relieve symptoms. Surgery may be necessary in refractory cases (Steichen et al 1988). Depending on the patient's findings and the surgeon's philosophies, surgery may entail releasing the posterior interosseous nerve within the radial tunnel and/or the lateral epicondyle. Good or excellent results have been reported in approximately 70–80% of cases (Roles and Maudsley 1972, Lister et al 1979, Werner 1979).

Superficial radial nerve

The superficial radial nerve is most commonly compressed at the wrist level or in the mid-forearm, where the nerve has an anatomic predisposition to compression; however, occasionally, it may be compressed in other locations such as near the elbow (e.g. by masses). At the wrist, the nerve passes subcutaneously, directly over the radial styloid. Here it is particularly vulnerable to external compression by objects such as handcuffs (Massey and Pleet 1978), bands, gloves, casts, and watchbands (Bierman 1959) and is referred to as 'cheiralgia paresthetica' (Ehrlich et al 1986) or Wartenberg's disease (Wartenberg 1932). The superficial radial nerve may also be injured directly (Linscheid 1965), iatrogenically, or indirectly from inflammation by tendonitis. In the distal third of the forearm, the nerve may be entrapped where it pierces the fascia approximately 6 cm proximal to the wrist crease (Dellon and Mackinnon 1986). The nerve is most susceptible in pronation to scissoring of the extensor carpi radialis

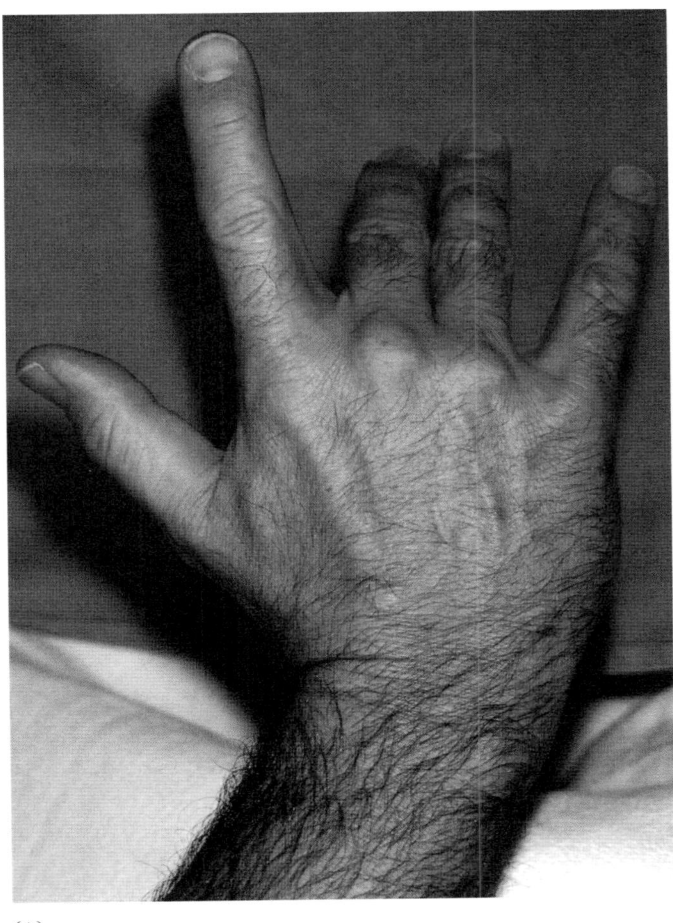

(A)

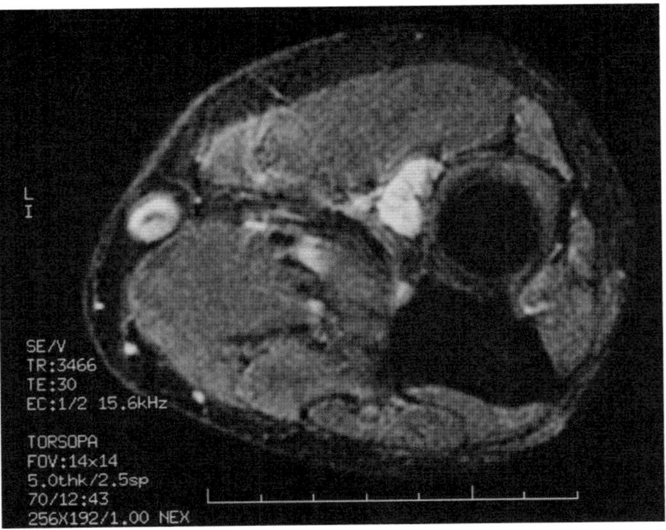

(B)

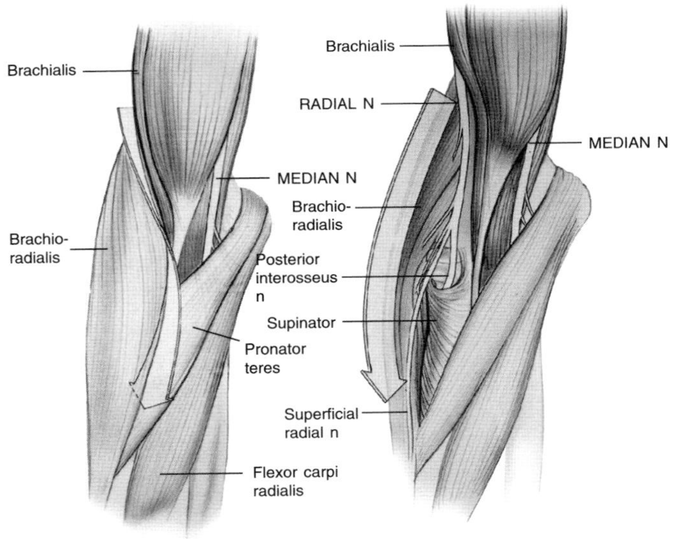

(C)

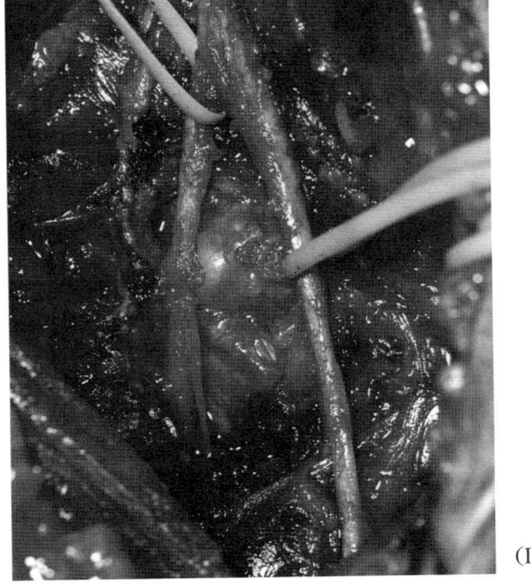

(D)

Figure 25.2

Partial posterior interosseous nerve syndrome. (A) This 44-year-old man presented with an 18-month history of weakness in his middle and ring fingers of the right hand ('sign of the horns'). He noted difficulty putting shaving cream on his face. He then developed weakness in the little finger as well. Examination revealed finger drop of the middle, ring, and little fingers at the metacarpophalangeal joints. Wrist dorsiflexion occurred in a radial direction and sensation was intact. Pressure over the radial head produced pain. (B) T2-weighted magnetic resonance image revealed a cystic mass in proximity to the radial head, displacing the posterior interosseous nerve. (C) A Henry approach was used to expose the posterior interosseous nerve. (Reproduced with permission from Spinner M (1978) *Injuries to the Major Branches of Peripheral Nerves of the Forearm*, 2nd edn. WB Saunders: Philadelphia.) (D) At surgery, the mass proved to be an extraneural ganglion originating from the radiocapitellar joint. The mass compressed the posterior interosseous nerve beneath the arcade of Frohse.

longus tendon under the brachioradialis tendon. This may be due to overuse/misuse in patients who perform repetitive forearm activities, such as using a screwdriver.

Patients with superficial radial nerve compression often complain of local pain that is maximal at the site of nerve injury. They experience paresthesias or dysesthesias and radiating pain in the autonomous zone of the superficialis radial nerve, i.e. the dorsum of the first web space. Symptoms are worse with wrist motion.

Physical examination demonstrates sensory abnormalities in the superficial radial nerve distribution. Percussion tenderness directly over the site of injury along the course of the nerve typically reproduces the radiating distal pain. In addition, the Finkelstein test, performed by palmar flexion of the wrist in an ulnar deviation (which was designed for De Quervain's disease), is a provocative maneuver for superficial radial nerve entrapment by stretching the nerve. Sustained pronation also may exacerbate symptoms (Dellon and Mackinnon 1986).

The superficial radial nerve entrapment can be mistaken for De Quervain's disease, or a lateral antebrachial nerve lesion (Mackinnon and Dellon 1985). Superficial radial nerve entrapment may coexist with these conditions (Rask 1978) as well as other common nerve entrapment lesions. Unfortunately, electrical studies are often not helpful in differentiating lesions. Nerve blocks of the superficial radial and lateral antebrachial nerves may help to distinguish between these lesions.

Non-operative treatment is often successful in decreasing or eliminating symptoms. This consists of avoidance of exacerbating activities or exposure to externally compressive objects. A trial of non-steroidal anti-inflammatory agents, steroid injections, or splinting can also be effective. Desensitization may lessen pain perception and local tenderness.

Surgical intervention is indicated for symptoms that are refractory to an adequate trial of non-operative therapy. External neurolysis is performed over the point of maximal tenderness, usually under local or regional anesthesia. When the lesion occurs between the extensor carpi radialis longus and brachioradialis tendons in the forearm, the fascia is released and the nerve is then able to glide in a free bed. In these cases, surgery is effective in approximately 80% of cases. Patients who have failed surgery or who have neuromas may benefit from neurectomy.

Digital nerve

Digital nerve compression most commonly occurs on the ulnar aspect of the thumb ('bowler's thumb') (Dobyns et al 1972, Belsky and Millender 1980). Digital nerve compression may also occur in other athletes such as baseball batters, tennis or racquetball players, or archers (Rayan 1992), or musicians such as string instrumentalists (Lederman 1989). The neural irritation results from direct pressure against a firm object, such as a bat, a racquet, a bow, or the neck of an instrument. Trauma to other digits may result in compression of the digital nerve by the transverse metacarpal ligament. Lesions of any digital nerve may also occur spontaneously from fibrous bands or masses (e.g. hyperplastic pacinian corpuscles, thrombosed aneurysms). Patients present with local pain and a sensory disturbance in the distribution of the nerve. There is no motor weakness as the innervation to the lumbricals occurs more proximally. Percussion tenderness over the nerve in the region of the metacarpophalangeal joint is characteristic. Hyperextension or adduction of the finger may aggravate symptoms. Symptoms often improve with reduced use of or decreased pressure against that side of the digit. Immobilization, non-steroidal anti-inflammatory agents, and steroid injections may relieve symptoms. Surgery is rarely necessary. Decompression alone or in combination with nerve transposition or local muscle flap may be necessary. Perineural fibrosis results from chronic compression.

References

Belsky M, Millender LH (1980) Bowler's thumb in a baseball player, *Orthopedics* **3**: 122–3.

Bierman HR (1959) Nerve compression due to a tight watchband, *N Engl J Med* **261**: 237–8.

Capener N (1964) Posterior interosseous nerve lesions, *J Bone Joint Surg* **46B**: 361.

Capener N (1996) The vulnerability of the posterior interosseous nerve of the forearm: a case report and an anatomical study, *J Bone Joint Surg* **48B**: 770–3.

Dellon AL, Mackinnon SE (1986) Radial sensory nerve entrapment in the forearm, *J Hand Surg* **11A**: 199–205.

Dobyns JH, O'Brien ET, Linscheid RL, Farrow GM (1972) Bowler's thumb – diagnosis and treatment: a review of seventeen cases, *J Bone Joint Surg* **54**: 751–5.

Ehrlich W, Dellon AL, Mackinnon SE (1986) Cheiralgia paresthetica (entrapment of the radial sensory nerve), *J Hand Surg* **11A**: 196–9.

Elgafy H, Ebraheim NA, Rezcallah AT, Yeasting RA (2000) Posterior interosseous nerve terminal branches, *Clin Orthop* **376**: 242–51.

England JD, Summer AJ (1987) Neuralgic amyotrophy: an increasingly diverse entity, *Muscle Nerve* **10**: 60–8.

Hartz CR, Linscheid RL, Gramser RR, Daube JR (1981) The pronator teres syndrome. Compressive neuropathy of the median nerve, *J Bone Joint Surg* **63A**: 885–90.

Hill NA, Howard FM, Huffer BR (1985) The incomplete anterior interosseous nerve syndrome, *J Hand Surg* **10**: 4–16.

Johnson RK, Spinner M, Shrewsbury MM (1979) Median nerve entrapment syndrome in the proximal forearm, *J Hand Surg* **4**: 48–51.

Kiloh LG, Nevin S (1952) Isolated neuritis of the anterior interosseous nerve, *BMJ* **1**: 850–1.

Kopell HP, Thompson WAI (1958) Pronator syndrome: a confirmed case and its diagnosis, *N Engl J Med* **259**: 713–15.

Lederman RJ (1989) Peripheral nerve disorders in instrumentalists, *Ann Neurol* **26**: 640–6.

Linscheid RL (1965) Injuries to radial nerve at wrist, *Arch Surg* **91**: 942–6.

Lister GD, Belsole RB, Kleinert HE (1979) The radial tunnel syndrome, *J Hand Surg* **4**: 52–9.

Mackinnon SE, Dellon AL (1985) The overlap pattern of the lateral antebrachial cutaneous nerve and the superficial branch of the radial nerve, *J Hand Surg* **10A**: 522–6.

Massey EW, Pleet AB (1978) Handcuffs and cheiralgia paresthetica, *Neurology* **28**: 1312–13.

Parsonage MJ, Turner JWA (1948) Neuralgic amyotrophy. The shoulder-girdle syndrome, *Lancet* **1**: 973–8.

Rask MR (1978) Superficial radial neuritis and de Quervain's disease, *Clin Orthop* **131**: 176–8.

Rayan GM (1992) Archery-related injuries of the hand, forearm and elbow, *South Med J* **85**: 961–4.

Roles NC, Maudsley RH (1972) Radial tunnel syndrome: resistant tennis elbow as a nerve entrapment, *J Bone Joint Surg* **54B**: 499–508.

Sharrard WJW (1968) Anterior interosseous neuritis. Report of a case, *J Bone Joint Surg* **50B**: 804–5.

Spinner M (1968) The arcade of Frohse and its relationship to posterior interosseous nerve paralysis, *J Bone Joint Surg* **50B**: 809–12.

Spinner M (1970) The anterior interosseous nerve syndrome. With special attention to its variations, *J Bone Joint Surg* **52A**: 84–94.

Steichen JB, Mulbry LW, Christensen AW (1988) Radial tunnel syndrome: clinical experience and results of treatment, *J Hand Surg* **13A**: 303.

Strachan JCH, Ellis BW (1971) Vulnerability of the posterior interosseous nerve during radial head resection, *J Bone Joint Surg* **53B**: 320–3.

Wartenberg R (1932) Cheiralgia paresthetica (isolierte neuritis des ramus superficialis nerve radialis), *Z Ges Neurol Psychiatr* **141**: 145–55.

Werner C-O (1979) Lateral elbow pain and posterior interosseous nerve entrapment, *Acta Orthop Scand Suppl* **174**: 1–62.

26 Nerve entrapment syndromes in musicians

R Tubiana

Nerve entrapment syndromes (NES) are common in musicians. However, their incidence varies according to the medical speciality of the reporting authors (Winspur 2002). These include 29% (Lederman 1989) to 48% (Charness 1992) of instrumentalists with a musculoskeletal disorder consulting in a Musician's Clinic run by a neurologist, 15% by an orthopaedist (Amadio and Russotti 1990) and even less by a rheumatologist (Wynn Parry 1998).

Almost all musical instruments can be associated with NES, especially if the way they are played involves non-physiological posture or movements; however, they mostly occur in flautists, pianists, guitarists, violinists and other string performers.

Almost all the peripheral nerves of the upper limb may be entrapped; however, there is also a wide variation in the relative incidence of specific entrapments according to different authors (Winspur and Wynn Parry 1997). The most common diagnoses of NES in our clinic are carpal tunnel syndrome (CTS) and thoracic outlet syndrome (TOS), then cubital tunnel syndrome and radial nerve entrapment in the lateral side of the elbow and of the proximal forearm, often co-existing with tennis elbow. However, the incidence of surgical treatment is different. The most common procedures are carpal tunnel releases, then cubital tunnel releases and radial nerve releases with tennis elbow and rarely TOS. In general, surgery is avoided in most cases of NES in musicians, and non-operative treatment is always used before resorting to surgical release.

Pathogenesis

Cumulative trauma, repetitive strain and long static periods in unnatural positions are usually incriminated (Mackinnon 1992). The most common aetiology is related to non-physiological postures and playing techniques, which can be corrected without surgery.

Carpal tunnel syndrome is more a compression neuropathy and ulnar nerve entrapment at the elbow is more a traction neuropathy (Millesi et al 1990). The final common pathway is local ischaemia of the nerve. Vasculitis is another cause of focal nerve pathology. It must be remembered that musicians are not immune from diabetes and other metabolic disorders, which do not respond to surgical decompression.

Clinical symptoms

In the early stages many nerve compressions produce only discreet symptoms. However, problems that cause relatively minor inconvenience for the general population may lead to severe loss in performance quality for the musician.

At this early stage, diagnosis is difficult, objective neurophysiological examinations will usually not yield any abnormalities. The most useful part of the evaluation comprises the history and symptoms provided by the patient.

Symptoms vary according to the nerve involved and the different stages of nerve compression. However, the diagnosis of nerve compression should be made before the classic triad of pain, paraesthesia and paralysis occurs.

Pain may be the only presenting symptom, but there are so many causes of arm pain in musicians that this symptom is insufficient for the diagnosis. Paraesthesia probably has more value, but it does not necessarily mean nerve compression. There is no pathognomonic test for nerve compression. However, constant paraesthesia in a defined anatomical area should provide a high index of suspicion, particularly if paraesthesiae are associated with a Tinel's sign. (When the nerve is tapped over the site of compression, pain is produced at that site and there is an electrical sensation radiating into the distal distribution of the nerve.) Physical findings should be elicited by positional provocative tests.

Clumsiness may be the first symptom, and the possibility of a focal dystonia, which is not uncommon in the musician population, must be considered. Focal dystonia has a far more serious prognosis than a NES and an incorrect surgical treatment, sometimes performed on a dystonic patient, would even worsen the condition. Focal dystonia in musicians is a painless motor control disorder of central origin. In the early stages it only occurs when playing: in the middle of a score, the instrumentalist can no longer control the movement of one or more fingers, usually the ulnar digits but when not playing, he can use his hand normally. The diagnosis of focal dystonia may be difficult when motor control disorders are still slight; it is subjective and based on some symptoms: focal dystonia is task-related, is painless, is prevalent in men; it appears in musicians over the age of 30, who despite all their efforts, cannot prevent a degradation in musical performance. No laboratory test is capable of distinguishing dystonia from other types of involuntary movement (Marsden 1991). The condition should be diagnosed by exclusion. Peripheral nerve compressions should be specifically sought and nerve conduction testing used in excluding these, particularly at the level of the ulnar nerve.

It seems that in some cases, nerve compression may precede or be associated with focal dystonia (Charness et al 1996).

Electrodiagnostic testing

Electrodiagnostic testing is essential for the diagnosis of nerve entrapment in the syndromes where direct measurement is easily achieved, such as CTS or cubital tunnel syndrome. For a long time, electrodiagnostic studies appeared to be of less value in the diagnosis of radial tunnel syndrome (Lawrence et al 1995); they are still considered of little value in TOS (Lederman 1994). Nerve conduction testing is not only useful for the diagnosis but also to assess the severity of the lesions. However, in the early stages of nerve entrapment in musicians, nerve conduction testing often fails to detect changes. Positional provocative tests are sometimes useful. In spite of the fallibility of these tests in early compression, *no surgical release should be made on the median cubital or radial nerves if nerve conduction testing is normal.* It is essential to confirm the clinical diagnosis preoperatively by positive electrodiagnostic tests.

The principal sites of NES in musicians and their treatment

As most NES in instrumentalists are caused by poor posture and playing techniques, no surgery should be considered until an effective trial of conservative care has been carried out (Box 26.1), including rehabilitation with a therapist skilled in the management of musicians, in combination with a music teacher for adjustment of technique and eventually modification of the instrument. The treatment is, of cause, influenced by the site of the entrapment (Nolan and Eaton 1989.

It is important to realize that several musicians have more than one nerve entrapment syndrome. In particular, TOS may have concomitant entrapment of the ulnar nerve at the elbow.

Box 26.1 *Conservative treatment of NES*

- Limitation of those activities that exacerbate the pain
- Modified positioning
- Anti-inflammatory drugs
- Breaking up practice sessions with periods of rest
- Rehabilitation with a musician's therapist in combination with a music teacher for adjustment of technique and eventually modification of the instrument

Cervical radiculopathy

Although muscular problems are the most common painful conditions at the neck, cervical pain may also result from skeletal disorders or nerve compressions. Cervical radiculopathies from diverse causes, such as cervical disc or osteoarthritic spur, were found in 3% of 226 instrumentalists with playing-related symptoms (Hochberg et al 2000). Violinists, violists (Figure 26.1) and flautists (Figure 26.2) in particular, rotate and tilt their head when playing.

Maintaining this position for several hours causes neck muscle contractions, as well as a narrowing of the foramina between the vertebrae where the spinal nerves exit. The C6, C7, C8 nerve roots are the most commonly affected, with resultant neck and arm pain. Careful assessment is made of the patient's posture when resting, when holding the instrument and in action. Raising the height of the chin rest in violinists (Figure 26.3), or the use of a curved mouthpiece on the flute (Norris 1992), help to correct the situation. Exercise, cervical traction, and steroid injections are often useful. Surgery is rarely indicated for severe and persistent pain.

Thoracic outlet syndrome (TOS)

Long-limbed musicians with sloping shoulders, with insufficient scapulothoracic muscle development, mostly women, are subject to compression of the lower roots of the brachial plexus (Figure 26.4 and 26.5). Symptoms are frequently dynamic, and worse with hand overhead, shoulder abduction, a position which tends to close the costo-clavicular space. This posture may be maintained for hours in some instrumentalists, particularly in those who perform standing. TOS may also be caused by carrying heavy musical instruments, such as a guitar, or accordion, or wind instruments, supported with a strap. Usually, the patient complains of pain, spreading down

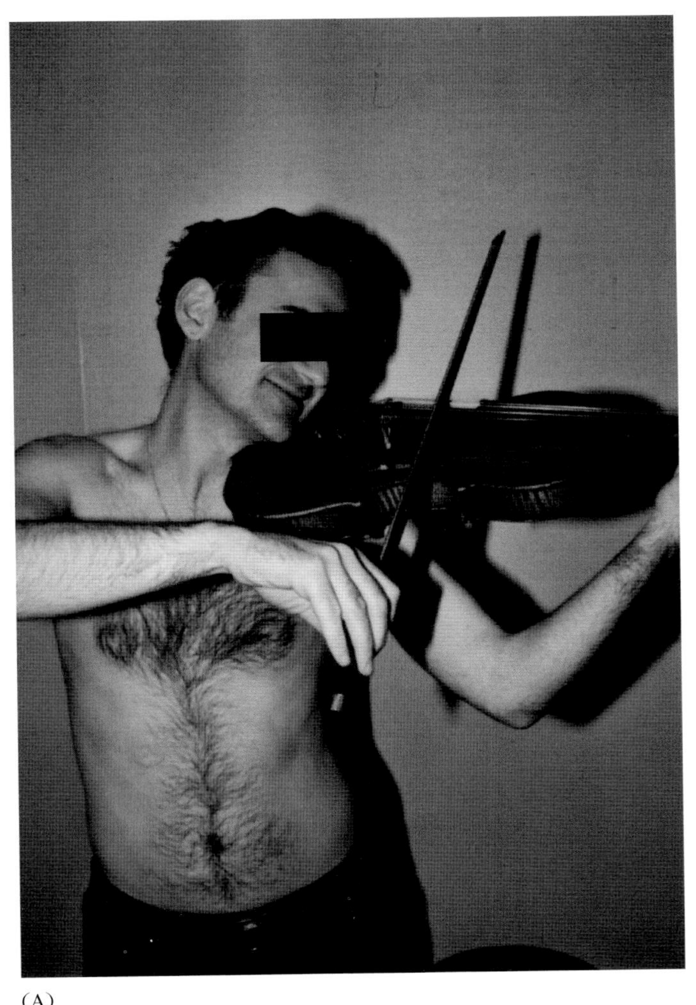

(A)

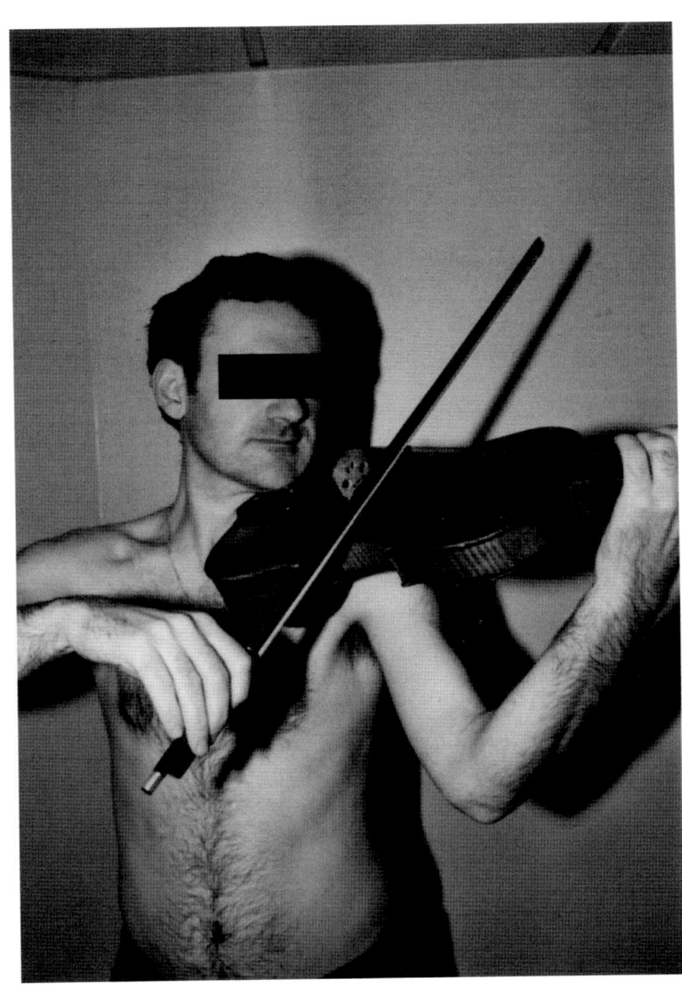

(B)

Figure 26.1
(A) Poor posture in a violist. (B) Correction of the position.

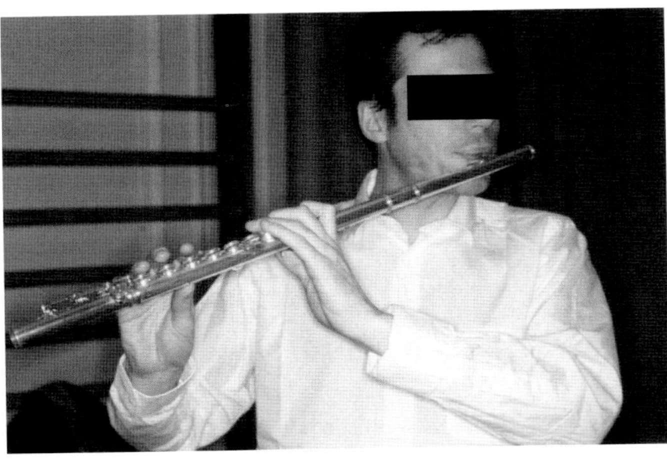

Figure 26.2
Flautist rotates and tilts the head, hypertension of right wrist (possible CTS), hyperextension of left index (digital nerve compression).

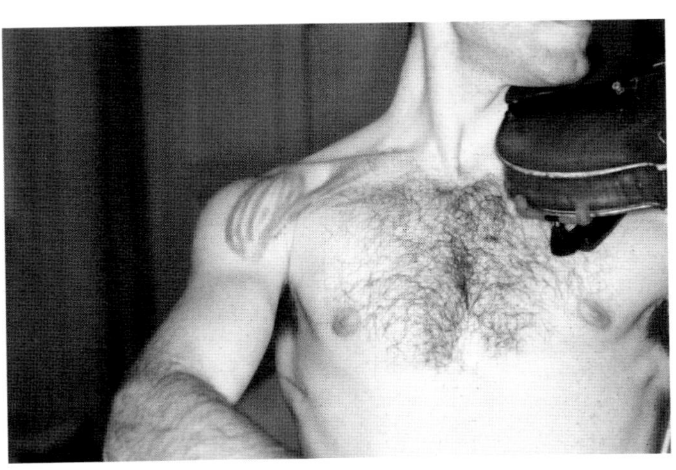

Figure 26.3
Raising the height of the chin rest in a violinist.

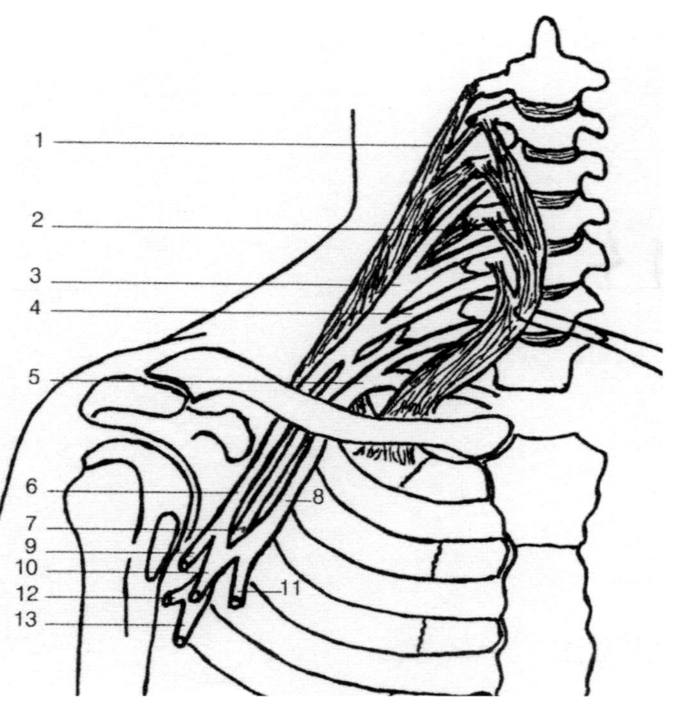

Figure 26.4

Course of the brachial plexus. The lower roots of the brachial plexus are subject to compression between the clavicle and the first rib. 1, Posterior and middle scalene muscles; 2, anterior scalene muscle retracted; 3, upper trunk of the brachial plexus; 4, middle trunk; 5, lower trunk; 6, lateral cord; 7, posterior cord; 8, medial cord; 9, musculocutaneous nerve; 10, median nerve; 11, ulnar nerve; 12, axillary nerve; 13, radial nerve. (From L. Poitevin in *The Hand* Vol 4, p. 334, WB Saunders 1993, with modifications.)

the inner aspect of the arm with paraesthesiae in the ring and little finger. The only objective findings are muscle tenderness in the root of the neck and occasional provocative testing by the overhead test in the 'surrender position'. The ulnar nerve supplies no sensation in the forearm, and if there is any sensory loss on the ulnar side of the forearm, the cause may well be found at the thoracic outlet (Wynn Parry 1998). The classic cervical rib is rarely present on X-rays of musicians. Nerve conduction tests have proved of little value in the diagnosis of TOS (Lederman 1993, 1994). Magnetic resonance imaging (MRI) angiography appears to be the most accurate method in the diagnosis of specific mechanical sources of TOS.

TOS in musicians can almost always be treated effectively by non-surgical procedures. Physiotherapy to improve the shoulder girdle musculature and correct poor posture and inappropriate movements is always indicated. Instrumentalists playing heavy instruments with neck straps should change to other types of support. Specific instrument modifications may be useful.

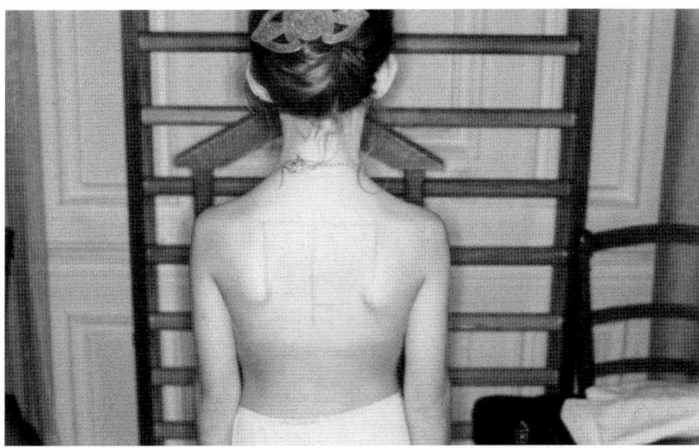

Figure 26.5

Morphology of a young female cellist with TOS.

In more than 100 musicians with TOS treated by re-education by our physiotherapist (Philippe Chamagne), only two cases had a surgical decompression after failure of the rehabilitation treatment, one of them had a cervical rib.

Median nerve entrapment

The median nerve is susceptible to compression at several points along its anatomic course. By far the most common entrapment syndrome in musicians, as in the general population, is CTS. However, in the forearm, fascial and vascular structures may impinge upon the nerve and may become clinically significant as a result of repetitive pronation/supination activities. They must be considered in cases of median nerve dysfunction where pathology in the carpal tunnel is not present.

Median nerve compression in the forearm

Anatomy

Median nerve anatomic relations in the forearm are complex, moreover, variations in nerve and musculoskeletal anatomy can result in abnormal pressures. From proximal to distal, the median nerve travels between the brachialis muscle and the lacertus fibrosus (Figure 26.6), then beneath the superficial head of pronator teres (Figure 26.7), then under the flexor superficialis arch (Figure 26.8). Entrapment can occur beneath the lacertus fibrosus or under the pronator and flexor superficialis fascial arches in any anatomic location. The anterior interosseous nerve is also at risk if it arises on the radial side of the median nerve rather than from a posterior origin (Mackinnon and Dellon 1988) (Figure 26.9).

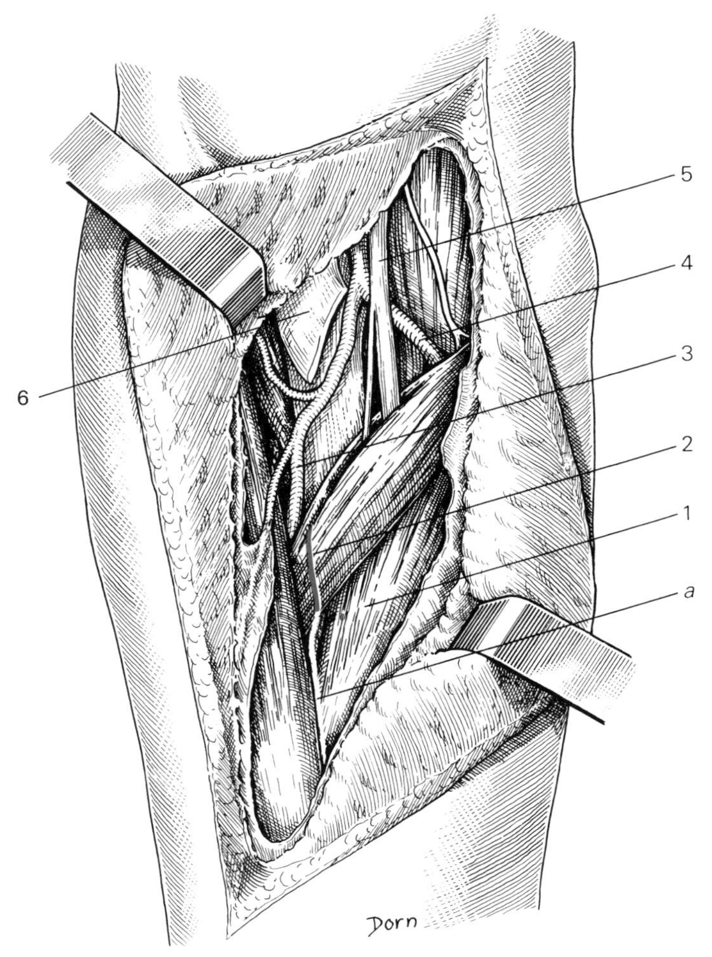

Figure 26.6
The median nerve in the proximal forearm. 1, flexor carpi radialis; 2, step cut in pronator teres; 3, radial artery; 4, ulnar artery; 5, median nerve; *a*, incision; 6, lacertus fibrosus divided.

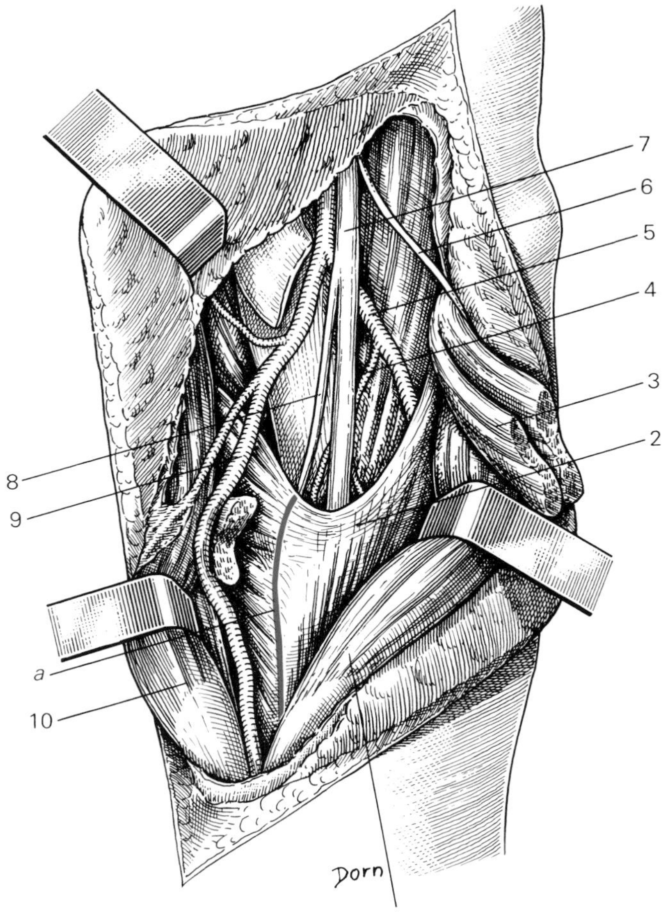

Figure 26.7
The median nerve travels under the superficial head of the pronator teres. 1, flexor carpi radialis; 2, flexor digitorum superficialis; 3, pronator teres, divided; 4, common interosseous artery; 5, ulnar artery; 6, branch to pronator teres; 7, median nerve; 8, anterior interosseous nerve; 9, radial artery; 10, brachioradialis; *a*, incision.

Compression by lacertus fibrosus

Discomfort in the left arm of violinists may be caused by compression of the median nerve beneath the lacertus fibrosus when they play with too much supination of the forearm. Mackinnon and Dellon (1988) have described a provocative test for lacertus fibrosus compression consisting of provocation of paraesthesiae in the median nerve distribution with elbow flexion and resisted supination. They have also described a resisted pronation test for the pronator teres syndrome.

Pronator teres syndrome

The pronator teres is the major pronator of the forearm and as such will tend to become hypertrophic by constant repetitive pronation movements of the right hand of violinists or flautists. Symptoms consist of muscle aches in the forearm and paraesthesiae in the median nerve sensory territory. The presence of a Tinel's sign will suggest compression neuropathy.

Anterior interosseous nerve syndrome

The anterior interosseous, a major branch of the median nerve, is the primary motor to the flexor pollicis longus muscle, the flexor profundus of the index and long fingers, and of the pronator quadratus. It has no cutaneous distribution.

Compression under the fascial arches will weaken the muscles supplied by this nerve. However, inability to flex distal interphalangeal joints of the thumb and index finger, characteristic of complete anterior interosseous nerve palsy, has never been described in a musician.

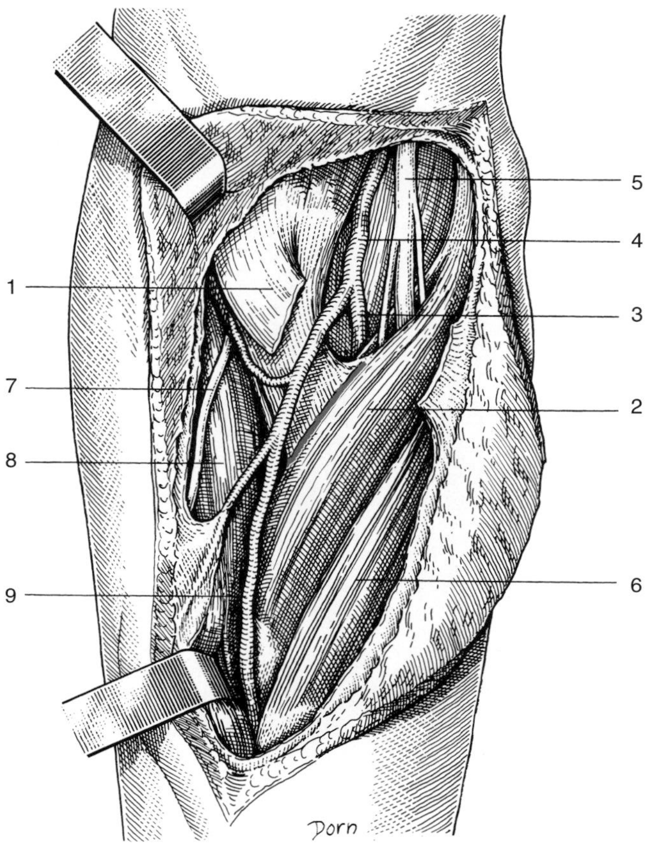

Figure 26.8

The median nerve under the flexor superficialis arch. 1, lacertus fibrosus = bicipital aponeurosis (divided); 2, pronator teres; 3, ulnar artery; 4, brachial artery; 5, median nerve; 6, flexor carpi radialis; 7, lateral cutaneous nerve of forearm; 8, brachioradialis; 9, radial artery.

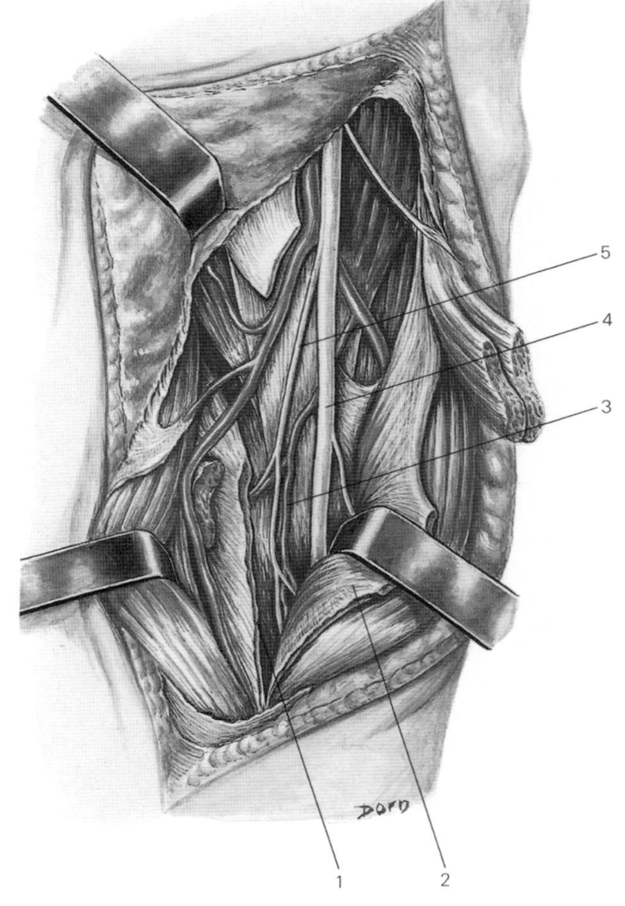

Figure 26.9

The anterior interosseous nerve. 1, flexor digitorum superficialis: divided border close to insertion into radius; 2, flexor digitorum superficialis, retracted; 3, anterior interosseous artery; 4, median nerve; 5, anterior interosseous nerve.

Modified positioning is the first treatment for median nerve compressions in the forearm of musicians.

Carpal tunnel syndrome (CTS)

CTS is a very common condition, especially in middle-aged females. CTS is a compression neuropathy involving the median nerve and localized at the wrist, producing a specific set of symptoms. The compression may occur because the rigid tunnel formed by the carpal bones and roofed by the unyielding transverse carpal ligament is too tight, or because the volume of tissue within the tunnel is too great. It is important to realize that when the wrist is in extreme flexion, the volume of the canal is reduced (Gelberman et al 1981). Repetitive hand motions can cause inflammation of the flexor tendons. In instrumentalists, repetitive finger flexion is often associated with poor posture of the wrist. Full pronation causes shifting of the flexor tendons against the median nerve (Figure 26.10).

The initial diagnosis of CTS is essentially based on interrogation of the patient. It is easy when there is a typical history of nocturnal pain, aching in the upper arm, and sensory disturbance limited to the median nerve distribution in the thumb, index and middle finger and the radial half of the ringer finger. There should not be any symptoms of dorsal numbness, nor in the thenar eminence, since the dorsal aspect of the lateral side of the hand is innervated by the radial nerve and the thenar eminence by the palmar cutaneous branch of the median nerve, which arises proximal to the carpal tunnel (Figure 26.11).

A Tinel's sign over the median nerve at the wrist and a positive provocative test with the wrist in complete flexion reproducing the paraesthesiae within 60 seconds (Phalen's test) are commonly used, but they are not totally specific (Katz et al 1990): 34% of patients with electrical signs of compression have negative results on Phalen's test and 20% of subjects without any clinical

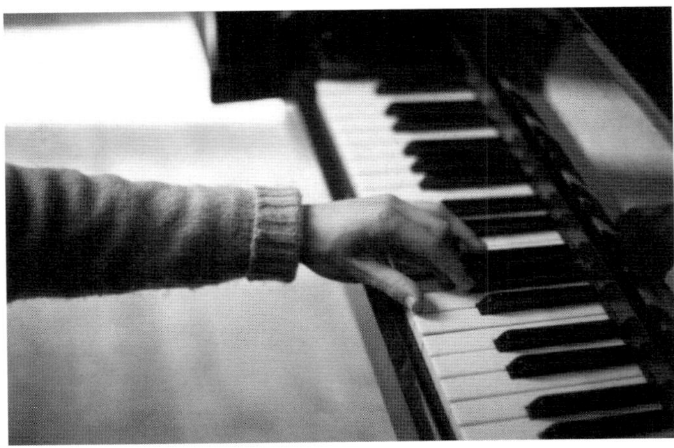

Figure 26.10
Full pronation with radial deviation of the wrist in a pianist.

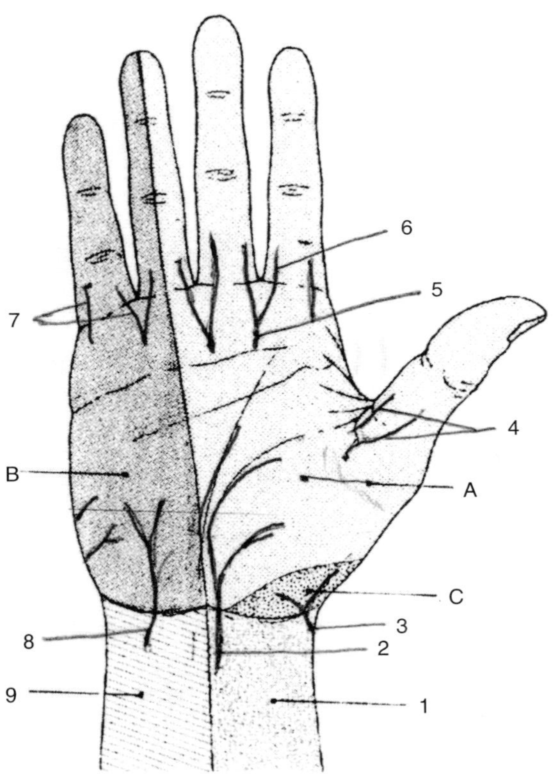

Figure 26.11
Cutaneous sensory distribution on the volar aspect of the hand. 1, lateral cutaneous nerve of forearm (musculocutaneous nerve); 2, palmar cutaneous branch of median nerve; 3, palmar cutaneous branch of radial nerve; 4, collateral nerves of the thumb; 5, palmar digital nerves from the median; 6, digital collateral nerves from the median; 7, digital collateral nerves from the ulnar nerve; 8, sensory nerve of the ulnar nerve; 9, median cutaneous nerve of the forearm (branch of the medial cord of the brachial plexus). (A) Median nerve cutaneous distribution, (B) ulnar nerve palmar territory, (C) radial nerve palmar territory.

symptoms have positive results on Phalen's test. In all cases, symptoms need to be confirmed by electrodiagnostic studies.

Winspur (1998) has classified CTS in musicians into three groups:

- classic idiopathic CTS
- acute positional CTS
- flexor tenosynovitis of the wrist.

Classic CTS
Idiopathie CTS is theoretically unrelated to performance and presents with classic pins and needles and pain at night. In musicians with early symptoms of the disease, relief can be achieved by using night splints and one or two steroid injections. However, when the condition is well established and electrical conduction tests are positive, surgical decompression is required.

Acute positional CTS
This group is composed of instrumentalists complaining of paraesthesiae and numbness in the median distribution when playing. They will not complain of nocturnal symptoms. Symptoms are caused by positional factors, particularly in guitarists with excessive flexion of the left wrist (Figure 26.12). Conduction tests are usually undisturbed and when the incorrect posture has been corrected, the symptoms disappear. Surgery, of course, is not indicated.

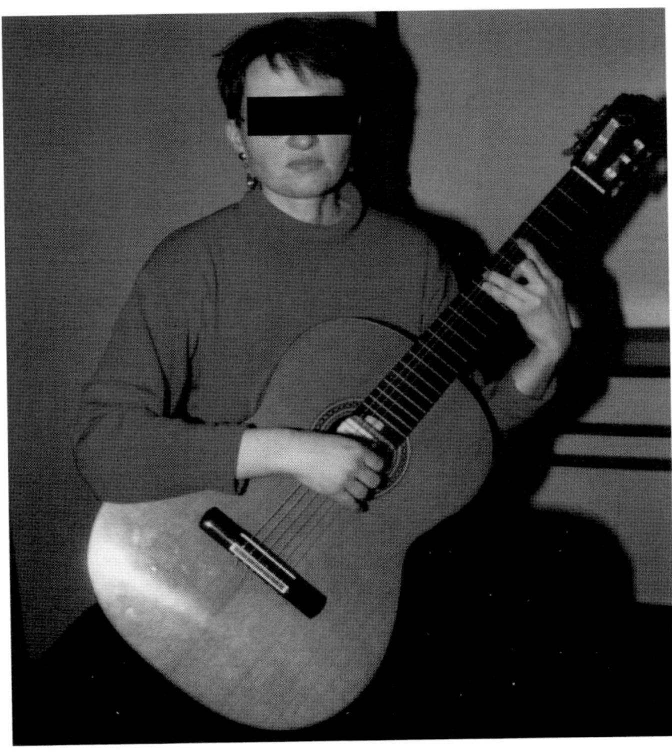

Figure 26.12
Guitarist with excessive flexion of the left wrist.

Flexor tenosynovitis of the wrist
In this group, paraesthesia in the median innervated fingers is associated with swelling of the flexor tendons. Symptoms are accentuated by playing and cease after a few hours rest or when the musician has a break from playing (e.g. during holiday periods).

Nocturnal symptoms are occasional but do not predominate. Examination shows swelling at the wrist, usually involving the long and ring flexor tendons. These tendons may be nodular and tender. Conduction tests are often undisturbed for a long time.

This disorder is mostly seen on both hands in keyboard players, or in the left hand of violinists, usually following periods of intensive playing.

These patients respond well to local steroid injection, splinting and relative rest. It may be necessary to modify either a practice regimen or the instrument interface. Surgery is not indicated unless nerve conduction tests become abnormal.

Surgical treatment

When surgery is decided, it should be done by an experienced surgeon so as to avoid complications which may be disastrous for the career of a professional musician. The open technique gives a clear visualization of the median nerve; however, the scar in the palm may remain sensitive for a long time, especially when the incision is too radial or when it crosses the wrist creases. The incision that we use follows the radial contour of the hypothenar eminence and avoids most of the cutaneous branches of the median and ulnar nerves (Figure 26.13). Endoscopic carpal tunnel release promises to be minimally invasive, with the chance of a rapid rehabilitation, and has some advantages in terms of pillar pain. However, the fear of the rare but disastrous possibility of serious nerve injury limits the indications for this procedure, and it should be done only by experts with great experience of this procedure (see Chapter 25). Postoperatively, we splint the wrist in slight extension for 10 days to minimize the chance of postoperative bowstringing of the flexor tendons, but patients are requested to move the fingers and thumb as soon as possible. A suitable repertoire can be selected for the initial return to play. Usually, musicians return to full-time playing 6–8 weeks after surgery.

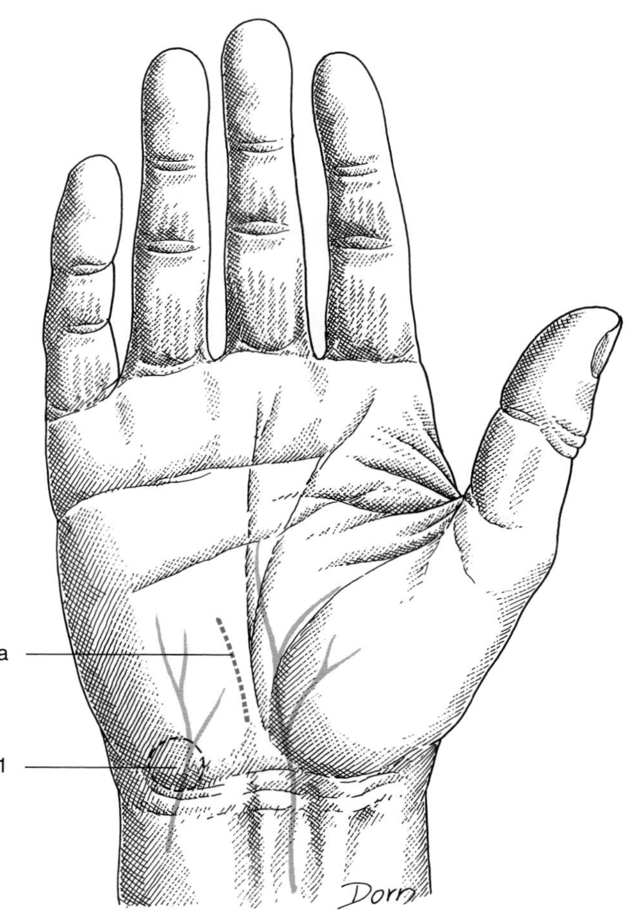

Figure 26.13
a: Incision for open carpal tunnel release. 1, pisiform.

Ulnar nerve entrapment

Ulnar nerve compressions in instrumentalists are mostly seen at the elbow level. However, rare distal entrapments in Guyon's canal or deep in the palm have been described in musicians.

Ulnar nerve entrapment at the elbow

Ulnar compression at the elbow is common in the left arm of string players. The selective involvement of the left arm in the string players with ulnar neuropathy

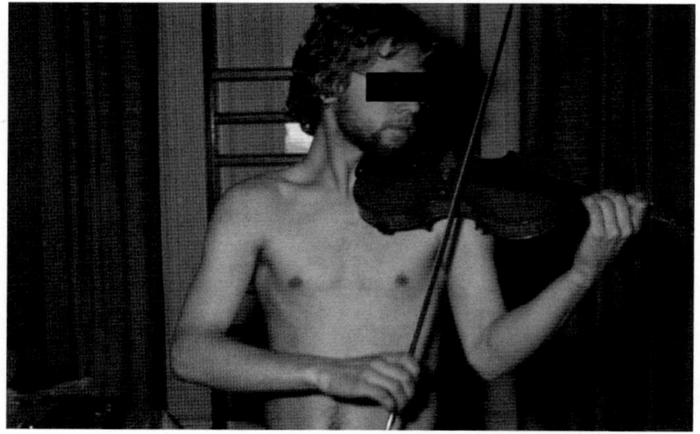

Figure 26.14
Violinist with ulnar nerve entrapment on the left side. The left arm sustains the instrument with marked elbow flexion and forearm supination.

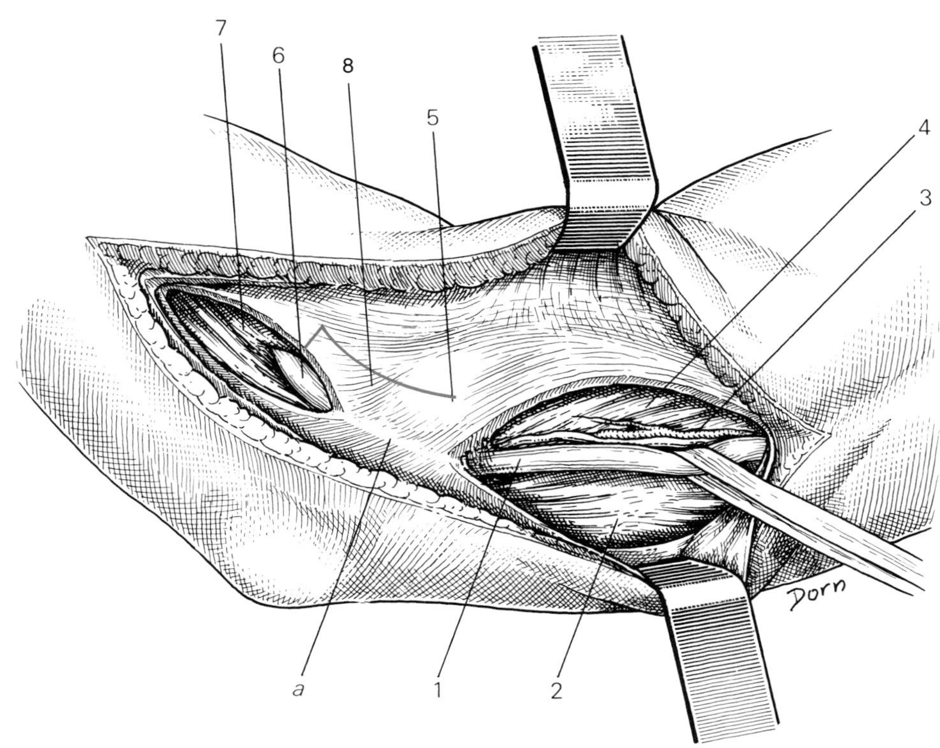

Figure 26.15

Ulnar nerve release at the elbow. The nerve is then transposed subcutaneously anterior to the medial epicondyle, being careful not to injure blood supply to the nerve and the flexor pronator muscles origin. 1, Ulnar nerve; 2, triceps; 3, superior ulnar collateral artery; 4, brachialis; 5, medial epicondyle; 6, ulnar nerve; 7, flexor carpi ulnaris; 8, a flap of fascia is prepared to make a pulley maintaining the nerve anteriorly to the medial epicondyle; *a*, incision in cubital tunnel.

suggests that sustained elbow flexion with finger movement (fingerboard left side) is more important than flexion-extension (bow right side) in the pathophysiology of this disorder (Charness 1987) (Figure 26.14).

The ulnar nerve passes round the medial epicondyle in the 'cubital tunnel'. The floor of the tunnel is made up of the joint capsule, the roof is formed by a dense, unyielding ligament. Ulnar nerve injury at the elbow is complex and multifactorial. The ulnar nerve may be entrapped at a variety of levels from the arcade of Struthers, proximal to the elbow, in the cubital tunnel, at the fibrous arch of the origin of the flexor carpi ulnaris and at the deep flexor pronator aponeurosis. The cubital tunnel retinaculum is the most common level in musicians. Because the ulnar nerve lies posterior to the axis of elbow flexion, it must stretch as the elbow flexes. During elbow motion, the ulnar nerve excursion proximal to the medial epicondyle can be as great as 10 mm, and distal to the epicondyle, as much as 6 mm (Wilgis and Murphy 1986). Limitation in ulnar nerve gliding, because of any constriction, can result in a traction neuropathy. When the elbow is flexed, the cubital tunnel is narrowed. Substantial flattening of the nerve normally occurs with elbow flexion. Flexing the elbow increases intraneural pressure within the cubital tunnel by two to three times. A greater increase in tunnel pressure was noted with elbow flexion, shoulder abduction and wrist extension (Pechant and Julius 1995). This is the motion that occurs in the violinist or cellist's right arm.

Stretching and compression interfere with intraneural circulation and this can produce localized ischaemia, oedema and ultimately fibrosis. Occupationally repetitive elbow flexion is a contributing factor in ulnar neuropathy. Also, valgus deformity of the elbow or instability in the post-epicondylar groove are other causes of ulnar neuropathy, particularly if there is loss of nerve gliding due to local inflammation. Positions of extreme elbow flexion are seen in the left arms of cellists and bassists. Violinists never flex as much as cellists but their left arm is twisted in supination, which puts an additional strain on the nerve.

Clinical symptoms include pain, which may occur in the inner aspect of the elbow, ulnar paraesthesiae, numbness and tingling in the ulnar side of the hand. Symptoms are aggravated by elbow flexion or by manual compression of the ulnar nerve at the elbow. Few musicians complain of weakness in daily activities; however, performance impairments may occur in the absence of sensory deficits, probably related to a mild degree of weakness, appreciated on examination of flexion of the little finger against resistance. In chronic cases, signs of muscle atrophy can be seen in the intrinsic muscles of the hand innervated by the nerve. Nerve conduction testing is most useful for the differential diagnosis with proximal and distal causes of ulnar neuropathy and with TOS.

Treatment of early cases should always be conservative. It consists of rehabilitation exercises, modification of playing posture with avoidance of prolonged elbow flexion, breaking up practice sessions with periods of rest, nerve mobilization exercises and night-time splinting at 40° of elbow flexion. In most cases surgery can be avoided. If no clinical and EMG improvement occurs after a few months, and particularly if the patient's musical performance is failing (Winspur 1998), a surgical

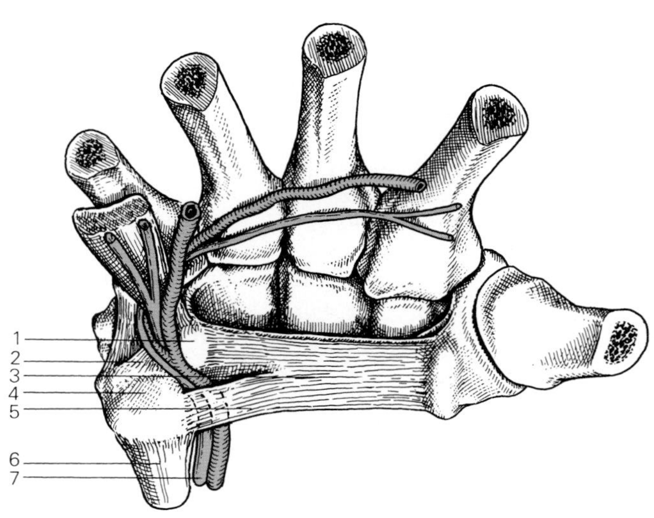

Figure 26.16

Distal entrapments of the ulnar nerve in the wrist and in the palm. 1, Hook of the hamate; 2, pisohamate ligament; 3, flexor retinaculum; 4, pisiform; 5, volar carpal ligament; 6, flexor carpi ulnaris; 7, ulnar neurovascular bundle.

release is considered. Surgical treatment includes in situ release, medial epicondylectomy and various types of transposition. In musicians, it seems preferable to use a subcutaneous transposition technique of the nerve (Figure 26.15) rather than a simple decompression, to prevent the constant traction associated with long periods of elbow flexion (Amadio and Beckenbaugh 1986). A pulley, with a flap of fascia, is made to hold the nerve in place (Tubiana 2001). With this technique of subcutaneous transposition, recovery is more rapid than after epicondylectomy or intramuscular or submuscular transposition, and the musicians can return to play within a few weeks after surgery (Dellon 1989, Amadio 1993, Nolan 1993.)

Distal entrapments of the ulnar nerve (Figure 26.16)

Ulnar nerve at Guyon's space

Ulnar nerve entrapment at the wrist has been reported in the left hands of flautists in dorsiflexion and radial deviation (Wainapel and Cole 1988) (see Figure 26.2). Patients may present painful dysaesthesiae in the ulnar aspect of the hand, sometimes associated with weakness of the ulnar innervated intrinsic muscles. A resting splint with the wrist in a physiological neutral position provided symptomatic relief in these reported cases.

Deep in the palm

Distal entrapment deep in the palm has also been reported in flautists (Wainapel and Cole 1988) or associated with a fractured hook of hamate.

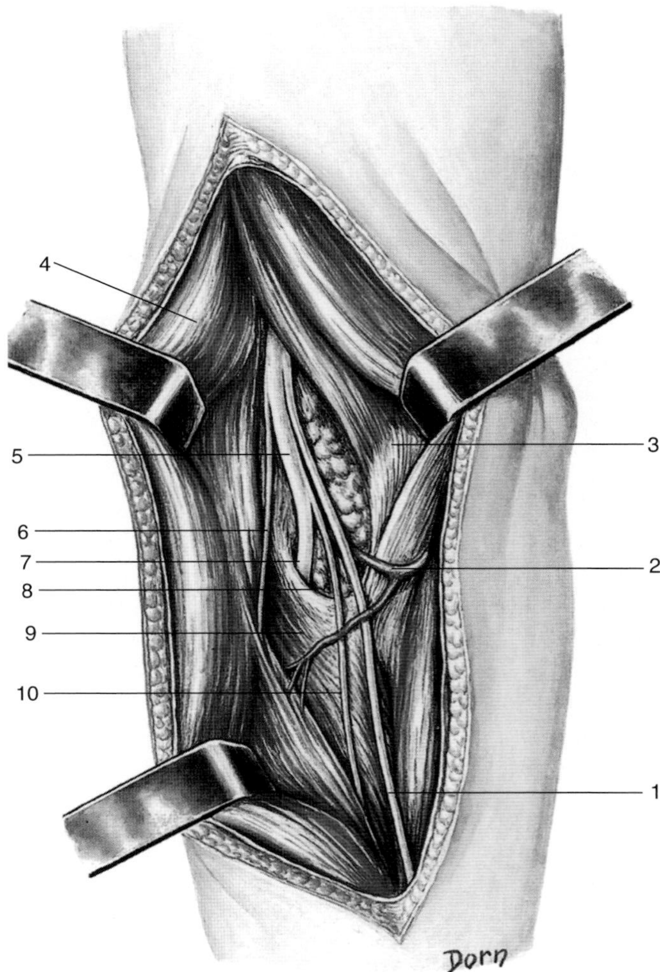

Figure 26.17

Division of the radial nerve at the elbow. 1, Sensory branch of radial nerve; 2, radial recurrent artery; 3, biceps and branchialis, retracted; 4, brachioradialis; 5, radial nerve; 6, branch to brachioradialis; 7, posterior interosseous nerve; 8, arcade of Frohse; 9, supinator; 10, branch to extensor carpi radialis brevis.

Radial nerve entrapments

The motor terminal branch of the radial nerve, the posterior interosseous nerve (PIN) can be entrapped at the elbow level, and the terminal sensory branch of the radial nerve can be compressed at the distal part of the forearm.

In fact, the problem is complex because entrapment of the motor branch at the elbow can cause a painful syndrome, the radial tunnel syndrome, which must be differentiated from the paralytic syndrome of the PIN, and also from lateral epicondylitis. On the other hand, the terminal superficial branch of the radial nerve can also, in rare cases, be compressed at the elbow (Moss and Switzer 1983). The different forms of radial nerve entrapments at the elbow (Figure 26.17) are described in detail in Chapter 23.

Paralytic forms

The motor posterior terminal branch of the radial nerve can be compressed by different structures at the elbow level. The syndrome was first described in 1905 by Guillain and Courtellement in a musical conductor who had his radial nerve compressed against the arcade of Fröhse of the supinator muscle. Deficits of motor function are variable, weakness of the extensor digitorum results in a deficit of metacarpophalangeal extension. To detect weakness of the extensor digitorum, one must maintain the wrist in extension to eliminate the tenodesis effect of wrist flexion (Comtet and Chambaud 1975). Extension of the interphalangeal joints and of the wrist is possible. Electrodiagnostic studies show abnormalities. This motor syndrome is rare but can exist in violinists, pianists or other musicians who require forceful repetitive work in pronation and supination, coupled with flexion and extension of the elbow. The constrictions can be an arcade of Fröhse or any anatomic anomaly in the radial tunnel.

Radial tunnel syndrome

The painful syndrome described by Roles and Maudsley (1972) is more often found in musicians than the paralytic syndrome. It has been reported to occur in the left forearm of violinists (Maffulli and Maffulli 1991) as well as in keyboard players and flautists (Charness et al 1985). At the onset, patients complain of pain located distal to the epicondyle on the lateral side of the forearm, radiating down the course of the radial nerve, toward the dorsum of the wrist. The pain may be relieved by shaking the hand. Instrumentalists present inability to perform fine finger movements with the usual speed and precision (Spinner and Amadio 2000). They may already present weakness of extension of one or more digits. At this stage, nerve conduction testing is of little value (Lawrence et al 1995). Diagnosis must be made on clinical grounds: direct tenderness of the nerve at the site of entrapment, especially if a Tinel's sign is present. Pressure 3–4 cm distal to the epicondyle on the radial point is painful; the degree of tenderness should be compared to pressure on the epicondyle. The study of resisted active supination, with the elbow flexed, then with the elbow in complete extension to put the nerve under more tension should bring out the pain.

Most authors still believe that electrodiagnostic studies are unreliable in radial tunnel syndrome (Younge and Moise 1994). However, Raimbeau (2002) has developed a protocol consisting of EMG study of several muscles innervated by the PIN and not only of the extensor digitorum, and a study of sensory and motor conduction velocities (see Chapter 23). This examination, although long and difficult, is necessary to confirm the diagnosis before any decision to carry out a surgical release.

Conservative treatment can be attempted: modifying positioning, with limitation of those activities which

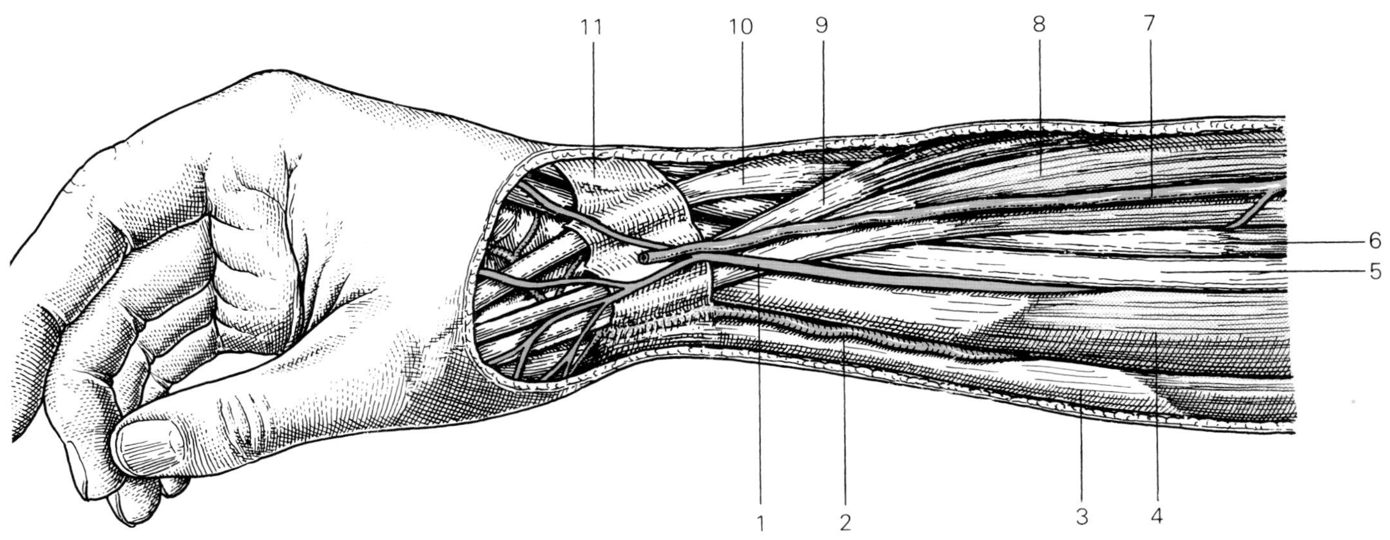

Figure 26.18
Entrapment of the superficial branch of the radial nerve. 1, Sensory branch of radial nerve; 2, radial artery; 3, flexor carpi radialis; 4, brachioradialis; 5, extensor carpi radialis longus; 6, extensor carpi radialis brevis; 7, cephalic vein; 8, abductor pollicis longus; 9, extensor pollicis brevis; 10, extensor pollicis longus; 11, extensor retinaculum.

exacerbate the pain, and anti-inflammatory medications (but steroid injections are not recommended for the treatment of radial tunnel syndrome). Exercises for rehabilitation should be controlled by a physiotherapist specializing in the treatment of musicians. If medical treatment is insufficient, the electrodiagnostic studies are repeated after about 6 months, especially if the initial EMG is normal. We believe like Raimbeau that 'since we are dealing with a painful syndrome without any consistent objective evidence to confirm the diagnosis, the decision to operate should not be made without alterations in EMG studies'.

The surgical release of the PIN is described in Chapter 23. I have never done a surgical release of a radial nerve for a paralytic syndrome in a musician. I have carried out three surgical procedures for persistent painful symptoms on the lateral side of the elbow and proximal forearm.

I had no EMG objective evidence of PIN entrapment because Raimbeau's protocol had not then been described, and clinically I was not able to differentiate a radial tunnel syndrome from a lateral epicondylitis, which is not uncommon in musicians. Steroid injections may improve epicondylitis; however, they cannot be used repeatedly as they have a degenerative effect, and lateral epicondylitis may coexist with a radial tunnel syndrome (Hagert et al 1977, Comtet et al 1985). In my ignorance I have decompressed the PIN and lengthened the conjoined tendon to relieve pressure on the supinator muscles. Results were satisfactory in two cases but the third patient had persistent pain.

Entrapment of the superficial branch of the radial nerve (Wartenberg syndrome)

The sensory branch of the radial nerve emerges from between the brachioradialis and extensor carpi radialis longus tendons at the distal part of the forearm. The combination of pronation and ulnar deviation often used by string players and pianists irritates the nerve squeezed by the two tendons and provokes pain over the first dorsal compartment, simulating de Quervain's disease (Figure 26.18).

Digital nerve compression

Digital neuritis may occur in any digit of instrumentalists who apply pressure on a digital nerve to support an instrument or pluck strings: e.g. the left thumb of French horn players, the left index finger of flautists (Cynamon 1981) while supporting the flute, the left index finger of violinists. Painful digital neuromas can occur in the pulp in harpists and cellists, for example (Patrone et al 1989).

In most cases, protective self-adhesive dressings are sufficient (Lederman 1989). The string tension should be altered by cellists, harpists and guitarists. Instrument adjustments or supports are available for flautists and horn players (Norris 1992). However, some painful pulp neuromas in the players of plucked string instruments should, in rare cases, be treated by surgical excision.

References

Amadio PC (1993) Diagnosis and treatment of ulnar nerve entrapment at the elbow and carpal tunnel syndrome in musicians, *Med Probl Perform Art* **8**: 53–60.

Amadio PC, Beckenbaugh RD (1986) Entrapment of the ulnar nerve by the deep flexor pronator aponeurosis, *J Hand Surg* **11A**: 83–7.

Amadio PC, Russotti GM (1990) Evaluation and treatment of hand and wrist disorders in musicians, *Hand Clin* **6**: 405–16.

Charness ME (1992) Unique upper extremity disorders of musicians. In: Millender LH, Louis DS, Simmons BP, eds, *Occupational Disorders of the Upper Extremity* (Churchill Livingstone: New York) 227–52.

Charness ME, Parry GJ, Markison RE (1985) Entrapment neuropathies in musicians, *Neurology* **35**: 74.

Charness ME, Barbaro NM, Olney RK, Parry GJ (1987) Occupational cubital tunnel syndrome in instrumental musicians, *Neurology* **37**: 115.

Charness ME, Ross MH, Shefner JM (1996) Ulnar neuropathy and dystonic flexion of the fourth and fifth digits: clinical correlation in musicians, *Mov Disord* **22**: 44–6.

Comtet JJ, Chambaud D (1975) Paralysie "spontanée" du nerf interosseux postérieur par lesion inhabituelle, *Rev Chir Orthop* **61**: 533–41.

Comtet JJ, Lalain JJ, Moyen B, Genety J, Brunet-Guedj E, Lazo-Henriïuez R (1985) Les épicondylalgies avec compression de la branche postérieure du nerf radial, *Rev Chir Orthop* **71** (Suppl II): 89–93.

Cynamon KB (1981) Flutist's neuropathy, *N Engl J Med* 305: 961.

Dellon AL (1989) Review of treatment results of ulnar nerve entrapment of the elbow, *J Hand Surg* **14A**: 688–700.

Gelberman RH, Hergenroeder PT, Hargens AR (1981) The carpal tunnel syndrome: a study of carpal canal pressures, *J Bone Joint Surg* **63A**: 380–3.

Gullain G, Courtellemont (1905) L'action du muscle court supinateur dans la paralysie du nerf radial, *Press Med* **18**: 50–2.

Hagert CG, Lundborg G, Hansen T (1977) Entrapment of the posterior interosseous nerve, *Scand J Plast Reconstr Surg* **11**: 205–12.

Hochberg FH, Hochberg NS (2000) In: Tubiana R, Amadio P, eds, *Medical Problems of the Instrumentalist Musician* (Martin Dunitz: London) 295–310.

Hochberg FH, Leffert RD, Heller MD, Merriman L (1983) Hand difficulties among musicians, *JAMA* **249**: 1869–72.

Katz JN, Larson MG, Sabra A et al (1990) The carpal tunnel syndrome: diagnostic utility of the history and physical examination findings, *Ann Intern Med* **112**: 321–7.

Lawrence T, Mobbs P, Fortems Y et al (1995) Radial tunnel syndrome, *J Hand Surg* **20B**: 454–9.

Lederman RJ (1987) Thoracic outlet syndromes. Review of the controversies and a report of 17 instrumental musicians, *Med Probl Perform Art* **2**: 87–91.

Lederman RJ (1989) Peripheral nerve disorders in instrumentalists, *Ann Neurol* **26**: 640–6.

Lederman RJ (1993) Entrapment neuropathies in instrumental musicians, *Med Probl Perform Art* **8**: 35–40.

Lederman RJ (1994) AAEM minimonograph #43: neuromuscular problems in the performing arts, *Muscle Nerve* **17**: 569–77.

Mackinnon SE (1992) Double and multiple crush syndromes, *Hand Clin* **8**: 369–95.

Mackinnon SE, Dellon AL (1988) *Surgery of the Peripheral Nerve* (New York: Thieme).

Maffulli N, Maffulli F (1991) Transient entrapment neuropathy of the posterior interosseous nerve in violin players, *J Neurol Neurosurg Psychiatr* **54**: 65–7.

Marsden CD (1991) Investigation and treatment of dystonia, *Med Probl Perform Art* **6**: 116–21.

Millesi H, Zoch G, Rath TH (1990) The gliding apparatus of peripheral nerve and its clinical significance, *Ann Hand Surg* **9**: 87–97.

Moss SH, Switzer HE (1983) Radial tunnel syndrome: a spectrum of clinical presentations, *J Hand Surg* **8A**: 441–20.

Nolan WB, Eaton RG (1989) Thumb problems of professional musicians, *Med Probl Perform Art* **4**: 20–2.

Nolan WB, Eaton RG (1993) Evaluation and treatment of cubital tunnel syndrome in musicians, *Med Probl Perform Art* **8**: 47–52.

Norris RN (1992) *The Musicians' Survival Manual* (MMB Music Co: St Louis).

Patrone NA, Hoppman RA, Whaley J, Schmidt R (1989) Digital nerve compression in a violinist with benign hypermobility: a case study, *Med Probl Perform Art* **4**: 91–4.

Pechant J, Julius I (1995) The pressure measurement in the ulnar nerve. A contribution to the pathophysiology of the cubital tunnel syndrome, *J Biomech* **8**: 75–80.

Raimbeau G (2002) Radial nerve compression at the elbow. In: Allieu Y, Mackinnon SE, eds, *Nerve Compression Syndromes in the Upper Limb* (Martin Dunitz: London) 141–60.

Roles NC, Maudsley R (1972) Radial tunnel syndrome: radial tennis elbow as a nerve entrapment, *J Bone Joint Surg* **54B**: 499–598.

Spinner RJ, Amadio PC (2000) Compression neuropathies of the upper extremities. In: Tubiana R, Amadio PC, eds, *Medical Problems of Instrumentalist Musicians* (Martin Dunitz: London) 273–94.

Tubiana R (2001) Peripheral nerve pathology. In: *Functional Disorders in Musicians* (Elsevier: Amsterdam) 127–32.

Wainapel SF, Cole JL (1988) The not-so-magic flute. Two cases of distal ulnar nerve entrapment, *Med Probl Perform Art* **3**: 63–5.

Wilgis EFS, Murphy R (1986) The significance of longitudinal excursion in peripheral nerves, *Hand Clin* **2**: 761–6.

Winspur I (1998) Surgical indications, planning and technique. In: Winspur I, Wynn Parry CB, eds, *The Musician's Hand: A Clinical Guide* (Martin Dunitz: London) 41–52.

Winspur I (2002) Musicians. In: Allieu Y, Mackinnon SE, eds, *Nerve Compression Syndromes of the Upper Limb* (Martin Dunitz: London) 179–94.

Winspur I, Wynn Parry CB (1997) The musician's hand, *J Hand Surg* **22B**: 433–40.

Wynn Parry CB (1994) Musicians suffer a variety of problems, *J Hand Surg* **19B** (Suppl 11–12).

Wynn Parry CB (1998) The musician's hand and arm pain. In: Winspur I, Wynn Parry CB, eds, *The Musician's Hand: A Clinical Guide* (Martin Dunitz: London) 5–12.

Younge DH, Moise P (1994) The radial tunnel syndrome, *Int Orthop* **18**: 368–70.

III Pediatrics

27 Hyponeurotization in spastic palsies (selective partial denervation)

Giorgio A Brunelli

Introduction

Spastic palsies are still a challenge to the surgeon. In fact the various surgical techniques of the so-called 'classical' surgery still end up in failure in a great number of patients. Spasticity depends on central neurological lesions involving the pyramidal system at various levels. (Lusskin et al 1968, Dujovny et al 1980). The etiology includes perinatal encephalitis, brain diseases in children, and vascular or traumatic hemiplegia in adults.

In children, brain lesions are generally stationary (non-evolutive), allowing reconstructive surgery. Sometimes lesions are present in asymmetric spastic quadriplegia. However, the main type depends on subcortical unilateral lesions affecting the pyramidal system and provoking motor impairment of the two limbs on the same side. The pyramidal lesion syndrome generally includes spasticity and motor problems of various types.

Spasticity takes the form of muscular hypertonia with exaggeration of myostatic reflexes with five classic characteristics:

1. Spasticity is 'elective', involving mainly pronator and flexor muscles as well as the adductor pollicis. It is responsible for the attitude in flexion pronation.
2. It is 'elastic'. In fact the attitude may be passively corrected by pulling the hand and fingers in extension with different levels of strength. On releasing the hand and the fingers they take up the pathological position again.
3. It persists at rest and it is worsened by voluntary movement, emotion, pain, and tiredness.
4. It is associated with hyper-reflexia.
5. It may be associated with synkinesias (global or elective synkinesias). Synkinesias and dyskinesias, if light, do not alter the diagnosis, or the prognosis, or the original indications of spastic palsies. Motor impairment in spastic palsies is not a real palsy, but a problem of the voluntary command which affects mainly the distal muscles.

In severe cases in adults, administration of baclofen, either orally or intrathecally (with pumps), may be useful; especially to allow the patient to stand or to improve the sitting position in a wheelchair. Baclofen is not used in children and its use seems disproportionate to improve the function of the hand. However, baclofen is especially effective in spasticity resulting from cord lesions, whereas it is less appropriate in cerebral palsies.

Extrapyramidal signs are often present: athetosis, chorea and even Parkinson-like syndrome. If extrapyramidal signs are predominant, surgery is contraindicated. Fibrous retractions may co-exist (which affects surgical indications). Sensory functions are also impaired, especially epicritic, tactile, proprioceptive and gnostic functions, whereas protopathic pain and thermic sensibility are preserved.

The rate of complications in children and the cost of implantable devices play a role in making a surgical and definitive treatment preferable.

Surgical treatment and indications

Surgery can be done with the aim of diminishing spasticity and deformity and improving hand dexterity.

Current treatment of spastic palsies includes:

1. tendon transfers
2. muscular release aimed at overcoming spasticity by cutting the proximal insertion of muscles
3. fasciotomies and septotomies
4. osteotomies
5. bone fusion (arthrodesis)
6. deafferentations (which try to reduce spasticity by removing the afferent stimuli).

Results of deafferentations are unpredictable, due to the difficulty of performing the neurotomy. Tendon transfers also give unpredictable results because of the possible

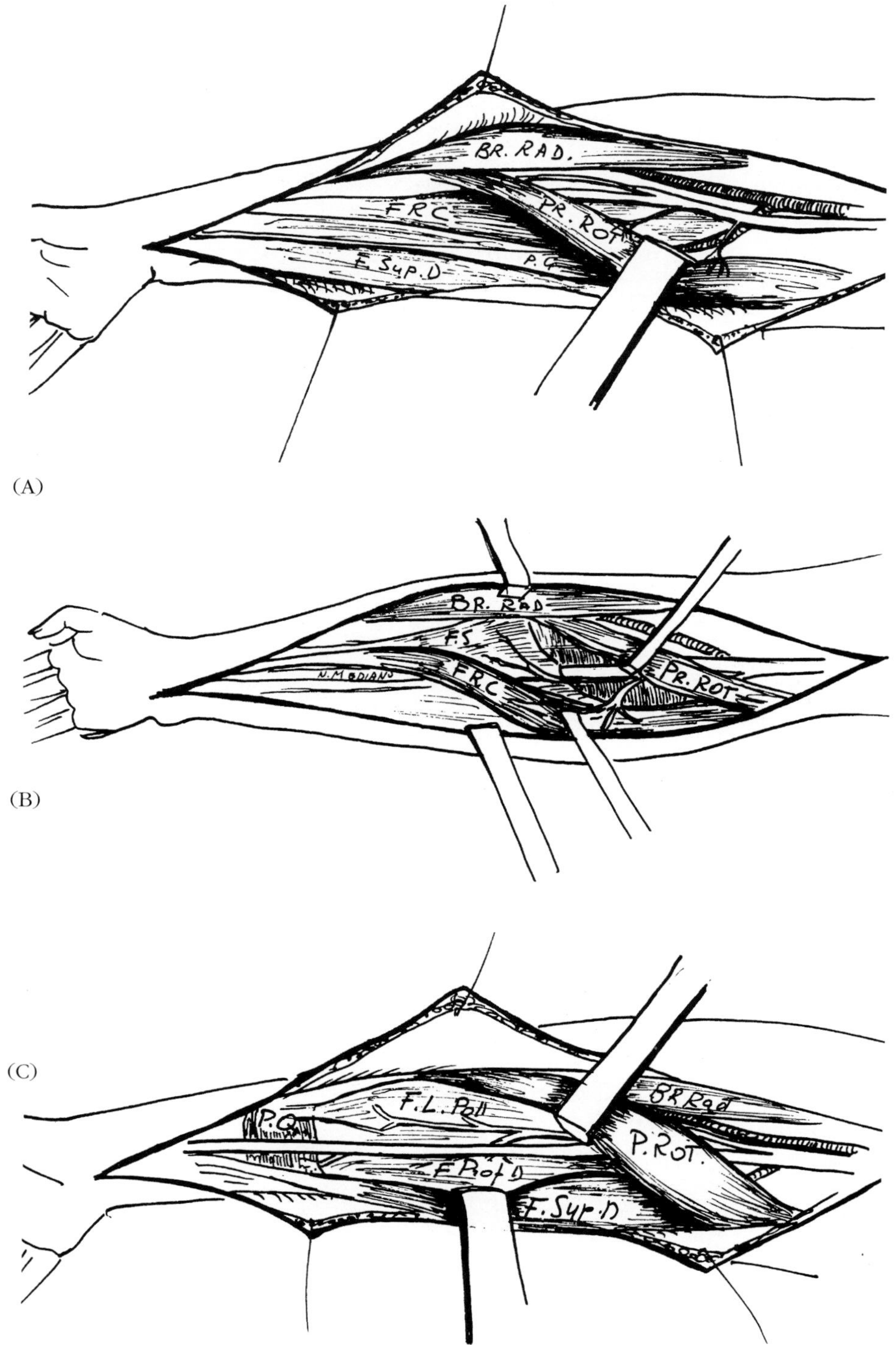

Figure 27.1

Scheme of the operation. (A) The pronator teres is retracted medially to reveal the branches of the median nerve to the muscles and to carry out selective denervation; (B) the pronator teres is retracted laterally and flexor carpi radialis (FRC) medially to show the motor branches for FRC and flexor digitorum superficialis (FS); (C) the flexor superficialis is retracted medially to show the flexor pollicis longus and flexor digitorum profundus and their motor branches.

muscular imbalance, as well as muscular release, whereas fasciotomies and septotomies seem to be more effective (in slight spastic palsies). Osteotomies and bone fusion may be useful in very severe cases.

None of the above-mentioned operations assures the solution of the problem, which is why selective neurotomy of motor nerves has attracted new interest. At the beginning of the twentieth century Stöffel (1913) conceived the idea of 'hyponeurotization', selectively denervating the spastic muscles by cutting at the elbow some of the fascicles destined to the muscles inside the median nerve (Stöffel's first operation) or later on, dividing the muscular branches (Stöffel's second operation, Tibbs et al 1981)

Stöffel's operations gave inconsistent results, due to the primitive conditions of surgery of his time (lack of anesthesia, antibiotics, electrical apparatus, etc.) and to poor knowledge of nerve physiology and biological data. The amount of data on nerve pathophysiology has greatly improved with the years, and together with microsurgery, this has allowed surgeons to take up Stöffel's idea again, changing the approach and improving the technique (Brunelli and Brunelli 1983).

The goal of hyponeurotization is to diminish the efferent impulses by such an amount as to eliminate spasticity, while still preserving the existing voluntary activity. The operation is performed under the operating microscope with the aid of intraoperative electrical stimulation, by substantially denervating the spastic muscles (Figure 27.1).

The approach has to be large enough to make it possible to check all the motor branches of all the spastic muscles.

The adoption phenomenon has to be carefully taken into consideration. In fact a lot of the denervated muscular fibers will exert a chemotactic effect on the remaining sound nerve fibers, which give out new branches. The latter 'adopt' the denervated muscular fibers and reinnervate them.

The following factors should be borne in mind:

- Indications are: disabling spastic palsies in cooperative patients.
- Favorable conditions as regards the patients are: attention, interpretation, cooperation, capability of speaking, seeing, hearing, motivation, and capability of voluntary grip and voluntary release even if seriously limited by spasticity.
- Contraindications are: muscular retractions, osseous deformities, athetosis, brain impairment.
- Partial indications require added operations. In fact retracted muscles require tenotomies (especially FCR and FCU).

A very careful repeated preoperative muscular test has to be done to determine a good approximation of which muscles depending on median and ulnar nerves have to be denervated and to what extent.

It is always difficult to decide the exact amount of denervation to perform. Sometimes it can be helpful to carry out a preliminary investigation by means of botulin toxin injected intramuscularly.

Tests are often affected by extrinsic and intrinsic conditions: weather, temperature, tiredness, emotion, etc.

The adoption phenomenon varies according to many factors: age, health, individuals, type of muscle, and type of surgical resection. Therefore, a second operation, to be done after the adoption phenomenon has finished, must always be planned 6 months later. This can require further denervation or even reconstructive procedures if the first denervation was too severe. Patients and their parents must be informed that a second operation must be done in 6 months.

Patients with athetosis, as well as those with insufficient intelligence and uncooperative individuals cannot be considered for this procedure.

According to the case the approach will involve the arm (to denervate the biceps and brachialis muscles), all the volar aspect of the forearm (to denervate the flexor and pronator muscles starting from the pronator teres down to the pronator quadratus), and the hand (to denervate intrinsic muscles and especially to remove the adductor pollicis muscle).

It is necessary to denervate the muscle by at least double what seems necessary, as the adoption phenomenon will lead to the desired result. If from the clinical point of view attenuation of half of the strength is required, the muscle has to be denervated by at least three-quarters as the quarter of spared nerve fibers will reinnervate around one-quarter of muscular fibers.

Selective denervation (Figure 27.2)

The median nerve is sought and recognized at the elbow, after dividing the lacertus fibrosus.

The pronator teres belly is retracted to inspect its motor branches. According to the severity of spasticity and to the foreseen adoption phenomenon, one-half, two-thirds or three-quarters of the fascicles going to the muscle are severed and removed over about 1 cm (to avoid spontaneous repair).

Denervation is done under magnification and with the help of repeated electrical stimulations. If there are three motor branches to a muscle it is easy to denervate one-third or two-thirds, but if there is only one motor branch, microsurgery is necessary to separate the fascicles, recognize them, and remove the desired amount of nerve.

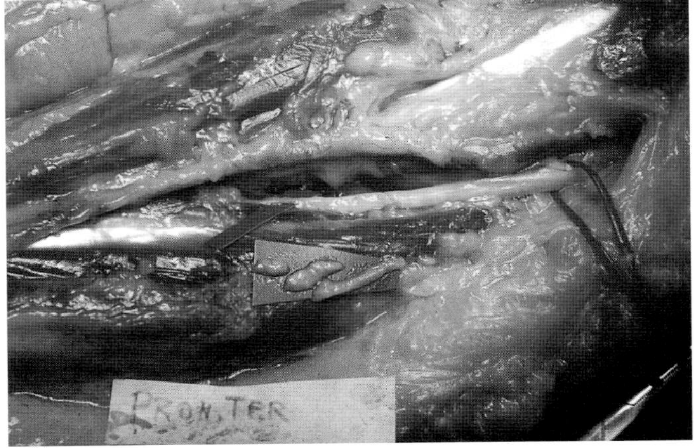

Figure 27.2
Example of selective denervation of pronator teres muscle.

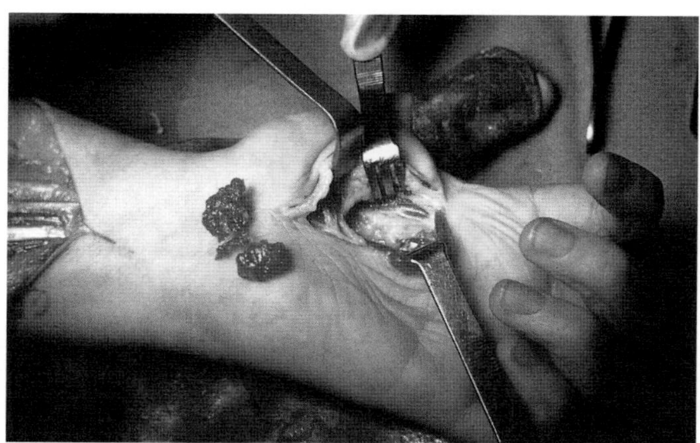

Figure 27.3
Example of myectomy.

Then the pronator teres is retracted upward and laterally whereas the flexor carpi radialis is pulled down and medially, so making it possible to see and denervate the branches to the flexor carpi radialis itself and to the flexor digitorum superficialis. The latter is then displaced laterally, allowing the denervation of the flexor digitorum profundus and flexor pollicis longus. In the lower part of the forearm the nerve to the pronator quadratus is found and hyponeurotized.

If necessary, in rare cases, the nerves to abductor pollicis brevis and opponens muscles are also partially divided and removed. Less frequently it may be necessary to carry out selective denervation of FCU and flexor digitorum profundus of the long and little fingers innervated by the ulnar nerve. These muscles are approached throughout the same incision used for the median nerve and are selectively hyponeurotized by the abovementioned technique.

As regards the intrinsic muscles innervated by the ulnar nerve, the adductor pollicis is generally the one which hinders most.

In the past I have done denervation at the Guyon canal and later on removal of the muscular branches under the muscle. I have learnt from experience that denervation leads to failures, because the adoption phenomenon takes place not only from the fibers of its own nerve, but also from surrounding muscles. Therefore, for many years I have removed the whole muscle (Figure 27.3). Adductor pollicis myectomy introduces the 'Froment sign', but it is the only surgery able to solve the 'thumb-in-palm' deformity which is peculiar to severe spastic hands. The Froment sign can be corrected with IF fusion of the thumb.

This is the standard operating protocol, but in some cases in which retraction is also present in addition to spasticity, tendon lengthening or tenotomies, or even arthrodesis may be added. Tenotomy is often necessary for flexor carpi radialis and ulnaris.

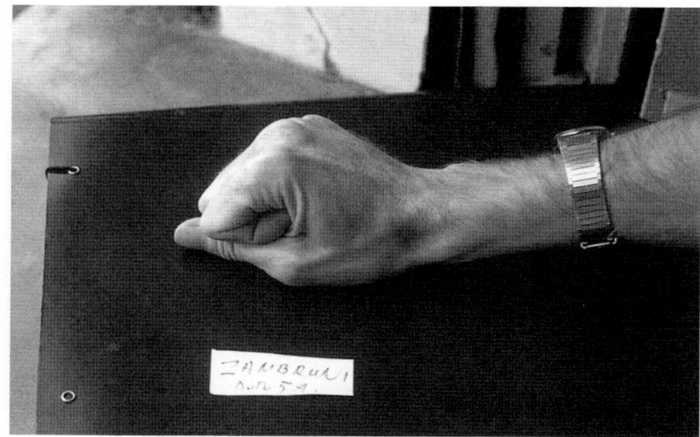

(A)

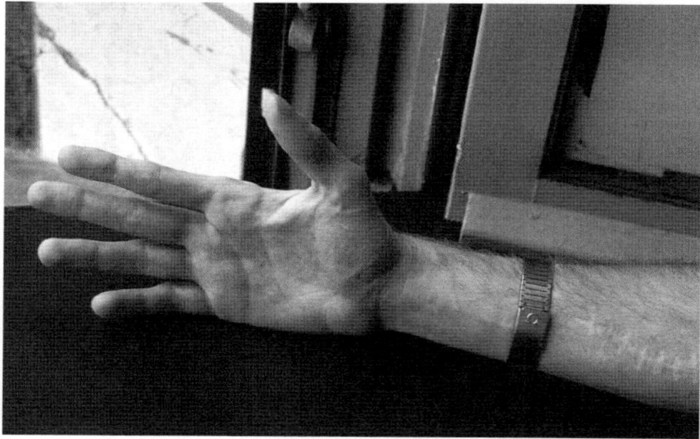

(B)

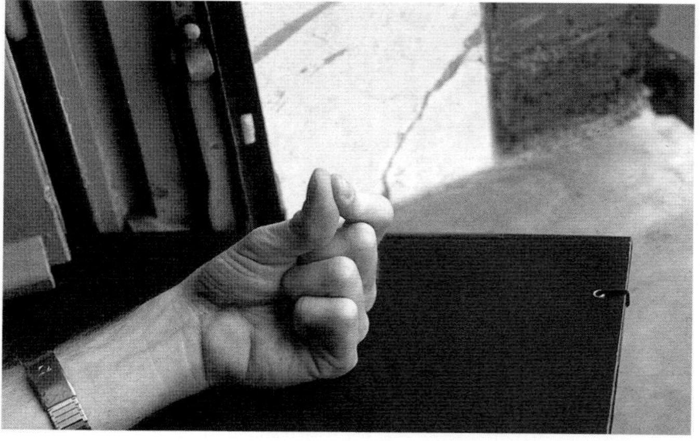

(C)

Figure 27.4
(A–C) Result in one patient at long-term follow-up. This patient became a doctor and practiced without any impairment.

After surgery a hypercorrecting splint forcing the finger in extension has to be worn for 45 days.

Generally the adoption phenomenon takes place within 45–60 days, restoring some muscular tone to the muscles which, after denervation, were more or less flabby. This phenomenon is generally complete in 4 months. Sometimes the result is good with the first operation; more often a second operation has to be done, at times to further denervate some muscles in which the adoption phenomenon was too effective, in rare cases to obviate a too generous denervation by means of tendon transfer to correct residual deformities (e.g. swan-neck deformity).

After the second operation a good result satisfying both patient and surgeon is generally obtained. In very rare cases (3 out of 60) a third operation had to be carried out. In general, results are better in young patients with perinatal spasticity of the upper limb. Less effective results are obtained in the lower limb or in adults with acquired hemiplegia.

Results

My series includes 60 hyponeurotizations in 30 years (57 of which of the upper limb). Only 5 were acquired adult hemiplegia; 43 cases required a second operation at 6 months; 2 cases needed a third operation.

Results differ according to the type and the severity of the lesion. A classification of results is impossible (Caldwell et al 1969) as they depend on so many factors: the number of muscles involved, the added retraction, the the patient's cooperation, etc.

I tried to evaluate the spasticity in four categories of severity in order to be able to score the improvement after the operation.

In cases with mild spasticity an almost perfect result can be achieved. One of our patients is practicing as a medical doctor (Figure 27.4), another became a priest and can give communion, and many have taken up manual jobs without handicap. Only one woman is not satisfied; she wanted a perfect result after a hemiplegia resulting from the removal of a brain tumor.

References

Brunelli GA, Brunelli F (1983) Selective microsurgical denervation in spastic paralyses, *Ann Chir Main* **2B**: 277–80.

Caldwell CB, Wilson DJ, Braun RM (1969) Evaluation and treatment of the upper extremity in the hemiplegic stroke patient, *Clin Orthop* **63**: 69–93.

Dujovny M, Laha RK, Yonas H (1980) Surgical management of spasticity, *Curr Probl Surg* **17**: 249–53.

Lusskin T, Nemunaitis J, Winer J, Grynbaum B (1968) Corrective surgery in adult hemiplegia, *Arch Phys Med Rehab* **49**: 437–42.

Stöffel A (1913) Treatment of spastic contractures, *Am J Orthop* **10**: 611–17.

Tibbs P, Young AB, Walsh JW, Bean JR (1981) Pharmacologic and surgical therapy for spasticity, *J Ky Med Ass* **79**: 359–62.

28 Surgery of the infantile spastic hand in cerebral palsy

Eduardo A Zancolli

Cerebral palsy may be defined as any disorder of neuromotor functions secondary to cerebral damage occurring prenatally, at birth or early in the postnatal period. Three principal types may be considered clinically: (1) pyramidal (spastic paralysis); (2) extrapyramidal (athetosis, ataxia, tremor and rigidity) and (3) mixed. Due to the involvement of the musculoskeletal system the lack of motor control is the greater handicap, whereas in others mental retardation, speed and sensory disturbances may be the most important impairments. About 60% of the patients have spastic paralysis, assumed to follow damage to the corticospinal tracts, producing a motor dysfunction that varies greatly in distribution and severity.

The purpose of this chapter is to discuss the surgical rehabilitation of the upper limb in the spastic paralytic type – particularly in infantile hemiplegia – where peripheral surgery yields its best results. In the great majority of cases, surgery considerably improves different functional grasps. Our experience is based on a series of 113 upper limb spastic cases operated on over a period of 33 years. The final results relate to 47 patients evaluated from a selected group of 91 patients (23% were hemiplegic). Of these cases, 84% had operations in the Rehabilitation Center of Buenos Aires (Argentina). Satisfactory results in hand position and movements were obtained in 92% of the most favourable cases – groups 1 and 2 of our classification system (Figure 28.1).

The spastic hand in patients with cerebral palsy presents one of the most complex problems in upper limb reconstructive surgery. This is because the pathology depends on lesions of the central nervous system and the severity of the motor imbalance and sensory impairment of the hand. In spite of these difficulties, upper extremity surgery has become an excellent aid in the management of the spastic hand when properly indicated and performed (Goldner 1955, 1975, Swanson 1968, Zancolli 1968, 1975, 1979).

Careful examination, testing and evaluation by the neurologist, the surgeon and the occupational therapist are of major importance in the selection of patients for surgical reconstruction.

Most poor surgical results are due to incorrect indications, poor patient selection and poor execution of surgical procedures. Our principal aim is to examine the surgical indications related to the general and local conditions and to develop the surgical techniques we prefer based on the clinical characteristics of upper limb pathology: elbow, forearm, wrist, fingers and thumb.

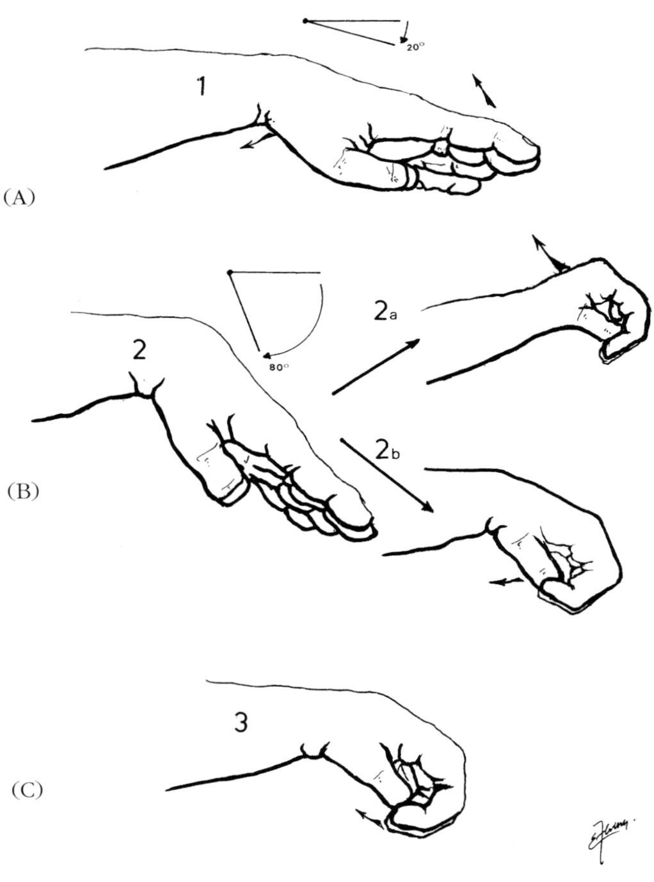

Figure 28.1

Grouping of wrist–finger deformities in the infantile spastic hand. (A) group 1; (B) group 2 and subgroups 2a and 2b; (C) group 3.

General preoperative evaluations

The principal evaluations that are important when selecting cerebral palsy patients who are suited to surgery are discussed below: i.e. aetiology, general neurological condition, type of neuromuscular disorder, extent of limb involvement, age and classification of hand deformity.

Aetiology

As noted, the lesion of the intercranial central nervous system may have its origin in pre-, peri- and post-natal periods. In our experience the perinatal brain damage is the most suited to peripheral reconstructive surgery when the patient is a spastic young hemiplegic.

Perinatal injuries have two main causes: trauma and anoxia at the time of birth. Prenatal cerebral palsy may be produced by congenital defects (rubella or other viral disease during the first 3 months of pregnancy) or erythroblastosis fetalis. These defects may produce ataxia or athetosis. Rarely is it familial. In many instances no specific aetiology can be found, and a development anomaly may be assumed. Postnatal lesions may be caused by infectious encephalitis (most frequent), meningitis convulsions in a very young child (intercranial haemorrhage) or injury.

Blumel et al (1960) found that most frequent lesions were due to trauma at birth (13%), anoxia (24%), prematurity (32%), congenital defects (11%) and postnatal damage (7%).

General neurological defects

Severe neurological defects are usually absent in the typical infantile spastic hemiplegia – the condition most adapted to reconstructive surgery of the upper limb. Surgery should be contraindicated when there are severe neurological alterations such as defects in speech, vision, hearing and mental retardation. These conditions are generally present in spastic, tetraplegia, extrapyramidal neuromuscular disorders, convulsions, manifest behavioural disorders, distractibility and learning disability. Mild alteration of the mental condition is not a surgical contraindication. Surgery is contraindicated when spasticity is markedly increased by emotional stimuli. In this latter condition it is very difficult to obtain a reasonable result even if the hand deformity is mild.

The patient must be capable of understanding the surgical goals and be sufficiently motivated to collaborate during postoperative re-education (Zancolli 1979).

Type of neuromuscular disorder

As noted above, patients with neuromuscular disorders can be classified into three types: spastic or pyramidal, extrapyramidal and mixed. It is important to study the principal clinical characteristics of each type of neuromuscular disorder when selecting candidates for reconstructive surgery.

Pyramidal type

In this type of neuromuscular disorder – the most frequent type of neuromuscular disorder in cerebral palsy – the classical deformity of the upper limb is characterized by a combination of spastic (pronator–flexor) and paretic or flaccid paralytic (extensor–supinator) muscles. This section will focus particularly on the principal clinical characteristcs of the spastic muscle.

- Spastic muscles through their hypertonicity produce the typical flexor–pronator deformity of the upper limb (Figure 28.2A).

  The most common posture is one of elbow, wrist and finger flexion with forearm pronation and the thumb in adduction or flexion–adduction. The wrist tends to deviate ulnarly. These deformities depend on the spasticity of the extrinsic muscles of the forearm and hand and particularly of the flexor–pronator muscular mass. Occasionally, spasticity produces some internal rotation contracture of the shoulder (Figure 28.2A). Flaccid paralysis or paresis affects the supinator–extensor muscles.
- It is typical of spastic muscle that its hypertonicity increases progressively as the muscle is gradually stretched passively.
- Spasticity is posturally and emotionally induced. It is rather constant except during sleep or under anaesthesia. Spasticity does not disminish with orthoses or manipulations.
- Synchronous activity or co-contraction (Samilson and Morris 1964) is a typical characteristic of the spastic muscle. Its clinical manifestation is represented by an abnormal reaction of the spastic muscles when the muscles are acting as antagonists. Antagonist spastic muscles remain electrically active on both flexion and extension of the involved part of the limb. A typical finding is the persistent activity of the flexor muscles of the wrist when complete finger and wrist extension are attempted, especially at the level of the flexor carpi ulnaris. Synchronous activity alters the normal grasping and release patterns of the hand.

  Co-contraction can be a favourable situation in some tendinous reconstructive procedures (Swanson 1968). Thus co-contraction favours active extension of the wrist after the transfer of a spastic FCU tendon to the extensors of the wrist. Under this condition, the co-contraction of the FCU produces wrist exten-

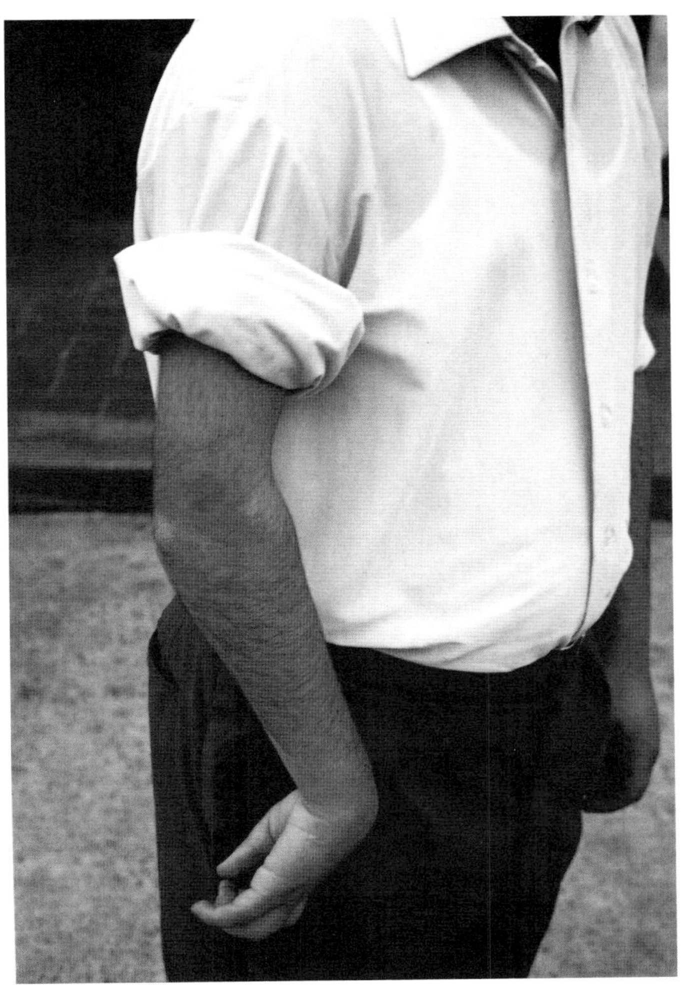

(A)

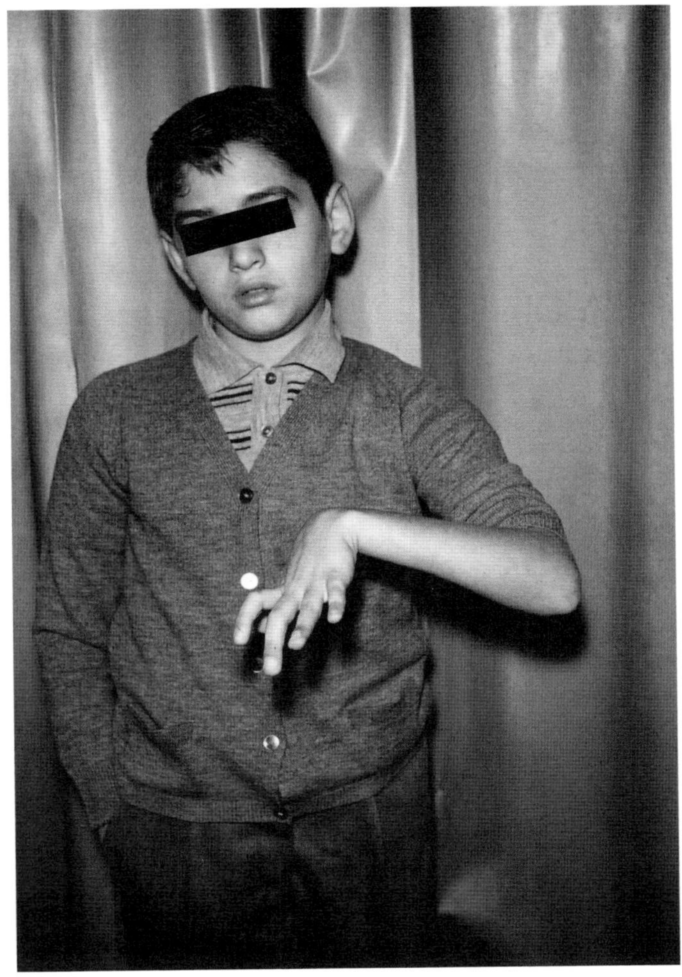

(C)

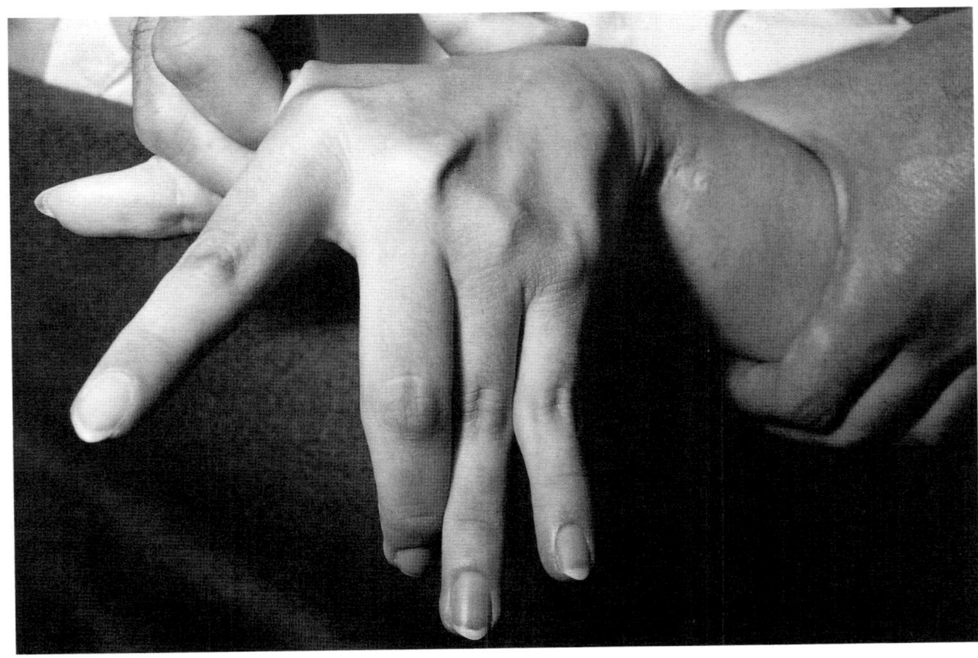

(B)

Figure 28.2

(A) Typical spastic hemiplegia with a flexor–pronator deformity of the upper limb.
(B) Extrapyramidal deformity of the hand in a quadriplegic athetoid patient. Fingers are deviated in opposite directions. Stretch reflex was absent. (C) Mixed deformity (extrapyramidal and pyramidal). Overactive stretch reflex and hypertonicity were present. These conditions allow soft tissue surgical reconstruction.

sion due to its synchronous activity (Green's procedure) (Green 1942).

- Overactive stretch reflex is one of the most useful manifestations in the diagnosis of spasticity. It is produced by failure of the normal muscle lengthening reaction on elongation by sudden passive stretching. As a result of the hyperactive stretch reflex, the spastic muscle contracts at the same point in the arc of motion each time a passive elongation manoeuvre is produced.

  This characteristic of the overactive stretch flex is absent in extrapyramidal neuromuscular disorders, but present in most of the mixed group, where spasticity is predominant over athetosis. Stretch reflex should be investigated for each muscle or group of muscles.

  Spasticity and overactive reflexes can be decreased by certain surgical procedures such as lengthening of distal tendons or release of proximal muscle insertions.

  Surgical reconstruction of the upper limb through soft tissue procedures, such as tenotomy and tendon transfer, is basically indicated in cases with pure spasticity and also in spastic patients where mild athetosis is combined with spasticity (mixed group).
- Myostatic contracture represents a secondary muscular fibrosis after a long-standing flexion contracture due to hypertonicity. This fibrosis is frequently seen in the flexor muscles of the wrist and digits. It is evaluated with the patient under general anaesthesia or peripheral nerve blocking. This muscular fibrotic retraction is not a contraindication to surgical reconstruction of the hand. Myostatic contracture is frequently observed during or after adolescence, particularly in permanent and severe contractures. It can be reduced preoperatively by physical methods of stretching with cast or braces. During surgery it can be eliminated by tenotomy, preserving muscular continuity.

Extrapyramidal type

The extrapyramidal type of neuromuscular disorder can be represented by athetosis, ataxia, tremor or rigidity. The most frequent extrapyramidal disorder is athetosis – it accounts for approximately 25%.

Athetosis, assumed to result from dysfunction of the basal ganglia, is characterized by the following:

- Abnormal, involuntary and poorly coordinated movements with varying degrees of tension (Figure 28.2B). The deformity decreases at rest and disappears during sleep, but it is accentuated by efforts to move or by any emotional or environmental stimulus. Typically the patient may show different asymmetrical finger deformities in the same hand; abnormal hand movements usually reduce if the patient is distracted.
- Delayed postural development. The disorder is usually generalized, but unilateral involvement can also occur. The most common aetiologies are neonatal anoxia and erythroblastosis fetalis.
- Hypotonus in infancy, which may change with growth to increased tonus in stress situations.
- Decreased reflexes in infancy, which may become hyperactive later.
- No tendency to muscular contracture.
- Absence of Hoffman reflex and stretch reflex.
- Frequently preserved tactile gnosis of the hand.

Soft tissue procedures carried out in the pure athetoid patient are absolutely contraindicated, as they may produce a new undesirable opposing deformity that may be totally uncontrollable by the patient. In this situation a transference of the initial distorted position to other muscle groups is produced. Soft tissue procedures are also contraindicated in other extrapyramidal muscular disorders such as chorea, ataxia, tremor and rigidity. In athetosis surgical procedures over bones (osteotomies) or joints (fusion) can be indicated.

Soft tissue procedures are also absolutely contraindicated in a young child with extrapyramidal hypotonus, which may change with growth to abnormal athetoid involuntary movements and increased tonus under emotional stimuli (Zancolli 1979).

Tremor is represented by involuntary movements that follow a regular rhythmic pattern in which flexor and extensor muscles contract alternately.

Ataxia is characterized by disturbed balance and equilibrium, lack of muscle coordination and hypotonia.

Rigidity is demonstrated by resistance to movement through the hand's entire range, and no exaggerated stretch reflex: both contracting muscles and their antagonists are affected. There is a tendency for diminished motion rather than abnormal motion.

Mixed type

The mixed type of neuromuscular disorder is a relatively common form. Most frequently spasticity is associated with athetosis and is characterized by a combination of hypertonus and abnormal movements (Figure 28.2C). Reconstructive surgery through soft tissue techniques may be indicated in the mixed type of neuromuscular disorder if hypertonicity and consequently the overactive stretch reflex are present and dominant.

Extent of limb involvement

Cerebral palsy can involve all four extremities as follows:

- Tetraplegia (both arms and both legs). Reconstructive surgery is rarely indicated in infantile tetraplegia, as these cases are frequently associated with severe neurological defects such as learning disability, extrapyramidal neuromuscular disorder, emotional instability, deficiency in motivation and cooperation, etc.

- Hemiplegia: one side of the body, usually with greater involvement of the upper limb. These cases usually offer the best local and general conditions for improving hand function and muscular balance and for correcting a pronator-flexor deformity.
- Diplegia: all four limbs, with the lower limbs much more severely involved than the upper limbs.
- Triplegia: three extremities, usually with both legs and one arm being affected.
- Monoplegia: single limb involvement.

Age

Surgical correction of spastic upper limb deformities is usually indicated after 6–7 years of age. Maturation of the central nervous system has occurred by this age, and the child is old enough to cooperate during postoperative rehabilitation. After adolescence, patients are generally not good candidates for reconstructive surgery, as they have usually accepted their cosmetic and functional problems.

Hand sensory impairment

Based on our experience (Zancolli and Zancolli 1987), all patients with a pure spastic neuromuscular disorder who are candidates for reconstructive surgery have some deficit of sensibility in proprioception (conscious control of position, motion and power) and stereognosia (ability to recognize objects by touch only). In the classical infantile hemiplegia with a pure spastic neuromuscular disorder the affected hand preserves the ability to recognize the physical characteristics of objects (shape, size, texture) or protective sensations (hot, cold, pain, pressure); but the patient is unable to name the objects because of cortical involvement. This is the typical condition in the spastic cases.

Defects in stereognosis (Twitchell 1966) are not a contraindication for attempting to improve hand motor function and appearance by surgery.

Only in cases where spasticity is combined with some athetoid component may hand sensibility be completely preserved.

Sensibility tests used in these patients are:

- pinprick test (protective sensation)
- recognition of size and shape of objects (differentiation of cubes from marbles by small children)
- Seddon's coin test (tactile gnosis): this is our preferred test during patient examination
- two-point discrimination (Moberg's paperclip test; tactile gnosis)
- position sense (proprioception or body position movement recognition).

Spastic hemiplegic children with stereognosis defects prefer to use the normal hand. They use the affected hand only when necessary for bimanual activities and always as an assistant limb. When sensibility is not affected (mixed group), better function can be obtained and independent function of the affected hand can be expected after reconstructive surgery.

In patients with severe sensory impairment, with loss of touch and pain sensations and permanently flexed digits, any attempt at functional restoration through surgery is ineffective. This is the situation with some stroke patients.

Upper limb deformity (pronator–flexor spastic contracture)

The typical flexion–pronation deformity of the spastic upper limb in cerebral palsy is characterized by:

- shoulder: unusual and very mild internal rotation contracture
- elbow: flexion contracture
- forearm: pronation contracture

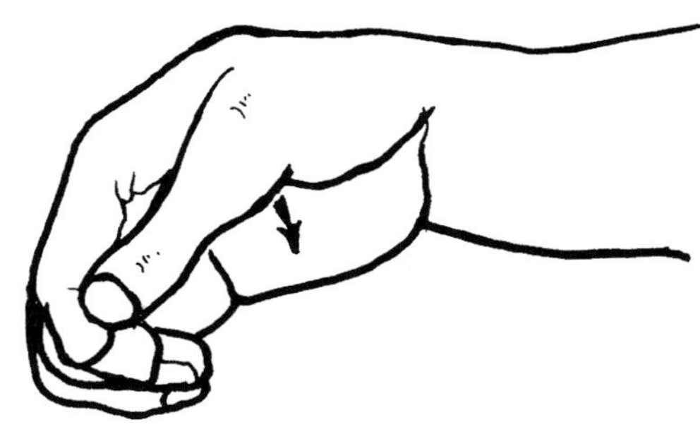

(A)

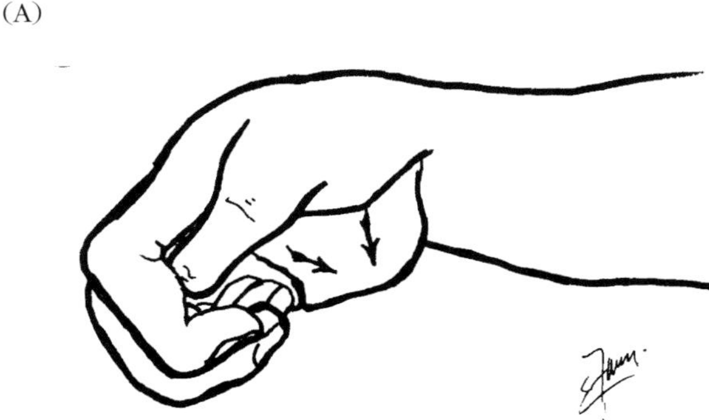

(B)

Figure 28.3

Spastic deformities of the thumb: (A) adduction; (B) flexion–adduction.

- hand:
  – wrist and fingers: flexion contracture of wrist and fingers, with occasional flexible swan-neck deformity (three groups) (Figure 28.1)
  – thumb: two types of deformities may be present: (1) adduction (adduction of the first metacarpal) and (2) flexion–adduction (thumb-in-palm deformity) (Figure 28.3).

All these deformities are variable in degree and reducibility by external manoeuvres.

Classification of hand deformity

Since our publications (Zancolli 1968, 1979, 1981, 1987), the spastic infantile hand has been classified into three groups. The classification is based on the voluntary ability of the patient to produce grasp and release patterns of the wrist and fingers (Figure 28.1). The surgical programme for the wrist and finger deformities is closely related to this classification.

Group 1

In this group flexion spasticity is minimal (Figure 28.1A). The patient can completely extend the fingers with a neutral position of the wrist or with <20° of wrist flexion. Spasticity is basically localized at the FCU muscle. The principal deficits in this group are the lack of complete active wrist dorsiflexion when the fingers are totally extended and the presence of thumb deformity (Zancolli and Zancolli 1987). The general appearance of the upper limb is satisfactory and the emotional influence on spasticity generally is usually mild or almost absent. Pronation spasticity of the forearm may be present.

Group 2 (Figure 28.1B)

In these patients, the fingers can also be actively extended (as in group 1), but only with >20° of wrist flexion. Spasticity is localized at the wrist and finger flexors. In severe cases of group 2 deformity the wrist needs to flex completely to permit complete or partial finger extension. Group 2 has two subgroups according to the functional condition of the extensor muscles of the wrist (2a and 2b). In subgroup 2a the patient can actively extend the wrist – partially or totally – with the fingers flexed. This means that the extensor muscles of the wrist are active and voluntarily controlled and that the main spasticity is localized in the flexor muscles of the fingers. In these cases, it is obviously unnecessary to perform tendon transfers to extend the wrist. In subgroup 2b the patient cannot actively extend the wrist with the finger flexed either because of flaccid paralysis of the wrist extensor muscles or because the flexor muscles are severely contracted. Tendon transfers to extend the wrist will be necessary in the cases with subgroup 2b deformity when the wrist extensors are paralysed.

Group 3 (Figure 28.1C)

Here the spasticity and deformity are very severe and localized at the flexor–pronator mass as in the other groups. The extensor muscles of the wrist and fingers are totally paralysed. The patient cannot extend the fingers even with maximal flexion of the wrist. Synergism is lost. This condition is the most difficult one to improve by reconstructive surgery. Release of all the spastic muscles of the upper limb is the only possibility in this group of patients.

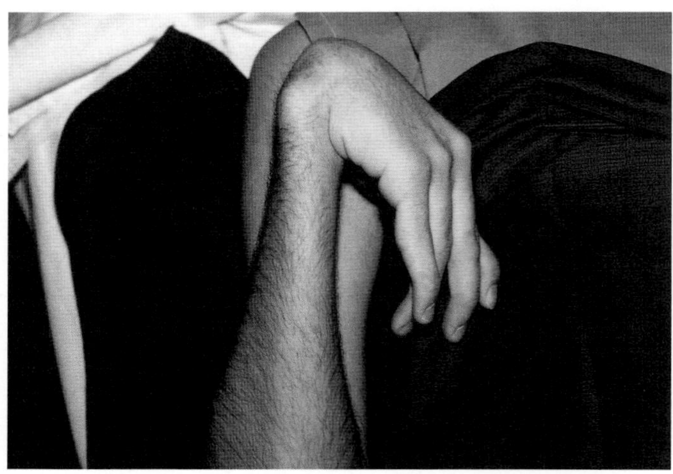

(A)

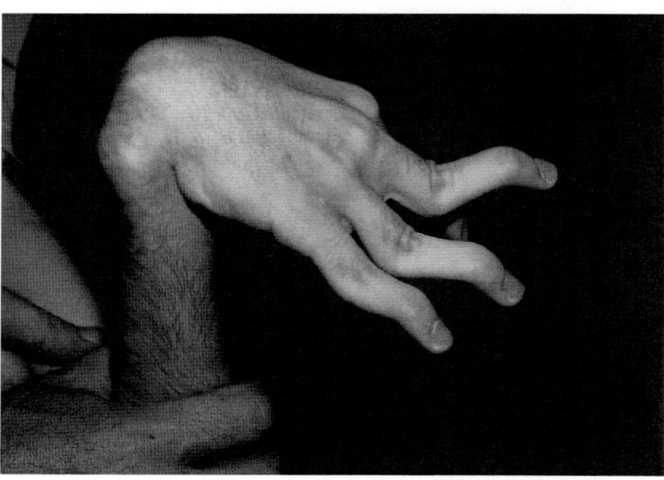

(B)

Figure 28.4

(A) Group 2b of hand spasticity. (B) During active finger extension the fingers' PIP joints hyperextended (swan-neck deformity of extrinsic type).

These three groups usually may be associated with: thumb contracture, elbow flexion contracture and pronation contracture of the forearm of variable degrees of severity. The degree of sensory impairment may vary from one group to another.

Swan-neck deformities may be present in all groups, but particularly in group 2 (Figure 28.4). These finger deformities reduce substantially after the flexion contracture of the wrist is corrected.

Surgical goals

The principal goals in surgical reconstruction of the spastic hand are directed to improve grasp and release patterns (between the wrist and digits), hand appearance and the psychological status of the patient and their family.

Prognosis

According to the classification described previously, basic hand functions in grasp (release and pinch functions) can be significantly improved in groups 1 and 2. In these cases it is possible to obtain: improved finger release with decreased flexion of the wrist; decreased flexion contracture of the elbow, wrist and fingers; decreased forearm pronation contracture and correction of thumb deformity to improve gripping and lateral pinch.

The main concept in surgical reconstruction of the spastic hand is that an improvement in the existing pattern of function can be achieved by improving the balance between the spastic pronator and flexor muscles and the normal or paretic-paralysed extensor and supinator muscles. Attempts to modify radically the existing patterns of activity (synergism) or overcorrection will usually produce a poor result. Only in very mild spasticity (group 1) is it possible to obtain normal complete and simultaneous extension of the wrist and fingers.

In group 3, surgery is indicated primarily to improve appearance, hygiene and comfort. This can be achieved by reducing the spasticity of the flexor–pronator muscles without, however, obtaining an acceptable voluntary hand release.

Adults and older patients with hemiplegia (of vascular origin) do not adapt well to hand reconstruction, because voluntary control of the wrist and fingers is usually absent. These patients generally cannot voluntarily flex the wrist to open the fingers, and consequently the digits are permanently closed and the hand is useless.

Surgical indications

According to the preoperative evaluations studied, the best candidates for reconstructive surgery are those with the following characteristics:

1. Spastic type of neuromuscular disorder.
2. Sufficient mental condition and emotional stability.
3. Low emotional influence on spasticity.
4. Infantile hemiplegia (especially perinatal).
5. Young patients (infantile or adolescent), ideally after 6–7 years of age, as training is more effective at this stage.
6. Basic sensibility, even with some impairment of proprioception and tactile gnosia.
7. Some voluntary control of the spastic muscles and voluntary ability to open the fingers in flexion (preserved synergism) (groups 1 and 2).

   It is important for the patient and the surgeon to have some type of voluntary control of the spastic muscles, and some voluntary ability to release and close the fingers for satisfactory results to be achieved through reconstructive surgery. Experience has shown that the most favourable cases for surgery are those in which it is possible to open the fingers by active flexion of the wrist. For this reason wrist arthrodesis should not be a primary option in typical spastic infantile hemiplegia, if the patient has the ability to extend the fingers through wrist flexion. Synergism between wrist and fingers should be preserved whenever possible. We only consider wrist fusion in atypical spastic conditions – residual deformities of failed previous operations – where tendon transfers or other soft tissue procedures are impossible to perform or are contraindicated, in reoperations and in some extrapyramidal neuromuscular disorders (Zancolli 1968) (Figure 28.5).
8. Capacity to concentrate and cooperate during the postoperative period.
9. Good motivation and family support.
10. Adequate behavioural patterns.
11. Good general neurological condition.

Spastic flexion–pronation deformity of the upper limb is the most adapted condition to indicate peripheral surgical reconstructive procedures. The surgical programme will depend on the severity and the type of deformity at the different levels of the upper limb.

The most common deformities that are corrected by reconstructive surgery are thumb deformities, flexion contracture of the wrist and fingers, flexion contracture of the elbow and pronation contracture of the forearm. In some cases swan-neck deformities of the fingers need to be corrected.

Surgery of the thumb is indicated to hold the digit out of the palm during grasp. The surgical procedures indicated depend on the type of deformity present; i.e. adduction or adduction–flexion contractures (thumb-in-palm deformity) (see Figure 28.3).

Flexion contracture of the elbow is common in the spastic upper limb and is frequently influenced by emotional stimuli. Correction of marked flexion contracture of the elbow improves the appearance and function of the hand.

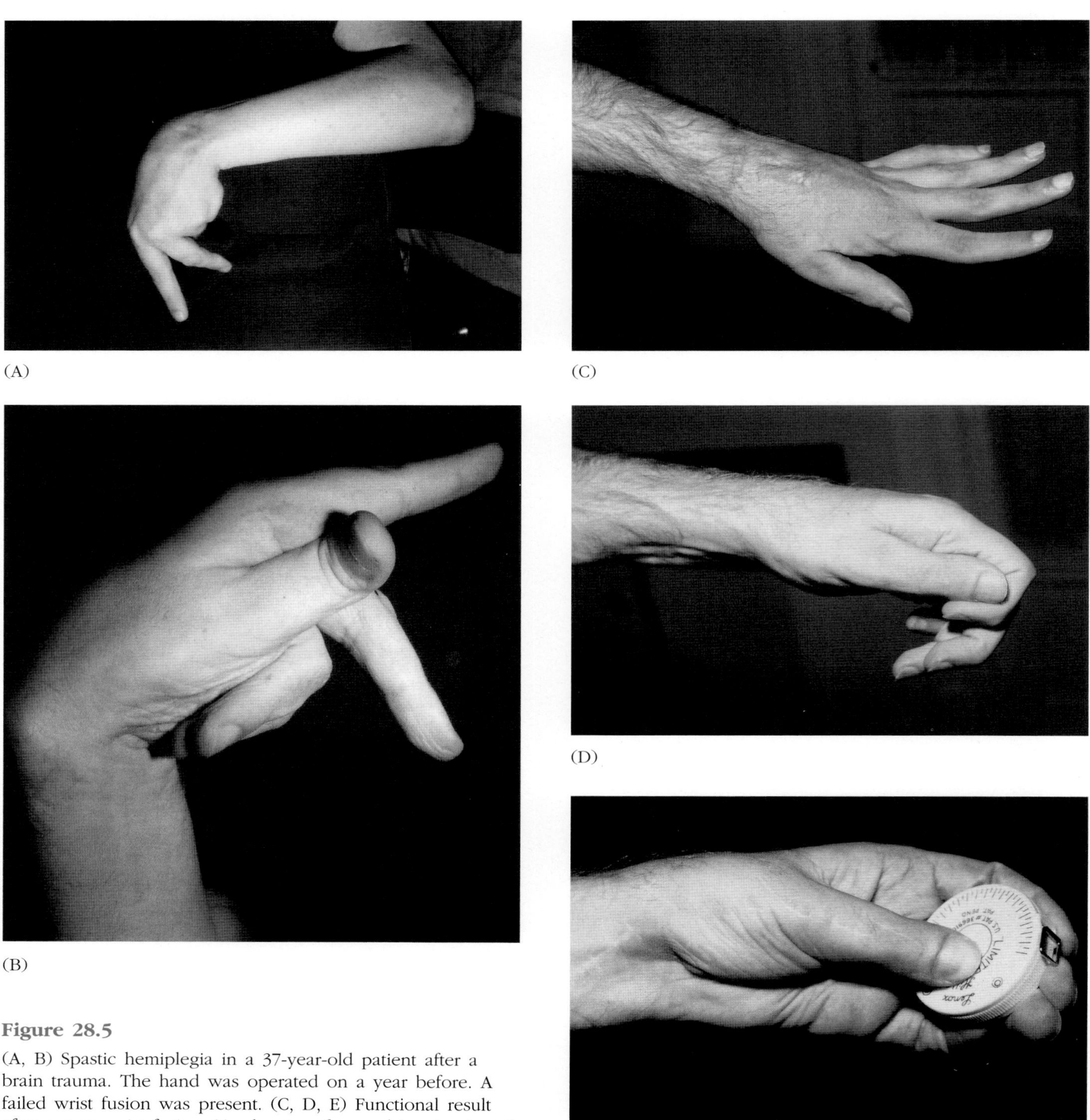

(A) (C) (D) (B) (E)

Figure 28.5

(A, B) Spastic hemiplegia in a 37-year-old patient after a brain trauma. The hand was operated on a year before. A failed wrist fusion was present. (C, D, E) Functional result after a new wrist fusion. Tendon transfers and tenotomies of the spastic muscles were performed.

Pronation contracture of the forearm is corrected when severe and when the patient has difficulty carrying out activities of daily living due to lack of supination. A mildly pronated forearm is a relatively useful position for hand function and its correction is not essential.

Flexion contracture of the wrist and fingers is corrected through surgical techniques based on the classification of hand deformity groups (1, 2 and 3). This indicates that during the preoperative examination it is of great importance to note the degree of wrist flexion needed to enable the patient to extend the fingers completely or partially. It is also important to note if the wrist can be extended with the fingers flexed (subgroups 2a or 2b). These tests demonstrate the degree of spastic-

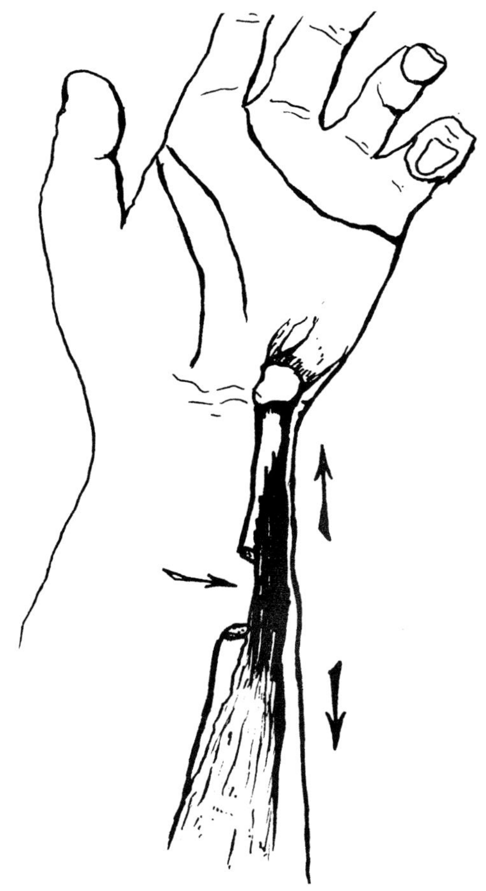

Figure 28.6
Flexor carpi ulnaris lengthening. Muscular continuity is preserved after excising part of the tendon. Indicated in mild spastic hand deformities (group 1).

ity of the flexor muscles of the wrist and fingers, the functional condition of the wrist extensors and the degree of voluntary control. This information is needed to correct the deformity, and the evaluation allows selection of the patient and the most appropiate surgical procedure for each patient.

It is of paramount importance to correct all the existing deformities of the upper limb (elbow, forearm and hand) at the same surgical procedure. A contracted thumb must be simultaneously corrected with the rest of the hand to allow better active extension of the fingers and lateral pinch grip.

Severe swan-neck deformities should be corrected in a secondary surgical stage. Severe spastic equinus foot should preferably be corrected before hand surgery with the aim to diminish diffusion of reflexes, to help with postoperative rehabilitation of the hand.

Surgical treatment

Surgical procedures which are usually indicated in the spastic hand due to cerebral palsy include: muscle release, tenotomy, fasciotomy, tendon lengthening, tendon transfer, capsuloplasty, tenodesis, arthrodesis, osteotomy and neurotomies. The selection of the procedure depends basically on the type and severity of the deformity, the type of neuromuscular disorder, the functional deficiencies, the age of the patient and the surgeon's preference. The following section will be confined to the author's preferred operative techniques.

Operative techniques

Flexion contracture of the wrist and fingers

This deformity basically results from the spasticity and occasional myostatic contracture of the flexor muscles of the wrist and fingers. The goal of surgery is to improve the opening of the hand without affecting voluntary closure of the digits and grasping functions. This is achieved by re-establishing the balance between the flexor and extensor muscles of the wrist and digits.

According to the grouping of hand deformities, our surgical programme to correct flexion contracture of the wrist and fingers is as follows.

Group 1

As already noted, the principal muscular co-contraction is located in the FCU. Our aim is to lengthen the FCU through a tenotomy in continuity. In this type of tenotomy the tendinous part is sectioned or partially excised, while preserving the continuity of the muscular fibres. After the release a passive stretching manoeuvre permits lengthening of the muscular unit. Tenotomy is located proximally to the distal end of the muscular belly (Figure 28.6).

If the wrist and finger flexor muscles and the pronator teres are spastic an aponeurotic release of the medial epicondyle muscles is added. This release is located 5 cm distally to the medial epicondyle. This technique is enough to release flexion contractures of the wrist and fingers in this group of patients. It is described in the technique described in group 2 of the spastic flexion-pronation deformity.

The treatment of the thumb deformity and occasional elbow flexion spasticity are described in subgroup 2b.

Group 2

Surgical technique in group 2 of flexion contracture of the fingers and wrist depends on their spasticity and the

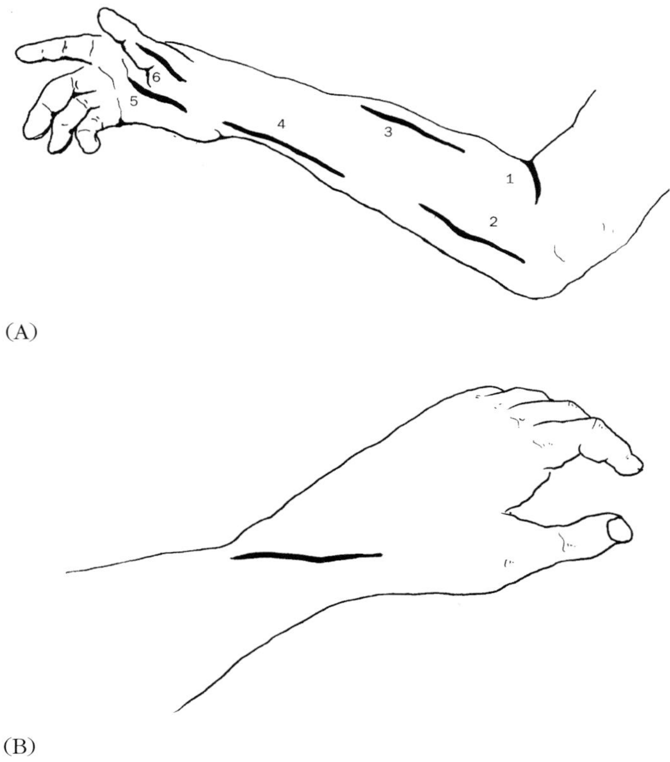

Figure 28.7

Incisions in group 2b. (A) 1, biceps release; 2, medial epicondyle aponeurotomy; 3, pronator teres approach (release of supination transfer); 4, flexor carpi ulnaris approach (transference to extensor carpi radialis brevis (ECRB) through the interosseous membrane); 5, adductor pollicis release; 6, metacarpophalangeal stabilization (sesamoid–metacarpal fusion). (B) Approach to ECRB tendon and extensor tendons of the thumb.

functional condition of the wrist extensor muscles (subgroups 2a and 2b).

Correction of spastic wrist and finger muscles is obtained by our technique of medial epicondyle aponeurotic release (Zancolli 1968, 1979). In subgroup 2b we advocate a tendon transfer to the paretic or paralytic extensor muscles of the wrist. Correction of spasticity producing flexion contracture of the elbow, pronation of the forearm and thumb deformities are treated separately.

Aponeurotic release of the medial epicondyle muscles

This is a very effective technique in cases with mild and median spasticity of wrist and finger flexor muscles. In this procedure spasticity is reduced because all the deep aponeurotic attachments of the medial epicondyle muscles are released at the proximal third of the forearm. The muscular fibres are left intact. Mild and median spastic cases are those in which preoperative voluntary finger extension is obtained with <70° of active wrist flexion (Figures 28.7 and 28.8).

In cases of severe spasticity or myostatic contracture of the wrist and finger muscles, where finger extension is only possible with >70° of wrist flexion, we add tendon release through selective tenotomies (preserving muscle continuity) of some retracted muscles (flexor digitorum superficialis and profundus and flexor carpi radialis).

This complementary release is located distally to the proximal aponeurotic release, approximately at the level of the musculotendinous functions in the middle of the forearm. Myostatic contracture is recognized under anaesthesia, where a passive extension manoeuvre is unable to obtain complete and simultaneous extension of the wrist and fingers.

In the aponeurotic release of the medial epicondyle muscles a transverse excision of the superficial fascia is made around the whole muscular mass. This is followed by a complete excision of all the septa that separate the muscles. Each septum is followed up to its deep end where the median and ulnar nerves covered by the muscles can be seen. The muscular bellies are left intact, particularly the FCU if this muscle is to be transferred to the extensor tendons of the wrist (subgroup 2b).

We do not advocate the classical muscular slide technique as described by Page (1923) (see also Inglis and Cooper 1966, White 1972). Using this technique it is difficult to calculate the degree of muscular release and consequently overcorrection could be the result, causing the fingers to lose flexion and grasp abilities. Another possible complication of an excessive muscular slide procedure is the loss of vascularization of the medial epicondyle muscular mass.

Tendon transfer of flexor carpi ulnaris to extensor carpi radialis brevis

This technique is indicated only when active wrist extensors are very weak or completely paralysed (subgroup 2b). Obviously it is not indicated in subgroup 2a, where active wrist extension is present (see Figure 28.1) In the classic Green's procedure (Green 1942, Green and Banks 1962), the FCU tendon is passed around the ulnar border of the wrist and is fixed to the extensor carpi radialis brevis tendon, as it is the major dorsiflexor of the hand. The goal is to obtain wrist extension and supination of the forearm. The other wrist flexors – flexor carpi radialis and palmaris longus – must remain in place to avoid undesirable permanent wrist hyperextension postoperatively.

The author has modified this procedure, preferring to pass the FCU through an ample window in the interosseus membrane (proximally to the pronator teres) and suture it to the extensor carpi radialis brevis tendon (see Figure 28.8). The tension of the transfer is calculated during surgery and is considered to be correct when the wrist maintains 20° of extension under the effect of gravity.

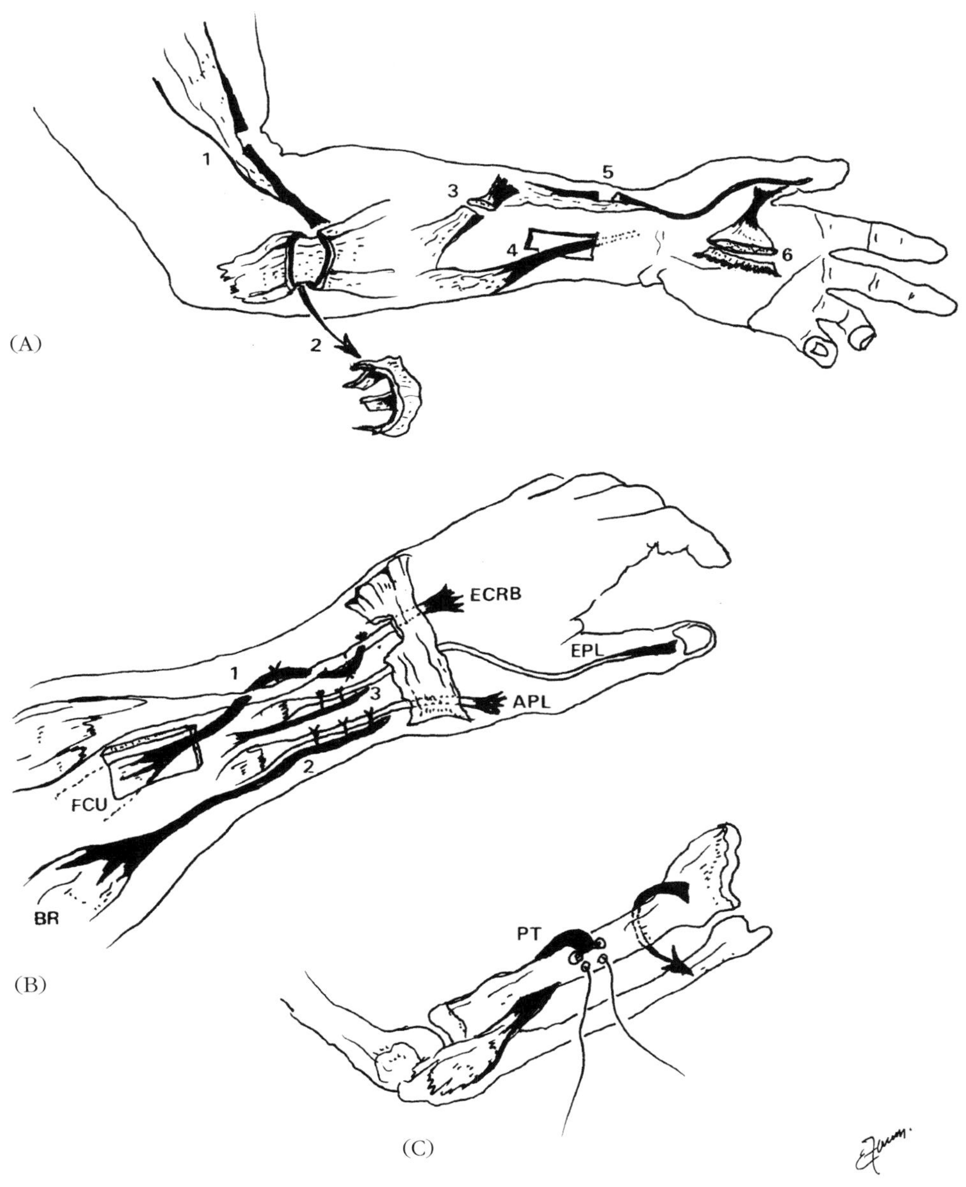

Figure 28.8

Surgical programme in subgroup 2b of spastic hand with thumb-in-palm deformity in a single surgical stage. (A) 1, Biceps lengthening in continuity; 2, excision of superficialis fascia and septae of medial epicondyle muscles; 3, pronator teres (PT) release in mild pronation contracture (pronator quadratus remains active); 4, transference of flexor carpi ulnaris (FCU) through the interosseous membrane to extensor carpi radialis brevis (ECRB); 5, lengthening in continuity of flexor pollicis longus (FPL) (avoid too much relaxation); 6, proximal adductor pollicis release. (B) 1, Transference of FCU to ECRB (partial excision of extensor retinaculum); 2, tranference of brachioradialis (BR) to abductor pollicis longus (APL); 3, transference – palmaris longus – to extensor pollicis longus (EPL) (too much tension should be avoided). Balance needs to be maintained between the lengthened FPL and the transferred EPL. Stabilization of the metacarpophalangeal joint of the thumb is frequently indicated to prevent MCP joint hyperextension. In cases with adduction contracture of the thumb the FPL tendon is left unreleased and the EPL is translocated radially. (C) Transference of pronator teres (PT) through the interosseous membrane to obtain forearm supination (volar view).

Group 3

In this group there is a permanent flexion contracture of the wrist and fingers, particularly under emotional stimuli, and it is impossible to open the hand voluntarily. The extensor muscles of the wrist and fingers are paralysed. These patients do have any kind of release and grasp pattern. Sensory function is usually seriously affected. Myostatic contracture is very frequent due to the severity of the spasticity and permanent flexed position of the hand.

The best indication for these patients is to obtain a release of all the upper limb flexed joints: elbow, forearm, wrist, fingers and thumb. This is accomplished by multiple tenotomies (with muscular continuity) of all the contracted muscles.

If the tenotomies are insufficient because of the severity of spasticity or myostatic contracture of the finger flexor muscles, then we advocate a technique that was described in 1957 (Zancolli 1957). The procedure consists in sectioning the flexor superficialis tendons distally, near the wrist, and the flexor digitorum profundus tendons are sectioned proximally at the mid-forearm level. The fingers are then extended to a median flexed position, and while maintained in this position, the proximal ends of the flexor superficialis tendons are sutured to the distal ends of the flexor digitorum profundus tendons with latero-lateral tenorraphies. The flexor tendons of the wrist are 'Z' lengthened. We initially advocated use of this procedure to correct pronounced flexion contractures of the wrist and fingers in severe segmentary arthrogryposis, but this technique can also be indicated in very severe group 3 cases of spastic hand in cerebral palsy. Braun et al described a similar procedure in 1974.

Flexion contracture of the elbow

Flexion contracture of the elbow is a common finding in the spastic upper limb and is frequently influenced by emotional stimuli. Correction of marked flexion contracture of the elbow improves the appearance and function of the upper limb. Flexor muscle origin release or aponeurotic release of the medial epicondyle muscles usually produces a partial correction of the deformity. Additional correction is obtained by tenotomy in continuity or 'Z' lengthening of the biceps tendon (Figure 28.8). Occasionally the lacertus fibrosus may be sectioned.

Pronation contracture of the forearm

Mild cases of forearm pronation spasticity which reduce passively preoperatively are improved by simple division of the distal tendon of the pronator teres (see Figure 28.8). In severe contractures the distal tendon of the pronator teres is rerouted around the radius through the interosseous membrane (procedure of Tubby, see Vulpius and Stoffel 1920) (Figure 28.8).

The distal end of the ulna was dorsally dislocated in three adolescent patients who had severe and fixed pronation contracture. In these cases it was necessary to perform complete release of the contracted interosseous membrane, the excision of the ulnar head and a distal radio-ulnar fusion. This technique fixes the forearm in 10° of pronation, which is a useful functional position for the hand.

Thumb deformities

Surgery is indicated to hold the thumb out of the palm during grasp and to permit lateral pinch. The surgical technique depends on the type of deformity: adduction or adduction flexion contracture (Figure 28.3) (Zancolli 1979, Zancolli and Zancolli 1981).

Adduction contracture

The adduction contracture of the thumb basically depends on spasticity of the adductor pollicis muscle. There is adduction contracture of the first metacarpal, but the metacarpophalangeal and interphalangeal joints are not flexed. Correction is obtained by a proximal release of the adductor pollicis muscle and reinforcement of the abductor pollicis longus.

This is obtained by sectioning its origin from the third metacarpal through a palmar incision, parallel to the proximal palmar crease (Matev 1963) (Figure 28.8A).

It is not necessary to release the origin of the lateral thenar muscles in a pure or predominant spastic thumb deformity. There is no spasticity of the lateral thenar muscles in a pure spastic neuromuscular disorder; this only occurs in athetoid or other extrapyramidal hands.

Reinforcement of the abductor pollicis longus is usually accomplished by transfer of the brachioradialis (McCue et al 1970) or by tendon plication (Matev 1963) or tenodesis of the abductor pollicis longus. In the latter, the proximal end of the abductor pollicis longus is fixed around the distal tendon of the brachioradialis. The best results are obtained by tendon transfers.

Adduction–flexion contracture (thumb-in-palm deformity)

The main deforming forces depend on the spasticity of the adductor pollicis and flexor pollicis longus muscles (Keats 1964). The most frequently used reconstructive procedures are: (1) release of the origin of the adductor pollicis from the third metacarpal; (2) lengthening of the flexor pollicis longus at its musculotendinous junction in the forearm, preserving the muscular continuity; (3) translocation of the extensor pollicis longus toward the radial aspect of the wrist; (4) reinforcement of the abductor pollicis longus and extensor pollicis longus by tendon transfers (motors: brachioradialis, palmaris longus, etc.).

It is very important to maintain some function of the flexor pollicis longus; overcorrection should be avoided.

When reinforcement of the extensor pollicis longus is indicated, but spasticity of the flexor pollicis longus is mild, the latter tendon is not lengthened. Stabilization of the metacarpophalangeal joint of the thumb, through fusion or capsuloplasty, is indicated when the joint is hypermobile in hyperextension (>2°). In arthrodesis in children, damage to the epiphyseal line can be avoided by the use of thin fixation pins. Metacarpophalangeal joint fusion alone, without proper release of flexion and adduction spasticity and without reinforcement of the extensor muscles, will not in itself eliminate the thumb-in-palm deformity.

Metacarpophalangeal capsuloplasty (Zancolli 1968, 1979, Filler et al 1976), is an excellent procedure for correction of hyperextension deformity of the joint. To accomplish a good joint stabilization the radial sesamoid is fixed to the neck of the first metacarpal in 10° of flexion (sesamoid–metacarpal synostosis) (Figure 28.9). General postoperative care includes immobilization for 5 weeks.

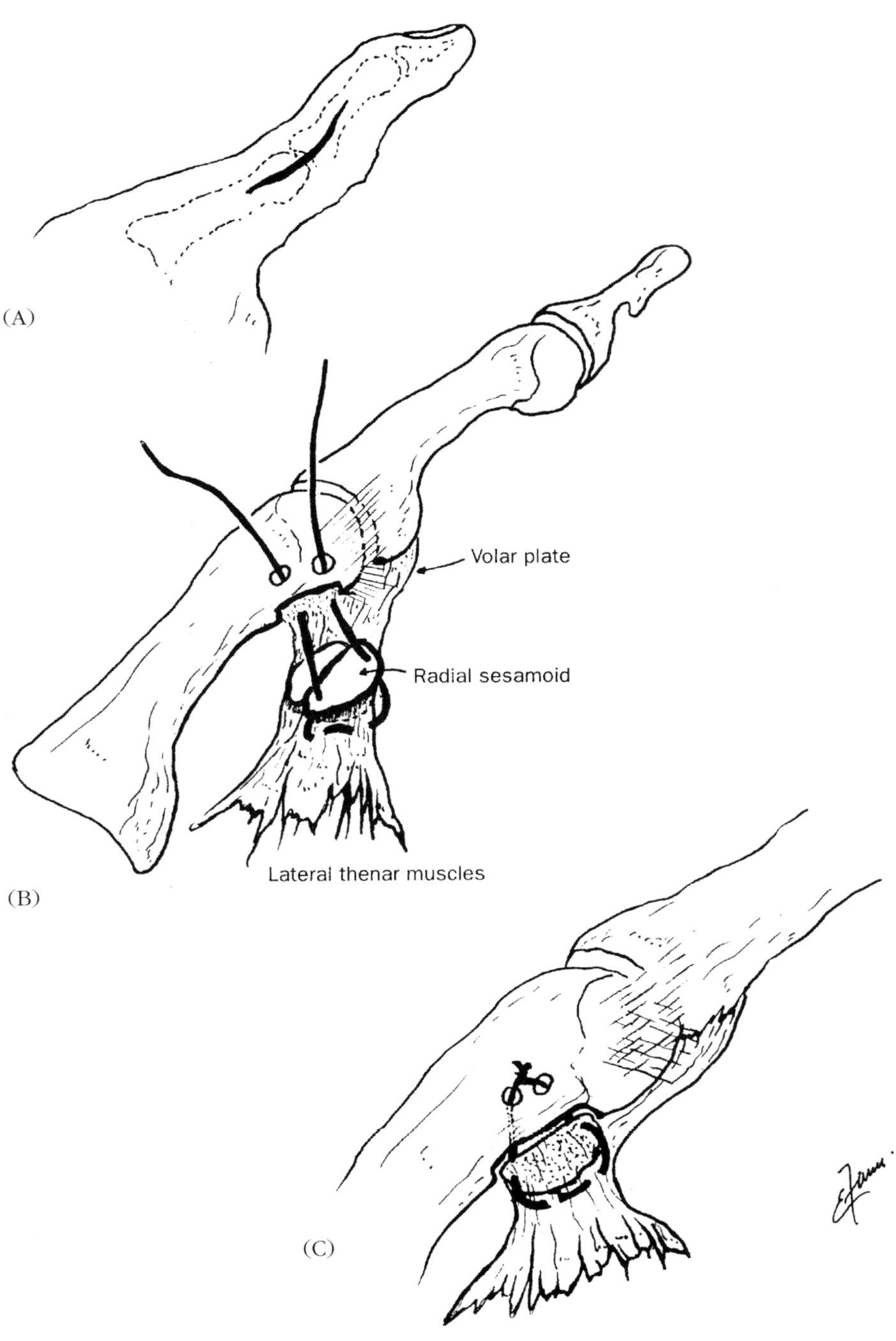

Figure 28.9

(A) Metacarpophalangeal hyperextension of the thumb. Radial side incision. (B) Sesamoid–metacarpal stabilization (synostosis). A strong suture fixes the radial sesamoid to the metacarpal neck. Sesamoid cartilage and cortical bone of the metacarpal neck are partially excised. (C) Sesamoid–metacarpal fusion with 5° of joint flexion.

Swan-neck deformity

Swan-neck deformity is relatively common in the hands of patients with cerebral palsy (Swanson 1960, 1982). This deformity depends on the effect of a permanent and pronounced flexed position of the wrist and the pull of the long extensor tendons during the patient's efforts to open the hand (Figure 28.4). These conditions are particularly present in group 2 of spastic flexion–pronation deformity. Under these functional conditions a progressive stretching of the finger's PIP joint volar plate is produced, associated with a flexion deformity of the DIP joint (dysfunction of the extensor apparatus). The finger's deformity frequently locks in extension, and the ability and force of pinch and grasp are impaired.

When the fingers show permanent and severe deformity after the release of the flexion spasticity of the wrist and fingers, a surgical correction of the finger deformity is indicated in a second surgical stage. This is a relatively uncommon indication in spastic cerebral palsy patients (Filler et al 1976).

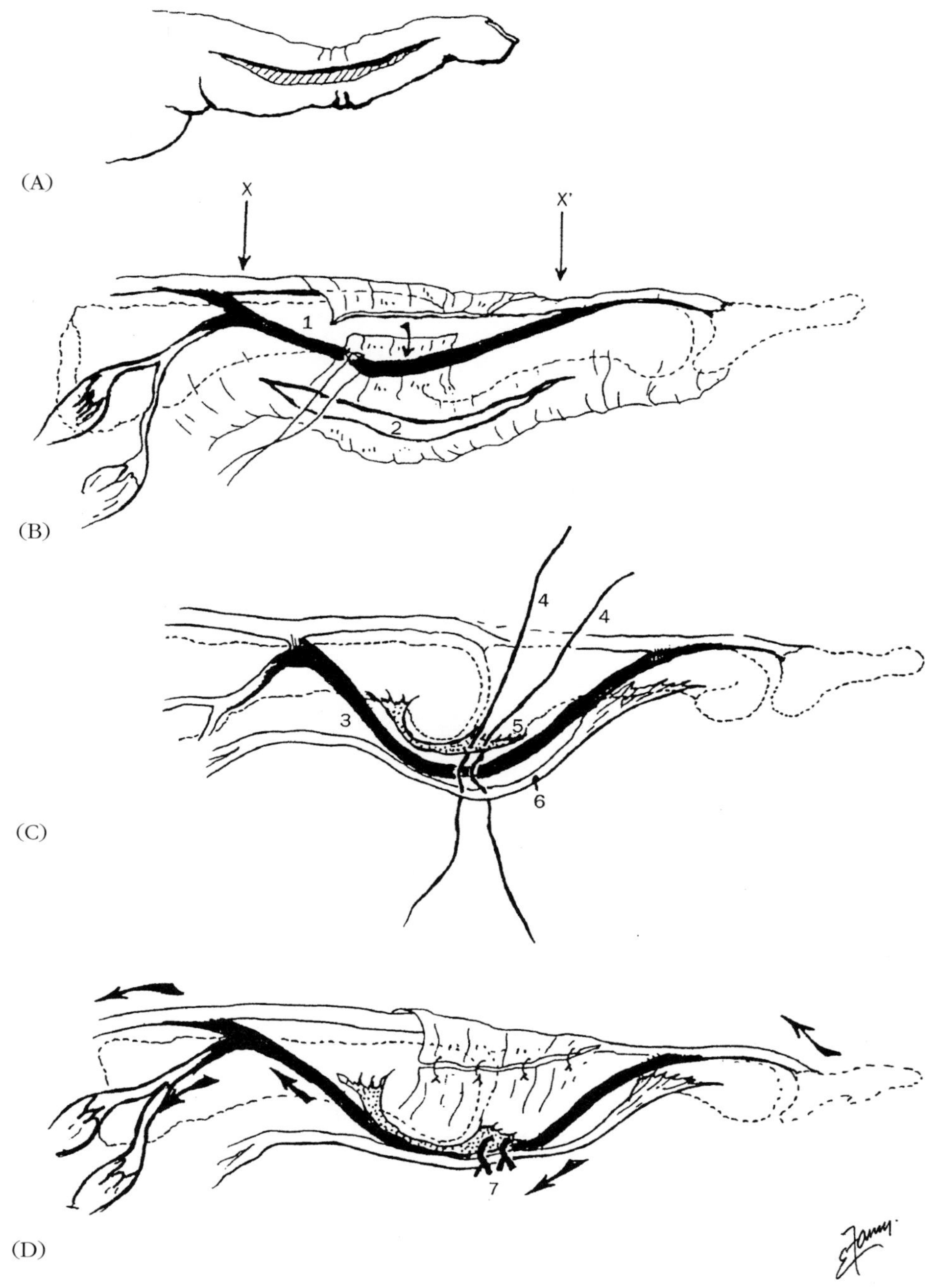

Figure 28.10

Correction of a flexible swan-neck deformity (Zancolli's technique). (A) Midlateral longitudinal incision on the radial side of the finger. (B) The lateral band (1) is dissected between the middle and the proximal phalanges. The proximal end of the dissected band is maintained in continuity with the lateral slip of the extensor tendon and the intrinsic tendons. The flexor tendon sheath is opened at the proximal interphalangeal (PIP) joint level (2). (C) The dissected lateral band (3) is translocated to the volar part of the finger and placed between the volar plate (5) and the flexor superficialis tendon (6). Two strong stitches (4) join the volar plate to the border of the chiasma of Camper, distally to the PIP joint level. These sutures maintain the lateral band volarly to the joint. (D) After the procedure, the finger must extend passively or actively – when local anesthesia is used – up to the neutral extension. The suture of the volar plate to the flexor superficialis represents a pulley for the transferred lateral band (7). During active finger extension the transferred band produces a simultaneous active stabilization of the PIP joint and an extension of the distal interphalangeal (DIP) joint. The lateral band in its new position is relatively shortened. In time the normal use of the finger will produce a relocation of the opposite lateral band to its normal position.

It is a frequent observation that swan-neck deformities improve spontaneously with correction of flexion contracture of the wrist, because this decreases the traction of the digital extensor tendons over the middle phalanx. In severe deformities correction is obtained by a procedure the author called the 'sling' operation (Zancolli 1975, 1982, 1986, 1991).

The procedure consists of the translocation of the radial side lateral band of the extensor apparatus into the flexor tendon sheath. The deformity and the incision are shown in Figure 28.10. The first step of the operation consists of freeing the extrinsic lateral extensor band of the affected fingers (radial side) between the middle third of the proximal phalanx and the middle third of the middle phalanx. The distal end of this tendinous sling remains attached to the extensor apparatus, and the proximal end continues the central extrinsic extensor tendon and the intrinsic muscles (radial interosseous and lumbrical). The second step consists of opening and exposing the fibrous sheath of the flexor tendons at the PIP joint level. In a third step the lateral band is rerouted volar to the joint, and introduced between the volar plate and the flexor superficialis tendon (Camper's chiasma). The lateral band is maintained in this position by two strong separate sutures (with the finger in 5° of PIP flexion) that unite the lateral border of the tendinous chiasma to the volar plate. These sutures are located distally to the PIP joint level at the base of the middle phalanx. The tendon sheath is closed. If the tension of the tendinous sling is correct the finger extends passively up to 5° of PIP flexion. If PIP flexion is greater (>5°) then the freeing of the lateral band is enlarged at its proximal and distal ends to reach the desired PIP position. If on the contrary there is some tendency to PIP joint recurvatum, stitches are applied at either end to tighten the sling. Flexion >5° of the PIP joint may produce a boutonnière deformity.

This technique represents the reconstruction of an active retinacular ligament. The activation of the tendinous sling by the action of the extensor tendons and the intrinsic muscles produces complete finger extension and corrects the hyperextension of the PIP joint.

The finger is immobilized in slight flexion for 1 week before active exercises begin. The results of this procedure have been very encouraging; however, the procedure cannot be used in cases with intrinsic paralysis.

Assessment of hand motor function

Grouping of the patients for results of surgery is obtained by precise examination of the upper limb functions (Zancolli and Zancolli 1987).

1. Study of the ability to open the hand. This is evaluated using wooden discs of different sizes (6, 8, 10, 12, 14, 16 and 18 cm), determining hand placement over the table; and measuring the degrees of wrist flexion that will enable the patient to extend the fingers.
2. Grasp and pinch patterns. The ability to grasp is evaluated through the use of spherical balls of 5, 8, 10 and 12 cm, and cylinders of 3, 5, 8, 10 and 12 cm. Tip pulp, lateral pinches and chuck three-digit pinch are examined during manipulation of different objects.
3. Speed, skill, voluntary control and coordination for prehension are functions examined by the pick-up test and by manipulating objects. Manipulation of toys by children can help the surgeon to make decisions on the indications for reconstructive procedures with the aim of improving both function and cosmesis. Coordination between both hands is studied.

Other evaluations include:

1. Grasp and pinch strength. The grip strength is measured with a dynamometer. (A sphygmomanometer may be used to record grip strength in

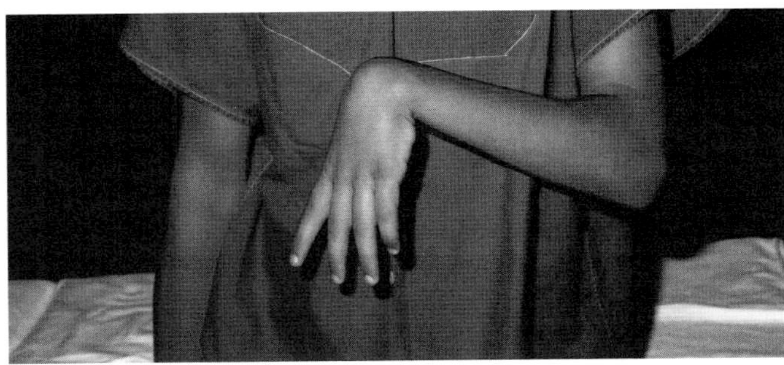

(A)

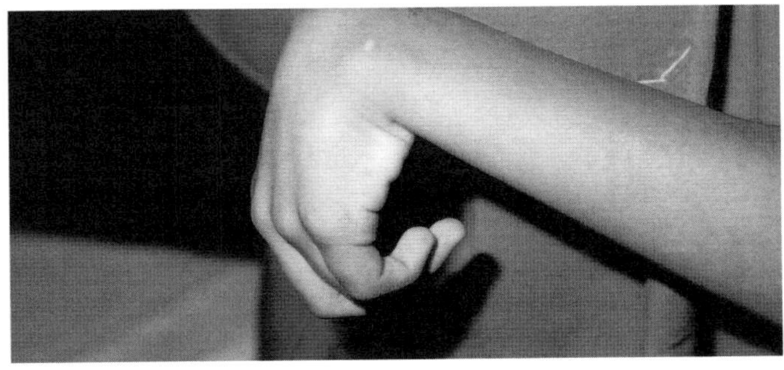

(B)

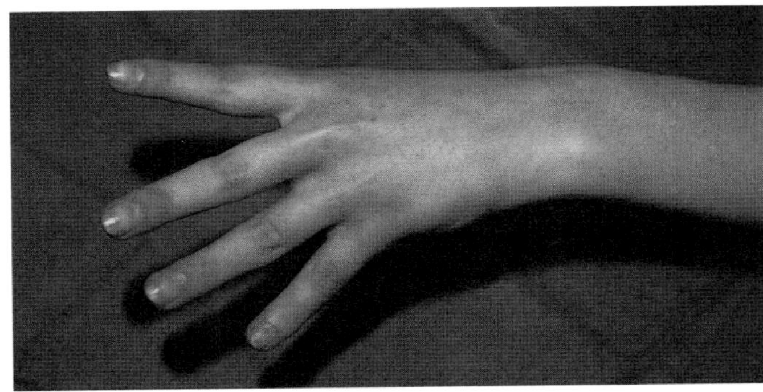

(C)

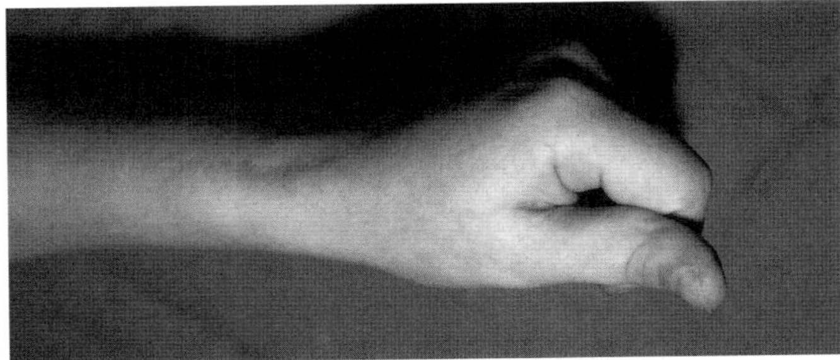

(D)

Figure 28.11

(A) Group 2b deformity of spastic hemiplegia in a 14-year-old boy. The fingers extend with 90° of wrist flexion. (B) Voluntary flexion of the fingers was present. Wrist extensors were paralysed. Thumb-in-palm deformity. (C) After surgical reconstruction (tenotomy of the spastic muscles and tendon transfers) the patient obtained simultaneous wrist and fingers extension. (D) Good lateral pinch and complete finger flexion were obtained. With better motor function the hand had improved sensory functions.

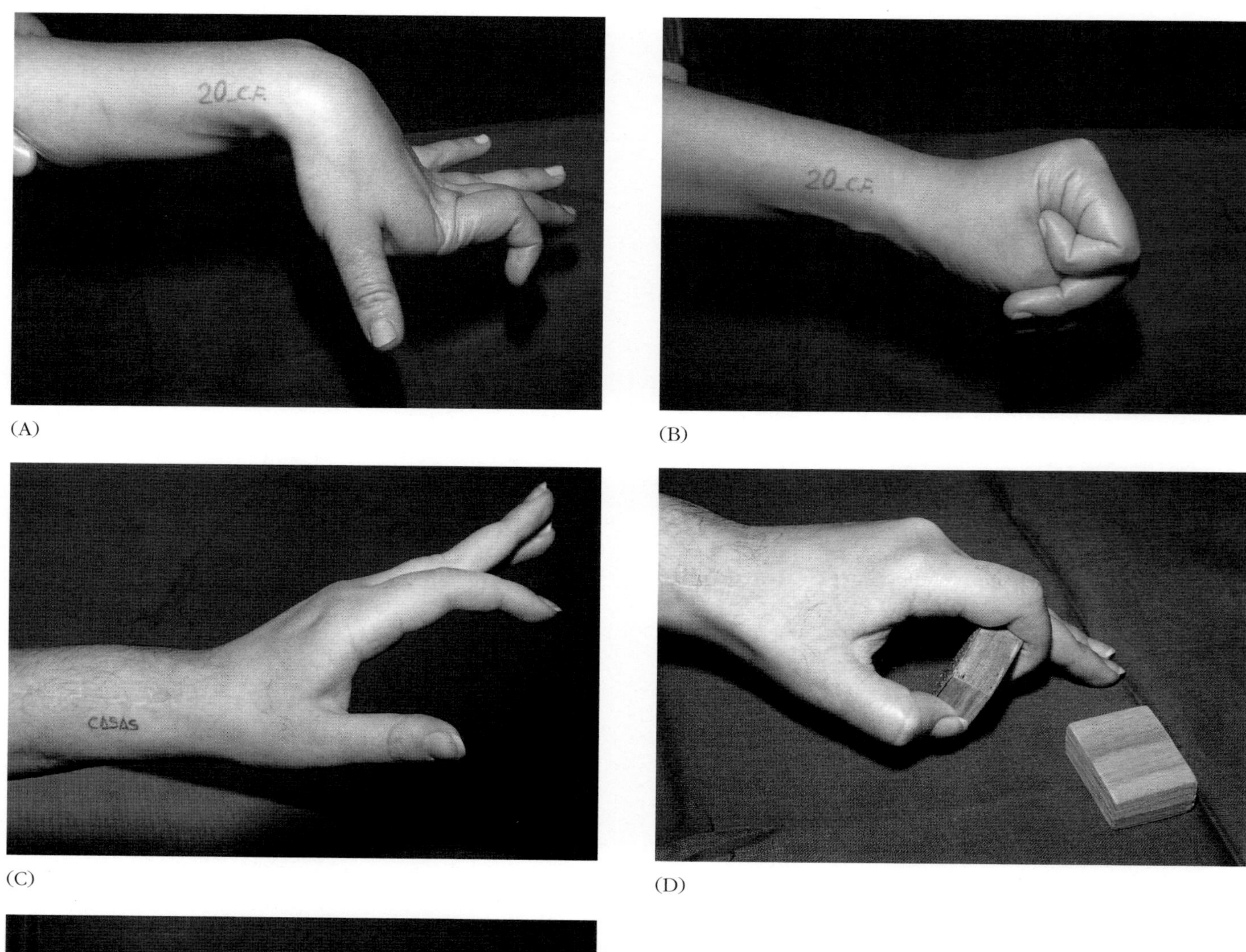

(A) (B) (C) (D) (E)

Figure 28.12

(A, B) Mixed neuromuscular disorder of the upper limb in an 18-year-old girl. Stretch reflex was overactive. Good voluntary control of movements and muscle hypertonicity were present. Group 2a hand deformity. The wrist extends when the fingers flex. Thumb-in-palm deformity. (C, D, E) Result after soft tissue surgical reconstruction. Good hand release, lateral pinch and thumb function were obtained.

weak hands.) A pinch meter is used to evaluate pinch strength.

2. Activities of daily living. These activities involve hygiene, dressing, writing and feeding.
3. Active and passive range of motion of all the upper limb joints: shoulder, elbow, forearm, wrist, fingers and thumb. The range of motion should be recorded on the principle that the neutral position equals 0° The patient is asked to straighten the fingers and to make a fist, to obtain a global idea of motion of all digits and to note limited motions or abnormal postures.

Results

Results after surgery can be classed as good, fair and poor as a basis for the assessment of hand function.

- Good:
  - complete digital extension with <20° of wrist flexion. In the best cases the wrist hyperextends with complete digital extension
  - complete elbow extension and almost complete forearm supination
  - good lateral pinch and grasping (thumb-in-palm deformity corrected)
  - good voluntary control of muscles.
- Fair:
  - complete digital extension with >20° of wrist flexion (reduced to the preoperative value)
  - partial elbow extension and forearm supination
  - weak and partial lateral pinch and grasping.
- Poor: hand function and deformities not improved with respect to the preoperative condition (passive hand).

We believe that good and fair results represent a very satisfactory improvement for this type of patients.

In the present author's surgical series (91 selected spastic patients) only 47 cases were evaluated in the final result (29 were females). The age at operation was over 7 years in the great majority of cases. According to the classification presented earlier, the number of patients was: group 1, 8 cases; group 2, 31 cases and group 3, 8 cases. The results were: group 1, 7 good and 1 poor; group 2, 19 good, 10 fair and 2 poor; group 3, 1 fair and 7 poor. The great majority of the patients in groups 1 and 2 felt that there was improvement in function and cosmesis of the hand (Figures 28.5, 28.11 and 28.12).

Three athetoid patients who had soft tissue procedures had a very poor result. The initial deformities were replaced by other deformities.

Conclusions

Selected patients with cerebral palsy can be helped by reconstructive surgery of the upper limb. The principal preoperative studies required for the selection of patients are: aetiology, general neurological conditions, type of neuromuscular disorder, topographic involvement, age, hand sensibility, type of deformity, patient motivation, cooperation, voluntary control of muscles, emotional influence on spastic muscle, and voluntary grasp and release patterns of the hand.

Although surgery cannot make a limb which was functionally poor into a perfect one, it can greatly improve the preoperative condition. Most poor surgical results are due to incorrect selection of patients or poor execution of the surgical procedures. The worst mistake is to perform soft tissue procedures – tendinous release or tendinous transfers – on patients with pure athetosis.

The surgical programme is organized according to the type and severity of the deformity (clinical groups).

The goal is to correct the deformities and to improve the muscular balance of the hand. It must be remembered that spastic muscle cannot be used for tendon transfer with the same efficiency as muscle in patients with a flaccid paralysis. Results were very satisfactory in 92% of all our patients in groups 1 and 2 and in 70% of all the patients in groups 1, 2 and 3.

References

Blumel I, Eggers GWN, Evans EB (1960) Genetic metabolic and clinical study on one hundred cerebral palsied patients, *JAMA* **174**: 860.

Braun RM, Guy TV, Roper B (1974) Preliminary experience wit)h superficialis-to-profundus on transfer in the hemiplegic upper extremity, *J Bone Joint Surg* **52A**: 466–72.

Filler BC, Stark HH, Boyes J (1976) Capsulodesis of metacarpophalangeal joint of the thumb in children with cerebral palsy, *J Bone Joint Surg* **58A**: 67–70.

Goldner JL (1955) Reconstructive surgery of the hand in cerebral palsy and spastic paralysis resulting from injury to the spinal cord, *J Bone Joint Surg* **37A**: 1141.

Goldner JL (1975) The upper extremity in cerebral palsy. In: Samilson RL, ed., *Orthopaedic Aspects of Cerebral Palsy* (Harper & Row: New York) 221–57.

Green WT (1942) Tendon transplantation of the flexor carpi ulnaris for pronation–flexion deformity of the wrist, *Surg Gynecol Obstet* **75**: 337–42.

Green WT, Banks HH (1962) Flexor carpi ulnaris transplant: its use in cerebral palsy, *J Bone Joint Surg* **44A**: 1343–52.

Inglis AE, Cooper W (1966) Release of the flexor pronator origin for flexion deformities of the hand and wrist in spastic paralysis, *J Bone Joint Surg* **48A**: 847–57.

Keats S (1964) Surgical treatment of the hand in cerebral palsy: correction of thumb-in-palm and other deformities, *J Bone Joint Surg* **47A**: 274.

McCue FC, Honner R, Chapman WC (1970) Transfer of the brachioradialis for hands deformed by cerebral palsy, *J Bone Joint Surg* **752A**: 1171–80.

Matev I (1963) Surgical treatment of the spastic 'thumb-in-palm' deformity, *J Bone Joint Surg* **45B**: 703–8.

Page CM (1923) An operation for the relief of flexion contracture in the forearm, *J Bone Joint Surg* **5A**: 233–4.

Samilsom SL, Morris JM (1964) Surgical improvement of the cerebral-palsied upper limb, *J Bone Joint Surg* **46A**: 1203–16.

Swanson AB (1960) Surgery of the hand in cerebral palsy and the swan-neck deformity, *J Bone Joint Surg* **42A**: 951–64.

Swanson AB (1968) Surgery of the hand in cerebral palsy and muscle origin release procedures, *Surg Clin North Am* **48**: 1129–38.

Swanson AB (1982) Surgery of the hand in cerebral palsy. In: Flynn YE, ed., *Hand Surgery*, 3rd edn (Williams & Wilkins: Baltimore) 476–88.

Twitchell TE (1966) Sensation and the motor deficit in cerebral palsy, *Clin Orthop* **46**: 55–62.

Vulpius O, Stoffel A (1920) *Orthopädisebe Operations Lebre* (Ferdinang Enke: Stuttgart).

White WF (1972) Flexor muscle slide in the spastic hand. The Max Page operation, *J Bone Joint Surg* **54B**: 453–9.

Zancolli EA (1957) Un nuevo método de corrección de las contrac-

turas congénitas de los músculos flexores digitales (alargamiento intetendinoso), *Prensa Méd Argentina* **44**: 279–8 1.
Zancolli EA (1968) *Structural and Dynamic Bases of Hand Surgery* (JB Lippincott: Philadelphia).
Zancolli EA (1975) *La Operación del "asa" en la Corrección de la Deformidad en "Cuello Cisne"*. 1st National Congress of the Spanish Society for Surgery of the Hand, 17–19 October 1975, Bilbao, Spain.
Zancolli EA (1979) *Structural and Dynamic Bases of the Hand Surgery*, 2nd edn (JB Lippincott: Philadelphia).
Zancolli EA (1982) *Management of Boutonniere and Swan-neck Deformities*, 25th Congress of the Japanese Society for Surgery of the Hand, 7–9 May 1982, Tokyo, Japan.
Zancolli EA (1986) *Panel on Soft Tissue Reconstruction in Rheumatoid Arthritis*. 41st Annual Meeting of the American Society for Surgery of the Hand, New Orleans.
Zancolli EA (1991) Surgical correction of flexible swan-neck deformity – volar translocation of the radial lateral band, *Curr Orthop* **51**: 230–2.
Zancolli EA, Zancolli ER (1987) Surgical rehabilitation of the spastic upper limb in cerebral palsy. In: *The Paralysed Hand* (Churchill Livingstone: New York) 153–8.
Zancolli EA, Zancolli ER (1981) Surgical management of the hemiplegic spastic hand in cerebral palsy, *Surg Clin North Am* **61**: 395–406.

29 Embryology and classification of the malformations

Toshihiko Ogino

Previous classification

Many statistical analyses of congenital hand deformities have appeared. However, it has been difficult to establish the true occurrence of these deformities and to compare one report with another, as the authors have used different classifications and the terminology is confusing. A standard classification and common terminology are needed, for discussion of congenital deformities. When congenital hand deformities are being diagnosed, giving the diagnostic term is equivalent to classifying the deformities. At the time of classifying the congenital deformities of the hand, some investigators think that they should be classified according to the finished form; and other think that, if at all possible, they should be classified according to the impairments occurring in pregnancy.

When babies with congenital hand deformities are seen, the observed form is used as the diagnostic name. The use of various Greek and Latin names to describe common deficiencies has only described an anomaly in another language. Using this method, diagnosis is easy. For example, the term syndactyly is used for accreted fingers, polydactyly for multiple fingers, macrodactyly for big fingers, and ectrodactyly for defective fingers. Taking ectrodactyly as an example, there are various types of ectrodactyly: those with constriction rings, those similar to amputation, those with dysplasia of the upper limb, and those with defects on the radial side or ulnar side of the upper limb. These deformities of digits are labeled as ectrodactyly, although the causes are divergent.

Numerous attempts have been made to classify ectrodactyly according to the genetic causes. Swanson et al (1968) reported a classification of congenital hand deformities based on the concept of embryological failure. Since then, modifications of this classification have been made, and this classification was adopted by the International Federation of Societies for Surgery of the Hand (Swanson 1976, Swanson et al 1983). In this classification, there are seven categories as follows: category 1, failure of formation of parts; category 2, failure of differentiation of parts; category 3, duplication; category 4, overgrowth; category 5, undergrowth; category 6, congenital constriction band syndrome; and category 7, generalized skeletal abnormalities. This classification has been used widely; however, it has some limitations. The biggest limitation occurs in the classification of ectrodactyly. To have a better understanding of the classification, it is necessary to clarify the normal and abnormal development of the hand.

Normal development of the hand

Limb bud

The development of the hand starts with the formation of the limb bud. The limb bud arises as an elevation of the ventrolateral side of the body wall and is covered by ectoderm; inside the bud there are evenly distributed pure mesenchymal cells (Figure 29.1A). On the tip of the limb bud, there is a confined thick ectoderm called the apical ectodermal ridge (AER). The signaling molecules from the AER regulate limb development by influencing cells in the mesoderm at the distal tip of the limb bud. This region is known as the progressive zone. Fibroblast growth factors (FGFs) expressed in the AER may have a role in controlling cell proliferation and/or in signaling to the progressive zone (Niswander et al 1993). AER implantation and ectopic FGF expression can induce extra limb development (Ohuchi et al 1997). The apical ectodermal ridge regulates the proximodistal sequence of the development of the hand. Progressive zone cells are also influenced by patterning signals from a small group of cells in the posterior margin of the limb bud, called the zone of polarizing activity (ZPA), which regulates the radio-ulnar sequence of the development of the hand.

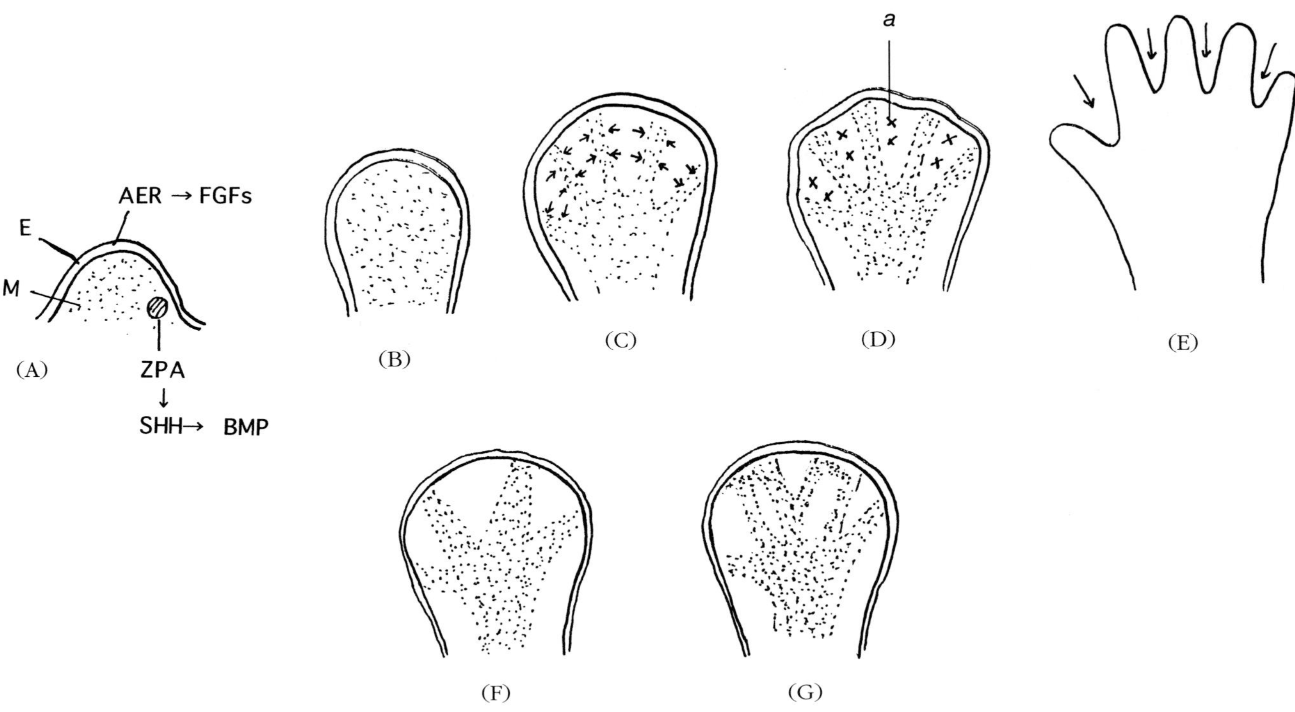

Figure 29.1

Development of the human upper limb. (A) E, ectoderm; M, mesoderm; AER, apical ectodermal ridge; ZPA, zone of polarizing activity; FGFs, fibroblast growth factors; *Shh*, sonic hedgehog; BMPs, bone morphogenetic proteins. FGFs are expressed in the AER and may control cell proliferation. *Shh* is expressed from ZPA and plays a crucial role in induction of the hand and digits by inducing the secretion of bone morphogenic proteins. (B) Limb bud enlarges. (C) Induction of digital rays; the proliferated mesenchymal cells move to the digital radiations. (D) Initial step for formation of the interdigital space; *a*, apoptosis. (E) Formation of the interdigital spaces. (F) Formation of osseous syndactyly due to abnormal induction of digital rays. (G) Formation of central polydactyly due to abnormal induction of digital rays.

Digital radiation

The limb bud becomes thicker and forms the hand plate (Figure 29.1B). Inside the hand plate, the mesenchymal cells increase in density and form digital radiations, which are equivalent to the digits. The increase of the mesenchymal cells during this period occurs mainly in the interdigital space. The increased mesenchymal cells in the interdigital space move to the digital radiation, and the overall density of the mesenchymal cells increases (Ohshio et al 1990) (Figure 29.1C).

The digital radiations are formed according to positional information established by signal centers such as the AER and ZPA. Sonic hedgehog (*Shh*) has been identified as a gene that contributes to the signal activities of the ZPA. *Shh* is expressed from ZPA and plays a crucial role in induction of hand and digits (digital rays) (Riddle et al 1993). *Shh* has been reported to induce the secretion of bone morphogenic proteins (BMPs), FGFs, and homeobox genes such as Hoxd-11 and 13. Homeobox genes are thought to control both cell proliferation and tissue patterning within the limb. There is a time-dependent sequential expression of growth factors and homeobox genes. However, the cellular and molecular mechanisms that control the induction of digital rays have remained unclear.

Joint

Within the digital radiation, centers of chondrification first appear in each presumptive skeletal element. BMPs stimulate condensed mesenchymal cells to differentiate to chondrocytes. When chondrocytes have reached the hypertrophic stage, they become surrounded by connective rings of flattened cells extending towards each of the bone rudiments. Between segments undergoing chondrification, the intervening undifferentiated tissue forms what is known as the interzone. Somewhat later, three distinct zones can be identified; i.e. a central loose layer between two denser zones. The central loose layer begins to undergo autolysis and liquefaction. In this layer, several small discrete cavities appear and form a joint cavity. The articular cartilage develops from dense layers of the interzone. Muscle contraction to move the joint and tendon gliding to conduct the force to the joint are necessary for further normal development of the joint. If the muscle contraction is disturbed by neurogenic factors or myogenic factors for a certain period, normal development of the joint does not occur.

Interdigital space

In the interdigital space, physiologic programmed cell death (apoptosis) occurs, and the interdigital chasm is formed (Figures 29.1D, E). Apoptosis is facilitated by BMP (Zou et al 1996). If apoptosis of the interdigital space does not occur, simple syndactyly results. In the human fetus, the formation of the limb occurs approximately 4 weeks after fertilization. The formation of the apical ectodermal ridge occurs at approximately 5 weeks, and the digital radiation approximately 6 weeks after fertilization. Then nail and fingerprints are formed and the final form of the hand is completed at 12–14 weeks after fertilization.

Teratogenic mechanisms of congenital defects of the digits

Congenital constriction band syndrome

As for the cause of the congenital constriction band syndrome, there are two main theories: the relationship with amnion and localized cell death. In the first theory, it is postulated that the pressure at the edge of the amnion on the limbs when the limb bursts out from the amnion causes the constriction by accretion of the amnion and the fetus due to the inflammation of the amnion. In the second theory, it is postulated that the ring is a developmental and hematogenous deficiency of the subcutis. Kino (1975) punctured the amniotic sac in rats and induced the constriction band syndrome in animal experiments. The results showed that bleeding inside the hand plate might cause the necrosis of the subcutaneous cells, which was associated with the abnormal shrinking of the wound. Controversially, Light and Ogden (1993) reported, 'The variable clinical manifestations of congenital constriction band syndrome support the concept of localized compression'. Although it is difficult to say that constriction band syndrome is caused by a single factor, this deficiency does appear after the formation of the digital rays. For this reason, constriction ring, acrosyndactyly, and amputation are classified into the same category in IFSSH classification, although their appearances are quite different from each other.

Longitudinal deficiency

The congenital deformity confined to the long axis of the upper limb is called longitudinal deficiency. In longitudinal deficiency, the absence of the finger of the ulnar side is called ulnar deficiency, and that of the digits of the radial side is radial deficiency. In ulnar deficiencies, absence of ulnar digits is sometimes associated with absence or hypoplasia of the ulna, and deformities of the elbow joint. On the other hand, in radial deficiency, the dysplasia of the thumb is sometimes associated with absence or hypoplasia of the radius. In radial or ulnar deficiency, the more severe the absence of the digits, the more likely is the dysplasia of the radius or ulna.

In animal experiments, if the antineoplastic drug busulfan is given to pregnant rats, radial deficiency and ulnar deficiency similar to that seen in clinical cases will be induced (Ogino and Kato 1988b). In the course of the development, if impairment is imposed on the fetus and deformation is induced, the period of the impairment is known as the critical period of the deformation. The critical periods for ulnar and radial deficiencies occur before the formation of the limb bud, and the critical period for ulnar deficiency occurs before that of radial deficiency (Kato et al 1990). If busulfan is given to different types of rats, the induced longitudinal deficiency will be different. It is possible that different aspects of drug receptiveness controlled by genes cause different types of longitudinal deficiencies.

During the period of limb bud formation in longitudinal deficiency, the cell deficiency was found at the ectoderm and mesoderm of the limb bud, the dead mesenchymal cells were distributed evenly, and there was no localized cell deficiency inside the limb bud. It then was clear that the absence of digits in longitudinal deficiency was not caused by the localized deficiency of the limb bud. When histologic figures were examined quantitatively in longitudinal deficiency, there were characteristics of the low density mesenchymal cells in the limb bud during the limb bud formation period, and the area of the development limb bud was small (Ogino and Kato 1998a). According to the above observations, it is possible that the inadequacy of the mesenchymal ingredients in the limb bud caused by the impairment before the formation of the limb bud is related to the cause of the absence of digits of longitudinal deficiency (Ogino and Kato 1993).

Cleft hand

In the impairment of the longitudinal axis, central deficiency has been used as the synonym for cleft hand. Barsky (1964) divided cleft hand into two types: typical and atypical. In the typical type, central digital rays are impaired: in the impaired position of the digits, there is always a uniform V-shaped deep interdigital cleft,

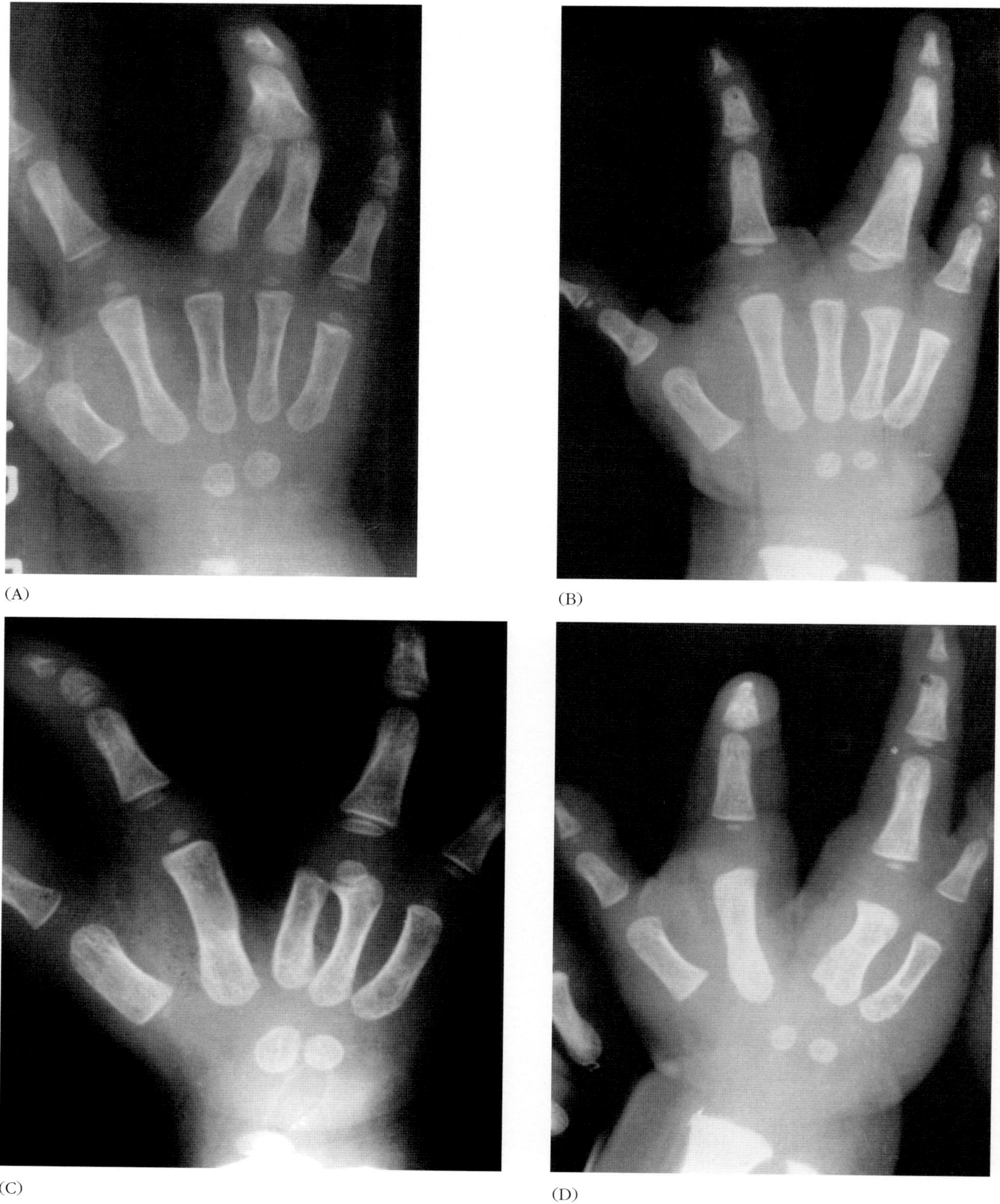

(A) (B) (C) (D)

Figure 29.2

Abnormal induction of digital rays: Relationship between osseous syndactyly and cleft hand. (A) Osseous syndactyly distal to the middle phalanx; (B, C) osseous syndactyly distal to the proximal phalanx; (D) osseous syndactyly distal to the metacarpus. The cases in which the fusion area extends as far as the proximal phalanx and metacarpal bone resemble typical cleft hand in appearance.

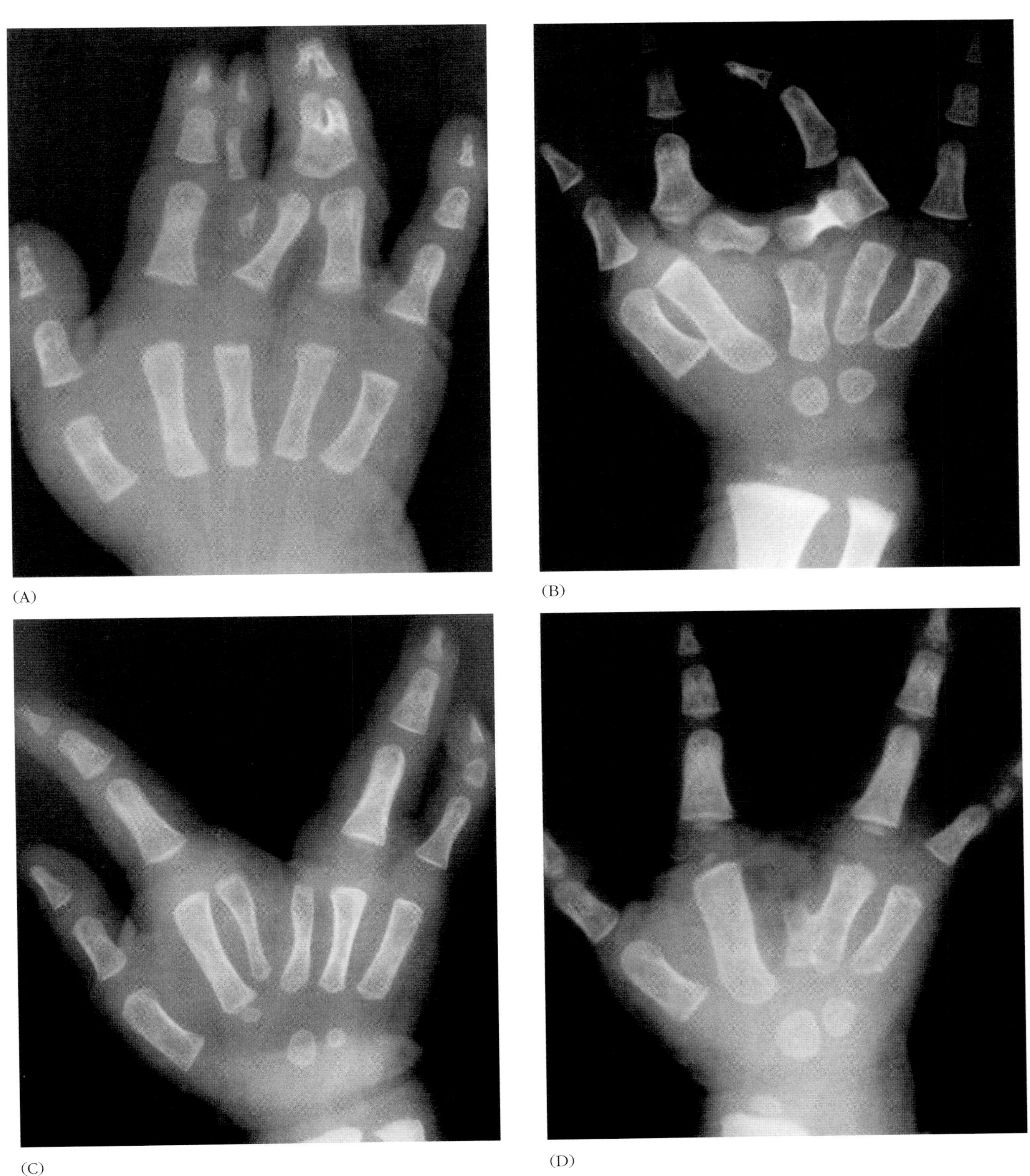

(A) (B) (C) (D)

Figure 29.3

Abnormal induction of digital rays: relationship between central polydactyly and cleft hand. (A) Polysyndactyly distal to the middle phalanx; (B) polysyndactyly distal to the proximal phalanx; (C, D) polysyndacty distal to the metacarpus. The cases in which the fusion area extends as far as the proximal phalanx and metacarpal bone resemble typical cleft hand in appearance.

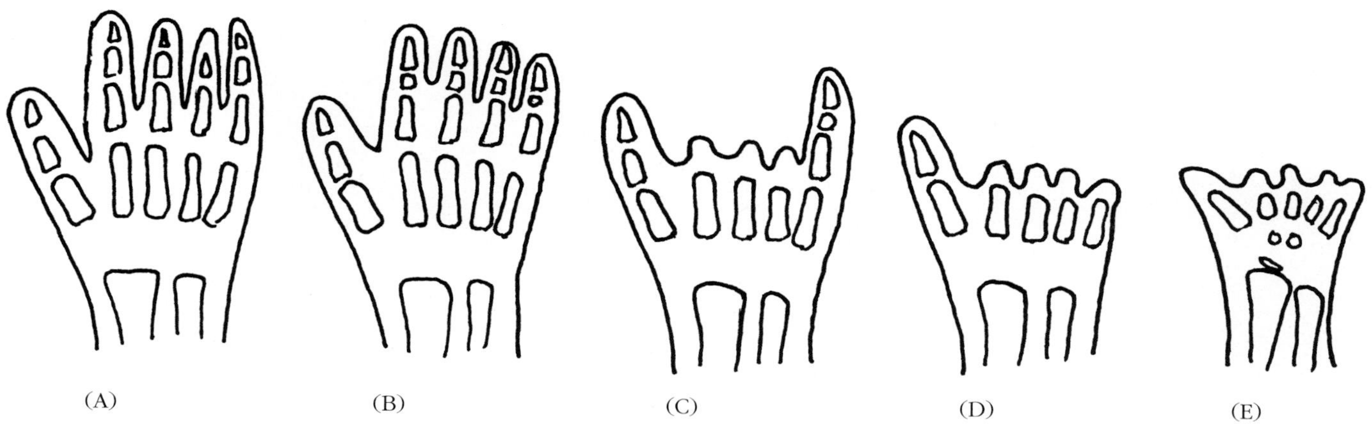

Figure 29.4

Transverse deficiencies Blauth and Gekeler's classification (1986) in parentheses: (A) peripheral hypoplasia type; (B) short webbed finger type (grade 1, short webbed fingers); (C) didactyly type (grade 2, atypical cleft hand); (D) monodactyly type (grade 3, monodactyly type); (E) adactyly type (grade 4, peromelia type).

whereas in the atypical type, there are usually vestigial digits in the same place. These two types are different categories of the congenital hand deformity, because typical cleft hand is a type of abnormal induction of the digital rays and atypical cleft hand is a type of so-called symbrachydactyly. On the basis of the same reasoning, the Congenital Committee of the International Federation of Societies for Surgery of the Hand urged that the term atypical cleft hand should not be used as the diagnostic name (unpublished data, Congenital Committee of the International Federation of Societies for Surgery of the Hand. Personal communication, 1992).

According to the analysis of clinical cases in recent years, cleft hand is a congenital deformity closely related to central polydactyly and syndactyly, and it is different from other absence of digits including longitudinal deficiency (Miura 1978). The cleft hand is a congenital deformity, similar to central polydactyly and syndactyly, that is caused by abnormalities during the induction of the digital rays in the developmental period of digital radiation (Ogino 1979) (Figures 29.1F, G). Based on this viewpoint, when radiographs of clinical cases are examined, in the case of osseous syndactyly between the middle and ring fingers and polydactyly of the middle finger, if the development of osseous syndactyly occurs in the proximal direction, then it will develop toward the cleft hand (Figures 29.2 and 29.3). In clinical cases, in the left and right hands of the same patient, the complicated combinations of central polydactyly, osseous syndactyly, and cleft hand do occur. Based on these observations, it is possible that cleft hand is a congenital deformity closely related to central polydactyly and syndactyly. Analysis of the laboratory-induced cleft hand indicates that if osseous syndactyly or polydactyly develop in the ring finger toward the proximal position, cleft hand will also develop. It is also clear that the time (critical period) in which the cleft hand appears is consistent with that of central polydactyly and syndactyly. A single cause affecting the limb bud in a certain receptive period of the development of the apical ectodermal ridge can induce the deformities. The changes of polydactyly and syndactyly caused by the abnormal induction of the digital rays may be found in the central deficiency. Therefore, when classifying congenital deformities of the hand based on genetics, central polydactyly, osseous syndactyly, and cleft hand may be grouped together and included in the same category of abnormal induction of digital rays (Ogino 1990).

Transverse deficiency (so-called symbrachydactyly)

In contrast to longitudinal deficiency, which occurs locally on the long axis of the upper limbs, the deformities across the upper limbs that are caused by dysplasia are known as transverse deficiencies. Originally the term transverse deficiency was synonymous with congenital amputation. In German-speaking areas, transverse deficiency is regarded as a congenital deformity in the same category as congenital amputation, atypical cleft hand, and brachysyndactyly, and these deformities are called symbrachydactyly by Blauth and Gekeler (1986). According to the classification of Blauth, grade 1 consists of short webbed fingers. Typical brachysyndactyly has middle phalanx shortage or middle phalanx

Table 29.1 *Classification of congenital hand deformities*

Category I: Failure of formation of parts (arrest of development)
A. Transverse deficiencies(so-called symbrachydactyly)
1. Peripheral hypoplasia type 2. Short webbed finger type
3. Tetradactyly type 4. Tridactyly type
5. Didactyly type 6. Monodactyly type
7. Adactyly type 8. Metacarpal type
9. Carpal type 10. Forearm type
11. Upper arm type
B. Longitudinal deficiencies
1. Radial deficiencies
①Dysplasia of the radius
Hypoplasia of the radius
Partial absence of the radius
Total absence of the radius
②Deformities of the hand
Five fingered hand (non-opposable triphalangeal thumb)
Hypoplastic thumb: Blauth's type 1, 2, 3, 4, 5
2. Ulnar deficiencies
①Dysplasia of the ulna
Hypoplasia of the ulna
Partial absence of the ulna
Total absence of the ulna
②Deformities of the hand
Hypoplasia of the little finger
Absence of 5th digital ray
Absence of 4th and 5th digital rays
Absence of 3rd, 4th and 5th digital rays
Absence of 2nd, 3rd, 4th and 5th digital rays
③Dysplasia of the elbow
Contracture of the elbow joint
Humero-radial synostosis
Radial head dislocation
C. Phocomelia
1. Complete type 2. Proximal type 3. Distal type
D. Absent tendons or muscles
E. Absent nail and skin

Category II: Failure of differentiation of parts
A. Synostosis
1. Humero-ulnar synostosis 2. Humero-radial synostosis
3. Radio-ulnar synostosis 4. Carpal coalition
5. Metacarpal synostosis
B. Radial head dislocation
C. Symphalangism.
1. Proximal type 2. Distal type 3. Combined type
D. Contracture
1. Soft tissue
a) Arthrogryposis multiplex
b) Pterygium cubitale
c) Trigger digit
d) Clasped thumb
e) Windblown hand
f) Camptodactyly (without other deformities)
Single digit type
Multiple digits type
g) Aberrant muscles
h) Muscle contracture
i) Swan-neck deformity
j) Nail deformity
2. Skeletal
a) Clinodactyly without shortening of the digit
b) Kirner's deformity
c) Delta bone
d) Madelung's deformity
E. Tumorous conditions
a) Hemangioma b) Arteriovenous fistula
c) Lymphangioma d) Neurofibromatosis
e) Juvenile aponeurotic fibroma.

Category III: Duplication
A. Thumb polydactyly
Wassel's classification type 1, 2, 3, 4, 5, 6
a) Floating type b) Thenar muscle hypoplasia type
c) Radially deviated type.
B. Polydactyly of the little finger
a) Floating type b) Others
C. Opposable triphalangeal thumb (without other anomalies)
D. Mirror hand
a) Typical mirror hand (ulnar dimelia)
b) Atypical mirror hand
E. Duplication of the whole limb
a) Complete type b) Incomplete type

Category IV: Failure of induction of digital rays
A. Soft tissue
1) Cutaneous syndactyly 2) Cleft of the palm
3) Camptodactyly
B. Skeletal
1) Osseous syndactyly 2) Central polydactyly
3) Cleft hand (absence of central finger rays)
4) Triphalangeal thumb
5) Cleft hand complex

Category V: Overgrowth
A. Macrodactyly
B. Hemihypertrophy

Category VI: Undergrowth
A. Microcheiria
B. Brachydactyly
C. Clinodactyly with shortening of the digit
D. Micronychia

Category VII: Constriction band syndrome
1. Constriction ring 2. Lymphedema
3. Acrosyndactyly 4. Amputation type

Category VIII: Generalized skeletal abnormalities and part of a syndrome

Category IX: Others
1. Unclassifiable case
2. Others

absence and cutaneous syndactyly. Grade 2 is called the atypical cleft hand, in which dysplasia of the central digital rays is severe, but complete absence of the fingers rarely occurs. There is no V-shaped depression in the palm of the cleft as found in the typical cleft hand. Grade 3 is the monodactyly type, in which the thumb remains and there are the vestigial fingers or vestigial nails. Grade 4 is the peromelia-type, congenital amputation in which all digits are impaired (Figure 29.4). Among the different types, there may be intertypes of deformities. In addition, there are some congenital deformities that can be found in all types: one-sided impairment; severe dysplasia of the central digital rays; bone dysplasia in the impaired digits, neighbored digits, or the entire impaired upper limb; and complications of the impairment of the pectoralis major muscle (Ogino et al 1989). According to these observations, the sequence of deformities from brachysyndactyly, or the atypical cleft hand, seems to be a morphological variant of transverse deficiency.

Classification of the upper extremity malformations (Table 29.1)

Based on clinical and experimental studies, the classification of congenital hand deformities proposed by IFSSH was modified by Ogino (1986). This classification has been updated and was adopted by the Japanese Society for Surgery of the Hand (1996).

In IFSSH classification, polydactyly is classified into duplication, syndactyly into failure of formation of parts, and typical cleft hand into failure of formation of parts. However, these congenital deformities may appear when the same teratogenic factor acts on an embryo at the same developmental period. Therefore, they are included in the same category of abnormal induction of digital rays in this classification. On the other hand, brachysyndactyly is classified into undergrowth, and transverse deficiency into failure of formation of parts, and there is no item of atypical cleft hand in IFSSH classification. However, brachysyndactyly, atypical cleft hand, or transverse deficiency seem to be developed as morphological variants of symbrachydactyly. Therefore, these deformities are included in the same concept of transverse deficiency as an item of failure of formation of parts.

Category I: Failure of formation of parts (arrest of development)

The category of failure of formation of parts is that group of congenital deficiencies noted by failure or arrest of formation of the limb, either complete or partial. It is subclassified into five types: transverse deficiency, longitudinal deficiency, phocomelia, absent tendons or muscles, and absent nail or skin.

Transverse deficiencies (so-called symbrachydactyly)

This category includes short webbed finger to amputation-like deformities. An anomaly belonging to this category usually has unilateral affection, hypoplasia of the adjacent digits and/or whole affected limb, and sometimes pectoral muscle absence is associated in every type.

- Peripheral hypoplasia type: While in the short webbed finger type, hypoplasia of the phalanx appears predominantly in the middle phalanges, in this type it appears predominantly in the distal phalanges. Therefore, in this type, hypoplasia of the distal phalanx or aplasia of the distal phalanx and absence of nails are common clinical features. Usually syndactyly is not associated with this type.
- Short webbed finger type: Short fingers and syndactyly are essential clinical features of this type. Brachymesophalangy, absence of the middle phalanx and/or absence of two phalanges – including middle phalanges in a single finger ray – are commonly observed.
- Tetradactyly type: All phalanges of one central digit are missing.
- Tridactyly type: All phalanges of two central digits are missing.
- Didactyly type: All phalanges of three central finger rays are missing.
- Monodactyly type: All phalanges of ulnar four digital rays are missing. There are one or two phalanges in the thumb.
- Adactyly type: All phalanges are missing.
- Metacarpal type: In addition to the absence of all phalanges, all or some part of the metacarpals are missing.
- Carpal type: All or some part of the carpals are missing.
- Forearm type: All or some part of the forearm bones are missing.
- Upper arm type: All or some part of the humerus is missing.

Longitudinal deficiencies

Radial deficiencies

The congenital deformities in which radial digits are hypoplastic or absent and the radius is hypoplastic or absent are classified as radial deficiency. The dysplasia of the thumb was classified in six types including five-fingered hand (non-opposable triphalangeal thumb) and five degrees of hypoplastic thumb by Blauth (1967) as follows: first degree, mild hypoplasia of the thenar muscles of the thumb; second degree, thenar muscle hypoplasia and adduction contracture of the thumb; third degree, hypoplasia or absence of the base of the first metacarpus; fourth degree, floating thumb; and fifth degree, total absence of the thumb. In contrast, dysplasia of the radius is classified into three types: total absence of the radius, partial absence of the radius, and hypoplasia of the radius. In radial deficiency, deformity of the hand and that of the forearm appear in various combinations. Therefore, deformities in this category must be expressed as a combination of hand and forearm deformities.

Ulnar deficiencies

The absence of the finger of the ulnar side is called ulnar deficiency. In severe ulnar deficiency, absence of the digits is sometimes associated with dysplasia of the ulna and/or elbow deformity. Hand deformities of ulnar deficiencies are classified into five types: hypoplasia of the little finger, absence of the little finger, absence of the two digital rays of the ulnar side, absence of the three digital rays of the ulnar side, and absence of the four digital rays of the ulnar side. Dysplasia of the ulna is classified into three types: total absence, partial absence, and hypoplasia of the ulna. The deformities of the elbow are classified into humeroradial synostosis, radial head dislocation, and flexion contracture of the elbow joint. In ulnar deficiencies, deformities of the hand, dysplasia of the ulna, and deformities of the elbow occur in various combinations. Therefore, deformities must be expressed as a combination of hand deformity, dysplasia of the ulna, and deformities of the elbow.

Phocomelia

The major manifestation of complete phocomelia is absence of the humerus and forearm bones: in the proximal type the humerus is absent, and in the distal type the forearm bones are absent.

Category II: Failure of differentiation of parts

Failure of differentiation or separation of parts is that category in which the basic unit of the hand and arm develops but the final form is not completed. In IFSSH classification, syndactyly is included in this category, but it appears as a result of abnormal induction of the digital rays. Therefore, syndactyly is excluded from this revised category. This category includes incomplete formation of the joint, contracture and deformity due to failure of differentiation, and tumor-like conditions including hamartomas.

Incomplete formation of the joint may result in synostosis, symphalangism, and congenital dislocation. Synostosis includes humero-ulnar synostosis, humeroradial synostosis, radio-ulnar synostosis, carpal coalition, metacarpal synostosis, and congenital radial head dislocation. Symphalangism is a congenital ankylosis of the finger joint: it includes ankylosis of the PIP joint (proximal type), ankylosis of the DIP joint (distal type), and a combination of proximal and distal types.

Contractures and deformities include arthrogryposis multiplex, pterygium cubitale, clasped thumb, windblown hand, camptodactyly, aberrant muscles, muscle contracture, swan-neck deformity, nail deformity, clinodactyly, Kirner's deformity, delta bone, and Madelung's deformity.

There are two types of camptodactyly. In single digit type, only a single digit is involved and usually the little finger is affected. Multiple digits type indicates multiple digit involvement. Camptodactyly-like deformity is often associated with cleft hand or thumb hypoplasia. These deformities must be classified according to the underlying conditions.

Hand deformity with aberrant muscles is a congenital deformity characterized by excessive muscle volume with unilateral hypertrophy of the upper extremity and particular deformity of the hand. In this deformity, there are many aberrant muscles and increase of the intermetacarpal and interdigital spaces. Crossing of the fingers and/or intrinsic plus deformity are sometimes observed.

In a case of muscle contracture, the range of motion of the joint, where the affected muscle is a mover, is limited. Usually the affected muscle has a short muscle belly and long tendinous portion. The excursion of the muscle is smaller than normal.

The congenital swan-neck deformity gives rise to the locking phenomenon after a few years of progressive laxity of the volar plate and the collateral ligaments, and becomes worse with aging.

Congenital hypoplasia or aplasia of the finger nail is classified into category I. Congenital nail deformity includes claw nail, hook nail, clam nail and circumferential nail.

Delta bone means that a triangular-shaped phalanx or metacarpal bone has an epiphysis which is located on the shorter side of the phalanx and runs from proximal to distal. Delta bone is often associated with other deformities, such as polydactyly and syndactyly. These cases must be classified according to the underlying conditions.

The majority of cases of Madulung's deformity are caused by hereditary dyschondrosteosis at the wrist. Those cases with mesomeric dwarfism must be classified into category 9.

Tumorous conditions include, hemangioma, arteriovenous fistula, lymphangioma, neurofibromatosis, and juvenile aponeurotic fibroma.

Category III: Duplication

In the IFSSH classification, radial, central, and ulnar polydactylies were included in this category, but central polydactyly appears as a result of abnormal induction of the digital rays and mostly it is associated with syndactyly. Therefore, central polydactyly is excluded from this category.

Thumb polydactyly can be subclassified according to Wassel's classification (1969), but there are other types, such as floating type, thenar muscle hypoplasia type, and radially deviated type. Polydactyly of the little finger is classified into floating type and others.

There is no item of triphalangeal thumb in IFSSH classification. There are two types of triphalangeal thumb: opposable and non-opposable. Non-opposable thumb is classified into radial deficiency. An opposable triphalangeal thumb might have formed as a result of incomplete fusion of the duplicated thumb (Ogino et al 1994); therefore, it is classified in this category. Opposable triphalangeal thumb is often associated with cleft hand with absence of the index finger. This type of triphalangeal thumb should be classified according to the underlying diseases.

In mirror hand, the thumb is always missing, but an excess number of fingers is present. In typical mirror hand, there are two ulnas and the radius is missing. In atypical mirror hand, there is no duplication of the ulna.

Category IV: Abnormal induction of digital rays

Manifestations of malsegmentation of the digital rays in the hand plate due to abnormal induction of digital rays are included in this category. Cleft of the palm means deep V-shaped excessive interdigital space. It appears as an isolated anomaly without absence of the central finger ray and mostly it is associated with absence of central finger rays. When the index finger seems to be missing, triphalangeal thumb is frequently associated. When only the single digit is preserved, it is necessary to distinguish it from the monodactyly type of transverse deficiency. In cleft hand, even if four digits are absent, hypoplasia of the retained digit, that of the the carpal bone or hypoplasia of the forearm bones do not exist. Clinodactyly and camptodactyly are sometimes associated with cleft hand. In such cases, associated clinodactyly and camptodactyly should not be classified into other categories, because these deformities seem to be a secondary change due to abnormal induction of the digital rays. In this category, hand deformity can be expressed as a combination of cutaneous syndactyly, cleft of the palm, camptodactyly, osseous syndactyly, central polydactyly, triphalangeal thumb, and absence of the central finger rays. A case with a complex combination of the manifestations can be called cleft hand complex.

Category V: Overgrowth

The whole limb or the digits may be affected by overgrowth. Overgrowth due to lymphangioma or hemangioma is classified according to the underlying disease. Most macrodactylies are associated with hypertrophy of fat and/or digital nerves.

Category VI: Undergrowth

Undergrowth is that category in which there is defective or incomplete development of the parts. This category is supplemental to category I, failure of formation of parts, and includes microcheiria, brachydactyly, clinodactyly with shortening of the digit, and micronychia.

Category VII: Constriction band syndrome

Congenital constriction band syndrome has four different expressions; i.e. constriction band, lymphedema, acrosyndactyly, and amputation. These expressions appear in various combinations. In the congenital constriction band syndrome, although the amputation may extend from the digital tip to the forelimb, or even to the proximal part of the limb, it is unique in that no bone dysplasia from the amputated part to the proximal occurs. Hand deformity should be expressed as a combination of constriction ring, lymphedema, acrosyndactyly, and amputation type.

Category VIII: Generalized skeletal abnormalities and part of a syndrome

Deformities in the hand may be a manifestation of a congenital syndrome or that of generalized skeletal abnormalities caused by osteochondrodysplasias.

Category IX: Others

This category includes unclassifiable cases.

References

Barsky AJ (1964) Cleft hand: classification, incidence and treatment. Review of the literature and report of nineteen cases, *J Bone Joint Surg* **46A**: 1707–20.

Blauth W (1967) Der hypoplastische Daumen, *Arch Orthop Unfall-Chir* **62**: 225–46.

Blauth W, Gekeler J (1986) Zur Morphologie und Klassifikation der Symbrachydaktylie, *Handchir Mikrochir Plast Chir* **8**: 161–95.

Japanese Society for Surgery of the Hand: Congenital Hand

Committee (1996) Manual for classification of congenital hand deformities, *J Jpn Soc Surg Hand* **13**: 455–67.
Kato H, Ogino T, Minami A et al (1990) Experimental study of radial ray deficiency, *J Hand Surg* **15B**: 470–6.
Kino Y (1975) Clinical and experimental studies of the congenital constriction band syndrome, with an emphasis on its etiology, *J Bone Joint Surg* **57A**: 636–43.
Light TR, Ogden JA (1993) Congenital constriction band syndrome. Pathophysiology and treatment, *Yale J Biol Med* **66**: 143–55 .
Miura T (1978) Syndactyly and split hand, *The Hand* **10**: 99–103.
Niswander I, Tickle C, Vogel A et al (1993) FGF-4 replaces the apical ectodermal ridge and directs outgrowth and patterning of the limb, *Cell* **75**: 579–87.
Ogino T (1979) Clinical and experimental study on the teratogenic mechanisms of cleft hand polydactyly and syndactyly, *J Jpn Orthop Assoc* **53**: 535–43.
Ogino T (1986) Congenital anomalies of the upper limb in our clinic – an application of modified Swanson's classification, *J Jpn Soc Surg Hand* **2**: 909–16.
Ogino T (1990) Teratogenic relationship between polydactyly syndactyly and cleft hand, *J Hand Surg* **15B**: 201–9.
Ogino T (1996) Congenital anomalies of the hand. the Asian perspective, *Clin Orthop* **323**: 12–21.
Ogino T, Kato H (1988a) Histological analysis of myleran induced oligodactyly of longitudinal deficiency, *Handchir Mikrochir Plast Chir* **20**: 271–4.
Ogino T, Kato H (1988b) Clinical and experimental studies on ulnar ray deficiency, *Handchir Mikrochir Plast Chir* **20**: 330–7.
Ogino T, Kato H (1993) Clinical and experimental studies on teratogenic mechanisms of congenital absence of longitudinal deficiencies, *Cong Anom* **33**: 187–96.
Ogino T, Minami A, Kato H (1989) Clinical features and roentgenograms of symbrachydactyly, *J Hand Surg* **14B**: 303–6.
Ogino T, Ishii S, Kato H (1994) Opposable triphalangeal thumb. Clinical features and results of treatment, *J Hand Surg* **19A**: 39–47.
Ohshio I, Ogino T, Nagashima K (1990) Investigation of DNA synthesis and cell condensation in the developing rat hand plate by the BrdU/anti-BrdU technique, *Cong Anom* **30**: 17–27.
Ohuchi H, Nakagawa T, Yamamoto A et al (1997) The mesenchymal factor, FGF 10, initiates and maintains the outgrowth of the chick limb bud through interaction with FGF 8, an apical ectodermal factor, *Development* **124**: 2235–44.
Riddle RD, Johnson RL, Laufer E et al (1993) Sonic hedgehog mediates the polarizing activity of the ZPA, *Cell* **75**: 1401–16.
Swanson AB (1976) A classification for congenital limb malformations, *J Hand Surg* **1A**: 8–22.
Swanson AB, Barsky AJ, Entin MA (1968) Classification of limb malformations on the basis of embryological failures, *Surg Clin North Am* **48**: 1169–79.
Swanson AB, Swanson GG, Tada K (1983) A classification for congenital limb malformations, *J Hand Surg* **8A**: 693–702.
Wassel HD (1969) The result of surgery for polydactyly of the thumb: a review, *Clin Orthop* **64**: 175–193.
Zou H, Niswander L (1996) Requirement for BMP signaling in interdigital apoptosis and scale formation, *Science* **272**: 738–41.

30 Ulnar deficiency

Dieter Buck-Gramcko and Rolf Habenicht

Ulnar deficiency is the most common term for the great variety of congenital deformities of the ulnar border of the hand and forearm, extending up to the shoulder. Synonyms are ulnar club hand, congenital absence or defect of the ulna, longitudinal arrest of development of the ulna, ulnar dysmelia, aplasia/hypoplasia of the ulna, and ulna hemimelia. This diversity of the terminology also reflects differences in the conception of which cases should be included. It seems to be logical to classify hands with a reduced number of digital rays (oligodactyly) as a first (slightest) group of ulnar deficiency, even if the ulna is normal, because all deformities at the ulnar border of the hand and arm are collected under this term. However, we have decided to omit discussion of the oligodactylous hand with a normal ulna – mainly in comparison with the radial club hand, to which thumb deformities will not belong if the radius is normal.

Incidence

Most authors have emphasized that deficiencies of the ulna are rare and much less frequent than the other longitudinal deficiencies of the arm; i.e. radial and central forms. Flatt (1994) saw only 34 patients with 'ulna hypoplasia' in his 2758 cases with congenital deformities, but 127 with radial club hands and 106 with central defects. Birch-Jensen (1949) reported 19 ulnar and 73 radial defects and stated the incidence at birth in Denmark to be 1:100,000. In these reports the ratio of ulnar to radial deficiencies is 1:3.7 or 3.8 respectively, while Carroll and Bowers (1977) mentioned a ratio of 1:10. In contrast to these data, in our own clinical series (which contains about the same number of patients as Flatt) there are 164 patients with ulnar, 223 with radial, and 89 with central deficiencies; with the number of involved arms being 200, 270, and 137 respectively. This means that ulnar deficiencies are not so rare as previously described, although in our group we have not included patients with a reduced number of digits (oligodactyly) without any hypoplasia of the ulna or patients with arms with transverse defects in the forearm level with some ulna deformations. These cases are counted as ulnar deficiencies by some authors.

Bilateral involvement is reported in about 25% of patients. Only in some of the bilateral cases is the deformity similar or even equal; in most patients the type of ulnar deficiency is quite different (Figure 30.1). The male

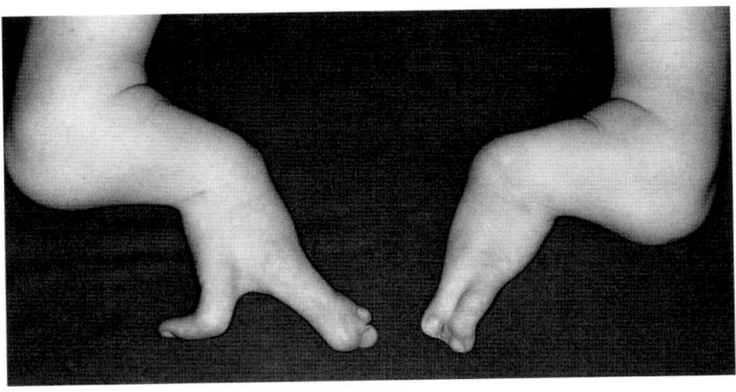

(A)

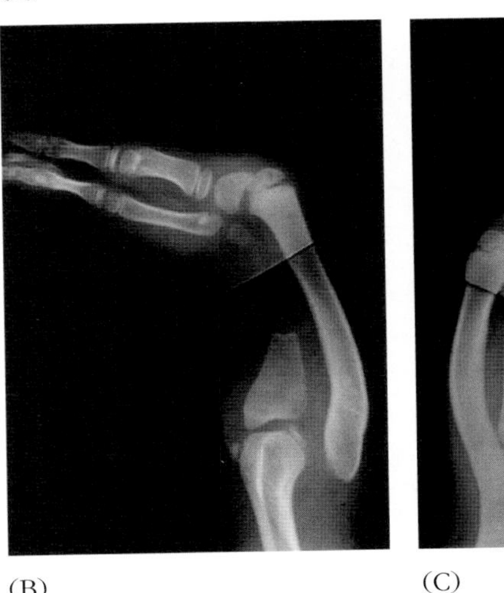

(B) (C)

Figure 30.1
(A) Ulnar deficiency with bilateral involvement. The type of deformity is different in the two arms: partial aplasia of the ulna in both sides, but in combination with congenital dislocation of the radial head (B) and with radiohumeral synostosis (C). In both hands oligodactyly is seen with syndactyly and rudimentary digital parts. The wrists show marked ulnar deviations and anomalies of the carpal bones (the radiograms are composed of two films).

to female ratio is approximately 3:2 in most series, but in our patients it is 2.3:1.

The cause of ulnar defects is unknown. Most cases are sporadic. There is an autosomal dominant inheritance in cases in which the ulnar deficiency is part of a syndrome, for instance the Cornelia de Lange syndrome or the FFU (femur-fibula-ulna) syndrome, described by Kühne et al (1967), which is the European synonym for the American PFFD (proximal femoral focal deficiency), described by Aitken in 1969. In our personal series there was a negative family history in all cases, with the exception of twin brothers who had bilateral identical deformities.

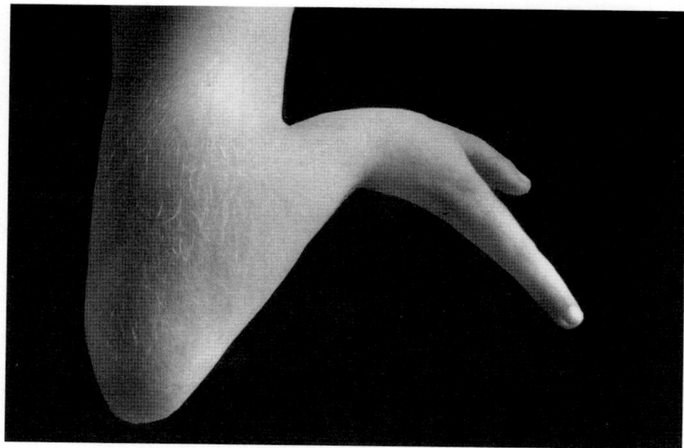

(A)

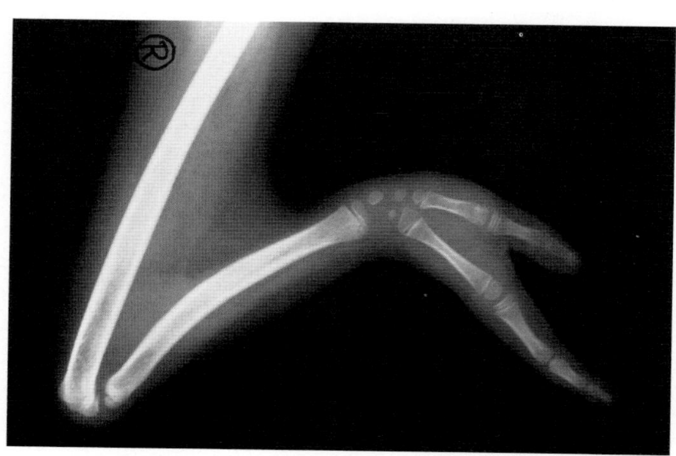

(B)

Figure 30.2

Severe fixed flexion contracture of the elbow with pterygium cubitale and aplasia of the ulna and the three ulnar digital rays.

Classification

There are at least a dozen classification systems, starting more than 100 years ago with Kümmel (1895) and ending in 1997 with Cole and Manske. Although several systems are based on combinations of the different deformities belonging to ulnar deficiencies, it is impossible to categorize all the details and their different combinations in a classification system. Therefore, all classifications must be incomplete in the anatomical description and have no or very little relation to the indication for surgical treatment. The best correlation is given in the classification by Cole and Manske (1997), but concerns only the radial border of the hand.

Clinical picture

The deformity involves all parts of the upper extremity to different extents and in various combinations, so that a separate description is given for these localizations.

Hand

The majority of ulnar deficiencies show an involvement of the hand. Most of the function of the patients with this malformation is determined by these deformities. There is no correlation between the hand anomalies and the extent of the wrist, forearm, and elbow deficiencies. The hand involvement is characterized by aplasia of one or more digits. Only in about 11% of patients is a full complement of digits present; only 17 (8.5%) in our own series of patients. In the 200 involved hands of our 164 patients, there are 31 hands with four fingers (15.5%), 87 with three fingers (43%), 48 with two fingers (24%), and 17 hands with only one finger (8.5%). The 33 hands with oligodactyly but a normal ulna are not included in these figures; in the majority of these hands, ring and little fingers are missing.

If a finger is counted as present, it does not mean that it is a normal digit. Many are hypoplastic; some do not have a metacarpal with the exception of an ossicle proximal to the metacarpophalangeal joint (see below) or have unstable joints and show anomalies of their tendons, especially the extensors. Hands with only one or two digits are often combined with severe flexion contractures of the elbow, pterygium cubitale, and complete absence of the ulna, as in the Cornelia de Lange syndrome (Figure 30.2).

Although it is primarily an ulnar-sided deformity, abnormalities of the thumb and the first web space were seen in a surprisingly high number of hands. With the exception of monodactylous hands (because such a digit cannot be defined exactly), a radial-sided involvement

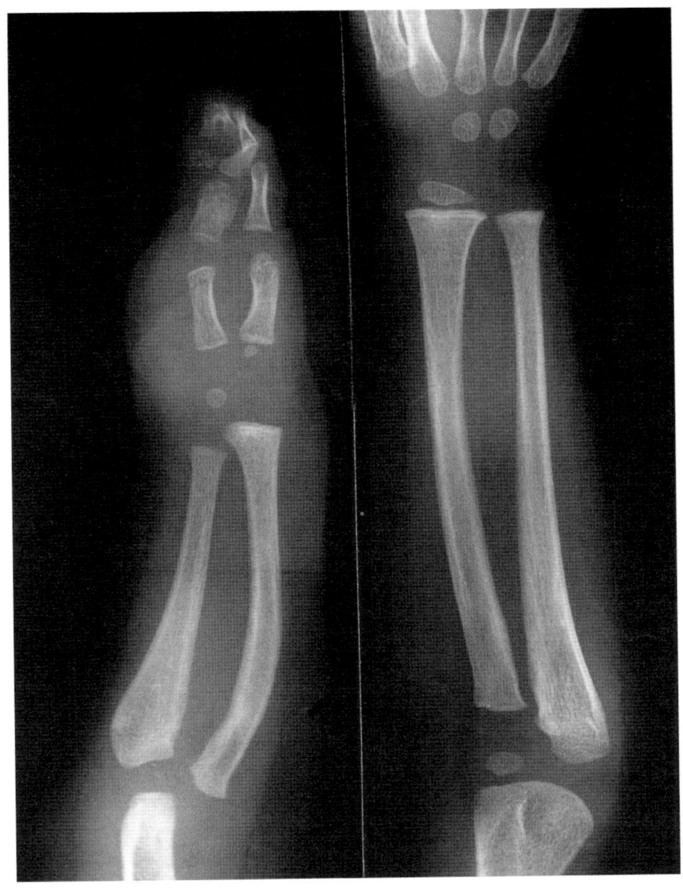

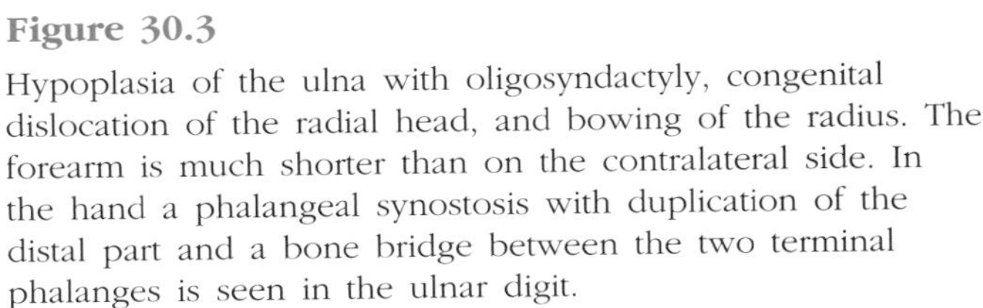

Figure 30.3
Hypoplasia of the ulna with oligosyndactyly, congenital dislocation of the radial head, and bowing of the radius. The forearm is much shorter than on the contralateral side. In the hand a phalangeal synostosis with duplication of the distal part and a bone bridge between the two terminal phalanges is seen in the ulnar digit.

was noted in 136 of 183 hands (74%). This consists of a narrowing of the first web or even complete syndactyly, and hypoplasia or aplasia of the thumb as well as its rotational deformity; so that the thumb is lying in the plane of the other digits. This percentage corresponds exactly with that reported by Cole and Manske (1997).

Additional digital parts were present in 25 hands (12.5%), mostly in hands with only two or three digits. Almost all are located at the distal phalangeal level. These additional bones sometimes look similar to duplicated phalanges (see Figure 30.3); in other hands, there are synostoses and bones with longitudinal bracketed epiphyses (Figure 30.4). In contrast, in many cases missing bones are noted: in 45 hands (22.5%) fingers with only two phalanges (thumb excluded) and in 11 (5.5%) a missing metacarpal in the presence of all three

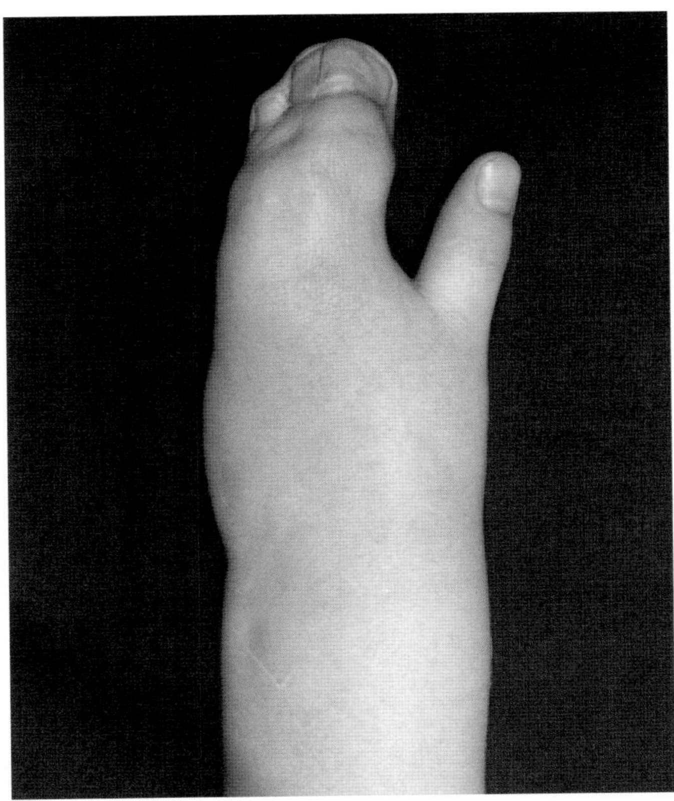

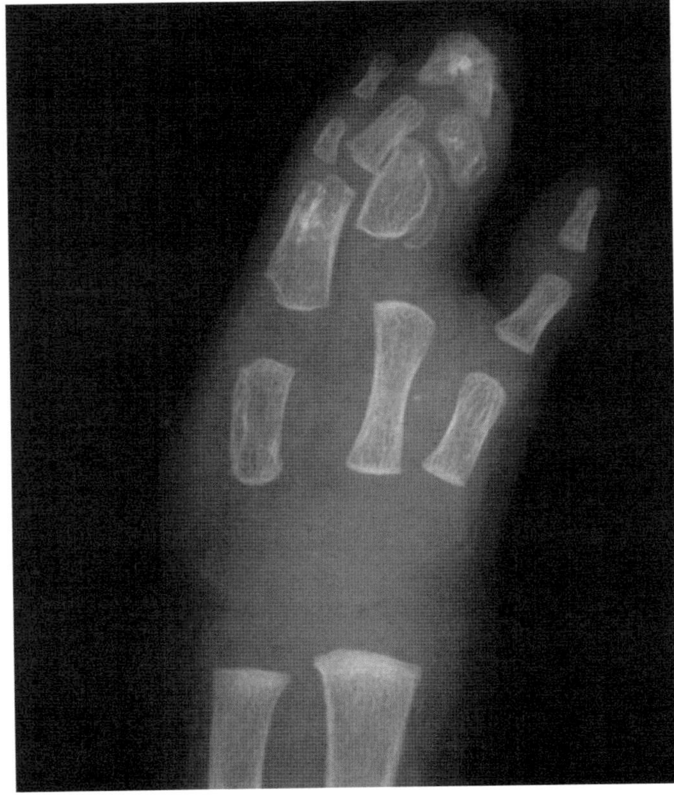

Figure 30.4
Additional bone deformities in a hand with oligosyndactyly: phalangeal synostoses, bones with longitudinal bracketed epiphyses, and terminal phalangeal bone bridges with common fingernails.

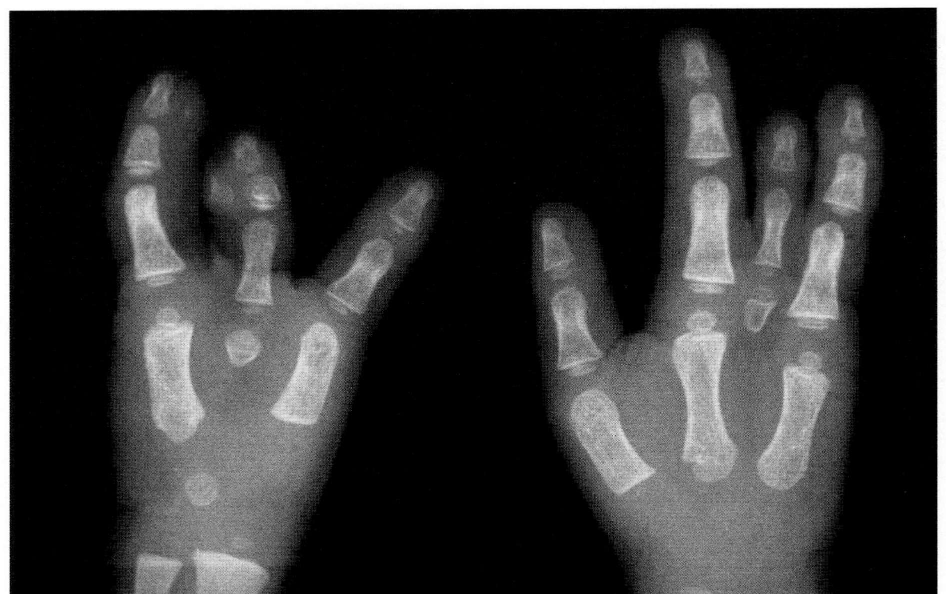

(A)

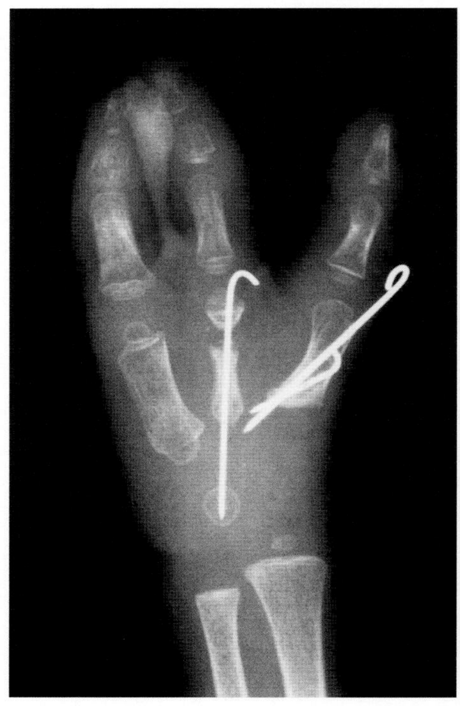

(B)

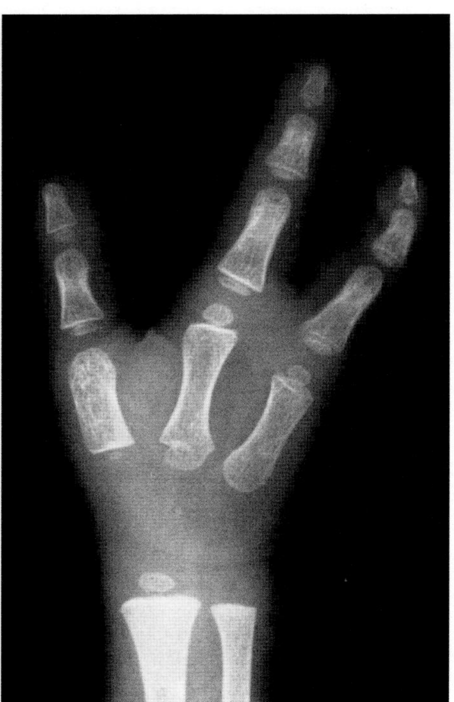

(C)

Figure 30.5
(A) Ulnar deficiency with missing metacarpals in both hands and an additional middle phalanx in the left index finger. (B) (C) Early result after amputation of the right incomplete digit and stabilization of the left index finger with bones from the ablated digit. (From Buck-Gramcko 1997, with permission.)

phalanges (see Figure 30.5). All the latter are seen in combination with syndactyly. Phalangeal deformations were noted as bones with longitudinal bracketed epiphyses in only five digits (plus one in a metacarpal), but as short triangular or trapezoidal middle phalanges (brachymesophalangia) in 38 hands (19%). Synostoses in different extents of the bone length were found in phalanges in 26 hands (13%) and in metacarpals in 23 (11.5%).

The most frequent soft tissue malformation in our patients with ulnar deficiencies was syndactyly. Sometimes it was only partial, but in the majority of the 92 hands (46%) the syndactyly was complete. A combination with bone bridges between the terminal

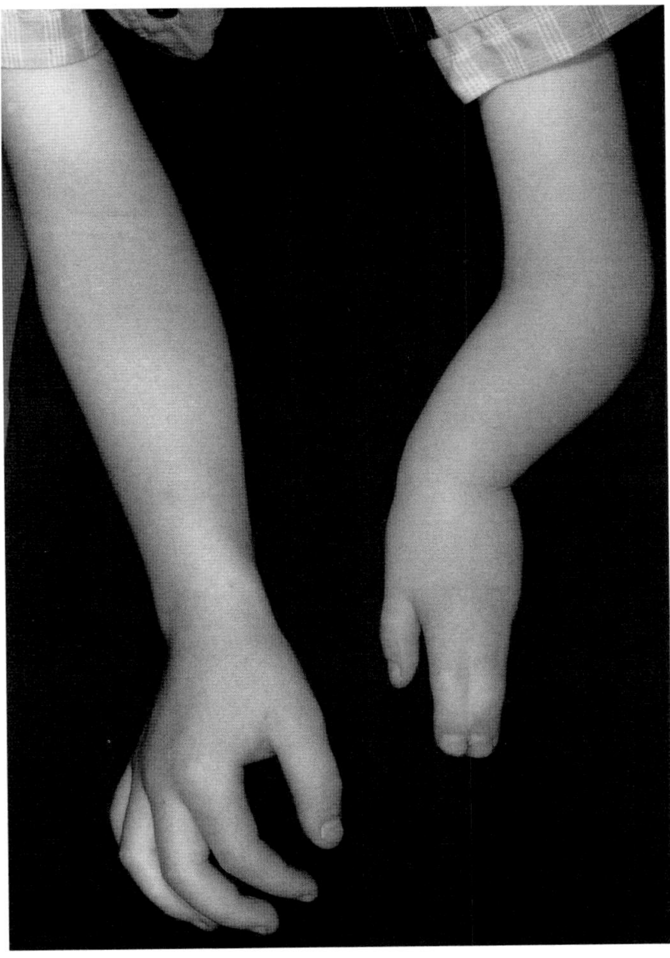

Figure 30.6
Shortening of the forearm in ulnar deficiencies; the radiogram of the arm is seen in Figure 30.9.

phalanges was often seen, especially in hands with only two fingers (as in Figures 30.3, 30.4 and 30.6).

Wrist

Precise information about the carpal bones in several congenital deformities has been known since the fundamental work of O'Rahilly (1951). In ulnar deficiencies the pisiform is almost always absent, while absence of other carpal bones is noted in correlation with the missing digital rays. In most cases the carpals show a delay in the appearance of their ossification centers. Synostoses of carpals are found in about 30–40% of cases. Because many patients are treated in their first years of life and not followed to an age with full carpal ossification, the exact frequency is not known. Sometimes, the shape of these synostotical carpal bones differs considerably from normal anatomy (see Figures 30.1, 30.7 and 30.8).

In many cases of partial or complete ulnar aplasia, there is an ulnar deviation at the wrist. This is caused both by bowing of the radius and by a slant of the distal articular surface of the radius (see Figures 30.8 and 30.9). Following the hypothesis that the slowly growing fibrocartilagenous anlage of the distal ulna tethers the distal radius and contributes to bowing of the radius, dislocation of its head, and ulnar slant of the articular surface with increase of the ulnar deviation, Riordan et al (1961) have recommended an early excision of the anlage. However, our experience and the observations of Broudy and Smith (1979) , Marcus and Omer (1984), and Johnson and Omer (1985) have shown that the excision of the anlage has only a minor effect on the ulnar deviation, which usually will not exceed 30°. Therefore it is our policy to excise the anlage only in progression of the deviation and to combine this procedure with a transposition of the tendon of the ulnar wrist flexor and extensor to the radial side of the wrist.

Forearm

The forearm deformities in ulnar deficiencies are easily differentiated into hypoplasia, and partial and complete aplasia of the ulna. These three basic types can be combined with all the different anomalies seen in the hand and at the elbow, but there is no correlation with the severity of the deformities in the different localizations.

Generally, the forearm is shorter than normal or than the unaffected arm respectively (Figure 30.6). This is not so pronounced in cases of ulna hypoplasia (Figure 30.10), but becomes more distinct when the radial head is dislocated (Figure 30.3). Particularly in patients with radiohumeral synostosis and aplasia of the ulna the forearm is severely shortened (see Figures 30.1 and 30.11).

The distribution of the three types in our clinical series shows that hypoplasia of the ulna is the most frequent of these deformities. As it was noted in 119 arms (59.5% of the 200 involved arms in 164 patients), hypoplasia is about twice as frequent as aplasia: 45 arms (22.5%) with partial aplasia and 36 arms (18%) with complete aplasia. In arms with ulna hypoplasia the number and particularly the severity of anomalies of the hand and the elbow are less than in most arms with ulna aplasia. The elbow is almost normal in its articular configuration and its range of motion in the majority of cases, even if the coronoid process is lower than normal (see Figure 30.10). The hypoplastic ulna was combined with congenital dislocation of the radial head in 25 arms (12.5% of all involved arms; 41% of all 61 dislocations) and with radiohumeral synostosis in 7 arms (3.5% of the 200

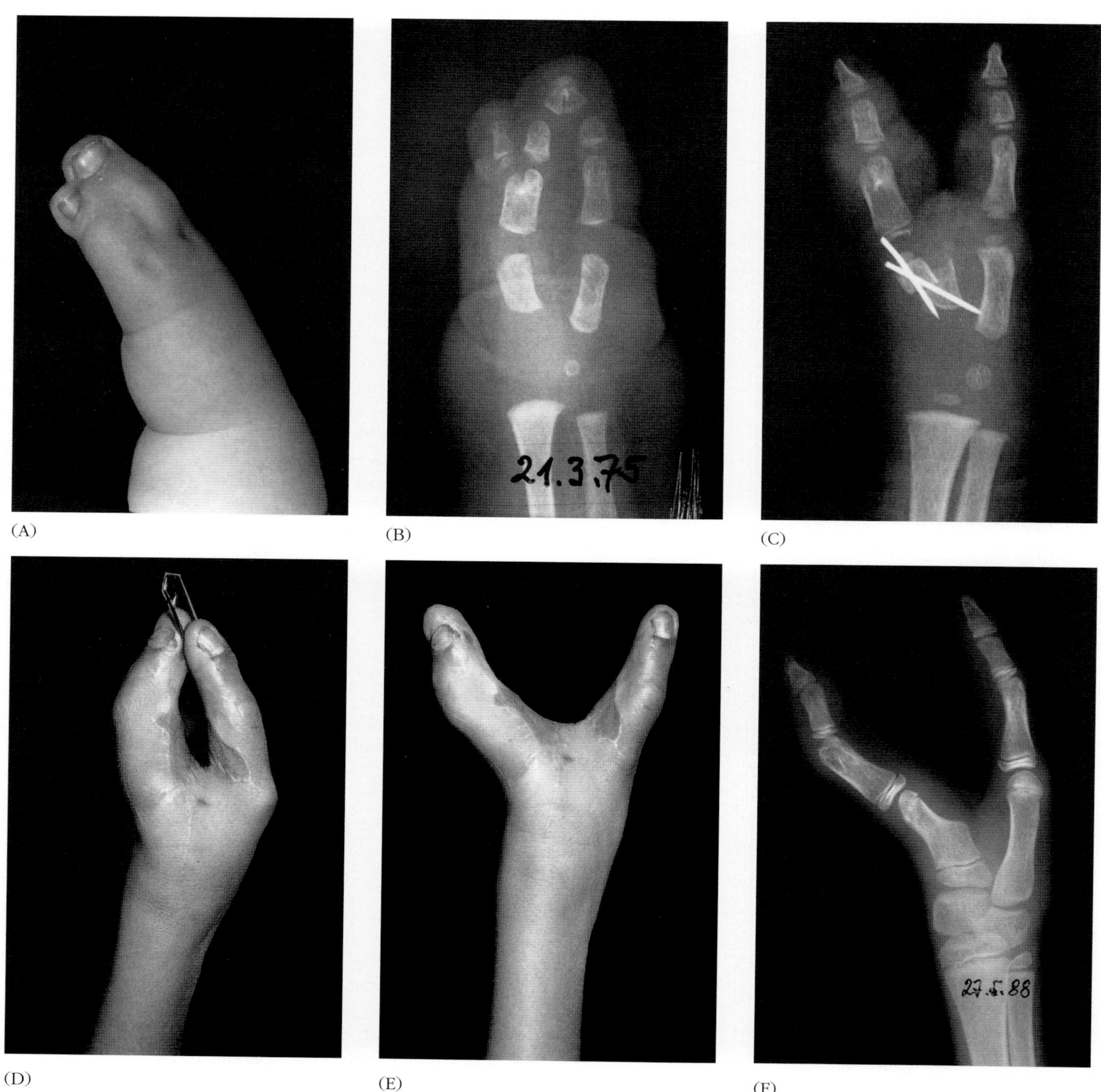

Figure 30.7

Ulnar deficiency with a small hand of two syndactylized digits with a distal bone bridge and an additional rudimentary radial digit with phalangeal synostosis (A) and (B). (C) Radiograph following syndactyly separation, removal of the additional bones and rotational angulatory osteotomy of the radial metacarpal. The result 13 years postoperatively shows a firm pinch (D) and a wide abduction of the two digits (E). (F) Note the configuration of the carpal bones in the radiograph. (From Buck-Gramcko 1997, with permission.)

involved arms; 20% of all 35 ankyloses) (see Figure 30.12).

In partial aplasia, the final extent of ossification of the ulna is often not determined in radiograms taken in the early years of life; in some patients the ossification of the fibrocartilagenous anlage occurs only in adolescence (Figure 30.9). A combination of ulna hypoplasia and radial head dislocation was found in 49% of cases (30

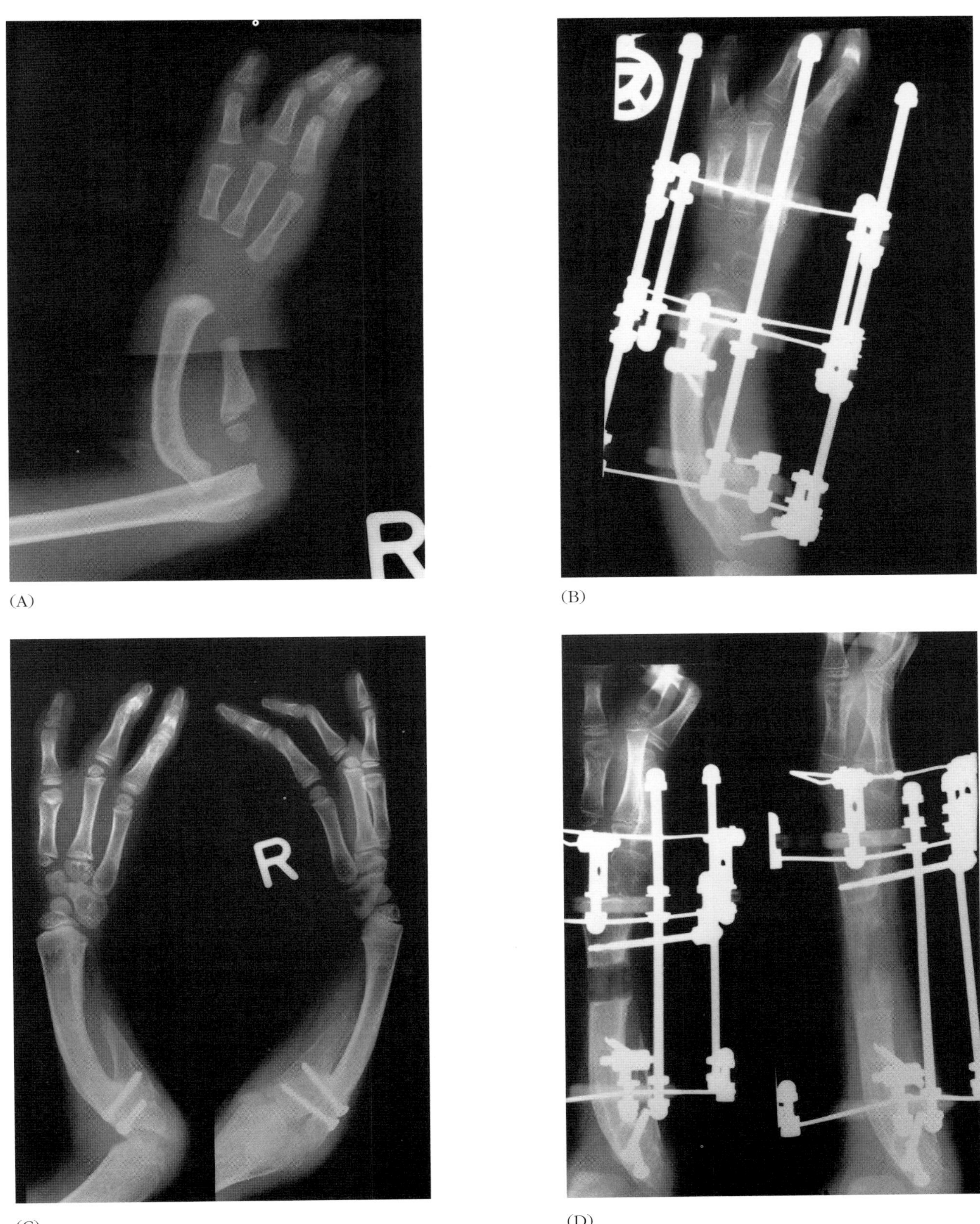

(A) (B) (C) (D)

Figure 30.8
Construction of a one-bone forearm in a patient with partial aplasia of the ulna, congenital dislocation of the radial head and oligodactyly (A). Distraction of the radius against the ulna (B) and fixation of the proximal radius to the ulna with two screws (C). Later a distraction lengthening of the whole forearm can improve the appearance (D).

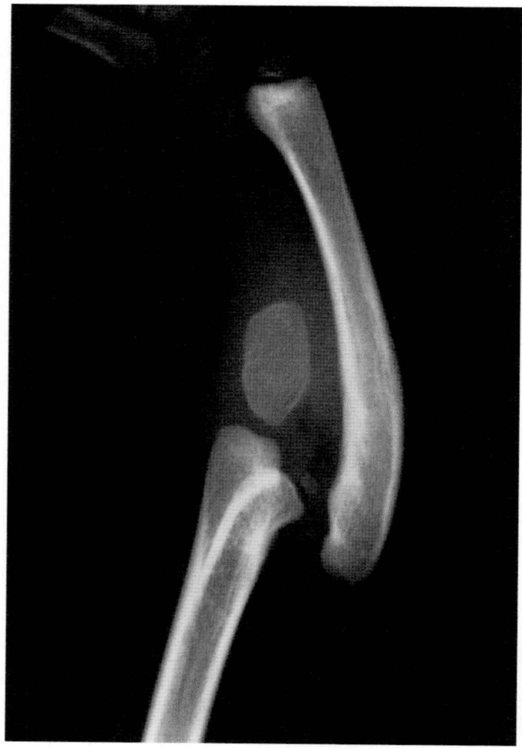

(A)

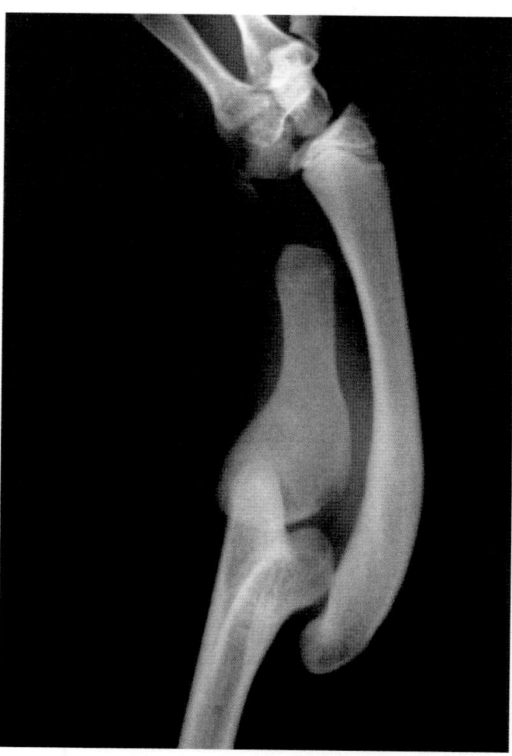

(B)

Figure 30.9

Partial aplasia of the ulna with dislocation of the radial head. The final ossification of the proximal part of the cartilagenous anlage occurred in some cases only during adolescence (A, at the age of 5, B, at 17 years).

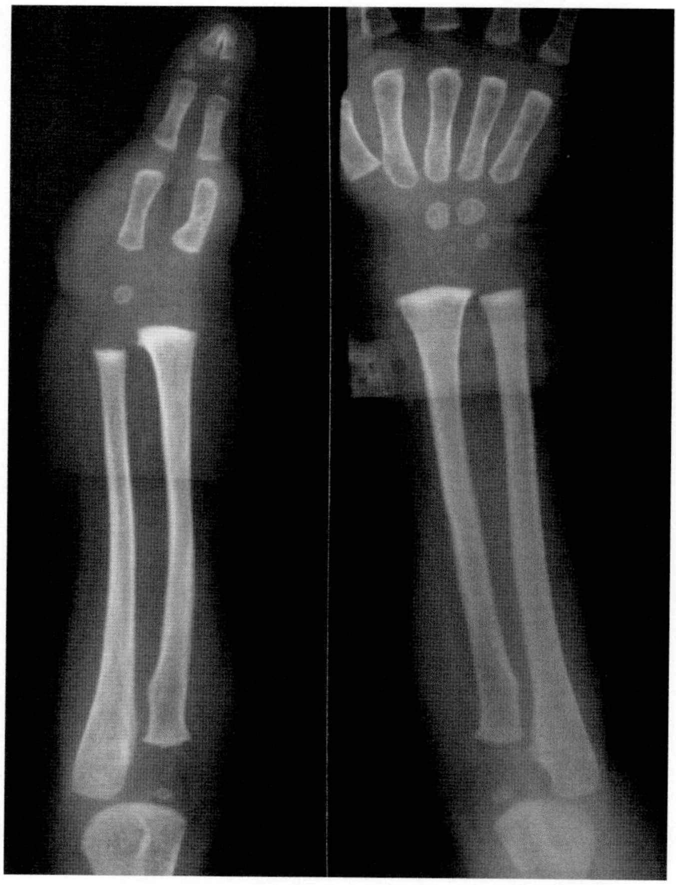

Figure 30.10

Hypoplasia of the ulna with oligosyndactyly. There is some shortening of the forearm; the ulna is slender and has a low coronoid process. Note also the brachymesophalangia in both digits.

of the 61 arms with these dislocations; 15% of all 200 involved arms). A radiohumeral synostosis was present in 10 arms with ulna hypoplasia (5% of all arms and 28.5% of the 35 arms with these synostoses).

The most severe deformity in ulnar deficiencies is the combination of complete aplasia of the ulna and radiohumeral synostosis (Figure 30.11). This will be discussed in the next paragraph, but the numbers should be given here. Such a combination was seen in our patients in 18 arms (9% of all 200 involved arms; 51% of all synostoses at the elbow). Another severe abnormality is the total absence of the ulna, with an unstable elbow joint, a slender radius, a hand with only one or two digital rays, and a severe flexion contracture of the elbow with pterygium, as shown in Figure 30.2. This deformity was found in 8 patients with 11 involved arms; two of these patients suffer from Cornelia de Lange syndrome.

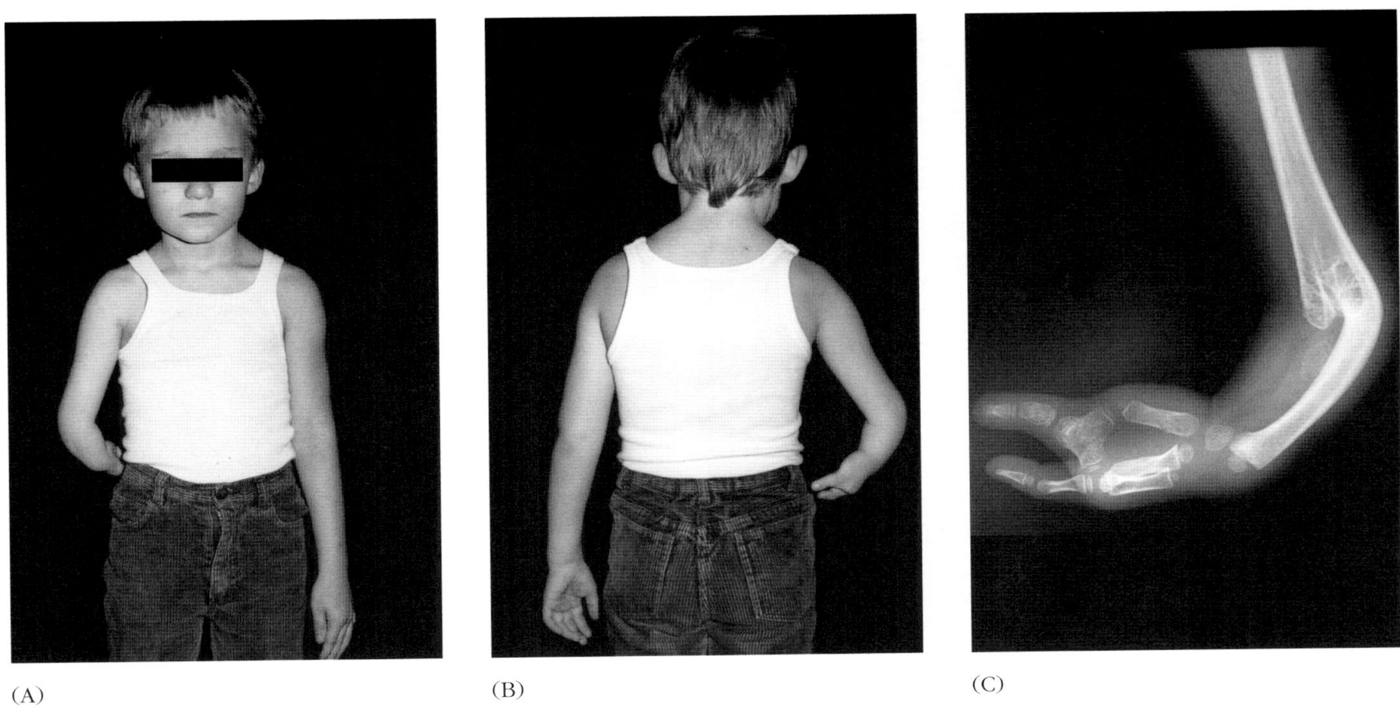

(A) (B) (C)

Figure 30.11
The most severe type of ulnar deficiency: aplasia of the ulna, radiohumeral synostosis with rotational angulatory deformity at the elbow, shortening of the forearm, and oligodactyly with a rare type of osseous syndactyly of the two ulnar digits. The position of the arm is typical for this deformity.

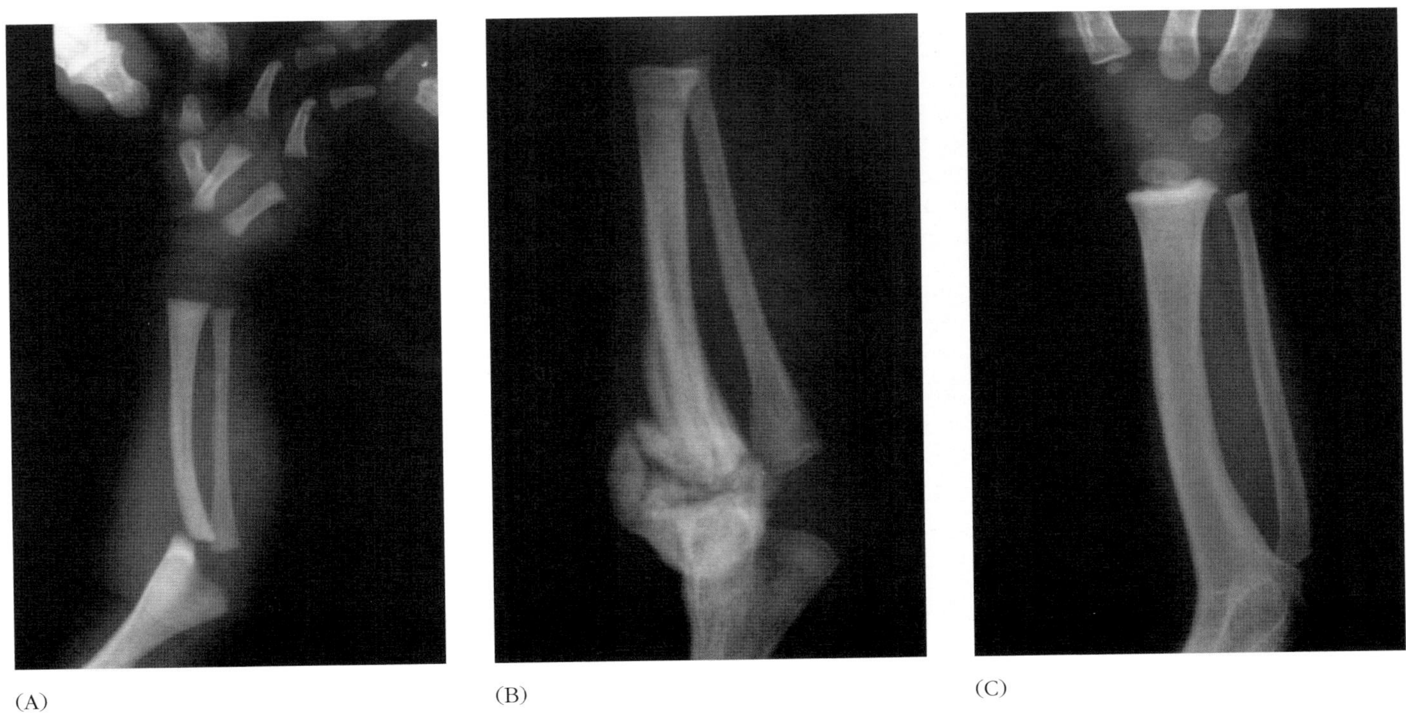

(A) (B) (C)

Figure 30.12
Fracture of a radiohumeral synostosis during delivery (radiogram 3 days later; A). Excessive callus formation in the elbow region of the non-immobilized arm 3 weeks later (B). Radiogram 2 years later with no signs of this injury (C).

In six arms there was also the rare combination of aplasia of the ulna and congenital dislocation of the head of the radius. In these cases there is an unstable elbow joint, although the range of active motion is fairly good.

Elbow

An almost normal configuration of the articular surfaces of the elbow joint is seen only in patients with hypoplasia of the ulna, but also in these cases the coronoid process is lower (see Figure 30.10). In all other types of ulnar deficiency there is some deformation, at least hypoplasia of all articular parts (see Figures 30.1–30.3, 30.9). The most severe form is an absence of any joints, radiohumeral synostosis or elbow ankylosis (Figure 30.11). This is always combined with an extreme shortening of the arm, mainly in the forearm; a rotational deformity in strong pronation; and a dorsal angulation at the elbow level. Any functional use of the hand – which always has a reduced number of digits – is possible only with compensatory rotation in the shoulder. Such a radiohumeral synostosis was seen in 34 of our 164 patients (20%) or in 35 of the 200 involved arms (17.5%); this means that one patient has a bilateral ankylosis of the elbow. The synostosis was combined with ulna hypoplasia in 7 arms (3.2%), with partial aplasia in 10 arms (5%), and with complete aplasia in 18 arms (9%).

Quite unusual changes were seen in one of our patients. He suffered from a fracture of a radiohumeral synostosis at the delivery (Figure 30.12 left), during the fracture healing a radiogram 3 weeks later showed an excessive callus formation (no immobilization of the tiny arm; Figure 30.11 centre), but 2 years later no signs of this trauma remained (Figure 30.11 right).

Congenital dislocation of the radial head is a frequent anomaly in ulnar deficiencies. In our patients it happened in 61 of the 200 involved arms (30.5%) and was combined with ulna hypoplasia in 25 arms (12.5%; 41% of all dislocations), with partial aplasia in 30 arms (15%; 49% of all dislocations), and with complete aplasia of the ulna in 6 arms (3%; 10% of all radial head dislocations).

Upper arm and shoulder

Although Masson et al (1995) found 19 patients (16%) with afflictions of the shoulder girdle, in most other reports the proximal part of the upper extremity is not mentioned. Even in our patients the data about the shoulder are incomplete; in the majority, the range of motion was normal. The reported anomalies include hypoplasia of the humerus and the glenoid, as well as hypoplasia of the muscles.

Associated anomalies

The reported frequency of further anomalies on parts of the child other than the involved extremity is quite variable. Masson et al (1995) found additional anomalies in 64 of their 116 patients (55%); the majority involved the musculoskeletal system. In our 164 patients, 43 (26%) have associated anomalies. More than half have the FFU syndrome (24 patients); one of them also suffered from hereditary cartilaginous exostosis. One patient each has neurofibromatosis, cardiac disease, esophageal atresia, anal atresia, or Fanconi anemia; the others have musculoskeletal anomalies.

Surgical treatment

There is no place for conservative treatment of ulnar deficiencies, not even for the often recommended splintage to prevent any progression in the ulnar deviation of the wrist. Experience has shown that it is useless and bothers both mother and child.

In our patients, as in most reports, the majority of operations were performed on the hand. Of 262 operative procedures, 242 (92.3%) were applied to the hand. The most frequent were syndactyly separations (63 hands), widening of the first web space (52 hands), rotational osteotomies of the first metacarpal (28 hands), or in cases of hands with only two fingers of both metacarpals (21 hands), and the removal of additional bones or rudimentary digits (36 hands). Many of these procedures were combined in one hand and performed in one stage. Usually, the result will improve the function considerably.

This is particularly impressive in oligodactylous hands with only two digits, bound together by complete syndactyly (see Figures 30.3 and 30.10). Often, some additional bones are seen in the distal part. It is possible to convert such a primitive 'paddle' into a pinching hand by several operations: syndactyly separation with excision of useless additional bones, rotational osteotomies of the radial or both metacarpals, and widening of the web space, created by syndactyly separation (Figure 30.7).

The most problematic procedure is rotational osteotomy at the metacarpal level. It is a successful and safe operation in cases of a hand with three digits, in which the thumb is not rotated and is lying in the plane of the other metacarpals. In combination with a widening of the first web space the new abducted and rotated position of the thumb is a permanent one, because the thenar muscles act in the same direction. This is quite

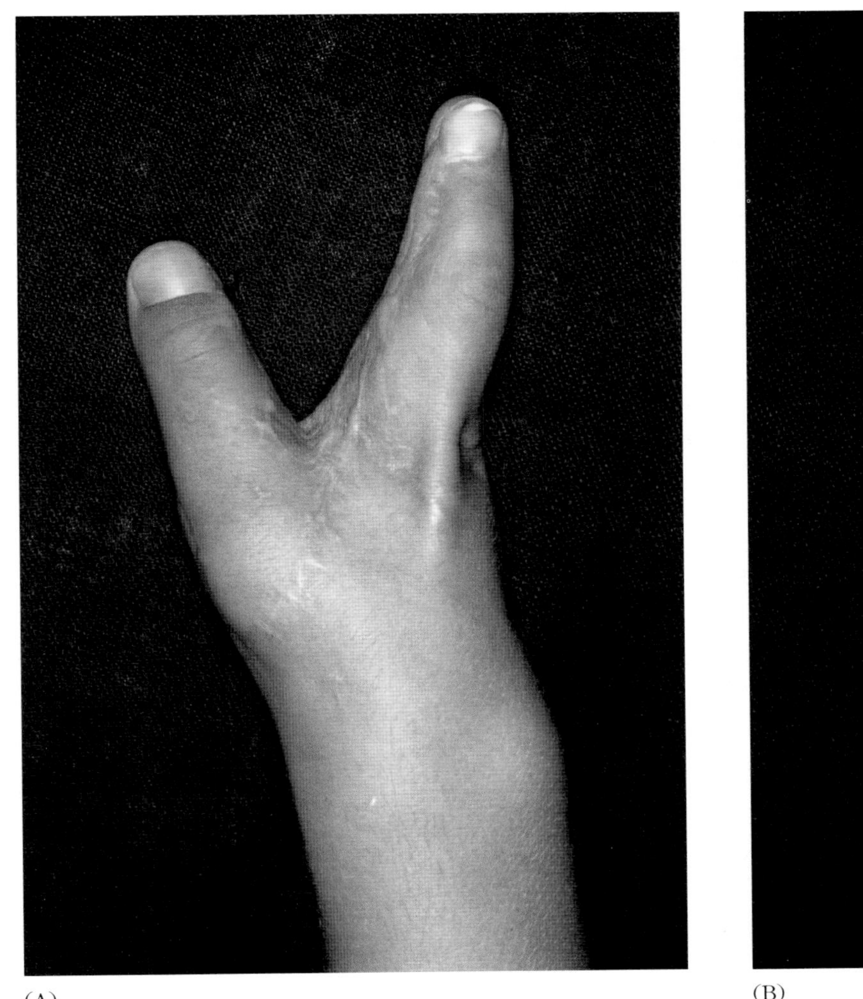

(A)

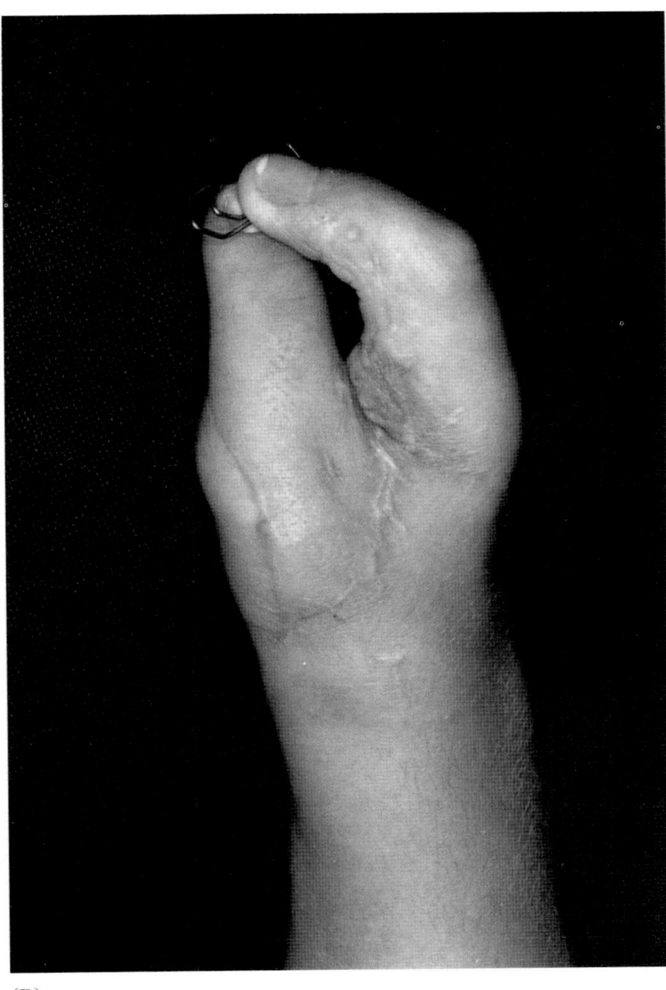

(B)

Figure 30.13
(A) Two-finger hand following syndactyly separation and two subsequent rotational osteotomies of both metacarpals without muscle transposition (performed elsewhere). (B) The result shows no adaequate rotation, so that a pulp-to-pulp pinch is not possible (compare this with the result in Figure 30.7).

different in a hand with only two digital rays; here a rotational osteotomy turns the distal skeletal elements, but increases the derotational action of the interossei. During further growth the pull of these muscles will direct the formation of new bone in a derotational sense, so that the two fingers again lie in the same plane (Figure 30.13). This can be prevented not only by sufficient bone rotation at the osteotomy site of at least 90°, but mainly by the transposition of the insertions of the interossei to the opposite side of the base of the proximal phalanx. In this way, the pull of the intrinsic muscles will act in the rotational sense and a permanent correction can be expected.

Syndactyly separation in these small hands with relative little skin can be facilitated by a new operative technique. Transverse soft tissue distraction – if necessary following division of a distal bone bridge – for some 5–6 weeks extends the skin so far that an almost direct wound closure is possible (Figure 30.14). It is important to allow the extended skin and the edema to 'settle' for about 2 weeks following the distraction period. We have developed special distraction devices that are particularly suitable for the small hands of children in their first years of life. Our present results with this technique are very satisfying.

Other operations performed in the hand include six pollicizations of the index finger in cases of absence of the thumb, 14 separations of metacarpal synostoses, and eight stabilizations of metacarpals with absence of their proximal three-quarters. One of the latter procedures is

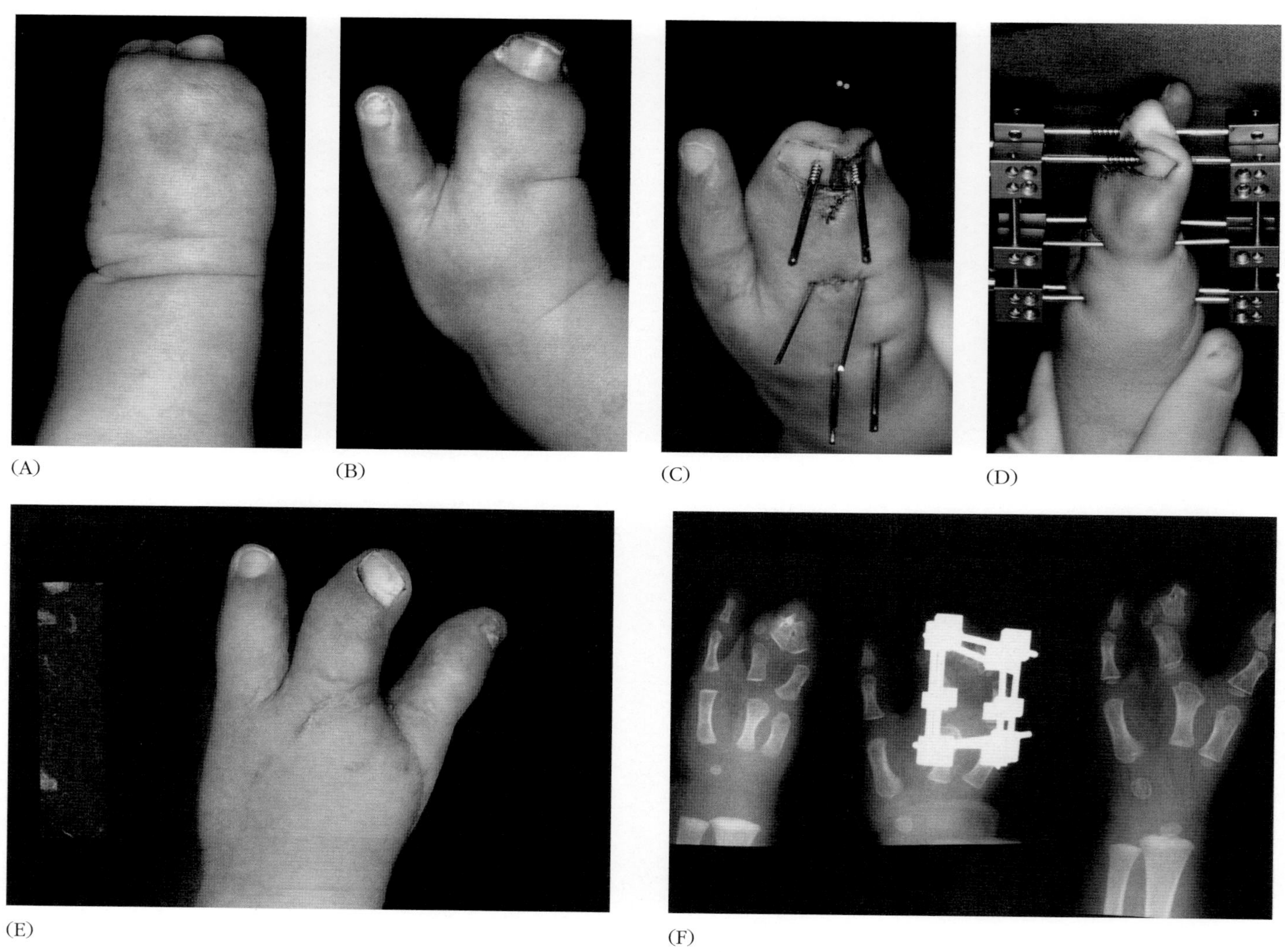

Figure 30.14

Facilitation of skin cover in syndactyly separation by transverse soft tissue distraction in a small hand with three incomplete digital rays (A). In a first stage the best finger (on the ulnar border) was separated (B). In the second stage the distal bone bridge between the two radial digits was divided and the threaded pins were inserted (C). Distraction was performed for 5–6 weeks by the completed device (D) and finally the syndactyly separated. A dorsal advancement flap was used for the cover of the widened new first web space (E). The three stages are also demonstrated in radiographs (F).

illustrated in Figure 30.5. In hands with two- or three-phalangeal fingers without a metacarpal, the presence or absence of flexor and extensor tendons and stable joints will determine the preservation or amputation of such a finger. In some bilateral cases it may be possible to combine both procedures: the amputation of the less functional finger (which would otherwise disturb the function of the whole hand) and the construction of a stable finger in the contralateral hand by using bone grafts from the amputated finger.

In the forearm the excision of the cartilagenous anlage remains controversial. We have done it seven times, three of them in combination with the construction of a one-bone forearm. To lessen the ulnar deviation forces, we have transposed the tendons of the ulnar wrist flexor and extensor to the radial side at the same session. Care was taken not to damage the ulnar nerve, which lies immediately anterior to the anlage.

The indication for the construction of a one-bone forearm in ulnar deficiencies was originally given only in the rare cases of unstable elbow and forearm. Nowadays, the modern technique of distraction lengthening can be combined successfully with this procedure (Figure 30.8). In a first stage, following division of the fibrous connections between radius and ulna and resection of the anlage, some longitudinal distraction of the whole radius against the ulna is performed. The dislocated radial head is brought into a better position; eventually a part of it has to be resected. The second stage is the osteosynthesis of the proximal parts of both forearm bones. Some years later a distraction lengthening of the one-bone forearm can be performed.

At the level of the elbow, the only valuable operation is the rotational angulatory osteotomy in cases of radiohumeral synostosis with rotational deformity of the whole arm (see Figure 30.11) The incorrect rotation as well as the dorsal angulation have to be corrected to bring the hand into a more functional position. The brachial artery and the nerves run very close to the bone at the osteotomy site and have to be protected very carefully.

References

Aitken GT (1969) *Proximal Femoral Focal Deficiency. A Congenital Anomaly* (National Academy of Science: Washington).

Birch-Jensen A (1949) *Congenital Deformities of the Upper Extremities* (Andelsbogtrykkeriet i Odense and Det Danske Forlag: Odense).

Broudy AS, Smith RJ (1979) Deformities of the hand and wrist with ulnar deficiency, *J Hand Surg* **4**: 304–15.

Buck-Gramcko D (1997) Ulnar deficiency. In: Saffar P, Amadio PC, Foucher G, eds, *Current Practice in Hand Surgery* (Martin Dunitz: London) 371–90.

Carroll RE, Bowers WH (1977) Congenital deficiency of the ulna, *J Hand Surg* **2**: 169–74.

Cole RJ, Manske PR (1997) Classification of ulnar deficiency according to the thumb and first web, *J Hand Surg* **22A**: 479–88.

Flatt AE (1994) *The Care of Congenital Hand Anomalies*, 2nd edn (Quality Medical Publications: St Louis).

Johnson J, Omer GE (1985) Congenital ulnar deficiency. Natural history and therapeutic implications, *Hand Clin* **1**: 499–510.

Kühne D, Lenz W, Petersen D et al (1967) Defekt von Femur und Fibula mit Amelie, Peromelie oder ulnaren Strahldefekten der Arme. Ein Syndrom, *Humangenetik* **3**: 244–63.

Kümmel W (1895) *Die Missbildungen der Extremitaeten durch Defekt, Verwachsung und Ueberzahl* (Th G Fisher & Co: Cassel).

Marcus NA, Omer GE (1984) Carpal deviation in congenital ulnar deficiency, *J Bone Joint Surg* **66A**: 1003–7.

Masson MV, Bennett JB, Cain TE (1995) Congenital absence of the ulna. Paper read at the 50th Meeting of the American Society for Surgery of the Hand, San Francisco, California, 15 September 1995.

O'Rahilly R (1951) Morphological patterns in limb deficiencies and duplications, *Am J Anat* **89**: 135–94.

Riordan DC, Mills EH, Alldredge RH (1961) Congenital absence of the ulna, *J Bone Joint Surg* **43A**: 614.

IV Inflammatory diseases

31 Rheumatoid arthritis
Pathogenesis of wrist and finger deformities

Raoul Tubiana

Introduction

Rheumatoid arthritis is a systemic disease which causes visceral, vascular, and nervous lesions. However, it is the synovial lesions in the joints and tendon sheaths that are the most constant feature of this affliction.

The synovial pannus

The most characteristic phenomenon is the presence of cellular infiltration in a hypertrophic synovial villus, comprising a majority of T lymphocytes plus lesser amounts of B lymphocytes and plasmocytes containing intracytoplasmic immunoglobulins. These cells are implicated in the initiation of the inflammatory process and destruction of osteoarticular structures. In addition to the destructive processes caused by immunologic reactions, the development of synovial pannus causes an increase in pressure within joints or tendon sheaths, leading to increased tension, thinning and then laxity within the fibrous structures, to which nutritional problems may be added.

Rheumatoid arthritis causes several deformities, these are most obvious in the wrist and hand. Surgical treatment is only one of the elements in the treatment of RA, and the hand is only one of the sites of the disease. Treatment of hand problems cannot be considered in isolation. It is necessary to evaluate not only the hands and wrists, but the entire patient.

Pathogenesis of the deformities of the rheumatoid wrist

The diversity of lesions, the existence of multiple distinct synovial joints, and the numerous tendon sheaths which surround the wrist, explain the variety of clinical problems that may occur at an early stage. Synovial proliferation provokes many different phenomena including capsular distension, osseous erosion, and

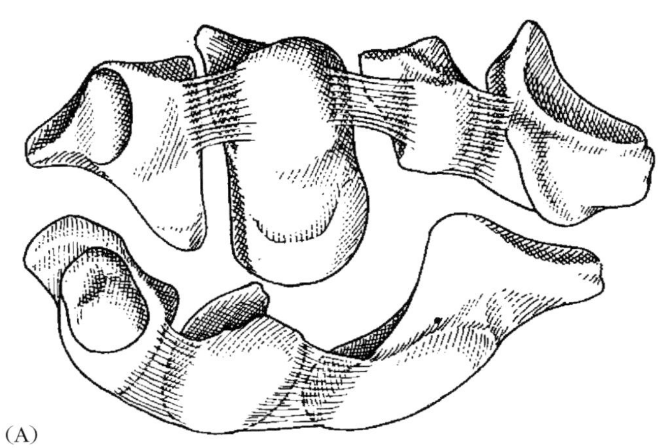

(A)

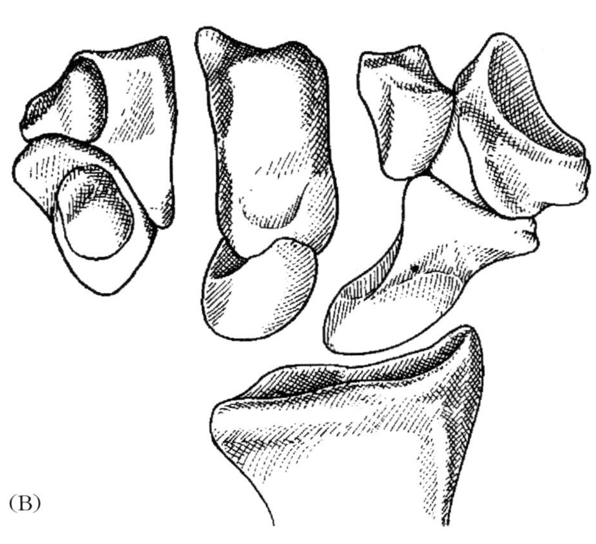

(B)

Figure 31.1

(A) The eight bones of the carpus are usually arranged into a proximal row and a distal row, although the scaphoid straddles the lunate-capitate interspace. (B) The concept of the three longitudinal parallel chains of bones: ulnar, central, and radial columns.

tendinous and ligamentous destruction, all of which may lead to a variety of deformities, that initially seem difficult to classify. In fact, these deformities are predictable when their processes of deformation are studied.

The concept of the carpal bones as chains of longitudinal parallel bones (Navarro 1937, Taleisnik 1985), where the proximal row is in an intercalated segment, allows a better understanding of the respective displacements of the bones during both normal and pathological movements (Figures 31.1A and B). This also allows a convenient classification of the deformities that can arise in rheumatoid arthritis of the wrist (Tubiana et al 1980). The deformities can be classified according to which group – ulnar, central or radial – is primarily affected.

Deformities of the ulnar side

Rheumatoid arthritis of the wrist most often starts on the ulnar side, in the sheath of extensor carpi ulnaris (ECU), at the distal radio-ulnar joint, and at the site of insertion of the postero-ulnar fibrous complex into the postero-ulnar angle of the radius (Figure 31.2). It is at these points, where the synovium forms cul-de-sacs and is well developed, that an abundant pannus of synovium is produced.

The fibrous structures weakened by the rheumatoid arthritis invasion are not able to stabilize the ulnar side of the wrist. The ulnar column of the carpus tends to slide anteriorly, leading to a rotation in supination of the carpus with respect to the distal extremity of the radius. Alternatively, the distal radio-ulnar joint may dislocate. The *posterior prominence of the ulnar head* is accentuated by the distension of the distal radio-ulnar joint, which is invaded relatively early by the pannus. A notch is often visible at the base of the ulnar styloid on the early X-rays.

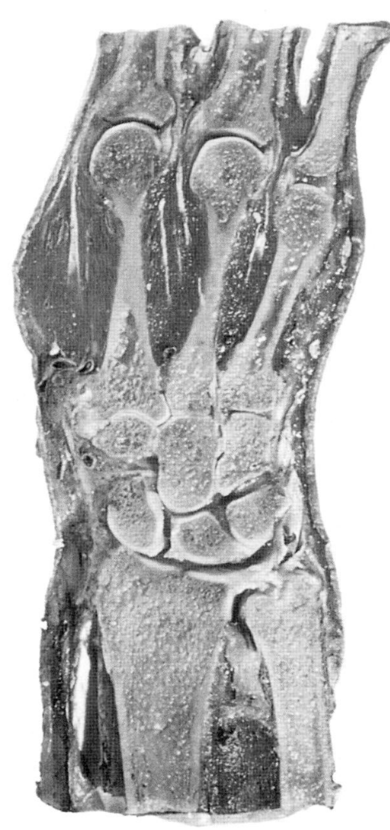

Figure 31.2
The triangular fibrocartilage complex; frontal section.

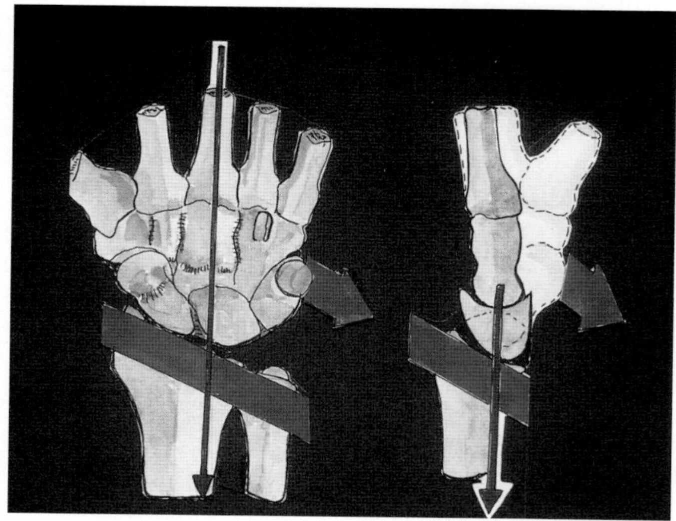

Figure 31.3
The radial joint surface, concave in both directions, presents a double obliquity facing both medially and anteriorly. If the capsuloligamentous structures are distended, the wrist tends to slide in these two directions.

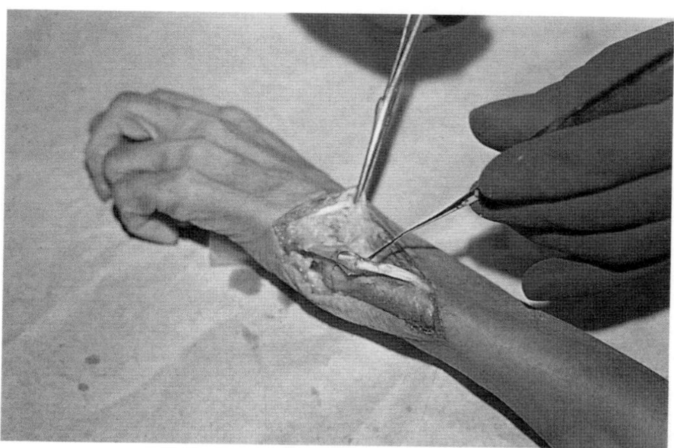

Figure 31.4
Volar displacement of the extensor carpi ulnaris tendon.

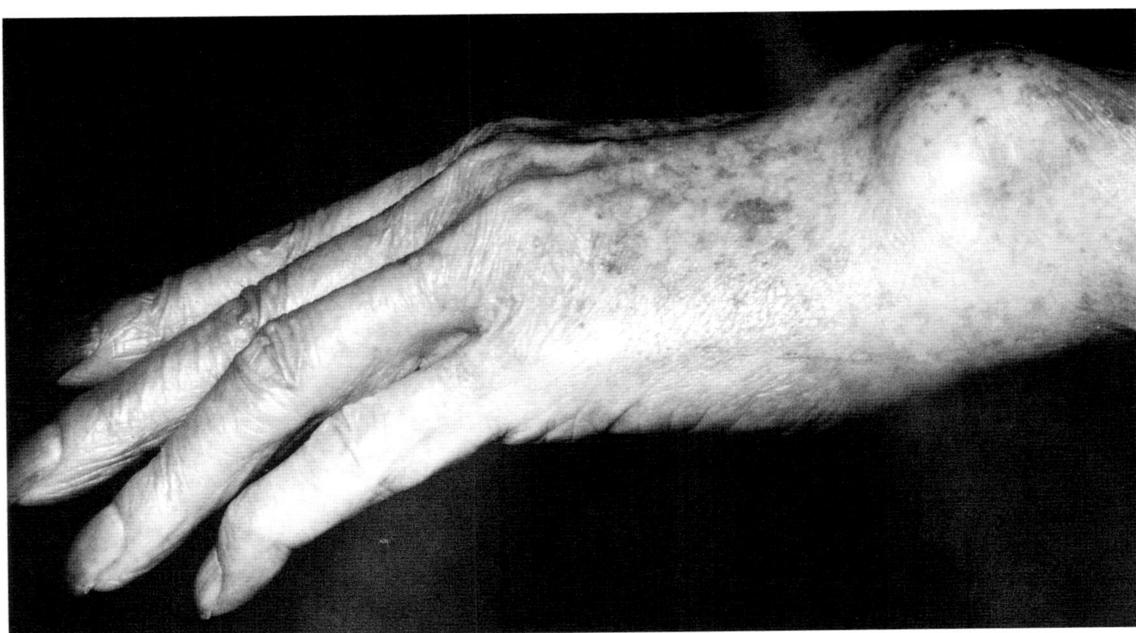

Figure 31.5
The posterior prominence of the subluxated ulnar head is accentuated by an anterior displacement of the ulnar part of the carpus. (Caput ulnae syndrome.)

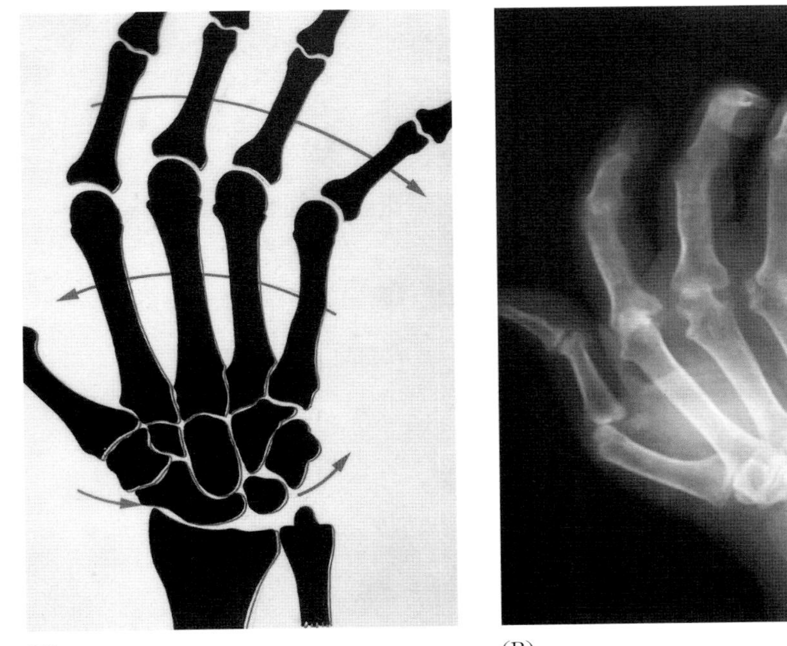

(A)

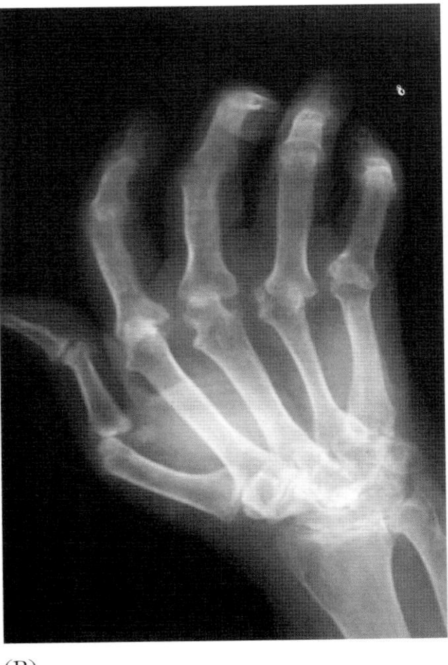

(B)

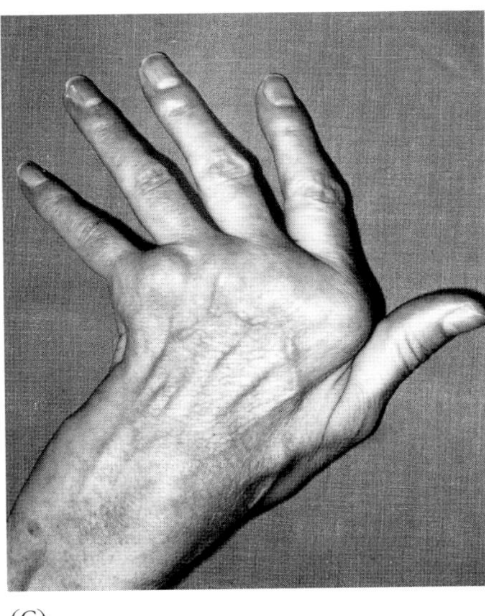

(C)

Figure 31.6
(A and B) Relationship between radial inclination of the carpometacarpal unit and ulnar deviation of the fingers. (C) Marked ulnar deviation of the fingers without deviation at the wrist level.

Invasion and weakening of the radio-ulnar triangular ligament result in the posterior displacement of the ulnar head, creating the 'caput ulnae' syndrome described by Backdahl (1963). The ECU tendon is normally held in a bony gutter by its tendon sheath, but once the sheath becomes distended by the pannus, the ECU tendon starts to progressively slide anteriorly. Being a wrist extensor, the ECU becomes a flexor and causes the ulnar side of the carpus to displace volarly.

Destabilization of the ulnar part of the carpus allows *ulnar translation of the carpus* (Figure 31.3). Destruction of the postero-medial structures, which are inserted onto the radius allows the flexor carpi ulnaris (FCU), reinforced by the ECU, to displace the ulnar column of

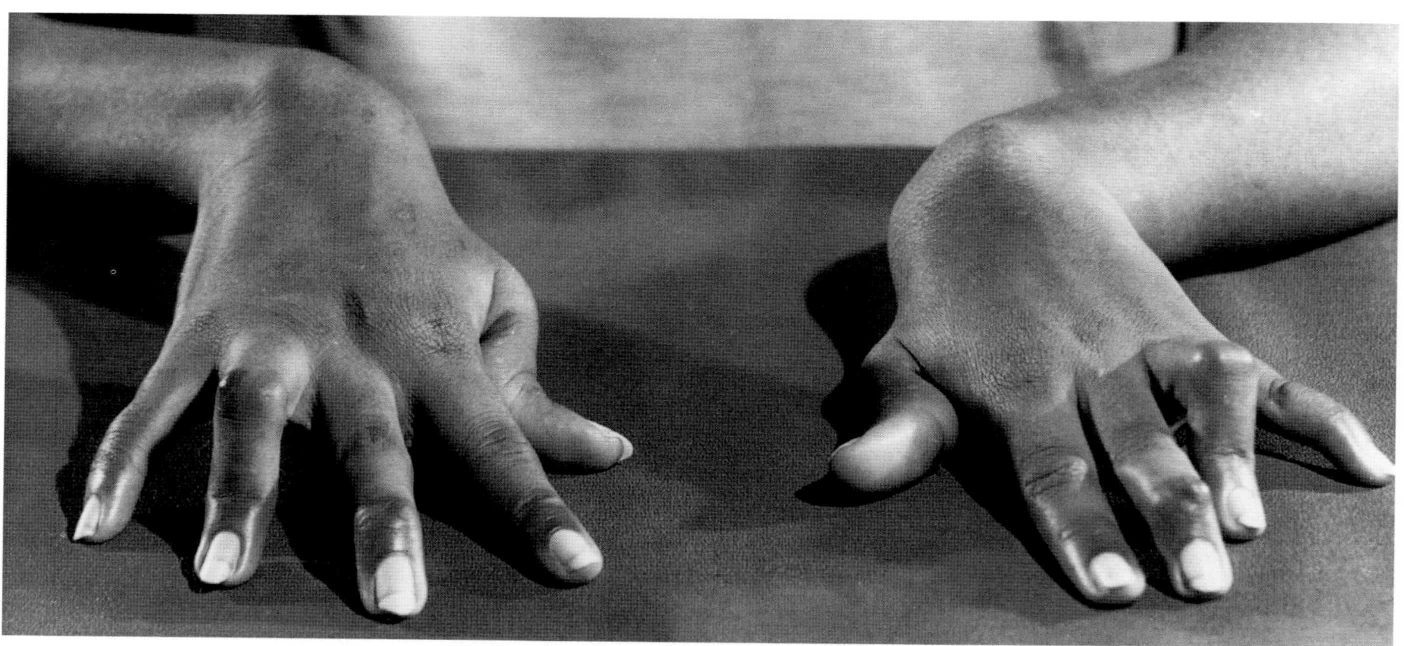

Figure 31.7
Reverse deviation. In juvenile arthritis, the wrist is often in ulnar deviation and the fingers in radial deviation.

the wrist volarly (Figure 31.4). The posterior subluxation of the ulnar head is often accentuated by an anterior displacement of the wrist (Figure 31.5) when the forearm is supinated. The extensor carpi radialis longus (ECRL), which now has no opposing force from the ECU, will draw the wrist and metacarpals into radial deviation. Shapiro (1968) established a correlation between the radial deviation of the carpometacarpal block and the ulnar deviation of the fingers according to the principle of Landsmeer's kinetic chain, in which the carpometacarpal block forms the intercalated segment between the radius and the phalanx (Figure 31.6) (Landsmeer 1960, 1968).

An inverse variation of ulnar deviation of the carpometacarpal block, which is seen in juvenile polyarthritis, may be accompanied by radial deviation of the fingers (Tubiana and Hakstian 1966) (see Figure 31.7). However, the deformities of the fingers often precede those of the wrist. This indicates that factors other than wrist deviation must be responsible for the deviation of the metacarpophalangeal (MP) joints. A study by Brahim et al (1980) confirms this proposition. In a series of 81 hands affected by rheumatoid arthritis, 93% of the wrists in radial deviation had coexisting radial deviation of the wrist. It can be concluded that in a rheumatoid hand, where the joints have lost their stability as a result of the rheumatoid synovitis, a lateral deviation of the carpometacarpal block may produce an opposite deviation of the fingers.

Posterior subluxation of the ulnar head threatens the extensor tendons. The prominence of the ulnar head, together with osteophytes, can produce *ruptures of most ulnar extensor tendons*, starting with the extensor digiti quinti (Figure 31.8). When this tendon is ruptured, the clinician must intervene to prevent subsequent rupture of the common digital extensors.

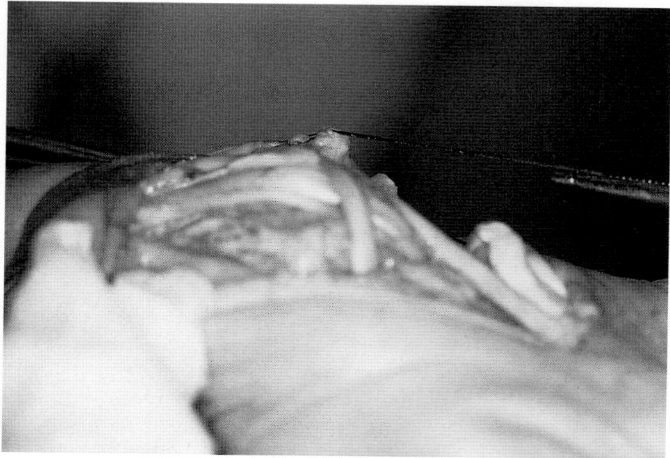

Figure 31.8
Prominence of the ulnar head with osteophytes producing ruptures of extensor tendons of the little finger.

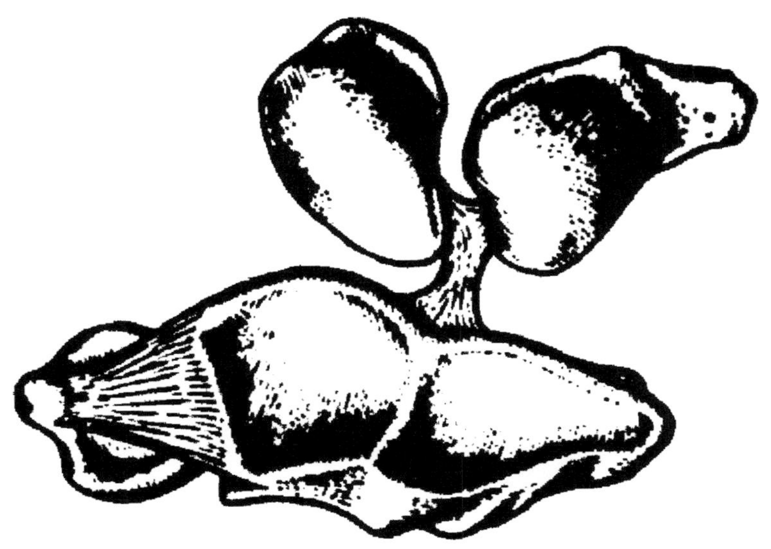

Figure 31.9
The radioscapholunate ligament.

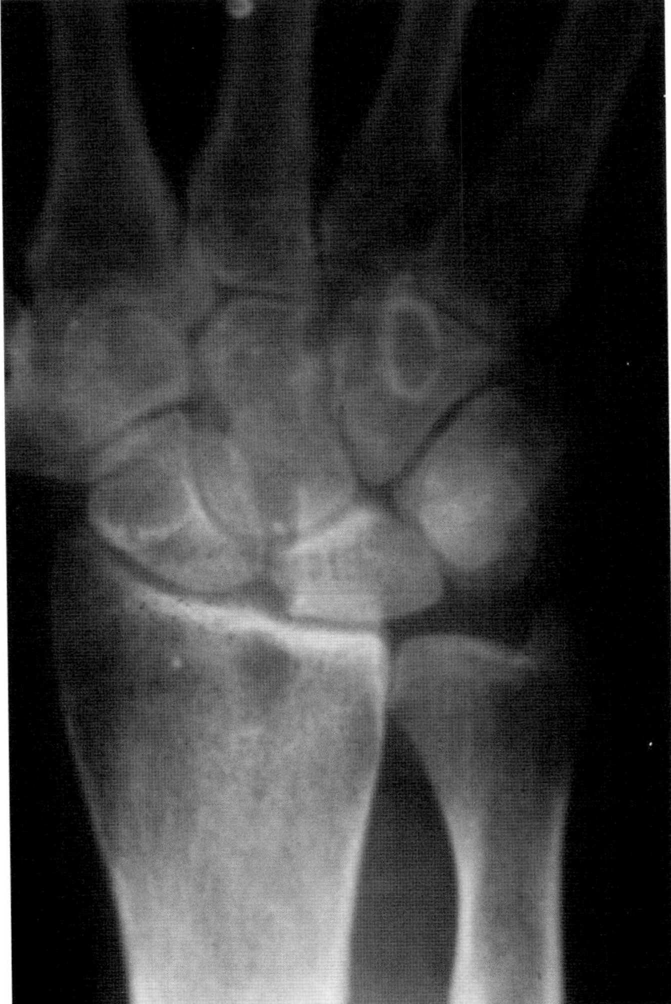

Figure 31.10
Geode in the radius at the insertion of the radioscapholunate ligament.

Central deformities

In the central forms, rheumatoid invasion often begins at the radial insertion of the radioscapholunate ligament of Testut and Kuentz (1923) (Figure 31.9) with its rich blood supply (Mannerfelt and Raven 1978). This is characterized by the appearance of geodes in the radius, the proximal pole of the scaphoid, and the lunate (Figure 31.10). The invasion of the ligament is followed by the destruction of the scapholunate interosseous ligament and is radiologically recognizable by the appearance of a scapholunate dissociation; it will produce a destabilization of the central column. On the frontal plane, the dissociation is accompanied by an ulnar translation and rotation of the lunate, which pushes the triquetrum distally and ulnarly (Figure 31.11). It is accepted that the lunocapitate joint is a weak point in the carpal structure (Poirier and Charpy 1926), as there are no ligaments

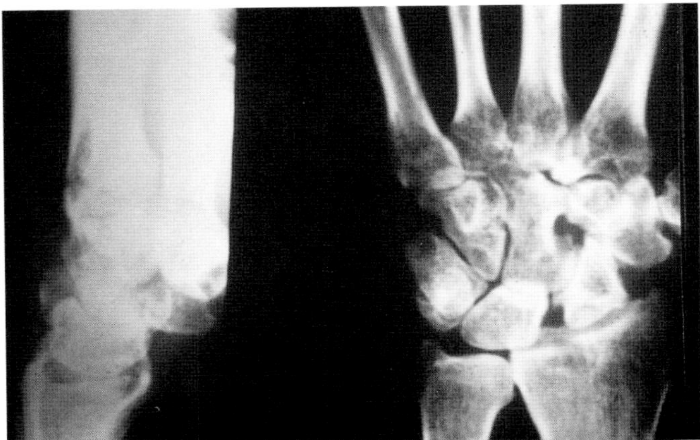

Figure 31.11
Scapholunate dissociation.

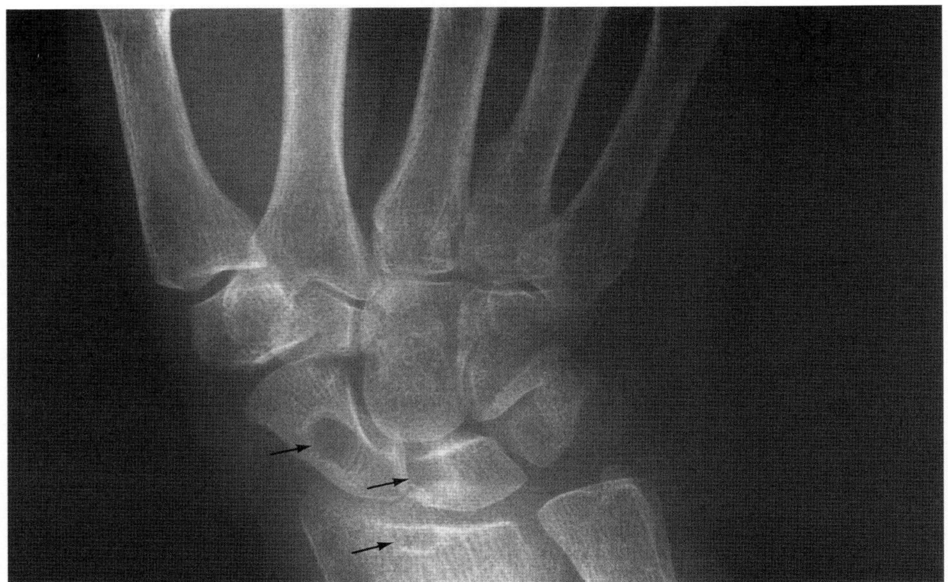

Figure 31.12

In spite of advance bony destruction in the radius, lunate, and scaphoid, the articular surface of the capitate is still normal.

between the two bones. It may be the lack of ligamentous insertion which protects the capitate from synovial erosion and the integrity of the articular surface of the capitate may be noted even in the advanced stages of rheumatoid arthritis deformities. This explains the fact that there is often longer preservation of the mid-carpal joint than of the radiocarpal joint (Figure 31.12).

Instability of the central column is shown by the opposing displacements of the lunate and the capitate, which has a concertina effect, most often with the lunate in flexion relative to the radius and the capitate in extension relative to the lunate (VISI deformity) (Linscheid and Dobyns 1971) (Figure 31.13). The DISI deformity (lunate

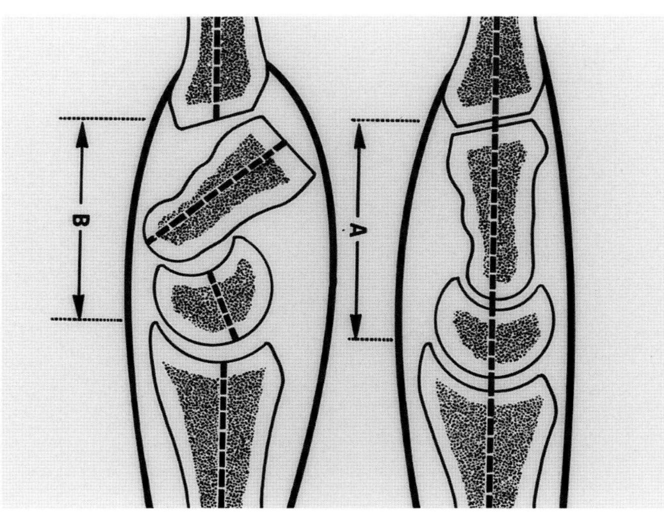

Figure 31.13

The VISI deformity is in part responsible for the loss of height of the carpus.

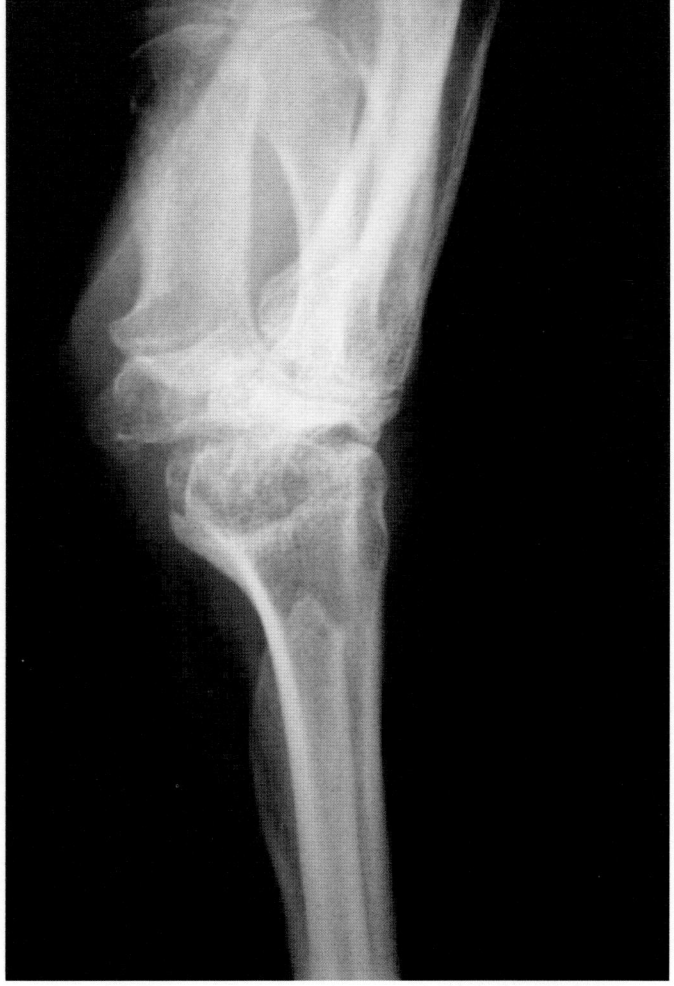

Figure 31.14

Severe destruction of the carpus.

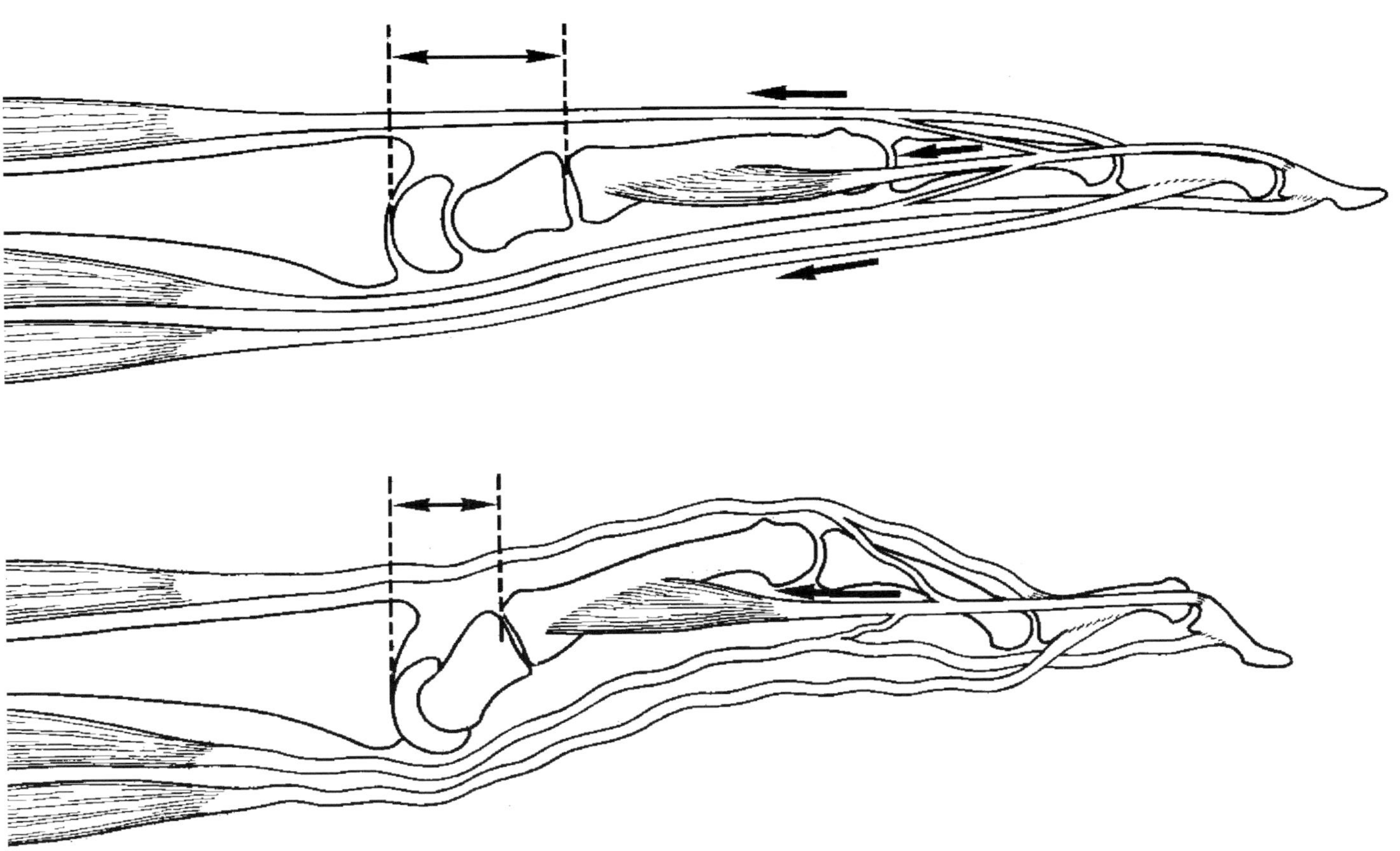

Figure 31.15
The loss of carpal height may be a cause of imbalance between the extrinsic muscles of the fingers and the intrinsic muscles, whose action is increased and may result in a swan neck deformity.

in extension) most often originates post-traumatically. The loss of height of the carpus, which results from these deformities and is aggravated by the bony destruction, creates an imbalance between the extrinsic and the intrinsic muscles (Figure 31.14). The tendons of the extrinsic finger muscles that cross the wrist are slack, and the reduction of effectiveness of the extrinsic muscles accentuates the effect of the intrinsic muscles. Shapiro (1982) saw this as a possible cause of a swan neck deformity in the fingers (Figure 31.15).

Erosion of the medial process of the radius opposite to the lunate precedes a collapse which sometimes embeds the carpus (Figure 31.16). A spontaneous radiolunate ankylosis before the collapse of the central column may limit the loss of height. Spontaneous or surgical arthrodesis of this type will ensure stability of the wrist, while reducing its mobility (Chamay et al 1983).

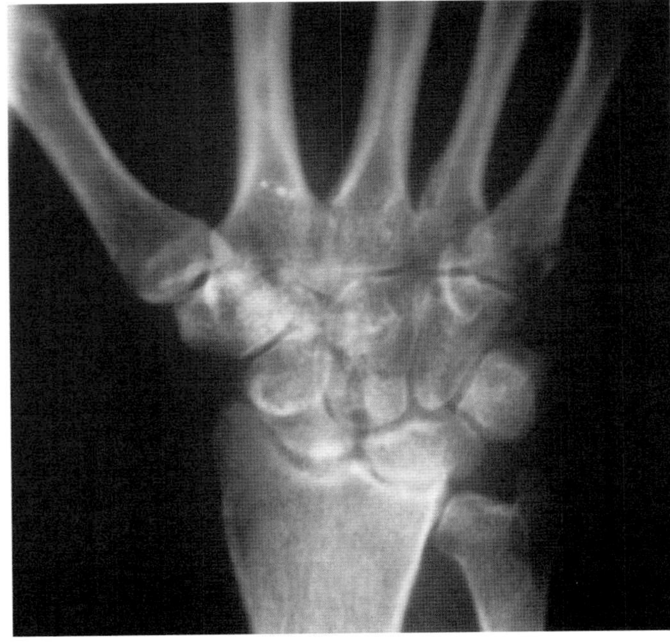

Figure 31.16
Spontaneous radioscapholunate embedding.

Radial deformities

Radiological signs in these forms are found in the radial styloid and especially in the waist of the scaphoid

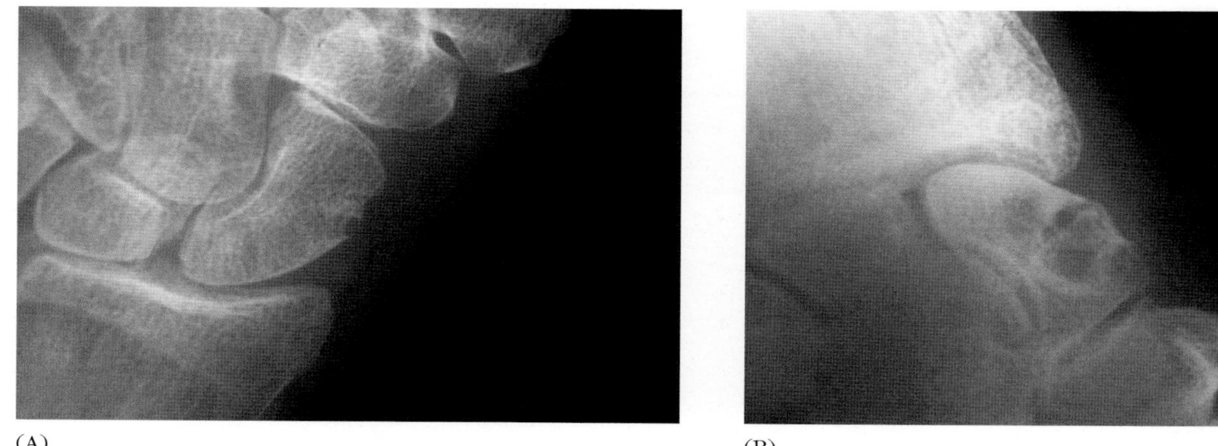

(A) (B)

Figure 31.17
(A) Radiological erosion in the waist of the scaphoid. (B) Radiologic progression of the lesions in the radial column of the carpus.

(Figure 31.17). The middle bundle of the radioscapho-capitate ligament crosses the scaphoid at this level. The scaphoid makes its normal rotational movements during radial and ulnar deviation of the wrist by pivoting around this strong ligament.

The destruction of the anterior ligamentous structures causes the scaphoid to rotate into a horizontal position and causes a loss of height of the radial column (Figure 31.18). The loss of stabilizing action between the two rows leads to a double zig-zag displacement, on both frontal and sagittal planes (VISI deformity; Linscheid and Dobyns 1971) (Figure 31.19). The proximal pole of the scaphoid is pushed posteriorly and the distal pole projects into the carpal tunnel and may come into

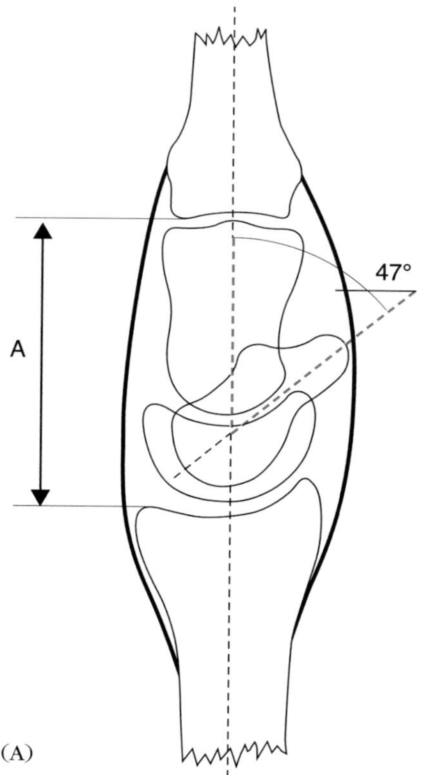

(A)

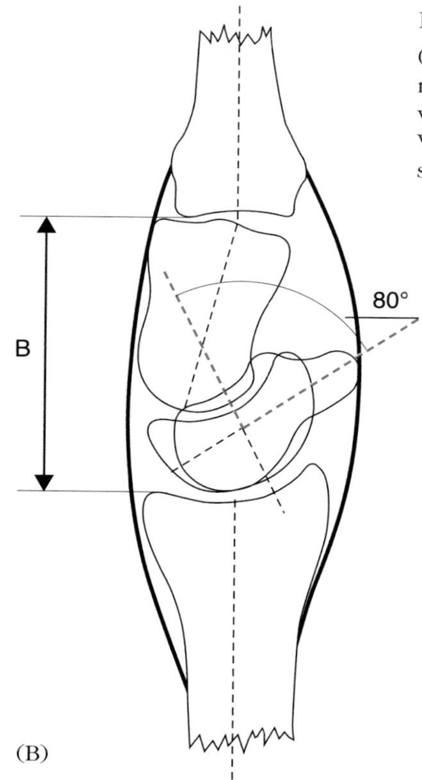

(B)

Figure 31.18
(A) Normally, the scaphoid makes an angle of about 47° with the longitudinal axis. (B) VISI deformity of the lunate, the scaphoid is rotated horizontally.

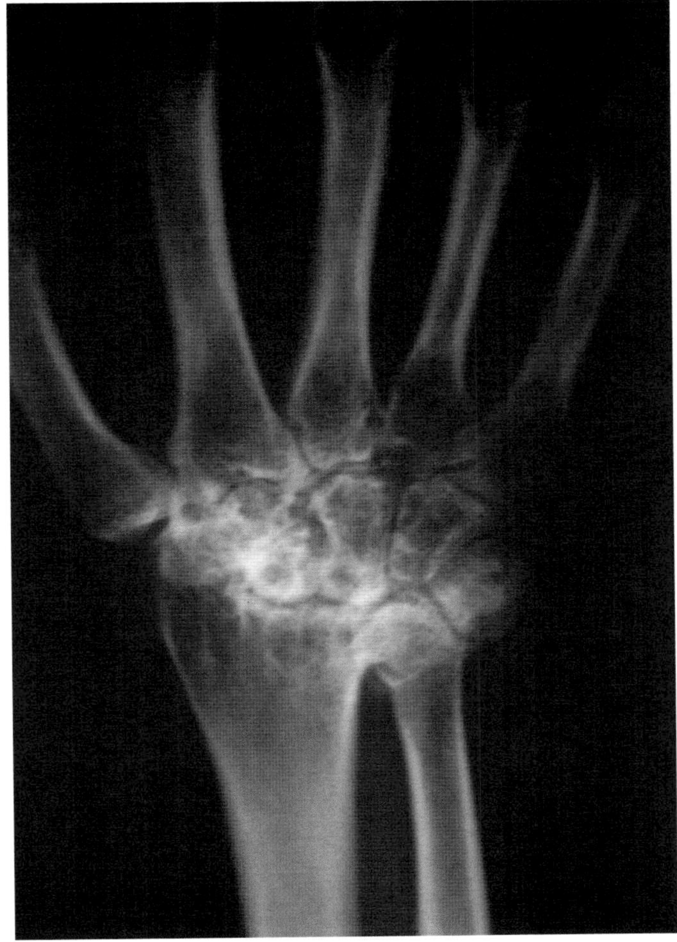

Figure 31.19
X-ray showing horizontalization of the scaphoid.

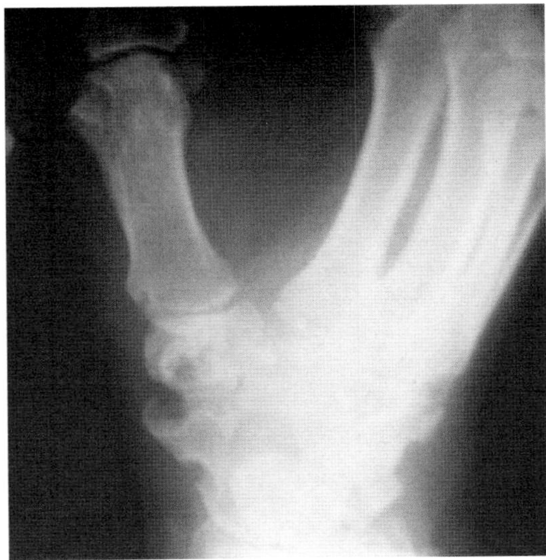

(A)

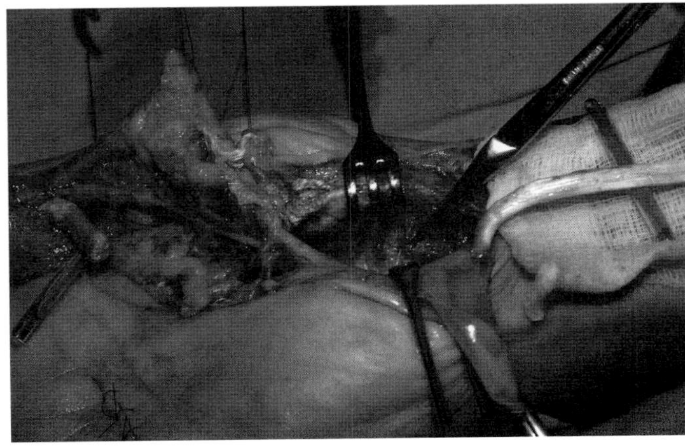

(B)

Figure 31.20
(A) Osteophyte of the horizontalized scaphoid causing (B) a rupture of the flexor pollicis longus tendon.

contact with the flexor pollicis longus tendon or even with the flexor digitorum profundus tendons and may lead to their rupture by abrasion (Mannerfelt 1969) (Figure 31.20). The erosion of the radial styloid will produce destruction of the anterolateral fibrous band which arises from here and leads to a destabilization of the wrist. The wrist will tend to slide anteriorly, down the radial slope, drawn by the preponderance of the strength of the finger flexors, which no longer have the opposing force of the extensor carpi ulnaris (Figure 31.21).

Associated deformities

These three initial sites of rheumatoid arthritis have been described to allow a schematic classification of wrist deformities. It is, however, clinically evident that the situation is much more complex and that there are often associations between the most characteristic deformities, including the following (Figure 31.22).

- Dorsal subluxation of the ulnar head.
- Palmar displacement in supination of the ulnar column of the wrist.
- Radial deviation of the carpometacarpal block.
- Ulnar translocation of the carpus.
- Concertina displacement of the carpal bones.
- Reduction in carpal height, caused by these deformities and osseous destruction.
- Anterior displacement of the wrist.

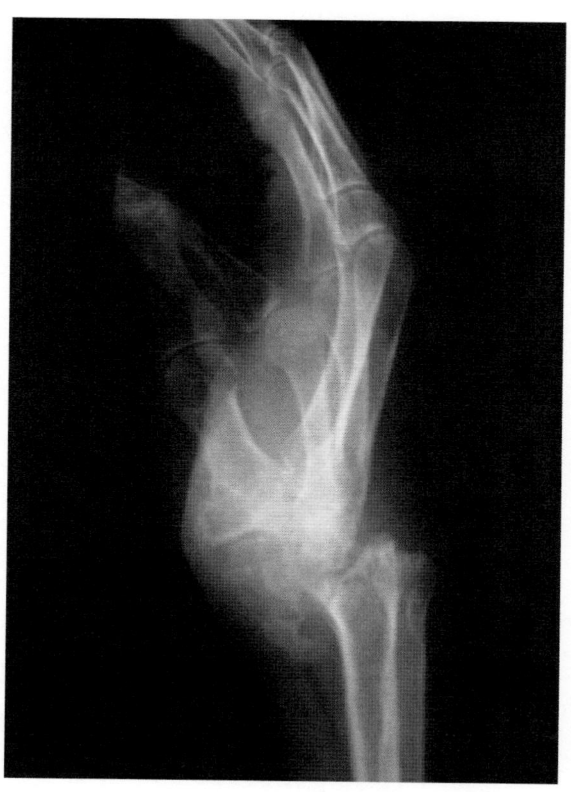

Figure 31.21
Volar subluxation of the carpus.

Natural history of the untreated rheumatoid wrist

The disease may progress towards stabilization of the wrist by fibrosis, which produces stiffness. With increasing stiffness the wrist becomes less painful. This may result in spontaneous fusion of the wrist or of the radiolunate joint: such stiffness is well tolerated in a functional position, i.e. in neutral flexion/extension and slight ulnar deviation. This will, however, require correction if it develops in marked flexion or radial deviation. Loss of prosupination constitutes a severe disability.

In other cases, the destruction of all fibrous structures causes an unstable, painful anterior dislocation of the wrist accompanied in the long term by a variable number of ruptures of the wrist and finger tendons.

It is important, from a therapeutic point of view, to anticipate at an early stage the evolution of rheumatoid disease in order to start the appropriate treatment of the wrist.

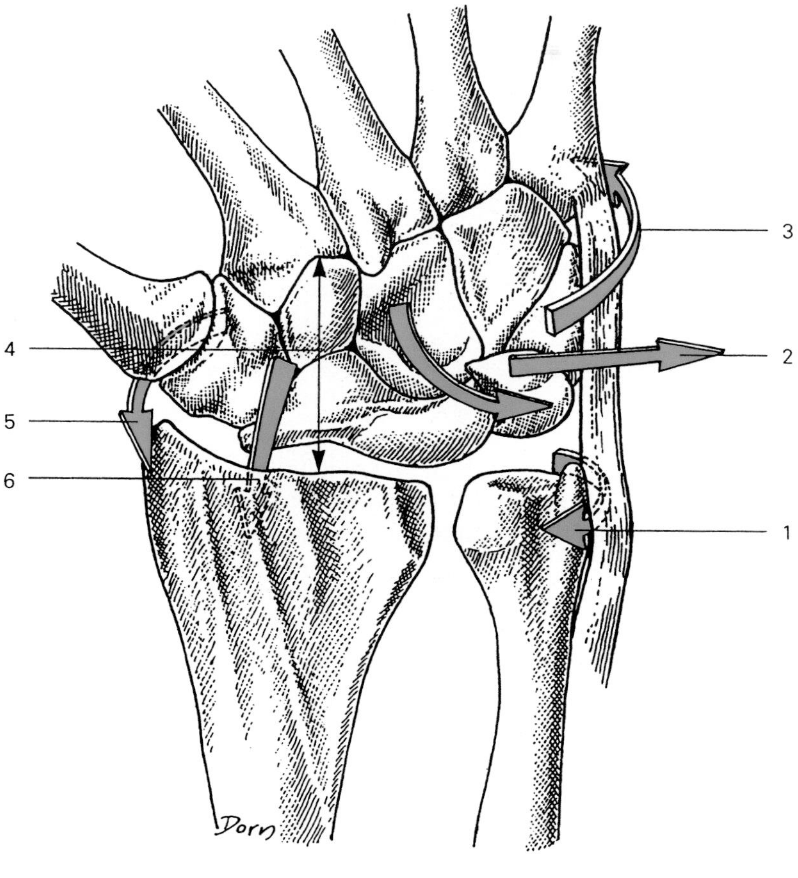

Figure 31.22
1 Dorsal subluxation of the ulnar head
2 Ulnar translocation of the carpus
3 Palmar displacement of the ulnar column of the carpus
4 Reduction in carpal height
5 Radial deviation of the carpometacarpal block
6 The carpus tends to slide volarly

Pathogenesis of long finger deformities

The complex and fragile musculotendinous balance of the hand and wrist is often altered by the rheumatoid process. The rheumatoid degenerative process may start at any of the three digital joints or at the wrist. Any resulting musculotendinous imbalance at one level of the osteoarticular chain may produce subsequent deformities of the neighboring joints.

Rheumatoid arthritis is the source of different patterns of finger deformities: intra-articular synovial hypertrophy will cause stretching of the supporting structures, invade the subchondral bone, and destroy the articular surfaces.

When the extensor mechanism is involved, the joint assumes a flexed position; when the volar plate is stretched, the joint will hyperextend.

The four most common finger deformities in rheumatoid arthritis are: mallet finger, swan neck, boutonnière and ulnar drift. None of these deformities is specific to rheumatoid arthritis, similar deformities can be caused by traumatic or neurologic lesions.

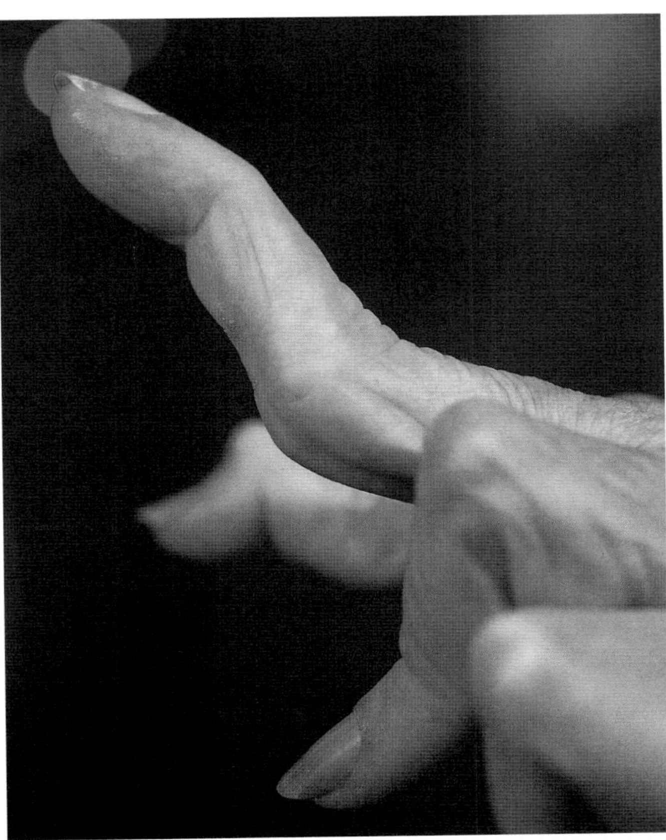

Figure 31.23
Three different deformities of finger are seen on the same rheumatoid hand: a boutonnière deformity, a swan neck deformity, and a mallet finger.

It is not uncommon to observe different kinds of finger deformities in the same hand, because of the initial localization of the rheumatoid process (Figure 31.23). It is therefore necessary to analyse the cause of each deformity for a specific treatment (see Chapter 36). These deformities are reinforced by muscle action during hand function, this explains why deformities often predominate on the dominant hand.

It should be remembered that rheumatoid arthritis is an evolutional disease and that the deformities can recur after treatment and can lead to other deformities.

Classification of finger deformities with musculotendinous imbalance

We use the same classification for rheumatoid deformities of fingers as already described for chronic musculotendinous imbalance in the fingers.

- Stage 1: there is no limitation of passive motion in any joint of the finger.
- Stage 2: limitation of motion in one joint is influenced by the position of another joint of the finger's multiarticular chain (tenodesis effect).
- Stage 3: fixed deformities. Limitation may be due to soft tissue contracture or adhesion. No articular surface alterations are seen on X-rays.
- Stage 4: fixed deformities. Radiography shows significant articular lesions.

Deformities at the MP joint level

Anatomical considerations

The MP joints allow flexion-extension and medial-lateral deviation associated with a slight degree of axial rotation; hence, their capsules are much looser than those of the interphalangeal articulations. The metacarpal condyle, which has a larger anteroposterior axis, articulates with the base of the proximal phalanx, which is smaller and concave and has a larger transverse axis. The surface of the glenoid cavity is amplified by the volar plate and can thus accommodate the metacarpal head. This arrangement allows great amplitude of movement, at the expense of stability, which is provided by the capsuloligamentous apparatus (Figure 31.24A, B and C).

The lax capsule is considerably reinforced by the radial and ulnar MP ligaments. These are relaxed in extension and tensed in flexion because of their eccentric insertions and the shape of the metacarpal head, which is narrower posteriorly and more prominent anteriorly. This explains why abduction-adduction movements of the MP joints are restricted in flexion and free in extension.

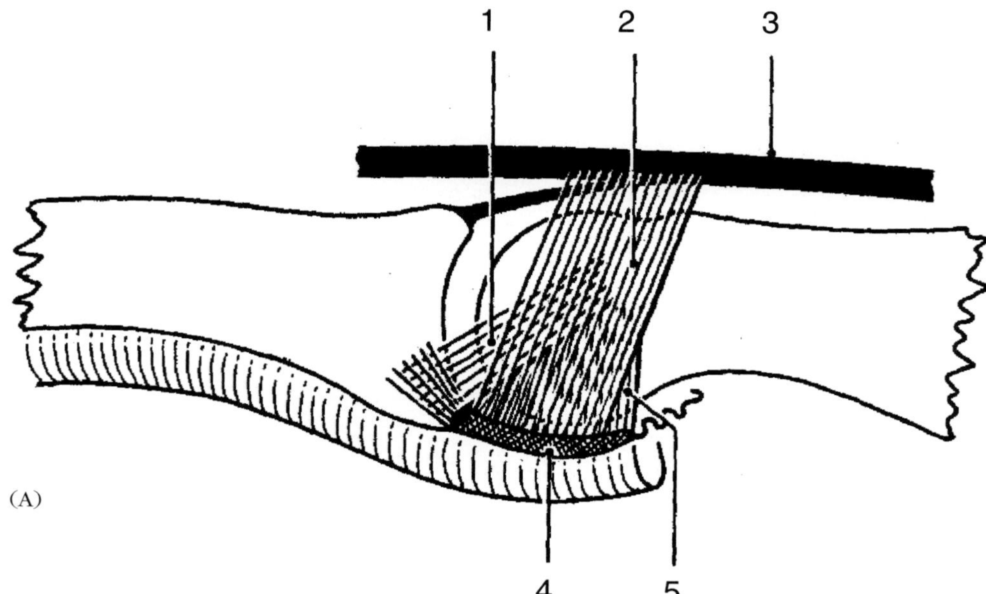

(A)

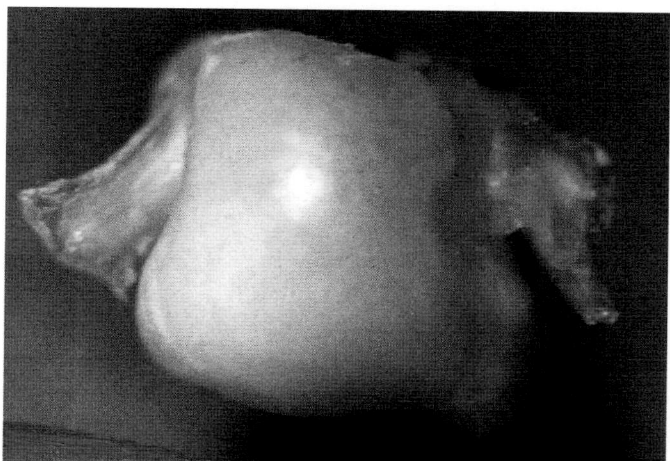

(B)

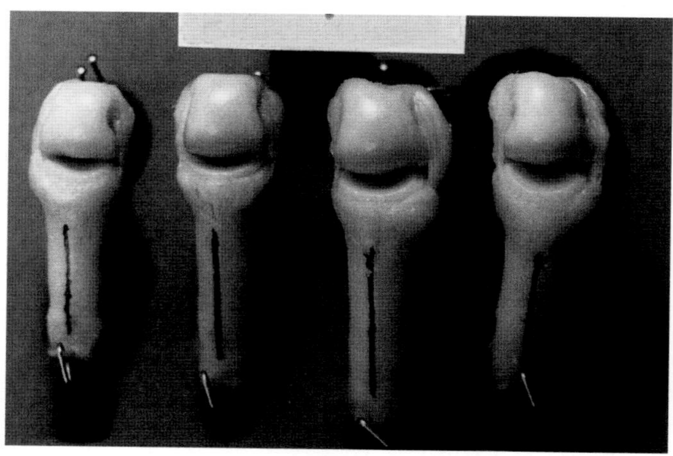

(C)

(D)

Figure 31.24

MP joint of the fingers. (A) 1, Collateral ligament; 2, sagittal band; 3, extensor tendon; 4, volar plate; 5, accessory collateral ligament. (B) The head of the index finger metacarpal is asymmetrical with a ridge on the ulnar side. (C) The radial collateral ligament of the index finger is longer than the ulnar. (D) The four finger joints. The shape of the metacarpal heads and the length and site of implantation of the collateral ligaments are all different. Note that there is no asymmetry on the fourth metacarpal head (Hakstian and Tubiana 1967).

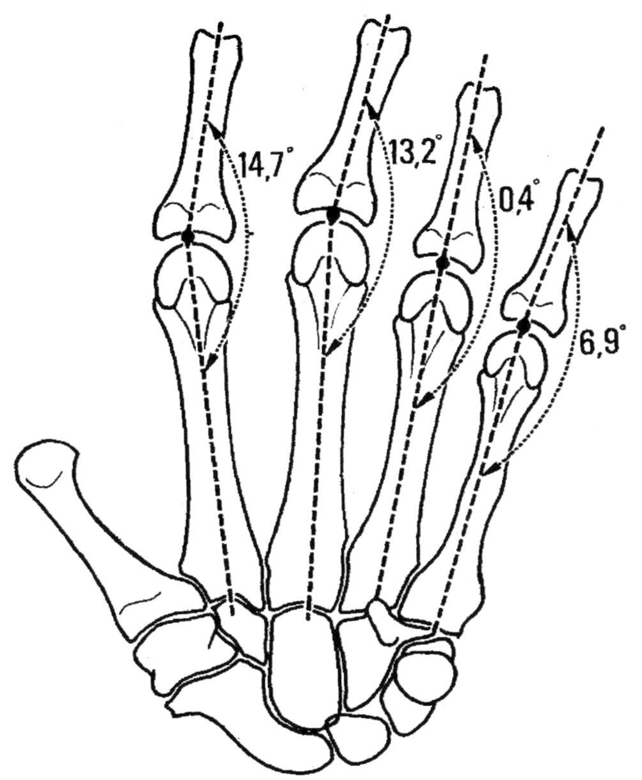

Figure 31.25
Normal ulnar deviation of the fingers in extension.

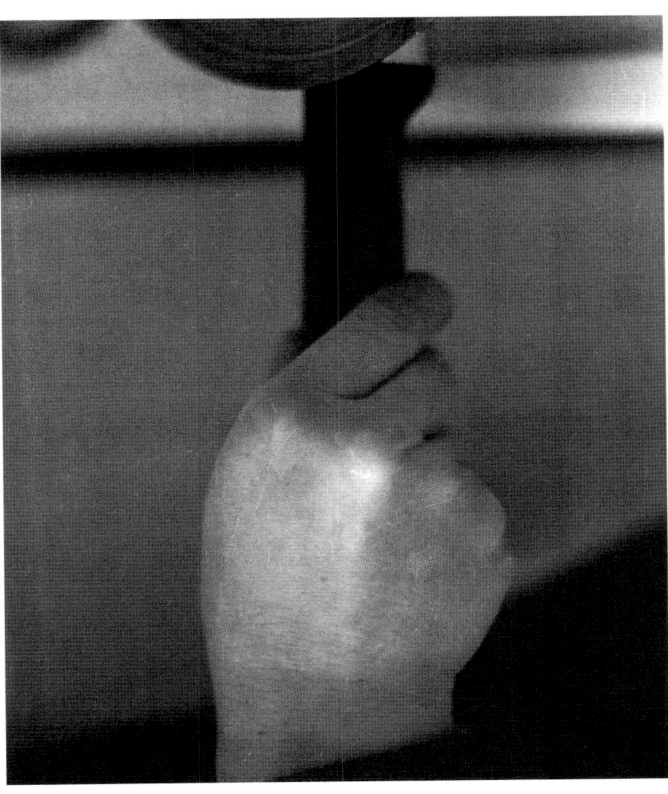

Figure 31.26
During the grasp, the MP joints of the fingers are flexed and in ulnar deviation.

The lateral accessory metacarpoglenoid ligaments suspend the volar plate, to which is attached the first pulley of the fibrous sheath of the flexor tendons. Any malalignment at the entrance of the fibrous sheath will have important repercussions on the deviation of the finger.

The deformities

The two main deformities at the MP level are:

- ulnar deviation of the fingers;
- volar subluxation of the base of the proximal phalanx.

According to Swanson, the MP joints are affected in 58% of cases involving the rheumatoid hand.

Ulnar deviation of the finger

There are normal physiological factors which favor ulnar inclination of the fingers at the MP level. These factors have different consequences in the different fingers. The inclination is most marked in the index finger, less in the middle and little fingers, and almost non-existent in the ring finger.

Articular effects
These are caused by the asymmetry of the metacarpal heads and the collateral ligaments (Hakstian and Tubiana 1967) (see Figure 31.24B and C). For example, the radial collateral ligament of the index finger joint is much longer than the ulnar collateral ligament and thus permits a greater ulnar than radial deviation. This can be shown by the normal ulnar deviation of the fingers in extension, on average 14.7° for the MP joint of the index finger, 13.2° for the long finger, 0.4° for the ring finger, and 6.9° for the little finger (Figure 31.25).

During the pinch grip, the MP joints are minimally flexed, and ulnar deviation of the index and long fingers is counteracted by action of the first and second dorsal interosseous muscles, which is more efficient when the MP joints are extended as a result of their lateral positioning. However, during the grasp, when the fingers are strongly flexed, these muscles have little control over lateral movement (Figure 31.26). In addition, the extensor loses its stabilizing effect because of the distal sliding of the interosseous hood (Figure 31.27). The fingers are positioned in ulnar deviation as a result of the configuration of the MP joints at the limit permitted by the collateral ligaments.

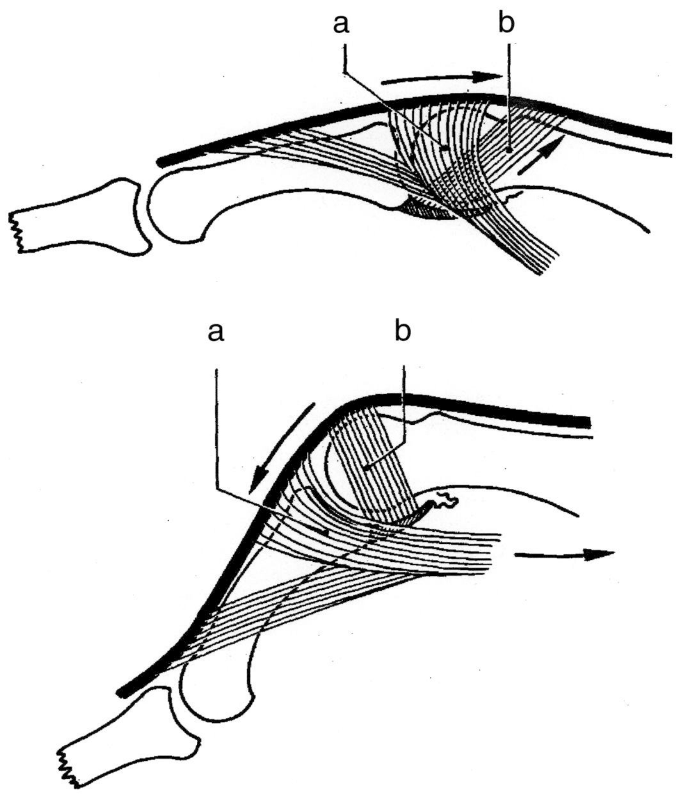

Figure 31.27

During flexion of the MP joint the interosseous hood slides distally.

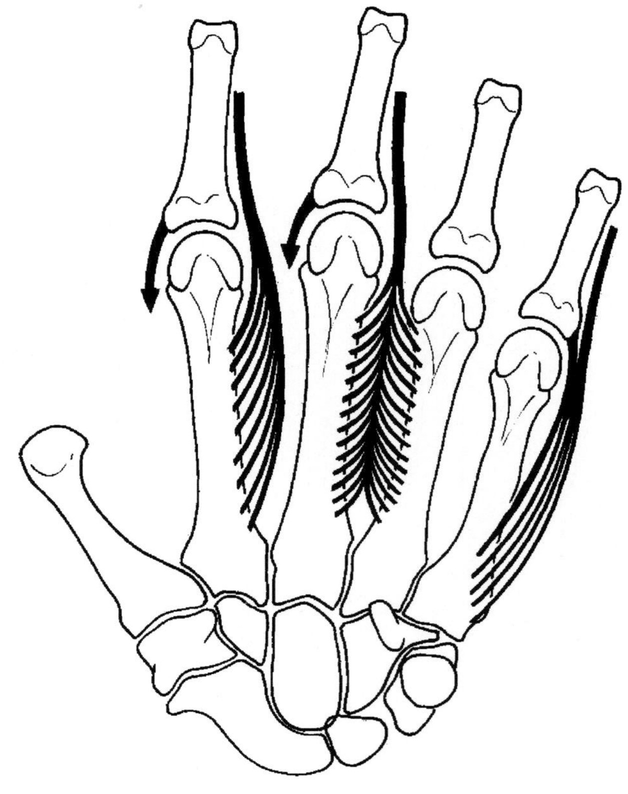

Figure 31.28

Action of the intrinsic muscles. The first palmar, third dorsal interosseous, and the abductor digiti minimi play an important role in ulnar deviation of the fingers.

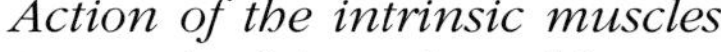

Action of the intrinsic muscles

Boyes (1969) and Backhouse (1968) have attributed a greater capacity to produce ulnar deviation to the intrinsic muscles that insert in the extensor hood than those inserting in the base of the proximal phalanx. Thus the first palmar and third dorsal interosseous muscles have, because of their more distal insertion (Figure 31.28), a greater ulnar deviating effect than the radial (first and second dorsal interosseous muscles), which have a more proximal bony insertion. Also, the lumbrical muscles of the index and middle fingers may be weakened by median nerve compression in the carpal tunnel. The predominant action of the powerful abductor digiti minimi muscle, which has no counterbalancing structure, plays an important role in ulnar deviation of the little finger.

Deforming effect of the extrinsic tendons

Long extensor and flexor tendons cross into the hand on the ulnar side of its longitudinal axis.

1. *Effect of the flexor tendons* (Smith et al 1964). The flexor tendons of the index and long fingers have an ulnar inclination at their point of entry into the fibrous flexor tendon sheath, leading to an ulnar deviation when the MP joints are unstable (Figure 31.29, see also Figure 31.33).

   The long finger is the first to be involved and, when flexed, the first signs of ulnar deviation can be found in this finger. The index finger is protected longer as a result of the powerful first dorsal interosseous muscle.
2. *Effect of the extensor tendons.* The transverse fibers of the interosseous hood are thinner on the radial than on the ulnar side. Exuberant dorsal synovitis tends to push between the extensor tendon and insertion of the intrinsic muscles on the radial is earlier than on the ulnar side. The slackening of the transverse fibers means that the tendon is no longer retained on the axis of the joint but is truly pushed to the ulnar side (Figure 31.30). Once off the summit, the displacement becomes self-perpetuating (Flatt 1966).

   Ulnar displacement of the extensor tendons, which is frequently seen, is probably not the initial cause of ulnar deviation of the fingers as was previously thought. However, displacement into the intermetacarpal space contributes to the fixation of this deformity.

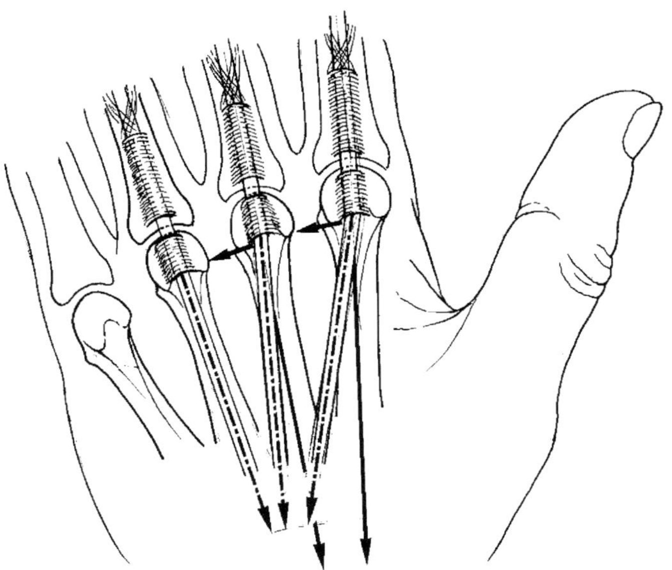

Figure 31.29
Deforming effect of the flexor tendons of the index and long fingers.

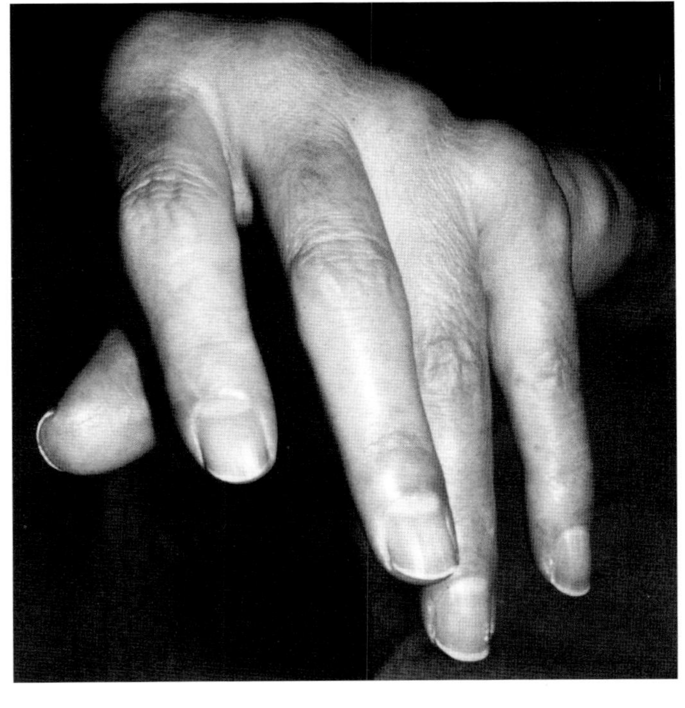

Figure 31.31
Palmar displacement of the two ulnar metacarpals.

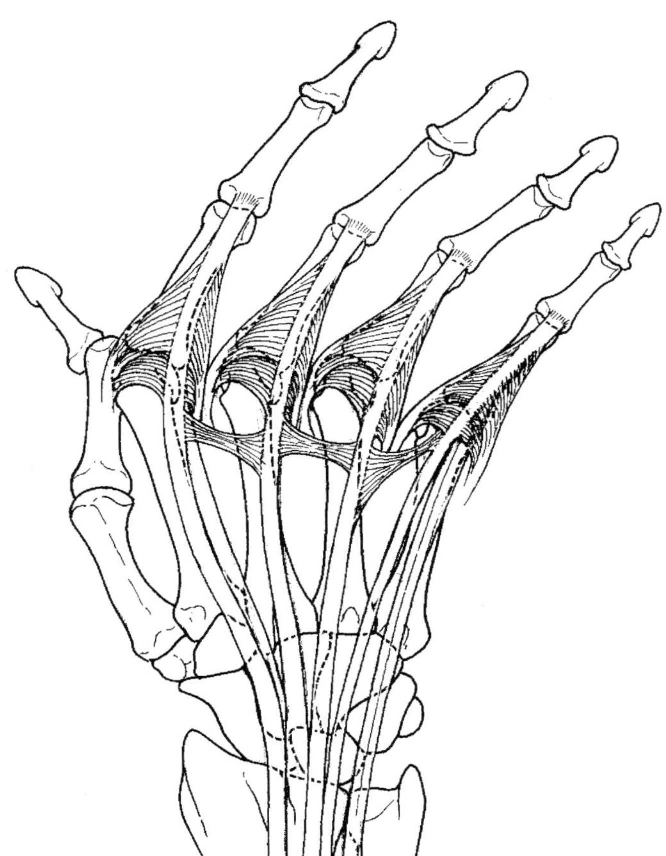

Figure 31.30
Ulnar sliding of the extensor tendons.

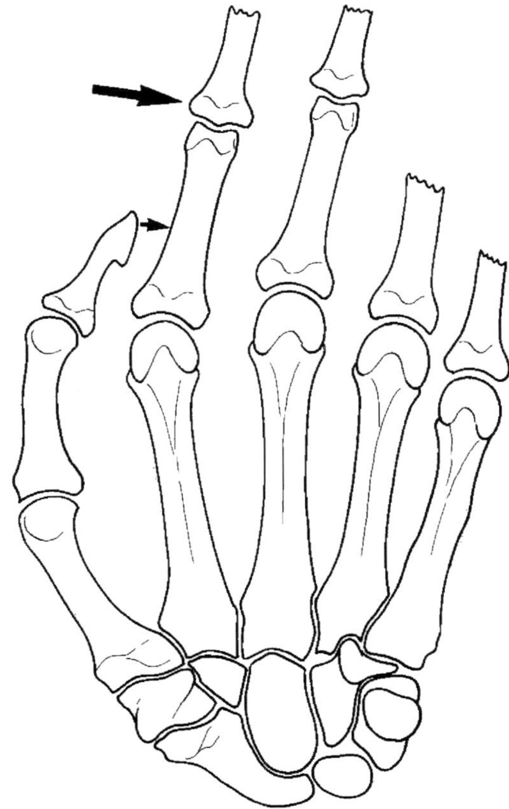

Figure 31.32
Pressure of the thumb on the fingers in lateral grip.

Table 31.1 *Ulnar deviation of the fingers*

Predisposing factors	*Structures opposing*
Normal physiologic factors	Radial collateral ligaments
• Metacarpal head asymmetry	Radial interosseous muscles
• Flexor tendons to index/long fingers	
• First palmar/and third dorsal interosseous muscles	
• Hypothenar muscles	
• Thumb pressure	
• Gravity	
Rheumatoid factors	
• Articular erosion	
• Weakening of capsuloligamentous structures	
• Intrinsic muscle contraction	
• Ulnar displacement of the extensor tendons	
• Radial inclination of the wrist	

3. *Metacarpal descent of fourth and fifth metacarpals.* Zancolli (1979) has emphasized the role of the anterior displacement of the two ulnar metacarpals (metacarpal descent) (Figure 31.31), which are pulled ulnarly by the two extensor tendons, united by their intertendinous connections.
4. *Extrinsic factors.* In lateral grip, the pressure of the thumb pushes the fingers ulnarly (Figure 31.32). Gravity also plays a role in ulnar deviation of the fingers when the hand is at rest and the forearm is in mid-pronation.

All of these factors do not lead to a pathologic deviation, when the capsuloligamentous structures are intact. As a result of rheumatoid arthritis, the metacarpal capsule becomes distended by synovial proliferation, and the collateral ligaments are stretched by subchondral erosions on the metacarpal head. This results in a laxity of the capsular ligamentous structures that allows a displacement of the flexor tendon sheath. Loss of capsular ligamentous support is the primary phenomenon that allows pathologic ulnar deviation to begin. It is apparent first in flexion because of the applied muscular traction and then becomes self-perpetuating because of the factors listed earlier, to which can be added radial deviation of the carpometacarpal block when this lesion pre-dates the MP lesions.

Volar subluxation of the base of the proximal phalanx

This deformity is frequently associated with ulnar deviation of the fingers. Once again, the initial phenomenon is proliferative articular synovitis, which leads to a distention of the capsuloligamentous structures. At the point of entry in the fibrous flexor sheath the flexor tendons exert a traction force that has two parts: one in a volar direction and the other (for the index and long finger) is ulnar (Figure 31.33). As long as the joint is stable, these forces exert their action on the stable metacarpal head, and thus no deformity is produced. The distention of the accessory collateral ligaments and the sagittal bands of the common extensor tendon allow volar displacement of the volar plate, which is fixed to the base of the proximal phalanx. The proximal part of the flexor tendon sheath (attached to the volar plate) moves, and the traction force is distally displaced with respect to the base of the proximal phalanx. This base, as opposed to the head of the metacarpal, is mobile and therefore is moved in ulnar deviation for the index and long fingers.

Table 31.2 *Volar subluxation of base of proximal phalanx*

Predisposing factors for subluxation	*Factors opposing subluxation*
Normal physiologic factors	Lateral accessory ligaments
• Flexor tendons	
• Intrinsic muscles	Volar plate
Rheumatoid factors	
• Articular erosions	
• Weakening of the capsule/ligament	
• Displacement of the flexor tendons	
• Intrinsic muscle traction	

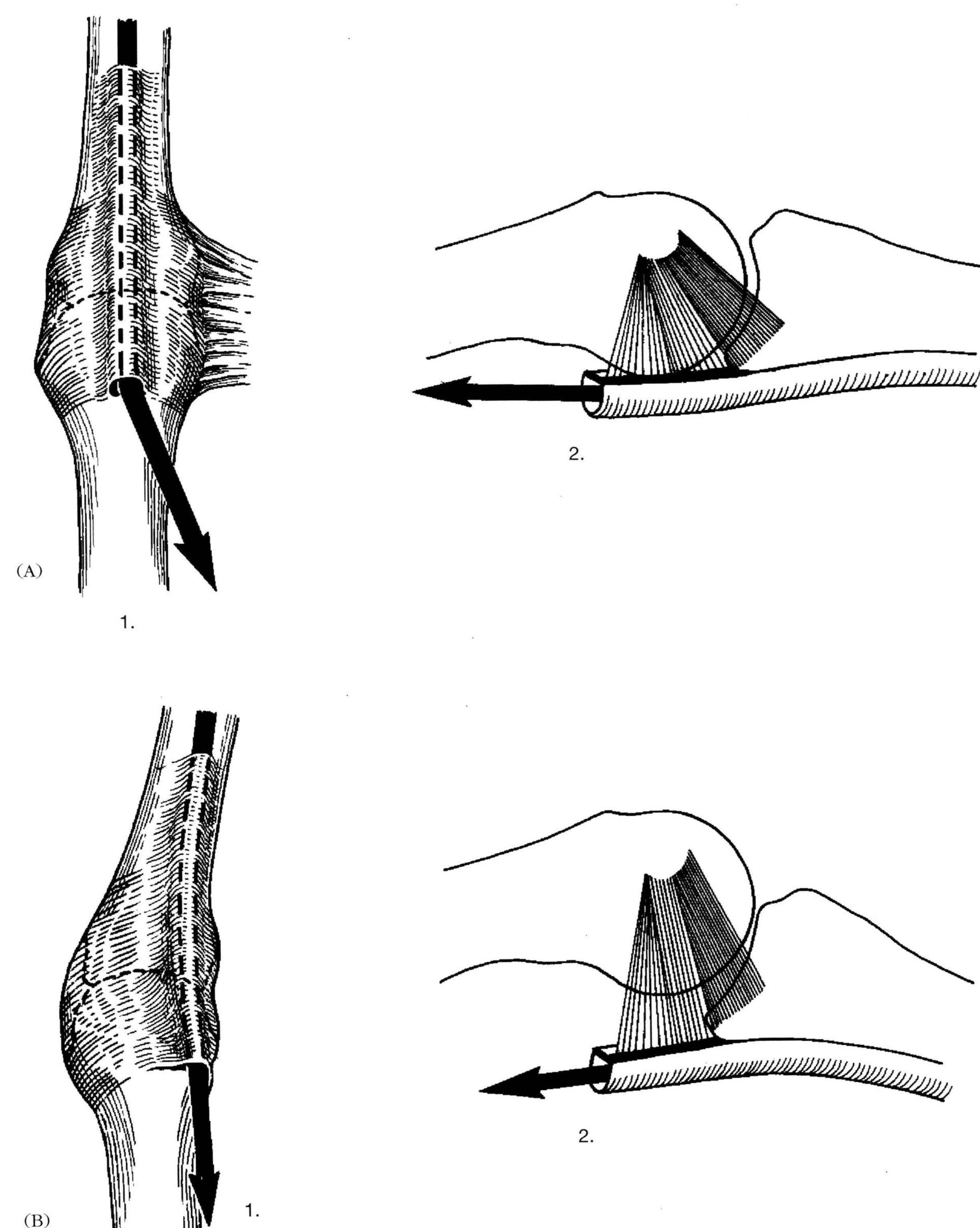

Figure 31.33

(A) Normal anatomy of the MP joint. 1, Anterior view showing the angulation of the flexor tendons of the index and long fingers as they enter into the pulley A1 of the flexor tendon sheath. The resultant ulnar deviation force has no effect on the joint as it is applied through resistant capsular and ligamentous structures to the metacarpal head. 2, Lateral view. The flexor tendon sheath is suspended on the volar plate. (B) In rheumatoid arthritis, the distention of the capsular and ligamentous structures invaded by the synovial pannus leads to a volar and ulnar displacement of the point of entry of the flexor tendons into the fibrous flexor sheath. 1, Anterior view. The resultant ulnar force tends to press on a mobile element (the base of the proximal phalanx) instead of the fixed metacarpal head, leading to an ulnar deviation of the index and long fingers. 2, Lateral view. For the same reasons, a volar subluxation of the base of the proximal phalanx occurs.

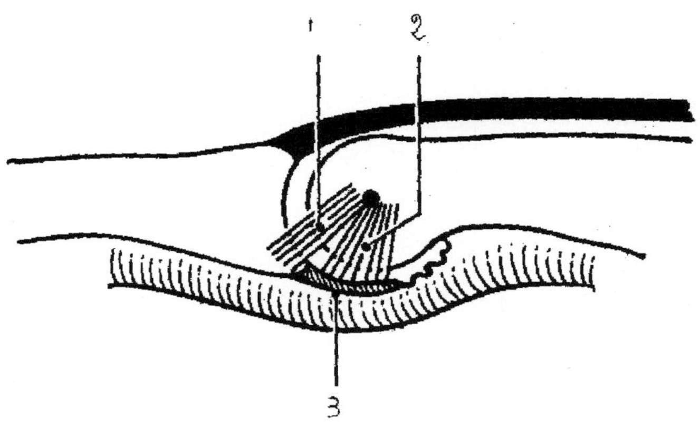

Figure 31.34
The PIP joint. 1, Collateral ligament; 2, accessory collateral ligament; 3, volar plate.

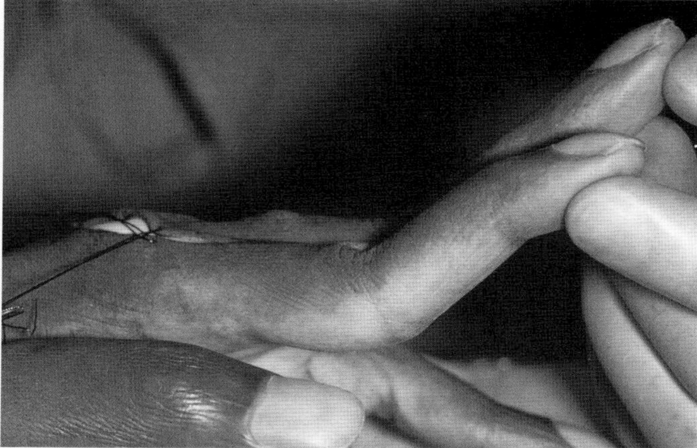

Figure 31.35
Rheumatoid swan neck deformity.

When the collateral ligaments are also distended, the base of the proximal phalanx subluxes volarly under the double action of both the long flexor tendons and the intrinsic muscles. This subluxation increases the traction of the extensor apparatus on the base of the middle phalanx, becoming one of the most frequent factors in the development of a swan neck deformity.

Deformities at the proximal interphalangeal joint level

Anatomical considerations

In contrast to the MP joints, which are only stable in flexion, the proximal interphalangeal (PIP) joints are stable throughout their range of movement. This is achieved by the trochlear shape of the articular surfaces and the arrangement of the connecting structures, as described below.

- Two strong symmetrical collateral ligaments that arise on the proximal phalanx near the axis of rotation of the joint and insert obliquely into the base of the distal phalanx (Figure 31.34).
- A thick volar plate which prevents hyperextension and has a thick distal insertion and two check ligaments proximally inserted on the middle phalanx.
- The fibrous flexor sheath, which is inserted on the volar plate and on the base of the phalanx immediately proximally and distally. This differs from the insertion at the MP joint, where the fibrous flexor sheath inserts on the volar plate and on the base of the proximal phalanx but not on the metacarpal.

This joint is therefore free to move in only one plane.

Deformities

There are essentially two types of deformity: the swan neck and the boutonnière. The site of the articular and peritendinous synovitis appears to be the factor that determines which of the two deformities will develop.

Swan neck deformity

The swan neck deformity is caused by excessive traction on the extensor apparatus inserted on the base of the middle phalanx, especially if the PIP joint is lax. Regardless of its origin, hyperextension of the PIP joint causes dorsal displacement of the lateral extensor tendons toward the midline. Their line of action being thus shortened, the tendons become lax, and their extensor effect on the distal interphalangeal (DIP) joint is lessened. At the same time, the flexor digitorum profundus tendon is stretched by hyperextension of the PIP joint, and the DIP joint is forced further into flexion (Figure 31.35). The result is the swan neck deformity, which combines hyperextension of the middle phalanx with flexion of the distal phalanx. Destruction or elongation of the oblique retinacular ligament heralds a loss of coordination of the IP joints. A reconstruction of its action is an essential part of the treatment of a swan neck deformity.

It is better to treat this condition early, before the deformity becomes fixed in extension and thus interferes with the grasp.

There are many lesions that may lead to such a deformity in rheumatoid arthritis, and the lesion may be at any point in the kinetic chain between the wrist and the distal phalanx.

1. *At the distal interphalangeal joint.* A rupture or elongation of the terminal part of the extensor tendon, leading to a mallet finger, with proximal

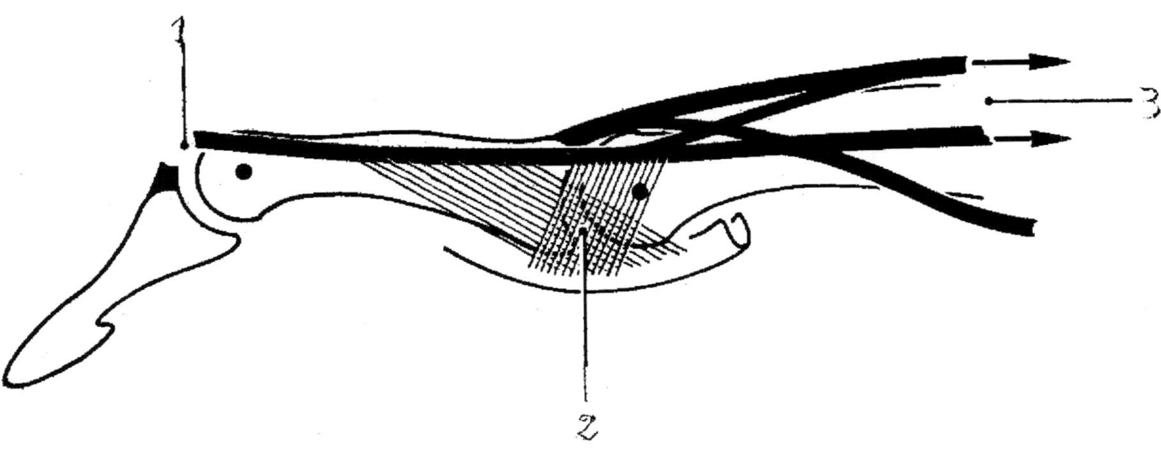

Figure 31.36
Swan neck deformity caused by a mallet finger. 1, Rupture of the terminal extensor tendon; 2, lax PIP joint; 3, proximal retraction of the extensor apparatus.

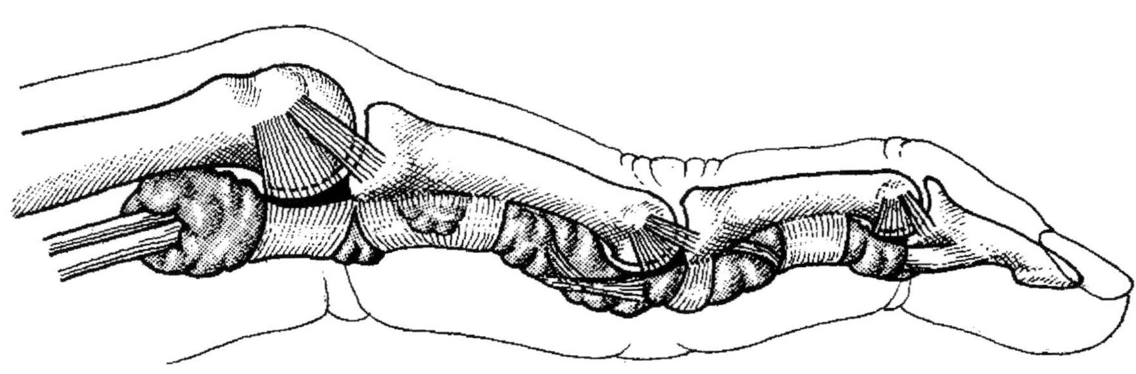

Figure 31.37
Flexor tenosynovitis with swan neck.

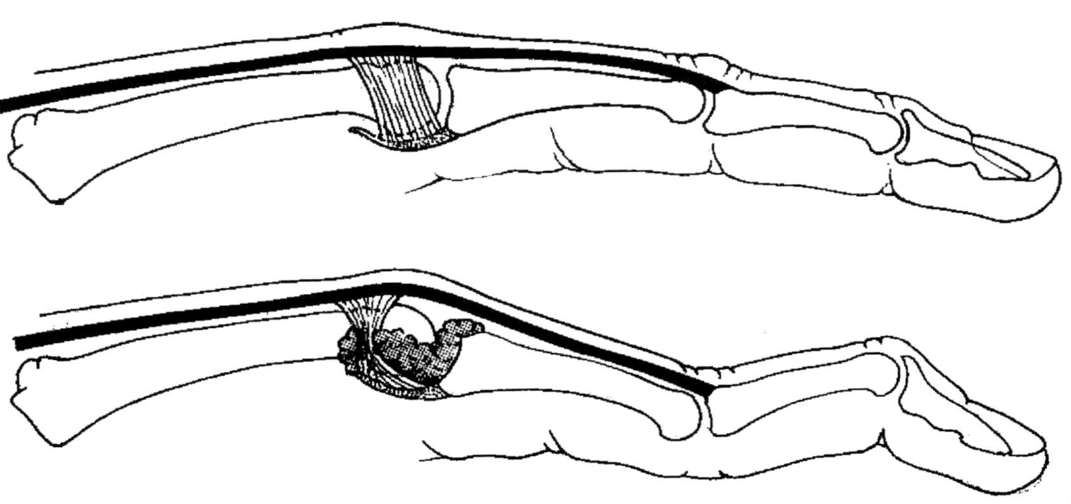

Figure 31.38
Swan neck caused by distention of the sagittal bands at the MP level.

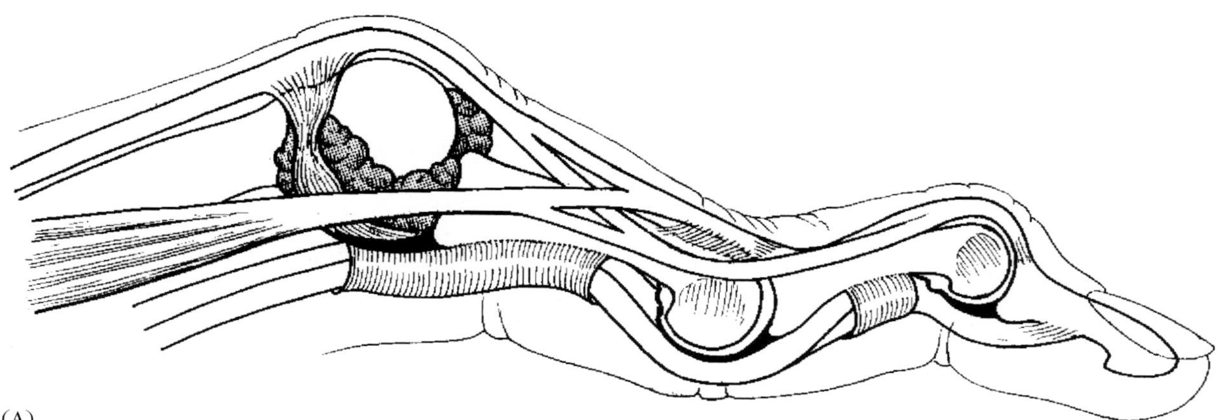
(A)

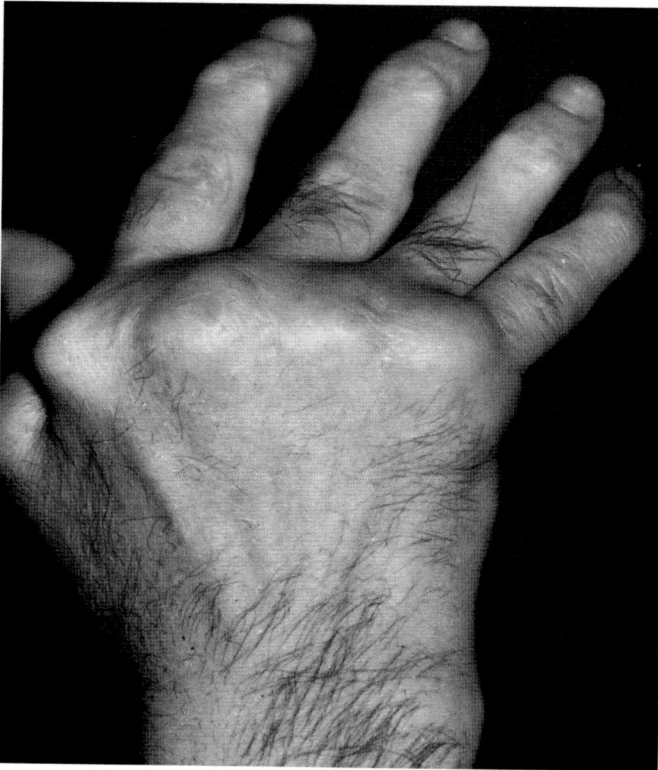
(B)

Figure 31.39

(A) Swan neck caused by subluxation of the base of the proximal phalanx. (B) Clinical case.

retraction of the extensor apparatus can be the cause of a swan neck deformity if the PIP joint is lax, as is often the case in rheumatoid arthritis (Figure 31.36).

2. *At the proximal interphalangeal joint.* Articular lesions may alter the structures that stabilize the PIP joint and normally prevent hyperextension. The initial phenomenon can be synovitis, often developing in the anterior part of the joint and extending in the flexor tendon sheath.

   Flexor tenosynovitis may lead to a limitation of flexion of the joint as a result of the volume of pannus and alteration of the sliding characteristics of the tendons within the sheaths (Figure 31.37). The patient will compensate for the loss of flexion at the PIP joint by using the intrinsic muscles that flex the MP joints. However, the intrinsic muscles are also extensors of the PIP joints; therefore, hyperextension of the PIP joints can occur if the joint structures are lax.

3. *At the MP joint.* Distention by rheumatoid pannus of the sagittal bands that constitute the proximal insertion of the central extensor tendon reinforces the action of the extensor tendon on the middle phalanx (Figure 31.38). Also, distention of the joint by synovitis can cause dorsal displacement of the axis of traction of the intrinsic muscles and thus reinforces their extensor action on the PIP joint.

   Flexion contracture of the MP joint, caused by contracture of the intrinsic muscles, or by volar subluxation of the base of the proximal phalanx, can reinforce the action of the intrinsic muscles on the extensor apparatus (Figure 31.39).

   Ulnar displacement of the extensor tendons at the MP joint level may increase traction on the base of the middle phalanx (Figure 31.40).

4. *At the wrist.* Chronic flexion of the wrist causes excessive traction of the extensor tendons. As already mentioned, bony shortening at the carpal level reduces the tension of the extrinsic tendons of the fingers. They become relatively too long (extrinsic minus), and an increased opposition of the power of the intrinsic muscles of the fingers may lead to an intrinsic plus deformity of the fingers (see Figure 31.15).

Boutonnière deformity

Synovial hypertrophy of the PIP joint stretches the extensor mechanism. Progressive elongation or avulsion of the central extensor tendon, inserted on the base of the middle phalanx, results in PIP flexion (Figure 31.41). The boutonnière deformity is a progressive condition. The distal phalanx becomes hyperextended as a result of proximal contracture of the extensor mechanism. The lateral extensor tendons slide volarly on the sides of the

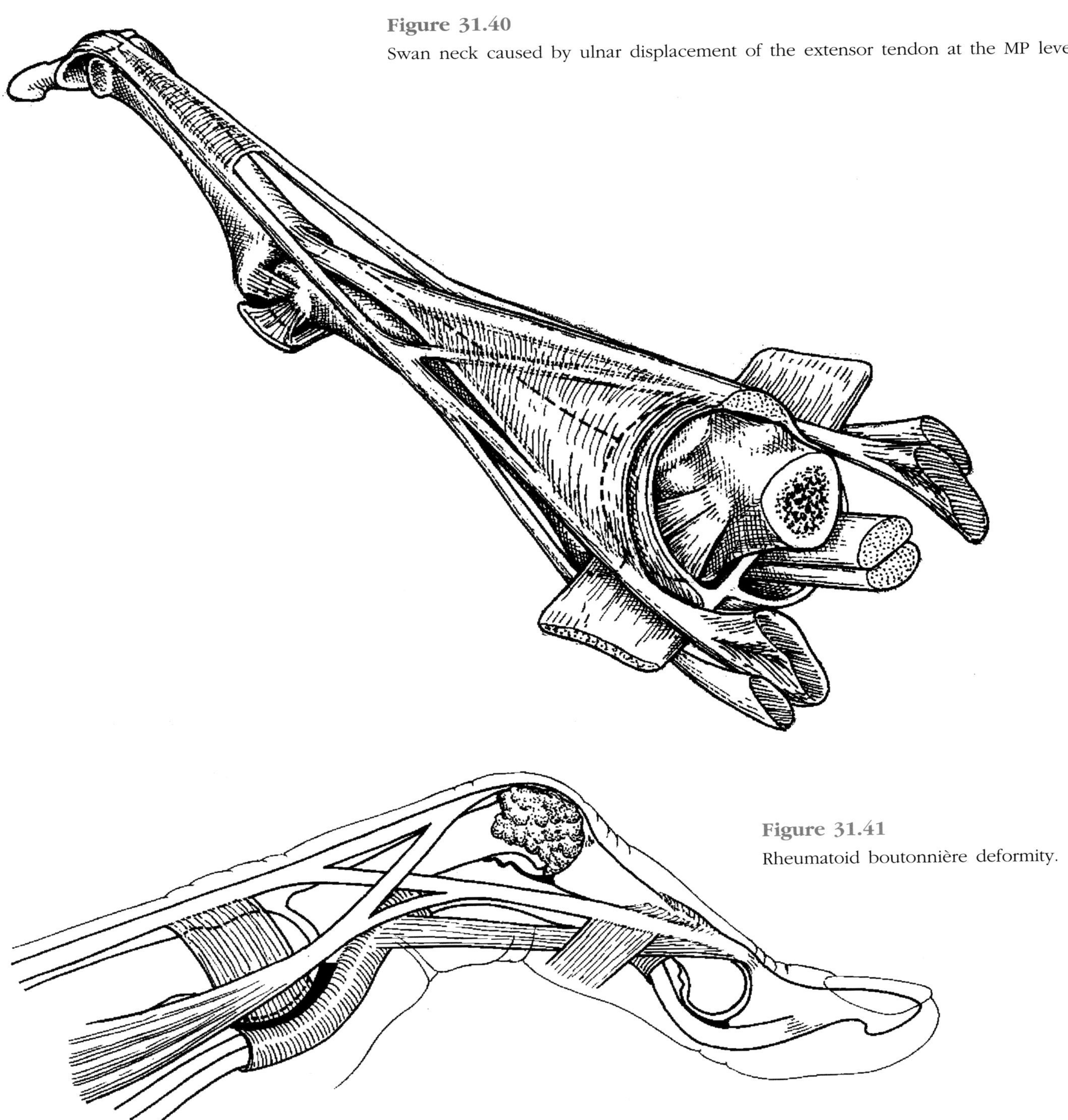

Figure 31.40
Swan neck caused by ulnar displacement of the extensor tendon at the MP level.

Figure 31.41
Rheumatoid boutonnière deformity.

PIP joint. When they pass volar to the axis of rotation of the joint, they increase its flexion. Proximal contracture of the extensor mechanism can put the MP joint in hyperextension.

Hyperextension of the distal phalanx is initially reducible, but becomes increasingly irreducible because of the contracture of the oblique fibers of the retinacular ligament; whereas the transverse fibers fix the displacement of the lateral extensor tendons.

Fixed hyperextension of the distal phalanx, as already mentioned (see Boutonnière deformity in the Chapter on Late extensor mechanism reconstruction) is an important functional step in the evolution of boutonnière deformity, because lack of flexion of the distal phalanx is often more disabling for prehension than lack of extension of the PIP joint. The distal phalanx is no longer used for grasping.

The deformity can be further aggravated by destruction of the articular surfaces.

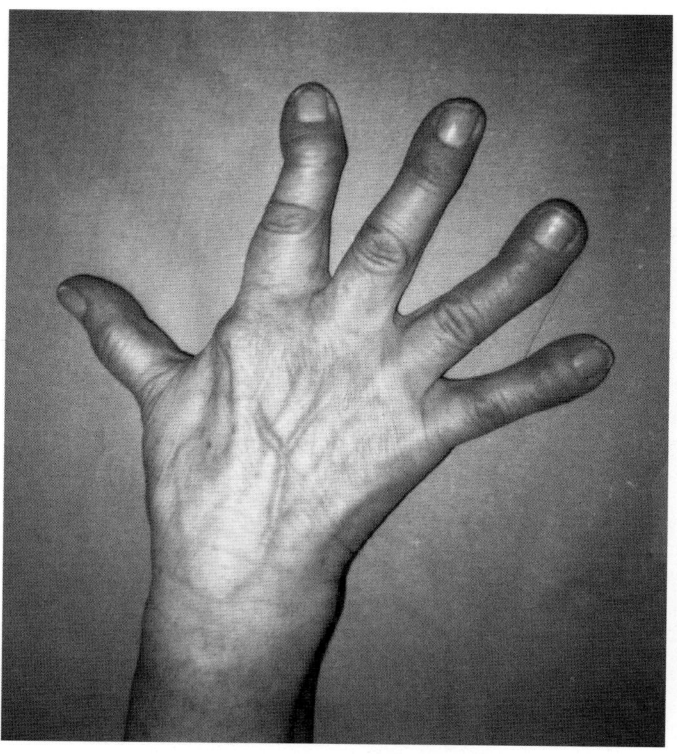

Figure 31.42

Lateral displacement of the distal phalanges of the index and ring fingers, associated with an adduction of the thumb metacarpal.

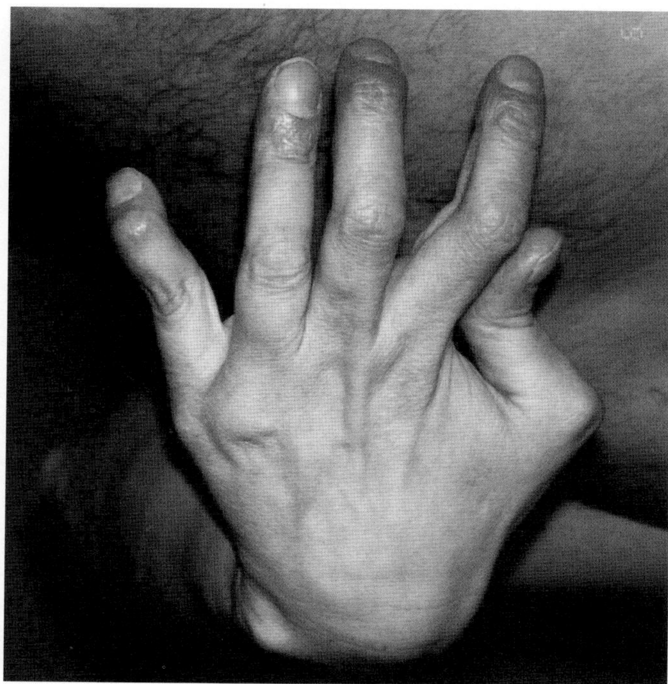

Figure 31.43

Thumb boutonnière deformity.

Deformities at the DIP joint level

Distal joint synovitis is less abundant than in the more proximal joints because of the smaller size of the joint and the absence of associated tenosynovitis. The DIP joint is not in contact with flexor tenosynovitis, as the flexor tendon sheaths end proximal to the joint.

Two types of deformity are found: mallet finger and lateral deviation.

Mallet finger

Flexion deformity is caused by a rupture or distension of the extensor tendon at the DIP joint because of articular synovitis. It can be expanded by bony shortening due to erosions, which increases the extension deficit at the DIP joint. If the PIP joint is lax, this deformity may lead to hyperextension of the PIP joint and a swan neck deformity (see Figure 31.36).

Lateral displacement

Bony erosion and external forces are responsible for lateral displacement of the DIP joint (Figure 31.42), mainly in an ulnar direction, associated or not with a

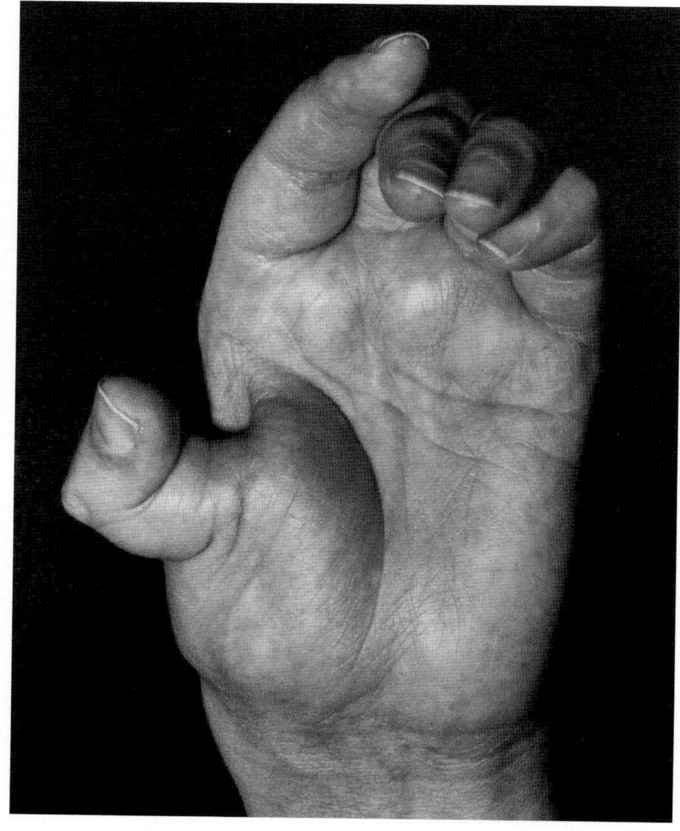

Figure 31.44

Thumb swan neck deformity.

mallet finger. It is necessary to note that such lateral deformities may be seen at other joints according to the destruction of the subchondral bone and the forces acting on those joints.

Pathogenesis of deformities of the thumb ray

The three joints of the thumb column are often the site of the rheumatoid process. Depending on the number and the different combinations of joints involved, many different types of thumb deformities have been described: the most common are the boutonnière and the swan neck. The indication for surgery at any level of this polyarticular chain must take into account the state of the other two joints.

Thumb metacarpal in abduction (boutonnière deformity)

The most frequent deformity is called a Z-thumb. Synovitis of the MP joint is the initial deformity, the capsule becomes distended on the dorsal aspect. Insertion of the extensor pollicis brevis is progressively destroyed, and the extensor pollicis longus tendon is displaced ulnarly; thus the extensor apparatus of the proximal phalanx is destroyed (Figure 31.43).

The flexion attitude of the proximal phalanx gradually becomes irreducible. However, all the strength of the extensor apparatus of the distal phalanx (intrinsic and extrinsic) is preserved, and the distal phalanx is displaced in hyperextension, partially compensating for the flexion of the proximal phalanx.

Thumb metacarpal in adduction

Less commonly (20% of cases), the deformity starts at the trapeziometacarpal joint and progressively produces a radial subluxation of the base of the thumb metacarpal. Functionally, these deformities with the thumb in adduction are more severe because the thumb web becomes contracted. Schematically two varieties of this deformity can be distinguished, depending on the deformation at the MP and IP joints. Sometimes, the MP joint is placed in flexion, and there is a compensatory hyperextension of the IP joint. More often, the hyperextension occurs at the MP joint, which loses its stability, and the IP joint goes into flexion, producing a distortion analogous to the swan neck deformity (Figure 31.44).

The simultaneous articular instability of the proximal and middle joints of the thumb is particularly disabling and difficult to treat.

References

Backdahl M (1963) The caput ulnae syndrome in rheumatoid arthritis, *Acta Rheumat Scan* **43**: 184.

Backhouse KM (1968) The mechanics of normal digital control in the hand and an analysis of the ulnar drift of rheumatoid arthritis, *Ann R Coll Surg Engl* **43**: 154.

Boyes JH (1969) The role of the intrinsic muscles in rheumatoid arthritis. In: Tubiana R, ed, *La Main Rhumatoïde* (Expansion Scientifique Française: Paris) 63.

Brahim B, Senac JP, Allieu Y (1980) Exploration radiologique de la main rhumatoïde après la résection de la tête du cubitus. A propos de 35 cas, *Ann Chir* **34**: 711–18.

Chamay A, Della Stante D, Vilasecca A (1983) L'arthrodèse radio-lunaire facteur de stabilité du poignet rhumatoïde, *Ann Chir Main* **2**: 5–17.

Flatt AE (1966) Some pathomechanics of ulnar drift, *Plast Reconstr Surg* **37**: 295.

Flatt AE (1995) *The Care of the Arthritic Hand* (Quality Medical Publishing: St Louis) 1–454.

Hakstian RW, Tubiana R (1967) Ulnar deviation of the fingers. The role of joint structure and function, *J Bone Joint Surg* **49A**: 299.

Kueny (1923) *Les geodes du semi-lunaire*, Thesis Lyon (Service Pr. Testut).

Landsmeer JMF (1960) Studies in the anatomy of articulation. II. Patterns of movement of bimuscular, biarticular systems, *Acta Morph Neerl Scand* **3**: 304.

Landsmeer JMF (1968) Les cohérences spatiales et l'équilibre spatial dans la région carpienne, *Acta Anatomica* **54**: 1–84.

Linscheid RL, Dobyns JH (1971) Rheumatoid arthritis of the wrist, *Orthop Clin North Am* **2**: 649.

Mannerfelt L (1969) On formation of bony spurs in the rheumatoid hand. In: *La Main Rhumatoïde*, Monographies du GEM (Expansion Scientifique Française: Paris) 121–2.

Mannerfelt L, Raven M (1978) Die Atiologie und Bedeutung der Radiuskrypte in rheumatischen Handgelenk. *Verh Dtsch Ges Rheumatol* **5**: 94–6.

Navarro A (1937) Anatomia y fisiologia del carpo. In: *Anales del Instituto Clinica Quirurgica y Chirurgia Experimental*, I, Montevideo, Uruguay: 162–250.

Poirier P, Charpy A (1926) *Traité d'Anatomie Humaine. Les Articulations* (Masson: Paris).

Shapiro JS (1968) Ulnar drift. A report of a related finding, *Acta Orthop Scand* **3**: 246.

Shapiro JS (1982) Wrist involvement in rheumatoid swan-neck deformity, *J Hand Surg* **7**: 484.

Smith EM, Juvinall RC, Bender LF, Pearson JR (1964) Role of the finger flexors in rheumatoid deformities of the metacarpophalangeal joints, *Arthr Rheum* **7**: 476.

Taleisnik J 91985) *The Wrist* (Churchill Livingstone: New York).

Taleisnik J (1992) The Sauvé–Kapandji procedure, *Clin Orthop Rel Res* **275**: 110–23.

Testut L, Latarjet A (1928) *Traité d'Anatomie Humaine*, vol 1 (Doin: Paris).

Tubiana R, Hakstian RW (1966) Le rôle des facteurs anatomiques dans les déviations cubitales normales et pathologiques des doigts. In: *La Main Rhumatoïde*, Monographies du GEM (Expansion Scientifiques Française: Paris) 11–21.

Tubiana R, Kuhlmann NJ, Fahrer M, Lisfranc R (1980) Etude de poignet normal et ses déformations au cours de la polyarthrite rhumatoïde, *Chirurgie* **106**: 257–64.

Zancolli E (1979) *Structural and Dynamic Bases of Hand Surgery*, 2nd edn (JB Lippincott: Philadelphia).

32 The rheumatoid wrist

Christian Dumontier

If wrist involvement reveals the rheumatoid disease in only 2.7% of patients, 35% of rheumatoid patients will suffer from problems with their wrists in the early stages. During their life, almost all patients will suffer from wrist problems, with bilateral involvement in 95% of cases. In two-thirds of the patients, wrist involvement will leave them with definitive sequelae (Clayton and Ferlic 1965, Eiken et al 1975, Allieu and Brahin 1977, Rasker et al 1980, Tubiana et al 1980, Brown 1984, Vahvanen and Patiala 1984, Wilson 1986, Flatt 1995). Surgery of the wrist represents between 20 and 40% of all operations performed on rheumatoid patients, as a stable, painless and well-aligned wrist is mandatory for the strength and function of the hand (Straub and Ranawat 1969, Linscheid and Dobyns 1971, Eiken et al 1975, Allieu and Brahin 1977, Nalebuff and Garrod 1984, Dennis et al 1986, Vicar and Burton 1986, Wilson 1986). Clinical symptoms and deformities will vary according to the predominant localization of the pannus (Tubiana et al 1980, Mannerfelt 1984). Synovial involvement of the wrist may involve three distinct anatomical compartments that are considered a surgical unit because their anatomical proximity: the radio-carpal joint, the distal radio-ulnar joint, and the synovial sheath of the extensor tendons under the extensor retinaculum.

Many techniques have been designed to produce improvements in patients but all act in two ways: removing the synovial pannus to remove pain and limit progression of the disease; and stabilizing the wrist to increase its function. Stabilization could be done with either soft tissue reconstruction, partial or total fusion, or articular replacement. Indications for the different techniques depend on the patient's needs and expectations, the disease (particularly its evolution), the efficacy of the medical treatment, and the surgeon's experience. This chapter describes the techniques that I have learnt and used with Professor Tubiana, and their recent evolution.

Synovectomies

In clinical practice, synovitis predominates on the dorsum of the wrist and involves one or more extensor tendon compartments with or without involving the distal radio-ulnar joint. Radio-carpal involvement is more difficult to appreciate but is associated with extensor tendon involvement in almost 95% of cases. Limited tendon synovectomies were performed in the late 1970s but this approach is largely debatable as the spontaneous evolution of the disease is unknown and other extensor compartments may be involved later. Most authors consider that synovectomy should be performed in one stage on the extensor tendons, the distal radio-ulnar joint, and the radio-carpal joint, where involvement is almost always associated.

Medical synovectomy

Medical synovectomy or synoviorthesis is a local treatment for a localized articular disease that does not resolve under medical treatment including anti-inflammatory drugs, corticosteroids, disease-modifying anti-rheumatic drugs, and local corticosteroid injections. Destruction and sclerosis of the synovial membrane is achieved with a radio-isotope. Radio-isotopes are used in colloidal preparations. The binding of the isotopes on colloids facilitates their phagocytosis and minimizes the extra-articular leakage. Extra-articular spread of the isotope is the major risk associated with radio-synoviorthesis and could lead to irradiation in the lymphatic and hepatic systems. X-Ray contrast medium is used to check the position of the needle in the joint and to show any communication with synovial tendon sheaths. Rhenium-186 is used at the wrist and complete recovery or marked improvement of local inflammatory symptoms has been reported in about 73% of cases at 2-year follow-up (Goldberg and Menkes 1995). However, synoviorthesis has limited indications in the wrist, as there is associated tendinous involvement in up to 95% of cases and this cannot be treated with synoviorthesis. Some attempts have been made to combine surgical synovectomy with synoviorthesis to limit recurrence of the pannus in the carpus, but the efficacy of this combination is unknown.

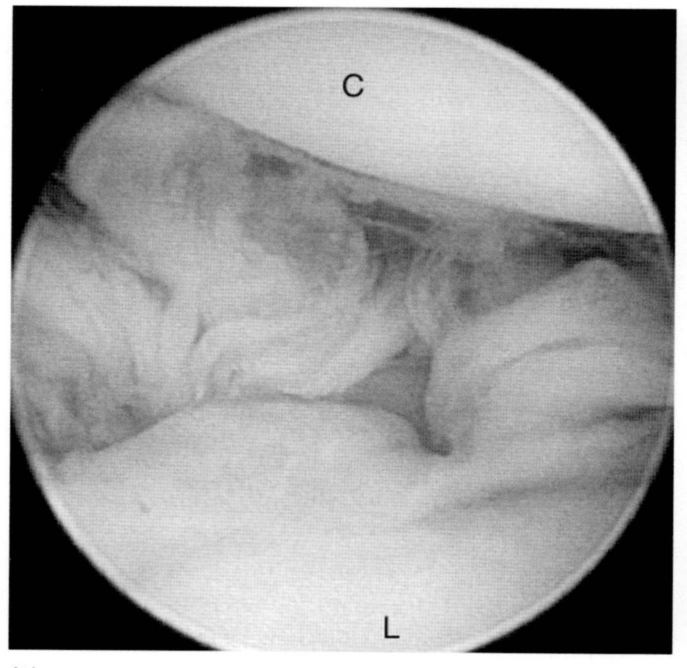

(A)

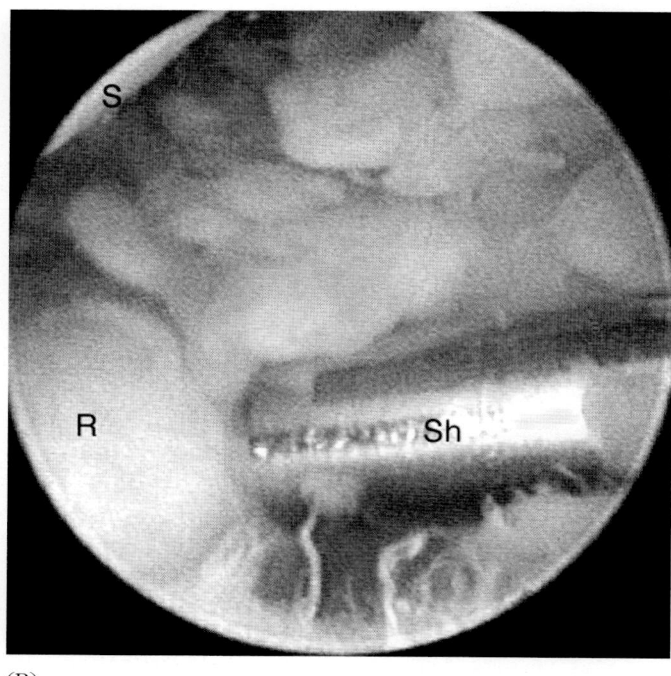

(B)

Figure 32.1

(A) Anterior synovitis viewed from the midcarpal joint. This synovitis is not accessible with open surgery. C, head of the capitate; L, inferior articular surface of the lunate. (B) Significant synovitis of the radio-scaphoid space removed with a shaver in the 3/4 portal. S, scaphoid; R, articular surface of the radius; Sh, shaver blade.

Surgical synovectomy

Surgical synovectomy alone is very rarely indicated, as synovectomy is only one part of a procedure that also includes wrist realignment and stabilization, as well as ulnar stump stabilization. However, new indications have appeared with wrist arthroscopy. Adolfsson and coworkers reported the efficacy of intracarpal wrist synovectomy in rheumatoid patients at 6 months and 3.8-year follow-up (Adolfsson and Nylander 1993, Adolfsson and Frisen 1997). It is possible, through the arthroscope (using the classic radio-carpal and midcarpal portal), to remove the synovial pannus in locations which are non-accessible with open surgery (pre-styloid ulnar recess, midcarpal joint especially the STT joint, etc.) (Figure 32.1). Patients with only intracarpal rheumatoid involvement are rare. In those patients, arthroscopic wrist synovectomy is a good indication. We have now chosen to perform arthroscopic wrist synovectomy as an alternative to open intracarpal synovectomy in stable, non-dislocated patients in association with open tendon and distal radio-ulnar joint synovectomy.

Synovectomy will be considered first, then stabilization techniques will be discussed.

Regional anesthesia is preferred to general anesthesia, as this limits the risk of cervical spine injuries and decreases the potential shock from corticosteroid depletion.

A large skin incision is mandatory to perform all the surgical steps. A longitudinal incision is preferred to a zig-zag incision in patients whose skin is very fragile. We favor an oblique incision extending from 2–3 cm proximal to the ulnar head and directed to the base of the second metacarpal (Figure 32.2A). Subcutaneous dissection should be minimal and at least two longitudinal veins should be preserved (Figure 32.2B). The distal sensory branches of the radial nerve, as well as the dorsal sensory branches of the ulnar nerve, should be preserved (Figure 32.3).

We usually incise the extensor retinaculum on the ulnar side as proposed by Clayton and Ferlic (1965) along the extensor carpi ulnaris tendon and a flap (5 cm wide) is raised, leaving the retinaculum attached to the first extensor compartment, which is usually free of disease (Kessler and Vainio 1966, Straub and Ranawat 1969, Tubiana 1990) (Figure 32.4).

Tenosynovectomy

All the extensor tendon compartments are opened successively. Synovial proliferation is usually maximum under and distal to the retinaculum (Clayton and Ferlic

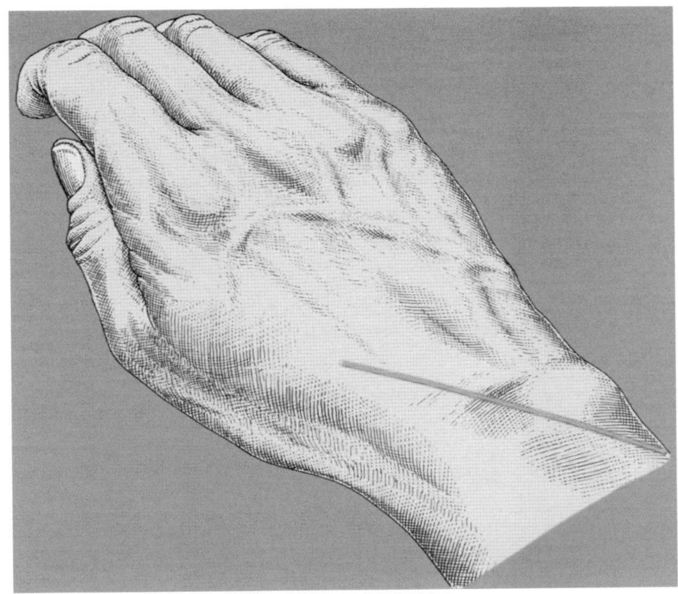

(A)

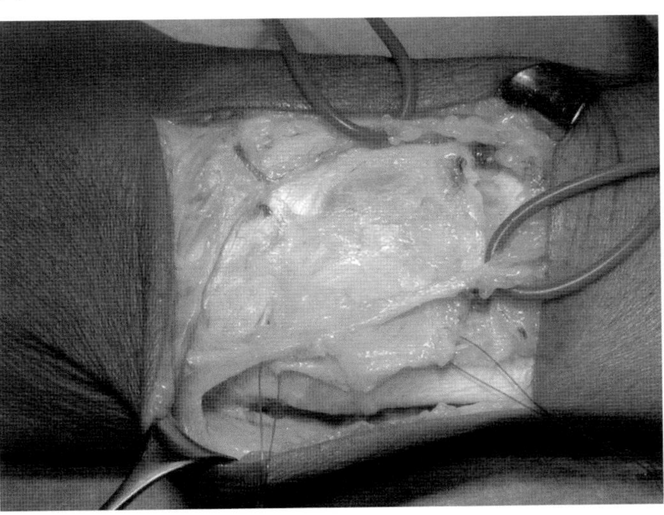

(B)

Figure 32.2

(A) Schematic drawing of the incision used by the author. A longitudinal incision is made from a point 2–3 cm above the ulnar head and is drawn to the base of the second metacarpal. (B) Subcutaneous dissection should preserve at least two longitudinal veins (places on laces). The retinaculum extensorum is open on the ulnar side, along the extensor carpi ulnaris tendon (seen at the bottom of the figure).

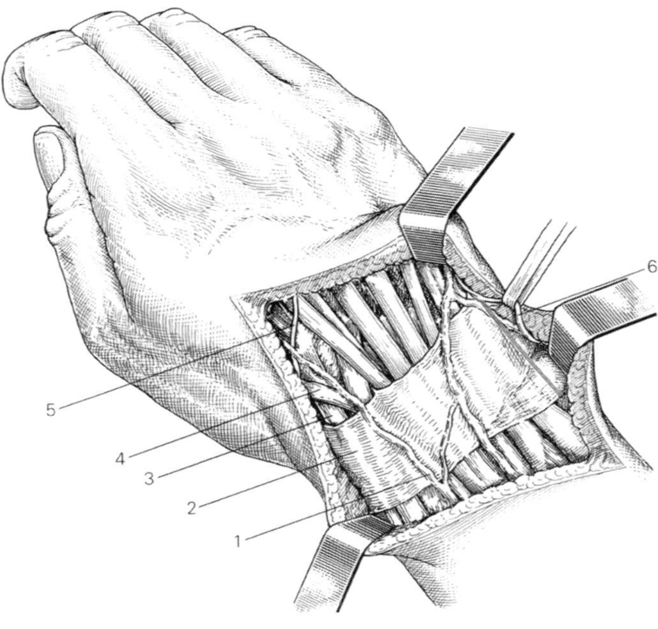

Figure 32.3

Subcutaneous dissection should preserve dorsal veins and cutaneous nerve branches. 1, dorsal veins; 2, retinaculum extensorum; 3, extensor carpi ulnaris tendon; 4, extensor pollicis longus tendon; 5, distal branch of the radial nerve; 6, dorsal cutaneous branch of the ulnar nerve.

1965, Backhouse et al 1971). Tendon decompression may, by itself, be an effective treatment for tendinous synovial proliferation (Abernethy and Dennyson 1979, Mannerfelt 1984). However, we prefer to perform a synovectomy of each individual tendon (Figure 32.5). Tenosynovectomy should be as complete as possible but should not weaken the extensors. Even if intratendinous proliferation is frequent (and we have observed this in almost 50% of our cases), postoperative ruptures are rare (Backhouse et al 1971, Millender et al 1974, Clayton and Ferlic 1975, Mannerfelt 1984, Brown and Brown 1988). Brown and Brown (1988) reported one postoperative rupture out of 44 intact tendons, one out of 42 tendons with synovial proliferation and three out of 43 repaired tendons. During this surgical step we always perform a resection of the distal branches of the posterior interosseous nerve, including its branches for the distal radio-ulnar joint (Figure 32.6).

Distal radio-ulnar joint synovectomy

This is the second step of the procedure. Distal radio-ulnar joint involvement occurs in 30% of patients (Figure 32.7). Radio-ulnar joint involvement includes weakness, pain during rotational movement, limited mobility in prono-supination, dislocation of the ulnar head (sometimes with tendon ruptures), and distal radio-ulnar joint synovitis. This is probably the most disabling location of the disease and the most dangerous for the function of the hand, as the extensor tendons may rupture on the dorsal dislocation of the ulnar head (Freiberg and Weinstein 1972, Mannerfelt 1984) (Figure

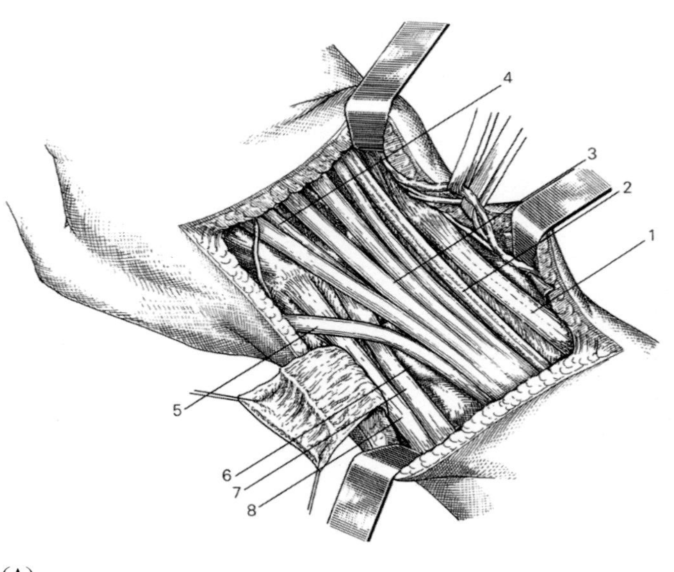

(A)

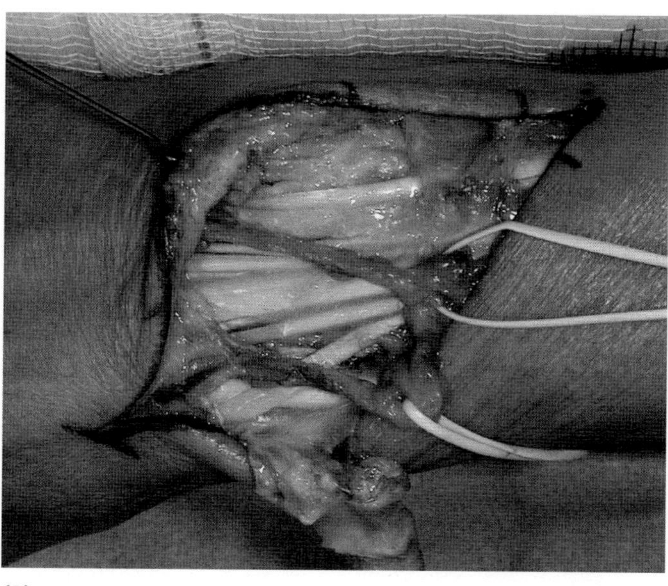

(B)

Figure 32.4

Opening of the retinaculum extensorum. (A) Schematic drawing. The extensor retinaculum is opened from the ulnar side, along the extensor carpi ulnaris tendon. Each extensor compartment is freed successively up to the first compartment, which is left intact. The two major technical difficulties are between the sixth and fifth compartment, where the extensor digiti minimi tendon is very deep to the distal radio-ulnar joint, and between the third and second compartment. 1, extensor carpi ulnaris tendon (sixth compartment); 2, extensor digiti minimi (fifth compartment); 3, extensor digitorum communis (fourth compartment); 4, extensor indicis proprius; 5, extensor pollicis longus tendon; 6, Lister's tubercle; 7, extensor carpi radialis brevis; 8, extensor carpi radialis longus. (B) Peroperative view.

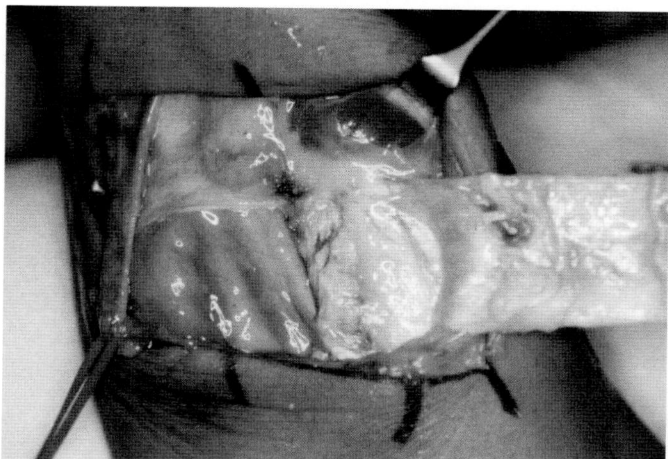

Figure 32.5

Preoperative view of the extensor tendon synovitis. Each tendon should be cleaned up with the knife, from the distal muscle fibers to the base of the metacarpals.

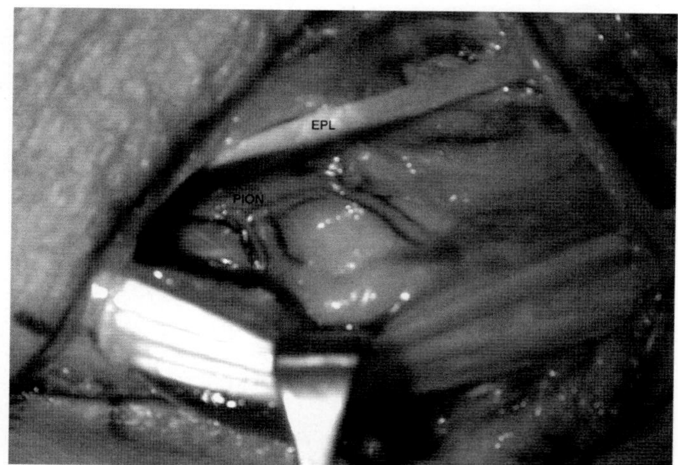

Figure 32.6

The posterior interosseous nerve runs deep to the extensor tendons of the fourth compartment along with a dorsal branch of the anterior interosseous artery. PION, posterior interosseous nerve; EPL, extensor pollicis longus.

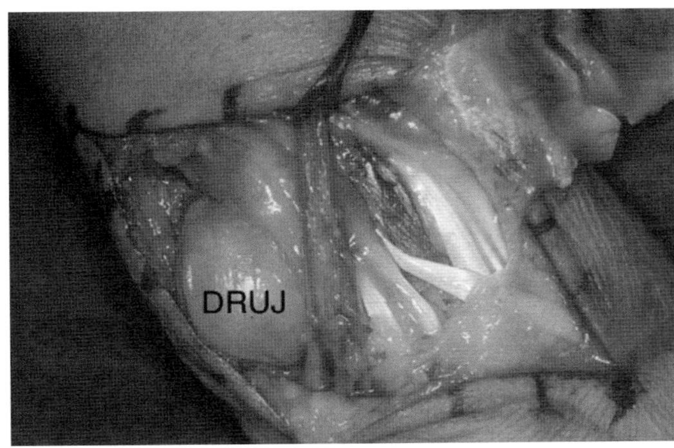

Figure 32.7
Distal radio-ulnar joint synovitis is very frequent and disabling. Note the importance of the synovitis. DRUJ, distal radio-ulnar joint.

32.8). The synovial proliferation predominates in the sacciform recess, which cannot be exposed without resecting the ulnar head. Resection of the ulnar head is mandatory to perform a distal radio-ulnar joint synovectomy correctly (Kessler and Vainio 1966, Eiken et al 1975, Allieu and Brahin 1977, Mannerfelt 1984, Flatt 1995).

Resection of the ulnar head limited to the length of the articular surface (Darrach's procedure) is the most frequently performed procedure (Figure 32.9). As the triangular fibrocartilage complex is usually one the first structures destroyed by the disease, it is also possible to perform a synovectomy of the ulnar side of the wrist after resection of the ulnar head (Flatt 1995). Technical variations of the Darrach's procedure – i.e. intra- or extra-periosteal resection, with or without preservation of the ulnar styloid – had no influence on the quality of the results (Dingman 1952). Darrach's resection has proved its efficiency in rheumatoid arthritis (Fraser et al 1999); however, there are two potential drawbacks. Firstly, instability of the ulnar stump may sometimes be a problem. Cast immobilization in supination is usually effective. The exact frequency of this instability is unknown: Edstrom et al (1975) reported no instability while others have reported up to 30% of unstable ulnar stumps (Rana and Taylor 1973, Jensen 1983b, Newman 1987). Instability is correlated to the amount of resection for some authors, but not for others (Rana and Taylor 1973). Finally, instability disappears with time in some series, but persists in others (Jensen 1983b, Newman 1987). From a practical point of view, very few patients complained of instability. However, the best treatment is stabilization during surgery. For a long time we used a strip of the extensor carpi ulnaris tendon, which is

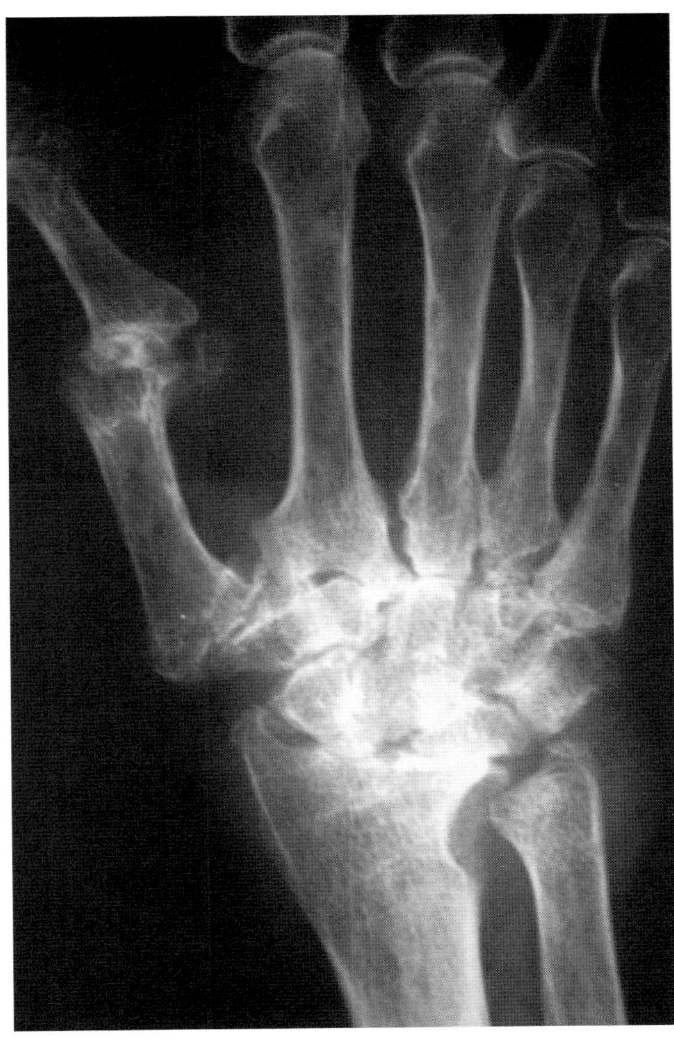

(A)

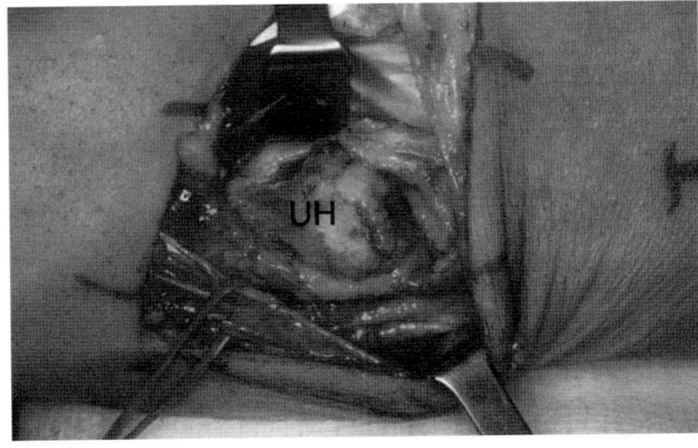

(B)

Figure 32.8
Distal radio-ulnar joint involvement. (A) Distal radio-ulnar joint synovitis is responsible for encroachment of the distal radius (Freiberg's sign). Freiberg's sign is associated with a high incidence of tendon rupture. (B) Spontaneous dorsal dislocation of the ulnar head is responsible for mechanical tendon attrition and rupture. UH, ulnar head.

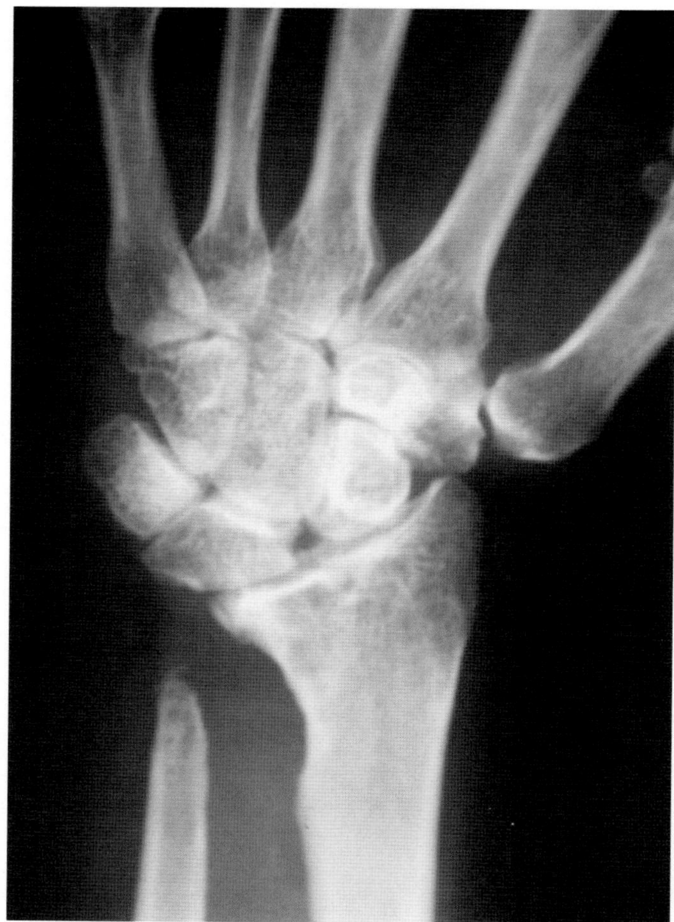

Figure 32.9

Radiological appearance of a wrist at 5 years after surgery. Note resection of the distal ulna (Darrach's procedure). Note also the sclerosis of the distal radius that indicates the ulnar stump instability with abutment against the radius (see also Figure 32.11).

passed through the stump from outside to inside, to cover the distal stump to avoid potential tendinous ruptures (Millender et al 1974, Abernethy and Dennyson 1979, Rasker et al 1980, Rowland 1984, O'Donovan and Ruby 1989, Leslie et al 1990) (Figure 32.10). More recently I changed the technique by using a strip of the flexor carpi ulnaris tendon, as a modification of Hui and Linscheid's procedure (Hui and Linscheid 1982). A second, volar incision is needed and the ulnar half of the flexor carpi ulnaris tendon is passed from volar to dorsal in the distal ulnar stump to exit on the dorsal surface. This technique both stabilizes the ulnar stump and corrects the supination deformity of the carpus. Clinical instability is usually present at rest, whatever the stabilization technique used and this explains why 80% of the patients present sclerosis of the medial side of the

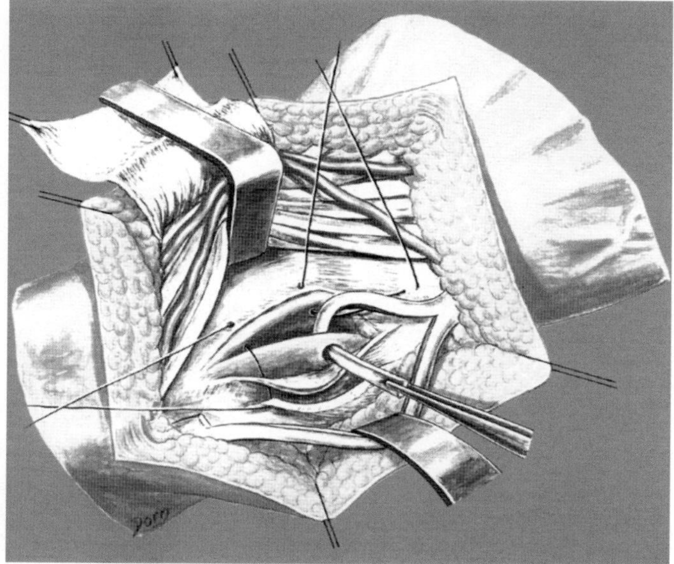

(A)

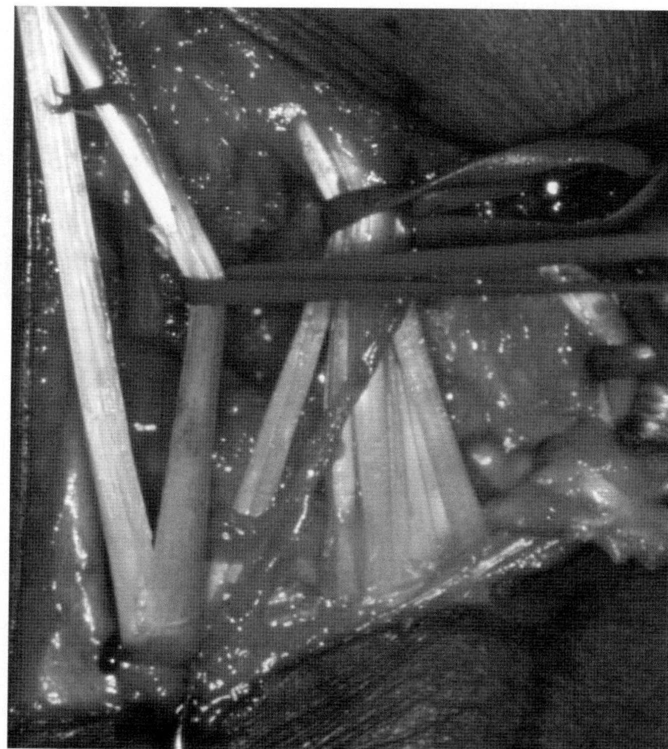

(B)

Figure 32.10

Stabilization of the ulnar stump with a strip of the extensor carpi ulnaris (ECU) tendon. (A) Schematic drawing showing the strip of the ECU tendon passing into the ulnar stump. Note that we usually perform the stabilization of the ulnar stump from outside to inside to protect the tendons from any bony spurs of the ulnar stump. Note also the sutures passing from the radius to the triquetrum to stabilize the carpus, and the suture passing from the radius to the medial side of the retinaculum extensorum to help stabilize the ulnar stump. (B) Peroperative view.

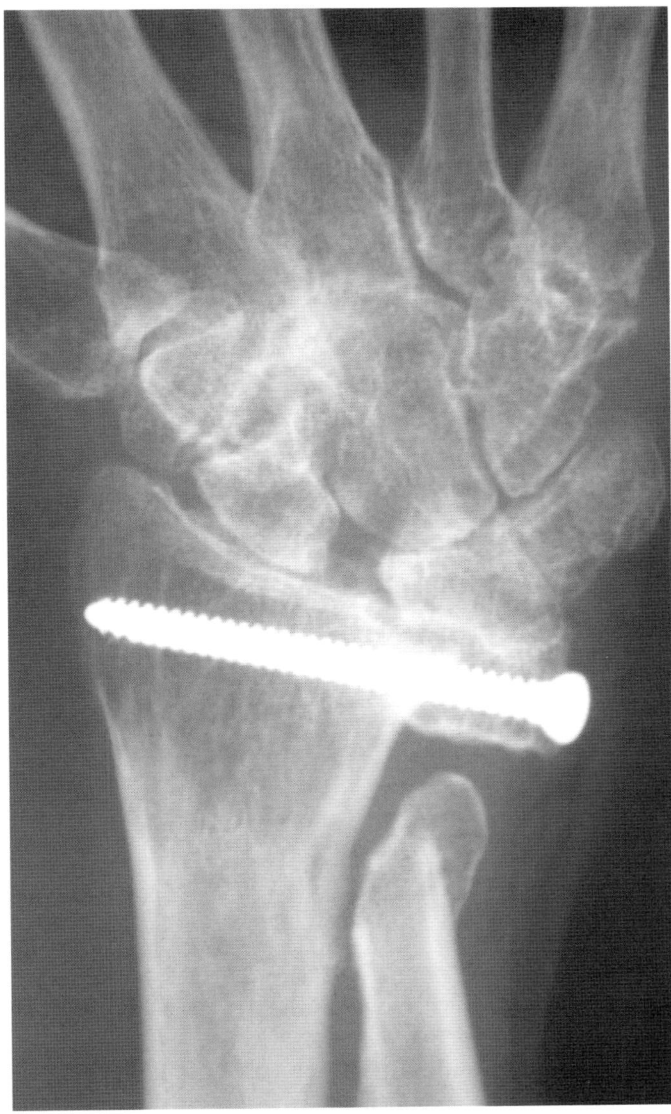

Figure 32.11
Severe ulnar translation of the carpus. Note that the lunate is medial to the radius and only articulates with the ulnar head. Note also the sclerotic changes of both the distal radius and the ulnar stump owing to the ulnar stump instability (patient had no symptoms). There is also severe scapholunate dissociation.

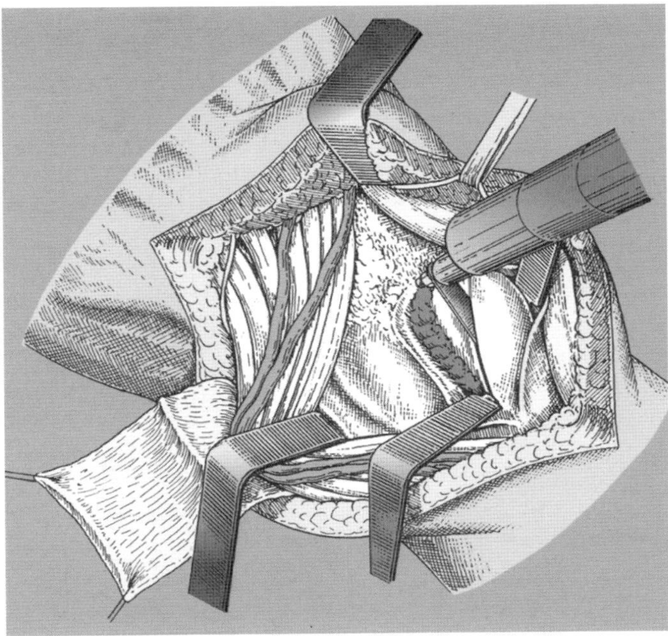

(A)

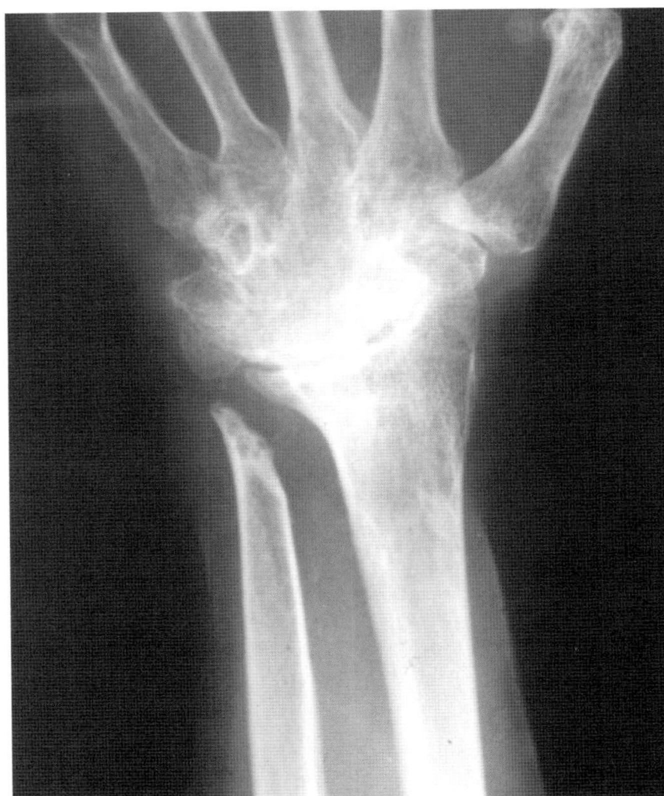

(B)

Figure 32.12
Bowers' osteotomy of the distal ulna. (A) Schematic drawing of the oblique osteotomy, which removes the entire articular surface of the distal ulna, keeping intact its medial side with the ulnar styloid. (B) Radiographic appearance of a Bowers' type osteotomy. Note the bony spur that has grown from the medial radius to perfectly mold the carpus and stabilize it.

radius on plain X-rays (Allieu and Brahin 1977, Newman 1987, O'Donovan and Ruby 1989) (Figure 32.9).

The other reported drawback of Darrach's procedure is a potential increase of ulnar carpal translation under the radius (Alnot and Leroux 1985). Postoperative ulnar translation and/or ulnar deviation of the wrist has been noted in all series, even after the Sauvé-Kapandji technique (Alnot and Fauroux 1992, Vincent et al 1993). This is due to the destruction of the radio-carpal ligaments by the disease and/or the destruction of the ulnar side of the radius (Backhouse et al 1971, Jackson et al 1974, Eiken et al 1975, Edstrom et al 1976, Allieu and Brahin 1977, Black et al 1977, Rasker et al 1980, Newman 1987, Alnot and Fauroux 1992, Fourastier et al 1992, Van Gemert and Spauwen 1994). In more advanced cases of the disease, ulnar head resection increases ulnar translation from about 2–3 mm in 10 years (Allieu and Brahin 1977). Van Gemert and Spauwen (1994) reported an ulnar translation of 5.3 mm in the operated patients with Darrach's resection, versus 3.7 mm in the non-operated group ($P < 0.05$) (Figure 32.11). After 5–9 years of follow-up mean difference between the wrists was 1.6 mm, while ulnar translation due to the disease itself was 3.7 mm. Ulnar translation is more pronounced if the ulnar side of the wrist is weakened by the disease (5 mm vs 2.1 mm) (Van Gemert and Spauwen 1994). Finally Jensen (1983b) reported one case of bony regrowth of the distal stump without functional impairment. We have frequently noted a thinning of the distal stump that is more probably secondary to remodeling than to an osseous regrowth. I now limit the indications for Darrach's resection to total or partial wrist fusion.

Tubiana (1990) chose to perform an oblique resection of the ulnar articular surface as in the Bowers' procedure, whenever possible (Bowers 1985). Bowers' resection is usually contraindicated when the triangular fibrocartilage complex is destroyed and this was the case in most of our patients. The principal advantage, in our opinion, is to facilitate stabilization of the ulnar stump by keeping it as long as possible (Figure 32.12). The retinaculum extensorum, which helps to stabilize the ulnar stump, is stronger in its distal part. Two sutures are made in the medial border of the distal radius that pass under the extensor tendons through the medial flap of the retinaculum extensorum (see also Figure 32.15B). Bowers' osteotomy and its equivalent, the matched ulna resection described by Watson (1986), also have their own complications: limitation of prosupination in case of inadequate resection or fracture of the distal stump if resection has been too generous.

This is why I prefer to carry out a Sauvé-Kapandji radio-ulnar arthrodesis (Figure 32.13). Synovectomy is achieved by rocking the ulnar head around the soft tissues of the medial part of the wrist. Resection of the ulna should be minimal (< 1 cm), as bony regrowth with limitation of prosupination mobility has only been reported in three patients, only one requiring surgery (Alnot and Leroux 1985, Alnot and Fauroux 1992). Proximal instability of the ulnar stump is theoretically more frequent than after a Darrach's procedure and has been reported in 21–62% of patients, some of them requiring secondary surgery (Vincent et al 1993, Taleisnik 1992). This high frequency of complications is very different from our experience, as well as that of Alnot and Fauroux (1992). None of our patients experienced either functionally disabling instability of the ulnar stump or bony regrowth. We always perform ulnar stump stabilization with the flexor carpi ulnaris (FCU) tendon nowadays. We believe that the carpal medial stabilization of the Sauvé-Kapandji technique is mostly theoretical, as ligamentous structures of the radio-ulnar joint are usually the first to be destroyed. The only stabilizing effect would be a bony buttress effect that is rarely observed (Vincent et al 1993) (see Figure 32.11).

However, the Sauvé-Kapandji technique has some advantages. It is indicated when the ulnar side of the radius is destroyed or in patients with an increased radial tilt, to prevent excessive ulnar deviation of the hand (see Figure 32.13). It increases the radial surface and helps to stabilize the carpus when it is lax (see Figure 32.11). It helps to stabilize the lunate when radiolunate arthrodesis is performed. It also provides better cosmetic results than those of ulna resection.

Radio-carpal and midcarpal synovectomy

We always perform an intracarpal synovectomy, as the radio-carpal joint is involved in 95% of patients presenting a tendinous synovitis and in 97% of patients presenting a distal radio-ulnar joint synovitis (Kulick et al 1981). For open surgery, we designed a U-shaped capsular flap with distal attachment (Figure 32.14). This flap is radially designed to respect the posterior radio-triquetral ligament (Tubiana 1990). Wrist flexion and axial traction facilitate synovectomy by opening the radio-carpal joint and especially the radioscaphoid joint where the synovial tissue is always abundant (see Figure 32.1). The synovium on the ulnar side is more easily removed through the distal radio-ulnar joint approach. Intraosseous invasion of the synovium, especially at the insertion site of the radioscapholunate ligament, must be carefully excised (Mannerfelt 1984). According to the literature, involvement of the midcarpal joint is less frequent but we always find synovitis in this joint and usually perform a midcarpal synovectomy (Hindley and Stanley 1991, Alnot and Fauroux 1992). We always perform a synovectomy of this joint; involvement seems rare from a review of the literature but is frequent in our experience (Mannerfelt 1984, Alnot and Fauroux 1992). Very few authors perform a synovectomy of the carpometacarpal joints (Allieu and Brahin 1977). Fourastier et al (1992) argued that intracarpal synovectomy can only be limited and may contribute to stiffness of the wrist. For those reasons they stated that no intracarpal synovectomy should be carried out during dorsal wrist synovectomy. It is true that intracarpal synovectomy contributes to stiffening of the wrist but we do not agree with the above proposal. It does not take into account the high frequency of intracarpal involvement as well as its role in the patient's pain. Furthermore, the choice of not opening the radio-carpal joint does not allow removal of the synovium of the radioscaphoid space, which in early involvement is responsible for the altered dynamics and the supination

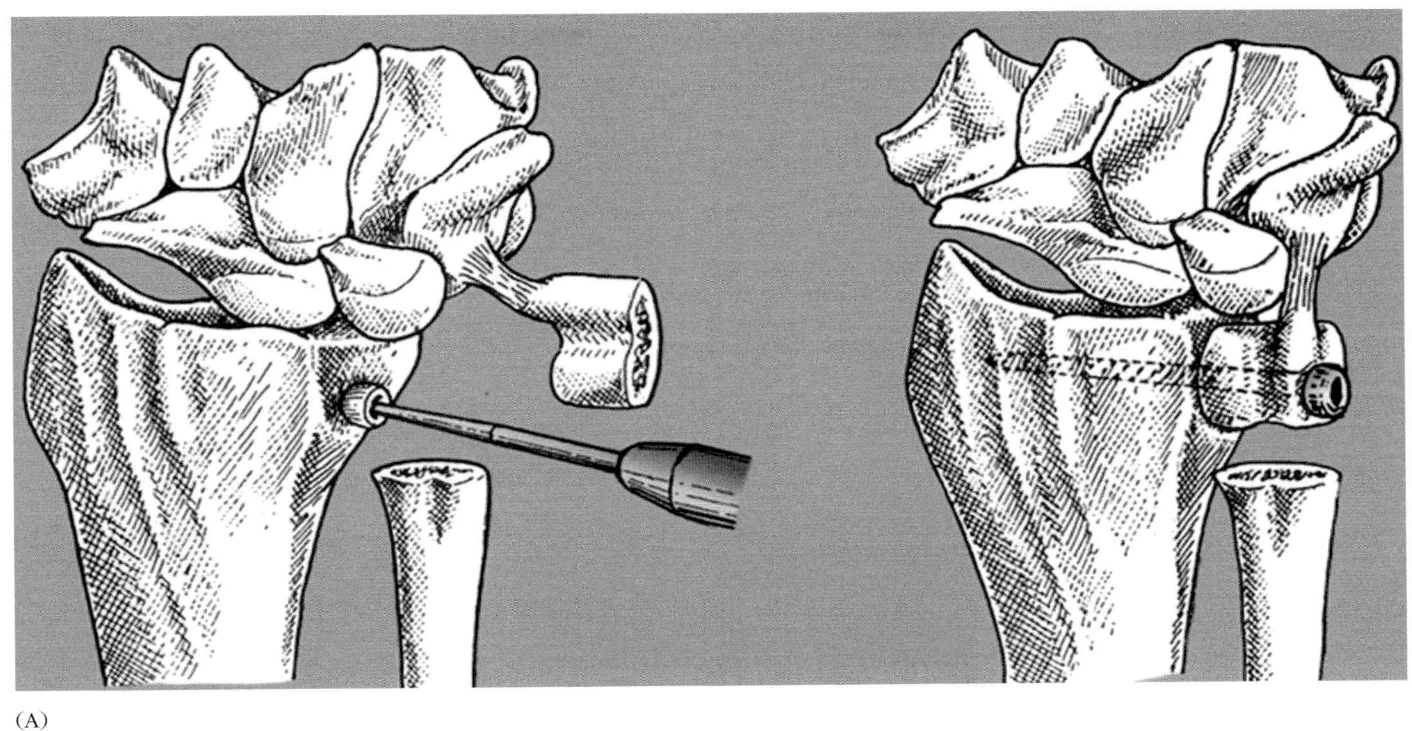

(A)

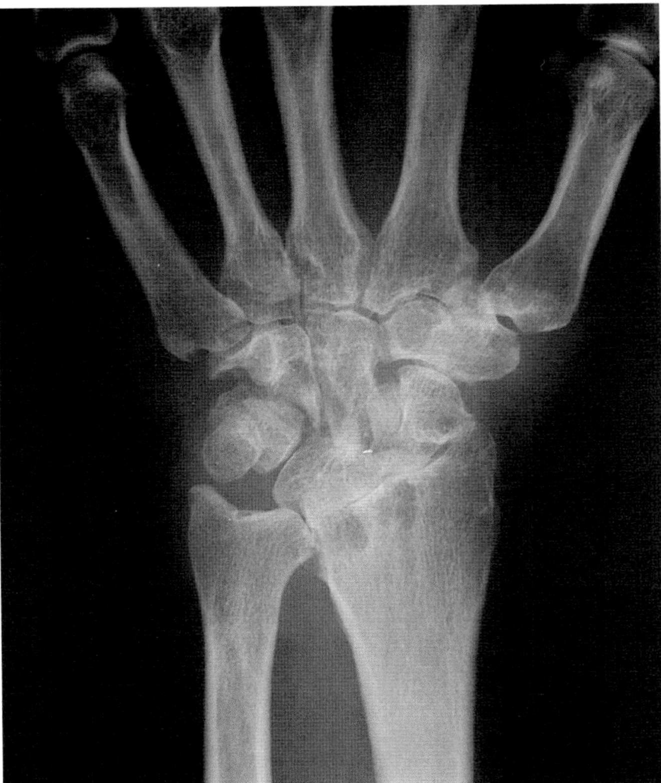

(B)

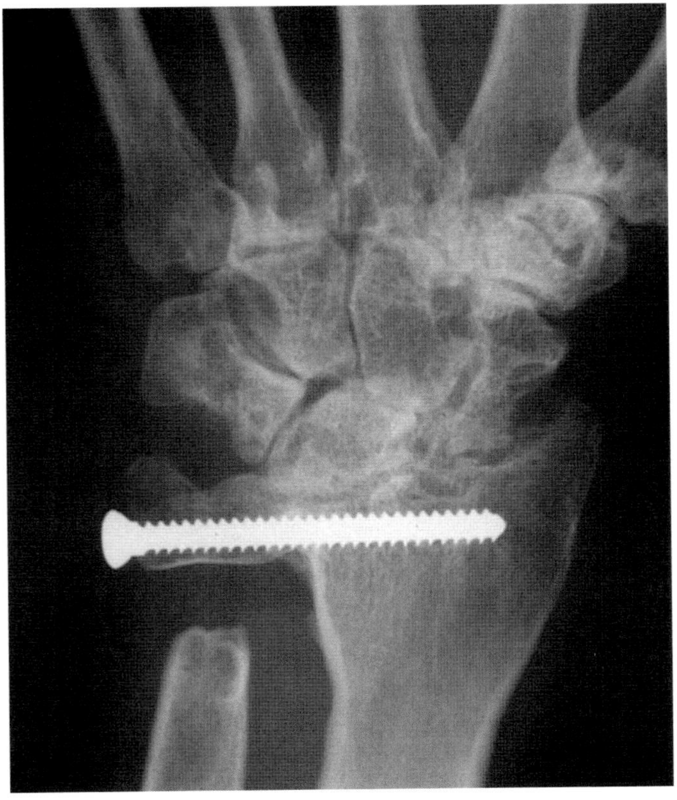

(C)

Figure 32.13

Sauvé-Kapandji procedure. (A) Schematic drawing of the Sauvé-Kapandji procedure. After cartilage removal of the sigmoid notch, the ulnar head is fixed in position. Note that <1 cm of ulnar diaphysis is to be removed, as distal as possible. (B) Preoperative AP view of a patient. Note the importance of the synovitis on the medial side of the radius with the huge cyst in the lunate fossa. In this type of patient, a Sauvé-Kapandji procedure is mandatory to avoid radius impaction with ulnar deviation of the carpus. (C) Postoperative appearance of a Sauvé-Kapandji distal radio-ulnar joint arthrodesis (same patient as in B).

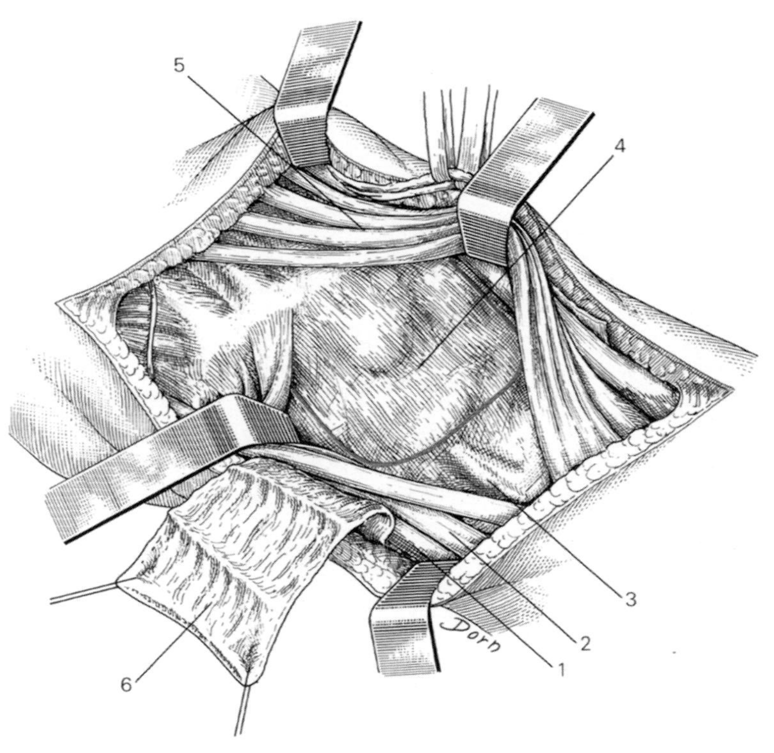

(A)

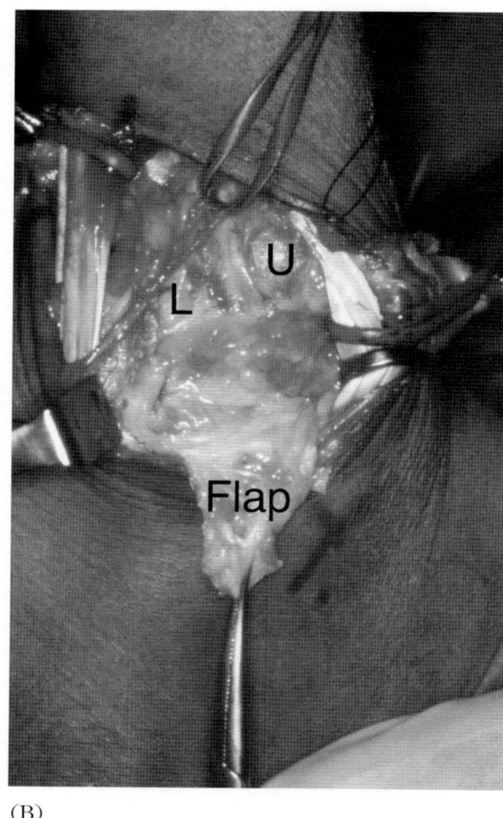

(B)

Figure 32.14

Intracarpal synovectomy. (A) Schematic drawing of the capsular flap designed to enter both radio-carpal and midcarpal joint. Note that the flap is radially drawn to respect the dorsal radio-triquetral ligament that is reconstructed or reinforced during the procedure. 1, extensor carpi radialis longus; 2, extensor carpi radialis brevis; 3, Lister's tubercle; 4, the capsular flap; 5, extensor digitorum communis tendons; 6, retinaculum extensorum. (B) Perioperative view. Note the importance of the intra-carpal synovitis. Flap, capsular flap; U, ulnar head; L, Lister's tubercle

deformity of the carpus. Moreover, the absence of intracarpal synovectomy precludes the radio-carpal stabilization, which is always done, except in patients with a stable and non-destroyed wrist, in whom arthroscopic synovectomy may be considered. It is during intracarpal synovectomy that the clinician can judge the reducibility of the carpus under the radius and the stabilization techniques that should be used. We believe that preoperative dynamic X-rays are of no help in evaluating the reducibility (Allieu and Brahin 1977).

Stabilization of the carpus under the radius

This is a fundamental step of the procedure. Ulnar dislocation correlated with poor results has been observed in 13–42% of wrist synovectomies without stabilization (Vahvanen and Patiala 1984, Ferlic and Clayton 1985). The first stabilizing technique, proposed by Straub and Ranawat (1969), was carried out with K-wires left in place for 6–8 weeks. This technique is only of historical interest, as it is close to a 'disguised' arthrodesis. Spontaneous arthrodesis has been observed in 43% of patients with this technique.

Soft tissue stabilization

We prefer to use a soft tissue stabilization technique that reconstructs the posterior radiotriquetral ligament (Tubiana 1990). Wrist deformity is corrected by placing the wrist in radial translation, ulnar deviation, and pronation. A non-absorbable suture is placed through the medial side of the radius to the triquetrum and sutured under tension while the deformity is corrected by an

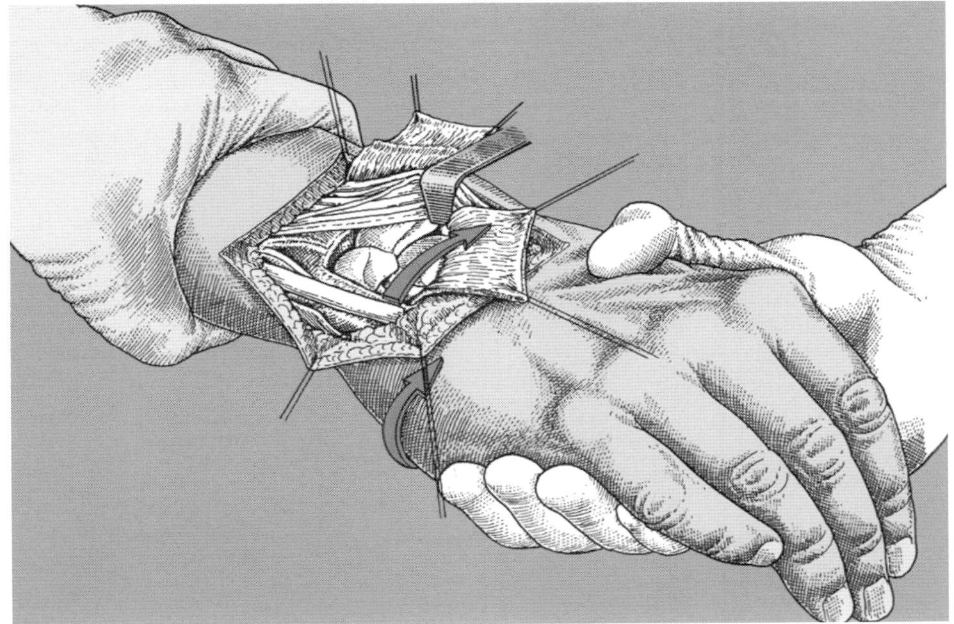

(A)

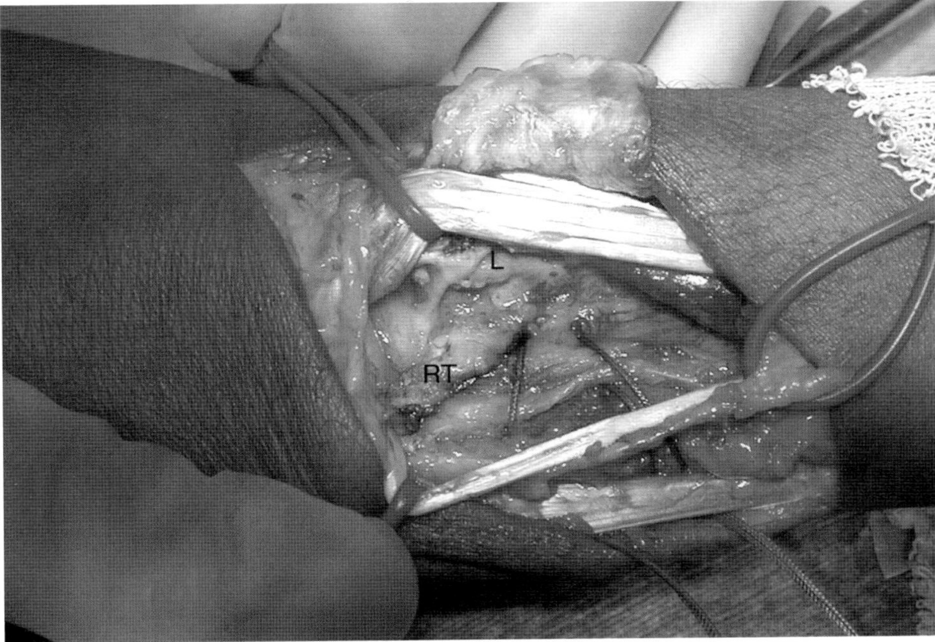

(B)

Figure 32.15

Correction of the deformity and soft tissue stabilization. (A) Schematic drawing of the different maneuvers to correct the deformity. Before sewing the sutures, the assistant must correct the ulnar translation, the radial inclination, and the supination deformity of the carpus. (B) Perioperative view of a soft tissue stabilization. Note the two sutures, one to reconstruct the radio-triquetral ligament (RT), and one to reinsert the capsular flap onto the Lister's tubercle (L). Note also the two sutures from the distal radius to the medial flap of the retinaculum extensorum that will help to stabilize the ulnar stump.

assistant (Figure 32.15). The dorsal capsule is sutured back to Lister's tubercle, which we always preserve. An isolated scapholunate dislocation is treated by placing one or two K-wires for 6–8 weeks, as proposed by Taleisnik (1989). However, in our experience early recurrence of the deformity is frequent, without apparent functional impairment (see Figure 32.11). In more advanced forms of the disease, it is sometimes necessary to stabilize the carpus by partial wrist arthrodesis. We always perform a Sauvé-Kapandji procedure with a soft tissue stabilization when there is an increased radial deviation of the radius or when the lunate fossa of the radius is attenuated by the disease (Hindley and Stanley 1991). In those particular cases, the tension of the reconstructed radiotriquetral ligament may destroy the lunate fossa of the radius, which will induce a major ulnar inclination of the carpus that is very unesthetic and functionally disabling.

Clinical results

Ninety per cent of patients were suffering preoperatively, with severe pain in three out of four. Pain relief is the most obvious effect of the procedure, as 66% of our patients had no pain postoperatively, even during exercises. On a visual scale, pain decreased from 7.17/10 preoperatively to 1.09 at the last follow-up. According to the literature, pain relief at rest is the rule and is maintained at follow-up in 80–95% of patients (Ansell et al 1974, Jackson et al 1974, Edstrom et al 1976, Kulick et al 1981, Thirupathi et al 1983, Mannerfelt 1984, Vahvanen and Patiala 1984, Bohler et al 1985, Wilson 1986, Allieu et al 1988, 1989, Linclau and Dokter 1988, Brumfield et al 1990, Ferlic et al 1991, Alnot and Fauroux 1992, Fourastier et al 1992). Less than 4% of the patients deteriorate, even in series without stabilization. In our experience, persisting pain was secondary to distal radio-ulnar impingement, or to recurrent synovitis of the radio-carpal or mostly the distal radio-ulnar joint.

Always present before surgery, synovitis was absent in 95% of our cases postoperatively. This disappearance of the synovitis explains the excellent pain relief reported in the literature in patients with extensive synovectomy (Clayton and Ferlic 1965, Millender et al 1974, Kulick et al 1981, Thirupathi et al 1983, Brown 1984, Vahvanen and Patiala 1984, Wilson 1986, Allieu et al 1988, 1989, Alnot and Fauroux 1992). Recurrence frequency is highly variable. Ferlic and Clayton (1985) reported no recurrence. Like many authors, we had between 4% and 5% recurrence of the synovitis (Straub and Ranawat 1969, Millender et al 1974, Edstrom et al 1976, Brown 1984, Wilson 1986, Fourastier et al 1992). Synovitis recurrence has been reported in 20% of patients by some authors (Kulick et al 1981, Allieu et al 1989, Brumfield et al 1990). All authors agree that the most aggressive forms are those most prone to recurrence. Alnot (1992) reported re-operation in 4% of his patients. However, only extensor or distal radio-ulnar joint synovitis are detected by a clinical examination. If radiological deterioration is considered, 80% of patients have a recurrence of carpal synovitis.

It is usual to say that surgery performed at an early stage will preserve or increase wrist mobility, as late surgery will stiffen the wrist (Alnot and Fauroux 1992, Fourastier et al 1992). In our experience, postoperative mobility was mostly correlated with preoperative mobility and not with the severity of the disease. Increased mobility in prono-supination was rather limited, as the preoperative mobility was usually preserved. However, patients were very pleased with the result, as prono-supination was now pain-free. Distal radio-ulnar joint synovectomy is so effective for reducing pain that Clayton and Ferlic (1975) claimed that it was the only useful procedure in wrist synovectomy. In the literature, a small gain of mobility in prono-supination is frequent (Rana and Taylor 1973, Rasker et al 1980, Kulick et al 1981, Jensen 1983a, Newman 1987, Taleisnik 1992); 80–90% of patients have complete mobility in prono-supination, whatever the technique used.

Extension and ulnar deviation, which are useful for placing the hand in a functional position, have been preserved in our experience (Figure 32.16). It is difficult to compare our results with the literature: without stabilization, a quarter of the patients had increased mobility, a quarter had decreased mobility and half were unchanged (Abernethy and Dennyson 1979, Jensen 1983a, Mannerfelt 1984, Vahvanen and Patiala 1984, Brown and Brown 1988, Alnot and Fauroux 1992, Fourastier et al 1992). Some authors have shown that loss of mobility was correlated with the evolution of the disease and the follow-up (Kulick et al 1981, Vahvanen

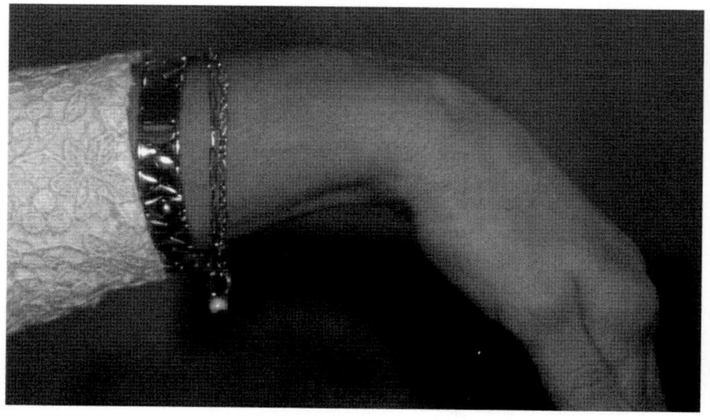

(A)

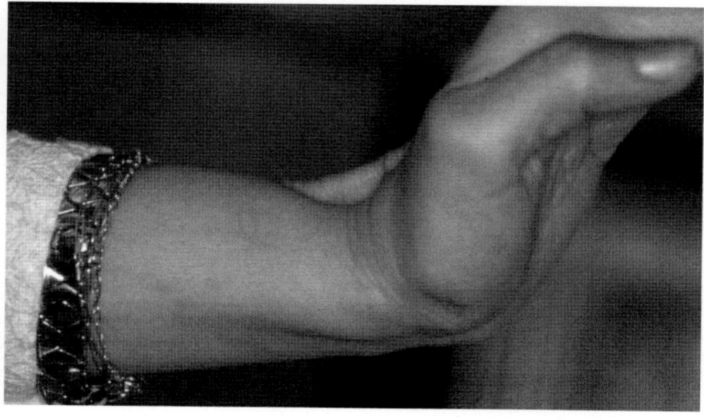

(B)

Figure 32.16

Postoperative results of wrist synovectomy with soft tissue stabilization. Note the bowstringing effect of the extensor tendons in this patient with good extension.

and Patiala 1984). After a stabilization technique, a flexion arc of 60° and a radial deviation arc of 20° are usually obtained (Vahvanen and Patiala 1984, Stanley and Boot 1989, Brumfield et al 1990).

Grip strength is directly correlated with a pain-free and stable wrist. According to the literature, strength increases between 30% and 40%, but it is difficult to appreciate, as the digital articulations are also involved and may deteriorate with time (Rana and Taylor 1973, Ansell et al 1974, Eiken et al 1975, Rasker et al 1980, Wilson 1986, Newman 1987, Allieu et al 1989, Stanley and Boot 1989). In our experience, strength was identical to the non-operated wrist and did not diminish with time. However, we found its measurement very disappointing as it does not only reflect wrist involvement. Most patients complained of loss of strength due to muscular atrophy, steroid therapy, other joint involvement (especially the thumb), limited use of the hand, and progression of the disease. From a practical point of view, once strength is lost it is never recovered.

We also tried to quantify the global function of the wrist by the performance of simple tasks such as holding a cup, pouring a liquid, opening a door. Like almost every other author who has attempted this, we have been disappointed, as it was impossible to test the wrist alone; other joints modified the results (Rana and Taylor 1973, Kulick et al 1981, Bohler et al 1985, Allieu et al 1989). On a maximum score of 30 points, patients had an average of 28 at 1 year follow-up and 26 at last follow-up. The wrist is no longer a problem in activities of daily living for the patients. According to Eiken et al (1975), 56% of patients are improved, 38% are unchanged and only 6% are worse in their performance of daily activities after surgery.

Radiological results

The different measurement systems described for the wrist, although very precise in their description, have been disappointing in our experience of the rheumatoid wrist. In more than 40% of our cases, especially in the most advanced, it was impossible to use the bony landmarks and in most of our cases, measurements appeared quite imprecise. Many authors have met the same problems and have abandoned or modified these techniques (Thirupathi et al 1983, Allieu et al 1989, Stanley and Boot 1989, Chamay and Della Santa 1991, Fourastier et al 1992). Shapiro's A1 angle, which measures the radial deviation of the carpus, changed from 119° preoperatively to 121° at the last follow-up, as in Brown's series (Brown 1984). Its apparent stability does not reflect the surgical correction of the deformity, as the frequent destruction of the lunate fossa of the radius or the existence of a radiolunate fusion had very often made measurements impossible. Moreover, this angle may be modified if the hand is not perfectly flat on the radiographical plate and it cannot help to predict the evolution of the wrist (Van Gemert and Spauwen 1994). Youm et al (1978) proposed criteria to evaluate the height of the carpus. More often than not, the destruction of the carpometacarpal joints and/or the metacarpophalangeal joint of the long finger made its measurement impossible. The technique of carpal height measurement proposed by Thirupathi et al (1983) seemed to us more easy to perform and in our series the mean loss of carpal height was 2 mm. Alnot and Fauroux (1992) considered that carpal height did not change with time, while Allieu et al (1989) and Thirupathi et al (1983) reported a carpal height loss of 4–5 mm. There is a linear loss of carpal height with time, which seems to be independent of the surgical techniques employed (Edstrom et al 1975, Thirupathi et al 1983, Allieu et al 1989, Stanley and Boot 1989).

Ulnar translation of the carpus is functionally very important but cannot be measured by Youm's criteria if the ulnar head has been resected. Allieu's or Chamay's criteria must be used, which utilize the radius as the reference point (Allieu et al 1989, Chamay and Della Santa 1991). In our experience, as in Allieu and Thirupathi's experience, deterioration is the rule and is almost linear with time. According to those authors, ulnar translation was of 1–3 mm at 5 years follow-up. In our more advanced cases, ulnar translation was 4 mm in 4 years and was 5 mm for Thirupathi et al (1983) with 7 years follow-up. The latter authors do not use any stabilization technique. There was no correlation between ulnar translation and clinical results. We found that Thirupathi's methods of measurement were more easy to use and we were able to achieve them in 95% of our patients (Thirupathi et al 1983).

Palmar subluxation is frequent but difficult to measure. Radiological measurements have shown palmar subluxation to be present in 43% of patients, with important variations: global anterior translation of the carpus or midcarpal anterior translation. Spontaneous radiolunate fusion has been observed with a frequency of between 10 and 25% (Black et al 1977, Kulick et al 1981, Chamay et al 1983, Vahvanen and Patiala 1984, Chamay and Della Santa 1991, Alnot and Fauroux 1992). It was present in 26% of our more advanced cases (Larsen 3 and above). Surgical synovectomy favors medial stabilization of the carpus, either by a spontaneous partial wrist fusion, or by the appearance of a bony spur on the medial side of the radius, which molds the proximal surface of the lunate (Eiken et al 1975, Gainor and Schaberg 1985) (see Figures 32.9 and 32.12B). Finally, even if inaccurate, Steinbrocker's or mostly Larsen's radiological classifications are the most useful for evaluation of the severity of the disease. However, their accuracy is limited by the stigmata of surgery and clinical evolution is still the best way to evaluate the results.

According to Vahvanen and Patiala (1984), 40% of patients had a radiological deterioration that was less important than the opposite wrist, while 56% had the same radiological evolution with 9 years follow-up. Comparison with the opposite wrist is in fact useless, as

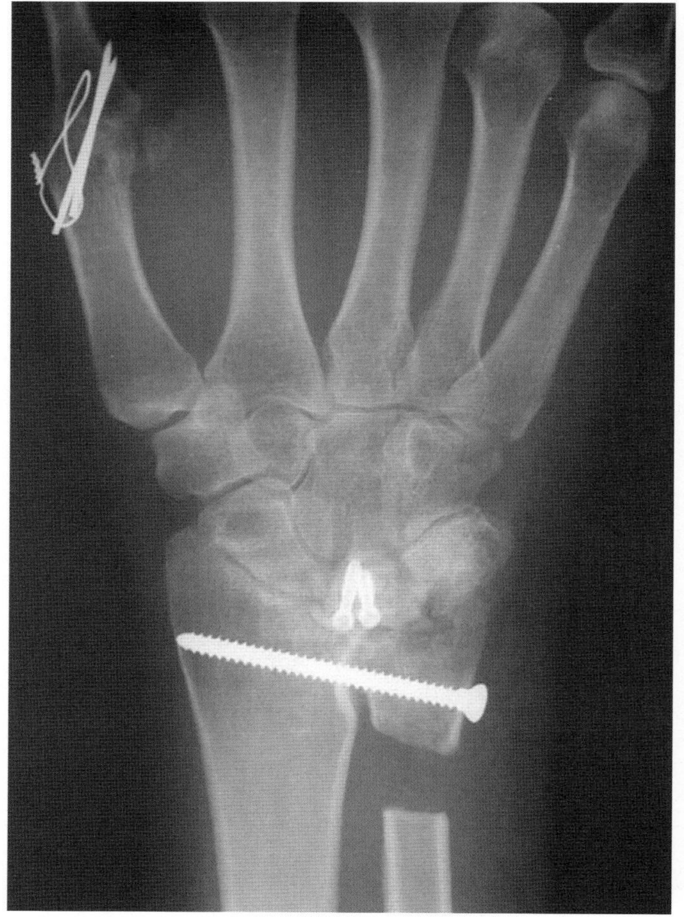

(A)

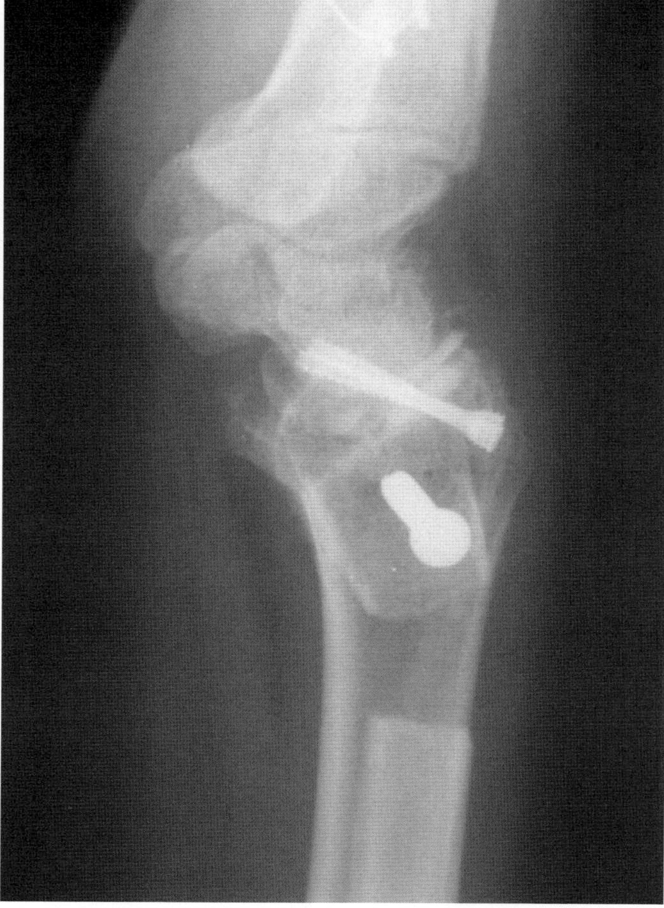

(B)

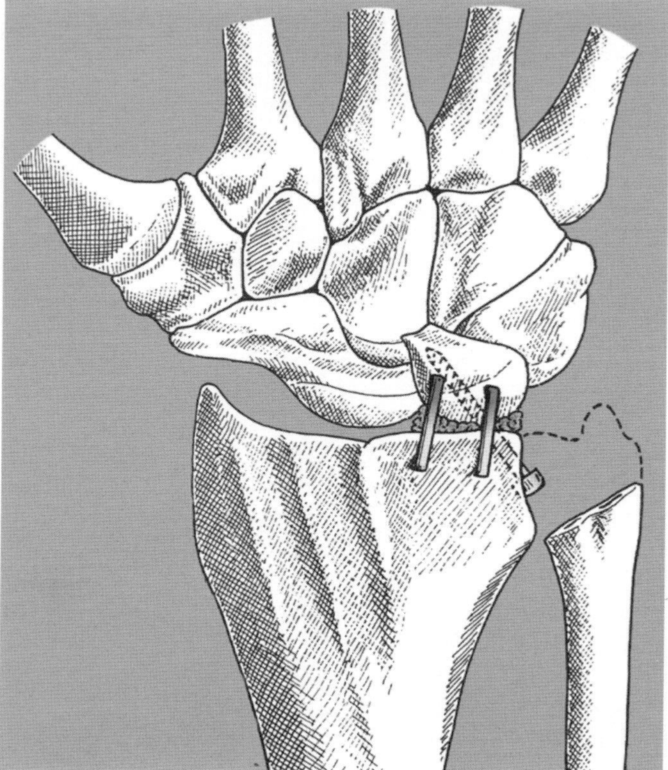

(C)

Figure 32.17

Radiolunate arthrodesis. (A) AP view of a radiolunate arthrodesis and a Sauvé-Kapandji technique. Note that the ulnar head is used to increase the amount of bony surfaces in contact. (B) Lateral view. (C) Schematic drawing of a radiolunate fusion. Note that a graft has been used so as not to increase the constraints on the scaphoid, which may be forced into flexion otherwise.

a symmetrical radiological involvement is noticed in only 30% of wrists, while the clinical evolution is symmetrical in 90% of wrists (Edstrom et al 1976). It is doubtful that surgery will change the radiological evolution of the wrist (Edstrom et al 1976, Bohler et al 1985). Finally, a radiological deterioration is obvious in every series, whatever the techniques used (Rana and Taylor 1973, Ansell et al 1974, Jackson et al 1974, Eiken et al 1975, Jensen 1983a, Torisu et al 1983, Newman 1987, Allieu et al 1989, Brumfield et al 1990, Alnot and Fauroux 1992, Della Santa and Chamay 1995). However, this radiological deterioration is not correlated with deterioration of the deformities and the wrist still remains aligned.

Partial wrist fusion

A radiolunate arthrodesis is indicated when the lunate fossa of the radius is destroyed or when the ulnar and/or volar carpal translation cannot be corrected. According to Chamay, radiolunate arthrodesis should be considered when the Bouman's index value falls below 0.80 (Bouman et al 1994, Chamay 1998). Another indication will be a severe ulnar drift of the metacarpophalangeal joints with severe radial inclination of the wrist. Radiolunate fusion will then help to correct the finger deformities (Chamay 1998). In all cases, there must be conservation of the carpal bone stock and preservation of the capitate and lunate articular cartilage. If Simmen types can be settled by successive measurement of the translation index (Simmen and Huber 1992), total wrist fusion is preferred in type III, and radiolunate fusion in type I and II (Della Santa and Chamay 1995).

The wrist joint can be opened by raising a rectangular capsulo-ligamentous flap from the distal radius, the lunate, the proximal pole of the scaphoid, and the capitate, to which it should remain attached. Good access to the radio-carpal and midcarpal joints is required, so that a synovectomy can be performed and the articular surfaces can be inspected (Chamay 1998).

The cartilage of the radiolunate joint is removed using rongeurs until cancellous bone is obtained on both surfaces. The lunate is reduced into an anatomical position and temporarily fixed with K-wires. An intra-operative X-ray is performed to verify the position before definitive fixation. It is often useful to control the lunate position from the ulnar side when an ulnar head resection has been performed.

The osteosynthesis may be performed by using oblique screws passing from the radius into the palmar part of the lunate or from the lunate into the anterior part of the radial epiphysis (Figure 32.17). Care must be taken not to violate the midcarpal joint. This may also be done by using two staples, two K-wires, or plate and screws. If there is insufficient bone stock, a bone graft can be carried out, using the ulnar head embedded between the radius and the lunate. If the lunate is still placed too ulnarly to the radius, Chamay (1998) recommended the use of a tooth-shaped graft screwed on the ulnar side of the radius, and placement of the graft into a prepared hole in the lunate. In these cases, we favor the association of radiolunate fusion with the Sauvé-Kapandji technique to facilitate bone healing.

When the normal bone shape of the carpal bones is preserved, the lunate should be fused in an anatomical position, thus correcting the radial deviation of the wrist. If the lunate is fused in an ulnar-translated position, the height determines the lateral deviation of the wrist (Chamay 1998). A radial inclination is favored by a high position, whereas a low position favors ulnar deviation. When the lunate is fixed in a high position (correcting the carpal collapse) the load that it must support is excessive, leading to a rapid deterioration of the capitolunate

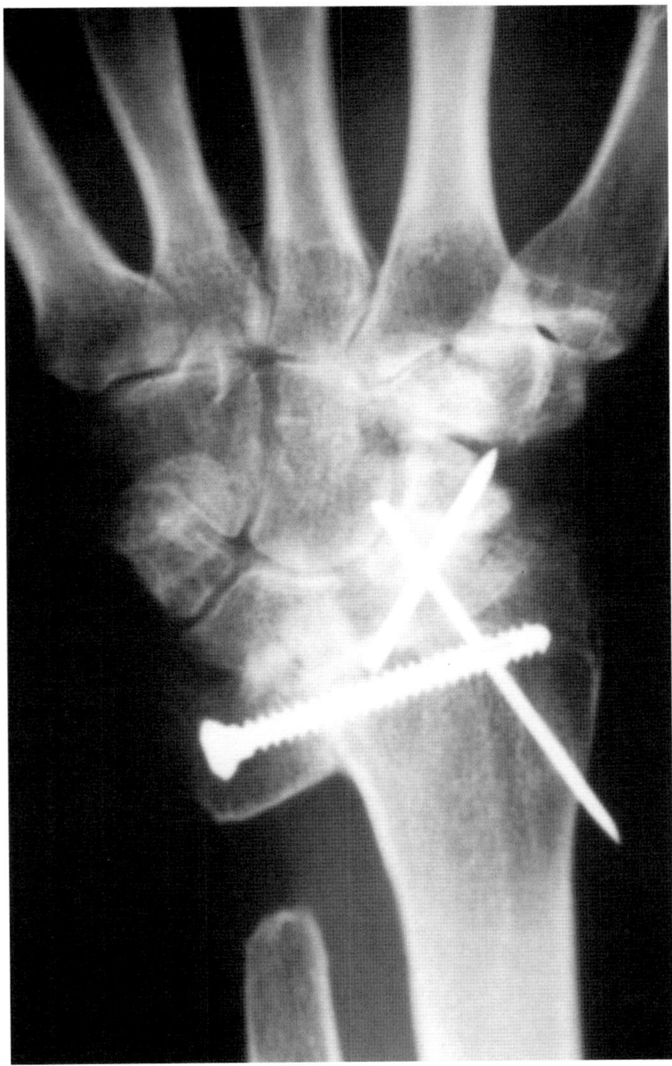

(A)

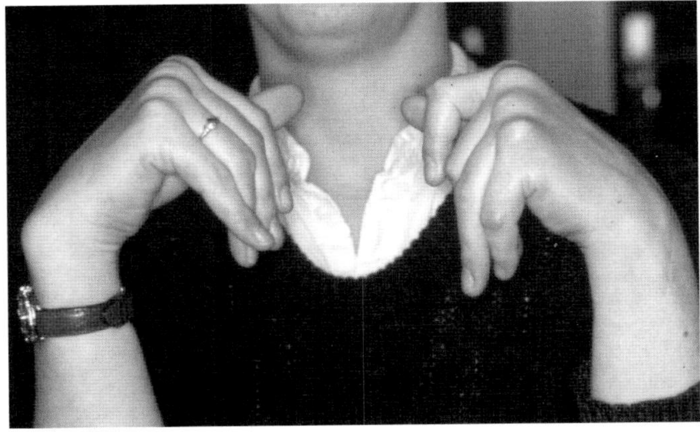

(B)

Figure 32.18

Radioscaphoid arthrodesis in a patient with severe ulnar translation of the carpus. Radiographic appearance (A) and clinical results in flexion, both wrists have been operated on with the same technique and the right hand also had Swanson's metacarpophalangeal joint prostheses (B).

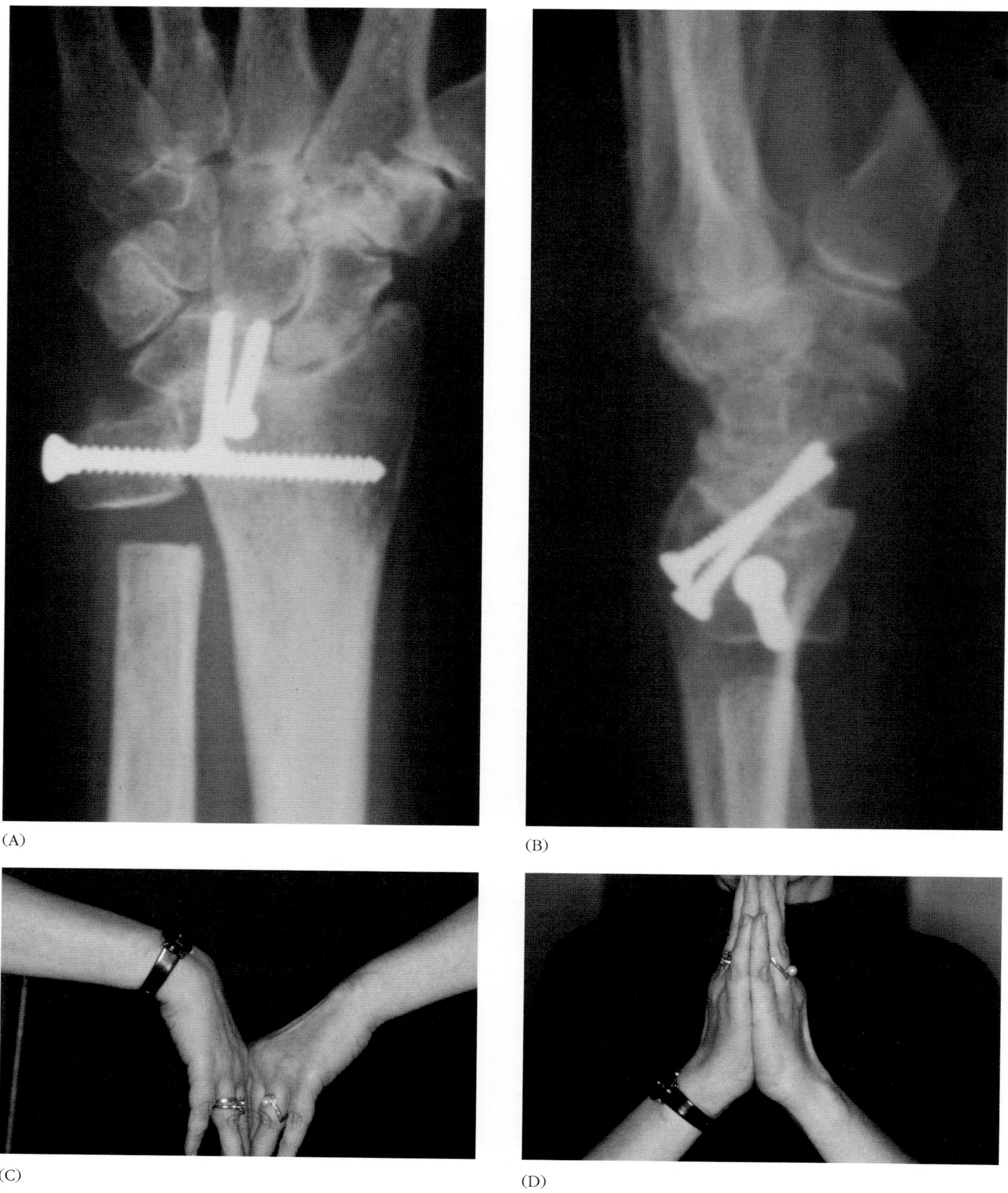

(A) (B) (C) (D)

Figure 32.19

Clinical results of a radiolunate arthrodesis with the Sauvé-Kapandji technique. AP (A) and lateral view (B). Note that if flexion is dramatically limited (C), wrist extension, which is essential for function, is maintained (D).

joint and radial angulation is not corrected. On the other hand, if the lunate is fixed in a low position (maintaining the carpal collapse), the load will be small, and the scaphoid will continue to occupy a flexed position with respect to the radius (Chamay 1998). If the lunate is deformed or the arthrodesis is performed with the lunate in a dorsally rotated position, carpal collapse is accentuated and lunocapitate instability is promoted with a limitation of wrist extension. Furthermore, if the lunate is deformed or fixed in a palmar position, carpal collapse and capitolunate instability are also accentuated and flexion of the wrist is limited. After reduction of the lunate on the radius a palmar bone spur can appear which may give rise to flexor tendon ruptures (Fourastier 1995).

Wrist immobilization in a plaster cast is necessary until bone healing takes place, between 4 and 8 weeks, depending on the quality of the bone and the type of osteosynthesis.

In more advanced cases, it is sometimes necessary to perform a radioscaphoid arthrodesis or even a radioscapholunate arthrodesis to stabilize the proximal row under the radius if the midcarpal joint is preserved. Radioscapholunate arthrodesis should be performed when the scaphoid is in a flexed position with its distal pole protruding anteriorly into the carpal tunnel, constituting a danger for the flexor tendons. Radioscapholunate arthrodesis will improve the midcarpal joint surfaces and the congruency of the scaphocapitolunate joint and partially corrects the radial deviation of the wrist (Figure 32.18). The scaphoid should be reduced until the longitudinal axis is approximately 60° relative to the axis of the radius. A plaster cast must be applied until there is bone fusion, which will be in 6–8 weeks, depending on the quality of the bone and the type of osteosynthesis.

We have no experience with the radioscapholunate arthrodesis associated with a midcarpal arthroplasty as proposed by Taleisnik (1987).

Results of radiolunate fusion are difficult to compare in different series. However, it seems from a literature review (Linscheid and Dobyns 1985, Stanley and Boot 1989, Chamay and Della Santa 1991, Della Santa and Chamay 1995) that:

- The average mobility in flexion-extension is 55° and in radial/ulnar deviation is 23°. Mobility is more limited after radioscapholunate fusion than after radiolunate fusion in Chamay's experience (Chamay 1998). However, we found that our patients had more stiffness than reported in the literature (Figure 32.19).
- The grasp is equivalent to that obtained after a total wrist fusion: 12 kg on the right, 9 kg on the left.
- Patients considered results as excellent in 69% of cases, fair in 18% and poor in 13%, often because of a recurrence of the rheumatoid arthritis.
- The radiolunate arthrodesis corrects the hand deformity with a beneficial effect on ulnar deviation of the fingers

Of 26 wrists reviewed at 5 years follow-up, all continued to deteriorate with time. All measurements showed an increase of ulnar translation and a decrease of carpal height. Two-thirds develop an osteoarthritic model of the midcarpal joint (Della Santa and Chamay 1995, Chamay 1998). Six patients were of Simmen type III and showed a rapid worsening of instability (Flury et al 1999). It is still debated whether or not partial wrist fusion gives better clinical results than total wrist fusion at long-term follow-up (Rittmeister et al 1999). In our experience we were a little disappointed with results in patients with osteoarthritic forms, as we found severe wrist stiffness in some patients. We rarely perform radiolunate fusion, except in patients with severe ulnar translation and limited midcarpal involvement.

Tendon transfers

Transfer of the extensor carpi radialis longus on the extensor carpi ulnaris was proposed initially by Clayton and Ferlic in 1974. Flatt (1995) has shown that this transfer is able to regain ulnar deviation, even in the more advanced cases. However, if carried out without stabilization this transfer will increase the ulnar translation of the carpus. We have performed this transfer in 8% of our patients and tend to perform the transfer with increasing frequency (Figure 32.20). This transfer corrects the supination deformity of the carpus and helps to control the radial deviation. It also helps to recenter the extensor carpi ulnaris tendon and, if carried out posterior to the extensor tendons, reconstructs a posterior strap, which limits the bowstringing effect. Bowstringing of the extensor tendons has been noted in 2% of our patients and has been reported in up to 25% of patients by some authors (Abernethy and Dennyson 1979, Linclau and Dokter 1988) (see Figure 32.16). Bowstringing is noticed more often in patients with a good extension and in patients without stabilization of the tendons (Clayton and Ferlic 1974, Boyce et al 1978, Abernethy and Dennyson 1979, Torisu et al 1983, Allieu et al 1988, Linclau and Dokter 1988, Taleisnik 1989, Flatt 1995). However, the extensor carpi radialis longus tendon transfer seems to have no effect on the ulnar translation of the carpus or the ulnar drift of the metacarpophalangeal joints (Boyce et al 1978, Fourastier et al 1992). Alnot and Leroux (1985) always transfer the extensor carpi radialis longus on the extensor carpi radialis brevis. Brown (1984) has proposed transferring the extensor carpi ulnaris on the extensor carpi radialis longus. This technique is dangerous if the extensor carpi radialis longus is very powerful, as it increases the radial deviation of the carpus. Brown's tenodesis is more effective for limiting palmar translation of the carpus (Brown 1984).

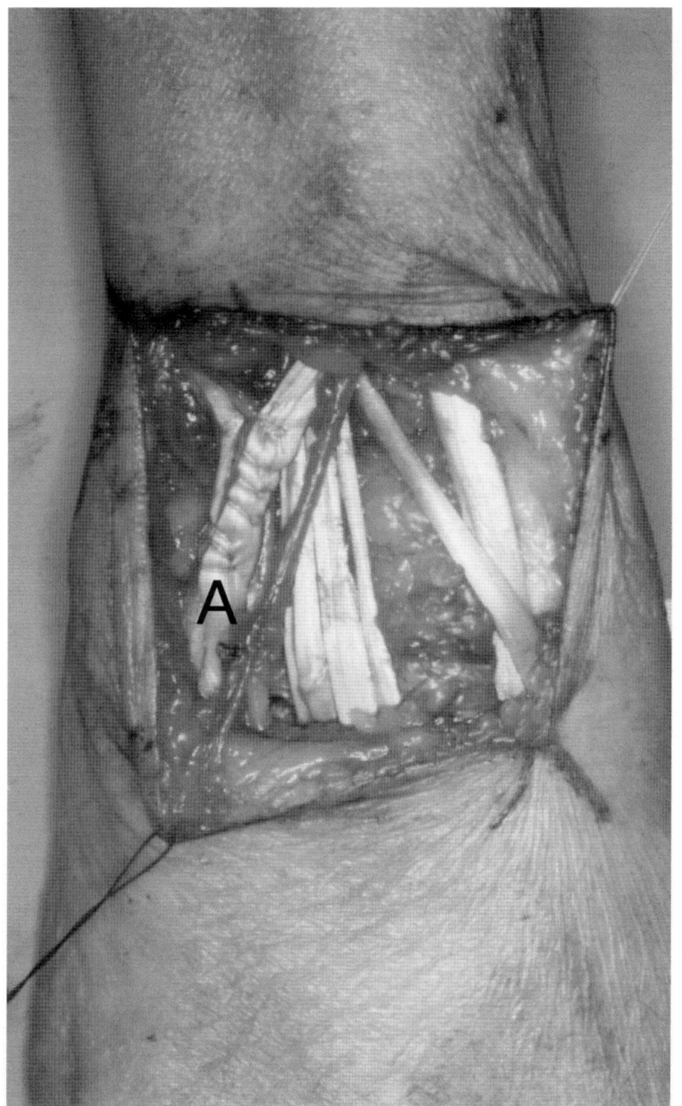

Figure 32.20

Extensor carpi radialis longus transfer on the extensor carpi ulnaris. A latero-lateral anastomosis (A) is carried out with absorbable running sutures. The extensor carpi radialis longus tendon is passed dorsally to the extensor tendon to act as a pulley for the extensor tendons.

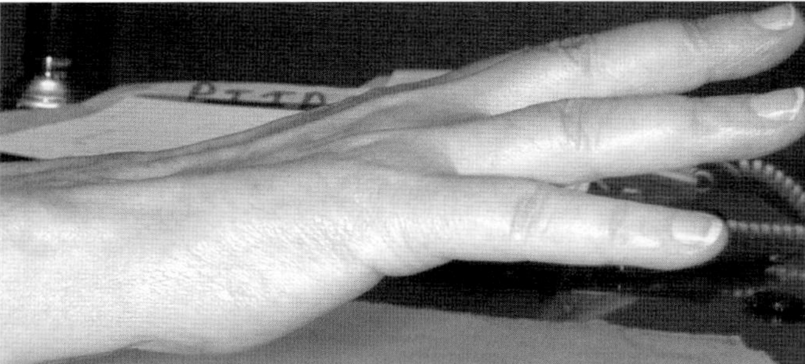

(A)

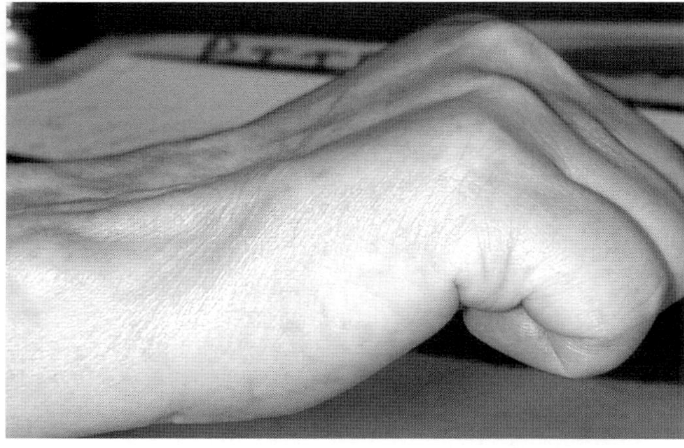

(B)

Figure 32.21

Clinical results of a latero-lateral anastomosis between the extensor digitorum communis of the fourth finger to the extensor digiti minimi (1-year follow-up).

Closure of the wrist

At the end of the procedure (i.e. after synovectomy and stabilization), tendon repair should be performed before closure. Tendinous lesions have been observed in 34% of our patients. Tendon ruptures are noticed in every series and their frequency increases with the evolution of the lesions (Linclau and Dokter 1988). The most frequently ruptured tendons were the extensor digiti quinti (12%) and tendons of the extensor digitorum communis (16%). Extensor pollicis longus and extensor carpi radialis longus ruptures were noticed in 6% of our patients. Very often there is a synovial infiltration of the tendons without rupture. Surgery protects the tendons from rupture, as we only had 1% of postoperative ruptures. This is also rarely reported in the literature (Millender et al 1974, Moore et al 1987, Newman 1987). Brumfield et al (1990) were the only authors to report a 5% postoperative rupture rate. We favor latero-lateral anastomosis for one or two ruptured tendons and transfer of the flexor digitorum superficialis of the fourth finger if three or more tendons are ruptured (Figure 32.21). If it is known before surgery that at least two tendons are ruptured, I now prefer to use an axial longitudinal incision, which facilitates the tendon sutures.

The retinaculum extensorum is placed under the extensor tendons, which provides the tendons with a smooth surface and protects them from the bony irregularities of the carpus. This also posteriorly displaces the tendons and increases their level arm. If the extensor carpi ulnaris is not stabilized by the transfer of the extensor carpi radialis longus, a strip of the retinaculum extensorum is sutured to itself around the tendon (Figure

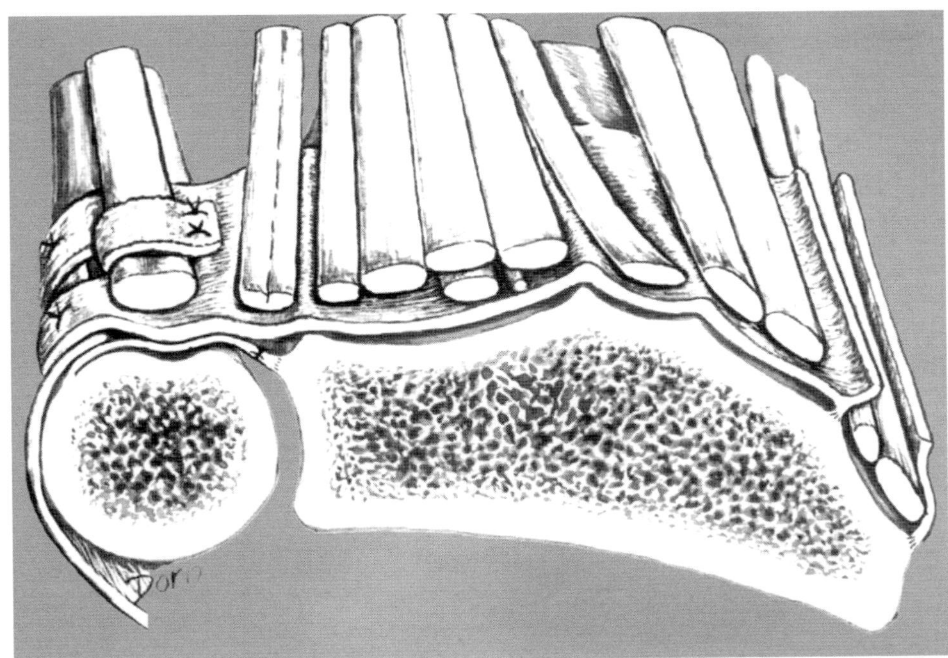

Figure 32.22
Schematic drawing of the extensor retinaculum passed under the extensor tendons to protect them from the bony surfaces. Note that a strip of the retinaculum can be used to dorsally replace the extensor carpi ulnaris if no tendon transfer is done.

32.22). The wrist is immobilized with a splint for 6 weeks. The wrist should be immobilized in neutral position and not in extension to avoid bowstringing of the tendons or stiffness in extension, which is very disabling. Drainage is used routinely.

Complications

Wound problems are the most frequent postoperative complications. Skin margin necroses are frequent if sinuous or zig-zag incisions are used and for that reason they are contraindicated. The frequency of skin problems varies according to the series but may be as high as 10% (Clayton and Ferlic 1965, Rana and Taylor 1973, Millender et al 1974, Eiken et al 1975, Edstrom et al 1976, Allieu and Brahin 1977, Abernethy and Dennyson 1979, Kulick et al 1981, Jensen 1983a, Taleisnik 1992, Van Gemert and Spauwen 1994, Flatt 1995). Dressings are usually sufficient for their treatment, but skin grafting or even local flaps may be necessary (Brunelli and Perrota 1996). Neuromas of the dorsal branch of the ulnar nerve is the second most frequent complication, as this nerve may be injured at the end of the procedure during reinsertion of the retinaculum extensorum (Rana and Taylor 1973, Eiken et al 1975, Rasker et al 1980, Van Gemert and Spauwen 1994). Superficial or deep infections are very rare, as are sympathetic dystrophies (Eiken et al 1975).

As regards changes in digital function, there is a strict correlation between alignment of the wrist and ulnar deviation of the metacarpophalangeal joints (Pahle and Raunio 1969). Correction of wrist deformity usually prevents finger deformation. If fingers were correctly aligned before surgery, 70% of them were still aligned after surgery of the wrist (Thirupathi et al 1983, Mannerfelt 1984, Chamay and Della Santa 1991, Fourastier et al 1992). However, if a metacarpophalangeal joint deformity exists, surgical correction of wrist deformity has little influence on finger deformity.

Total wrist arthrodesis

In large but old series, wrist arthrodesis represented 11–12% of all upper limb surgery in patients with rheumatoid arthritis and 4.5% of all operations (Vahvanen and Kettunen 1977). However, absence of mobility is a true handicap for sophisticated tasks needing dexterity – especially in rheumatoid patients, where both upper limbs are frequently affected. Consequently total wrist fusion is now less frequently indicated, as partial wrist fusion and arthroplasties could be an alternative. The main indication for total wrist fusion is intractable pain or persistent synovitis but other influencing factors are as follows (Mannerfelt and Malmsten 1971, Clayton and Ferlic 1975, Nalebuff and Garrod 1984):

- Severe destruction of the carpus, making soft tissue stabilization or partial fusion unrealistic.
- Extensive extensor tendon rupture, especially extensor carpi radialis longus and brevis.
- Patients who will need crutches or a stable wrist for work.

- Failure of a previous wrist operation.
- Previous wrist infection.

All 'historical' techniques have been employed for wrist fusion and have been abandoned, as they needed at least 3 months in a cast (Haddad and Riordan 1967, Debeyre and Goutallier 1970, Carroll and Dick 1971, Eiken et al 1975, Vahvanen and Kettunen 1977, Lenoble et al 1993), and had a high percentage of complications (Clendenin and Green 1981). As spontaneous wrist fusion is frequent in rheumatoid arthritis, many authors have tried internal stabilization techniques to limit the immobilization time needed (Clayton and Ferlic 1965, Mannerfelt and Malmsten 1971, Nalebuff and Garrod 1984). Clayton and Ferlic (1965) added a stabilization using a Rush pin to a radial bone graft.

Total wrist fusion is only the stabilization technique that will be used at the end of a procedure that also includes tenosynovectomy, distal radio-ulnar joint (DRUJ) synovectomy and stabilization techniques, which have been described before. However, when a total wrist fusion is planned a longitudinal, axial incision is preferred as it can be extended to the metacarpals where pins are introduced. Second, a Darrach's procedure is usually the only technique used at the DRUJ when total wrist fusion is performed and the ulnar head is often used as a bone graft (Clayton and Ferlic 1975).

Surgical techniques

Mannerfelt used an intra-medullary Rush pin with an anti-rotation staple (Mannerfelt and Malmsten 1971, Mannerfelt 1972, 1992). Articular surfaces are freshened and any persisting cartilage is removed. Excision of the radial styloid is frequently needed to correct wrist alignment. A Rush pin is introduced through the ulnar side, into the diaphysis of the third metacarpal and pushed back into the radial shaft as high as possible to obtain three points of a fulcrum (Figure 32.23). Manual compression of bony surfaces is maintained with one or two staples. At the end of the procedure, the surgeon will bend the Rush pin to obtain the correct position of fusion. The curved part of the Rush pin is covered, if possible, with the periosteum and interosseous muscle insertions. Immobilization in a cast for 1 month only is proposed. Many variations have been described: using the second metacarpal which is usually bigger and more in the functional axis of the hand (Mikkelsen 1980); introducing the Rush pin on the radial side of the third metacarpal (Koka and D'Arcy 1989); not using bone graft or staples, with identical results (Koka and D'Arcy 1989). Basically, the surgeon will adapt his technique to the patient's wrist deformity to choose the best introductory point. In Learmonth's experience, Rush pins were mostly introduced in the third metacarpal (Learmonth et al 1992).

To limit the need for immobilization and the complications of Mannerfelt's technique, Millender has proposed the use of a Steinmann pin, which is stiffer and requires that total wrist fusion is done in a neutral position of flexion-extension (Millender and Nalebuff 1973, Nalebuff and Garrod 1984). The radius is prepared first with the largest size possible, usually a 2.7 or 3.2 mm Ø, which

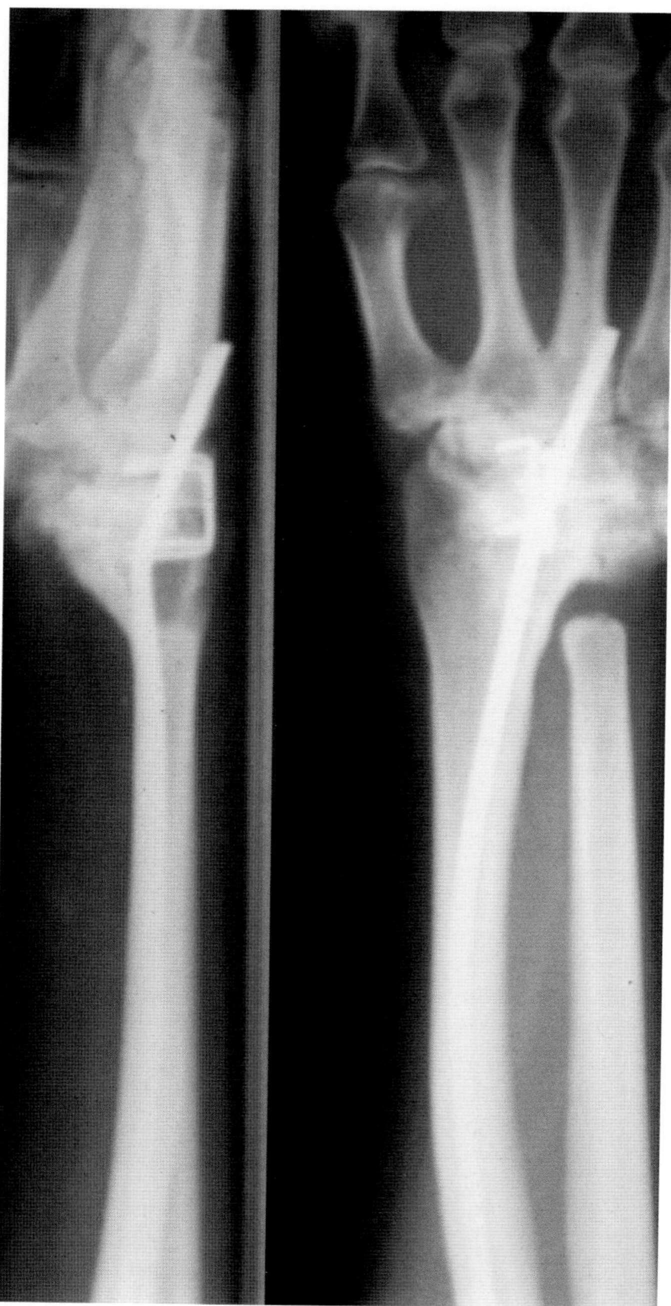

Figure 32.23

Mannerfelt's total arthrodesis using one Rush pin and two staples. The pin is introduced first, and bent at the end of the procedure to obtain the desired alignment. This may break the metacarpals.

determines the length of the pin (Figure 32.24). The Steinmann pin is then introduced into the carpus and exits into the second or third intermetacarpal space (Nalebuff and Garrod 1984). The pin is then pushed back into the radius with a hammer, so as not to perforate the cortices, and buried down under the skin up to the level of the metacarpal neck (Nalebuff and Garrod 1984). A staple may be used to stabilize the carpus in rotation and immobilization for 2 weeks is usually enough.

A variation of this technique was introduced by Stanley and Hullin (1986), who used a 2-cm incision over one metacarpal head and did not operate on the carpus. Clinical and radiological results seemed identical (Christodoulou et al 1999).

Nalebuff et al (1988) quoted Feldon for using two small Steinmann pins (2–2.8 mm Ø), which blocks rotational movements of the carpus and avoids the need for staples. One pin is introduced into the second metacarpal space, one into the third (Nalebuff et al 1988). However, with this technique it is more difficult to obtain a good compression of the articular surfaces (Figure 32.25).

Total wrist fusion with plates is another option (Larsson 1974, Rehak et al 2000). Even in those patients whose skin is very fragile, and in whom the plate tends to project under the skin, Howard et al (1993) showed that the plate fixation was as efficient in term of consolidation, and did not increase the complication rate. No immobilization is needed, and bone graft is not necessary owing to the quality of the fixation (Larsson 1974). Larsson always removed the plate, not because of any problems, but to maintain the mobility of the carpometacarpal joints that are not included in the fusion in his technique.

Technical problems

Carpometacarpal joints

Fusion of the carpometacarpal joints is still debated. Spontaneous fusion is rare, even if 40% of the joints are radiographically involved after a few years of evolution (Vahvanen and Kettunen 1977, Hämäläinen et al 1992).

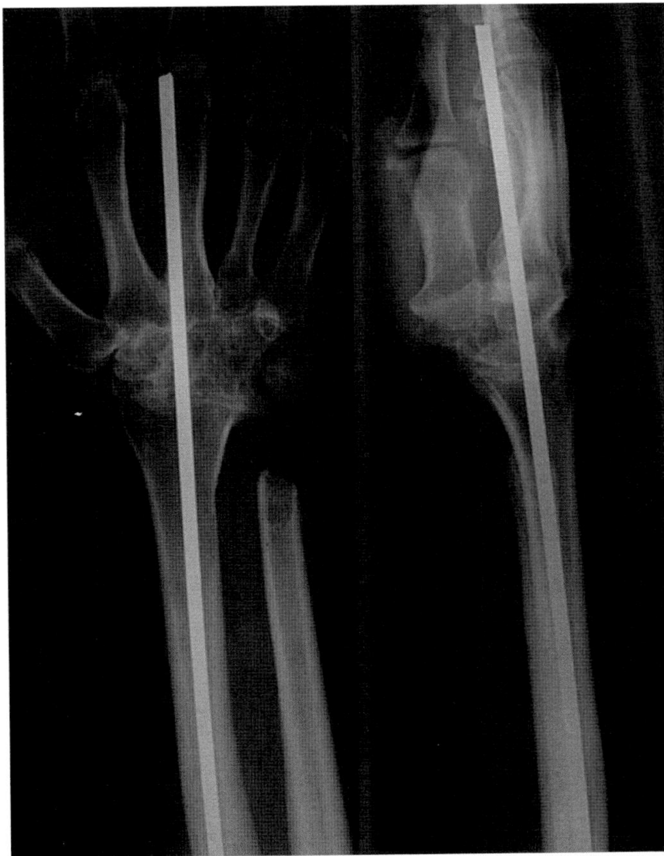

Figure 32.24
Millender's total wrist arthrodesis technique with one Steinmann pin. Note that the Steinmann pin is too anterior and too long in this patient, who did not complain of any symptoms relating to the pin.

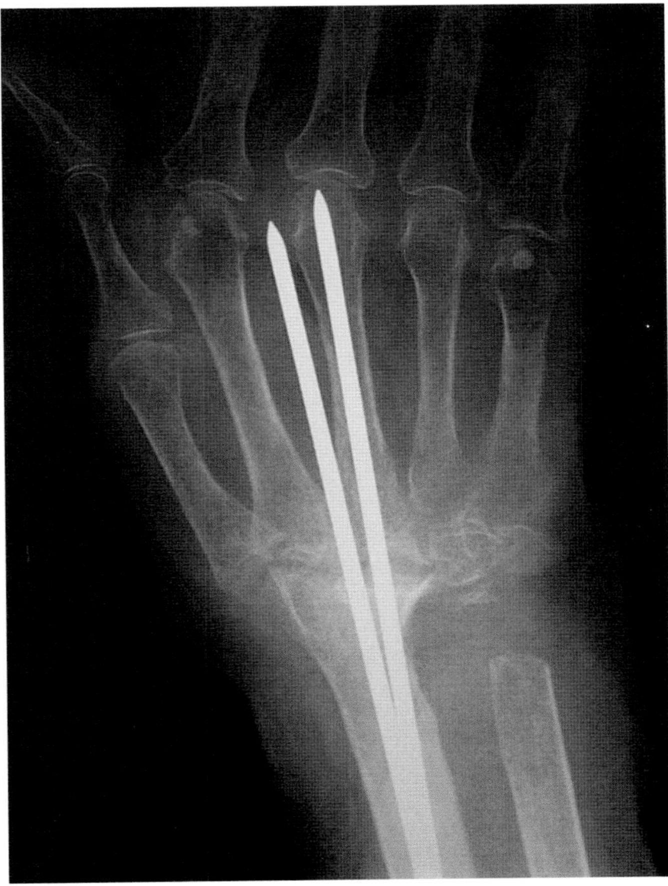

Figure 32.25
Feldon's total wrist arthrodesis technique with two thin Steinmann pins. Note that the carpus has entirely disappeared in this patient.

After wrist fusion, about 40% of the carpometacarpal joints will fuse spontaneously (Vahvanen and Kettunen 1977, Shak 1982). Clayton recommended fusing the carpometacarpal joints, as secondary flexion deformity has been reported at this level after wrist fusion (Clayton and Ferlic 1965, Shak 1982). As regards the literature, the results seem to be identical whether or not the carpometacarpal joints are fused (Rechnagel 1971, Lenoble et al 1993).

Bilateral involvement

Bilateral wrist fusions are rare indications. Even if they have a poor reputation, the rare series reported little discomfort for daily activities, including hygiene care, and this is in agreement with our experience (Rayan et al 1987, Kobus and Turner 1990).

Secondary wrist fusion

A secondary procedure is needed after wrist synovectomy in 2–5% of cases (Kulick et al 1981, Thirupathi et al 1983, Mannerfelt 1984, Vahvanen and Patiala 1984, Bohler et al 1985, Brumfield et al 1990). Most techniques with preservation of wrist mobility do not increase the technical difficulty; however, after partial wrist arthrodesis, it is often difficult to use an intra-medullary pin, or to place it properly. In these particular cases, plate fixation or tension-band wiring techniques may be useful

Wrist positioning

This is the most debated problem. Carroll and Dick (1971) stated that a slight dorsiflexion was useful on the dominant hand, with a neutral position on the non-dominant hand in bilateral wrist fusion. Straub and Ranawat (1969) favored a neutral position on the dominant hand and slight flexion on the non-dominant hand. In the frontal plane, the wrist should be in a neutral position or slight ulnar deviation, as radial inclination of the wrist increases the fingers' ulnar drift (Pahle and Raunio 1969, Vahvanen and Kettunen 1977). As regards literature results, most patients are fused in a position close to neutrality in flexion-extension and in radial-ulnar inclination (Carroll and Dick 1971, Eiken et al 1975, Vahvanen and Kettunen 1977, Mikkelsen 1980, Rayan et al 1987, Kobus and Turner 1990, Barbier et al 1999, Christodoulou et al 1999).

Complications of wrist arthrodesis

Skin leakage

This is quite frequent in those patients whose skin is fragile. It is more frequent if zig-zag incisions are used and has been reported in up to 10% of cases (Clayton and Ferlic 1965, Carroll and Dick 1971, Rana and Taylor 1973, Larsson 1974, Eiken et al 1975, Mikkelsen 1980, Shak 1982, Mannerfelt 1992). The leakage is treated with skin dressings, but local flaps have been needed in some series (Mannerfelt 1992, Brunelli and Perrota 1996).

Median nerve injuries

Median nerve injuries have been reported with Mannerfelt's technique in up to 28% of patients (Mannerfelt and Malmsten 1971, Eiken et al 1975, Ekerot et al 1983, Kobus and Turner 1990, Learmonth et al 1992, Mannerfelt 1992). Most often they are secondary to a cam effect due to the bulging of the anterior margin of the radius (Eiken et al 1975, Ekerot et al 1983, Kobus and Turner 1990). This cam effect is more frequent in patients with anterior carpal translation.

Pseudarthrosis and fixation failure

Millender and Nalebuff (1973) reported pin removal in 12 patients in a series of 60. This complication has disappeared when the pins have been sunk deep to the metacarpal space and a staple has been added on the radio-carpal joint. About 10% of patients had trouble with their fixation device (Mikkelsen 1980, Kobus and Turner 1990, Learmonth et al 1992). Pseudarthrosis, which was reported as between 2 and 10% with previous techniques, is very rare with the intra-medullary rod techniques (Pahle and Raunio 1969, Carroll and Dick 1971, Mannerfelt and Malmsten 1971, Mannerfelt 1972, Millender and Nalebuff 1973, Eiken et al 1975, Vahvanen and Kettunen 1977, Millender and Philips 1978, Mikkelsen 1980, Shak 1982, Ekerot et al 1983, Nalebuff et al 1988, Koka and D'Arcy 1989, Barbier et al 1999).

Miscellaneous complications

Postoperative infection or tendon adhesions have been reported in 2% of patients (Mannerfelt and Malmsten 1971, Mannerfelt 1972, Millender and Nalebuff 1973). Fracture of the metacarpal is specific to Mannerfelt's technique and its frequency has been reported to be 16% in some series (Shak 1982, Koka and D'Arcy 1989). Usually the metacarpal healed during the period of immobilization.

Metacarpal joint stiffness is possible if the intramedullary pin is introduced too distally in the metacarpal (Mikkelsen 1980). Stiffness is more frequent if tendon transfers have been done for tendinous rupture, as the tenodesis effect disappears with the fusion (Millender and Nalebuff 1973).

Results

Pain relief is always good, with satisfactory results in 80–93% of patients (Straub and Ranawat 1969, Mannerfelt and Malmsten 1971, Millender and Nalebuff 1973, Larsson

1974, Eiken et al 1975, Vahvanen and Kettunen 1977, Koka and D'Arcy 1989). Ulnar stump instability is the main cause of poor results (Straub and Ranawat 1969, Shak 1982). Persisting mobility between carpal bones may also be responsible for poor results (Chantelot et al 1997). Strength improvement is usual but most patients still complain of limited grip strength (Millender and Nalebuff 1973, Larsson 1974, Eiken et al 1975, Millender and Philips 1978). Functional impairment seems limited but some patients complained of difficulties with small objects (toothbrush, spoon, or knives) or reaching objects placed on shelves (Mannerfelt and Malmsten 1971, Millender and Nalebuff 1973, Eiken et al 1975). Objective testing with the Jebsen-Taylor test showed abnormal values in 75% of tasks (Kobus and Turner 1990). Comparative testing has shown that both wrists were in the lower range of the Jebsen's test but that there were no statistically significant differences between the fused wrist and the non-fused wrist (Barbier et al 1999).

Arthroplasties

Resection arthroplasties

If it is necessary to preserve mobility in the radio-carpal joint it is possible to either model the radio-carpal joint as proposed by Allbright or to use an interposition tissue. Silastic interposition arthroplasty has been abandoned (Allieu et al 1988). A few authors used either the retinaculum or the capsule (Kulick et al 1981, Thirupathi et al 1983, Torisu et al 1983). However, most of the remodeling arthroplasties are designed as an arthrodesis without fixation and early motion (Ryu et al 1985, Gellman et al 1989, Biyani and Simison 1995). In fact, the fusion rate is very high (60%) and an arthrodesis is usually observed in advanced cases with a limited preoperative mobility. Finally, long-term results are disappointing, as most of the patients with persistent mobility have pain (Gellman et al 1989). We believe that these techniques should be abandoned even if some technical improvement, e.g. wrist distraction, has been proposed (Skoff 1999). In the most advanced cases in which the first row is entirely dislocated volarly and cannot be replaced under the radius, we prefer to resect the proximal row, as initially proposed by Straub and Ranawat (1969). Proximal row carpectomy always gives poor results if carried out alone and must always be associated with a stabilization technique (Ferlic et al 1991, Culp et al 1993).

Swanson radio-carpal implant arthroplasty

The Swanson implant has been widely used since its first description in 1973 and early reports were enthusiastic. However, radiological deteriorations were subsequently observed: fractures, dislocation of the implant, osteolysis resulting in an unstable and destroyed wrist, silicone synovitis, and radial impaction of the implant (Figure 32.26). With longer follow-up radiological deterioration was substantial, with almost 100% complications (Comstock et al 1988, Allieu 1998). However, 50–70% of patients were satisfied owing to the absence of pain and their limited functional requirements (Comstock et al 1988, Allieu 1998, Schill et al 2001). One-third to half of the patients had pain and/or major wrist instability because of implant breakage (Jolly et al 1992, Schill et al 2001). Active mobility is limited, with a flexion-extension arc of 40–50° (Comstock et al 1988, Jolly et al 1992, Schill et al 2001). About one-third of patients had their implant revised, and survivorship analysis showed rapid deterioration in the first 5 years (Fatti et al 1986, Vicar and Burton 1986, Comstock et al 1988, Jolly et al 1992, Allieu 1998). Even if totally abandoned because of its high incidence of complications, the Swanson implant seems to function in 50% of patients at long-term follow-

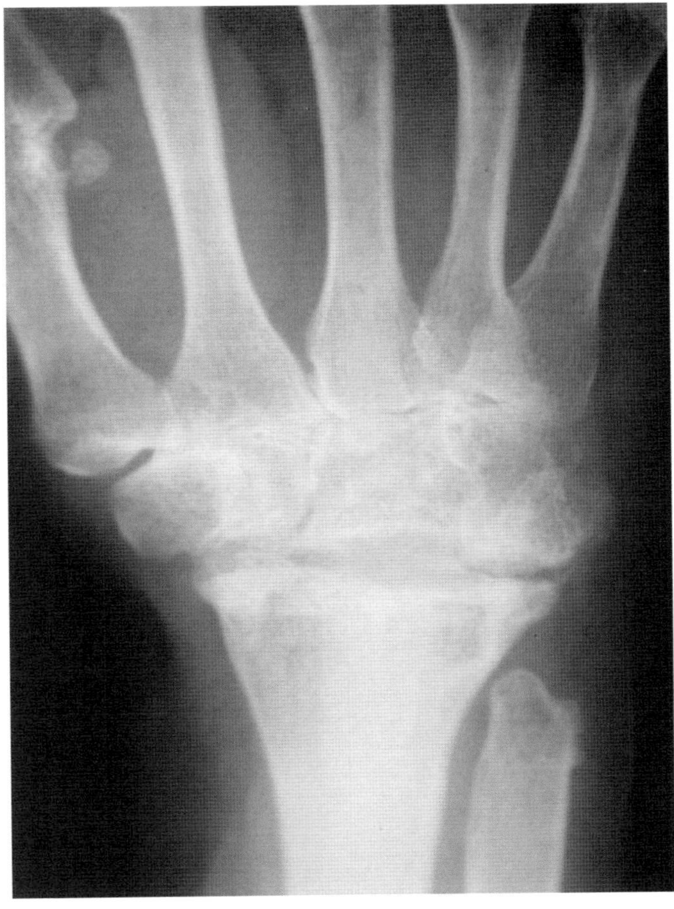

Figure 32.26
Swanson implant with subsidence, osteolysis, and fracture of the implant. Note that the wrist is still well-aligned.

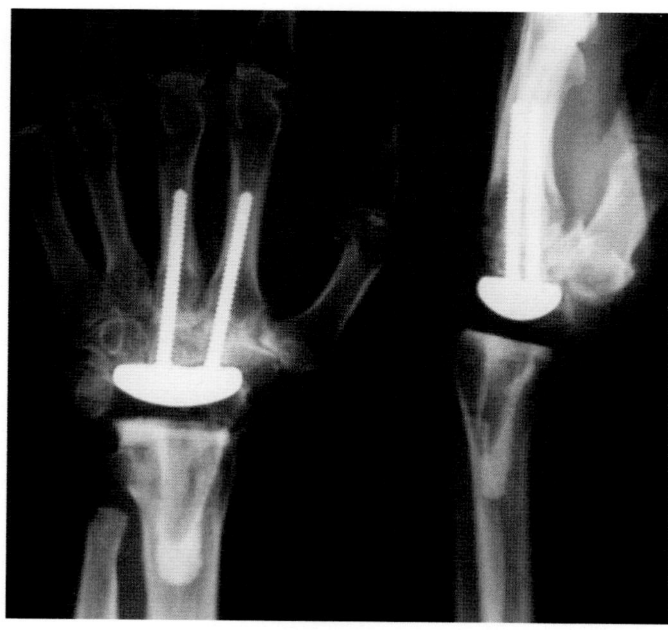

Figure 32.27
Total wrist arthroplasty (Guepar type). The patient has an excellent clinical result and her wrist is well-aligned and functional. However, she has limited mobility.

up and could still be indicated in elderly and low-demand patients. The addition of 'grommets' recommended by Swanson failed to eliminate any of these complications. The surgical technique will not be detailed here.

Total wrist prostheses

We have little experience with total wrist prosthesis (Figure 32.27). In the literature, the results seem to be impressive. Clinical results are good to excellent and most patients are pain-free and have an arc of mobility in flexion-extension of about 40–70° and radio-ulnar deviation of 30° (Figgie et al 1990, Cobb and Beckenbaugh 1996, Radmer et al 1999). Most patients had improved performance of daily living activities, but 16% were made worse (Meuli and Fernandez 1995). Grip strength decreased or remained unchanged in one series (Meuli and Fernandez 1995) and improved in another (Radmer et al 1999). Satisfactory results have been reported in only 50% of patients (Courtman et al 1999). However, literature review shows a complication rate of 30–60% at 6-year follow-up, with loosening, implant failure, and infection. Implant loosening gave an overall survivorship of 83% at 5-year follow-up (Cobb and Beckenbaugh 1996).

If functional results are far superior to those of alternatives such as arthrodesis or biologic arthroplasty, as stated by promoters, there is still an unacceptable loosening rate and difficulties in achieving proper balance. To date we believe that a reliable arthroplastic technique has not yet been achieved and research continues in specialized centers.

References

Abernethy PJ, Dennyson WG (1979) Decompression of the extensor tendons at the wrist in rheumatoid arthritis, *J Bone Joint Surg [Br]* **61**: 64–8.

Adolfsson L, Frisen M (1997) Arthroscopic synovectomy of the rheumatoid wrist. A 3.8 year follow-up, *J Hand Surg [Br]* **22**: 711–13.

Adolfsson L, Nylander G (1993) Arthroscopic synovectomy of the rheumatoid wrist, *J Hand Surg [Br]* **18**: 92–6.

Allieu Y (1998) Surgical treatment of the rheumatoid wrist. A series of 603 rheumatoid wrists operated between 1968 and 1994. In: Allieu Y, ed, *The Rheumatoid Hand and Wrist* (Expansion Scientifique Française: Paris) 63–79.

Allieu Y, Brahin B (1977) [Surgery of the "dorsal wrist" in rheumatoid arthritis: synovectomy and reaxation of the corpus], *Ann Chir* **31**: 279–89.

Allieu Y, Lussiez B, Desbonnet P, Benichou M (1988) [Current status of surgery of the rheumatoid wrist], *Acta Orthop Belg* **54**: 170–7.

Allieu Y, Lussiez B, Asencio G (1989) [Long-term results of surgical synovectomies of the rheumatoid wrist. Apropos of 60 cases], *Rev Chir Orthop Reparatrice Appar Mot* **75**: 172–8.

Alnot JY (1992) [Apropos of ulnar translocation of the carpus after surgery of the rheumatoid wrist. Review of 54 cases], *Rev Chir Orthop Reparatrice Appar Mot* **78**: 491–2.

Alnot JY, Fauroux L (1992) [Synovectomy in the realignment-stabilization of the rheumatoid wrist. Apropos of a series of 104 cases with average follow-up of 5 years], *Rev Rhum Mal Osteoartic* **59**: 196–206.

Alnot JY, Leroux D (1985) Realignment stabilization synovectomy in the rheumatoid wrist. A study of twenty-five cases, *Ann Chir Main* **4**: 294–305.

Ansell BM, Arden GP, Harrison SH (1974) The results of ulna styloidectomy in rheumatoid arthritis, *Scand J Rheumatol* **3**: 67.

Backhouse KM, Kay AGL, Coomes EN, Kates A (1971) Tendon involvement in the rheumatoid hand, *Ann Rheum Dis* **30**: 236–42.

Barbier O, Saels P, Rombouts JJ, Thonnard JL (1999) Long-term functional results of wrist arthrodesis in rheumatoid arthritis, *J Hand Surg [Br]* **24**: 27–31.

Biyani A, Simison AJ (1995) Fibrous stabilization of the rheumatoid wrist, *J Hand Surg [Br]* **20**: 143–5.

Black RM, Boswick JA Jr, Wiedel J (1977) Dislocation of the wrist in rheumatoid arthritis. The relationship to distal ulna resection, *Clin Orthop* **124**: 184–8.

Bohler N, Lack N, Schwagerl W et al (1985) Late results of synovectomy of wrist, MP and PIP joints. Multicenter Study, *Clin Rheumatol* **4**: 23–5.

Bouman HW, Messer E, Sennwald G (1994) Measurement of ulnar translation and carpal height, *J Hand Surg [Br]* **19B**: 325–9.

Bowers WH (1985) Distal radio-ulnar joint arthroplasty: the hemiresection-interposition technique, *J Hand Surg [Am]* **10**: 169–78.

Boyce T, Youm Y, Sprague BL, Flatt AE (1978) Clinical and experimental studies on the effect of extensor carpi radialis longus transfer in the rheumatoid hand, *J Hand Surg [Am]* **3**: 390–4.

Brown FE (1984) Wrist deformity in rheumatoid arthritis extensor carpi ulnaris tendon transfer, *Ann Plast Surg* **13**: 121–5.

Brown FE, Brown ML (1988) Long-term results after tenosynovectomy to treat the rheumatoid hand, *J Hand Surg [Am]* **13**: 704–8.

Brumfield R Jr, Kuschner SH, Gellman H, Liles DN, Van Winckle G (1990) Results of dorsal wrist synovectomies in the rheumatoid hand, *J Hand Surg [Am]* **15**: 733–5.

Brunelli F, Perrota R (1996). Les complications cutanées des synovectomies du poignet dans les polyarthrites rhumatoïdes. In: Tubiana R, ed, *Traité de Chirurgie de la Main*, vol. 5 (Masson: Paris) 425–32.

Carroll RE, Dick HM (1971) Arthrodesis of the wrist for rheumatoid arthritis, *J Bone Joint Surg [Am]* **53**: 1365–9.

Chamay A (1998) Radiolunate and radioscapholunate arthrodesis in rheumatoid wrist. In: Allieu Y, ed, *The Rheumatoid Hand and Wrist* (Expansion Scientifique Française: Paris) 35–47.

Chamay A, Della Santa D (1991) Radiolunate arthrodesis in rheumatoid wrist (21 cases), *Ann Chir Main Memb Super* **10**: 197–206.

Chamay A, Della Santa D, Vilaseca A (1983) Radiolunate arthrodesis. Factor of stability for the rheumatoid wrist, *Ann Chir Main* **2**: 5–17.

Chantelot C, Le Coustumer F, Fontaine C, Migaud H, Duquennoy A (1997) [Arthrodesis of the wrist in inflammatory arthropathy. Effects of fusion of intracarpal joint spaces on functional results], *Ann Chir Main Memb Super* **16**: 198–206.

Christodoulou L, Patwardhan MS, Burke FD (1999) Open and closed arthrodesis of the rheumatoid wrist using a modified (Stanley) Steinmann pin, *J Hand Surg [Br]* **24**: 662–6.

Clayton ML, Ferlic DC (1965) Surgical treatment at the wrist in rheumatoid arthritis, *J Bone Joint Surg [Am]* **47A**: 741–50.

Clayton ML, Ferlic DC (1974) Tendon transfer for radial rotation of the wrist in rheumatoid arthritis, *Clin Orthop* **100**: 176–85.

Clayton ML, Ferlic DC (1975) The wrist in rheumatoid arthritis, *Clin Orthop* **106**: 192–7.

Clendenin MB, Green DP (1981) Arthrodesis of the wrist – complications and their management, *J Hand Surg [Am]* **6**: 253–7.

Cobb TK, Beckenbaugh RD (1996) Biaxial total-wrist arthroplasty, *J Hand Surg [Am]* **21**: 1011–21.

Comstock CP, Louis DS, Eckenrode JF (1988) Silicone wrist implant: long-term follow-up study, *J Hand Surg [Am]* **13**: 201–5.

Courtman NH, Sochart DH, Trail IA, Stanley JK (1999) Biaxial wrist replacement. Initial results in the rheumatoid patient, *J Hand Surg [Br]* **24**: 32–4.

Culp RW, McGuigan FX, Turner MA, Lichtman DM, Osterman AL, McCarroll HR (1993) Proximal row carpectomy: a multicenter study, *J Hand Surg [Am]* **18**: 19–25.

Debeyre J, Goutallier D (1970) [Arthrodesis of the wrist by intracarpal iliac graft], *Presse Med* **78**: 1993–4.

Della Santa D, Chamay A (1995) Radiological evolution of the rheumatoid wrist after radio-lunate arthrodesis, *J Hand Surg [Br]* **20**: 146–54.

Dennis DA, Ferlic DC, Clayton ML (1986) Volz total wrist arthroplasty in rheumatoid arthritis: a long-term review, *J Hand Surg [Am]* **11**: 483–90.

Dingman PVC (1952) Resection of the distal end of the ulna (Darrach operation), *J Bone Joint Surg [Am]* **34A**: 893–900.

Edstrom B, Lugnegard H, Syk B (1975) X-ray changes in connection with late synovectomy of the hand in rheumatoid arthritis, *Scand J Rheumatol* **4**: 92–6.

Edstrom B, Lugnegard H, Syk B (1976) Late synovectomy of the hand in rheumatoid arthritis, *Scand J Rheumatol* **5**: 184–90.

Eiken O, Haga T, Salgeback S (1975) Assessment of surgery of the rheumatoid wrist, *Scand J Plast Reconstr Surg* **9**: 207–15.

Ekerot L, Jonsson K, Eiken O (1983) Median nerve compression complicating arthrodesis of the rheumatoid wrist, *Scand J Plast Reconstr Surg* **17**: 257–62.

Fatti JF, Palmer AK, Mosher JF (1986) The long-term results of Swanson silicone rubber interpositional wrist arthroplasty, *J Hand Surg [Am]* **11**: 166–75.

Ferlic DC, Clayton ML (1985) Synovectomy of the hand and wrist, *Ann Chir Gynaecol Suppl* **198**: 26–30.

Ferlic DC, Clayton ML, Mills MF (1991) Proximal row carpectomy: review of rheumatoid and nonrheumatoid wrists, *J Hand Surg [Am]* **16**: 420–4.

Figgie MP, Ranawat CS, Inglis AE, Sobel M, Figgie HE 3rd (1990) Trispherical total wrist arthroplasty in rheumatoid arthritis, *J Hand Surg [Am]* **15**: 217–23.

Flatt AE (1995). *The Care of the Arthritic Hand* (Quality Medical Publishing: St Louis).

Flury MP, Herren DB, Simmen BR (1999) Rheumatoid arthritis of the wrist. Classification related to the natural course, *Clin Orthop* **366**: 72–7.

Fourastier J (1995) [Rupture of the flexor tendons after partial arthrodesis of carpus in the rheumatoid wrist], *Ann Chir Main Memb Super* **14**: 224–8.

Fourastier J, Langlais F, Colmar M (1992) [Ulnar translocation of the carpus after surgery of the rheumatic wrist. Review of 54 cases], *Rev Chir Orthop Reparatrice Appar Mot* **78**: 176–85.

Fraser KE, Diao E, Peimer CA, Sherwin FS (1999) Comparative results of resection of the distal ulna in rheumatoid arthritis and post-traumatic conditions, *J Hand Surg [Br]* **24**: 667–70.

Freiberg RA, Weinstein A (1972) The scallop sign and spontaneous rupture of finger extensor tendons in rheumatic arthritis, *Clin Orthop* **83**: 128–30.

Gainor BJ, Schaberg J (1985) The rheumatoid wrist after resection of the distal ulna, *J Hand Surg [Am]* **10**: 837–44.

Gellman H, Rankin G, Brumfield R Jr, Chandler D, Williams B (1989) Palmar shelf arthroplasty in the rheumatoid wrist. Results of long-term follow-up, *J Bone Joint Surg [Am]* **71**: 223–7.

Goldberg D, Menkes CJ (1995) La main rhumatoïde. In: Tubiana R, ed, *Traité de Chirurgie de la Main*, vol. 5 (Masson: Paris) 170–97.

Haddad RJ Jr, Riordan DC (1967) Arthrodesis of the wrist. a surgical technique, *J Bone Joint Surg [Am]* **49A**: 950–4.

Hämäläinen H, Kammonen M, Lehtimäki M et al (1992) Epidemiology of wrist involvement in rheumatoid arthritis. In: Simmen BR, Hagena FW, eds, *The Wrist in Rheumatoid Arthritis* (Karger: Basel) 1–7.

Hindley CJ, Stanley JK (1991) The rheumatoid wrist: patterns of disease progression. A review of 50 wrists, *J Hand Surg [Br]* **16**: 275–9.

Howard AC, Stanley D, Getty CJ (1993) Wrist arthrodesis in rheumatoid arthritis. A comparison of two methods of fusion, *J Hand Surg [Br]* **18**: 377–80.

Hui FC, Linscheid RL (1982) Ulnotriquetral augmentation tenodesis: a reconstructive procedure for dorsal subluxation of the distal radio-ulnar joint, *J Hand Surg [Am]* **7**: 230–6.

Jackson IT, Milward TM, Lee P, Webb J (1974) Ulnar head resection in rheumatoid arthritis, *Hand* **6**: 172–80.

Jensen CM (1983a) [Rheumatoid arthritis of the wrist joint. A review of surgical possibilities], *Ugeskr Laeger* **145**: 2511–16.

Jensen CM (1983b) Synovectomy with resection of the distal ulna in rheumatoid arthritis of the wrist, *Acta Orthop Scand* **54**: 754–9.

Jolly SL, Ferlic DC, Clayton ML, Dennis DA, Stringer EA (1992) Swanson silicone arthroplasty of the wrist in rheumatoid arthritis: a long-term follow-up, *J Hand Surg [Am]* **17**: 142–9.

Kessler I, Vainio K (1966) Posterior (dorsal) synovectomy for rheumatoid involvement of the hand and wrist. A follow-up study of sixty-six procedures, *J Bone Joint Surg [Am]* **48**: 1085–94.

Kobus RJ, Turner RH (1990) Wrist arthrodesis for treatment of rheumatoid arthritis, *J Hand Surg [Am]* **15**: 541–6.

Koka R, D'Arcy JC (1989) Stabilisation of the wrist in rheumatoid disease, *J Hand Surg [Br]* **14**: 288–90.

Kulick RG, De Fiore JC, Straub LR, Ranawat CS (1981) Long-term results of dorsal stabilization in the rheumatoid wrist, *J Hand Surg [Am]* **6**: 272–80.

Larsson SE (1974) Compression arthrodesis of the wrist. A consecutive series of 23 cases, *Clin Orthop* **99**: 146–53.

Learmonth ID, Grobler G, Jaffe R, Heywood AWB (1992) Arthrodesis of the wrist for inflammatory arthritis. In: Simmen BR, Hagena FW, eds, *The Wrist in Rheumatoid Arthritis* (Basel: Karger) 122–7.

Lenoble E, Ovadia H, Goutallier D (1993) Wrist arthrodesis using an embedded iliac crest bone graft, *J Hand Surg [Br]* **18**: 595–600.

Leslie BM, Carlson G, Ruby LK (1990) Results of extensor carpi

ulnaris tenodesis in the rheumatoid wrist undergoing a distal ulnar excision, *J Hand Surg [Am]* **15**: 547–51.
Linclau L, Dokter G (1988) Operative treatment of dorsal lesions of the wrist in rheumatoid arthritis, *Acta Orthop Belg* **54**: 185–8.
Linscheid RL, Dobyns JH (1971) Rheumatoid arthritis of the wrist, *Orthop Clin North Am* **2**: 649–65.
Linscheid RL, Dobyns JH (1985) Radiolunate arthrodesis, *J Hand Surg [Am]* **10**: 821–9.
Mannerfelt L (1972) [New technique for arthrodesis of the wrist in the treatment of rheumatoid arthritis. Technique not requiring external immobilization], *Rev Chir Orthop Reparatrice Appar Mot* **58**: 471–80.
Mannerfelt L (1984) Surgical treatment of the rheumatoid wrist and aspects of the natural course when untreated, *Clin Rheum Dis* **10**: 549–70.
Mannerfelt L (1992) Total arthrodesis of the wrist. In: Simmen BR, Hagena FW, eds, *The Wrist in Rheumatoid Arthritis* (Karger: Basel) 116–21.
Mannerfelt L, Malmsten M (1971) Arthrodesis of the wrist in rheumatoid arthritis. A technique without external fixation, *Scand J Plast Reconstr Surg* **5**: 124–30.
Meuli HC, Fernandez DL (1995) Uncemented total wrist arthroplasty, *J Hand Surg [Am]* **20**: 115–22.
Mikkelsen OA (1980) Arthrodesis of the wrist joint in rheumatoid arthritis, *Hand* **12**: 149–53.
Millender LH, Nalebuff EA (1973) Arthrodesis of the rheumatoid wrist. An evaluation of sixty patients and a description of a different surgical technique, *J Bone Joint Surg [Am]* **55**: 1026–34.
Millender LH, Philips C (1978) Combined wrist arthrodesis and metacarpophalangeal joint arthroplasty in rheumatoid arthritis, *Orthopedics* **1**: 43–8.
Millender LH, Nalebuff EA, Albin R, Ream JR, Gordon M (1974) Dorsal tenosynovectomy and tendon transfer in the rheumatoid hand, *J Bone Joint Surg [Am]* **56**: 601–10.
Moore JR, Weiland AJ, Valdata L (1987) Tendon ruptures in the rheumatoid hand: analysis of treatment and functional results in 60 patients, *J Hand Surg [Am]* **12**: 9–14.
Nalebuff EA, Garrod KJ (1984) Present approach to the severely involved rheumatoid wrist, *Orthop Clin North Am* **15**: 369–80.
Nalebuff EA, Feldon PG, Millender LH (1988) Rheumatoid arthritis in the hand and wrist. In: Green DP, ed, *Operative Hand Surgery* (Churchill Livingstone: New York) 1655–766.
Newman RJ (1987) Excision of the distal ulna in patients with rheumatoid arthritis, *J Bone Joint Surg [Br]* **69**: 203–6.
O'Donovan TM, Ruby LK (1989) The distal radio-ulnar joint in rheumatoid arthritis, *Hand Clin* **5**: 249–56.
Pahle JA, Raunio P (1969) The influence of wrist position on finger deviation in the rheumatoid hand. A clinical and radiological study, *J Bone Joint Surg [Br]* **51**: 664–76.
Radmer S, Andresen R, Sparmann M (1999) Wrist arthroplasty with a new generation of prostheses in patients with rheumatoid arthritis, *J Hand Surg [Am]* **24**: 935–43.
Rana NA, Taylor AR (1973) Excision of the distal end of the ulna in rheumatoid arthritis, *J Bone Joint Surg [Br]* **55**: 96–105.
Rasker JJ, Veldhuis EF, Huffstadt AJ, Nienhuis RL (1980) Excision of the ulnar head in patients with rheumatoid arthritis, *Ann Rheum Dis* **39**: 270–4.
Rayan GM, Brentlinger A, Purnell D, Garcia-Moral CA (1987) Functional assessment of bilateral wrist arthrodeses, *J Hand Surg [Am]* **12**: 1020–4.
Rechnagel K (1971) Arthrodesis of the wrist joint. A follow-up study of sixty cases, *Scand J Plast Reconstr Surg* **5**: 120–3.
Rehak DC, Kasper P, Baratz ME, Hagberg WC, McClain E, Imbriglia JE (2000) A comparison of plate and pin fixation for arthrodesis of the rheumatoid wrist, *Orthopedics* **23**: 43–8.
Rittmeister M, Kandziora F, Rehart S, Kerschbaumer F (1999) [Radiolunar Mannerfelt arthrodesis in rheumatoid arthritis], *Handchir Mikrochir Plast Chir* **31**: 266–73.
Rowland SA (1984) Stabilization of the ulnar side of the rheumatoid wrist, following radio-carpal Swanson's implant arthroplasty and resection of the distal ulna, *Bull Hosp Jt Dis Orthop Inst* **44**: 442–8.
Ryu J, Watson HK, Burgess RC (1985) Rheumatoid wrist reconstruction utilizing a fibrous nonunion and radio-carpal arthrodesis, *J Hand Surg [Am]* **10**: 830–6.
Schill S, Thabe H, Mohr W (2001) [Long-term outcome of Swanson prosthesis management of the rheumatic wrist joint], *Handchir Mikrochir Plast Chir* **33**: 198–206.
Shak SV (1982) Arthrodesis of the wrist by the method of Mannerfelt. A follow-up of 19 patients, *Acta Orthoped Scand* **53**: 557–9.
Simmen BR, Huber H (1992) The rheumatoid wrist: a new classification related to the type of the natural course and its consequence for surgical therapy. In: Simmen BR, Hagena FW, eds, *The Wrist in Rheumatoid Arthritis* (Karger: Basel) 13–25.
Skoff H (1999) Palmar shelf arthroplasty, the next generation: distraction/interposition for rheumatoid arthritis of the wrist, *Plast Reconstr Surg* **104**: 2068–72, 2073.
Stanley JK, Boot DA (1989) Radio-lunate arthrodesis, *J Hand Surg [Br]* **14**: 283–7.
Stanley JK, Hullin MG (1986) Wrist arthrodesis as part of composite surgery of the hand, *J Hand Surg [Br]* **11**: 243–4.
Straub LR, Ranawat CS (1969) The wrist in rheumatoid arthritis. Surgical treatment and results, *J Bone Joint Surg [Am]* **51**: 1–20.
Taleisnik J (1987) Combined radio-carpal arthrodesis and midcarpal (lunocapitate) arthroplasty for treatment of rheumatoid arthritis of the wrist, *J Hand Surg [Am]* **12**: 1–8.
Taleisnik J (1989) Rheumatoid arthritis of the wrist, *Hand Clin* **5**: 257–78.
Taleisnik J (1992) The Sauve-Kapandji procedure, *Clin Orthop* **275**: 110–23.
Thirupathi RG, Ferlic DC, Clayton ML (1983) Dorsal wrist synovectomy in rheumatoid arthritis – a long-term study, *J Hand Surg [Am]* **8**: 848–56.
Torisu T, Masumi S, Aso K (1983) Utilization of the extensor retinaculum in the radio-carpal joint of rheumatoid wrists, *Clin Orthop* **181**: 179–85.
Tubiana R (1990) Technique of dorsal synovectomy on the rheumatoid wrist, *Ann Chir Main Memb Super* **9**: 138–45.
Tubiana R, Kuhlmann N, Fahrer M, Lisfranc R (1980) Etude du poignet normal et ses déformations au cours de la polyarthrite rhumatoïde, *Chirurgie* **106**: 257–64.
Vahvanen V, Kettunen P (1977) Arthrodesis of the wrist in rheumatoid arthritis. A follow-up study of 62 cases, *Ann Chir Gynaecol* **66**: 195–202.
Vahvanen V, Patiala H (1984) Synovectomy of the wrist in rheumatoid arthritis, related diseases. A follow-up study of 97 consecutive cases, *Arch Orthop Trauma Surg* **102**: 230–7.
Van Gemert AM, Spauwen PH (1994) Radiological evaluation of the long-term effects of resection of the distal ulna in rheumatoid arthritis, *J Hand Surg [Br]* **19**: 330–3.
Vicar AJ, Burton RI (1986) Surgical management of the rheumatoid wrist – fusion or arthroplasty, *J Hand Surg [Am]* **11**: 790–7.
Vincent KA, Szabo RM, Agee JM (1993) The Sauve-Kapandji procedure for reconstruction of the rheumatoid distal radio-ulnar joint, *J Hand Surg [Am]* **18**: 978–83.
Watson HK, Ryu JY, Burgess RC (1986) Matched distal ulnar resection, *J Hand Surg [Am]* **11**: 812–17.
Wilson RL (1986) Rheumatoid arthritis of the hand, *Orthop Clin North Am* **17**: 313–43.
Youm Y, McMurthy RY, Flatt AE, Gillespie TE (1978) Kinematics of the wrist. I. An experimental study of radial-ulnar deviation and flexion-extension, *J Bone Joint Surg Am* **60**: 423–31.

33 Extensor tenosynovitis

Raoul Tubiana

Dorsal tenosynovitis is a pathologic proliferation of the normal dorsal tenosynovium surrounding the extensor tendons beneath the dorsal retinaculum. Nine extensor tendons are located beneath the dorsal retinaculum, within six separate anatomical compartments (Figure 33.1).

The disease most frequently involves the digitorum communis and extensor pollicis longus (EPL) and manifests as a non-painful, non-tender soft mass extending along the course of the extensor tendons and usually bulging beneath the inferior border of the extensor retinaculum. However, it may occur either ulnarward or radially and may affect the tendons on each side of the hand. Extensor tendon function is usually not impaired and any associated pain is provoked by carpal or radioulnar involvement. The main complication of dorsal tenosynovitis is extensor tendon rupture.

Dorsal tenosynovectomy, with retinacular relocation and distal ulna excision when indicated, is a proven method to prevent tendon rupture. Recurrence of tenosynovitis is possible, but rare. Tenosynovectomy is indicated wherever tenosynovitis persists for more than 6 months despite appropriate medical treatment.

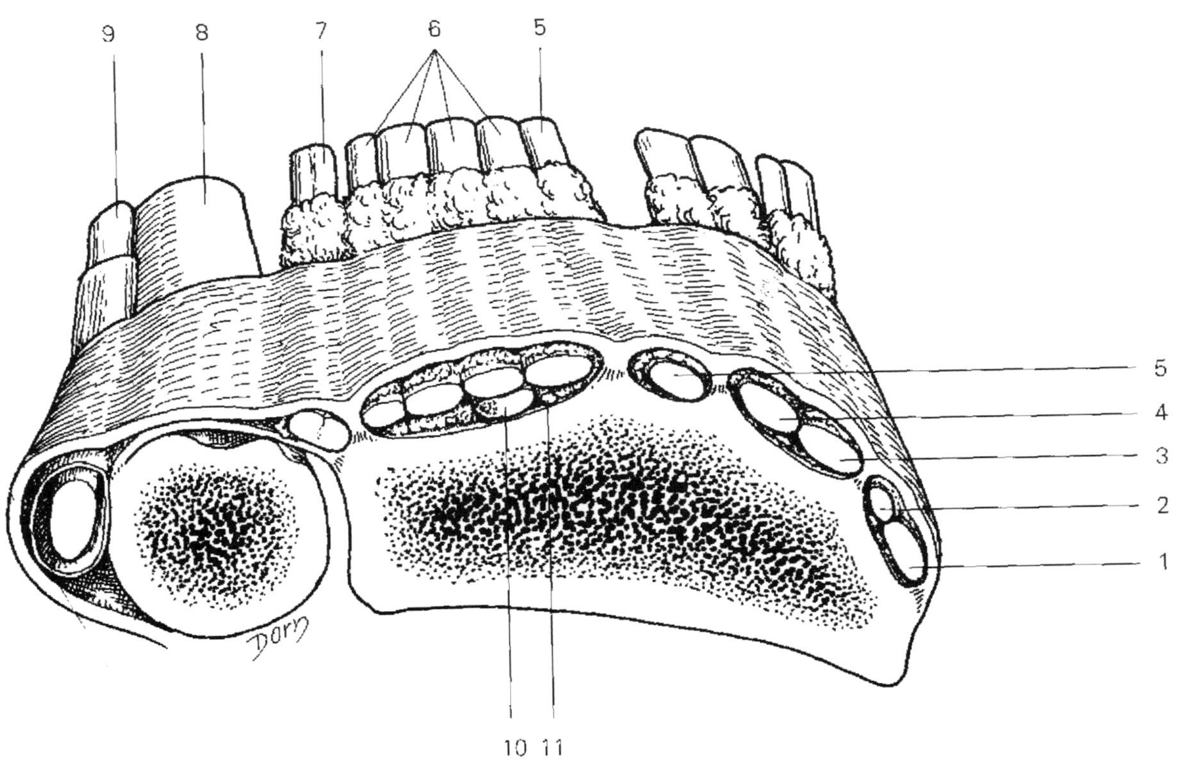

Figure 33.1
1, APL; 2, EPB; 3, ECRL; 4, ECRB; 5, EPL; 6, EDC; 7, EDM; 8, ulna; 9, ECU; 10, EIP; 11, posterior interosseous nerve.

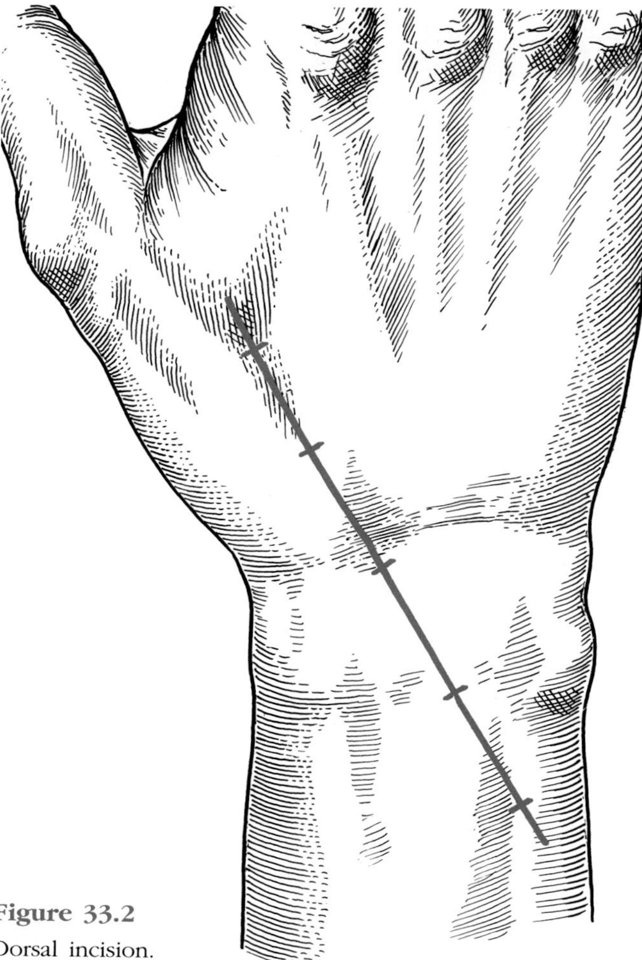

Figure 33.2
Dorsal incision.

Dorsal tenosynovectomy

Extensor tenosynovectomy is rarely performed alone, but is usually combined with synovectomy of the distal radio-ulnar joint and a wrist synovectomy.

Incision

Our preferred incision is a dorsal oblique incision, extending from a point 4 cm proximal to the ulnar styloid, directed towards the base of the index finger metacarpal. This obliquity minimizes the risk of an incision directly over the longitudinal axis of the extensor tendons (Figure 33.2). Also, this exposure facilitates the ulnar excision and stabilization. Only straight incisions are made. Zig-zag or curved incisions are dangerous on the thin, fragile dorsal skin of the rheumatoid patients. The incision is taken down to the extensor retinaculum and the skin flaps are retracted by means of traction sutures. The superficial branches of the ulnar and radial nerves are protected and retracted (Figure 33.3).

It is important to preserve one or two dorsal longitudinal veins, to avoid postoperative venous stasis. These are dissected and retracted with soft slings.

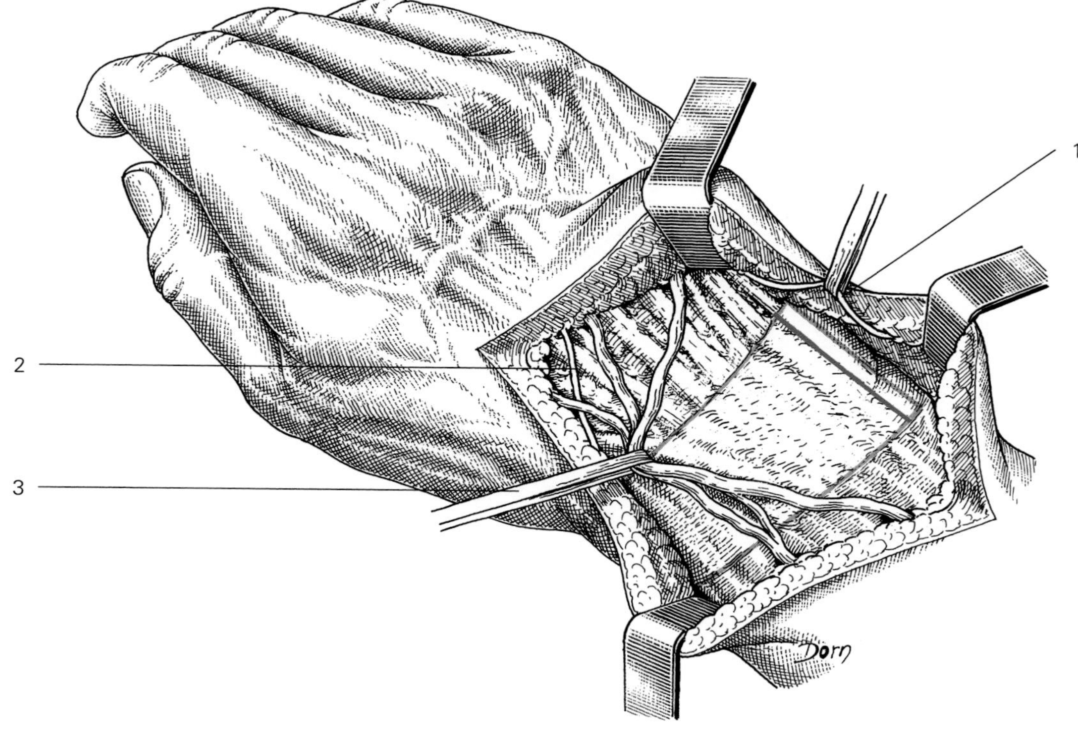

Figure 33.3
1 A dorsal branch of the ulnar nerve
2 Superficial branch of the radial nerve
3 Dorsal longitudinal veins are retracted

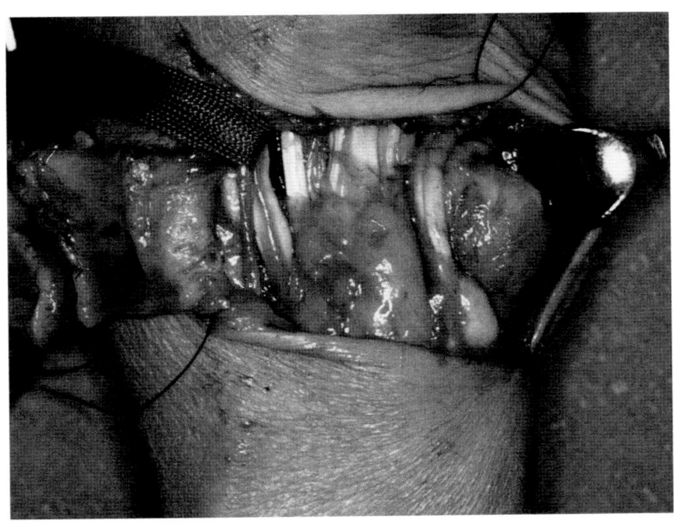

Figure 33.4
The extensor retinaculum is divided at the level of the ECU tendon. A 5-cm wide strip is raised. The vertical fibrous septa are divided and the retinacular flap is reflected radially, exposing the extensor tenosynovitis.

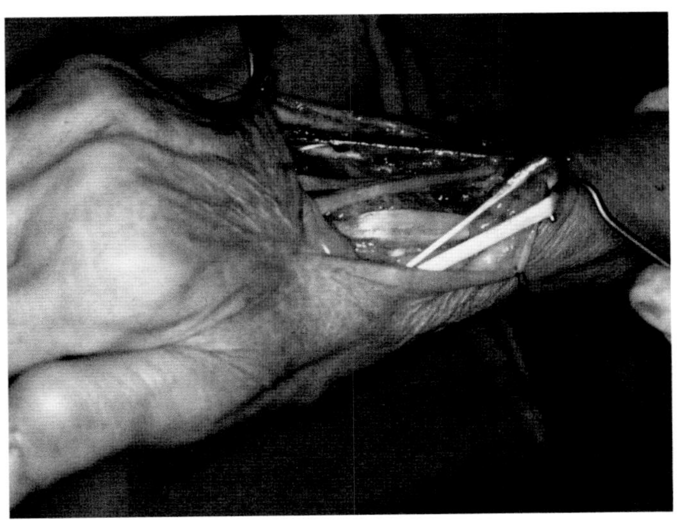

Figure 33.5
The extensor tendons are tested after the tenosynovectomy.

Opening of the extensor retinaculum

The extensor retinaculum may be opened in a different manner. It can be incised over the digital extensors and then reflected radially and ulnarwards. We prefer to incise the retinaculum longitudinally into the sixth compartment at the level of the extensor carpi ulnaris (ECU) tendon.

A 5-cm wide strip is carefully raised and reflected radially, exposing in order, five of the six dorsal compartments (Figure 33.4). Care is taken to protect the extensor pollicis longus (EPL) as it changes direction distal to Lister's tubercle.

A separate longitudinal incision in the retinaculum may be required to provide exposure of the tendons of the abductor pollicis longus (APL) and extensor pollicis brevis (EPB) when necessary.

Tenosynovectomy

Hypertrophic synovium surrounding each extensor tendon is systematically removed with small scissors (Figure 33.5).

The sheath of the ECU tendon is opened and cleared of synovium. Occasionally the tenosynovitis is seen to have invaded into the tendon, in which case it should be removed with fine synovectomy forceps, avoiding damage to the tendon as far as possible (Figure 33.6). The distal radio-ulnar joint and the wrist joint are evaluated.

If tendon rupture is imminent, reefing of the tendon or side-to-side suture is carried out. After tenosynovectomy is completed, any additional indicated surgery is carried out.

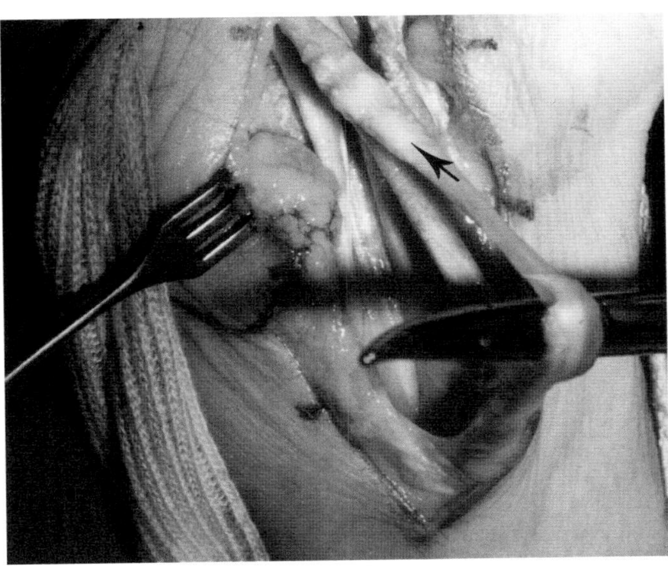

Figure 33.6
Tendons invaded by rheumatoid granulation.

Resection of the posterior interosseous nerve

We routinely resect the posterior interosseous nerve. The extensor carpi radialis tendons and EPL are retracted radially, and the extensor digiti minimi (EDM) and

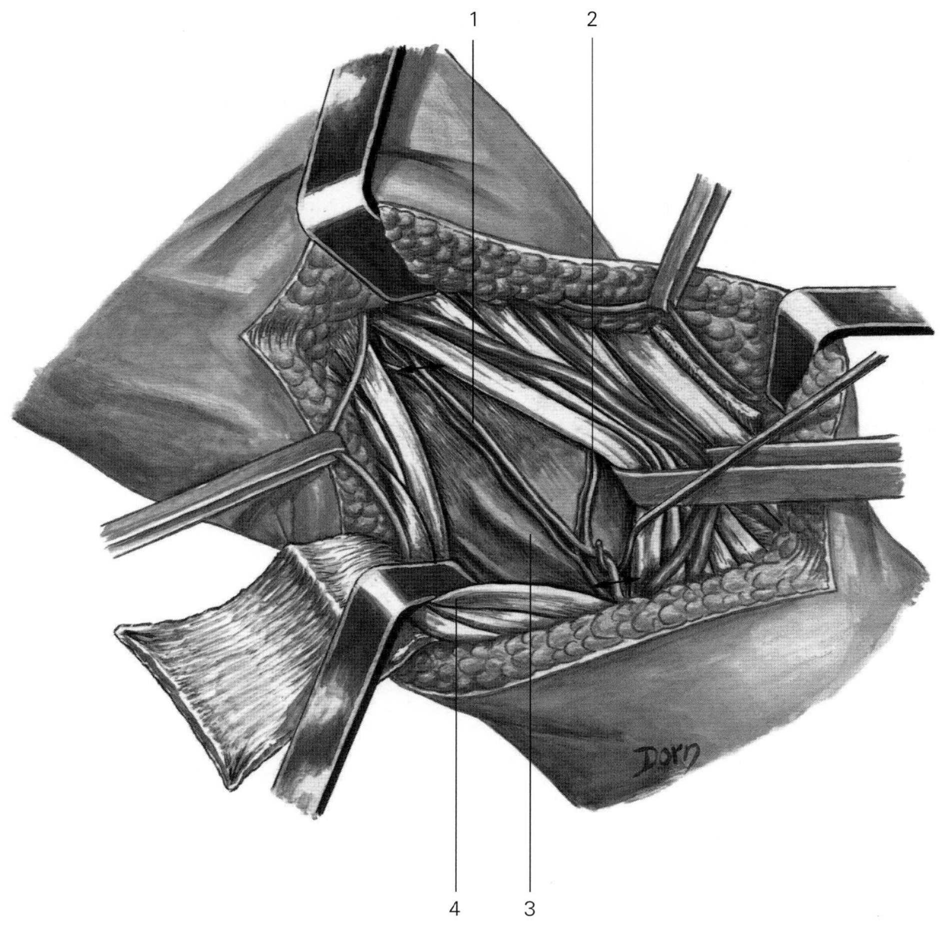

Figure 33.7

Resection of the posterior interosseous nerve (1) and the branches supplying the distal radioulnar joint (2). (3) Lister's tubercle. (4) EPL tendon.

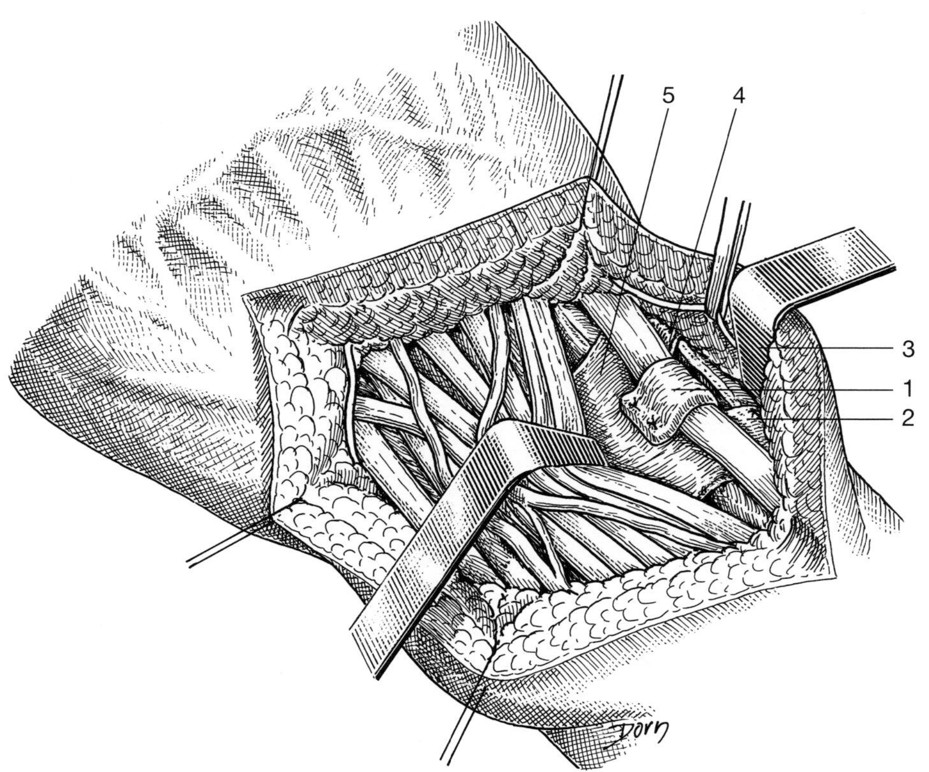

Figure 33.8

Transposition of the transverse portion of the dorsal retinaculum deep to the extensor tendons. Its ulnar extremity is divided into three slips, the middle slip is used as a pulley for the dorsalization of the ECU tendon (1).
(2) The proximal slip is passed posterior to the ulna and sutured to the antebrachial fascia.
(3) Oblique portion of the extensor retinaculum.
(4) The distal slip is passed volarly to the ECU tendon and sutured to the oblique portion of the extensor retinaculum.
(5) Transverse portion of the dorsal retinaculum transposed deep to the extensor tendons.

extensor digitorum communis (EDC) are retracted ulnarwards (Figure 33.7). The posterior interosseous nerve courses through the fourth compartment, initially beneath the extensor indicis proprius (EIP) and then between this tendon and the EPL. It is easily located on the ulnar side of Lister's tubercle. A 4–5-cm long segment of the nerve is resected, proximal to the wrist, sufficient to include the small branches supplying the distal radioulnar joint.

Transposition of the dorsal retinaculum

The dorsal retinaculum is passed deep to the extensor tendons. It provides a gliding plane for the tendons, protects them from bony irregularities of the carpus, and reinforces the wrist capsule (Figure 33.8). We use the ulnar extremity of the transposed retinaculum for the stabilization of the ulnar part of the carpus and for the dorsalization of the ECU tendon (see also Figure 38.4).

Some surgeons use a part of the dorsal retinacular flap, passed dorsally over the extensor tendons to prevent bowstringing. In fact bowstringing is rare after dorsal wrist synovectomy because rheumatoid wrists hardly reach 50° of extension.

Closure and postoperative care

The tourniquet is removed before closure to permit meticulous hemostasis and to prevent hematoma formation and skin complications. The wound is closed in two layers. Small drains are left in place. A bulky dressing is applied with the wrist splinted in neutral position. The fingers are left free, and active movements encouraged, except in cases requiring tendon repairs.

Complications

Skin problems and extensor tendon ruptures are the most frequent postoperative complications.

Skin problems are usually seen in patients with thin, fragile skin, caused by vasculitis and long-term steroid therapy. The wound may be slow to heal and occasionally there are dehiscences and superficial necroses despite all the operative precautions. When this occurs, the extensor tendons become exposed and may slough. In cases of especially thin skin with the possibility of skin necrosis, the extensor retinaculum may be placed superficial to the tendons to act as a barrier.

Most of these necroses are limited and can be treated conservatively by gentle debridement. The skin will generally re-epithelialize within 3–4 weeks. While the wound is healing, the metacarpophalangeal (MP) joints must be immobilized in a functional position to prevent extensor tendon lag. However, proximal interphalangeal joint motion should be allowed.

There were 417 dorsal wrist synovectomies performed at the Institut de la Main between 1987 and 1992. Skin wound healing complications appeared in 20 patients. Slight wound dehiscence developed in 12 wrists, which responded to local wound care. In eight other cases, deep necrosis developed which required debridement and skin cover. Skin grafts were not thought to be appropriate because of the nature of the bed or because of the general state of the patients' skin. None of the currently available ulnar-sided skin flaps was considered appropriate because of the disruption of the vascular axis located in the ulnar side, after excision of the ulnar head and the dissection and moving of the ECU. Five cases were treated by means of an island flap vascularized by the distal branch of the radial artery. In two cases a kite flap was used (Figure 33.9); and in one case of more extensive necrosis a Chinese flap as required based on the radial artery (Brunelli et al 1999).

Extensor tendon ruptures

Extensor tendon ruptures are quite often associated with rheumatoid wrists at the wrist level. They are more frequent than flexor tendon ruptures. They are caused by attrition against a prominent bone spur (Vaughan-Jackson 1948) or direct invasion by hypertrophic synovitis associated with ischemic necrosis.

At the wrist level the extensor tendons, with their synovial sheaths, pass under the dorsal retinaculum on the back of the wrist before diverging toward the digits.

The most common extensor tendon ruptures are those to the digital extensors of the little finger at the distal end of the ulna and to the EPL at Lister's tubercle. The pathologic process causing the rupture will affect the other extensor tendons. Thus extensor tendon ruptures constitute an indisputable indication for surgery, not only to repair the tendon but also to prevent other ruptures. A synovectomy should be performed as soon as possible, in association with a careful removal of any bony prominence that might have been responsible for tendon attrition.

Extensor tendon ruptures are usually treated by adjacent sutures, tendon transfers, joint fusion, and occasionally by tendon bridge grafts. Direct repair between the tendon ends is rarely possible because of the rheumatoid lesions and the proximal muscle retraction.

Ruptures of the EPL

These ruptures are usually located at Lister's tubercle. Interphalangeal motion is still possible through the intrinsic muscles. One should not be misled by the presence

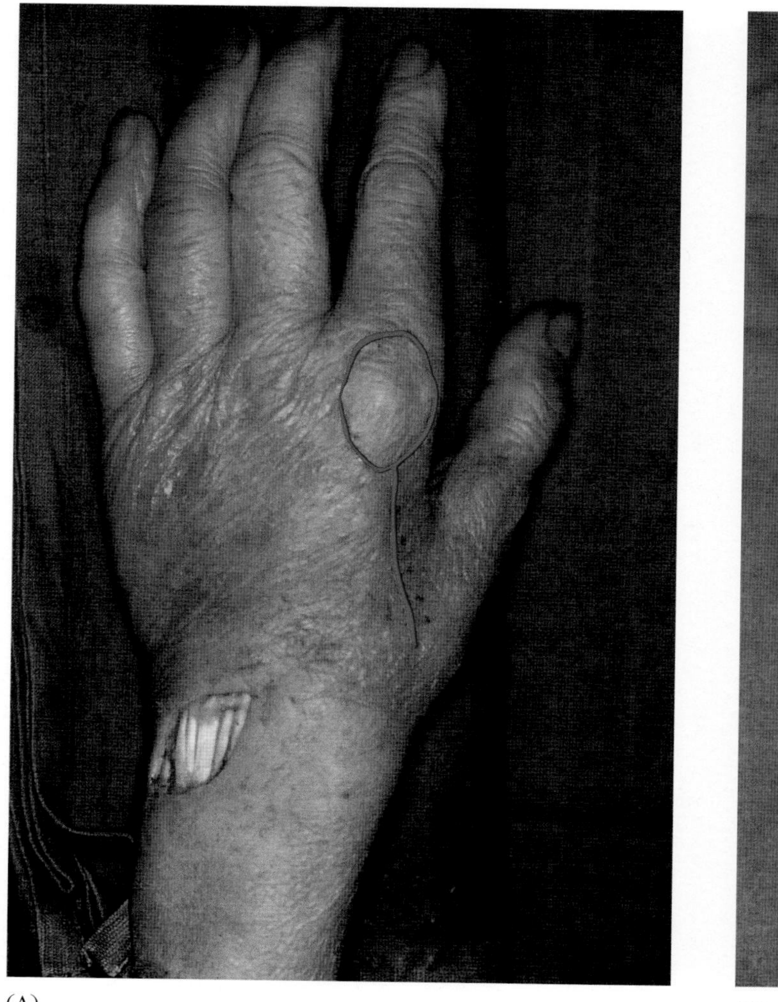

(A)

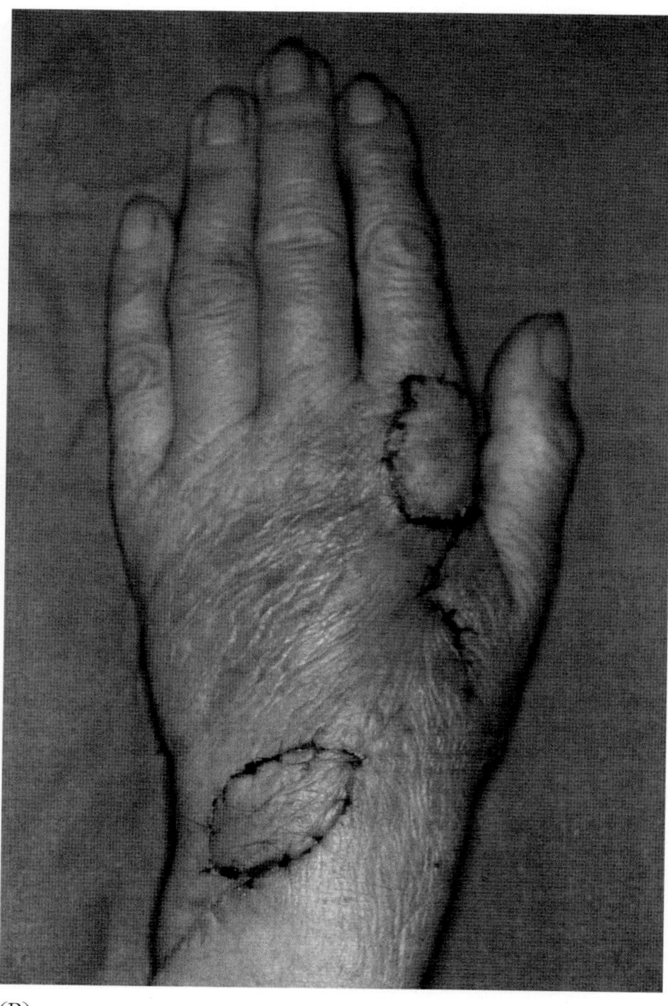

(B)

Figure 33.9

(A) Skin necrosis at the level of the dorsal wrist incision; drawing of the kite flap. (B) Subcutaneous transposition of the kite flap; skin graft on the donor site (Brunelli et al 1999).

of extension movements at the distal thumb phalanx. The impossibility for the patient of moving the thumb ray into retroposition, with the thumb in abduction, is the sign of EPL rupture (Figure 33.10).

Exploration is effected through a curved longitudinal incision. The gap between the two tendon extremities is usually important. A tendon graft from the palmaris longus (PL) can be a solution. Most authors use an EIP tendon transfer (Figure 33.11).

The EIP is an excellent tendon to use because it is an in-phase transfer, the excursion is the same as the ruptured tendon, and the disability produced in the index finger is minimal.

A curved longitudinal incision is made on the ulnar side of the head of the second metacarpal. The EIP and EDC are isolated. The ulnarly located EIP is freed and

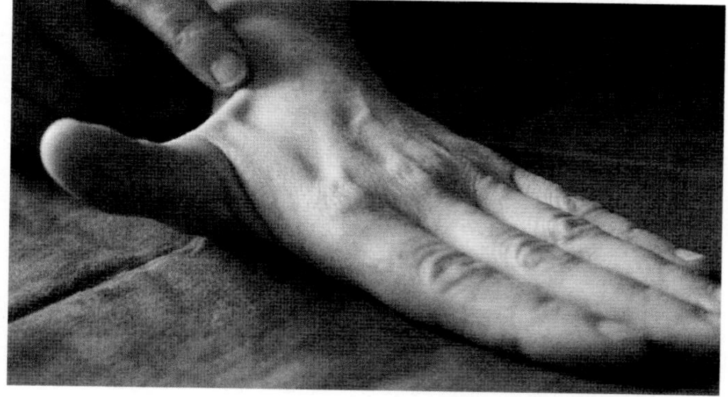

Figure 33.10

Only the EPL is capable of effecting active retroposition of the thumb column.

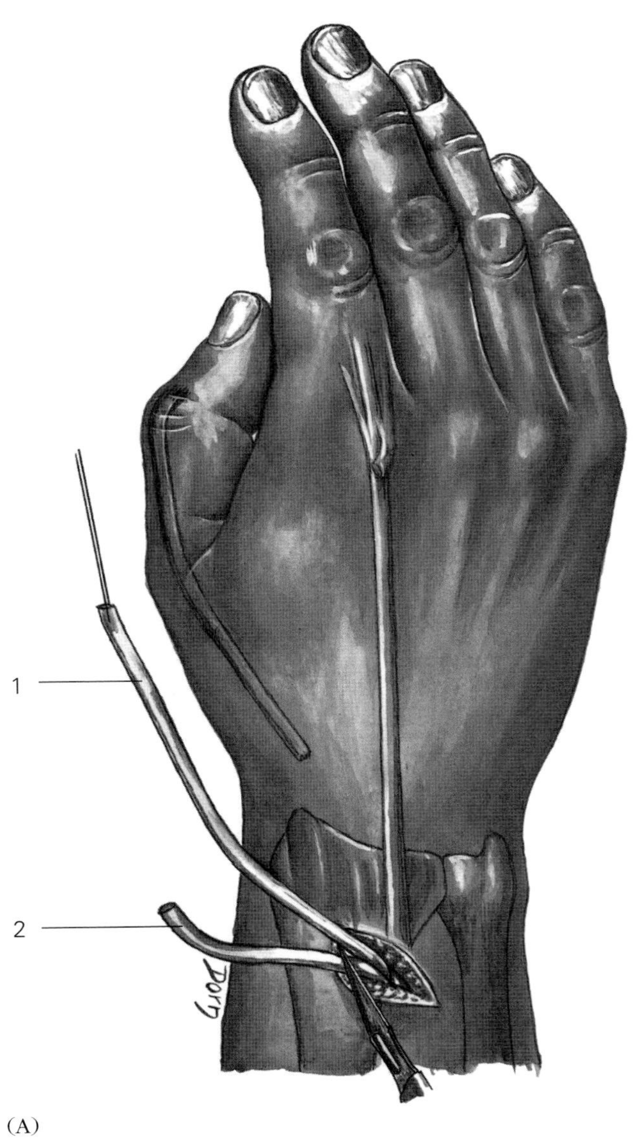

(A)

1
2
3

(B)

Figure 33.11

Rupture of the EPL. EIP tendon transfer.

1 EIP
2 Proximal stump

The EIP tendon is passed through the distal stump of the EPL and is woven into the extensor mechanism at the MP joint level.

divided 1 cm proximally of its junction with the EDC. The distal stump of the EIP is sutured to the index EDC tendon.

A second incision is made just proximal to the wrist dorsal retinaculum. The EIP is easily identified at the wrist because it has the most distal muscle belly. It is delivered with traction to the proximal wound. A third curved incision is made on the radial side of the MP joint of the thumb.

The EIP tendon is then directed subcutaneously over the thumb MP joint. Nalebuff (1969) advises not connecting the transfer with the distal stump of the ruptured tendon, but passing the EIP tendon directly to the MP joint level and weaving it into the extensor mechanism. The transfer should be sewed in tightly because it will stretch when motion begins.

Finger extensor tendon ruptures

The site of ruptures is usually at the wrist level; however, it may be more distal when the rupture is caused by invasion of the tendon by synovitis.

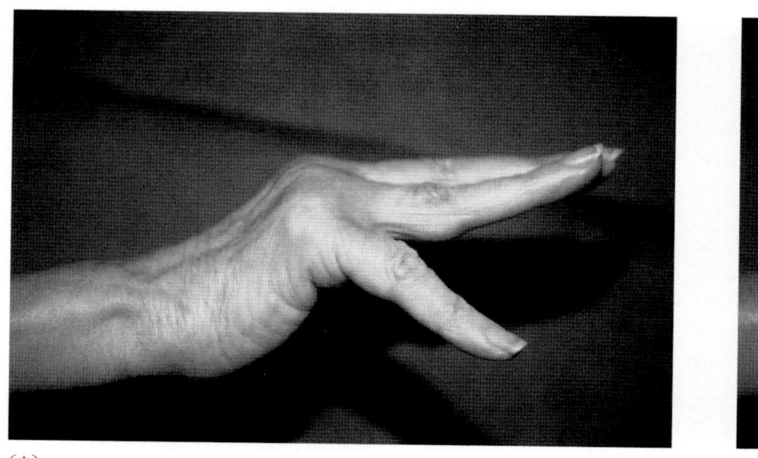
(A)

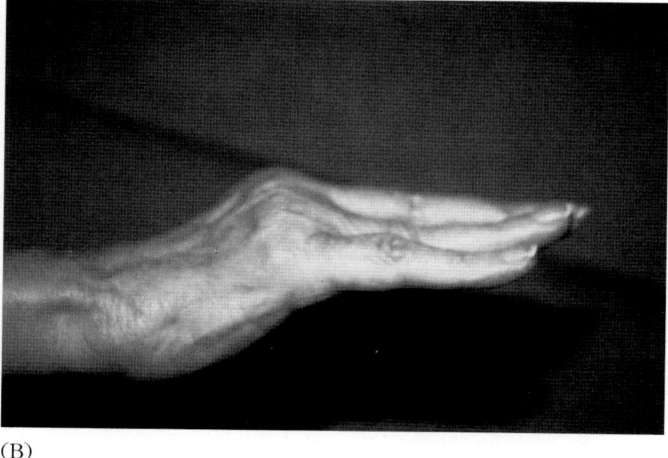
(B)

Figure 33.12
(A) Subluxation of extensor tendons of the little finger simulating a tendon rupture. (B) The little finger is placed in passive extension.

Single rupture to the little finger

Rupture of the extensor tendons of the little finger is most common, and is often the prelude to ruptures of the extensor tendons of the ring finger and then of the other finger extensor tendons. The diagnosis of rupture of the finger extensor tendons relies on the defect of active extension of the proximal phalanx. The middle and distal phalanges can be extended by the interosseous muscles. The diagnosis of rupture of the extensor tendons in the little finger is not always made, for the defect in extension of the finger may be caused by subluxation of the tendon. To make this diagnosis, the finger is placed in passive extension, and the patient is asked to maintain this position (Figure 33.12). If the patient is unable to do this, there is probably a rupture. When possible, one can also flex the wrist, which, as a result of a tenodesis effect, will extend the finger if there is a luxation but not if there is a rupture.

Adjacent side-to-side suture is the best procedure when the distal stump is long enough (Figure 33.13). If side-to-side suture cannot be done, the best solution is then transfer of the EIP to the ruptured tendon. The EIP is an excellent tendon to use because it is an in-phase transfer, the excursion is the same as the ruptured tendon, and the disability produced in the index finger is minimal.

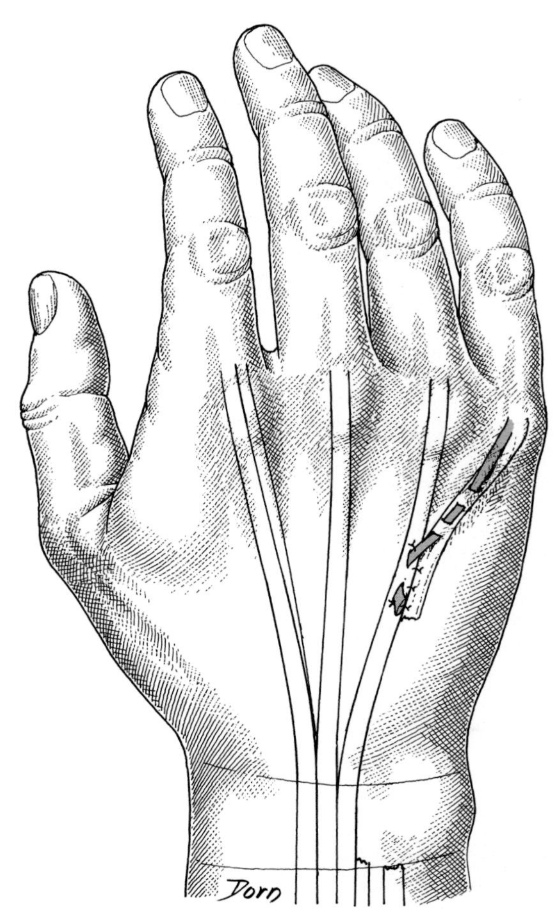

Figure 33.13
Rupture of the extensor tendons of the little finger. Adjacent side-to-side suture.

Double rupture to the ring and little fingers

This is the most common double rupture (Figure 33.14), usually on the basis of attrition. The EIP is transferred to the fifth extensor tendon and the ring EC tendon is sutured side-to-side to the long EC tendon.

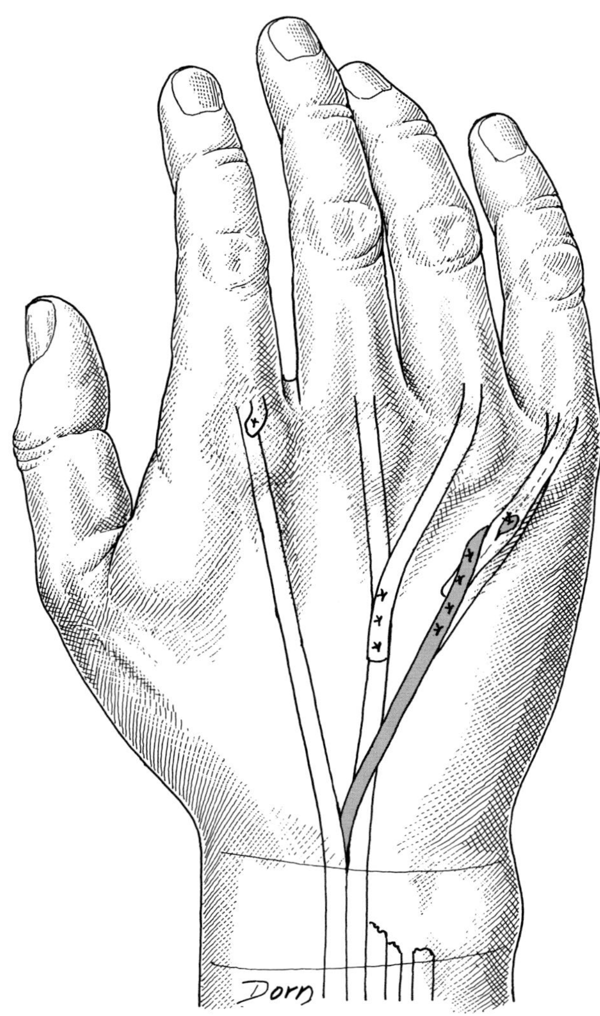

Figure 33.14

Double rupture of extensor tendons. The EIP tendon is transferred to the fifth extensor tendons. the fourth EDC tendon is sutured to the third.

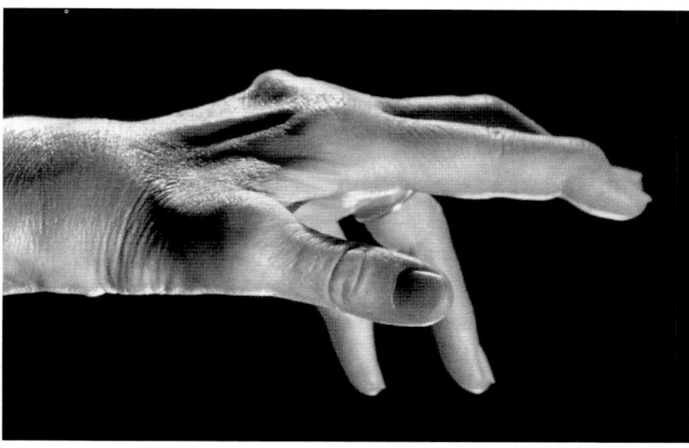

Figure 33.15

Rupture of extensor tendons of the ring and little fingers.

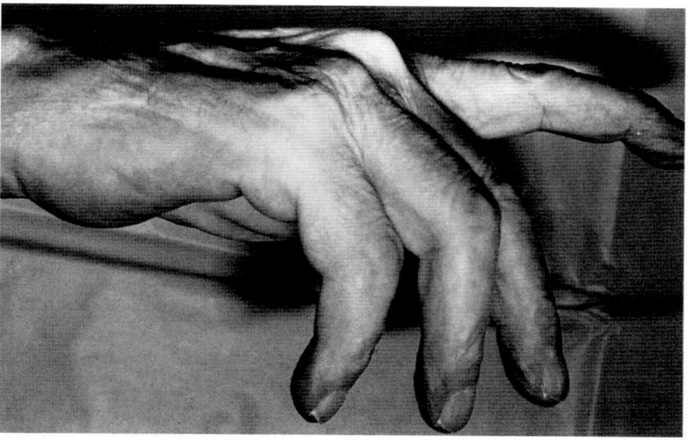

(A)

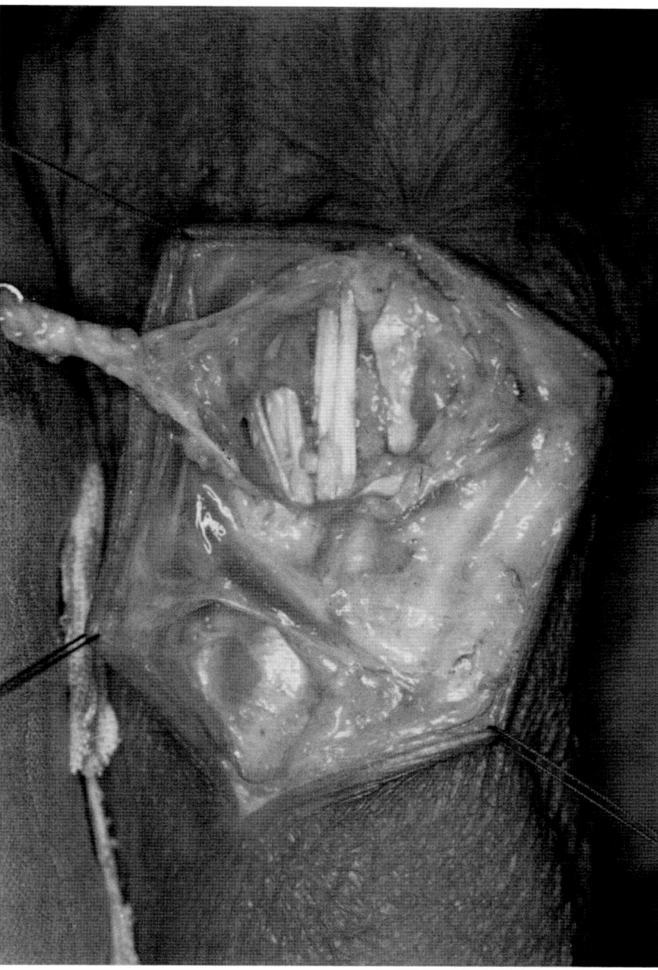

(B)

Figure 33.16

Triple rupture. Only the index finger can be extended.

Because of the extensive dissection, a suction drain should always be applied before skin closure.

Postoperative physiotherapy is initiated very early, after the first dressing and removal of the drain 2–3 days postoperatively. Active and passive motion are camed out several times a day, and a dynamic flexion splint is often necessary.

Flexor tendon rupture

Unlike extensor tendons, flexor tendon ruptures are not frequent in rheumatoid arthritis. In Moore's series of tendon ruptures in the rheumatoid hand (Moore et al 1987) there were only 12 ruptures of flexor tendons (20%).

Diagnosis is often difficult in the rheumatoid context, as tendon synovitis, stiffness and joint deformities are often present. Their first description was by Laine and Vainio (1955). Since Mannerfelt and Norman's series of 25 cases in 1969, the largest reported series is by Ertel et al in 1988 (115 flexor tendon ruptures in 45 patients).

The tendon most exposed to rupture is the FPL. Spontaneous hyperextension of the thumb interphalangeal joint suggests the rupture, which is confirmed by the inability to actively flex the distal phalanx.

Ruptures are less frequent in the finger flexors. Flexor tendons of the index finger may occur with or follow the rupture of the thumb flexor, sometimes misleading the diagnosis towards an interosseous nerve palsy. Rupture is less frequent in the little finger tendons, and very infrequent in the central digits.

Like flexor synovitis, flexor tendon rupture must be sought every time one examines a rheumatoid patient as they often go unnoticed, especially in advanced cases with finger deformities and stiffness. Not only should it be treated, but most of all subsequent rupture of other tendons should be prevented.

Sometimes, during an active finger flexion, the patient feels a painful snapping sensation radiating to the forearm, and may notice a subsequent modification in the pinch grip.

Clinical examination tests each finger and thumb flexor specifically (Figure 34.6), but a rupture can still be masked by synovitis. The tenodesis test is then useful: passive motion of the wrist in flexion and extension does not modify the position of the involved finger in a case of flexor tendon rupture. Brunelli's test (compression of the flexor mass in the forearm) is also negative in case of a rupture, but sometimes examination is extremely difficult because of severe associated deformities (e.g. swan-neck). Ultrasound and MRI may be helpful in such cases, but the associated synovitis, frequently invading the tendons, may give false positive results.

Two types of mechanisms lead to tendon rupture: attrition due to a progressive tendon wear on a bony protuberance, and invasion of the tendon by synovitis, or a rheumatoid nodule, which weakens it to rupture. Flatt (1995) stresses the role of tendon avascular necrosis in the pathogenesis of these ruptures.

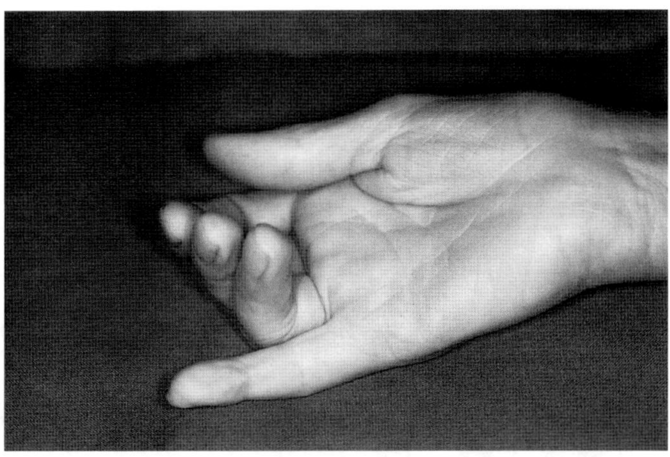

Figure 34.6
Rupture of FPL, and of both flexor tendons of the little finger.

Attrition

Described by Vaughan-Jackson in 1959, attrition is the most frequent type of rupture (Ertel and Millender 1987). It always takes place at the wrist: progression of rheumatoid arthritis leads to carpal joint arthritis, with sharp bone spurs which, when anterior, may perforate the volar capsule, and come into contact with a flexor tendon. Repeated motion progressively wears the tendon, which finally ruptures during an ordinary movement.

The most frequent cause of attrition is a scaphoid spur which ruptures the FPL. Owing to rheumatoid arthritis, the scaphoid progressively assumes a horizontal position, the scapho-trapezial joint becomes arthritic, and a sharp bony spur develops at the distal part of the tubercle: this is the classic 'critical corner' described by Mannerfelt (Mannerfelt and Norman 1969) (Figure 34.7). Once the FPL has ruptured, the flexor digitorum profundus (FDP) of the index finger comes into contact with the spur, and if left untreated, soon ruptures in turn, followed by either the flexor digitorum superficialis (FDS) of the index finger or the FDP of the middle finger. Other sites of attrition are the trapezius or the anterior border of the distal radius. Less frequently the unciform process of the hamate, or the distal edge of the ulna (Craig and House 1984) are responsible for the rupture of the FDP to the little finger. We treated a patient who presented with a double rupture of the FPL on the scaphoid and of the

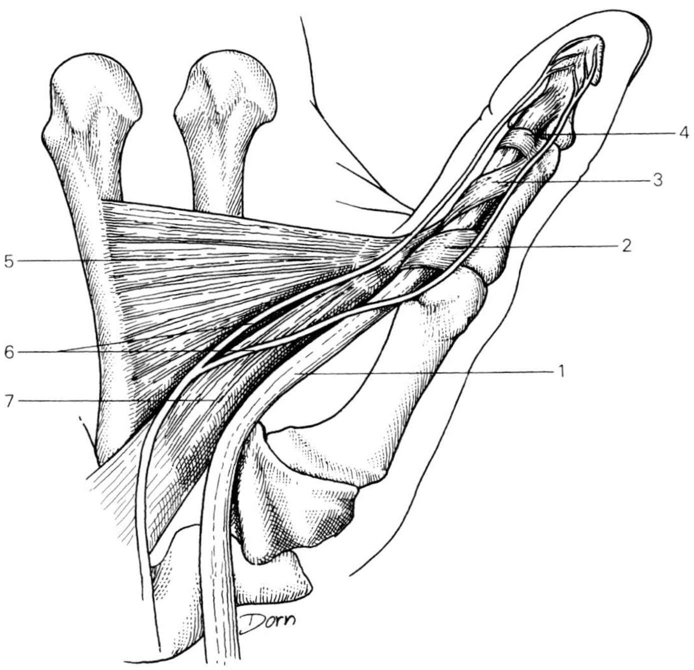

Figure 34.7
Mannerfelt's critical corner.
1 flexor pollicis longus
2 A_1 pulley
3 oblique pulley
4 A_2 pulley
5 transverse head of adductor pollicis
6 digital nerves
7 oblique head of adductor pollicis

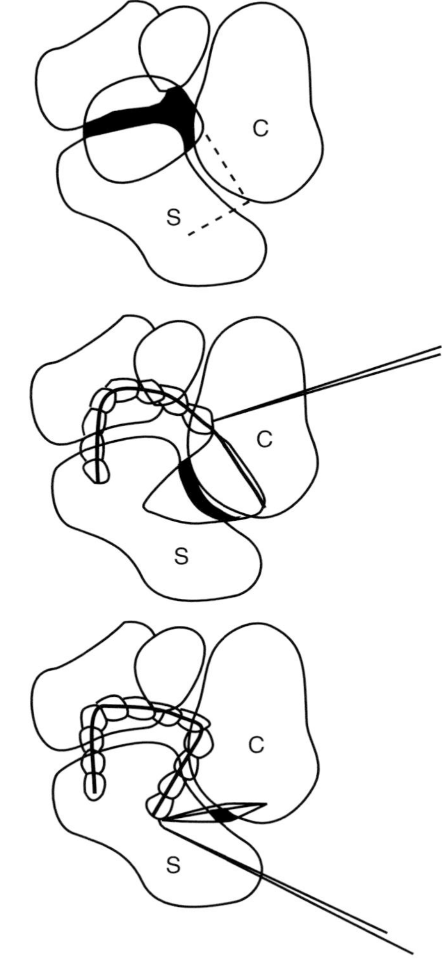

Figure 34.8
Repair of the capsular tear (Ertel).

little finger FP on the unciform process. Zangger and Simmen (1993) have described a case of rupture of the tendons of the index and middle fingers on the tilted lunate.

These attrition ruptures may occur without any synovitis, and the rupture is then easily diagnosed, and the site of the rupture is usually easily identified with standard X-rays showing the bony spur.

Treatment of tendon ruptures in rheumatoid arthritis, regardless of their cause, must be planned with regard to the patient's general status (age, duration of rheumatoid arthritis, medical treatment, other locations of the disease, use of a walking stick) and local status (delay since rupture, number of ruptured tendons, associated finger joints involvement).

When recent, the rupture requires urgent treatment, to prevent further ruptures of adjacent tendons. The goal of surgery is both to restore finger flexion and to protect other tendons. Once the flexor retinaculum has been incised and the median nerve has been protected, a complete synovectomy of all flexor tendons is performed first, which allows visualization of any tendons that have ruptured. It is not uncommon to find more ruptures than suspected clinically.

Inspection and palpation of the floor of the carpal tunnel reveal the bony spur responsible for the rupture. This is removed piecemeal with a rongeur, then the capsular tear is repaired. It is rarely possible to perform a direct suture of the tear, and a local flap, such as that suggested by Ertel (1989), is performed (Figure 34.8). Tendon repair can seldom be performed by direct suture of the tendon, because it is always dilacerated.

In isolated tears of the FPL one can either perform an intercalated graft, or a transfer of the ring finger flexor superficialis. The former is preferred in recent ruptures, when the muscle has a satisfactory excursion. The palmaris longus, when present, is used as a graft source. Feldon et al (1993) have emphasized the following technical point: tendon–graft sutures must be performed away from the carpal tunnel, to avoid adhesions in the canal. Transfer of the FDS to the ring finger is preferred in older ruptures with a retracted muscle–tendon unit, provided that the FDP is healthy. One may also choose to leave the tendon unrepaired and perform a thumb interphalangeal arthrodesis when the interphalangeal joint is already stiff, or painful and radiologically arthritic. The thumb metacarpophalangeal (MP) joint must also be evaluated preoperatively: any previous instability is likely to be increased by the restoration of a strong pollici-digital pinch, and needs to be addressed, either with a ligamentoplasty, or with an arthrodesis.

In isolated ruptures of another tendon, this can be treated by a direct lateral suture of the distal stump to the tendon of the adjacent finger. This useful procedure restricts digital independence, and is therefore preferred for repair of the ulnar finger tendons.

In ruptures of several tendons, one may resect the ruptured FDS, and use them as tendon grafts to repair the ruptured FDP tendons.

In these cases of attrition ruptures, there is usually no or little associated synovitis, and the result of repairs is usually quite satisfactory provided that there is no joint stiffness.

Invasion

Ruptures occur here in a very different environment. The diffuse tenosynovitis makes the diagnosis of a rupture very difficult. Signs of synovitis are predominant (pain, anterior swelling, crepitus, trigger fingers, lack of active flexion), and each tendon must systematically be examined carefully for rupture. The diagnosis is particularly difficult for FDS ruptures, as they usually go totally unnoticed by the patient, whereas rupture of the FDP produces some decrease of grasp strength and of finger dexterity. The clinical tests described earlier are very useful here, but beware of a false tenodesis effect created by adhesion of the ruptured tendon to an adjacent healthy one.

The site of rupture may also be very difficult to localize when the tenosynovitis is widespread. MRI studies are not always contributive. In such cases, surgical exploration should start at the wrist level, as this is the most frequent site of rupture (wrist 50%, palm 25%, fingers 25%). Incisions are performed in the same manner as for synovectomy, longitudinally oriented in a zigzag fashion which can be prolonged as required.

The first surgical step is tenosynovectomy of all involved flexor tendons. The type of repair depends on the patient's general and local status, as in attrition ruptures.

In isolated ruptures of the FPL, the strategy is identical to that for attrition ruptures.

In tendon ruptures in the wrist or palm, only FDP tendons are usually repaired, either with intercalated grafts from the resected FDS, or by lateral suture to an intact neighbouring tendon. Isolated rupture of an FDS is usually left unrepaired. Isolated ruptures of an FDP are repaired only if the distal interphalangeal (DIP) joint is intact (except in cases of simultaneous rupture of the FDS). If the DIP joint is arthritic, one will preferably perform a tenodesis to the FDS or an arthrodesis of the distal joint.

Tendon ruptures in the finger are difficult to treat, and the results of repair are often unsatisfactory.

- In isolated rupture of one finger tendon, the primary goal of surgery is to protect the other tendon of this finger, by performing a complete synovectomy. If the superficialis is ruptured, it is not repaired. If the profundus is ruptured tenodesis or arthrodesis provide more dependable results than a graft of the profundus through the intact superficialis. This last procedure leads to a high rate of failures (50% in Ertel's series, Ertel 1989), and should be restricted to young and motivated patients.
- If both tendons are ruptured, poor results should be anticipated. Surgical repair usually requires a two-stage tendon graft, owing to the poor quality of the osteo-fibrous canal. This sophisticated procedure, which gives inconstant results even in post-traumatic cases, should be restricted to young motivated patients with supple digital joints. In the remainder, one will preferably perform an arthrodesis of both the proximal interphalangeal (PIP) and DIP joints, provided that the MP joint is mobile.

Conclusion

Surgical repair of flexor tendons in rheumatoid arthritis often produces disappointing results. Thus one must focus on prevention of ruptures, including:

- clinical examination for any sign of flexor tenosynovitis each time one sees a rheumatoid patient;
- surgical treatment of flexor synovitis when it does not subside after 6 months of appropriate medical treatment;
- excision of all threatening bone spurs in the carpal tunnel;
- systematic examination of all patients for flexor tendon rupture, and if present, rapid surgery to avoid further ruptures.

References

Craig EV, House JH (1984) Dorsal carpal dislocation and flexor tendon rupture in rheumatoid arthritis. A case report, *J Hand Surg* **94**: 261–4.

Ertel AN (1989) Flexor tendon ruptures in rheumatoid arthritis, *Hand Clin* **5**: 177–90.

Ertel AN, Millender LH (1987) Flexor tendon involvement in patients with rheumatoid arthritis. In: Hunter JM, Schneider LH, Mackin EJ, eds, *Tendon Surgery in the Hand* (CV Mosby: St Louis) 370–84.

Ertel AN, Millender LH, Nalebuff EA et al (1988) Flexor tendon ruptures in rheumatoid arthritis, *J Hand Surg* **13A**: 860–8.

Feldon P, Millender LH, Nalebuff EA (1993) Rheumatoid arthritis in the hand and wrist. In: Green D, ed, *Operative Hand Surgery*, 3rd edn (Churchill Livingstone: Edinburgh) 1587–690.

Flatt AE (1995) *The Care of the Arthritic Hand*, 5th edn (Quality Medical Publishing: St Louis) 206–17.

Laine VAI, Vainio KJ (1955) Spontaneous ruptures of tendons in rheumatoid arthritis, *Acta Orthop Scand* **24**: 250–7.

Mannerfelt N, Norman O (1969) Attrition ruptures of flexor tendons in rheumatoid arthritis caused by bone spurs in the carpal tunnel, *J Bone Joint Surg* **51B**: 270–7.

Moore JR, Weiland AJ, Valdata L (1987) Tendon ruptures in the rheumatoid hand: analysis of treatment and functional results in 60 patients, *J Hand Surg* **12**: 9–14.

Vaughan-Jackson OJ (1959) Attrition ruptures of tendons as a factor in the production of deformities in the rheumatoid hand, *Proc R Soc Med* **52**: 132–4.

Zangger P, Simmen BR (1993) Spontaneous ruptures of flexor tendons secondary to extreme DISI deformity of the lunate in rheumatoid wrist, *Ann Chir Main* **12**: 250–5.

35 Arthroplasties and arthrodeses of the fingers

Caroline Leclercq

Metacarpophalangeal joint arthroplasties

Among the many prostheses that have been developed since the 1960s (Egloff 2000), only one has stood the test of time so far, and remains the gold standard for metacarpophalangeal (MP) joint arthroplasty, more than 30 years after being introduced by Alfred Swanson (Swanson 1968, Swanson and de Groot Swanson 1984): the one-piece silicone implant. This flexible hinge prosthesis acts as a spacer and produces local encapsulation. Although it has drawbacks, related mainly to a limited range of motion, and a risk of fracture over the long term, its overall results in rheumatoid patients are still more satisfactory than two-piece prostheses. The latter, whether constrained or not, have had many problems including instability, recurrence of the deformity, bone fracture or erosion, cement loosening, and contracture.

Research is still ongoing with one- and two-piece prostheses, and some preliminary results seem promising (Beckenbaugh 1999, Moller et al 1999).

Technique

The surgical steps for MP joint arthroplasty in rheumatoid patients have been thoroughly described (Swanson 1972, Millender and Nalebuff 1973).

The joint is approached through a gently curved longitudinal incision on the dorsum of the MP area. If two adjacent joints are operated, a single longitudinal incision may be used. If more than two joints are operated a transverse incision is preferred, located on the dorsum of the metacarpal necks (Figure 35.1).

The dorsal veins and sensory nerves are located and protected in the web spaces. Then the juncturae tendinum are divided longitudinally. In the fourth web a dividing extensor communis tendon to the fourth and fifth fingers must not be confused with a juncturum.

Next, each ulnar interosseous muscle is dissected, its tendon is divided at the MP level and marked with a suture.

Each joint is then approached through a longitudinal incision of the extensor hood on its ulnar aspect (Figure 35.2). The capsule is detached from the extensor hood, then incised longitudinally in the same area.

The synovitis is then removed, taking care to keep the capsule intact, and the joint is inspected. At this stage of the disease, there is usually wide destruction of the cartilage on both surfaces, and anterior subluxation of the proximal phalanx.

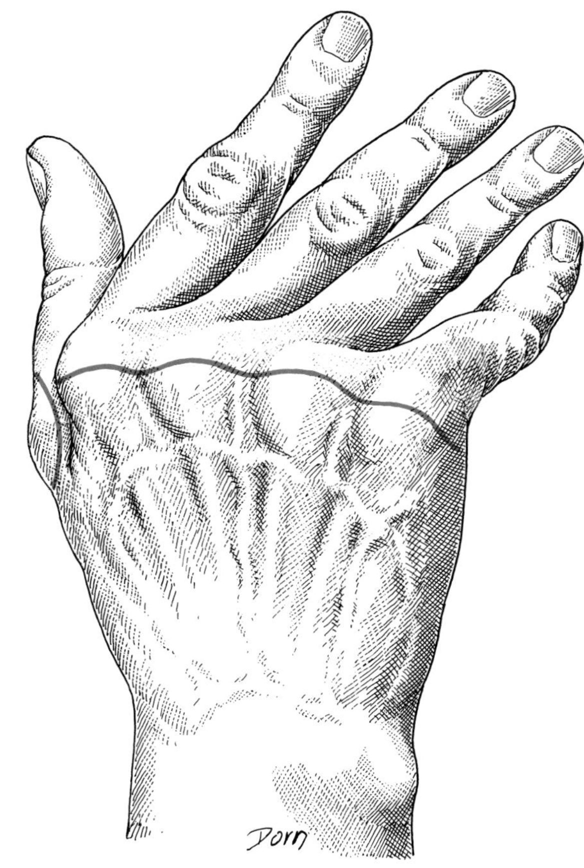

Figure 35.1

Transverse incision for multiple MP joint arthroplasties.

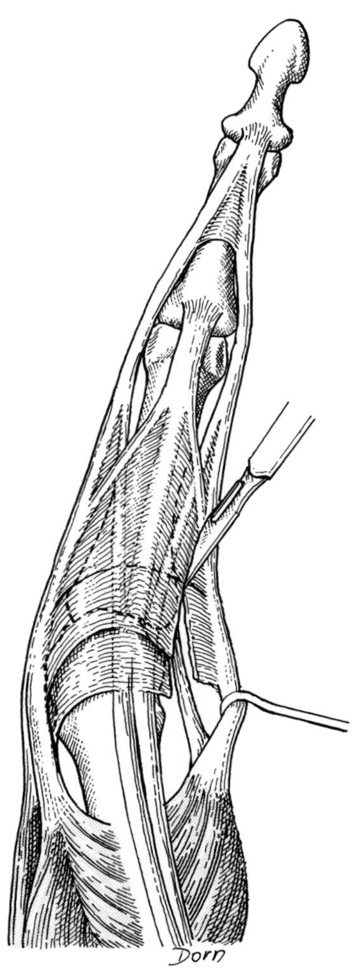

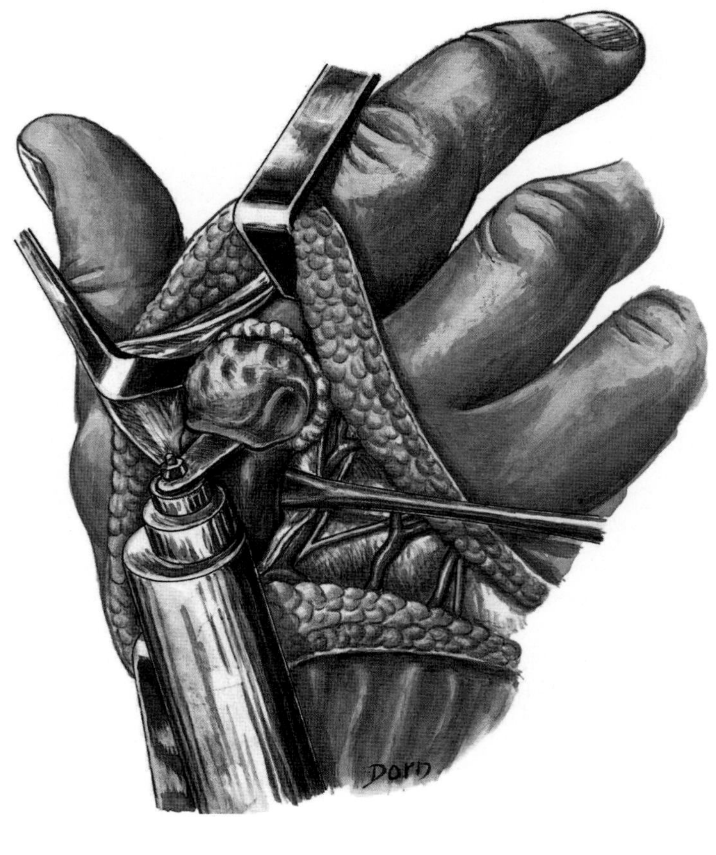

Figure 35.3
Resection of the metacarpal head.

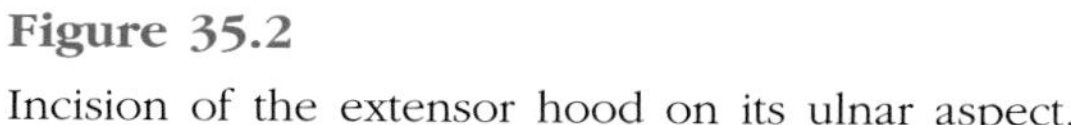

Figure 35.2
Incision of the extensor hood on its ulnar aspect.

Each joint is then approached through a longitudinal incision of the extensor hood on its ulnar aspect (Figure 35.2). The capsule is detached from the extensor hood, then incised longitudinally in the same area.

The synovitis is then removed, taking care to keep the capsule intact, and the joint is inspected. At this stage of the disease, there is usually wide destruction of the cartilage on both surfaces, and anterior subluxation of the proximal phalanx.

The two collateral ligaments are then divided at their metacarpal insertion, and the radial ligament is marked with a suture.

The joint is subsequently dislocated, and the metacarpal neck is prepared for section. This is performed with a power-driven oscillating saw, at the junction of the head and the neck of the metacarpal (Figure 35.3). The line of section is transversal, oriented slightly radially when there is a significant ulnar drift of the fingers. Synovectomy of the anterior part of the joint is then performed. If there is marked volar subluxation of the proximal phalanx, an anterior capsular release must also be performed.

Through the same approach, when required, a limited flexor tendon synovectomy may be carried out.

Next the metacarpal and phalangeal shafts are prepared for implantation. This is best performed with hand-driven tools, as the bone cortex is fragile and may easily rupture. Rasps of increasing size remove the cancellous bone and adapt the shaft to the shape of the prosthesis.

The trial implants are then used to determine the appropriate size. A large enough implant should be used so that the stem fits loosely within the medullary canal, and the collar abuts against the bony edges of the metacarpal and the phalanx. Flexion of the joint should be smooth and easy, if it is not, then the anterior capsular release should be completed, and if this is not sufficient, the metacarpal shaft should be shortened by a few millimetres.

Before inserting the prosthesis, a drill hole is created on the dorso-radial aspect of the metacarpal shaft and a suture is prepared for reattachment of the radial collateral ligament. If the ligament has become too weak, it can be augmented with the radial half of the palmar plate, which is detached proximally, then transferred dorsally around the joint to the dorso-radial aspect of the

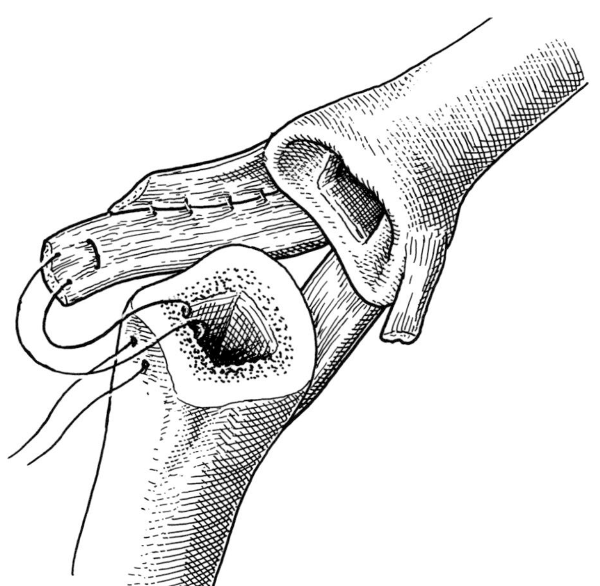

Figure 35.4
The weak radial collateral ligament is augmented with the radial half of the palmar plate. The suture for reattachment to the metacarpal is placed before implant insertion.

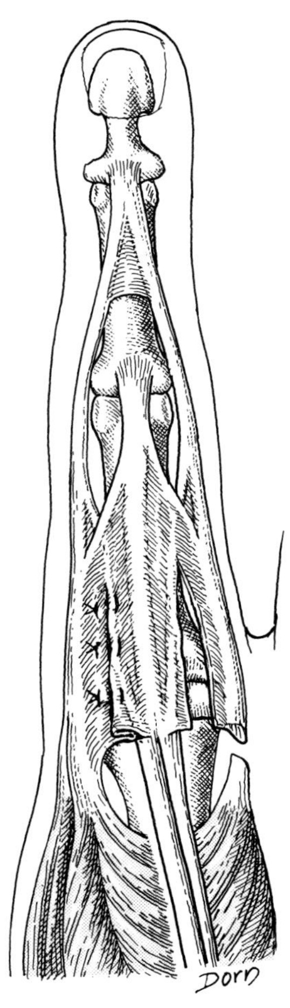

Figure 35.5
Plication of the radial part of the extensor hood.

joint (Swanson et al 1985b, Tubiana 1999) (Figure 35.4).

The operative area is then rinsed thoroughly to remove any bone debris, and the prosthesis is implanted.

The radial collateral ligament suture is tied, and the capsule is closed with absorbable sutures. If there was marked preoperative ulnar drift of the fingers, each ulnar interosseous muscle is transferred to the radial aspect of the adjacent MP joint (Oster et al 1989). Next the ulnar collateral ligament and the extensor hood incisions are sutured back.

The joint is then tested for stability of the extensor apparatus. If there was marked synovitis of the MP joint, the extensor hood is usually slackened, and the extensor tendon subluxes ulnarly during joint flexion. Stabilizing procedures include either plicating the radial part of the extensor hood (Figure 35.5), or performing a tendon-plasty with the ulnar half of the extensor tendon.

The skin is closed in a layers over a suction drain and a bulky dressing is applied.

Postoperative regimen

The suction drain is removed on the second or third postoperative day. The initial dressing is removed after a few days. Gentle active flexion is initiated by the physiotherapist at this stage. To encourage motion at the MP joint level, an external splint blocking PIP joint motion may be added during exercises (Nalebuff 1984). Provided that wound healing is satisfactory and oedema is limited, a dynamic extension splint is applied to all involved fingers, in extension and radial deviation.

After 1 month the splint is discontinued during the day, and active extension and passive motion are added. After 6 weeks, lateral motion is initiated, as well as independent finger motion. Physiotherapy is usually discontinued after the third postoperative month.

Results

Relief of pain is usually achieved in all patients, although this is difficult to evaluate when there are other adjacent painful foci.

MP joint range of motion, when compared with the preoperative range, is not significantly improved, but the overall arc is changed to a much more functional range of motion (Kirschenbaum et al 1993, Hansraj et al 1997) (Figure 35.6). However, with time there seems to be some degree of loss of MP joint motion (Wilson et al 1993).

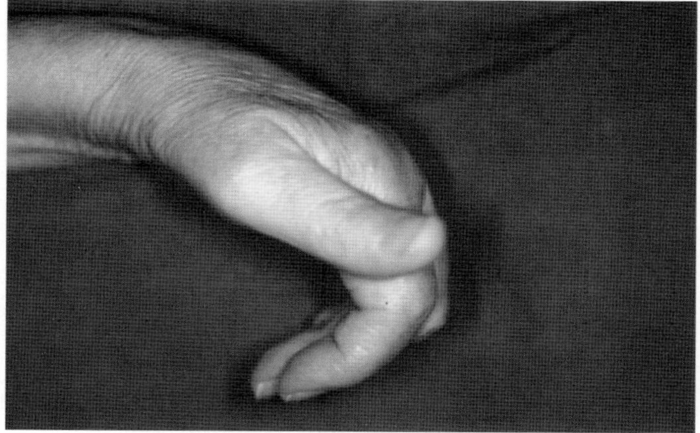

(A)

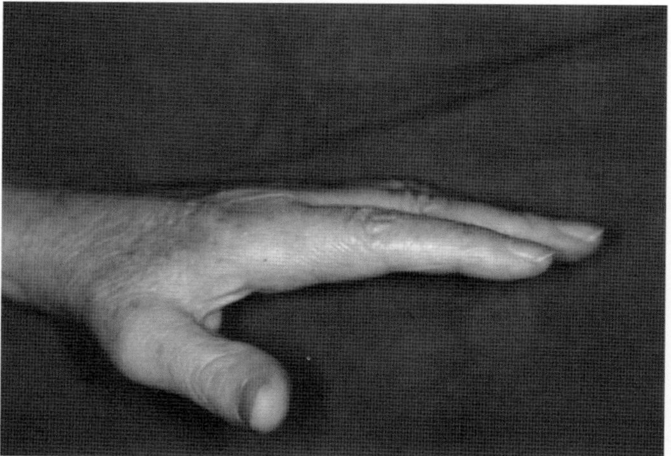

(B)

Figure 35.6
Clinical result 8 months postoperatively: (A) maximal MP joint flexion; (B) maximal MP joint extension.

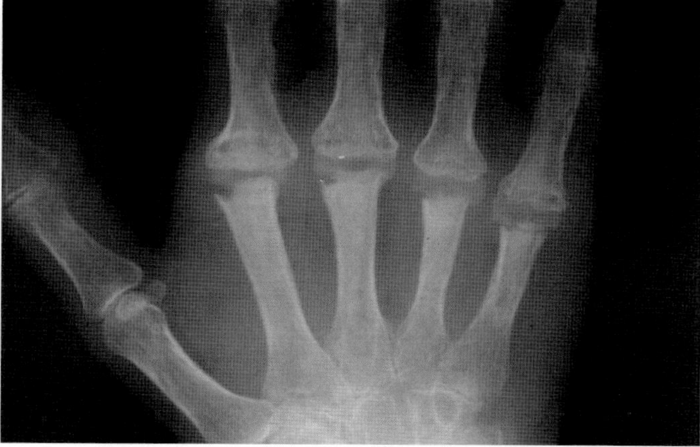

Figure 35.7
Radiographic result 6 months postoperatively. Note bone remodelling of the distal metacarpal.

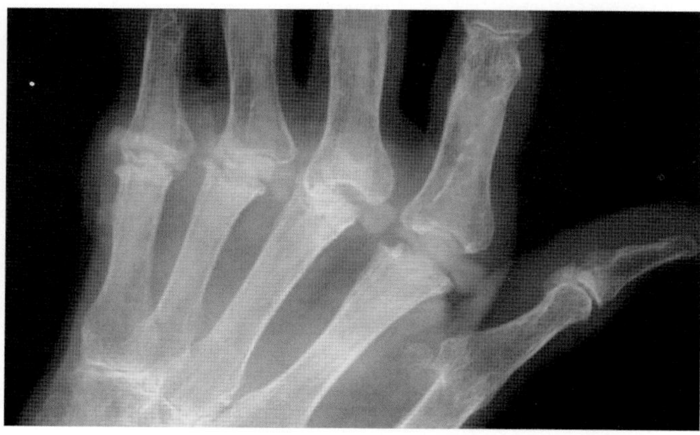

Figure 35.8
Routine X-rays at 12 years follow-up: the patient did not complain of either pain or reduction of the range of motion, although most implants are broken and worn out.

Radiographic follow-up indicates some bone remodelling (Swanson et al 1986), with newly formed cortical shell around the implant, thickening of the cortical bone, shortening of the metacarpal but no shortening of the proximal phalanx (Figure 35.7).

Complications

Several complications have been described after the use of silicone arthroplasties of the MP joint (Foliart 1995), but their incidence remains low.

Fractures of the implant

Fractures of the implant have been reported to occur in as many as 50% of cases (Kay et al 1978), and as rarely as 0.8% (Swanson 1972). Their frequency has gone down since more resistant silicone elastomer (HP) has been available. They seem to be more frequent with the Sutter implant than the Swanson implant (Bass et al 1996). In more recent large series, it was reported to occur in 5–15% of cases (Gellman et al 1997). The fracture usually occurs at the implant collar; because of encapsulation around the prothesis, it is often clinically silent, and revealed only by X-rays. It should be suspected when there is a recurrence of the ulnar drift, or a shortening of the finger. It does not necessarily require replacement of the implant, as in a number of cases it does not interfere with function (Figure 35.8).

Grommets developed by Swanson to protect the flexible hinge from bony edges and thus avoid abrasion and tears leading to implant fracture and silicone wear particles (Swanson et al 1997) have not gained much popularity and do not seem to help solve this problem.

Siliconitis

Since a report by Peimer and Medige in 1986 there has been concern about the possible spreading of silicone particles around the implant, leading to an aggressive giant cell synovitis. This complication has been described mainly for implants around the wrist, and has led to a progressive disaffection with this type of implant in the wrist (including the thumb carpometacarpal joint). However, surprisingly, it seems to affect the finger MP joint implants only rarely in rheumatoid patients. Aptekar et al described one case in 1974, and one case of silicone-induced adenopathy was reported by Groff et al in 1981.

Infection

Infection is a rare complication of silicone implants at the MP joint: Millender et al (1975) reported only 0.5% infection in 2000 implants, and Gellman et al (1997) only 3% deep infections. This complication usually requires removal of the prosthesis.

Recurrence of ulnar deviation

If the soft tissue deformities are not corrected, ulnar deviation is very likely to recur (Bieber et al 1986: 100% recurrence). But even when intrinsic tendons are crossed-transferred, and extensor tendons are realigned, this is susceptible to reattenuation and recurrence of the deformity with time (Blair 1984, Wilson et al 1993).

Despite all these complications, patient satisfaction is reported to be high in all series.

Indications

Replacement arthroplasty is indicated when the MP joints present with cartilaginous destruction and related symptoms (pain, limitation of motion, joint deformity) or long-standing synovitis that is non-responsive to an appropriate medical treatment.

In a number of cases, patients display several localizations of the disease which require surgery, and careful planning needs to be done. Hand procedures should be performed after the more proximal joints of the upper limb, and particularly after wrist procedures, so as not to create tendon imbalance. If lower limb surgery requiring the postoperative use of walking aids needs to be performed, this should also be done before hand procedures, so as to avoid excessive strain on freshly operated hands.

Proximal interphalangeal joint arthroplasties

Proximal interphalangeal (PIP) joint replacement has been performed for many years in rheumatoid arthritis. Many different types of prostheses have been used, including the following.

- *Silicone prosthesis.* This flexible hinge prosthesis developed by Swanson in 1968 is by far the most popular in rheumatoid patients. Other designs have been produced more recently: Sutter's implant with a broader hinge and shorter stems and Niebauer prosthesis surrounded with Dacron in order to promote adhesion.
- *Hinge prostheses.* Initially developed by Brannon, then by Flatt (1961), hinge prostheses have been progressively abandoned because of the many complications encountered (hinge breakage, loosening, cortical fracture). Newer concepts have evolved towards a better quality hinge, and methyl-metacrylate cementing of the stems.
- *Semi-constrained prostheses.* This type of implant was developed in the PIP joint by Condamine et al (1988).
- *Unconstrained prostheses.* These prostheses were developed in the 1980s (Lindscheid et al 1979), initially they were metal-polyethylene and cemented, more recently they have been made of pyrocarbon and non-cemented. They require preservation or reconstruction of good quality collateral ligaments, which may be a problem in rheumatoid patients.

Surgical approach

The PIP joint can be entered dorsally, laterally or palmarly.

- The *dorsal approach* was initially the most popular. A dorsal curvilinear incision is performed about the PIP joint. After protecting dorsal veins and nerves, the joint is approached through a central longitudinal incision through the central extensor tendon, but the tendon insertion on the basis of the middle phalanx is left untouched (Figure 35.9). The joint may also be approached through a dorso-lateral incision between the central tendon and the lateral band (Figure 35.10). This approach bears the inconvenience of a weakening of the extensor apparatus. It is particularly indicated in cases where there is a boutonnière deformity.
- The *lateral approach* is performed through the ulnar side of the joint, so as to preserve the radial collateral ligament. The joint is approached between the central and the lateral band of the extensor tendon, then the ulnar collateral ligament is detached distally, leaving a short distal ligament stump for later reinsertion. The joint can then usually be dislocated laterally. In some cases it may be necessary to cut the distal insertion of the central extensor band and of the palmar plate. Care must be taken while

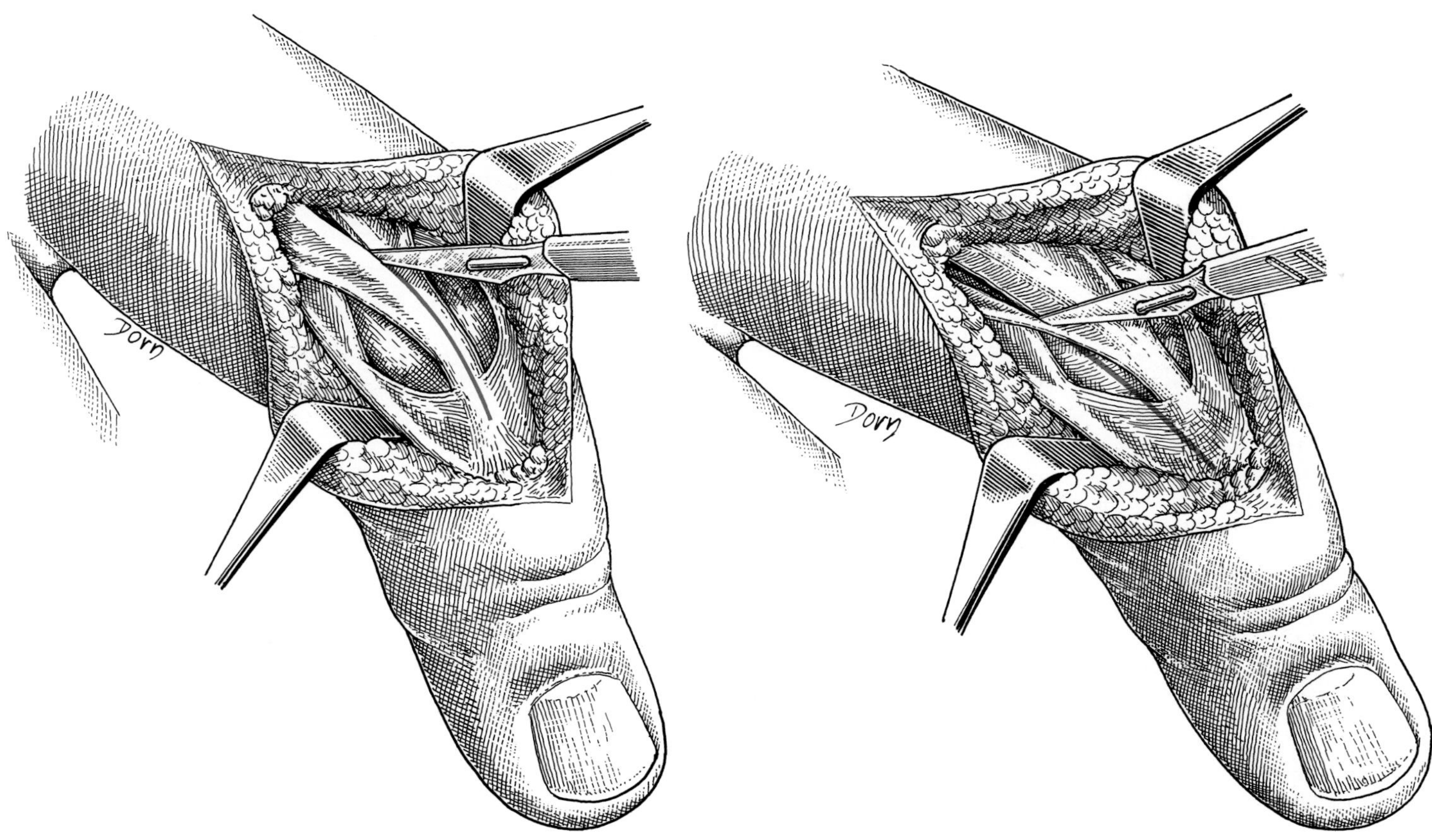

Figure 35.9
Longitudinal incision through the central tendon.

Figure 35.10
Incision between the central and the lateral extensor tendons.

manipulating the joint, so as not to pull on the ulnar collateral neurovascular bundle.

- The *palmar approach* is technically more demanding, because of the flexor tendons which get in the way. The skin is incised in a zigzag manner, and the cruciate pulley facing the PIP joint is incised. The flexor tendons are retracted laterally, and the palmar plate is then incised proximally (check-reins) and laterally in a U shape. The joint can then be dislocated palmarly. It may be necessary to free the collateral ligaments from their distal insertion on the middle phalanx. This approach is useful when there is associated synovitis, or a flexion contracture due to adhesions of the flexor tendons.

Surgical technique (silicone implant)

Whatever approach has been performed, the first step of the procedure is a PIP joint synovectomy. This is completed once the proximal phalangeal head has been removed. Lateral ligaments are freed as required, then the proximal phalangeal head is cut transversally and removed. The base of the middle phalanx is not usually removed unless there is marked persistent stiffness. Any significant bony spur is removed.

The phalangeal shafts are then prepared in the same manner as for MP joint implants. The largest possible implant is used, provided that there is full passive motion of the joint, and the stems fit completely inside the bone shaft, with the hinge resting on the cortical edge. Before implant insertion any necessary transosseous ligament or extensor tendon reinsertion is prepared.

Lateral stability is then tested. If it is insufficient, the collateral ligaments must be reinforced accordingly. Part of the palmar plate may be used, as recommended by Swanson et al (1985a) (Figure 35.11).

Associated deformities of the PIP joint must be corrected during the procedure.

Swan-neck deformities are best approached through a dorsal curvilinear incision (Figure 35.12). The extensor apparatus is tenolysed, and the lateral tendons are mobilized laterally. It may be necessary to lengthen the central tendon in severe deformities. In such an event, the joint may be approached through a zigzag or a V-Y incision of the central band (Figure 35.13). The flexor

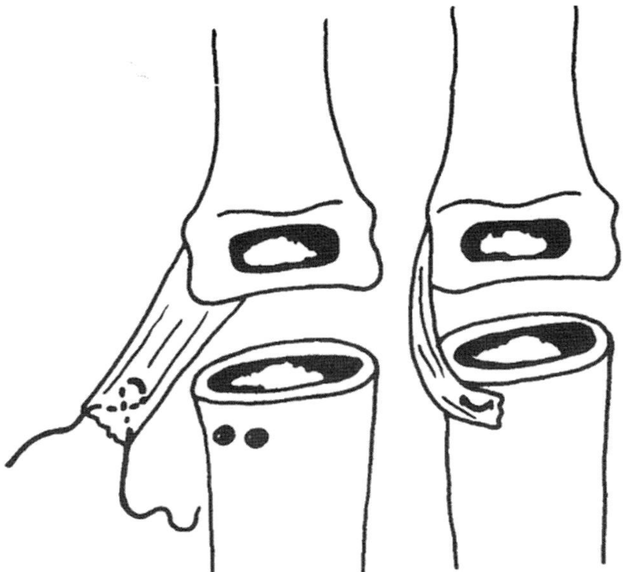

Figure 35.11
Replacement of the attenuated radial collateral ligament with the radial half of the palmar plate.

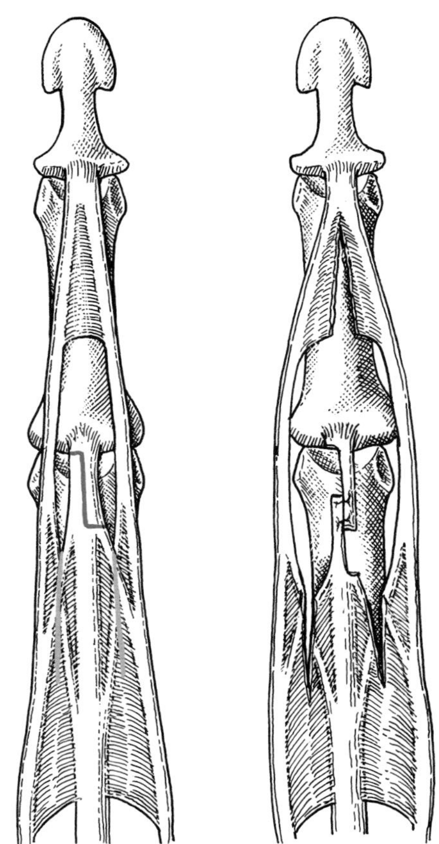

Figure 35.13
In severe swan-neck deformities, the central tendon may require lengthening.

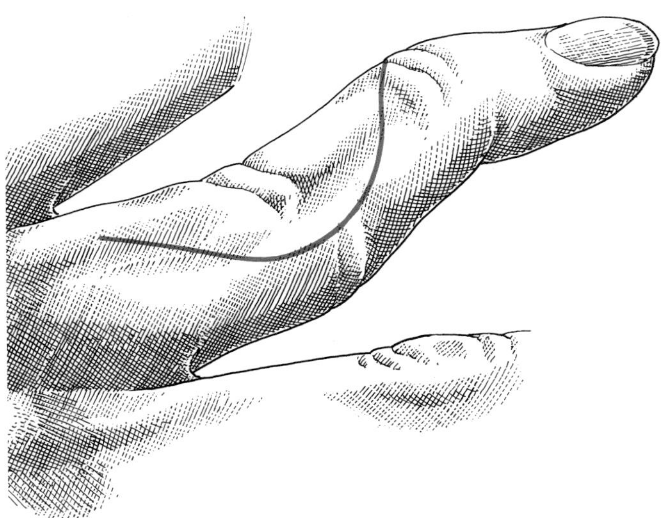

Figure 35.12
Dorsal curvilinear incision for swan-neck deformities.

apparatus must be checked for associated flexor synovitis which could be the cause of the swan-neck deformity. In severe cases, there may be a skin defect at the end of the procedure. This can be treated by leaving the distal part of the incision open (Nalebuff 1999) (Figure 35.14). If the DIP joint is permanently flexed, this can be addressed by a K-wire in extension, or in more severe cases by a tenodermodesis.

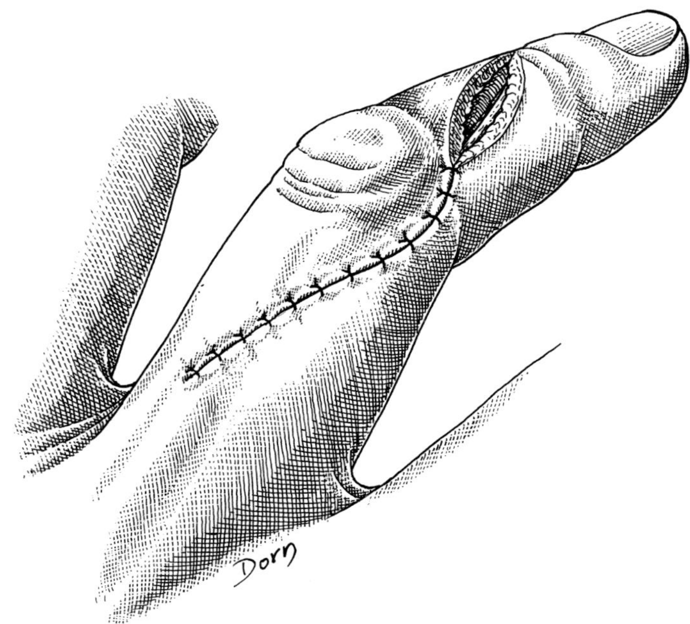

Figure 35.14
The distal third of the incision, over the middle phalanx, is left open.

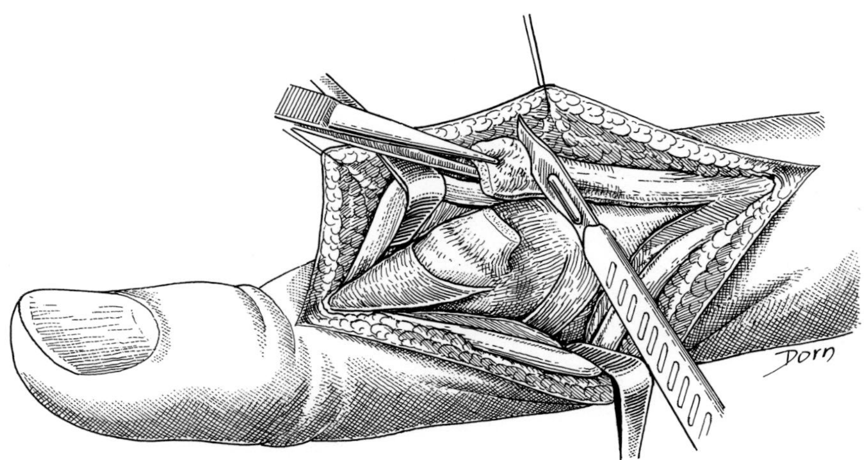

Figure 35.15
The central tendon is detached distally, then shortened by about 3 mm.

Boutonnière deformities are also best approached dorsally. The central tendon is detached from the middle phalanx, and will be shortened and reinserted at the end of the procedure (Figure 35.15). If it is attenuated, it must be supplemented by a tendonplasty or a graft. The lateral bands are carefully tenolysed, and mobilized dorsally. If the deformity is severe, it may be necessary to shorten the proximal phalanx considerably to make room for the implant. The distal interphalangeal (DIP) joint is gently manipulated in flexion. If this is ineffective, a distal tenotomy may be indicated.

Postoperative care

The hand is immobilized in a bulky dressing for a few days, then gentle active motion is initiated, and a dynamic extension splint is applied. Lateral motion is not allowed for a minimum of 3 weeks, and more if collateral ligaments have been reconstructed. If flexion remains limited after 3 weeks, a flexion splint is alternated with the extension splint. In swan-neck deformities, the finger is maintained in slight flexion for 4–6 weeks, and only flexion exercises are allowed during that period.

In boutonnière deformities, the PIP joint is immobilized in full extension for 10 days, whereas the DIP joint is actively flexed. Then PIP motion is initiated, with a splint in extension between exercises for 4 more weeks.

Results

After silicone PIP joint implants, an average range of motion from 10° in extension to 60° in flexion may be anticipated.

When there is an associated swan-neck deformity, PIP joint hyperextension has been reported to recur in 25% of cases; however, some motion in flexion is gained (Swanson 1972).

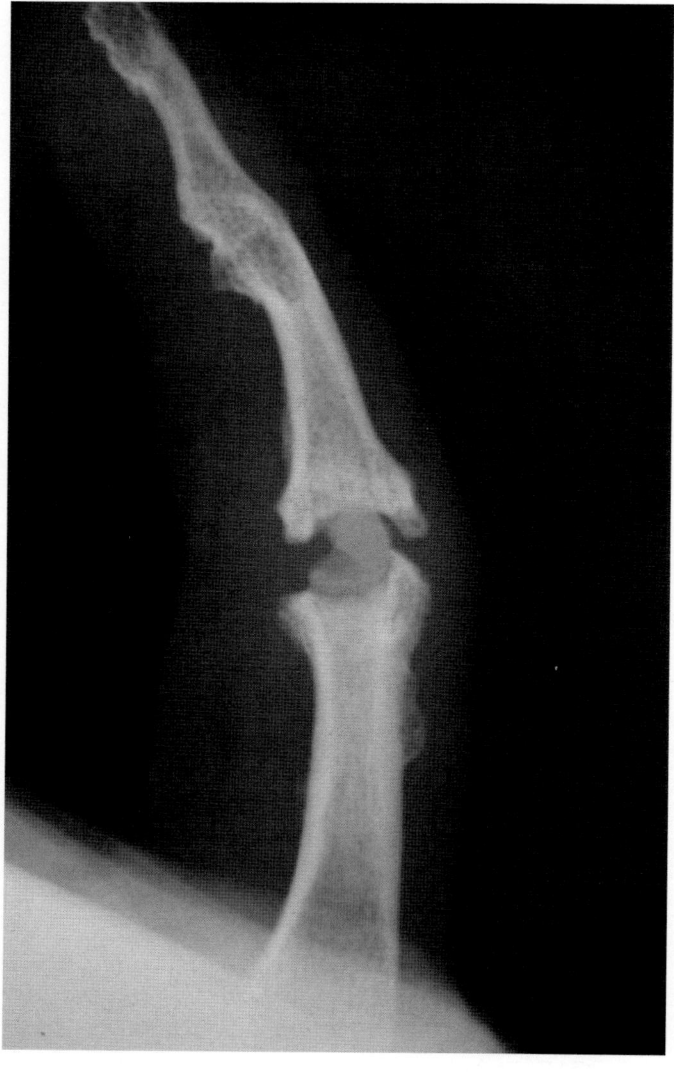

Figure 35.16
Radiographic aspect of a PIP joint Swanson implant at 2 years: progressive sinking of the implant into the bone on either side.

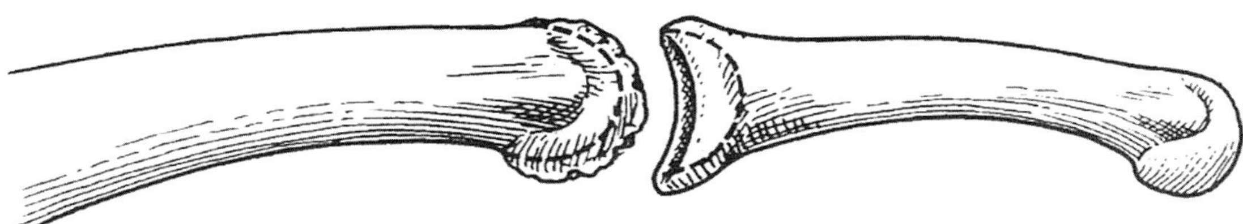

Figure 35.17
Ball and socket technique for PIP joint arthrodesis.

When there is a boutonnière deformity, surgery usually results in a displacement of the arc of motion towards extension, with no significant improvement in the range of motion (Swanson et al 1985a, Ferlic 1989).

Long-term results evolve towards a progressive reduction in the range of motion of the PIP joint, with a 30% loss after 2–3 years. The radiographic aspect evolves towards cortical eroding of the bone adjacent to the hinge, and progressive embedding of the implant (Figure 35.16).

Fractures of the implants have been reported, with rates similar to those for MP joints.

In 1986, Peimer and Medige reported 18 cases of reactive synovitis in patients with a silicone implant in the hand or wrist, including 4 PIP implants; but none of them except for one, were young and active patients without rheumatoid arthritis. Indeed, it seems that this complication is much less frequent in rheumatoid patients who have a lower demand, and limited motion.

Ulnar deviation should be anticipated if the attenuated radial collateral ligaments were not augmented at the time of surgery. This is particularly a risk in radial fingers because of the repeated lateral strain exerted by the thumb during pinch.

Indications

See below, indications for PIP joint arthrodesis.

PIP joint arthrodesis

Surgical technique

The optimal approach for PIP joint arthrodesis is dorsal, as it provides a clear view of all structures, and the clinician does not have to worry about weakening the extensor central tendon.

After division of the collateral ligaments and dislocation of the joint, a complete synovectomy is performed, with removal of all bone spurs. The proximal phalangeal head is shortened as required, depending on joint stiff-

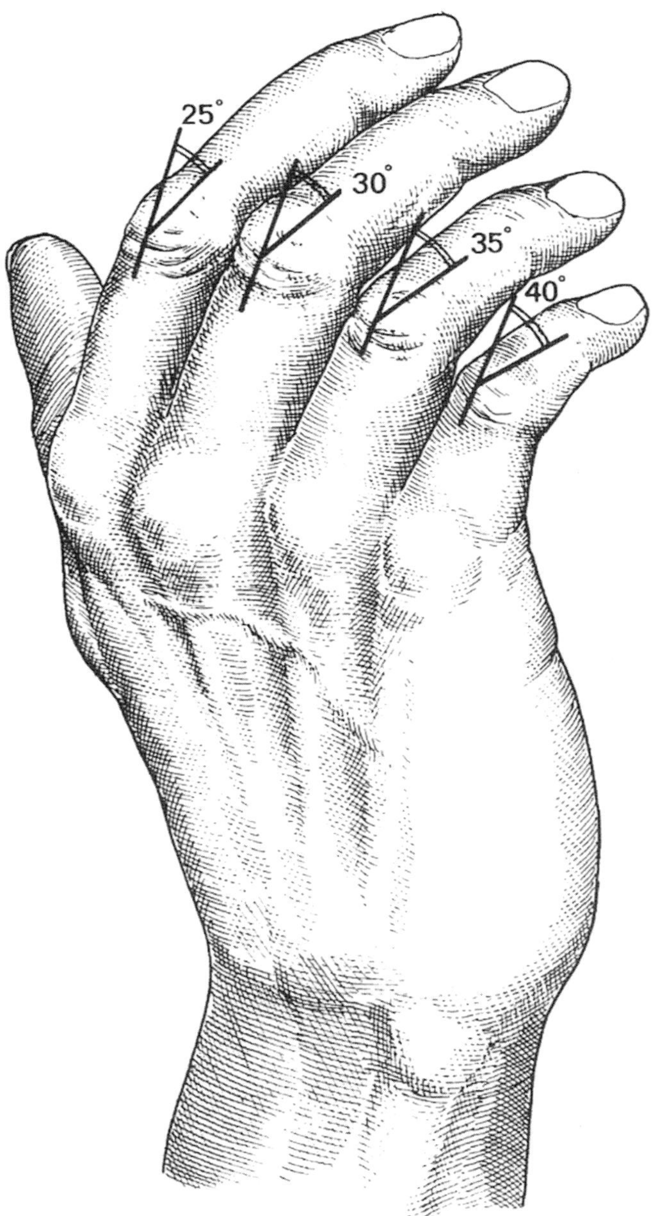

Figure 35.18
Positioning of PIP joint arthrodesis in each finger.

ness, and the middle phalangeal cartilage is removed. In rheumatoid patients it is difficult to create two flat surfaces with the perfect angle, and it is usually more appropriate to create a ball and socket type of joint in these patients (Tubiana 1985) (Figure 35.17).

The functional position of immobilization varies according to the finger, from 25° flexion for the index finger to 40° for the little finger (Figure 35.18). However, this may depend on other factors, such as the status of adjacent joints.

Various methods of fixation have been described: for example, K-wires (Figure 35.19), screws, staples and tension band wiring (Fig 35.20). Jones and Stern (1994) state that most of the methods produce satisfactory results as long as there is careful preparation and close opposition of the cancellous surfaces, but Leibovic and Strickland (1994) found a significantly higher number of non-unions with Kirschner wires than with Herbert screws or tension band in rheumatoid patients.

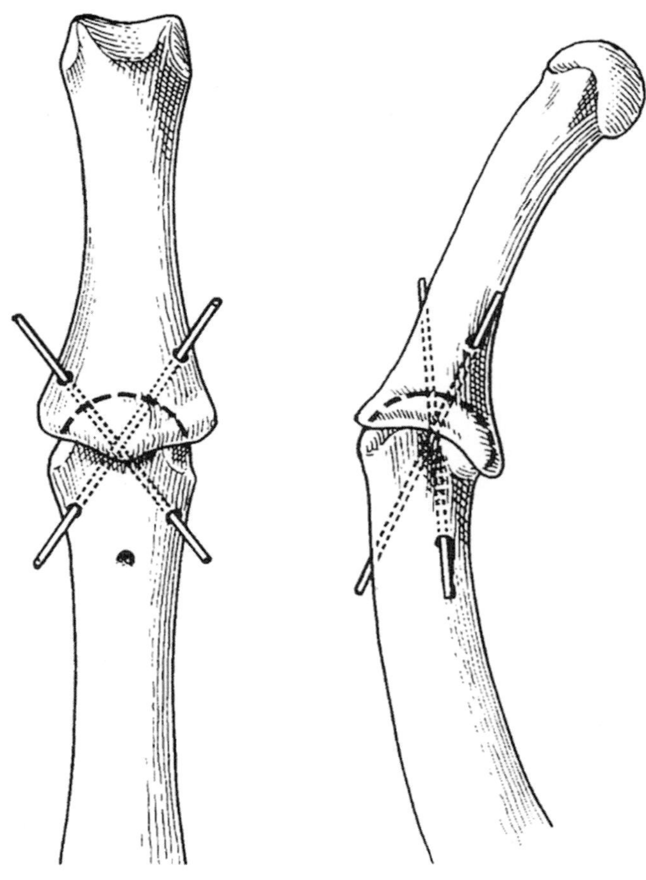

Figure 35.19
Fixation of arthrodesis with crossed K-wires.

Results

PIP joint arthrodesis is not as easy a procedure as it may seem, especially in the rheumatoid patient where the bone stock is scarce and fragile. Positioning the joint at the proper angle may prove difficult in view of deformities of adjacent fingers. The most bothersome complication in that respect is positioning the joint in lateral deviation, which produces overlapping of the fingers in flexion.

Bone fusion may take longer in rheumatoid patients, but overall the rate of non-unions remains low (Granowitz and Vainio 1966).

Indications

Arthroplasty and arthrodesis of the PIP joint are not indicated before joint arthritis reaches the stage of Larsen III degenerative changes. Respective indications for each of these two procedures depend upon a number of factors:

- The finger involved. Arthrodesis is usually preferred for the index and long fingers, because they require lateral stability, whereas arthroplasty is more indicated for the ring and little fingers, which require some flexion for hand grip.
- Adjacent joints. If the adjacent MP joint requires an arthroplasty, then an arthrodesis will be preferred at the PIP joint level.
- Peri-articular structures. An arthrodesis is more indicated if the collateral ligaments, especially the radial ligaments, are severely attenuated, or if the joint is stiff in severe flexion (i.e. boutonnière deformity).

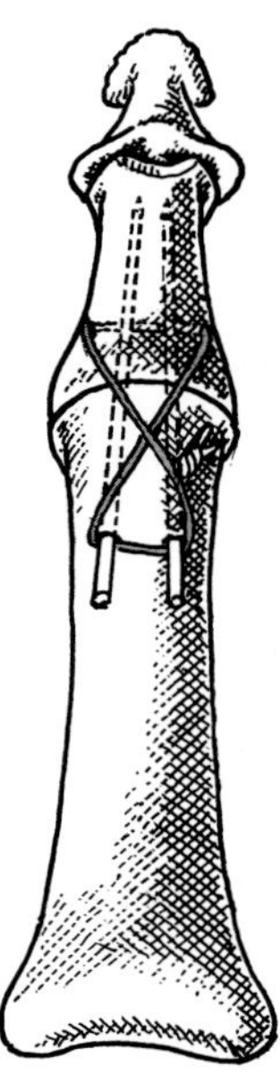

Figure 35.20
Tension band procedure: this produces compression at the arthrodesis site.

- Flexor tendons. Rupture of the flexor tendons of the involved finger contraindicate an arthroplasty, but flexor synovitis does not, although it will necessitate simultaneous treatment.

References

Aptekar RG, Davie JM, Cattell HS (1974) Foreign body reaction to silicone rubber. Complication of a finger joint implant, *Clin Orthop* **98**: 231–2.

Bass RL, Stern PJ, Nairus J (1996) High implant fracture incidence with Sutter silicone metacarpophalangeal joint arthroplasty, *J Hand Surg [Am]* **64**: 813–18.

Beckenbaugh RD (1999) The development of an implant for the metacarpophalangeal joint of the fingers, *Acta Orthop Scand* **70**: 107–8.

Bieber EJ, Weiland AJ, Volenec-Dowling S (1986) Silicone-rubber implant arthroplasty of the metacarpophalangeal joints for rheumatoid arthritis, *J Bone Joint Surg [Am]* **68**: 206–9.

Blair WF, Shurr DG, Buckwalter JA (1984) Metacarpophalangeal joint implant arthroplasty with a Silastic spacer, *J Bone Joint Surg Am* **66**: 365–70.

Condamine JL, Benoit JY, Comtet JJ, Aubriot JH (1988) Proposed digital arthroplasty critical study of the preliminary results, *Ann Chir Main* **7**: 282–97.

Egloff D (2000) Flexible silicone implant arthroplasties. In: Simmen B, Allieu Y et al, eds, *Hand Arthroplasties* (Martin Dunitz: London) 295–300.

Ferlic DC (1989) Boutonnière deformity in rheumatoid arthritis, *Hand Clin* **5**: 215–22.

Flatt AE (1961) Restoration of rheumatoid arthritis finger joint function: interim report on trial of prosthetic replacement, *J Bone Joint Surg [Am]* **43**: 753–74.

Foliart D (1995) Swanson silicone finger joint implants: a review of the literature regarding long-term complications, *J Hand Surg [Am]* **20A**: 1.

Gellman H, Stetson W, Brumfield RH Jr, Costigan W, Kuschner SH (1997) Silastic metacarpophalangeal joint arthroplasty in patients with rheumatoid arthritis, *Clin Orthop* **342**: 16–21.

Granowitz S, Vainio K (1966) Proximal interphalangeal arthrodesis in rheumatoid arthritis, *Acta Orthop Scand* **37**: 301–10.

Groff GD, Schned AR, Taylor TH (1981) Silicone-induced adenopathy eight years after metacarpophalangeal arthroplasty, *Arthritis Rheum* **24**: 1578–81.

Hansraj KK, Ashworth CR, Ebramzadeh E et al (1997) Swanson metacarpophalangeal joint arthroplasty in patients with rheumatoid arthritis, *Clin Orthop* **342**: 11–15.

Jones BF, Stern PJ (1994) Interphalangeal arthrodesis, *Hand Clin* **10**: 267–75.

Kay A, Jeffs J, Scott J (1978) Experience with silastic prostheses in the rheumatoid hand, *Ann Rheum Dis* **37**: 255–8.

Kirschenbaum D, Schneider LH, Adams DC, Cody RP (1993) Arthroplasty of the metacarpophalangeal joints with use of silicone-rubber implants in patients who have rheumatoid arthritis. Long-term results, *J Bone Joint Surg [Am]* **75**: 3–12.

Leibovic SJ, Strickland JW (1994) Arthrodesis of the proximal interphalangeal joint of the finger: comparison of the use of the Herbert screw with other fixation methods, *J Hand Surg [Am]* **19**: 181–8.

Linscheid RL, Dobyns JH, Beckenbaugh RD, Cooney WP 3rd (1979) Proximal interphalangeal joint arthroplasty with a total joint design, *Mayo Clin Proc* **54**: 227.

Millender LH, Nalebuff EA (1973) Metacarpophalangeal joint arthroplasty utilizing the silicone rubber prosthesis, *Orthop Clin North Am* **4**: 349–71.

Millender LH, et al (1975) Analysis of infections after silicone rubber prosthesis in the hand, *J Bone Joint Surg [Am]* **57**: 724.

Millender LH, Nalebuff EA, Hawkins RB, Ennis R (1975) Infection after silicone prosthetic arthroplasty in the hand, *J Bone Joint Surg Am* **57**: 825–9.

Moller K, Sollerman C, Geijer M, Branemark PI (1999) Osseointegrated silicone implants. 18 patients with 57 MCP joints followed for 2 years, *Acta Orthop Scand* **70**: 109–15.

Nalebuff EA (1984) The rheumatoid hand. Reflections on metacarpophalangeal arthroplasty, *Clin Orthop* **182**: 150–9.

Nalebuff EA (1999) The rheumatoid hand. In: Tubiana R, ed, *The Hand*, vol 5 (Saunders: Philadelphia) 258–68.

Oster LH, Blair WF, Steggers CM (1989) Crossed intrinsic transfers, *J Hand Surg* **6**: 963–71.

Peimer CA, Medige J (1986) Reactive synovitis after silicone arthroplasty, *J Hand Surg [Am]* **11**: 624–38.

Swanson A (1968) Silicone rubber implants for replacement of arthritic or destroyed joints in the hand, *Surg Clin North Am* **48**: 113–27.

Swanson AB (1972) Flexible implant arthroplasty for arthritic finger joints: rationale, technique, and results of treatment, *J Bone Joint Surg [Am]* **54**: 435–55.

Swanson AB, de Groot Swanson G (1984) Flexible implant arthroplasty in the rheumatoid metacarpophalangeal joint, *Clin Rheum Dis* **10**: 609–29.

Swanson AB, Maupin BK, Gajjar NV, Swanson GD (1985a) Flexible implant arthroplasty in the proximal interphalangeal joint of the hand, *J Hand Surg [Am]* **10**: 796–805.

Swanson AB, de Groot Swanson G (1985b) Flexible implant arthroplasty in the upper extremity. In: Tubiana R, ed, *The Hand*, vol 2 (Saunders: Philadelphia) 576–620.

Swanson AB, Poitevin LA, de Groot Swanson G, Kearney J (1986) Bone remodeling phenomena in flexible implant arthroplasty in the metacarpophalangeal joints. Long term study, *Clin Orthop* **205**: 254–67.

Swanson AB, de Groot Swanson G, Ishikawa H (1997) Use of grommets for flexible implant resection arthroplasty of the metacarpophalangeal joint, *Clin Orthop* **342**: 22–33.

Tubiana R (1985) Arthrodesis of the fingers. In: Tubiana R, ed, *The Hand*, vol 2 (Saunders: Philadelphia) 698–702.

Tubiana R (1999) Rheumatoid arthritis. In: Tubiana R, Gilbert A, Masquelet AC, eds, *Atlas of Surgical Techniques of the Hand and Wrist* (Martin Dunitz: London) 377–445.

Wilson YG, Sykes PJ, Niranjan NS (1993) Long-term follow-up of Swanson's silastic arthroplasty of the metacarpophalangeal joint in rheumatoid arthritis, *J Hand Surg [Br]* **18**: 81–91.

36 Treatment of rheumatoid finger deformities

R Tubiana

Rheumatoid arthritis is the source of frequent finger deformities. The basic pathology is hypertrophy of synovium. Within the joint, it stretches the supporting structures, invades the subchondral bone and destroys the articular surfaces. On tendons, it forms nodules that are invasive and lead to a tendon rupture.

Different patterns of deformities are possible. When the extensor mechanism of a finger joint is involved, the joint assumes a flexed position; when the volar plate is stretched, the joint will hyperextend.

In a digital osteo-articular chain, any deformity at one joint will cause tendino-muscular imbalance and results in deformities in the adjacent joints (Tubiana 1969).

A better understanding of the mechanism of finger deformities, described in a preceding chapter (see Chapter 31 Rheumatoid arthritis) will help in the indications for an appropriate treatment. However, one must remember that rheumatoid arthritis is an ongoing process and progressive disease may deteriorate the benefits of surgery.

The four most common finger deformities are ulnar lateral deviation at the metacarpophalangeal (MP) level, swan-neck and boutonnière at the proximal interphalangeal (PIP) level, and mallet finger at the distal interphalangeal (DIP) joint. None of these deformities is specific to rheumatoid arthritis, and they have already been described in Chapter 33 (Late reconstruction of the extensor tendons). The treatment is in many ways similar to that for traumatic deformities of the fingers. However, they differ on two essential points: there is much less scar tissue in rheumatoid deformities, and tendons and articular surfaces are very often invaded by rheumatoid synovitis. The main differences between a traumatic and a rheumatoid deformity are the importance of scarring in traumatic cases and the progressive evolution of rheumatoid arthritis. According to the initial lesion of the rheumatoid arthritis in the three finger joints, different deformities may coexist in neighbouring fingers of the same hand (Figure 36.1). The existence of rheumatoid lesions makes a medical treatment of rheumatoid arthritis imperative. Great strides have been made in the medical treatment of rheumatoid arthritis and in the prevention of finger deformities.

We have adopted a common four-stage classification in the evolution of the lesions for all three finger deformities (see Chapter 2).

Ulnar deviation

Ulnar deviation of the fingers is so common in rheumatoid patients that it is often considered synonymous with rheumatoid arthritis. However, it is also seen in other conditions such as arthrogryposis, polio and Parkinson's disease.

In fact, there is a normal ulnar inclination of the fingers at the MP joints, due to a number of anatomical factors, which have already been described in the chapter on pathogenesis of finger deformities. These factors have different consequences in each finger: the inclination is most marked in the index finger, less in the middle and little fingers, and almost non-existent in the ring finger. The ulnar inclination is normally limited by the capsulo-ligamentous resistance and by the action of the interosseous muscles.

In rheumatoid arthritis the weakness of these stabilizing elements allows the ulnar inclination to be accentuated, resulting in pathological ulnar deviation.

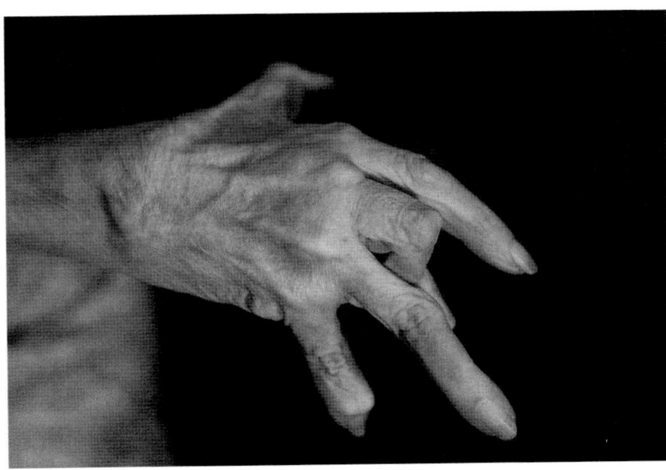

Figure 36.1

Different finger deformities may occur on the same hand. Here, there are a boutonnière on the middle finger, a swan-neck on the thumb and a mallet finger on the little finger.

Treatment of rheumatoid ulnar deviation

It is necessary to treat both the rheumatoid lesions and the MP deformity. In many patients, ulnar deviation of the fingers is associated with a radial deviation of the wrist (see Figure 2.41). The persistence of a radial wrist deviation will cause the recurrence of the MP ulnar deviation.

Correction at the wrist level should precede the MP correction.

Synovectomy of the MP joint must always be associated with the treatment of the deformity. We use the four-stage classification as a guide to the indications for treatment.

Stage 1: No limitation of passive motion in any finger joint

The deviation is passively reducible. The articular surfaces are normal. There is no deformity of the PIP joint. Surgery is rarely indicated at this stage.

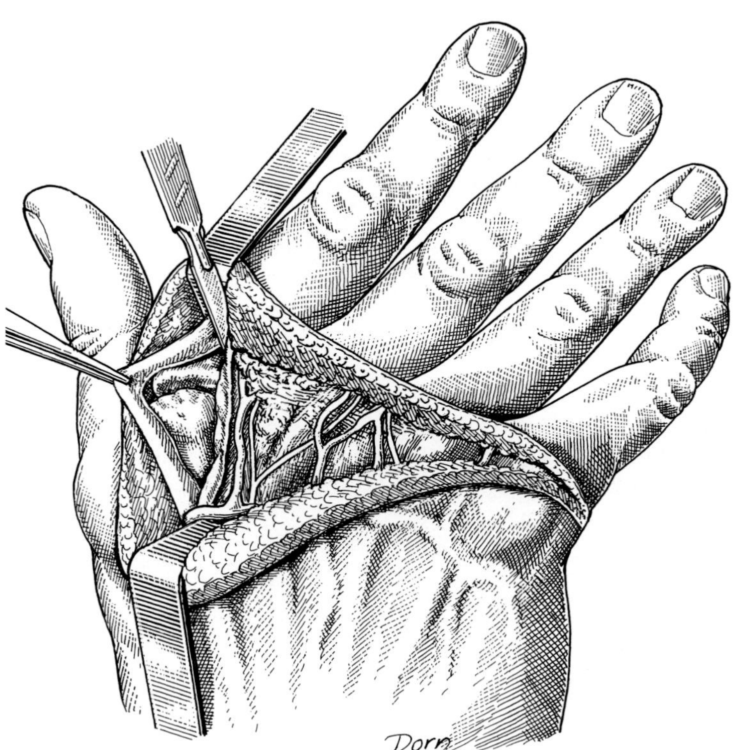

Figure 36.2

MP joint synovectomy. On the dorsal aspect of the MP joint of the middle finger, the extensor tendon is subluxated on the ulnar side. The extensor mechanism is exposed. The proliferating synovium has herniated dorsally on the radial side of the tendon. On the index, a longitudinal incision is made in the ulnar-side sagittal band. The capsule is opened and synovectomy performed

A local treatment of injections of steroid derivatives may be repeated two or three times. Injections of chemical or radioactive substances (erbium 162) have been used in some rheumatoid centres.

In case of repeated recurrences a surgical synovectomy may be indicated. However, indications for synovectomy alone are limited because they also have a high incidence of recurrences.

MP joint synovectomy

A transverse undulating incision over the dorsum of the metacarpal heads is performed when multiple MP joints are involved. A longitudinal incision is used when synovectomy is performed on a single finger. Care is taken to preserve the dorsal veins and nerves located within fat pads in the interdigital spaces. The extensor mechanism is exposed. The extensor tendon is usually subluxated on the ulnar side of the joint. The extensor tendon is mobilized by incising the extensor hood on the ulnar side.

The extensor mechanism is carefully separated from the underlying capsule, often disrupted by the rheumatoid synovitis. The extensor tendon is retracted radially. We try not to divide too distally the extensor hood, so that the flexion of the joint will not be weakened.

The joint capsule is incised longitudinally. Synovitis is excised. The recess under the collateral ligaments is cleaned with a small curette. Traction applied to the finger will allow partial volar synovectomy (Figure 36.2).

The dorsal capsule may be left open. The radial fibres of the extensor hood are reefed to realign the tendon over the middle of the joint.

Stage 2: Limitation of motion in one joint is influenced by the position of another joint

Ulnar deviation of the finger may increase traction of the subluxated extensor tendon on the base of the middle phalanx and produce a swan-neck deformity (Figure 36.3).

Surgical correction is indicated before the deformity becomes fixed. The extensor tendon should be realigned over the middle of the MP joint. In patients without MP joint subluxation, resection of the oblique fibres of the interosseous hood at the level of the proximal phalanx, as described by Littler (1954), restores flexion of the distal phalanges when the proximal phalanx is held in extension (see Figure 2.36).

Stage 3: Fixed ulnar deviation; articular surfaces intact

A soft tissue release is performed in conjunction with MP joint synovectomy and often with an MP joint arthroplasty. The resection of the metacarpal head will help in reducing the intrinsic muscle tightness.

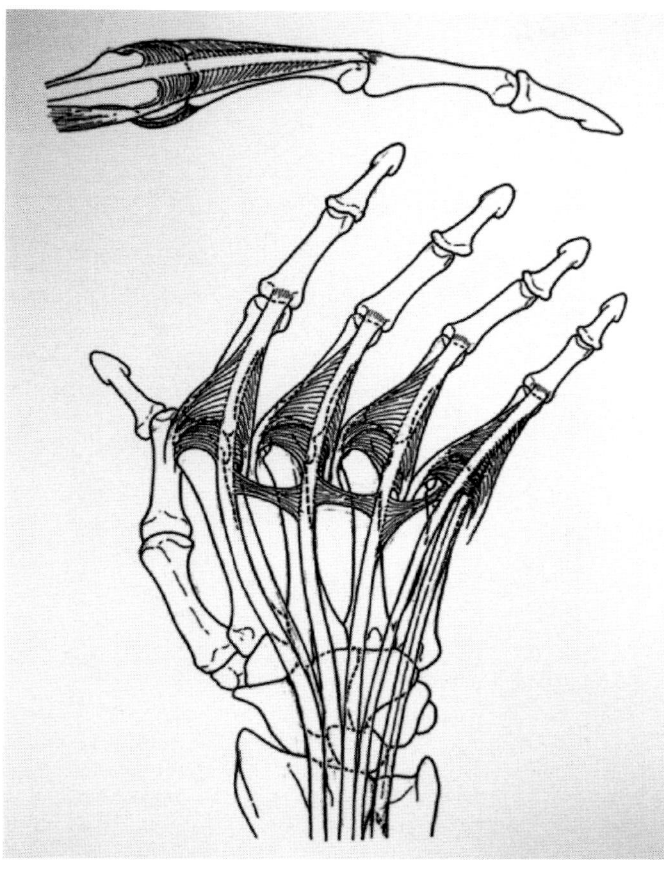

Figure 36.3
Ulnar deviation of the fingers increases traction of the subluxated extensor tendons on the base of the middle phalanges.

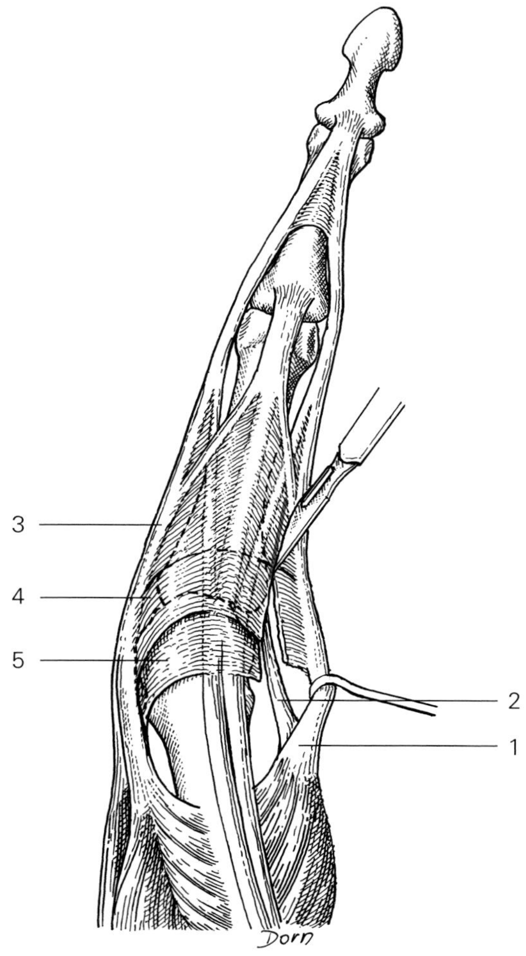

Figure 36.4
Intrinsic release.
1 Ulnar intrinsic tendon
2 Bony attachment of the intrinsic tendon
3 Oblique fibres of the hood
4 Transverse fibres of the interosseous hood
5 Sagittal band

Soft tissue release

The entire ulnar side of the extensor mechanism is exposed. The different structures are divided one after the other, step by step; first the ulnar-side sagittal band, then the transverse and oblique fibres of the extensor hood (Figure 36.4). It must not be forgotten that the intrinsic musdes are the primary flexors of the MP joint and it is important to preserve them when possible.

If necessary, the ulnar intrinsic tendon is pulled up into the wound with a blunt hook, and sectioned at the myotendinous junction for persistent flexion contracture (Figure 36.5). The bony attachment of the intrinsic tendon may be divided as well. However, because the ulnar intrinsic muscles of the index finger normally apply a supinatory force to this digit, they may be preserved, to avoid a postoperative pronation whenever possible (Swanson 1973).

In the little finger, the abductor digiti minimi (ADM) tendon is always exposed on the ulnar aspect of the fifth MP joint, with a blunt hook. The dorsal branch of the digital nerve and the ulnar neurovascular bundle are protected. Only the ADM tendon is sectioned. The flexor digiti minimi (FDM) tendon is preserved because it is an important flexor of this joint (Flatt 1983).

In addition to the intrinsic release, Straub (1960) recommends a cross-intrinsic transfer to prevent recurrent ulnar drift. The intrinsics released from the ulnar side of the index, long and ring fingers are transferred to the radial aspect of the adjacent fingers. We have no experience of this procedure.

Stage 4: Luxation of the MP joint (Figure 36.6)

MP joint arthroplasty is indicated, especially when there is a marked flexion deformity of the MP joints.

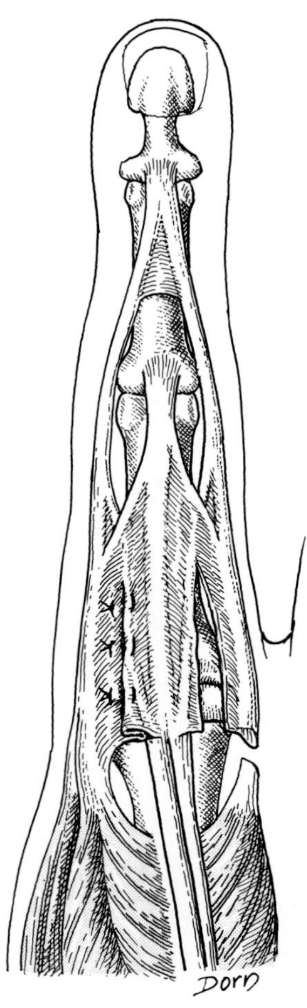

Figure 36.5

Realignment of the extensor tendon. The radial fibres of the hood are reefed, and eventually the ulnar intrinsic tendons divided, to realign the extensor tendon.

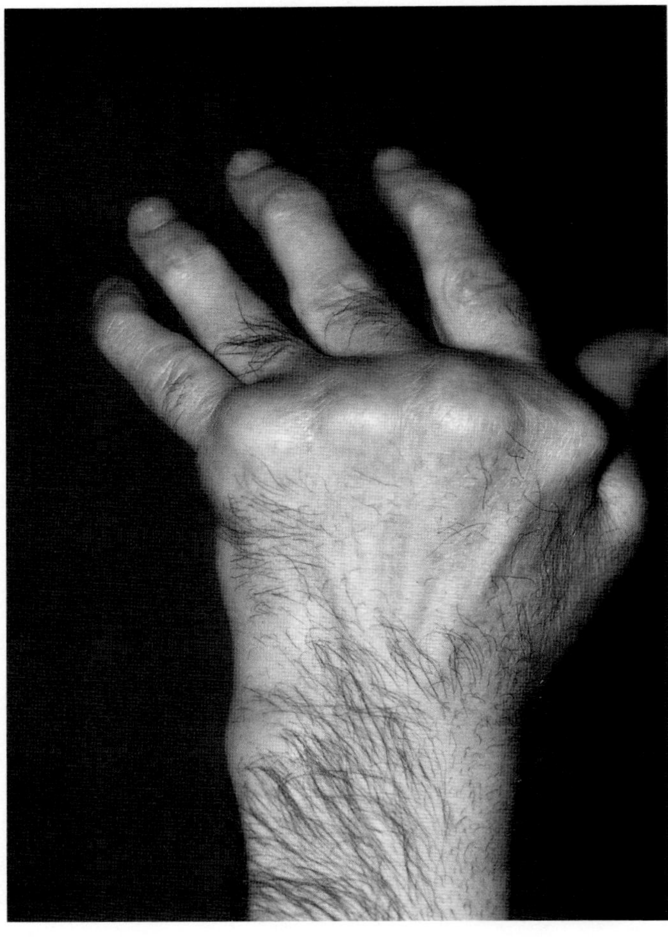

Figure 36.6

Rheumatoid hand with luxation of the MP joints and ulnar deviation of the fingers.

Many MP joint arthroplasty techniques have been proposed. The most commonly used procedure is the Swanson silicone implant (Figure 36.7) (Swanson 1968).

Rheumatoid swan-neck deformity

The swan-neck deformity is caused by excessive traction on the extensor apparatus inserted on the base of the middle phalanx, especially if the PIP joint is lax. Hyperextension of the middle phalanx is combined with flexion of the distal phalanx (Figure 36.8).

Swan-neck deformity represents the end result of muscular imbalance caused by rheumatoid lesions at different sites (see Chapter 3 on Pathogenesis of swan-neck): at the MP joint (articular synovitis with volar subluxation of the proximal phalanx, intrinsic muscle contracture); at the PIP joint (rupture of the volar plate, flexor tendon synovitis, rupture of the flexor digitorum superficialis (FDS) tendon); at the DIP (mallet deformity); or even at the wrist joint (a flexion contracture may cause excessive traction on the extensor digitorum communis (EDC) tendons).

It is necessary to treat the rheumatoid lesions responsible for the deformity at their different levels, and it is also necessary to treat the deformity (Nalebuff 1989).

The functional disturbance associated with this deformity is related to the loss of flexibility at the PIP joint, therefore, it is important to treat swan-neck deformity at an early stage to prevent stiffness of the PIP joint in extension.

Corrective splinting and exercises are used at all stages, alone or in conjunction with surgery. Many surgical procedures have been proposed. They should be

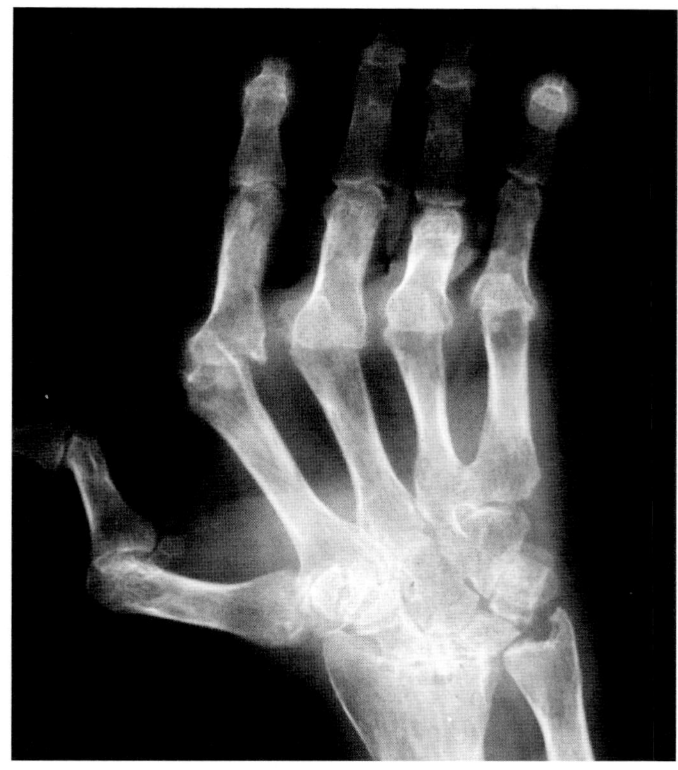

(A)

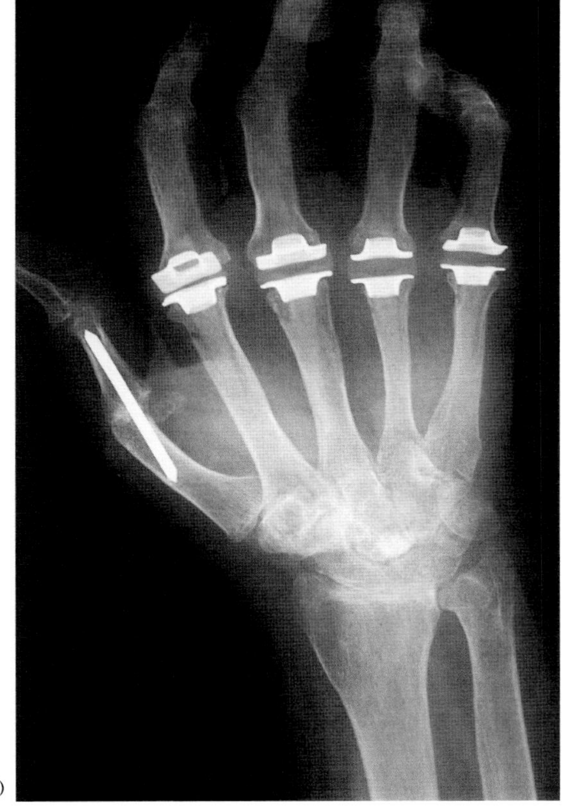

(B)

Figure 36.7

MP joint arthroplasties with Swanson's silicone implants and grommets. (A) Preoperative view. (B) MP finger joint arthroplasties and MP thumb fusion.

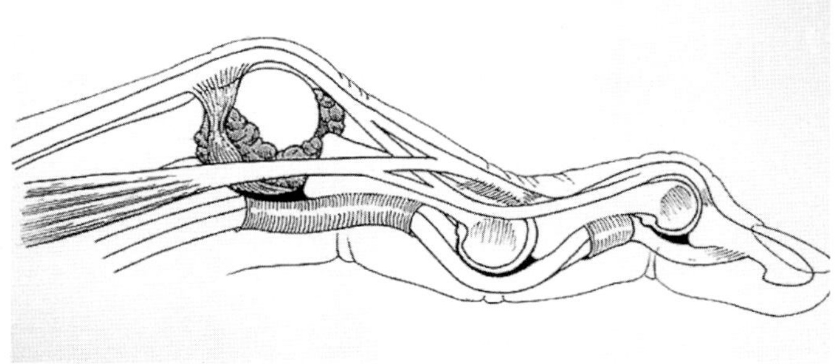

Figure 36.8

Rheumatoid swan-neck deformity. One of the most common causes of rheumatoid swan-neck deformity is MP joint synovitis.

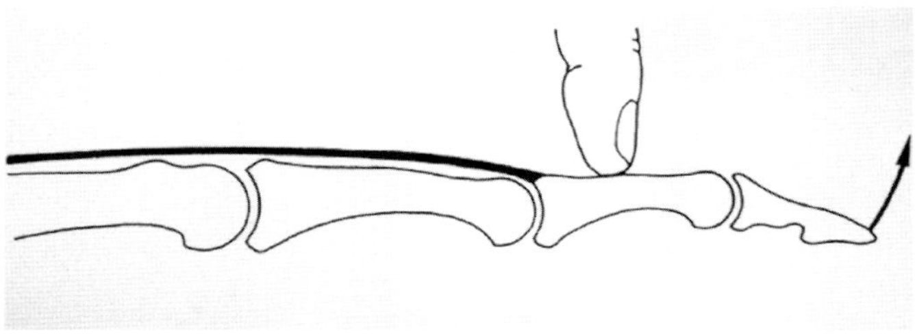

Figure 36.9

Swan-neck deformity, stage 1. If PIP joint hyperextension is prevented, DIP joint flexion is corrected.

carefully selected and the classification in four stages will help, as a guide.

Stage 1

There is no limitation of passive motion in any finger joint (limitation of active PIP flexion would be in favour of a flexor tendon synovitis).

The treatment is aimed at correcting the dynamic imbalance at the two interphalangeal joints. If PIP joint hyperextension is prevented, DIP joint flexion is corrected (Figure 36.9).

Several procedures have been used to correct PIP joint hyperextension in rheumatoid swan-neck deformity. In all cases synovitis of the flexor tendon is treated first.

Tenotomy of the central extensor tendon

This tenotomy (Fowler 1949), rarely performed, is theoretically the most physiological procedure to re-establish an equilibrium between the extensor's forces.

The tenotomy of the central extensor tendon at the distal extremity of the proximal phalanx will result in a diminution of tension at the PIP joint. The risk of creating a reverse deformity, the boutonnière deformity, is avoided if the other fibrous structures maintaining the two lateral extensor tendons in dorsal position at the level of the PIP joint are preserved, i.e. the spiral fibres and the transverse retinacular ligament (see Figure 2.15).

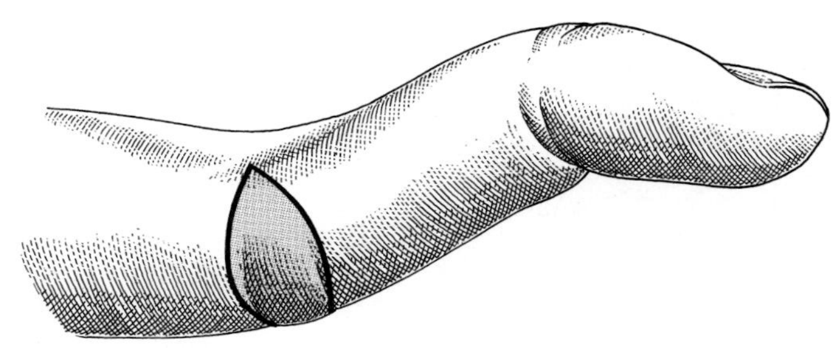

Figure 36.10
Dermadesis.

Dermadesis

An elliptical wedge of skin is removed from the volar aspect of the PIP joint (Figure 36.10). The subcutaneous venous network should be preserved. Care is taken not to open the underlying flexor tendon sheath. The skin defect is closed with the PIP joint in at least 25° of flexion. This is the simplest procedure, but recurrences of joint hyperextension are frequent and dermadesis is usually carried out in conjunction with other procedures.

In flexor superficialis tenodesis, one slip of the FDS is divided 2 cm proximal to the PIP joint, but is left attached distally (Figure 36.11). This slip will act as a check-rein against extension. The proximal attachment can be made at the flexor tendon sheath. An attachment into the bone is much stronger and is indicated on spastic hands.

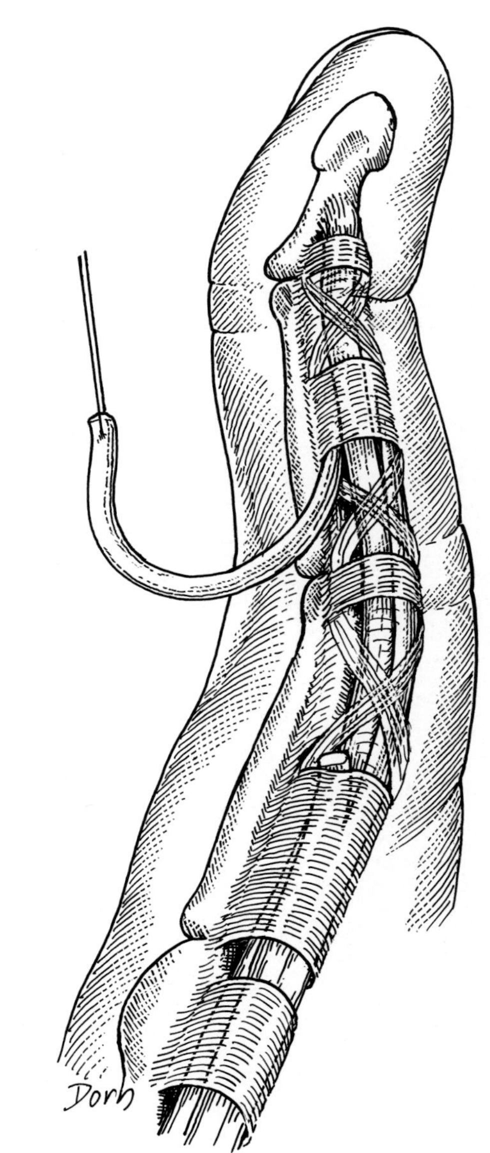

Figure 36.11
Flexor superficialis tenodesis. The FDS slip is detached proximally to the PIP joint, then reattached at the flexor tendon sheath or into the distal extremity of the proximal phalanx, with the PIP joint in 20° of flexion.

Stage 2

The three finger joints have a complete passive mobility; however, one joint has a limitation of motion influenced by the position of another joint. The chapter on 'Late extensor apparatus reconstruction' has already described the two mechanisms responsible for the deformity: oblique retinacular ligament release and interosseous muscle contracture. These lesions can be seen in rheumatoid hands.

Distal joint fusion in extension is particularly indicated when the mallet deformity is primary and is associated with a swan-neck.

Oblique retinacular ligament reconstruction

Two ingenious techniques are proposed to prevent hyperextension of the PIP joint, while extending the distal joint: Littler's oblique retinacular ligament reconstruction (Littler and Eaton 1967) and Zancolli's lateral extensor tendon translocation (Zancolli, personal communication, 1986).

Littler and Eaton (1967) described the reconstruction of an oblique retinacular ligament using the ulnar lateral extensor tendon divided at the musculotendinous junction at the base of the proximal phalanx and rerouting volar to Cleland's ligament at the PIP joint. Several procedures have been successively described (see Figure 2.33).

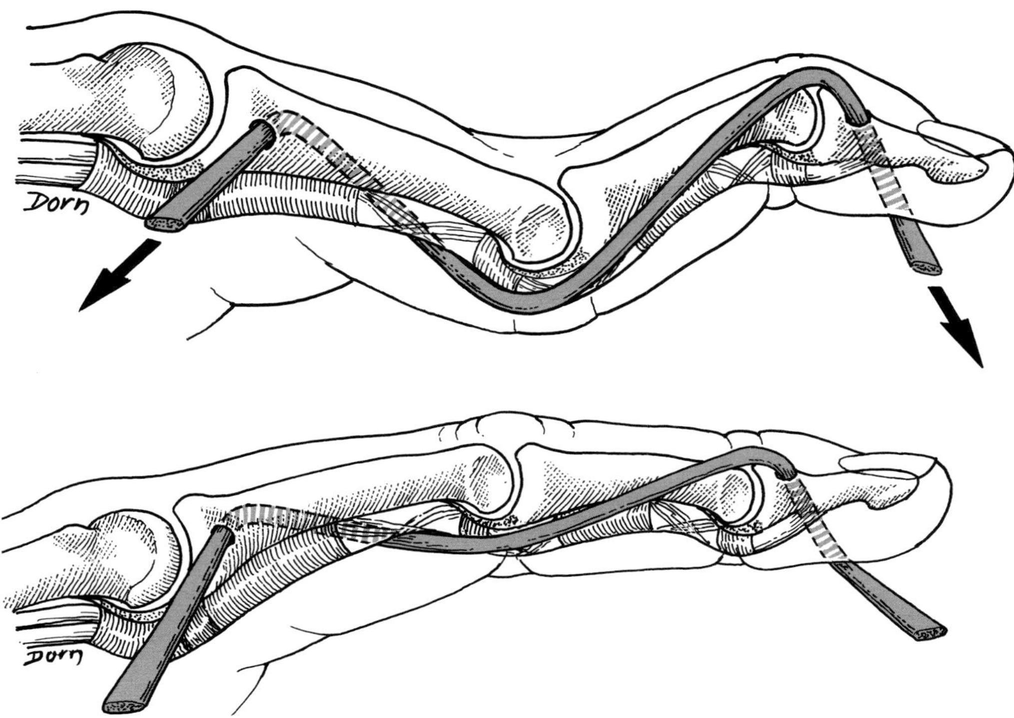

Figure 36.12
Spiral oblique retinacular ligament reconstruction.

For a more secure repair of a rheumatoid swan-neck deformity with extensor tendons of poor quality, it seems preferable to use a slender tendon graft (Figure 36.12) to construct an anterior spiral check-rein. Both extremities of the graft transfix the skeleton (Thomson et al 1978).

Zancolli (1986) liberates the lateral extensor tendon on the radial side of the finger. This tendon is then subluxated volarly in front of the volar plate of the PIP joint and is maintained in this position by fixation of the volar plate to the FDS tendon, distally in relation to the joint (Figure 36.13).

Intrinsic tightness

Intrinsic tightness restricts PIP joint flexion with the MP joint extended or radially deviated. Intrinsic tightness is more often seen in patients with an MP joint subluxation; the PIP joint hyperextension is secondary (Figure 36.14). However, intrinsic tightness can also be seen in rheumatoid patients with swan-neck deformity without MP joint deformity. The Bunnell–Finochietto test indicates the intrinsic muscle contracture (see Figure

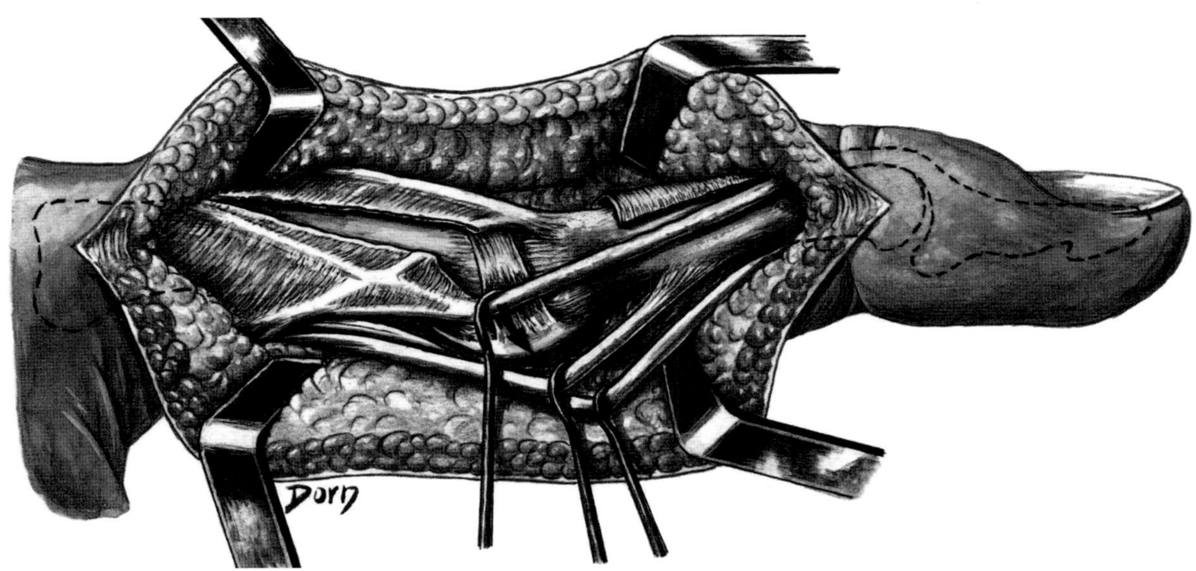

Figure 36.13
Zancolli's translocation of the lateral extensor tendon.

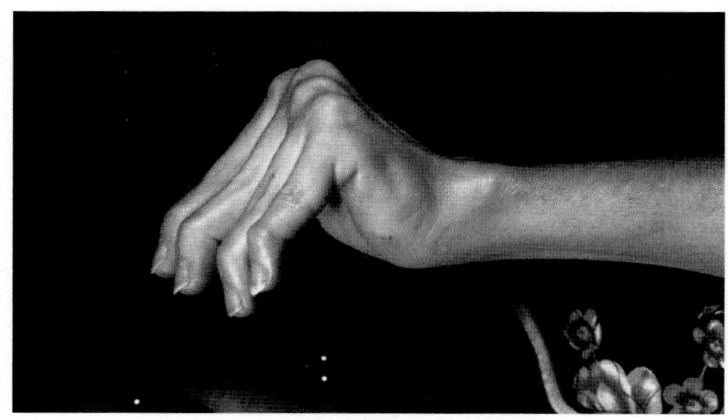

Figure 36.14
Swan-neck deformity with MP joint subluxation and intrinsic tightness.

2.35). In patients with swan-neck and associated MP joint deformity, a metacarpal joint arthroplasty with resection of the metacarpal head will lengthen the intrinsic muscles and an ulnar intrinsic muscle release will reduce the risk of recurrence of tightness.

In patients without MP joint subluxation, resection of the oblique fibres of the interosseous hood at the level of the proximal phalanx, as described by Littler (1954), restores flexion of the distal phalanges when the proximal phalanx is held in extension (see Figures 2.35 and 2.36).

Stage 3

There is joint stiffness at this stage, articular surfaces are intact on X-rays. There is permanent limitation of joint motion. In the rheumatoid swan-neck deformity, the PIP articular surfaces are preserved for a longer time than in a rheumatoid boutonnière deformity because the joint is usually not directly involved by the synovitis.

PIP joint manipulation

Nalebuff (1998) has shown that it is often possible to gently manipulate the PIP joint into flexion. If the joint is flexed and splinted in flexion, the tight soft tissues will stretch.

A limiting factor to passive correction is usually the skin. This limitation has been overcome by making an associated skin oblique relaxing incision just distal to the PIP joint (see Figure 2.40). The skin release is left open and will close in 3 weeks.

Soft tissue release

When the deformity cannot be corrected by manipulation, one should proceed to a soft tissue release with tenolysis of the extensor apparatus and mobilization of the lateral extensor tendons from the central tendon in order to recover their normal volar shift. Then gentle manipulation into flexion often achieves functional flexion of the PIP joint (see Figure 2.39). It is rarely necessary to release the collateral ligaments or to lengthen the central tendon. An exploration and assessment of the flexor tendons may be made through a palmar incision to ensure that their excursion is normal.

The use of soft tissue release is often associated with MP joint arthroplasty. This procedure is necessary if there is subluxation of the base of the proximal phalanx, to prevent a recurrence of the swan-neck deformity. In these patients the PIP joint is held in flexion by a K-wire. This allows the postoperative exercises to concentrate on MP and DIP joint flexion. The K-wire is removed after 4 weeks. A long careful follow-up with a splinting and exercise programme is necessary to avoid recurrence of the deformity.

Stage 4

There is joint stiffness with intra-articular alterations at this stage. In these patients, a salvage procedure is needed: arthroplasty or arthrodesis. The choice between these two procedures is influenced by the finger involved, the status of the adjacent joints and the flexor tendons.

PIP joint arthroplasty

A PIP joint arthroplasty is preferable, particularly for the ring and little fingers if the adjacent joints and tendons are in good condition. We prefer an ulnar lateral approach that respects the lateral collateral ligament for a swan-neck PIP arthroplasty (Figure 36.15). A longitudinal incision is made within the lateral extensor tendon at its inferior margin. The transverse retinacular ligament along with the inferior margin of the lateral extensor tendon is reflected volarwards. This will facilitate the closure. The periosteum of the proximal and middle phalanges is in continuity with the volar plate and may be elevated together from the volar aspect of these phalanges (Saffar 1997).

PIP arthrodesis

A PIP joint arthrodesis may be preferable in the index and middle fingers because lateral stability is more important in these digits. We also favour PIP joint fusion if the MP joints require arthroplasty and when the tendons are in poor condition. The degree of flexion increases toward the little finger and varies from 20° to 40°.

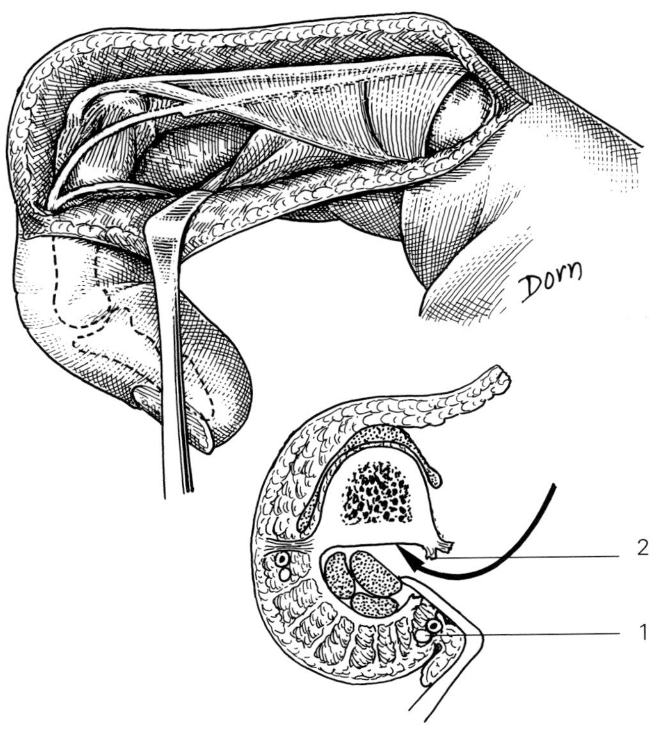

Figure 36.15
Lateral approach for PIP joint arthroplasty.
1 Neurovascular bundle, retracted volarly
2 Cleland's ligament, incised and retracted

Rheumatoid boutonnière deformity

Unlike the rheumatoid swan-neck deformity, which may originate at any of the digital joints, a boutonnière deformity originates at the PIP joint level.

Synovial hypertrophy of the PIP joint stretches the extensor mechanism. Progressive elongation or avulsion of the central extensor tendon, inserted on the base of the middle phalanx, results in PIP flexion (Figure 36.16). The boutonnière deformity is a progressive condition. The distal phalanx becomes hyperextended as a result of proximal retraction of the extensor mechanism. The lateral extensor tendons slide volarly on the sides of the PIP joint. When they pass volar to the axis of rotation of the joint, they increase its flexion. Proximal contracture of the extensor mechanism can put the MP joint in hyperextension.

Contracture of the retinacular ligaments, of the volar plate and of the collateral ligaments contributes to the fixation of the deformity. The deformity can be further aggravated by destruction of the articular surfaces.

With boutonnière deformity, the functional loss caused by a moderate PIP joint flexion remains less important than the PIP joint stiffness in extension of the swan-neck. For this reason, in the early stages, the treatment should involve minimal risk. Paradoxically, it is the distal deformity, the lack of DIP flexion which is, in most cases, more disturbing than the PIP flexion.

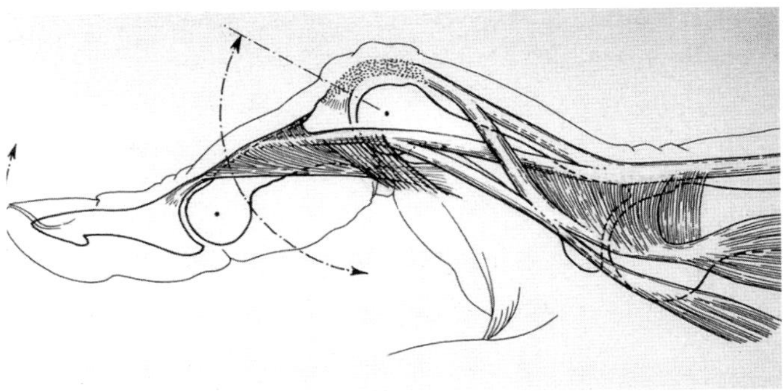

Figure 36.16
Boutonnière deformity.

Rheumatoid boutonnière, like the rheumatoid swan-neck deformity, is classified in four stages. This four-stage classification takes into account not only the PIP joint but also the DIP joint.

Stage 1: No limitation of passive motion in any finger joint (Figure 36.17)

The patient has only a slight lag of PIP joint extension. Full grasping ability is maintained, the functional loss is minimal. The flexibility of the distal joint improves as the PIP joint is flexed.

Synovectomy of the PIP joint is the first aim of the treatment at this stage. Usually a conservative treatment with a combination of local injections, splintage in extension at the PIP level and active flexion exercises of the DIP, over a period of at least 2 or 3 months, is attempted (see Figure 2.19).

For most authors no surgery is indicated at this stage. However, an extensor tenotomy of the distal extensor tendon, developed by Fowler (1949) and reported by Dolphin (1965), may restore the balance of extensor forces at the level of the two interphalangeal joints.

The risk of a mallet finger deformity is increased when the tenotomy is too distal, it seems preferable to perform the tenotomy of the terminal extensor tendon proximal to the distal insertions of the oblique retinacular ligament or even at the level of the lateral extensor tendons (see Figure 2.21).

Extensor tenotomy is preferably performed under local anaesthesia in order to observe the patient's function immediately.

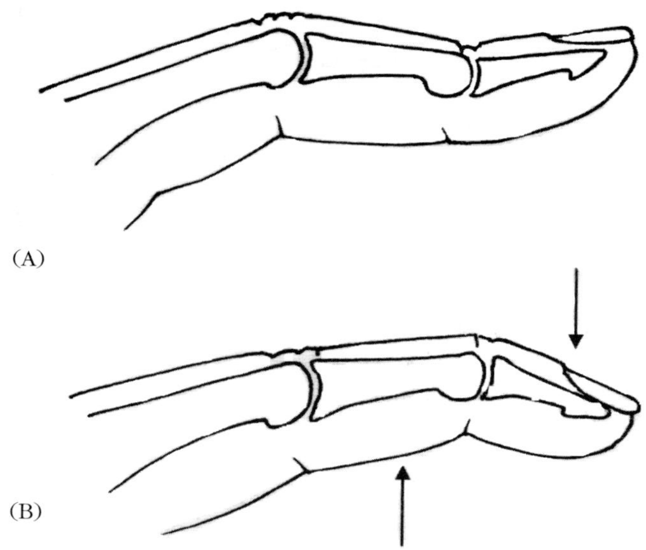

Figure 36.17

Boutonnière deformity, stage 1. (A) The deformity. (B) The distal phalanx can be flexed passively while the middle phalanx is maintained in extension.

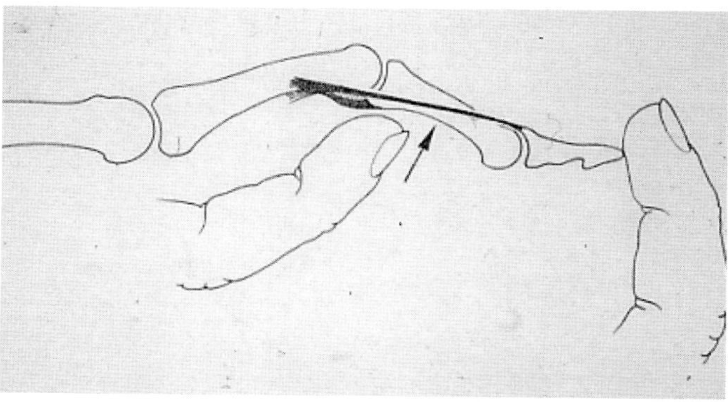

Figure 36.18

Boutonnière deformity, stage 3. Contracture of the PIP volar plate and the oblique retinacular ligaments.

Stage 2: Tenodesis effect

When the middle phalanx is maintained in extension, flexion of the distal phalanx is not possible. The retinacular test is positive (see Figure 2.17). The specific treatment is partial resection of the contracted oblique retinacular ligament. This is rarely performed on a rheumatoid boutonnière deformity; a tenotomy of the distal extensor tendon seems more appropriate for the restoration of the extensor mechanism balance.

Stage 3: Limitation of PIP and DIP joint motion with articular surfaces intact

Soft tissue contracture limits PIP and DIP joint motion (Figure 36.18):

1. Contracture of PIP volar plate and accessory collateral ligaments limit extension of the joint.
2. Contracture of oblique retinacular ligaments limits DIP joint flexion.
3. Proximal retraction of the extensor apparatus causes hyperextension of MP joint.

However, PIP joint flexion is still possible and the main functional loss is caused by the lack of DIP flexion excluding terminal pinch grip.

It is tempting to treat both the synovitis and the extensor imbalance surgically. However, in a rheumatoid patient, tendons are often in poor condition, the extensor mechanism has stretched out and there is a risk of jeopardizing existing function, particularly PIP joint flexion, for a small gain.

Before surgery, a conservative treatment is always necessary at this stage. The joint synovitis is treated by local injection. It is very important to be able to correct the deformities passively before the restoration of extensor apparatus is attempted. The use of corrective splints aims to reduce the flexion contracture of the PIP joint and, when combined with active mobilization of the DIP joint, causes distal traction on the extensor apparatus (see Figure 2.20). As progress is made, the splint can be altered.

Procedures aimed at rebalancing the extensor apparatus should only be attempted if the interphalangeal joint contractures are passively corrected preoperatively. If, in spite of an adequate conservative programme, complete passive correction is not obtained, it is wise to renounce attempts to repair the extensor apparatus and to be content with a distal extensor tenotomy when useful PIP joint flexion is still possible.

Oblique tenotomy of the lateral extensor tendons (Figure 36.19)

An oblique incision is made on the dorsum of the middle phalanx.

The proximal portion of the extensor apparatus is freed with a blunt spatula passed under the lateral tendons, then the two lateral extensor tendons are divided obliquely.

Usually, complete flexion of the distal phalanx is obtained without dividing the lateral border of the tendons into which the oblique retinacular ligament is inserted.

The obliqueness of the tendon division allows lengthening of the distal extensor apparatus without loss of contact between the ends of the divided tendons.

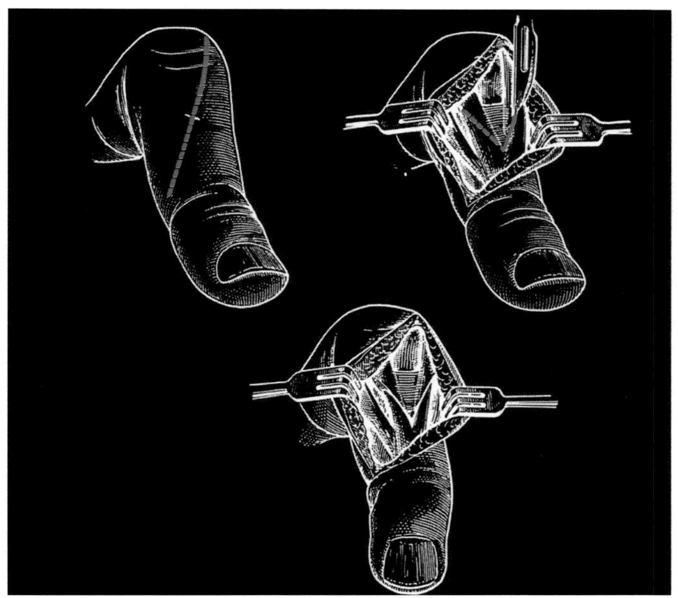

Figure 36.19
Oblique tenotomy of the lateral extensor tendons. (A) Incision. (B) The two lateral extensor tendons are divided obliquely. (C) Flexion of the distal phalanx. The obliqueness of the tendon division allows lengthening of the distal extensor apparatus without loss of contact between the ends of the divided tendons.

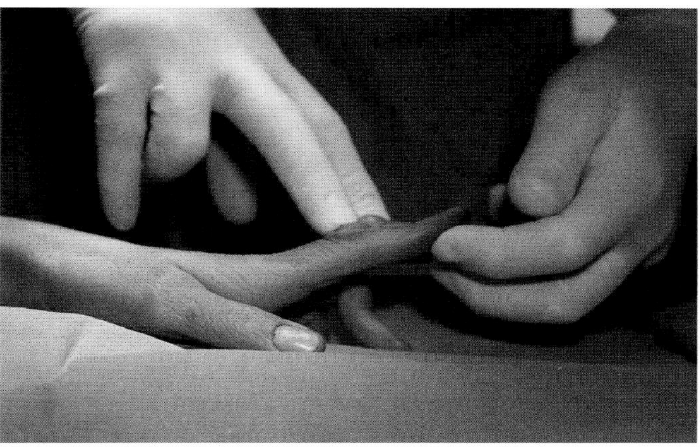

Figure 36.20
The deformity has been passively corrected preoperatively.

A splint holds the PIP joint in as much extension as possible and the DIP joint in neutral position. Active mobilization of the distal phalanx is started after 1 week. A splint holds the distal phalanx in extension between exercises, for 2 more weeks.

Extensor mechanism reconstruction

The procedure has already been described in the chapter on traumatic extensor tendon lesions (see Figures 2.24–2.28). The advantage in rheumatoid lesions is that there is less scar tissue, but the tendons are often invaded by synovitis. Of course, the freedom of the flexor tendons must be assured before the restoration of the extensor apparatus.

Both the extension defect of the PIP joint and the flexion defect of the DIP joint must be corrected preoperatively (Figure 36.20).

The lateral extensor tendons are subluxated volarly; they are freed to relocate dorsally (Figure 36.21A–D).

The fibrous scar of the central tendon is resected for about 3 mm, care being taken to preserve the distal insertion of the tendon at the base of the middle phalanx. The PIP joint is held in extension by an oblique K-wire. The shortened central tendon is sutured.

An oblique tenotomy of the lateral extensor tendons is performed. The distal phalanx is flexed. The elongated lateral extensor tendons are replaced in their physiological dorsal position. They are sutured to one another at their distal ends. Sometimes, it is possible to save the triangular lamina, which is overlapped onto the lateral extensor tendons and then fixed with several fine sutures (Figure 36.22).

The finger is immobilized with a volar splint. The K-wire is removed after 2 weeks, the PIP is held in extension on a splint for 6 weeks, but the distal phalanx is allowed to move actively (Figure 36.23).

Stage 4 Fixed boutonnière deformity with lesions of the articular surfaces

The only two alternatives when the flexion deformity at the PIP level is very severe are fusion or arthroplasty of the PIP joint. Arthroplasties with implant require active flexor tendons and an extensor apparatus that can recover after reconstruction. They are sometimes indicated in selected cases on the ring and little finger on one hand in patients who have severe bilateral boutonnière deformities. Arthrodesis is the best solution when the extensor apparatus is largely destroyed, associated with a distal extensor tenotomy.

When several fingers present deformities, often of different types, one must assess the functional needs of the patient and establish a programme of correction for the two hands that allows both grasping and precision grip.

Rheumatoid mallet finger

Rheumatoid mallet fingers are caused by synovitis at the distal joint. The terminal extensor tendon adheres and

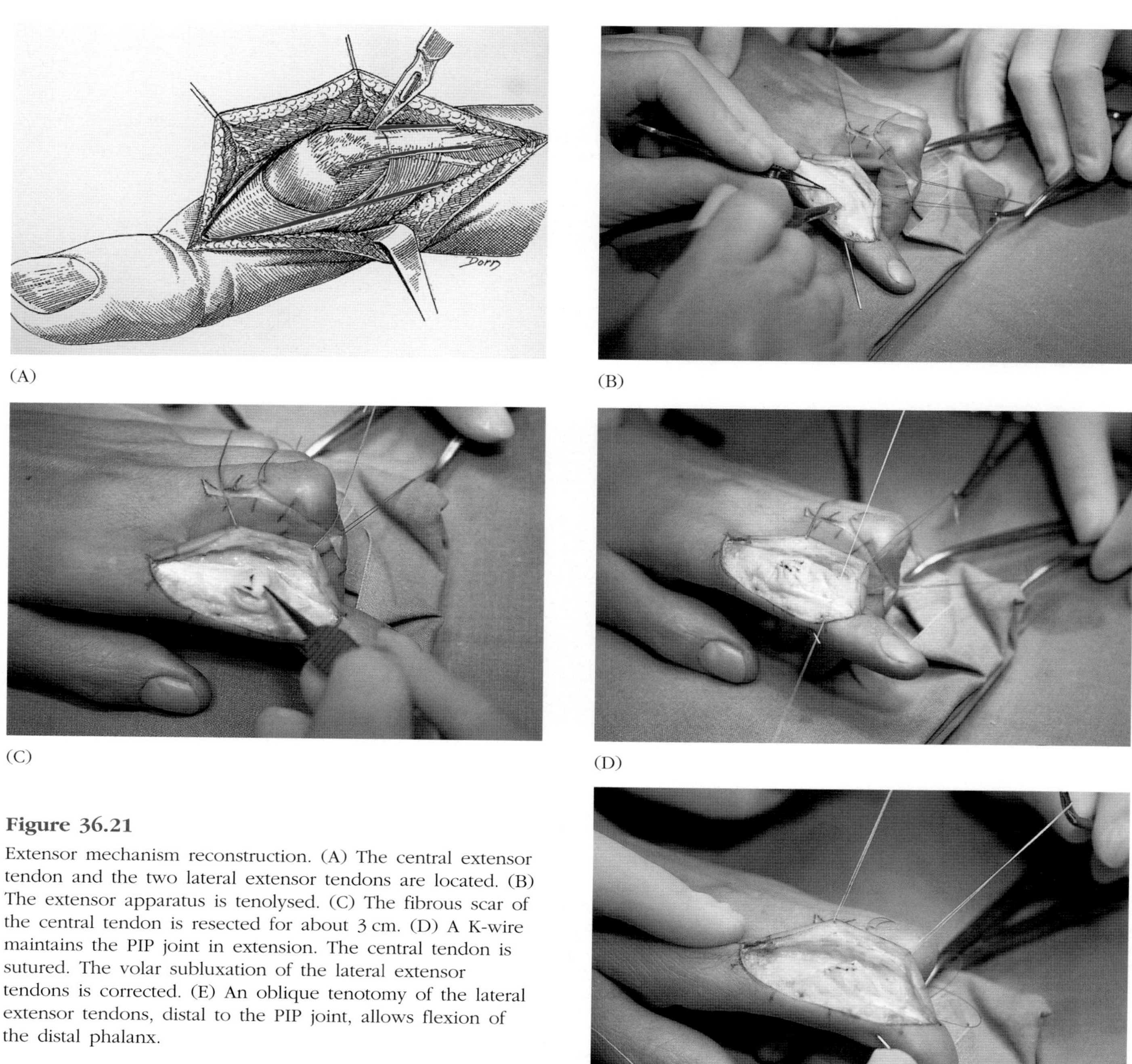

Figure 36.21

Extensor mechanism reconstruction. (A) The central extensor tendon and the two lateral extensor tendons are located. (B) The extensor apparatus is tenolysed. (C) The fibrous scar of the central tendon is resected for about 3 cm. (D) A K-wire maintains the PIP joint in extension. The central tendon is sutured. The volar subluxation of the lateral extensor tendons is corrected. (E) An oblique tenotomy of the lateral extensor tendons, distal to the PIP joint, allows flexion of the distal phalanx.

blends with the joint capsule and inserts across the width of the dorsal aspect of the base of the distal phalanx. Progressive elongation or avulsion of this tendon has two important functional repercussions:

- inability to extend the distal phalanx;
- proximal retraction of the extensor apparatus, reinforcing its action on the middle phalanx.

If the PIP joint is lax, which is common in rheumatoid hands, its secondary hyperextension results in a swan-neck deformity. For this reason, even if the functional handicap is not severe, a distal joint synovitis in a rheumatoid patient should be treated – by local injections, splintage or surgery.

The rheumatoid mallet finger can also be classified in four stages.

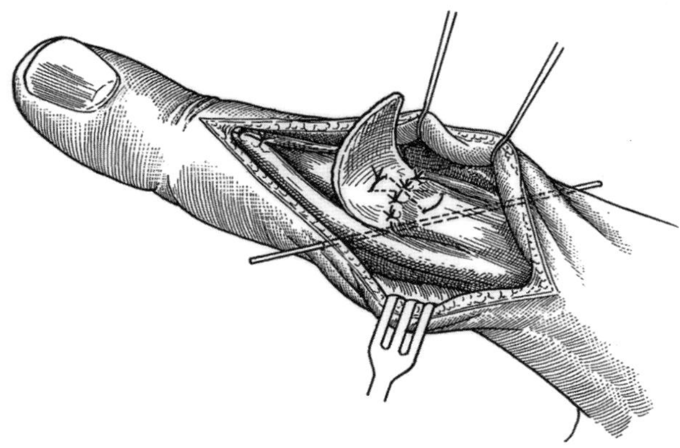

(A)

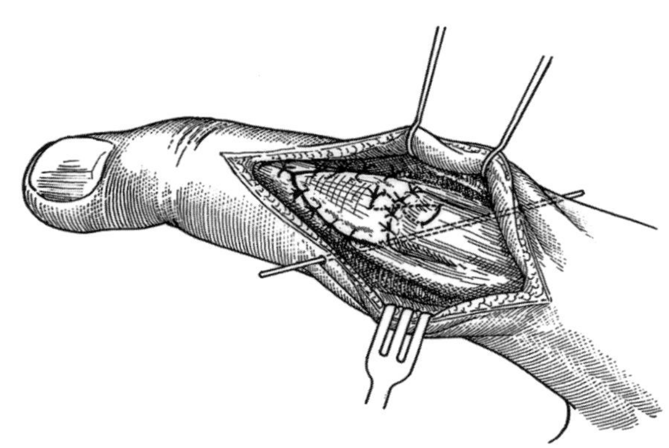

(B)

Figure 36.22
(A) Sometimes it is possible to preserve the triangular lamina. (B) The triangular lamina is overlapped and sutured on the lateral extensor tendons.

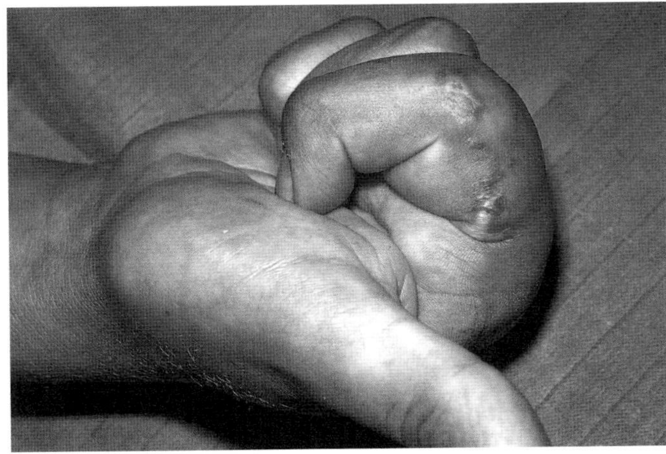

Figure 36.23
Result of procedure shown in Figure 36.22.

Stage 1

- DIP flexion deformity with no limitation of active and passive motion at the PIP and DIP joints.
- Uninterrupted immobilization of the DIP joint in extension for 10 weeks. Night splinting is continued for several weeks (Figure 36.24).

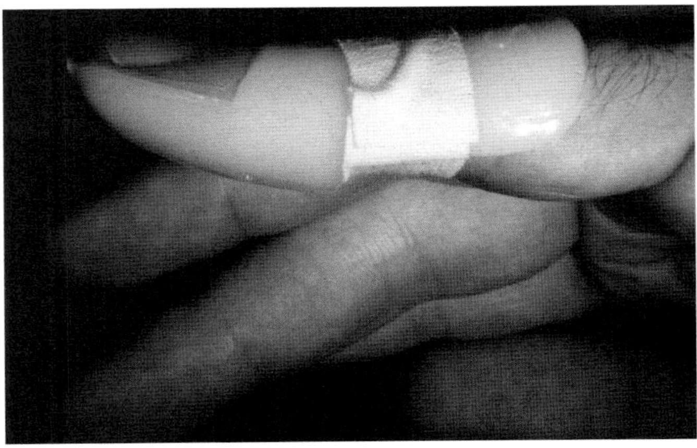

Figure 36.24
Rheumatoid mallet finger, stage 1. Uninterrupted splint immobilization of the distal phalanx in extension for at least 10 weeks.

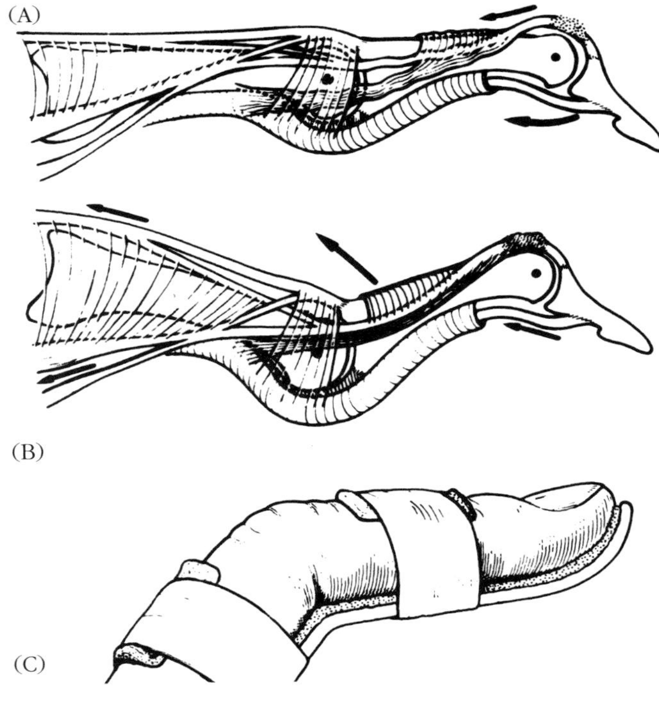

Figure 36.25
Mallet finger. (A) Stage 1. (B) Stage 2. Mallet finger with hyperextension of the PIP joint. (C) It is important to prevent stiffness in hyperextension of the PIP joint.

Stage 2

- Tenodesis effect. DIP joint flexion with PIP joint hyperextension.
- Splinting is the first treatment (Figure 36.25).
- A tenotomy of the central extensor tendon has been advocated by Fowler (1949) (see stage one of swan-neck deformity).
- Littler's spiral oblique retinacular reconstruction is another technique for correction of the two interphalangeal joints.

Stages 3 and 4

- Fixed deformity.
- Persistent symptomatic deformity may benefit from fusion of the distal joint in about 10–30° of flexion (the degree of flexion increases toward the little finger).

References

Dolphin JA (1965) Extensor tenotomy for chronic boutonnière deformity of the finger – Report of two cases, *J Bone Joint Surg* **47A**: 161.

Flatt AE (1983) *Care of the Arthritic Hand*, 4th edn (Mosby: St Louis).

Fowler B (1949) Extensor apparatus of the digits, *J Bone Joint Surg* **31B**: 477.

Littler JW (1954) quoted in Harris C, Riordan DC, Intrinsic contracture in the hand and its surgical treatment, *J Bone Joint Surg* **36A**: 10–20.

Littler JW, Eaton RG (1967) Redistribution of forces in the correction of the boutonnière deformity, *J Bone Joint Surg* **49A**: 1267–74.

Nalebuff EA (1989) The rheumatoid swan-neck deformity, *Hand Clin* **5**: 203–14.

Nalebuff EA (1998) The rheumatoid hand: surgical techniques. In: Tubiana R, ed, *The Hand*, Vol 5 (WB Saunders: Philadelphia).

Saffar P (1997) Proximal interphalangeal joint midlateral approach. In: Saffar P, Amadio PC, Foucher G, eds, *Current Practice in Hand Surgery* (Martin Dunitz and CV Mosby: London and St Louis).

Straub LR (1960) The etiology of finger deformity in the hand affected by rheumatoid arthritis, *Bull Hosp Joint Dis* **21**: 322–9.

Swanson AB (1968) Silicone rubber implants for replacement of arthritic or destroyed joints in the hand, *Surg Clin North Am* **48**: 1113–27.

Swanson AB (1973) *Flexible Implant Resection Arthroplasty in the Hand and Extremities* (CV Mosby: St Louis).

Thomson JS, Littler JW, Upton J (1978) The spiral oblique retinacular ligament (SORL), J *Hand Surg* **3**: 482–7.

Tubiana R (1969) The mechanism of deformities of the fingers due to musculotendinous imbalance. In: Tubiana R, ed, *La Main Rhumatoïde* (Expansiion Scientifique Française: Paris) 141.

Zancolli EA (1979) *The Structural and Dynamic Bases of Hand Surgery*, 2nd edn (JB Lippincott: Philadelphia) 305–60.

37 The rheumatoid thumb: surgical treatment

Dominique Le Viet and Christian Allende

The thumb column is one of the most frequently affected sites in rheumatoid arthritis; involvement occurs in 60–81% of patients with rheumatoid arthritis (Clayton 1962, Brewerton 1966, Ratliff 1971, Eiken 1972, Inglis et al 1972, Salgeback et al 1976, Brumfield and Conaty 1980, Swanson et al 1981, Nalebuff 1984, Tubiana and Toth 1984, Alnot 1987). Thumb deformities are often associated with deformities of the fingers and wrist and, once the decision to proceed with surgical treatment has been made, not only should the involved joints of the hand and wrist be considered, but the entire upper extremity must be addressed. When determining appropriate treatment for the rheumatoid thumb, all extrinsic (soft tissue) as well as intrinsic (bone and joint) factors contributing to thumb function must be assessed. We will describe the different thumb lesions commonly found in rheumatoid arthritis, their mechanisms and the different surgical treatments.

Anatomy

The thumb consists of three joints: trapeziometacarpal (TMC), metacarpophalangeal (MP) and interphalangeal (IP). The scaphotrapezial joint has classically been included in the wrist. The IP joint allows only flexion and extension motion; flexion is produced by the flexor pollicis longus (FPL) and extension by the extensor pollicis longus (EPL); these movements are reinforced by the expansion of the internal and external thenar muscles.

The MP joint allows not only flexion and extension (amplitude can be quite variable from one subject to the next), but it also allows small lateral movements, specifically in radial deviation and a small degree of derotation, which allows an effective pulp-to-pulp pinch between the thumb and the fingers.

Flexion of the MP joint is performed by the flexor pollicis brevis (FPB); this explains the fact that with flexion there is radial deviation and some associated pronation. Extension is performed by the extensor pollicis brevis (EPB), which inserts into the base of the proximal phalanx by fine expansions. Extension is reinforced by the EPL; which is attached to the EPB by crossed fibres that mix with the joint capsule (Le Viet and Lantieri 1993).

The TMC joint is the most important joint for opposition. Due to its unique saddle shape, movements in flexion, extension, abduction and adduction are all possible (Duparc et al 1971, Bettinger and Berger 2001).

The capsule alone does not ensure contact between the articular surfaces, because it has been shown that with distraction a distance of at least 3 mm may separate the articular surfaces. This relative instability of the TMC joint is due in part to the diagonal orientation of the dorsal and palmar ligaments. The principal ligamentous stabilizer is the intermetacarpal ligament that is found in the distal part of the commissure in-between the first two metacarpals. The capsule is reinforced by the oblique posteromedial ligament, which holds the articulation in the back. The oblique anteromedial ligament originates from the crest of the trapezium and crosses the joint in the front. The straight anterolateral ligament seats directly on the anterolateral part of the joint. It is important to realize that there is no lateral ligament; this explains the frequent lateral subluxation of the TMC joint. In addition, during opposition there is a natural tendency toward subluxation of the TMC joint, due to the effect of traction of the medial adductor pollicis on the medial sesamoid and the lateral traction of the abductor pollicis longus (APL) at the base of the proximal metacarpal.

Anatomo-pathology of the deformities

Thumb deformities in rheumatoid arthritis can be divided into two groups depending on whether the first metacarpal has been displaced in abduction or in adduction. This results in a Z-deformity of the thumb that is equivalent to the boutonnière deformity, which is the most frequent deformity; or it can lead to an adductus thumb or a thumb with a swan-neck deformity, which represents only 20% of lesions (Figure 37.1).

Several authors have proposed classifications for the deformities of the first column based on the anatomopathology. Ratliff (1971) proposed a four-stage classifi-

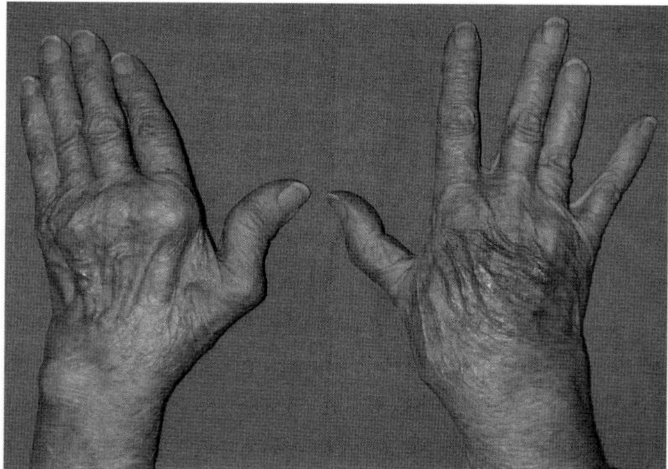

(A)

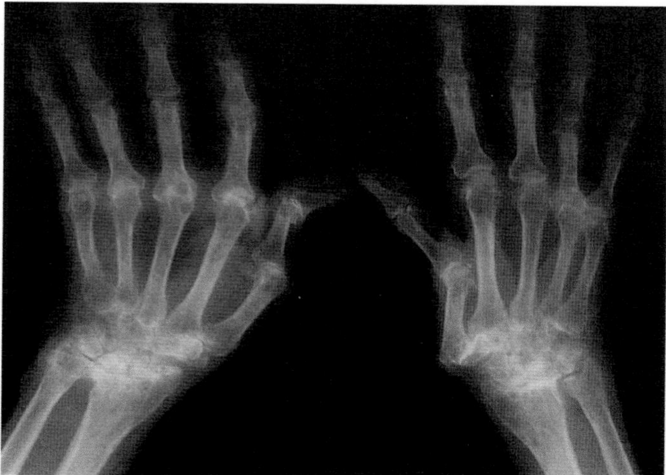

(B)

Figure 37.1

(A,B) The rheumatoid thumb deformities; bilateral involvement, clinical and X-ray appearance. Z-thumb on the left hand and adductus thumb on the right.

Box 37.1 *Ratliff's four-stage classification*

Group 1: Z-thumb or boutonnière deformity
Group 2: Unstable thumb
Group 3: Adductus thumb
Group 4: Deformity secondary to tendon ruptures
- FPL
- EPL

Box 37.2 *Nalebuff's six-stage classification*

Type 1: Boutonnière deformity, extrinsic minus deformity divided into three stages
Type 2: Association of adductus and boutonnière thumb
Type 3: Adductus thumb deformity
Type 4: Abduction deformity at the MP joint
Type 5: MP hyperextension
Type 6: Bony destruction and unstable thumb

Box 37.3 *Alnot's four-stage classification of Z-thumb*

Stage 1: Reducible MP flexion, with normal or subnormal X-rays
Stage 2: Reducible MP flexion, with normal or subnormal X-ray appearance at the MP joint and destruction or dislocation at the IP joint
Stage 3: Destroyed or dislocated MP joint with irreducible flexion, and a normal or subnormal IP joint
Stage 4: Destroyed and dislocated MP and IP joints with irreducible deformation

cation that corresponded to different clinical forms (Box 37.1). Nalebuff (1984) proposed a six-stage classification (Box 37.2). Alnot (1987) described a four-stage classification for the Z-thumb deformation, combining damage to the MP and IP joints (Box 37.3). These different classifications have the advantage of being able to evaluate the results based on the initial deformity, but they are unable to assess an evolving condition. In addition, with the exception of Ratliff's classification, they do not take into consideration associated ruptures of flexor or extensor tendons of the first column.

We will describe the anatomo-pathologic deformities of the Z-thumb and then the adductus thumb.

Z-thumb

This is the most common deformity of the thumb, representing approximately 80% of thumb deformities in rheumatoid arthritis. The first sign is synovitis of the MP joint that progressively distends the dorsal capsule. The distal band of the EPB gradually lengthens and the EPL subluxates over the ulnar border of the MP joint. Initially this deformity is reducible, but with time it becomes fixed and the dislocation of the EPL (into which the adductor expansions are inserted) produces a progressive hyperextension of the IP joint (Figure 37.2). This hyperextension is at first reducible, but it also becomes fixed with time.

This Z-deformity of the thumb is equivalent to a boutonnière deformity of the long fingers, the main difference is that the EPB does not subluxate over the radial border of the MP joint, but becomes progressively distended by the dorsal synovitis and becomes ineffective. Along with this tendon misalignment, there are

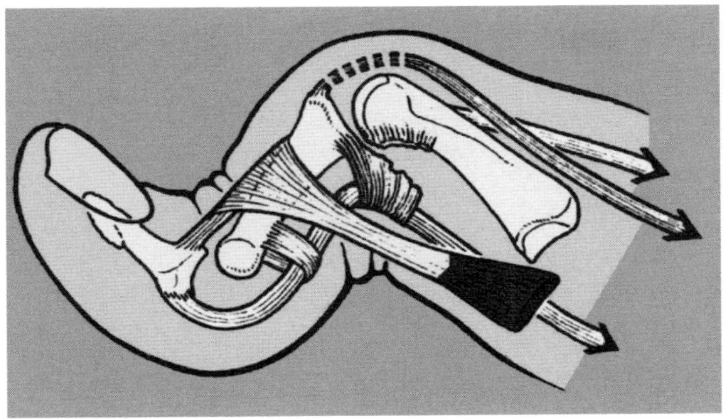

Figure 37.2
Physiopathology of the Z-thumb. Note EPB distension, dislocation of the EPL and traction from the adductor expansion over the distal portion of the EPL.

often associated intra-articular changes that can affect both the MP and the IP joints to different degrees. There is frequently an associated radial deviation of the distal phalanx that is secondary to the instability of the IP joint, which is pushed radially during pinch (Figure 37.3). Z-deformity of the thumb is usually associated with ulnar deviation of the long fingers at the MP joints (see Figure 37.10A), and can significantly compromise pinch.

Adductus deformity

The adductus deformity of the thumb (also called swan-neck deformity of the thumb), has its origin at the TMC joint. This lesion is much more rare than the Z-deformity described above.

The base of the first metacarpal subluxates dorsally and radially because of synovial distension of the TMC joint and traction of the APL (Cooney et al 1977) (Figure 37.4); followed promptly by lesions at the TMC joint.

This subluxation of the base of the first metacarpal produces an adduction contracture of the thumb, which is a serious lesion because it leads to narrowing of the first web space. It produces, secondarily, an adaptive hyperextension deformity of the MP joint by progressive distension of the palmar plate; this hyperextension is at first reducible but with time the deformity stiffens. It is not until the final stages that one finds the classic adductus deformity of the thumb that includes subluxation of

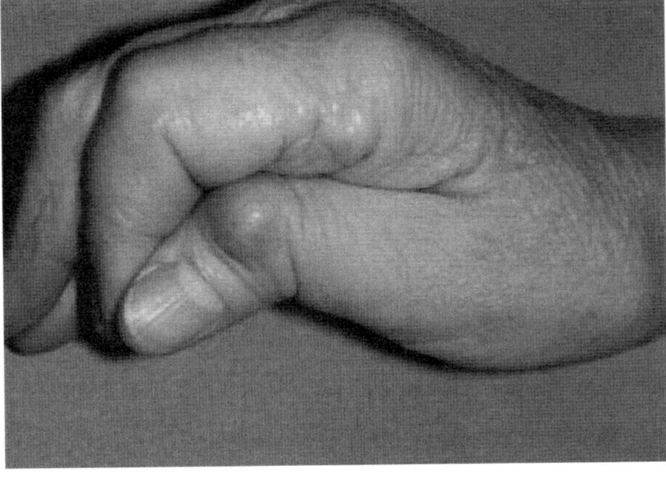

Figure 37.3
Radial displacement of the unstable IP joint, made evident during pinch.

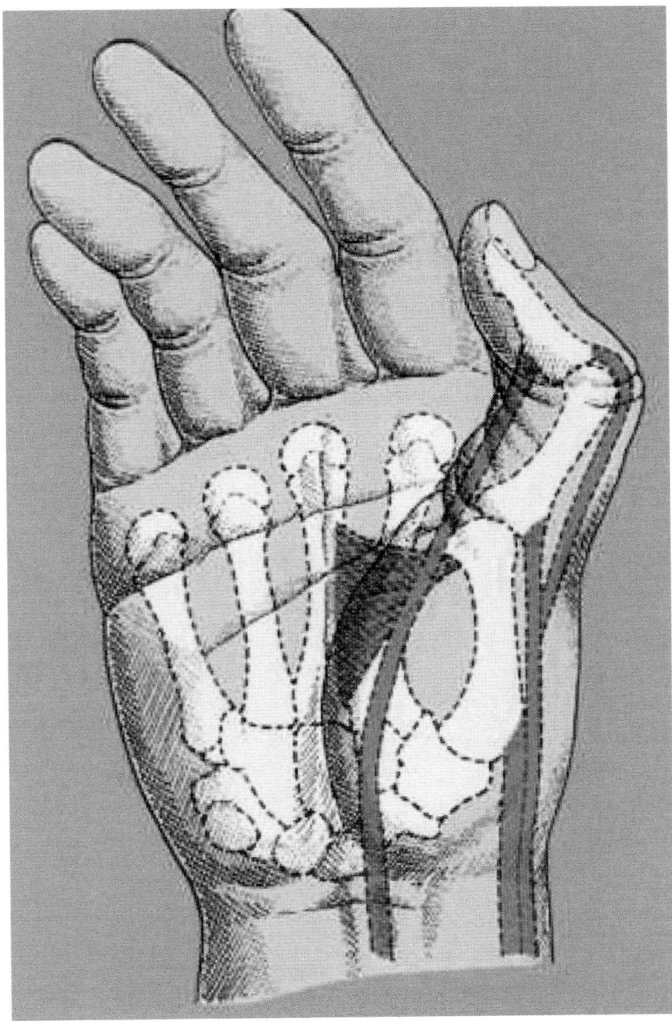

Figure 37.4
Physiopathology of the adductus thumb. Note that the base of the first metacarpal subluxates dorsally and radially because of the synovial distension of the TMC joint and the traction of the APL.

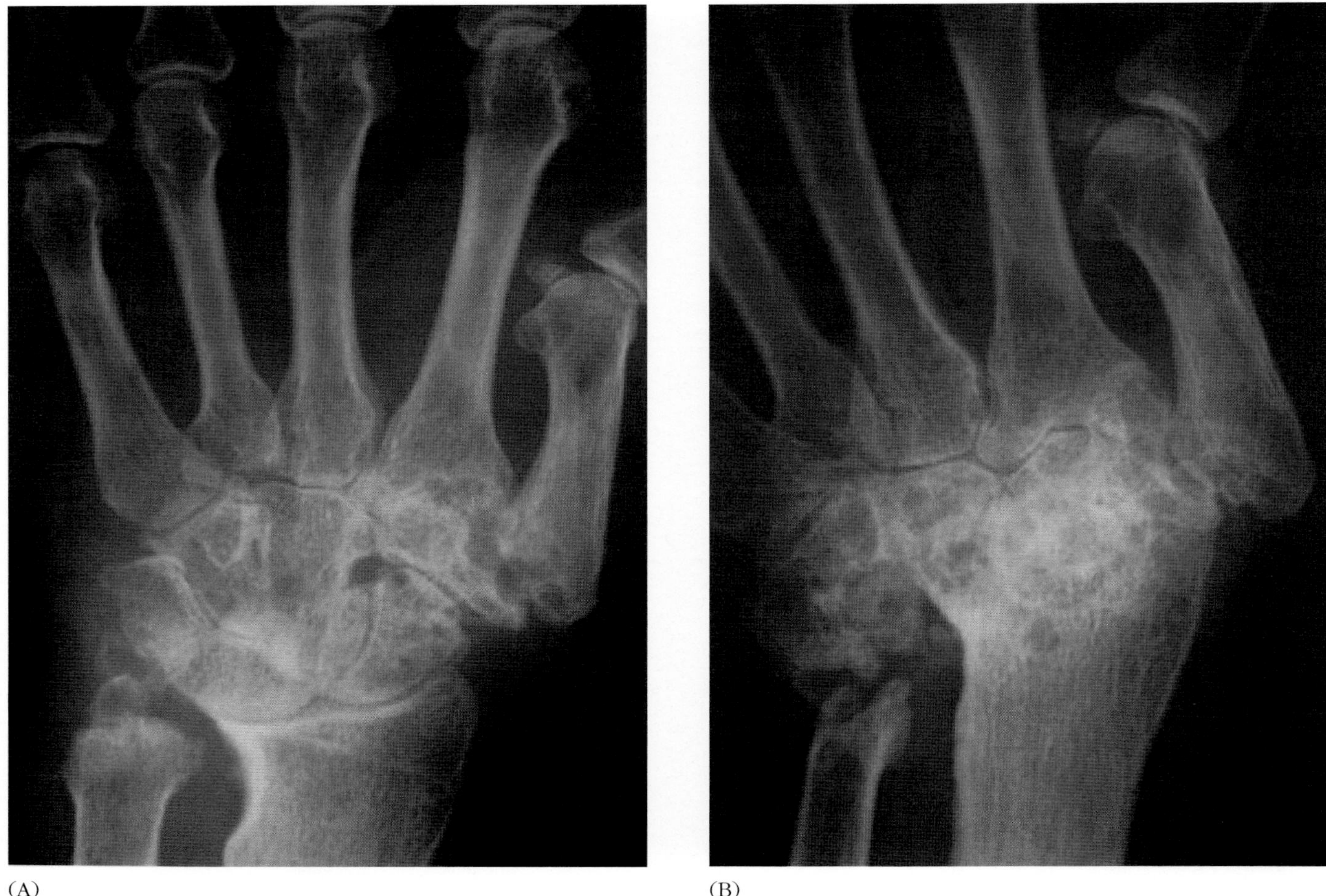

Figure 37.5
X-Ray evolution in adductus thumb deformity. (A) The distance between the radius and first metacarpal is conserved. (B) After 5 years, there is evident impaction of the first metacarpal over the radius styloid.

the TMC joint, a reactive hyperextension of the MP joint and flexion of the IP joint (Figure 37.5). In the adductus deformity, the EPL is not subluxated over the ulnar border of the joint, but remains attached with the EPB.

Tendinous lesions of the extrinsic muscles

Parallel with the above deformities, one can see rupture of the tendons of the extrinsic muscles of the thumb (Moore et al 1987, King and Tomaino 2001); these are essentially the EPL and the FPL.

Different factors can lead to rupture; it can be related to direct invasion of the tendon by synovial pannus (Backhouse 1969, Feldon et al 1993), compression of the tendon producing ischaemia, or an attenuation related to constant friction over prominent bony spurs.

The FPL is particularly at risk at the level of the scaphotrapezial joint (Mannerfelt and Norman 1969, Ertel et al 1988, Mannerfelt 1988, Walker 1993). In fact this area has been named the 'critical corner of Mannerfelt' (Figure 37.6); it is where the FPL changes direction with an angulation of 30°. An associated deviation of the carpus with a more horizontal scaphoid may allow its inferior pole, which is often irregular, to irritate and progressively damage the FPL (Figure 37.7). This irregular inferior pole seats in the floor of the carpal tunnel under the radioscaphocapitate ligament. The projection of the lunate at the floor of the carpal tunnel may lead to rupture of the flexor tendons to the fingers (Zangger and Simmen 1993).

Diagnosis of a rupture of the FPL tendon is often quite obvious, and there is often a sudden inability to flex the IP joint of the thumb. However, in patients with significant joint destruction and with stiffness of the IP joint, or a fixed hyperextension deformity as in the adductus

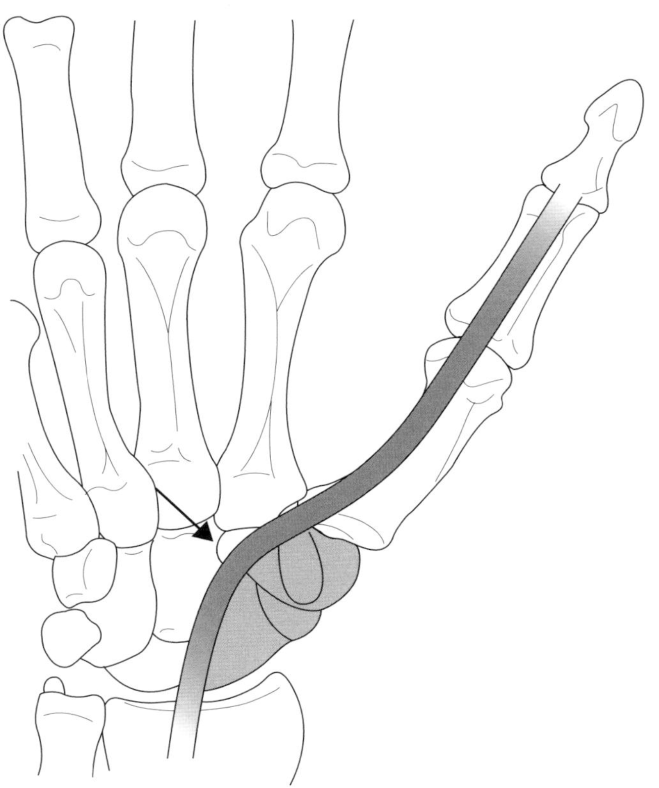

Figure 37.6
Critical corner of Mannerfelt.

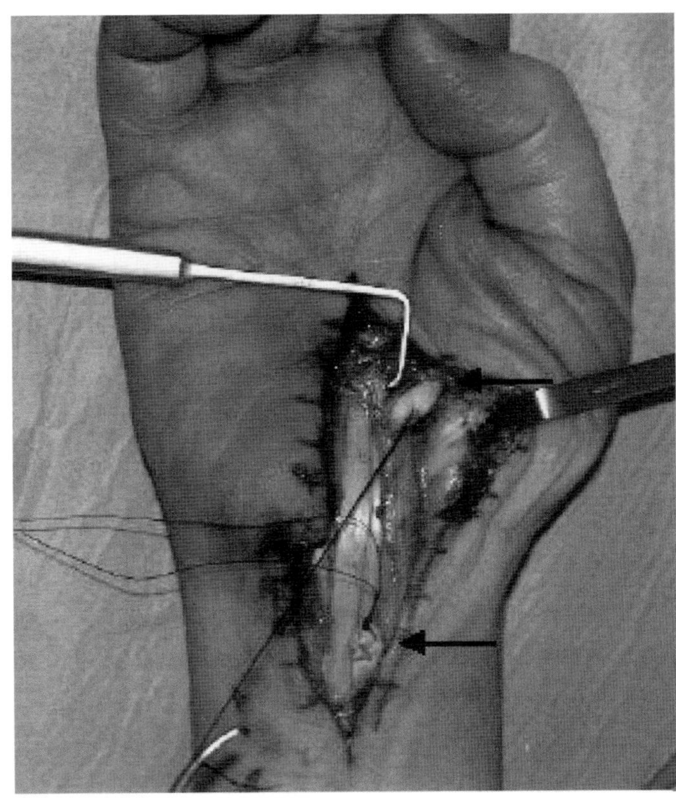

Figure 37.7
FPL rupture.

deformity of the thumb, diagnosis of tendon rupture may be more difficult. The treatment will vary according to the functional limitation and the condition of the various joints of the thumb column, particularly the flexibility of the IP joint. Rupture of the EPL is relatively frequent in rheumatoid arthritis (Harris 1951). This lesion often occurs at the level of Lister's tubercle in the third dorsal extensor compartment; at this level, the EPL is in a tight osteofibrous canal, often infiltrated with synovial pannus; here it changes direction by approximately 30°. This rupture is often heralded by a painful tenosynovitis and there is often tenderness along the extensor tendon sheath, especially at Lister's tubercle. Pain with resisted extension of the thumb should make one think of tenosynovitis of the EPL. If this is diagnosed before rupture of the tendon, corticosteroid injections are contraindicated; corticosteroids risk weakening the integrity of an already fragile tendon. In this case the only effective treatment is rest and splinting with a volar forearm brace. If conservative treatment fails, opening and debridement of the third extensor compartment, synovectomy of the EPL and radial displacement of the tendon are indicated.

Unfortunately, these lesions are often not diagnosed until the tendon ruptures. Function loss is variable; the function of the IP joint in flexion as well as the residual force of the EPB (as long as the EPL is not subluxated ulnarly) may partially compensate for the rupture of the EPL tendon.

Bony lesions of the thumb

Bony lesions are difficult to schematize, because involvement of the TMC, MP and IP joints can be quite variable. Classically these lesions can be evaluated following the four-stage radiological classification of Steinbrocker et al (1949) or the six-stage classification of Larsen et al (1977). We will review these deformities elsewhere in the surgical treatment.

Surgical treatment

As with all rheumatoid conditions, the decision to proceed surgically is best made as part of a multidisciplinary decision. One must consider the age, profession, evolution of the rheumatoid arthritis and the patient's response to medical treatment. The goal should be to reduce pain, improve function, prevent osteo-articular destruction, correct the deformities and finally to improve the aesthetic aspect of the hand. The indication for surgery is based on the clinical examination, the biological factors and the radiographic progression.

Primarily we recommend isolated interventions such as articular synovectomy, tendon sheath synovectomy, tendon repair and localized arthrodesis. Secondarily, we recommend the treatment of the more global thumb deformities; i.e. the Z-deformity of the thumb (also called boutonnière deformity) and the adductus thumb (also called a swan-neck deformity).

Articular synovectomies

Their indication is rare, isolated and most frequently at the MP joint of the thumb. The synovectomy must be as complete as possible, so as to eliminate the pain caused by the distension caused by the synovial proliferation, and to limit the osteo-articular destruction caused by the pannus, and protect the tendons, which because of this synovitis may subluxate, distend and possibly rupture. However, it has not been proven that a simple synovectomy can change the natural history of the rheumatoid disease. In effect, if the first goal, which is to decrease pain, is achieved, then it is hoped that it will also help prevent progressive destructive lesions within the joint. In effect, this synovitis may recur; however, this new synovitis usually contains fewer cells and fewer vessels with an inflammatory component that is less marked. The main indication for a synovectomy of the MP joint is usually a dorsally distended joint that is resistant to medical therapy.

A longitudinal incision is made dorsally, centred over the MP joint. This is usually made over the radial border of the joint. Once the skin has been incised, the sensory nerves are dissected and retracted laterally. The lateral and medial flaps are minimally manipulated and are held with traction sutures anchored to the skin. The first step is to evaluate the dorsal synovitis. The extensor brevis tendon should also be evaluated, it is often distended but in the correct location. The EPL is often subluxated ulnarly at the level of the MP joint.

This synovitis may travel in the space between the EPB and EPL dorsally. It can also be seen laterally through the sagittal bands.

Once the exposure is complete, the approach passes between the EPB and EPL via a longitudinal incision. These two tendons are retracted out of the way. If the capsule of the MP joint is intact, it is preferable to preserve it by making a longitudinal incision. With the help of a Freer elevator, the hypertrophic synovium is detached at the level of the metacarpal neck. The synovectomy is started with a blade at the metacarpal neck and proceeds distally to the base of the proximal phalanx. During the distal synovectomy, one must be cautious not to proceed too far distally, so as to avoid disrupting the insertion of the EPB on the proximal phalanx.

Once the dorsal synovectomy has been completed, one can assess the medial and lateral collateral ligaments of the MP joint. These ligaments must be respected to prevent future instability of the joint. Placing traction at the level of the proximal phalanx allows the completion of the intra-articular synovectomy. The synovium hidden in the recesses of the medial and lateral collateral ligaments at the level of the metacarpal neck can be excised by using a synovial rongeur.

Once the synovectomy has been completed, the capsule should be closed if possible. The EPB and EPL should be returned to their anatomic locations. The ulnar subluxation of the EPL should be reduced. This synovectomy through a dorsal incision is unfortunately always incomplete, because it is not possible to access the anterior synovial recesses of the palmar plate. Eventually, a second volar synovectomy may need to be added.

A synovectomy of the MP joint of the thumb in rheumatoid arthritis is indicated in isolated synovitis of the MP joint resistant to medical treatment, without intra-articular destruction and without palmar subluxation of the base of the proximal phalanx.

Arthrodesis of the MP joint

Arthrodesis of the MP joint is certainly the best arthrodesis at the level of the hand. It reliably abolishes pain, provides stability, corrects deformities and restores good pinch strength (Stanley et al 1989).

The incision and exposure are the same as for MP synovectomy. After passing between the EPB and EPL, the joint is progressively dislocated. The medial and lateral collateral ligaments are excised. Instead of a chevron osteotomy, which in our opinion shortens the thumb too much, we prefer to shape the metacarpal head in a circular fashion and to form a socket in the base of the proximal phalanx until good subchondral bone is reached. This allows good contact and allows control of the flexion, which should be between 15 and 20°. Because of the loss of automatic pronation with flexion of the MP joint, it seems preferable to place the arthrodesis in a little pronation to allow satisfactory opposition between the thumb and the other digits. The flexion of the joint should be discussed with the patient before the intervention. This can be done with the aid of specific braces that allow variable degrees of flexion of the MP joint. The patient should be asked which amount of flexion leads to the least amount of handicap. Usually the amount of flexion preferred by the patient is between 15 and 20° at the MP joint.

Fixation of the arthrodesis can be achieved by a number of methods (parallel K-wires with cerclage, simple cerclage, crossed K-wires, micro-screws, resorbable screws or staples) (Figure 37.8).

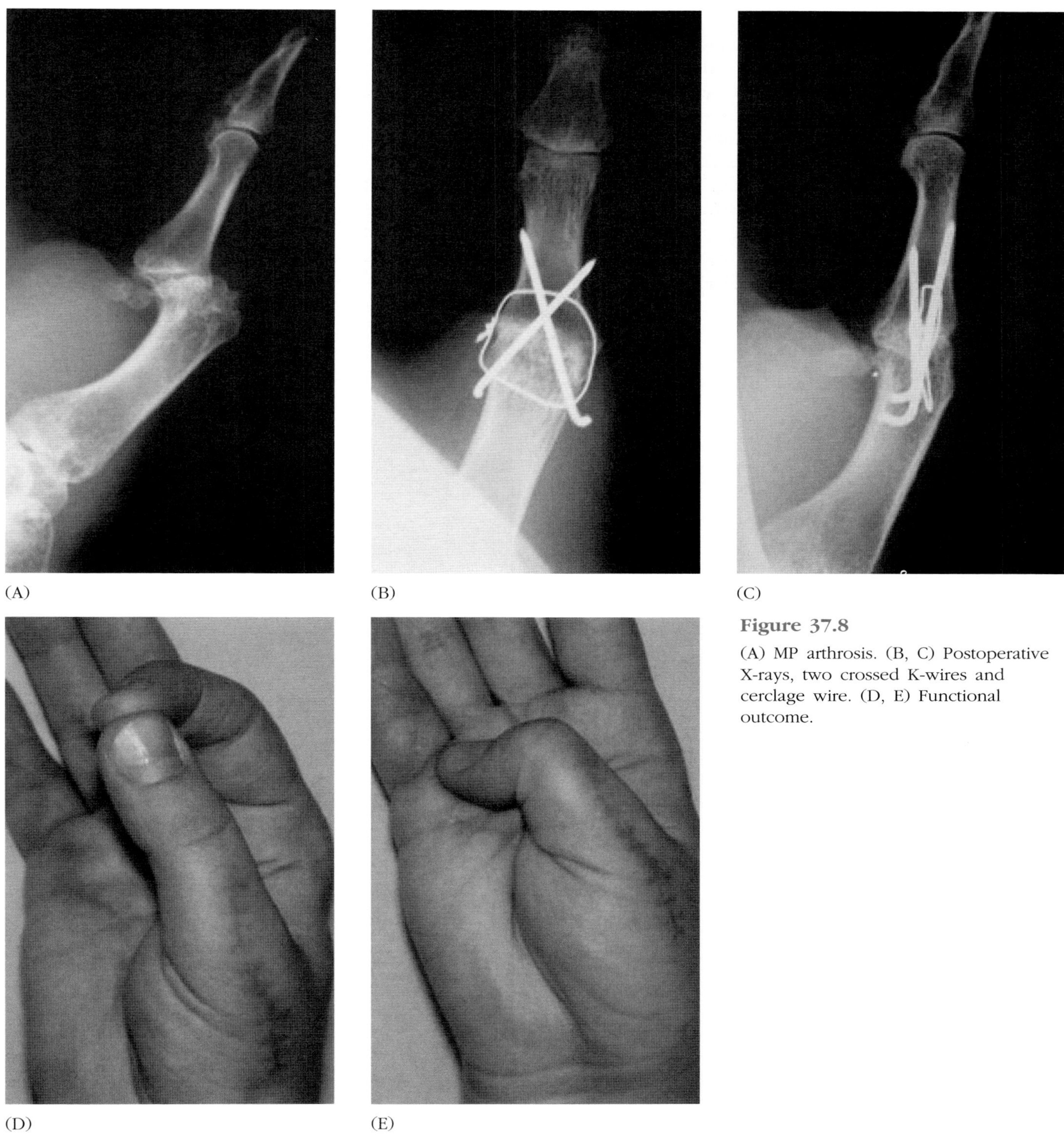

Figure 37.8
(A) MP arthrosis. (B, C) Postoperative X-rays, two crossed K-wires and cerclage wire. (D, E) Functional outcome.

Union usually occurs between 5 and 6 weeks. During this time, an orthosis that protects the MP joint is worn. This orthosis must allow immediate mobilization of the IP joint, as to decrease the risk of adhesions of the EPL at the level of the fusion. Immobilization of the MP joint does not suppress the TMC and the IP joints if they are preserved.

We will discuss briefly the fusion of the IP joint. This is the only therapeutic option if this joint is destroyed, painful or malaligned; it is usually performed through a medial dorsal incision along the proximal phalanx and extended in a T shape at the level of the IP joint. The EPL is detached at its distal extent, leaving a small tendinous band at the base of the distal phalanx that will allow its reattachment at the end of the procedure. The surgery starts with a dorsal synovectomy; then the joint is dislocated as the lateral and medial collateral ligaments are sectioned, the head of the proximal phalanx and the base of the distal phalanx are resected, until there is good subchondral bone. The fusion is placed in 10–15° of flexion and some pronation, especially if the MP joint is not functioning normally. Fixation of the fusion is variable, but as with the MP joint, one axial K-wire can be used, followed by a second oblique wire that prevents rotation. The technique finishes with the reinsertion of the EPL of the thumb and skin closure.

Synovectomy of the EPL and/or tendinous repair

Synovectomy of the EPL may be proposed in the face of synovitis protruding from the dorsal extensor retinaculum that is resistant to medical therapy. This synovitis, as mentioned previously, is the only one that should not be infiltrated locally with corticosteroids because of the risk of tendon rupture at the level of Lister's tubercle.

In the case of persistent synovitis with pain at resisted extension of the thumb, a synovectomy should be suggested before frank rupture of the tendon occurs.

The incision is sinus-shaped and should be centred over the third dorsal extensor compartment at the level of the flexion creases of the wrist. Once the skin incision has been made, the cutaneous branches of the radial sensory nerves should be retracted. The third compartment should be opened and the EPL should be removed from its sheath. Using vessel loops, the synovectomy is performed using sharp dissection with a scalpel.

If after completing the synovectomy, there are nodules in the tendon, these should be excised by carefully opening the tendon and removing the nodules. The tendon should then be closed using 7–0 suture.

Once the synovectomy has been completed, there are two possible approaches to the placement of the tendon. Some authors advocate keeping the EPL outside its osteofibrous sheath; this gives the tendon a more direct radial direction subcutaneously and avoids the 30° angulation that usually occurs at Lister's tubercle, and has the advantage of reducing the irritation of the tendon. Unfortunately, it decreases the power of thumb extension due to the radialization and the possible bowstringing. Personally, we prefer to remove Lister's tubercle, remove the fibrous sheath between the second and third compartments and place the EPL in the second dorsal extensor compartment on top of the extensor carpi radialis longus (ECRL) and brevis (ECRB) (Figure 37.9). The dorsal extensor retinaculum is repaired over the second and third extensor compartments. This reduces the risk of compression of the EPL and assures normal function of the EPL.

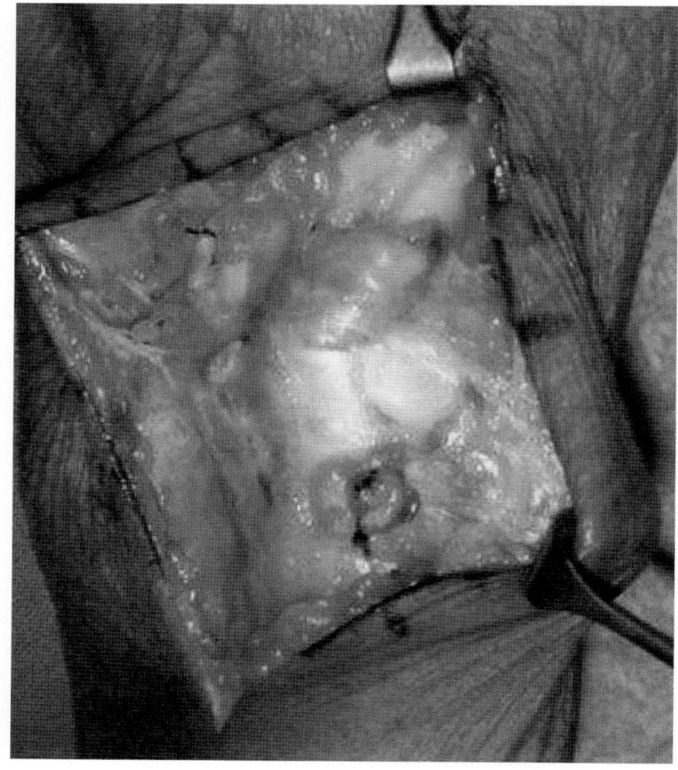

(A)

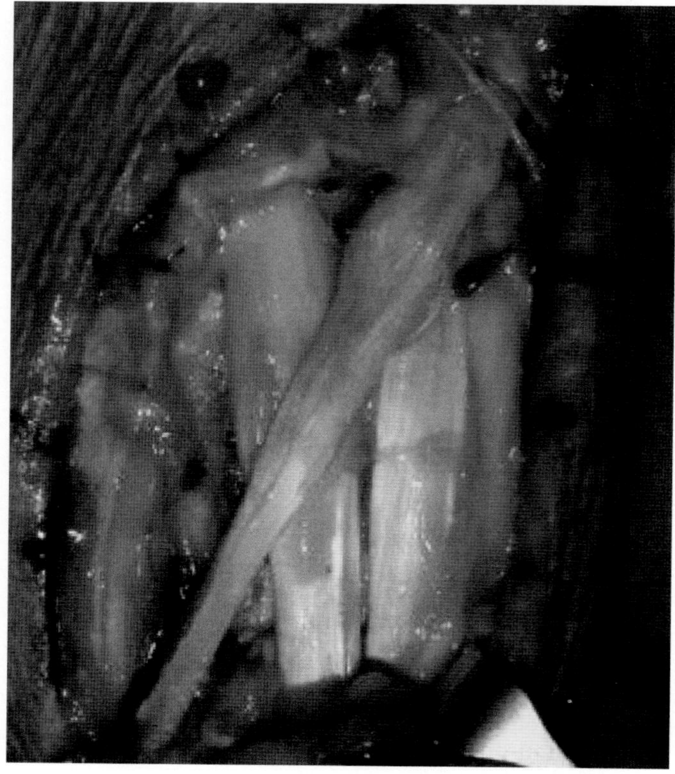

(B)

Figure 37.9

(A) EPL synovitis. (B) Resection of Lister's tubercle, and rerouting of the EPL in the second compartment over the ECRL and ECRB tendons.

In case of rupture of the EPL, we prefer to place a graft in-between the proximal and distal edges of the ruptured tendons when possible. For this graft to be effective, the proximal edge should not be retracted and the tendon must be mobile when traction is placed on the proximal edge. We prefer this technique to a tendon transfer because tendons must be preserved for possible future use in rheumatoid arthritis.

If the proximal edge is retracted or ineffective, we have the choice between the classic transfer of extensor indicis to the EPL and eventually arthrodesis of the IP joint – particularly useful when motion at the IP joint is limited or when the joint is already destroyed.

Synovectomy of the FPL and/or tendon repair

Isolated FPL synovectomy is exceptionally indicated; it usually presents as a component of a global flexor tendon synovitis or it is secondary to a rupture of the FPL (Millender and Nalebuff 1975, Ferlic and Clayton 1978).

The surgical approach is over the volar forearm at the level of the wrist flexion crease, often in a zigzag-type Bruner fashion. This approach allows a synovectomy of the digital flexor sheath of the thumb in the carpal tunnel, which is usually associated with a synovitis that envelops all the superficial and deep digital flexors in the carpal tunnel. If there is an extensive palmar digital synovitis of the FPL, a second incision needs to be made starting 3 cm distal to the flexion crease of the MP joint of the thumb, and is also classically made in a zigzag fashion according to Bruner. The synovectomy is performed carefully, and A1 and A2 pulleys are respected. It is often difficult to keep the oblique pulley located at the level of the proximal phalanx where there is an expansion of fibres of the thumb adductor.

Once the synovectomy has been completed, if there is a prominence over the scaphoid tubercle that has eroded the medial portion of the floor of the carpal tunnel, this osteophyte should be removed. Once the excision is complete, the capsule should be reapproximated either directly, or with a flap.

If the FPL is ruptured, then we use a short interpositional graft taken from the palmaris longus tendon, if present.

Some authors are reluctant to place an avascular graft in a zone of inflammation and prefer to transfer the FDS of the ring finger. It should be understood that if the IP joint of the thumb shows destructive changes or is stiff, then it is often preferable to proceed with an arthrodesis. The IP joint should be placed in 15° of flexion.

Z-deformity or boutonnière deformity of the thumb

The Z-deformity of the thumb is by far the most frequent deformity seen in rheumatoid arthritis. The initial lesion is a progressive distension of the dorsal capsule, secondary to synovial proliferation; this distends the distal insertion of the EPB and often leads to progressive ulnar subluxation of the EPL (Terrono and Millender 1990, Terrono et al 1990).

If the disease is in the early stages, a dorsal approach to the capsule with reinsertion of the EPB can be considered, but this is only very rarely possible. In reality, the EPB alone does not have sufficient strength to ensure extension of the MP joint and, in addition, these patients are often seen in later stages of the disease. The technique used is the one proposed by Nalebuff (1984), which consists of removing the distal insertion of the EPL and refixing it with the EPB at the base of the proximal phalanx (Figure 37.10). The thenar muscles that attach to the distal lateral part of the EPL perform extension of the IP joint. If these expansions cannot be conserved, they should be reinserted. The dorsal fixation of the EPL to the base of the proximal phalanx can be accomplished by transosseous sutures, by bone anchors, or by a transosseous tunnel as described by Harrison and Ansell (1974). It can also be sutured to the dorsal capsule as described by Nalebuff (1984). The MP joint should be immobilized in a volar forearm-based splint. The joint should also be temporarily pinned in extension for 1 month. If reinsertion of the thenar muscles is not necessary, then mobilization of the IP joint can be started early, once the pain has diminished.

Concerning the indications for the Z-thumb, the four-stage classification of Alnot (1987) corresponds best with the different lesions that can be found and allows definition of the therapeutic indications:

- In stage I: painful reducible flexion of the MP joint with little or no joint involvement. At this stage the repair according to Nalebuff (1984) is recommended; it is understood that this repair is always associated with a synovectomy as described above. The patient must be informed that this procedure allows some recuperation of extension; this is due to the tension of the EPL as well as the temporary pinning of the joint. However, there is often a flexion deficit that rarely exceeds 30°. The patient must also be warned that the deformity or the synovitis may recur, and that if there is a recurrence, then the salvage procedure is a fusion of the MP joint.
- In stage II: reducible flexion deformity of the MP joint associated with minimal MP joint destruction, associated with IP joint dislocation or destruction. This is the indication for the Nalebuff procedure along with a fusion of the IP joint, performed after a synovectomy of the IP joint. The position of the arthrodesis is usually 15° of flexion and 15° of pronation. The arthrodesis is usually performed with one long axial intramedullary K-wire passed from the distal phalanx; the K-wire is advanced into the proximal phalanx and then crosses the MP joint, holding the joint in extension. A second oblique K-wire is

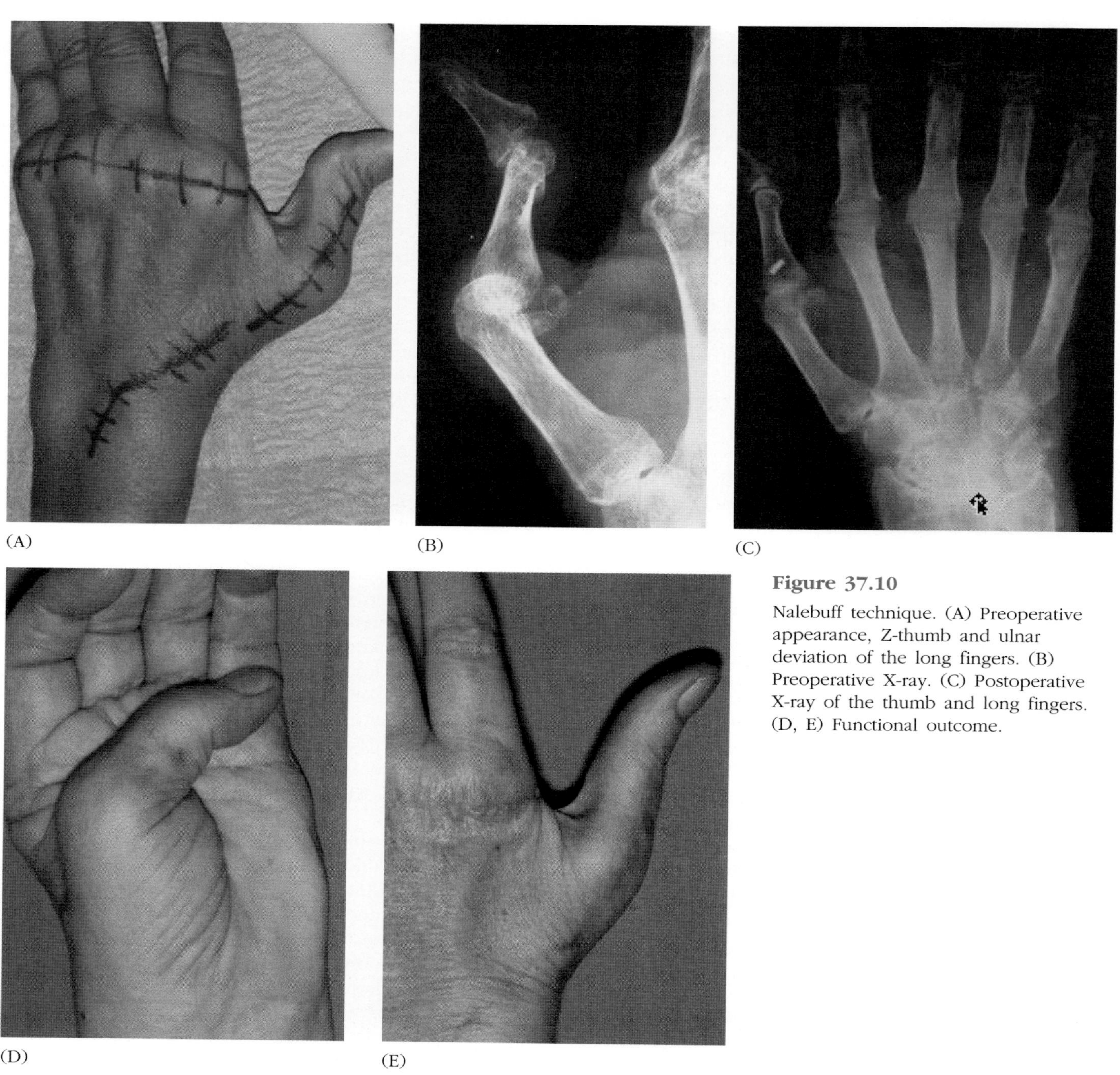

(A) (B) (C)

(D) (E)

Figure 37.10

Nalebuff technique. (A) Preoperative appearance, Z-thumb and ulnar deviation of the long fingers. (B) Preoperative X-ray. (C) Postoperative X-ray of the thumb and long fingers. (D, E) Functional outcome.

passed across the joint to control rotation. The axial K-wire is removed 1 month postoperatively.

- In stage III: rigid flexion with destruction of the MP joint, and the IP joint is preserved. At this stage the treatment consists of an arthrodesis of the MP joint after adequate synovectomy. The position of the fusion is in 20° of flexion with 15° of pronation. As mentioned above, this procedure often gives excellent results. However, certain authors such as Figgie et al (1990) propose joint replacement with a Swanson silicone prosthesis instead of fusion. Figgie et al reported a series of 43 patients followed with a Swanson prosthesis. The mobility averaged 25° and in general results were satisfactory.
- In stage IV: destruction of the MP and IP joints. Certain authors (Alnot 1987, Toledano et al 1992, Wilson et al 1993) propose a fusion of the IP joint associated with a Swanson arthroplasty of the MP joint. The justification for this technique is that arthrodesis of both the MP and IP joints of the thumb leads to a very stiff thumb, and transfers all the stress to the TMC joint. The other justification is

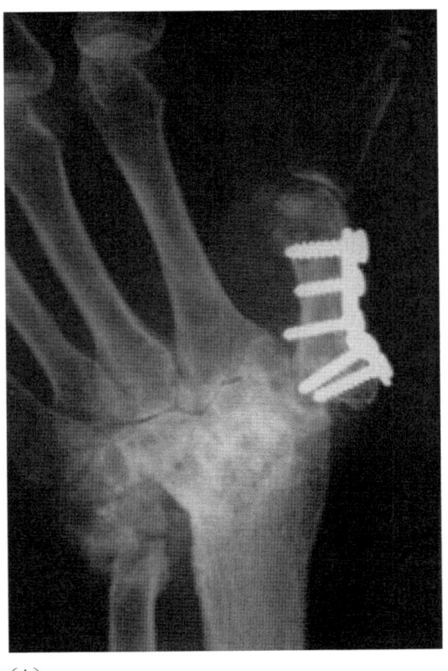
(A)

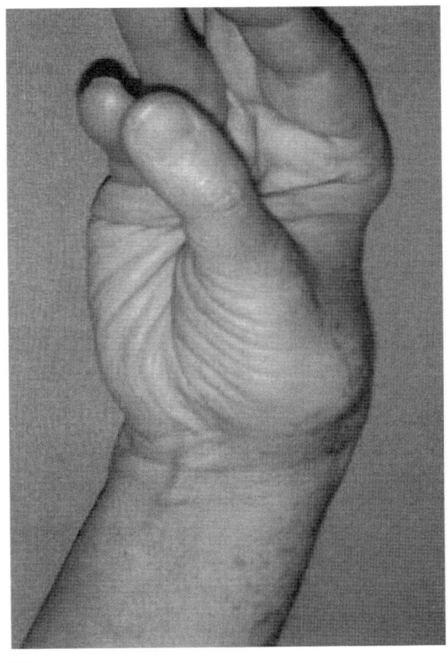
(B)

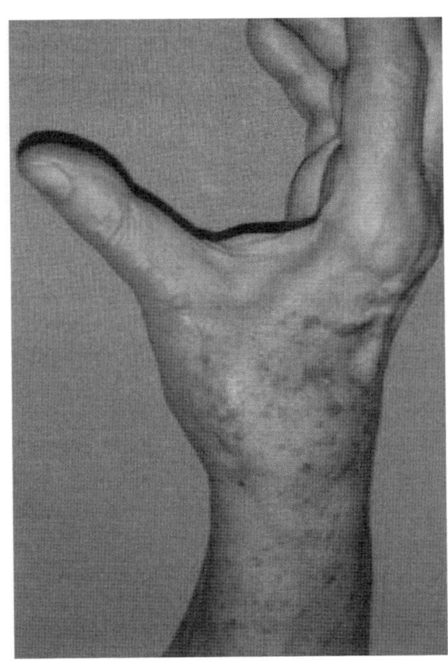
(C)

Figure 37.11
(A) Abduction osteotomy for adductus thumb. (B, C) Functional outcome.

that double arthrodesis shortens the thumb and makes pinch very difficult. Personally, we prefer to proceed with an arthrodesis of both the MP and IP joints as long as the TMC joint is preserved. In this case, bone graft is needed in order to ensure stability and to restore the length of the thumb. In effect, the Swanson prosthesis, which does not maintain lateral stability and in our opinion only gives fair results, is inferior to the arthrodesis; especially when grip strength is considered.

In conclusion, surgery for the Z-deformity of the thumb always begins with consideration of the MP joint. A synovectomy is always performed and this can be associated with tendon transfers like those according to Nalebuff (1984) if the MP joint is preserved. If the MP joint is destroyed, then one may proceed with an arthrodesis or Swanson prosthesis. As regards the IP joint, if it is damaged, the only solution is an arthrodesis.

Adductus deformity or swan-neck deformity of the thumb

In this deformity, which is much more rare in rheumatoid arthritis, the starting point is at the TMC joint. This joint, distended with synovium, subluxates by the forces of the adductor pollicis and under the effect of digital pinch. There is a secondary contracture of the adductor. This deformity represents only about 20% of the thumb deformities seen in rheumatoid arthritis. The surgical indications are relatively rare. This lesion is well tolerated from a functional standpoint because of the compensatory hyperextension of the MP joint.

If there is an indication for surgery, it must always start with the treatment of the adductus deformity of the first metacarpal. The options include:

- An advancement of the APL, which is fixed distally to the first metacarpal to increase the power of abduction.
- Release of the adductor at the level of the medial sesamoid; however, this may destabilize the first metacarpal. It is often preferable to release the adductor from the third metacarpal.
- Regarding eventual treatment of the skin, it is rare that an adductus deformity of the thumb evolves to a fixed skin contracture significant enough to warrant a Z-plasty or trident procedure.
- Finally, in certain cases, one can consider an abduction osteotomy at the base of the first metacarpal (Figure 37.11) as proposed by Wilson (1973) for the treatment of carpometacarpal (CMC) arthritis.

Once the adduction deformity of the first metacarpal has been corrected, an intervention at the level of the TMC joint can be considered. It must be realized that for the rheumatoid adductus deformity, there are currently few satisfactory interventions known at this level.

Fusion of the TMC joint is contraindicated because it limits the most important joint in the thumb column (Müller 1949); and in addition there are often adjacent lesions of the MP and IP joints.

The different arthroplasties that have been suggested have not proven to be effective at the level of the TMC joint.

- Prostheses of the TMC joints are indicated only exceptionally. The first described was that by Caffiniere (1974). Often the bone stock, especially that of the trapezium, is quite weak and there is the possibility of deterioration of the adjacent scaphoid. In addition, if there is a hyperextension of the MP joint or an arthrodesis, the constraints placed on this prosthesis risk significant early wear and failure (Rosenthal et al 1983).
- As regards Swanson silastic implants (Swanson et al 1981, Wilson et al 1993) and the condylar implant (Ashworth et al 1977, Howard et al 1985), bony resection is less, but these implants have a tendency to subluxate, and there is the risk of progression of the deterioration at the level of the trapezium in the case of a condylar implant, or at the level of the scaphoid in the case of a trapezial implant. There is also the risk of silicone synovitis, especially when the implants are placed under compression.

Trapeziectomies with or without associated tendinous interposition (Gervis 1949) or ligamentoplasty (Froimson 1970, Eaton and Littler 1973) are also not frequently indicated (Dell et al 1978). In patients with limited bone stock, complete resection of the trapezium should be avoided because in cases of secondary destruction of the scaphoid, there is a risk of the first metacarpal articulating directly with the radius. If it is decided to proceed with a trapeziectomy, then we recommend a partial trapeziectomy in order to conserve bone stock. In the cases in which a trapeziectomy is performed, a ligamentoplasty must be performed. The most common ligamentoplasty is that described by Eaton and Littler (1973), which involves taking half of the flexor carpi radialis and leaving it attached to its distal insertion at the base of the second metacarpal; the tendon is passed parallel to the articular surface of the proximal phalanx. The remaining part of the tendon is interposed in the space between the scaphoid and the metacarpal according to the technique of Froimson (1970), after securing the transposition to the lateral part of the metacarpal. Many other stabilization techniques have been described including that of Tubiana (1997), which uses a lateral slip of the ECRB pedicled on its distal insertion at the dorsal base of the second metacarpal; the tendon is then passed in an oblique fashion at the base of the first metacarpal, and it is sutured where it exits from the lateral cortex of the first metacarpal to the APL, which is released and advanced distally onto the first metacarpal. The rest of the tendon is then interposed in the space between the scaphoid and the first metacarpal. Sutures are placed in the medial and dorsal aspect of the capsule.

In addition to correcting the TMC joint, the MP joint that is in extension must always be considered. If the hyperextension is fixed with associated intra-articular destruction, the only solution is a fusion of the MP joint. If this hyperextension is irreducible but the joint is preserved, a capsulorrhaphy or a fusion of the sesamoidometacarpal joint can be attempted. This fusion is protected temporarily with a K-wire from posterior.

When the IP joint is involved, the only solution is an arthrodesis.

In summary, the indications for surgery of the adductus deformity of the thumb are quite rare. The main indications involve a painful deformity or functional incapacity, which is quite rare as the functional impairment secondary to an adductus thumb is usually quite well tolerated.

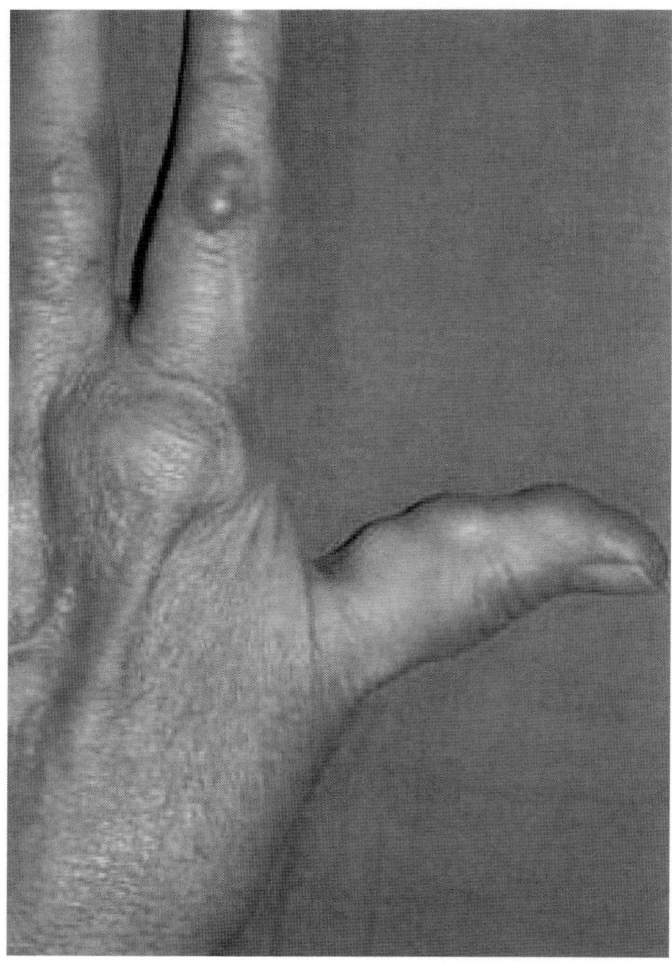

Figure 37.12
Rheumatoid nodules.

Rheumatoid nodules

Cutaneous rheumatoid nodules are part of the extra-articular aspect of the disease. They are often described as being associated with a strongly seropositive disease that is usually quite aggressive. They are more frequently seen in patients treated with methotrexate. These are irregular nodules that have a hard consistency and are mobile with respect to the deep tissues but are often adherent to the dermis. They are often not painful, but become bothersome because of their large volume. If located next to a joint, they can limit flexion due to their size. Usually these nodules are well tolerated and their excision is rarely required. If they are very large and trapped in the pulp of the thumb or the first or second web space, they may interfere with fine pinch or grasp. This may be a reason for excision (Figure 37.12). The patient must always be warned about the possibility of recurrence and the risk of incomplete excision. If this nodule is adherent to the dermis, the skin must be excised in order to achieve a complete excision, this is often not possible and leads to an incomplete excision. The only indication for excision in the thumb is if the lesion is large or limits function.

Conclusion

Surgical treatment for the rheumatoid thumb must be integrated in the whole treatment of the rheumatoid patient. The objective must be to regain pinch between the thumb and the other digits.

Precise analysis of the deformities is essential in order to decide the surgical treatment best suited to the patient. This decision is best made in consultation with the medical team, taking into consideration the functional demands of the patient and their reaction to treatment. Although it is better not to divide treatments, we think it is preferable to treat the long fingers in a first intervention, and to schedule the surgical intervention on the thumb once the results in the long fingers have been obtained. In effect, once the flexion at the level of the long fingers has been reached, the intervention at the level of the thumb can be planned, so as to re-establish a useful thumb opposition. This treatment most often involves correction of the Z-deformity of the thumb, and is based on the involvement of the joint. Treatment at the initial stages gives satisfactory results with the understanding that recurrence of the deformity might occur.

References

Alnot JY (1987) Le pouce rhumatoïde, *Ann Chir Main* **6**: 67–78.

Ashworth CR, Blatt G, Chuinard RG, Stark HH (1977) Silicone rubber interposition arthroplasty of the carpo-metacarpal joint of the thumb, *J Hand Surg* **2**: 145–57.

Backhouse KM (1969) Rheumatoid tenosynovial involvement, *Hand* **1**: 7–8.

Bettinger PC, Berger RA (2001) Functional ligamentous anatomy of the trapezium and trapeziometacarpal joint (gross and arthroscopic), *Hand Clin* **17**: 151–68.

Brewerton DA (1966) The rheumatoid hand, *Proc R Soc Med* **59**: 225.

Brumfield RH, Conaty JP (1980) Reconstructive surgery of the thumb in rheumatoid arthritis, *Orthopaedics* **3**: 529–33.

Caffiniere JY (de la) (1974) Prothèse totale trapézo-métacarpienne, *Rev Chir Orthop* **60**: 299–308.

Clayton ML (1962) Surgery of the thumb in rheumatoid arthritis, *J Bone Joint Surg [Am]* **44**: 1376.

Cooney WP, Chao EYS (1977) Biomechanical analysis of static forces in the thumb during hand function, *J Bone Joint Surg* **59A**: 27–36.

Dell PC, Brushart TM, Smith RJ (1978) Treatment of trapezio-metacarpal arthritis: results of resection-arthroplasty, *J Hand Surg* **3**: 243–9.

Duparc J, Caffiniere JY (de la), Pineau H (1971) Approche biomécanique et cotation des mouvements du premier métacarpien, *Rev Chir Orthop* **57**: 3–12.

Eaton RG, Littler JW (1973) Ligament reconstruction for the painful thumb carpometacarpal joint, *J Bone Joint Surg* **55A**: 1655–66.

Eiken O (1972) Aspects of rheumatoid hand surgery, *Acta Orthop Belg* **38**: 53–9.

Ertel AN, Millender LH, Nalebuff E, McKay D, Leslie B (1988) Flexor tendon ruptures in patients with rheumatoid arthritis, *J Hand Surg* **13A**: 860–6.

Feldon P, Millender LH, Nalebuff EA (1993) Rheumatoid arthritis in the hand and wrist. In: Green DP, ed, *Operative Hand Surgery*, 3rd edn (Churchill Livingstone: New York) 1587–690.

Ferlic DC, Clayton ML (1978) Flexor tenosynovectomy in the rheumatoid finger, *J Hand Surg* **3**: 364–7.

Figgie MP, Inglis AE, Sobel M, Bohn WW, Fisher DA (1990) Metacarpal-phalangeal joint arthroplasty of the rheumatoid thumb, *J Hand Surg* **15A**: 210–16.

Froimson AI (1970) Tendon arthroplasty of the trapezio-metacarpal joint, *Clin Orthop* **70**: 191–9.

Gervis WH (1949) Excision of the trapezium for osteoarthritis of the trapezo-metacarpal joint, *J Bone Joint Surg* **31B**: 537–9.

Harris R (1951) Spontaneous rupture of the tendon of extensor pollicis longus as a complication of rheumatoid arthritis, *Ann Rheum Dis* **10**: 298–306.

Harrison SH, Ansell BH (1974) Surgery of the rheumatoid thumb, *Br J Plast Surg* **27**: 242–7.

Howard FM, Simpson LA, Belsole RJ (1985) Silastic condylar arthroplasty, *Clin Orthop* **195**: 144–50.

Inglis AE, Hamlin C, Sengelmann RP et al (1972) Reconstruction of the metacarpophalangeal joint of the thumb in rheumatoid arthritis, *J Bone Joint Surg [Am]* **54**: 704–12.

King JA, Tomaino MM (2001) Surgical treatment of the rheumatoid thumb, *Hand Clin* **17**: 275–89.

Larsen A, Dale K, Eck M (1977) Radiographic evaluation of rheumatoid arthritis and related condition by standard reference films, *Acta Radiol Diagn* **18**: 481–91.

Le Viet D, Lantieri L (1993) Luxation cubitale du long extenseur du pouce. Etude anatomique et clinique, *Ann Chir Main* **12**: 173–81.

Mannerfelt LG (1988) Tendon transfers in surgery of the rheumatoid thumb, *Hand Clin* **4**: 309–16.

Mannerfelt L, Norman O (1969) Attrition ruptures of flexor tendons in rheumatoid arthritis caused by bony spurs in the carpal tunnel, *J Bone Joint Surg* **51B**: 270–7.

Millender LH, Nalebuff EA (1975) Preventive surgery: tenosynovectomy and synovectomy, *Orthop Clin North Am* **6**: 765–92.

Moore JR, Weiland AJ, Valdata L (1987) Tendon ruptures in the rheumatoid hand: analysis of treatment and functional results in 60 patients, *J Hand Surg* **12A**: 9–14.

Müller GM (1949) Arthrodesis of the trapezio-metacarpal joint for osteoarthritis, *J Bone Joint Surg* **31B**: 540–4.

Nalebuff EA (1984) The rheumatoid thumb, *Clin Rheum Dis* **10**: 584–608.

Ratliff AH (1971) Deformities of the thumb in rheumatoid arthritis, *The Hand* **3**: 138–44.

Rosenthal DJ, Rosenberg AE, Schiller AL, Smith MJ (1983) Destructive arthritis due to silicone. A foreign body reaction, *Radiology* **149**: 69–72.

Salgeback S, Eiken O, Haga T (1976) Surgical treatment of the rheumatoid thumb, *Scand J Plast Reconstr Surg Hand Surg* **10**: 153–6.

Stanley JK, Smith EJ, Muirhead AG (1989) Arthrodesis of the metacarpo-phalangeal joint of the thumb: a review of 42 cases, *J Hand Surg* **14**: 291–3.

Steinbrocker O, Traeger GH, Batterman RC (1949) Therapeutic criteria in rheumatoid arthritis, *JAMA* **140**: 659.

Swanson AB, Swanson GD, Watermeier JJ (1981) Trapezium implant arthroplasty. Long-term evaluation of 150 cases, *J Hand Surg* **6A**: 125–41.

Terrono A, Millender L (1989) Surgical treatment of the boutonniere rheumatoid thumb deformity, *Hand Clin* **5**: 239–48.

Terrono A, Millender L, Nalebuff E (1990) Boutonniere rheumatoid thumb deformity, *J Hand Surg [Am]* **15**: 999–1003.

Toledano B, Terrono AL, Millender LH (1992) Reconstruction of the rheumatoid thumb, *Hand Clin* **8**: 121–9.

Tubiana R (1997) Indications chirurgicales de la polyarthrite rhumatoïde de la main. In: Tubiana R, ed, *The Hand*, Vol 5 (WB Saunders: Philadelphia).

Tubiana R, Toth B (1984) Rheumatoid arthritis: clinical types of deformities and management, *Clin Rheum Dis* **10**: 521–48.

Walker LG (1993) Flexor pollicis longus rupture in rheumatoid arthritis secondary to attrition on a sesamoid, *J Hand Surg* **18A**: 990–1.

Wilson JN (1973) Basal osteotomy of the first metacarpal in the treatment of arthritis of the carpo metacarpal joint of the thumb, *Br J Surg* **60**: 854–8.

Wilson YG, Sykes PJ, Niranjan NS (1993) Long-term follow up of Swanson silastic arthroplasty of the metacarpophalangeal joints in rheumatoid arthritis, *J Hand Surg* **18B**: 81–91.

Zangger P, Simmen BR (1993) Spontaneous ruptures of flexor tendons secondary to extreme DISI deformity of the lunate in rheumatoid wrist, *Ann Chir Main* **12**: 250–5.

38 Indications for surgical treatment of the rheumatoid hand and wrist

Raoul Tubiana

The multiplicity of factors that need to be considered in the surgical treatment of rheumatoid lesions of the hand and wrist make the indications difficult, best served in centers specialized in the treatment of these lesions.

Factors affecting the indications

They can be divided into three groups:

- Clinical evolution of the disease.
- Local state.
- General state of the patient.

Clinical evolution of rheumatoid arthritis

The clinical state of rheumatoid arthritis and the response to medical treatment are of great importance. A poorly controlled illness causes rapid progress of the destructive lesions and thus local recurrences.

The majority of patients with rheumatoid arthritis have slowly evolving manifestations. However, there are some forms with rapid articular destruction. For a long time it has been considered impossible to predict the severity of rheumatoid arthritis at its onset. Recent studies have attempted to find prognostic indicators of the evolution of the disease. Some factors predicting unfavorable outcome can be mentioned.

Signs of unfavorable prognosis

Early signs pointing to a severe form of rheumatoid arthritis are clinical, radiological, and biochemical.

- Acute polyarticular onset with a large number of swollen joints.
- Early and important functional impact.
- Positive biochemical tests for inflammation, i.e. high sedimentation rate and high C-reactive protein (CRP).
- High rate of rheumatoid factors (RF) (latex agglutination and Rose–Waaler tests).
- Early destructive joint lesions.
- Eventually, extra-articular manifestations.

Several ongoing studies allow the hope that genetic markers can be correlated with the severity of the disease. The HLA-DRBI locus genes may be a prognostic factor for severe rheumatoid arthritis.

Early recognition of the severe form is of obvious interest in establishing the therapeutic indications. It would allow a rapid introduction of aggressive medical treatment; increase of controls; and the start of a protective occupational therapy program, including the use of splints to prevent joint deformities. It would also allow the use of early surgical synovectomy associated with bony rather than ligamental stabilization.

Local state

The local state of hand and limb is of prime importance. The information gained from the clinical examination and radiographs should be borne in mind, while also noting any intractable pains, tenosynovitis, persisting articular synovitis, or stiffness and articular instability. As a general rule, rheumatoid arthritis affects several joints in the limb, and the indications for surgery in one joint can be established only while keeping in mind the state and mobility of the joints above and below and, in a more general way, the mobility of the limb itself considered as a functional chain. In these pluri-articular lesions, the clinician must try to identify the disabling effect of each joint, and the possible compensatory mechanisms that are occurring, so as to identify the site of the most disabling problem.

General state of the patient

Age, sex, occupation, hobbies, functional or aesthetic concerns, and patient cooperation are among the factors that can influence the choice of surgical treatment.

The place of surgery

Recent progress in medical treatment has tended to diminish the place of surgery in the treatment of rheumatoid arthritis. The joint inflammation associated with rheumatoid arthritis may result in severe joint damage if left untreated or inadequately treated. However, important progress is being made. Earlier diagnosis and treatment, and the development of new strategies aiming at a tight control of the inflammatory process by using methotrexate at appropriate dosage, combination therapy and, if needed, biologic agents that neutralize critical elements such as TNF which plays a key role in the inflammation cascade and the promotion of joint destruction, are leading to a revision of the expectations in terms of preservation or restoration of function. So, the need for surgery will probably decrease in the future. If joint synovitis and tenosynovitis remain after 6 months, despite general medical treatment, local treatment should be added to the general treatment.

Local treatments usually consist of injection of steroid derivatives into the affected joints or synovial sheaths of flexor tendons. Such injections should be avoided around the extensor tendons because of their fragility. In any case, this treatment should not be continued indefinitely because there is a risk of precipitating tendon and articular cartilage destruction.

If there is no improvement, or if improvement only lasts for a few weeks, surgical treatment is indicated.

Surgical priorities

Surgical treatment should take into account various priorities. Tendon rupture represents an urgent indication for surgery, not only to repair the tendon but also to prevent other ruptures. In decreasing order of importance, the other priorities are as follows.

- Suppression of pain.
- Improvement of function. A deformity in itself does not constitute an indication for surgery. We often see rheumatoid hands with severe deformities with a quite remarkable function. Conversely, some non-apparent joint stiffness can be very disabling.
- Prevention of destruction.
- Correction of deformity. A distinction should be drawn between those deformities that are not very disabling when still not too pronounced (ulnar drift of the fingers or boutonnière deformity) and those that instead lead to stiffness in extension of the PIP joint (swan neck deformity).
- Although improvement in function is the primary aim, it should not be forgotten that many rheumatoid patients are very concerned about the appearance of their hands and desire esthetic improvement.

When a surgical option is decided, an essential point should always be borne in mind: rheumatoid arthritis is a developing systemic disease that can invade all connective tissue covered by synovial membrane. This characteristic dominates the indications for surgery and means that a final result is never achieved.

Potential value of the proposed operations

Numerous techniques have been described in the preceding chapters. All these operations are far from having the same value. The value can be established only by a series of criteria. Souter (1979) has established an ingenious index for each operation used in the treatment of the rheumatoid hand with respect to its effect on pain, function, prophylactic value, esthetic improvement, and negative effects (e.g. loss of mobility by arthrodesis) (Table 38.1).

Synovectomies

The removal of diseased synovium constitutes the most effective local treatment of rheumatoid arthritis. This can be done at an early stage in the hope of stopping the process of destruction and to prevent the invasion of tissues covered by synovium.

At a more advanced stage the synovectomy should be combined with methods of correcting the deformity and of stabilization. We can distinguish between synovectomy around tendons or tenosynovectomy, and synovectomy of joints.

Table 38.1 *Index for each operation used in the treatment of the rheumatoid hand (Souter 1979)*

Operation	*Index value (%)*
Thumb MP joint arthrodesis	85
Extensor tendon tenosynovectomy plus resection of the ulna head	83
Wrist synovectomy and stabilization	73
Flexor tendon synovectomy	68
PIP joint arthrodesis	68
Thumb IP joint arthrodesis	68
MP joint arthroplasty	65
Correction of swan neck deformity	65
Finger(s) MP and IP joint synovectomy	53
PIP joint arthroplasty	43
Correction of boutonniére deformity	35

MP, metacarpophalangeal; IP, interphalangeal; PIP, proximal interphalangeal. Long-term postoperative reviews allow more precise evaluation of each of these operations.

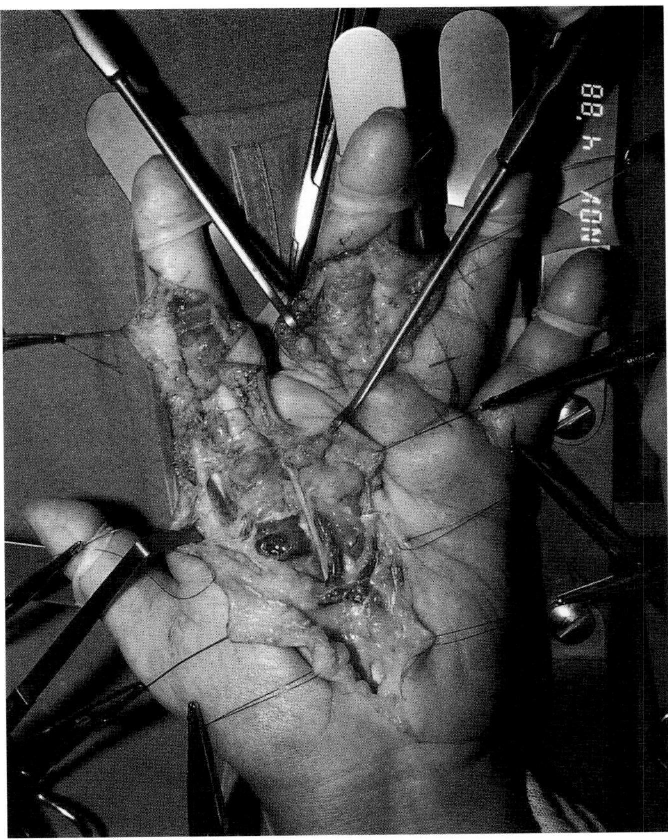

Figure 38.1
Flexor tendon tenosynovectomy.

Tenosynovectomies

The removal of diseased synovium facilitates the free gliding of the tendons in the zones of the wrist and in the fingers, where the flexor and extensor tendons run in narrow fibro-osseous canals (Figure 38.1). Mobility and strength are increased. Pain caused by associated nerve compression is relieved. Furthermore, tenosynovectomy is a proven method to prevent tendon rupture.

Recurrence of tenosynovitis is possible, but rare. Tenosynovectomies are indicated wherever tenosynovitis persists for more than 6 months despite appropriate medical treatment.

Joint synovectomies

Joint synovectomies have less value than tenosynovectomies. A distinction should be made between synovectomy of the finger joints and that of the wrist.

Synovectomies of the finger joints (Figure 38.2)

These procedures generally give a good result with respect to pain. Movement may be a little decreased

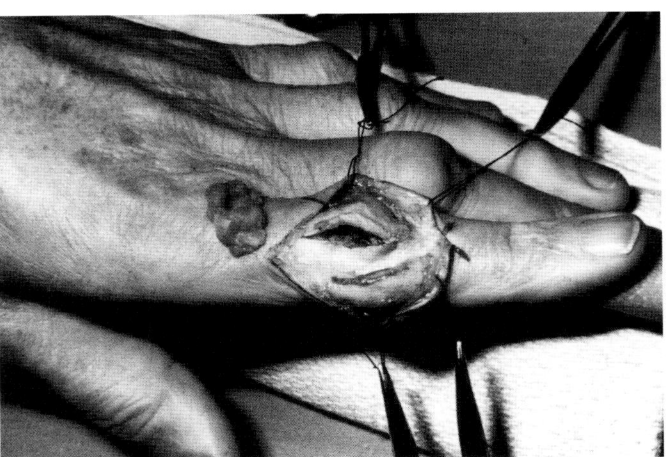

Figure 38.2
Synovectomy of the PIP joint.

postoperatively, but often power is increased. The percentage of recurrence varies from author to author, but it is well established that it occurs in an appreciable number of cases. It seems that recurrence depends on a series of factors, the most important of which include:

- The extent of the synovectomy, the choice of the approach, and the operative technique.
- Early intervention before the formation of bony cysts.
- Recurrence usually happens with new inflammatory attacks, and these arise because of either insufficient medical treatment or a particularly aggressive form of the disease.

Thus joint synovectomy has only a braking action on the disease process in the long term and is more effective if it is done early, before any bony invasion.

Wrist synovectomies

Synovectomy of the wrist is seldom performed alone these days. As a rule, it is performed with a dorsal tenosynovectomy, resection of the distal ulna, and realignment and stabilization of the wrist by various methods. It is difficult to establish the potential value of one surgical procedure when it is associated with several others. This association of several procedures gives good clinical results as regards pain and function. Extension and ulnar inclination of the wrist are usually preserved, whereas flexion and radial inclination are greatly reduced; prono-supination is improved. It is important to note that the wrist does not need a large range of

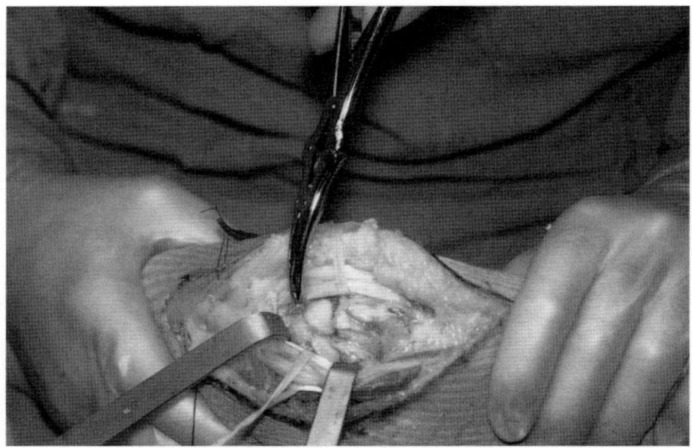

Figure 38.3

Wrist joint synovectomy. A dorsal approach does not allow a complete wrist joint synovectomy.

movement in flexion and extension to be useful. It needs to be stable and pain-free with an extension of 20–30°, flexion of 10°, and ulnar deviation of 10°, but with as much pronation and supination as possible.

This section aims to assess the value of each procedure that is usually designated 'wrist synovectomy'.

The usefulness of synovectomy of the wrist joint, which is a partitioned joint and difficult to treat (Figure 38.3), was doubted for a long time, when this procedure was performed alone and recurrences were frequent. The extensor tenosynovectomy is an important step. Transposition of the extensor retinaculum (Figure 38.4) protects the extensor tendons from any recurrence of synovitis; it reinforces the dorsal joint capsule, and its suture to the fibrous complex at the ulnar aspect of the wrist significantly improves the stability of the ulnar side of the wrist.

The resection of the distal section of the ulna (Figure 38.5) allows a complete synovectomy of the distal radio-ulnar joint that would otherwise be impossible. It has an obvious action in preventing tendon ruptures. The extent of resection of the distal ulna should be limited to the ulnar head and must allow, in the absence of elbow lesions, the re-establishment of as much prono-supination as possible, which gives significant functional improvement. Resection of the distal ulna, despite its apparent benefits, has been blamed for accentuating ulnar translocation of the carpus. This point of view is still debated (Fourastier et al 1992, Van Gemert et al 1994).

The principal fibrous structures that stabilize the wrist on the medial side consist of the triangular fibrocartilaginous complex and its expansions on the ulnar side of the wrist. The triangular ligament is destroyed early in the disease by the invasion of rheumatoid tissue, so that the ulnar head becomes unstable and subluxes. It is unlikely that conservation of the ulnar head, especially when it is subluxed, can play a significant part in the stabilization of the wrist. Indeed, it is common to find an ulnar translocation of the carpus despite conservation of the ulnar head. It seems that the rheumatoid process contributed more to ulnar dislocation than resection of the distal ulna.

We think, like Black et al (1977), that it is the destructive process at the ulnar border of the radius rather than resection of the distal ulna that leads to carpal translocation. However, Gainor and Schaberg (1985) found a correlation between marked ulnar translocation and excision that exceeded 2 cm of the distal ulna.

Procedures for stabilization of the wrist have certainly improved the results, by preventing deterioration.

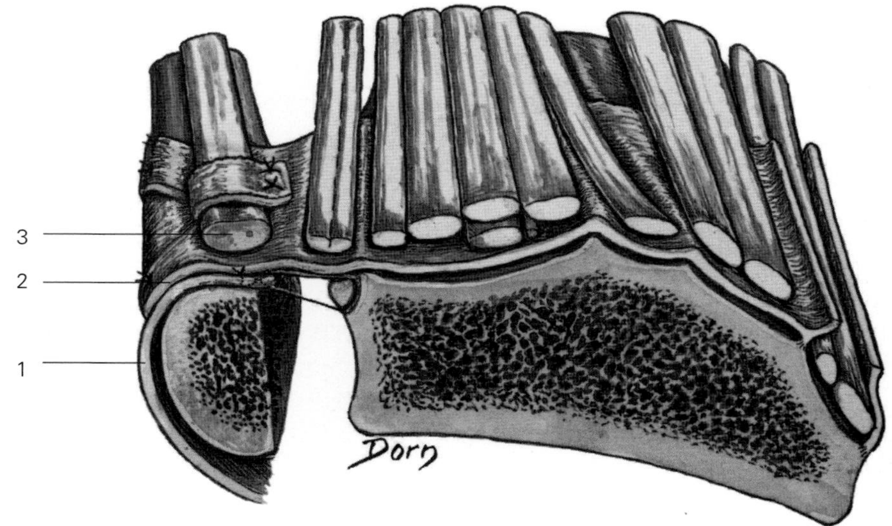

Figure 38.4

Transposition of the dorsal retinaculum deep to the extensor tendons. This transposition: (a) protects the extensor tendons from recurrence of synovitis, (b) reinforces the dorsal joint capsule, (c) its ulnar extremity improves the stabilization of the ulna shaft, and (d) allows dorsalization of the ECU tendon.

1 Oblique portion of the dorsal retinaculum
2 Transverse portion of the dorsal retinaculum
3 ECU tendon dorsalized by means of a pulley constructed from a slip of the dorsal retinaculum

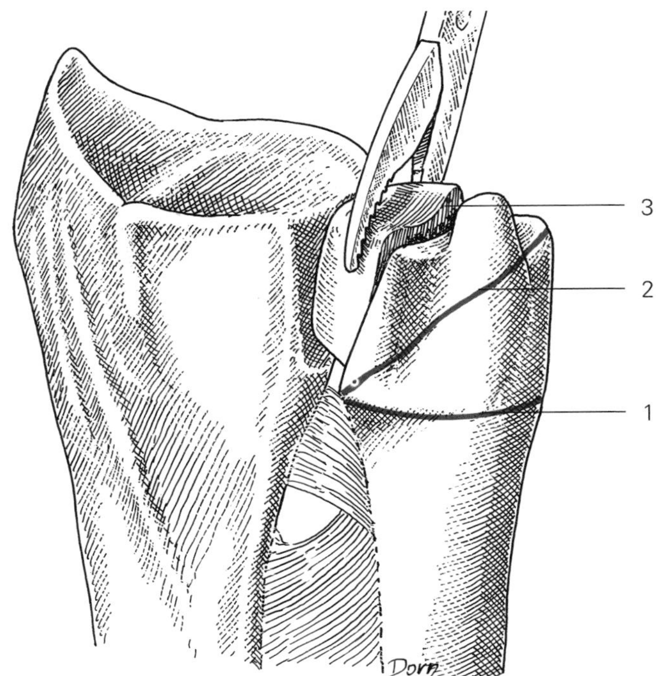

Figure 38.5

Resection of the distal ulna.

1 Transverse Darrach's procedure, just proximal to the distal radioulnar joint
2 Oblique resection including the ulnar styloid (type 2)
3 Oblique Bower's type 3 resection

Reconstruction of the capsulo-ligamentous ulnar structures give good results when the longitudinal axis of the wrist is preserved and the evolution of the disease is slow (Figure 38.6).

The Sauvé–Kapandji procedure (Figure 38.7), which is routinely performed by some surgeons in association with a wrist synovectomy, increases by an appreciable amount the area of the distal radial articular surface and support of the translocating ulna. It may have a stabilizing effect on the carpus, particularly in early cases of wrist synovectomies when the ligaments inserted on the ulnar head are still preserved. The main advantage of this procedure is cosmetic, owing to the conservation of the ulnar head ledge.

Partial radio-carpal arthrodesis between the radius and the lunate is a more effective stabilizer (Figure 38.8). It is indicated when ulnar and/or volar carpal translation cannot be corrected and an intra-articular correction of the radio-carpal joint is needed. It is preferable to try to correct the position of the lunate before its fixation.

Radioscapholunate arthrodesis (Figure 38.9) is indicated in more advanced cases with destruction of cartilage of the radioscaphoid joint or when the scaphoid is in a flexed position with its distal pole protruding into the carpal tunnel. The longitudinal axis of the scaphoid should be reduced and fixed at 60° relative to the axis of the radius.

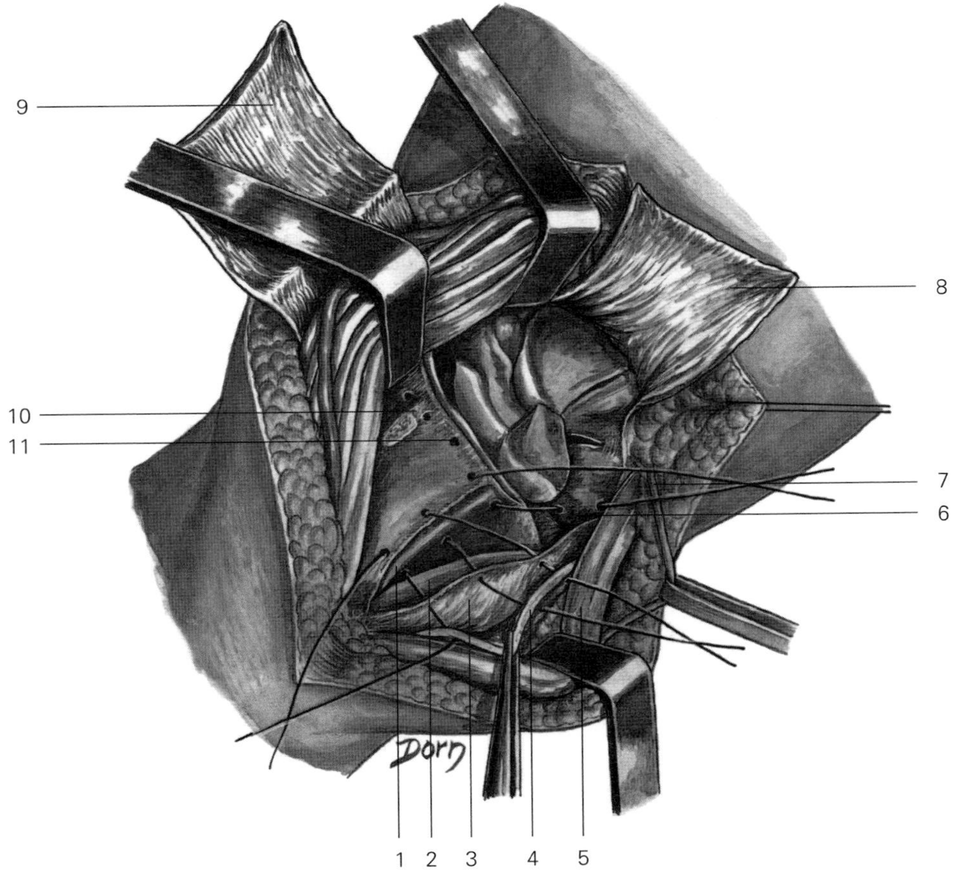

Figure 38.6

Capsulo-ligamentous stabilization.

1 Posteromedial border of the radius
2 Distal ulna after oblique type 2 resection
3 Distal radioulnar part of the dorsal retinaculum
4 Oblique ulnar part of the dorsal retinaculum
5 ECU tendon
6 Triquetrum
7 Dorsal sensory branch of the ulnar nerve
8 Wrist dorsal capsule
9 Transverse part of dorsal retinaculum
10 Lister's tubercle
11 Holes in the posterior border of the articular surface of the radius for suture of the wrist capsule
12 Three holes are drilled in the posteromedial border of the radius, permitting passage to three strong non-absorbable transosseous sutures. The distal suture is fixed through the triquetrum bone in order to correct supination of the carpus

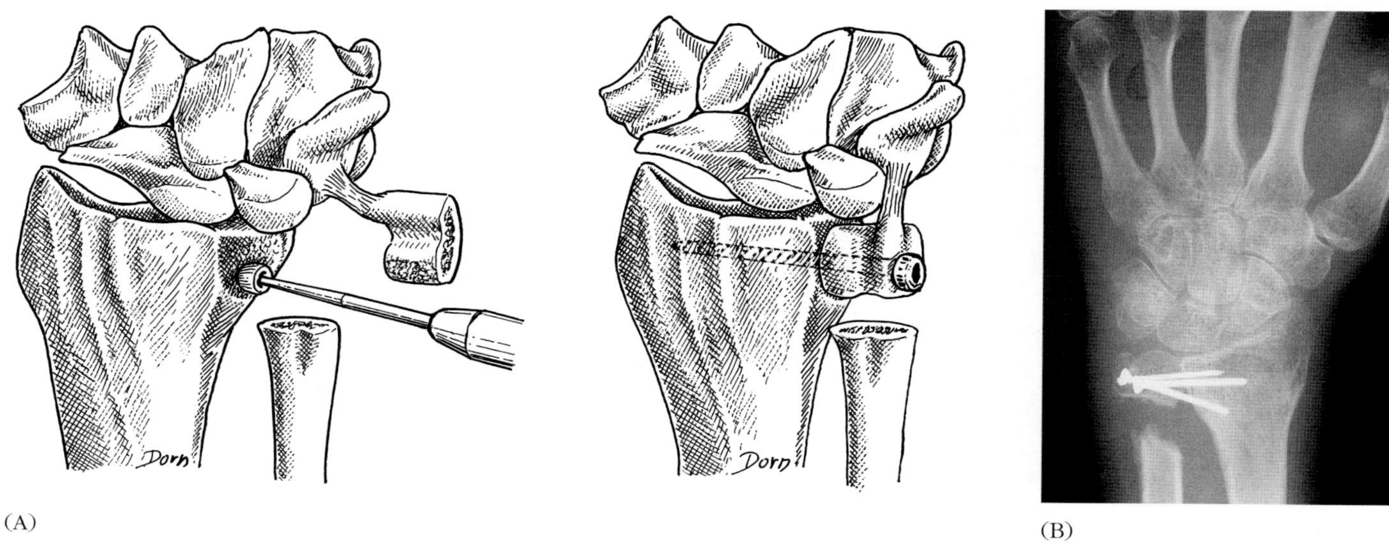

(A) (B)

Figure 38.7

Sauvé–Kapandji procedure. (A) Technique. (B) If the resection of the distal ulna is too proximal, there is a risk of symptomatic instability of the proximal ulnar stump.

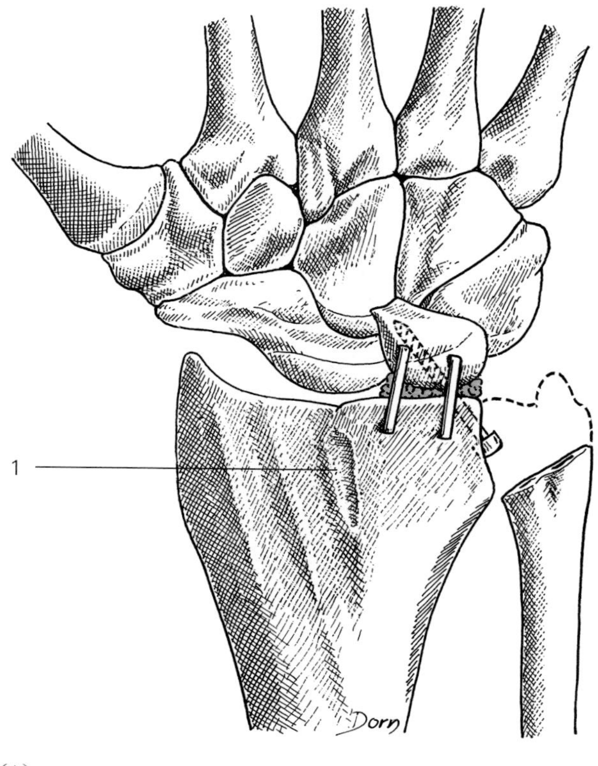

(A)

Figure 38.8

Radiolunate arthrodesis. (A) Technique of Chamay et al (1983). (B) Clinical case.

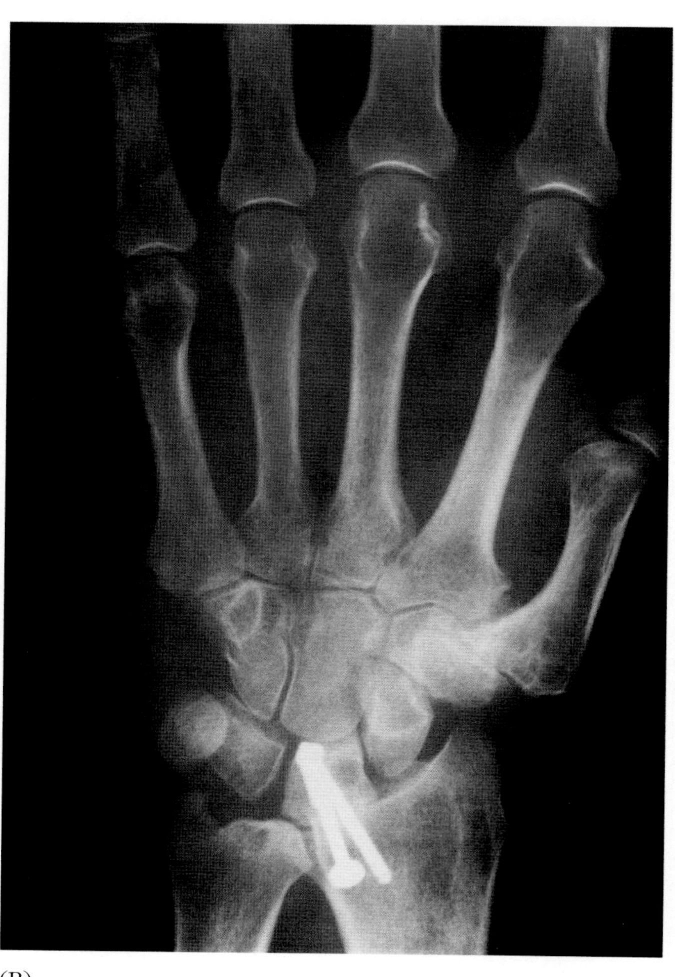

(B)

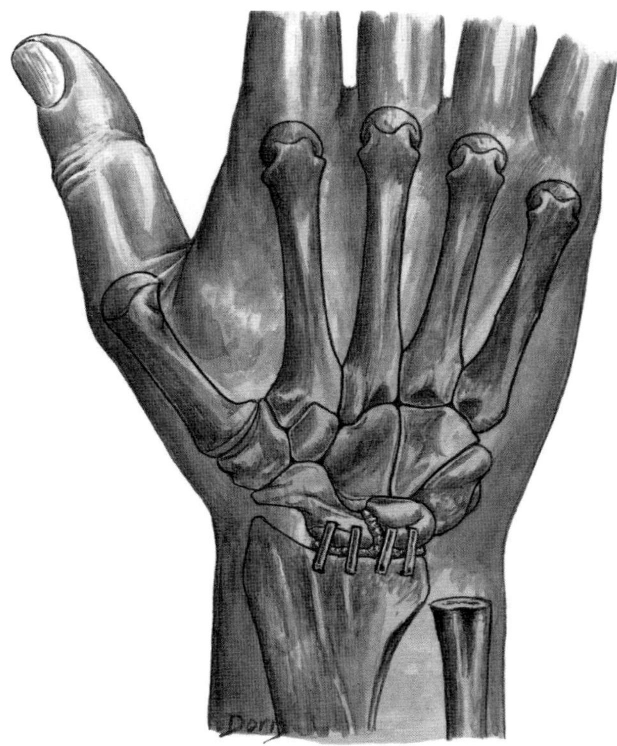

Figure 38.9
Radioscapholunate arthrodesis.

Partial radiocarpal arthrodesis is an alternative to complete wrist fusion when the midcarpal joint is preserved.

We know that the head of the capitate is often well preserved in the rheumatoid wrist, with its cartilage. Risk of late deterioration of the midcarpal joint remains.

Radiological follow-up of the radiolunate arthrodesis, with a mean of 5 years, by Della Santa and Chamay (1995) compared operated and non-operated wrists in the same patients. The progression of carpal collapse was the same in the two groups and ulnar translocation was found to be slowed down. However, partial radiocarpal arthrodesis is unable to protect the wrist in rapidly destructive forms of the rheumatoid disease (group 3 in Simmen and Huber's classification (Simmen and Huber 1992).

All long-term studies of more than 10 years show a discrepancy between radiographic appearances which continue to deteriorate, and the usual absence of pain, and useful function, even if there is a more pronounced limitation of movements.

Only 2–6% of patients followed over a period of 10 years needed arthrodesis, according to Mannerfelt's figures and a multicenter study (Mannerfelt 1984, Gschwend and Kentsch 1985). Compared with the opposite side, which was not subjected to synovectomy, we can say that precious time can be saved and unnecessary operations can be avoided.

Synovectomy with denervation and stabilizing techniques has become our basic operation for rheumatoid wrists.

Arthroplasties

The term arthroplasty covers a number of different types of operations that aim to mobilize a joint and includes resection arthroplasty, flexible hinge implant, and total joint prosthesis. Whatever the joint, an arthroplasty cannot function unless the flexor and extensor tendon apparatus is active and mobile.

Resection arthroplasties

Resection arthroplasties are difficult to stabilize. Even the resection of the distal ulna should not exceed 2 cm because of the risk of symptomatic instability to the proximal ulnar stump, as evidenced by a clunk on rotation of the forearm. Some authors have noticed this ulnar clunk in more than 17% of patients after the Sauvé–Kapandji operation (Taleisnik 1992, Vincent et al 1993).

Total wrist replacement

Total wrist replacements, whether cemented, covered with porous coating to promote osseous integration or fixed with screws, are all associated with specific problems. They only have limited indications especially in rheumatoid arthritis, because of the poor quality of the bony support.

Silastic implants

The flexible silastic implants designed by Alfred Swanson (1972) have supplanted most of the other forms of arthroplasties in rheumatoid hands. The addition of a flexible implant to a classic resection arthroplasty maintains the alignment of the bony extremities but is not capable of correcting a deformity or guaranteeing stability in the same way as an articular prosthesis. All deformity should be corrected before the implant is inserted. Any stability is achieved only by the formation of a fibrous neocapsule around the spacer and by ligamentous reconstruction.

Although such stability is insufficient for a young manual worker, in older subjects with polyarticular rheumatoid arthritis it allows good functional readaptation. The effect on pain is excellent and mobility can be achieved in a useful range. Unfortunately complications such as wear, breaking, dislocation, bony resorption, and incarceration limit the indications for these implants. The use of titanium grommets may help; they appear to

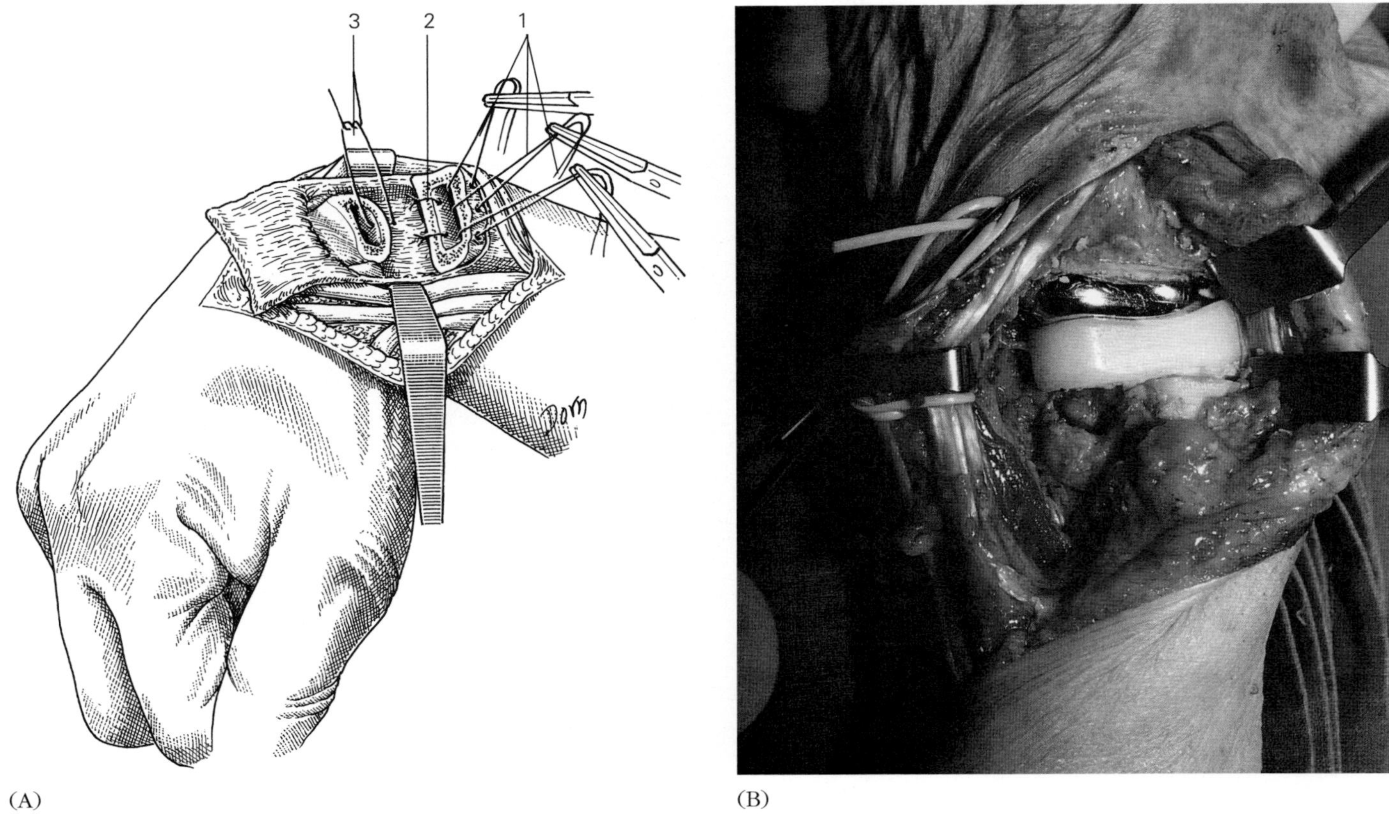

(A) (B)

Figure 38.10
(A) Wrist arthroplasty with flexible implant. (B) The implant is protected by a titanium grommet.

prolong the life of the implant by delaying implant fracture (Figure 38.10).

However, as time passes, a progressive alteration in the radiological appearance – for which there is no immediate clinical correlation – is seen. The deterioration of results in the long term may also be due to progression of the disease and aging of the patient. The frequency of these complications varies greatly among the different authors and the site of the implant.

It seems probable that surgical technique has a great influence. A correction of deformities by rebalancing soft tissues before the placement of implants, a perfect placement of the implant within the skeleton, the absence of wires and sutures throughout, are all factors that can improve the longevity of the implant (Stanky and Tobat 1993). On the other hand, implants are more vulnerable when they are exposed to shear forces. One must avoid excessive loads, like those produced by crutches or sticks, or excessive mobility at the arthroplasty site. All these possibilities explain the results that vary according to the patient and surgeon.

Long-term results also vary according to the site of the implant (Wilson et al 1993). Implants in the fingers have been shown to be much better tolerated than those at the wrist (Figure 38.11). The wear is slower and the fracturing of the implant is often compatible with the conservation of a satisfactory functional activity. The implants can be replaced (Figure 38.12).

Complications at the wrist are more frequent, occur earlier and are more extensive. The most worrying complication is probably the tissue reaction, showing the appearance of bony cysts that have developed around silicone wear particles, sometimes distant to the implant.

Silicone synovitis has been mostly found after a wrist bone replacement, they can be seen infrequently after a wrist arthroplasty, and rarely at the finger level. However, the existence of these complications has reduced the indications for these implants, mainly at the wrist level and in young patients.

Joint arthrodesis

Joint arthrodeses have multiple advantages: there is no pain from fixed joints, any deformity is corrected, recurrence is prevented, and both stability and strength of grip are improved. However, benefits are gained at the expense of joint mobility. The functional value of joint mobility differs considerably according to the joint.

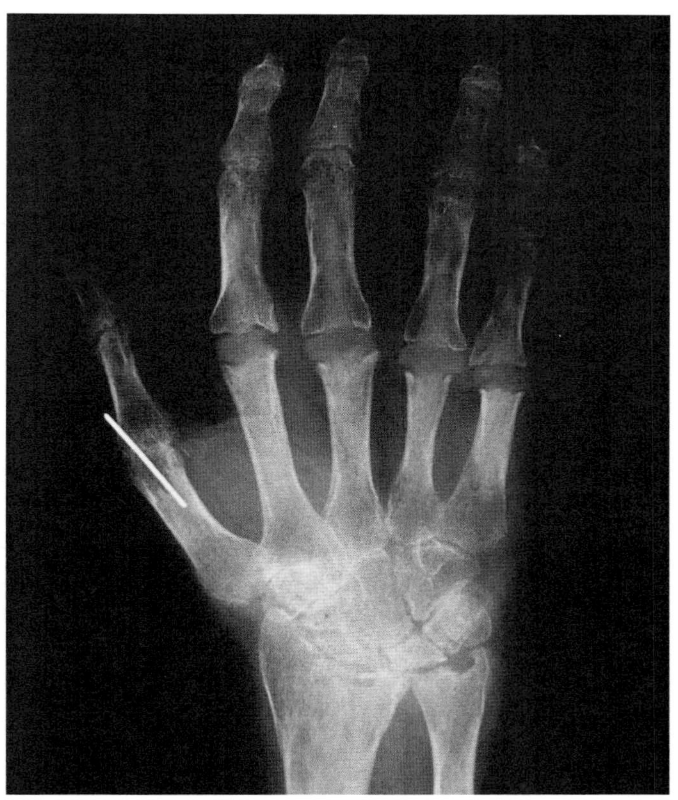

Figure 38.11
MP joint arthroplasties associated with a thumb MP joint fusion.

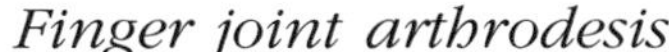

Finger joint arthrodesis

The joint in the hand in which loss of movement is felt the least is the metacarpophalangeal (MP) joint of the thumb, especially when the proximal and distal joints of the thumb retain their movement. Thus arthrodesis of the MP joint of the thumb is an excellent operation and is often indicated. However, it is essential that the length of the thumb ray is not overly diminished. The loss of length in a finger causes less functional problems than in the thumb and often may produce a functional benefit.

Loss of movement at the level of the distal interphalangeal (DIP) joint alters precision grip, but good function in the fingers can be maintained when the proximal interphalangeal (PIP) joints have a useful range of movement. The DIP joints should not be fixed in more than 15–30° of flexion according to the fingers.

Fusion in flexion of the PIP joint limits the ability to grip large objects but is well tolerated if the MP joint is mobile. Arthroplasty of the MP joint is often associated with a PIP joint arthrodesis.

Arthrodesis of the MP joints of the fingers produces major disabilities, as much when done in extension (limiting the grasp) as when done in flexion (preventing the gripping of large objects). Thus it is rarely performed.

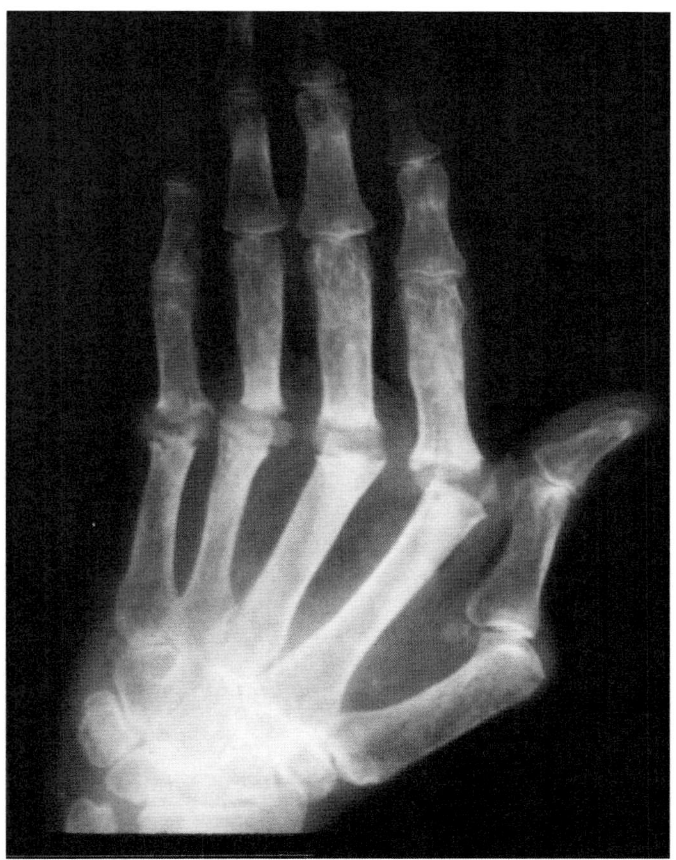

(A)

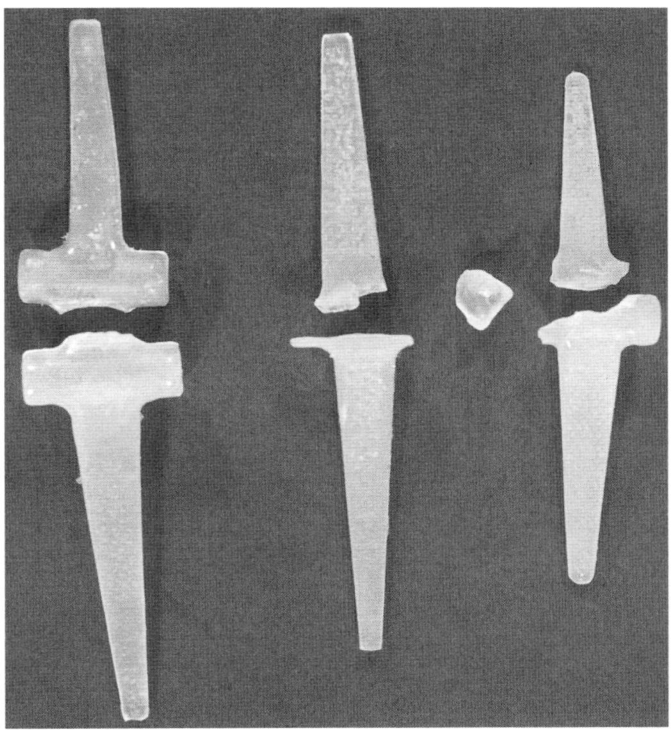

(B)

Figure 38.12
(A) Rupture of MP joint implants, (B) the ruptured implants.

Arthrodesis of the trapeziometacarpal joint at the base of the thumb is seldom indicated in rheumatoid arthritis. When the first metacarpal is fixed in opposition, it loses a large part of its functional value, because the movements required in grasping must come from the unstable MP joint, which is then pushed into hyperextension.

Total wrist arthrodesis

Total wrist arthrodesis eliminates pain at this level, and improves the strength and stability of the joint that determines the position of the hand. In addition, an arthrodesis of the wrist is usually easier to obtain in rheumatoid wrists (Figure 38.13). Against this fusion is the loss of flexion–extension movements, giving an active tenodesis effect and augmenting the action of finger flexion and extension. This effect is particularly useful after the repair or transfer of digital tendons, which is often necessary in rheumatoid hands. Furthermore, these patients often have involvement of the other joints of the limb and of the other wrist, considerably increasing the functional handicap experienced at the level of the hand. It must be remembered that a stiff, non-painful shoulder may become painful after wrist arthrodesis.

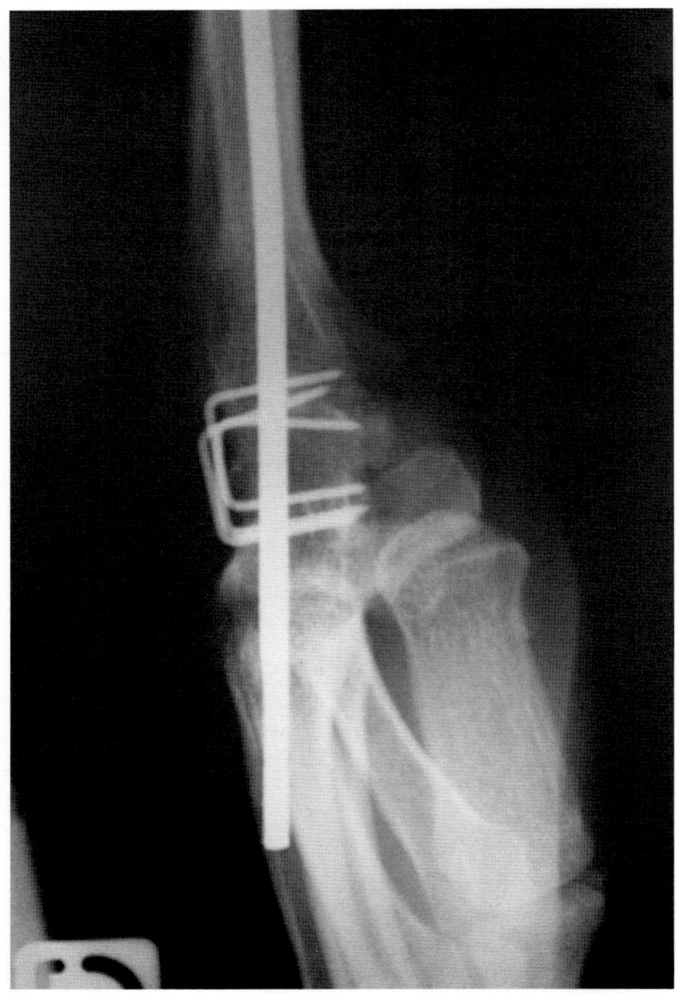

Figure 38.13
Wrist arthrodesis (Mannerfelt technique).

Indications for the various procedures

These indications are changing and will continue to do so as long-term results become available and surgical techniques improve.

At the level of the wrist joint

For a long time, we have had at our disposal three types of operation for rheumatoid wrists: synovectomy, arthroplasty, and complete arthrodesis. Each operation had its specific indication. Tenosynovectomy of the extensor tendons associated with wrist synovectomy was used at an early stage, on a well aligned wrist. Arthroplasty and arthrodesis were indicated when the carpus was displaced and the articular surfaces were damaged. Arthroplasty was preferable to arthrodesis when the state of the tendons allowed active mobilization of the wrist.

During the last decades, there has been a considerable evolution in surgical techniques and their indications (Allieu 1996). Two factors have contributed to this evolution. Long-term study of synovectomy with stabilization of the wrist has often shown the persistence of clinical improvement after more than 10 years. However, despite a promising start arthroplasty has displayed numerous complications and no longer seems so attractive.

The good results obtained after early synovectomy of the wrist have encouraged us to extend its indications

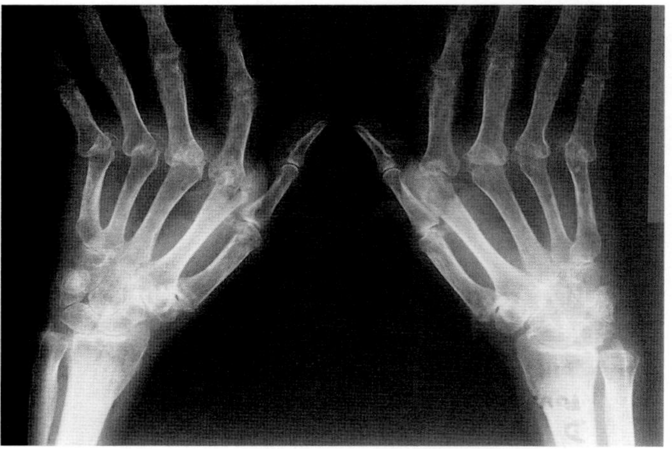

Figure 38.14(a)
Bilateral wrist synovectomy at an advanced stage.

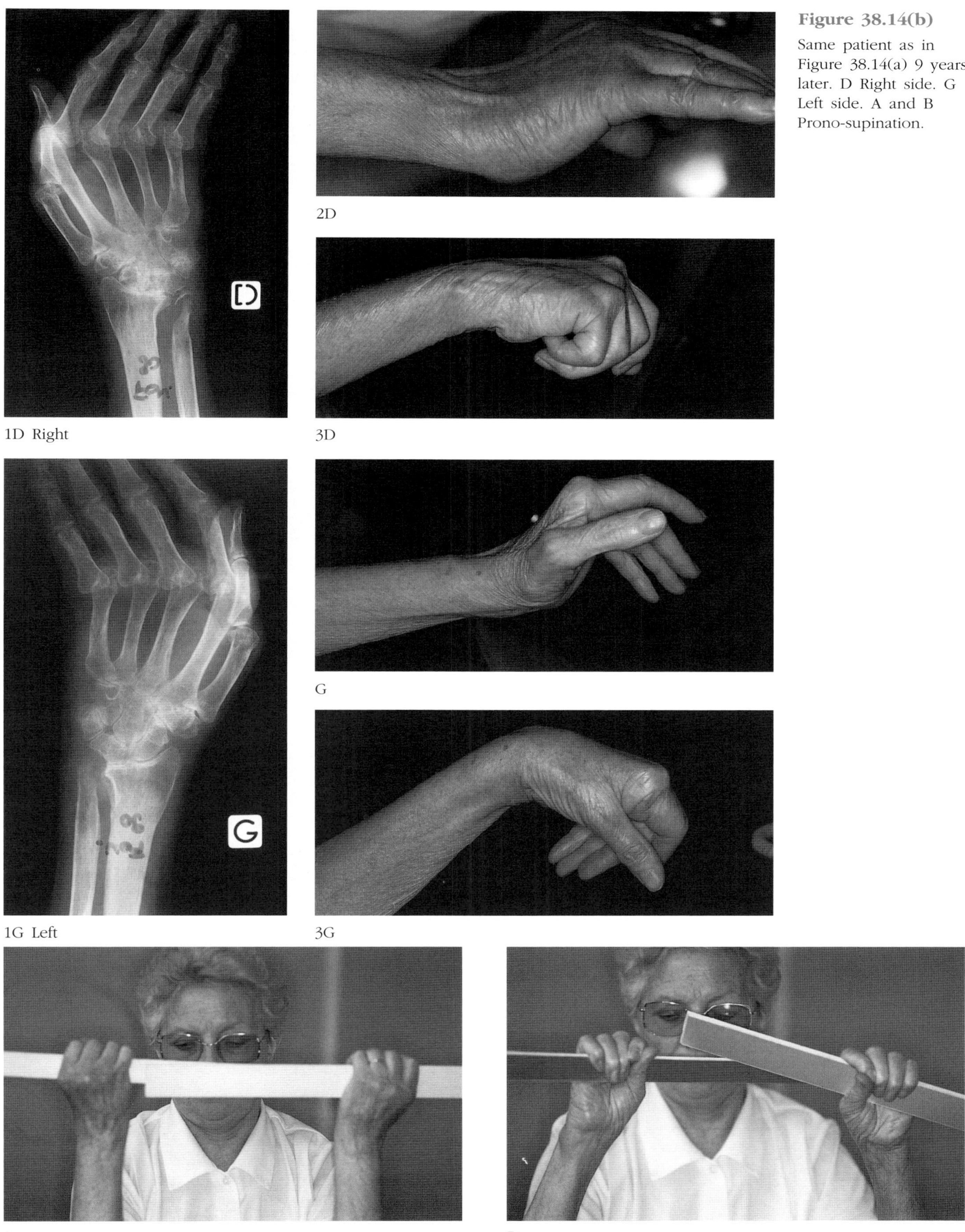

Figure 38.14(b)

Same patient as in Figure 38.14(a) 9 years later. D Right side. G Left side. A and B Prono-supination.

and to practice it at an advanced stage in association with other stabilizing procedures that are adapted as the case demands (Figure 38.14).

Thus synovectomy with denervation and stabilizing techniques has become our basic operation for rheumatoid wrists (Tubiana 1990). However, the surgical indication should take into account several factors, as described below.

The local state

This necessitates clinical and radiological examination. The clinical state of the wrist is evaluated according to the degree of pain, quantity of synovitis, state of the skin, mobility and stability of the wrist, and any deformities. The radiological examination does not always coincide with the clinical examination.

Radiologic examination is so important that attempts have been made to classify lesions based on the radiologic appearances, to clarify the indications for surgery. Thus the Wrightington classification (Hodgson et al 1989) includes four groups of increasing severity based solely on radiologic criteria and corresponding to different, specific operative indications. This classification relies on existing radiologic changes but has no prognostic indicators. The classification used at the Schulthes Clinic in Zurich is more ambitious (Simmen and Huber 1992). It is based on the type of radiologic change rather than the extent of the lesions. The analysis of series of radiographs taken as the disease progresses has allowed the authors to describe three types of change, requiring different treatments. Group 1 proceeds to a spontaneous ankylosis; group 2, in which osteoporosis as subchondral rheumatoid lysis is accompanied by the sclerotic signs of a degenerative arthritis, but the wrist remains aligned, and a synovectomy is indicated; and group 3, in which the progress is rapid and the wrist quickly becomes deformed with an accompanying loss of stability. Loss of the carpal height and progressive ulnar translation allow progress to be followed on graphs. The changes are most rapid in group 3 (disintegration) rather than in group 1 or 2, and this group requires an early bony stabilization.

Despite the great interest in these and other radiologic classifications, it seems that the indications for surgery should not rely solely on radiographic changes. It is necessary to include other factors, such as the morbidity of the disease and the effect of medical treatment. If progress of the rheumatoid disease is slow, the disease is well controlled, and the longitudinal axis is well maintained, we usually perform surgical synovectomy with the prophylactic aims of preventing tendon ruptures and nerve compression, resecting bony prominences or spurs, and facilitating the stabilization of the wrist after synovectomy. At an early stage a ligamentoplasty or a Sauvé–Kapandji procedure is used in women for cosmetic reasons; at more advanced stages when carpal displacement is not reducible without the help of a surgi-

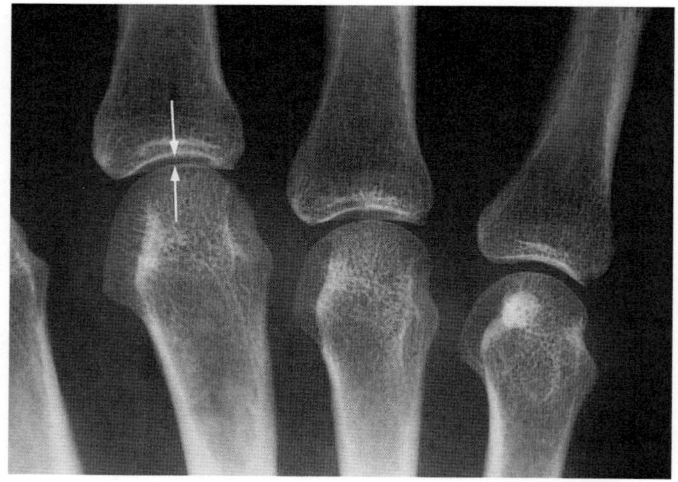

(A)

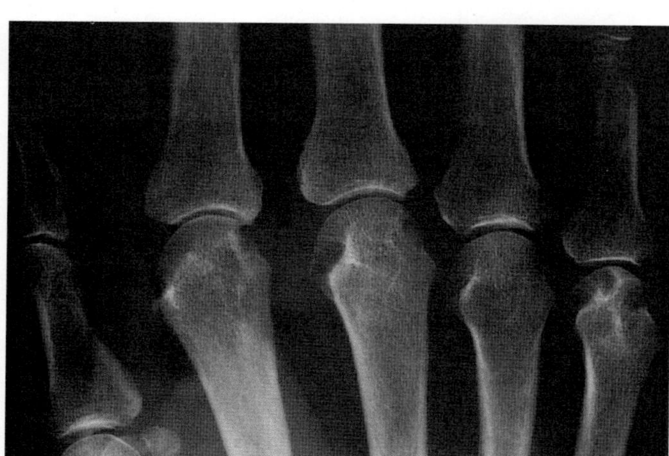

(B)

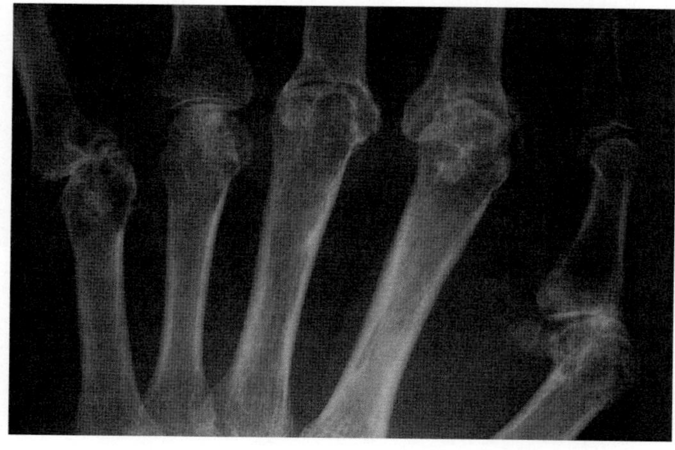

(C)

Figure 38.15

Evolution of MP joint rheumatoid lesions. (A) An early stage, synovitis without articular surface lesion. Synoviorthesis is used. (B) Subcartilaginous erosions. Even if the granulomatous synovitis is surgically removed, recurrence is extremely frequent. (C) Natural evolution of the lesions: joint destruction.

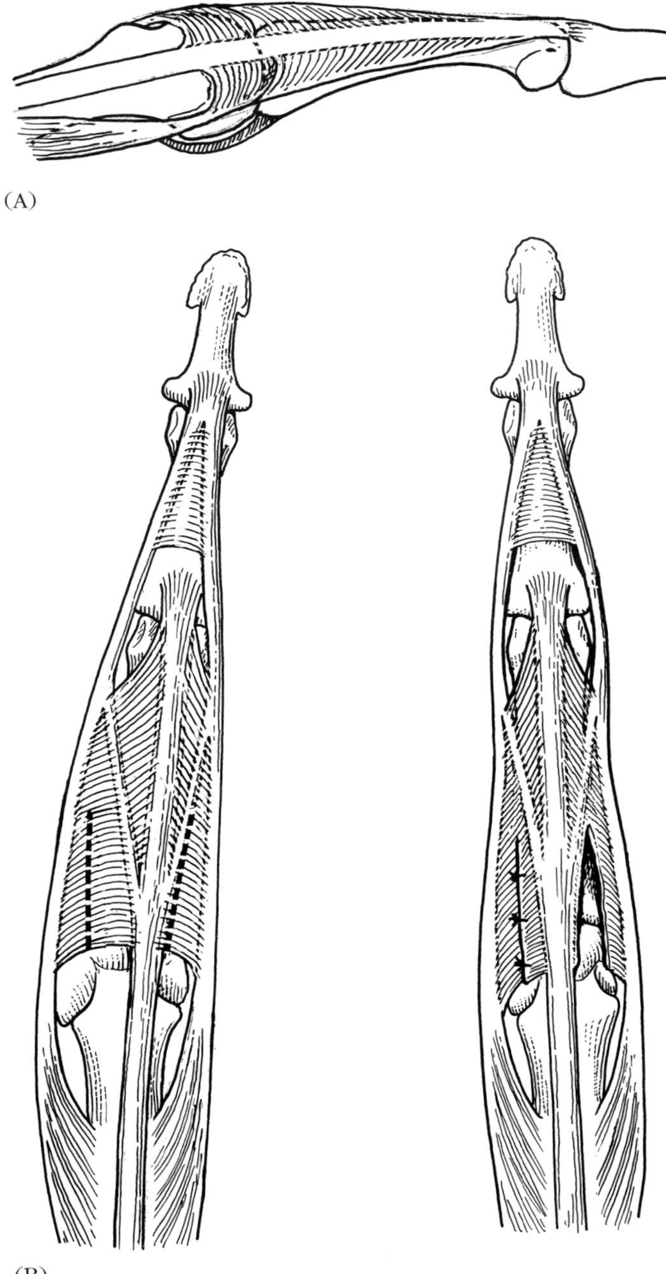

Figure 38.16
(A) Ulnar subluxation of the extensor tendon; (B and C) corrected by plasty of the radial fibers of the extensor hood.

cal bony procedure, a radiolunate arthrodesis is indicated.

Alternatively, if the progression of the disease is poorly controlled by the medical treatment, with bony destruction, we would consider synovectomy associated with partial radio-carpal arthrodesis or even a total wrist arthrodesis when the bony destruction is rapidly progressive.

Proximal row carpectomy

Proximal row carpectomy is another alternative when the aim is to conserve a limited mobility of the wrist and when the midcarpal joint is considerably destroyed. This operation, practiced only when there is significant destruction of the first row (which is subluxed anterior to the radius), consists of a bony realignment rather than a strict procedure.

Wrist arthroplasty with an implant

Arthroplasty with an implant is reserved for the elderly who are not permanently using sticks or crutches and whose extensor carpi radialis tendons are sufficient to allow extension of the wrist. Furthermore, the diaphysis of the second or third metacarpal must be fairly wide to accommodate the tail of the implant. Here also there may be a discrepancy between the radiographic appearance of the wrist – which is often alarming – and the absence of pain.

Total wrist arthrodesis

The range of applications for this procedure has decreased, but it still has some useful indications, particularly the following:

1. In patients with destroyed wrists who need to use sticks or crutches.
2. When there is a carpal dislocation in association with a rupture of the extensor tendons of the wrist.
3. In cases of failure of arthroplasty when revision surgery and replacement of the implant or prosthesis cannot be performed easily.
4. In cases of bilateral lesions, on one side, with the aim of achieving one stable, strong wrist, especially if the patient is relatively young.

At the finger joints

The three finger joints, with three phalanges, constitute a multiarticular chain, and a deformity at one level may alter the balance of the whole finger. We use a classification in four stages, already mentioned, as a guide for the therapeutic indications at each joint level (see Chapter 3 and Chapter X).

At the MP joint level

When there is synovitis of the MP joint without articular surface lesions, synoviorthesis is used. Synoviorthesis is the destruction of the synovium by a chemical or radioactive substance. In case of recurrence, another injection can be done or a surgical synovectomy, when MP joint synovitis is associated with finger deformities. Indications for surgical synovectomy alone are limited because of the high incidence of recurrence (Figure 38.15). Rheumatoid deformities at this level are essentially ulnar deviation and flexion deformity (see Chapter 36).

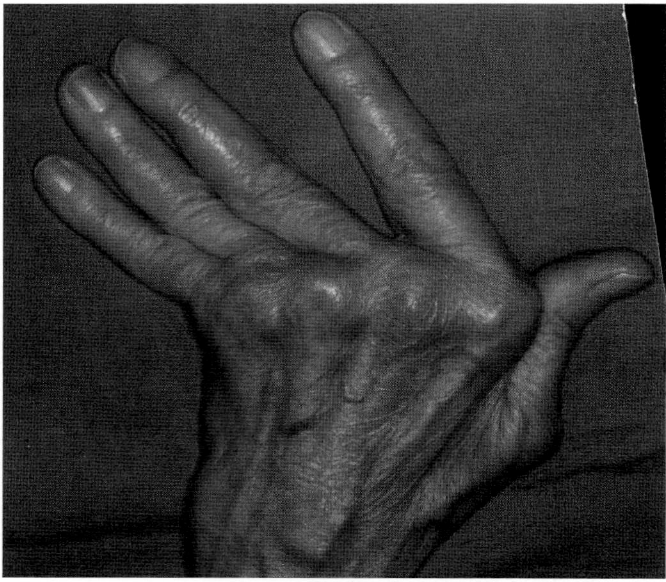

Figure 38.17
Swan neck deformities associated with ulnar deviation of the fingers.

Lateral deviation

Lateral deviations of the fingers in adults are almost exclusively ulnar. Radial deviation of the fingers is seen in juvenile arthritis, often associated with an ulnar deviation of the wrist (Figures 38.16, 38.17 and 38.18).

MP joint flexion deformity

MP joint flexion deformity may be caused by intrinsic muscle contracture or MP joint lesions.

Very often MP flexion deformity is associated with MP joint subluxation and intrinsic tightness. This is a good indication for an MP joint arthroplasty, especially when MP flexion is associated with a swan neck deformity (Figure 38.19).

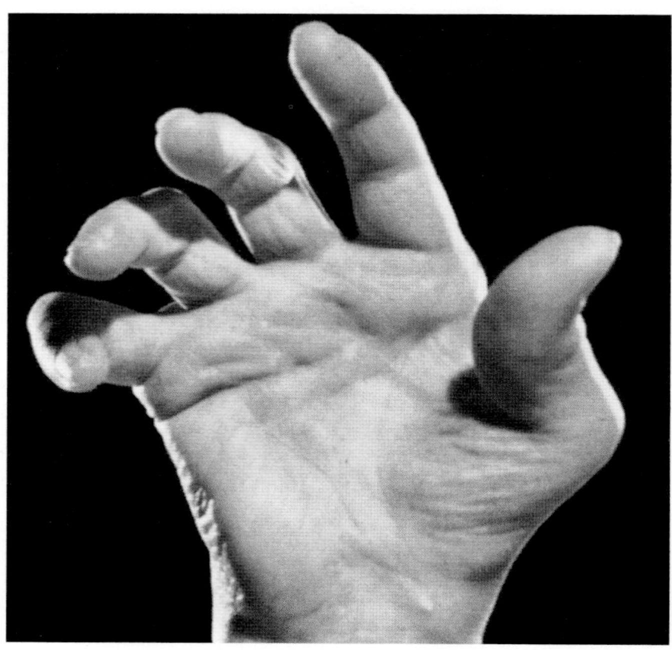

Figure 38.18
Ulnar deviation of the fingers on a rheumatoid hand, associated with a boutonnière deformity of the thumb.

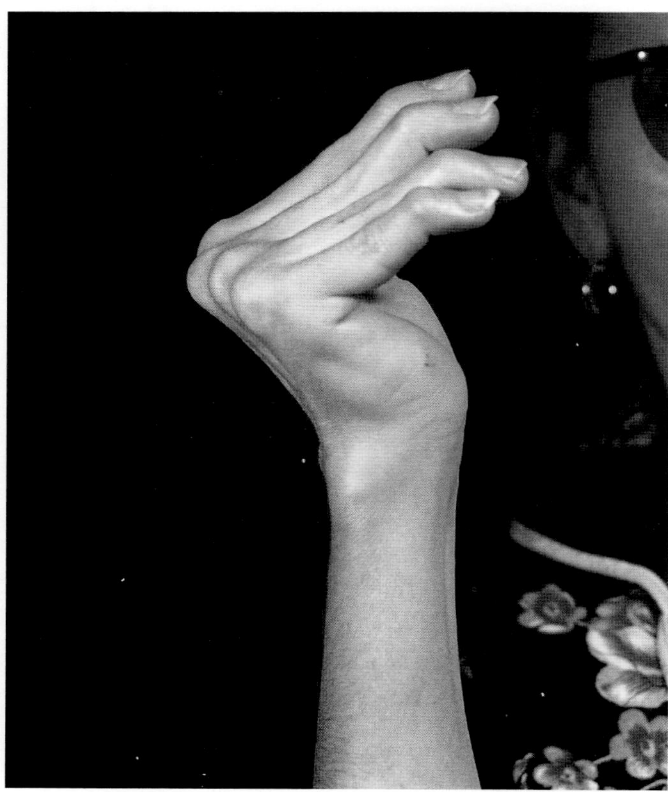

Figure 38.19
Flexion deformity of the MP joints.

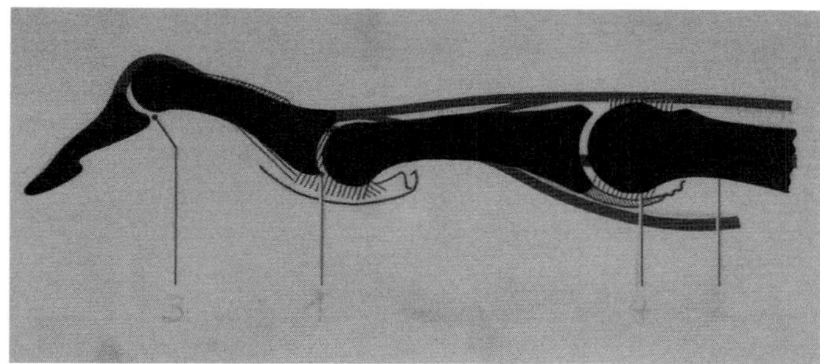

Figure 38.20

Swan neck deformity. 1, DIP joint; 2, transverse retinacular ligament; 3, sagittal band; 4, metacarpal.

At the proximal interphalangeal joint level

Surgical synovectomy is performed when the synovitis is associated with a deformity that needs surgical correction. Two deformities seen at this level in the course of the rheumatoid arthritis are the boutonnière and swan neck deformities (see Chapter 36, Pathogenesis of long finger deformities); they are progressive conditions. Corrective splinting and exercises are used at all stages, alone or in conjunction with surgery; they constitute an essential step before any operation. Many surgical procedures have been proposed for both boutonnière and swan neck deformities; they should be selected carefully taking into account the discomfort experienced by the patient and the possibilities for repair.

Rheumatoid swan neck deformity (Figure 38.20)

It is important to treat swan neck deformity at an early stage to prevent stiffness of the PIP joint in extension. It is also necessary to treat the cause of the deformity.

- **Stage 1.** There is no limitation of passive motion in any finger joint. The treatment is aimed at correcting the dynamic imbalance at the two IP joints. In all cases synovitis of the flexor tendons is treated first and the PIP joint laxity must be corrected to prevent recurrence of the deformity. Several procedures have been described (see Chapter 36); the simplest is flexor superficialis tenodesis.
- **Stage 2.** Limited PIP motion is influenced by MP joint position with a tenodesis effect. Indications for intrinsic muscle release have been described.
- **Stage 3.** There is fixed deformity, articular surfaces are intact. Contracture of the extensor apparatus, dorsal skin, and later, para-articular structures, fix the deformity. Nalebuff and Terrono (1999) have shown that gentle manipulation into flexion, associated with splinting, and an exercise program, may progressively correct the deformity. If not, the clinician should proceed to a dorsal soft tissue release, followed by a PIP joint tenodesis to prevent recurrence of the deformity.
- **Stage 4.** PIP articular surfaces are destroyed. The only two options are arthroplasty or fusion of the PIP joint. The choice mostly depends on the condition of the other two finger joints.

Rheumatoid boutonnière deformity

- **Stage 1.** No limitation of passive motion in any finger joint.

  Splinting in extension at the PIP level, combined with active flexion exercises of the DIP is indicated.

  Extensor tendon tenotomy has been suggested by Fowler in an attempt to restore the balance of extensor forces. This procedure is combined with dynamic splinting.
- **Stage 2.** Tenodesis effect. When the middle phalanx is maintained in extension, flexion of the distal phalanx is not possible.

(A)

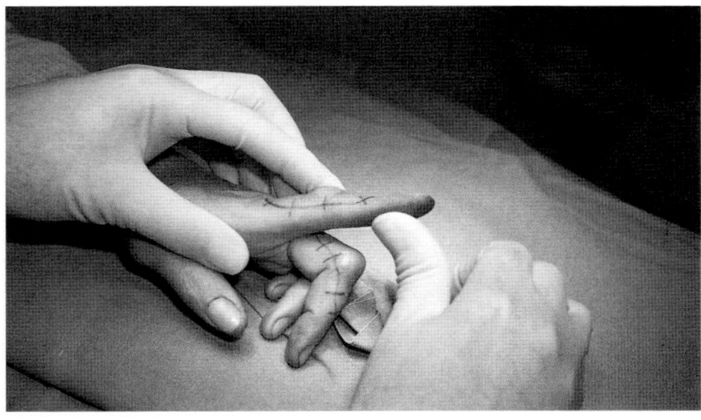

(B)

Figure 38.21

Rheumatoid boutonnière deformities of the fingers. (A) Before rehabilitation; (B) complete passive correction of the deformity has been obtained by exercises and splintage.

Surgical treatment theoretically consists of partial resection of the contracted oblique retinacular ligament to correct the distal joint hyperextension. This procedure is rarely performed separately on a rheumatoid boutonnière deformity. A tenotomy of the lateral extensor tendons at the level of the middle phalanx seems most appropriate for the restoration of the extensor mechanism balance.

- **Stage 3.** Fixed deformity with articular surfaces intact. Flexion of the PIP joint is possible, but total extension is limited. In addition, flexion of the DIP joint is not possible. The distal phalanx is precluded for prehension. This is the main functional disability and its treatment is a priority.

Indications for surgery should be evaluated cautiously and candidates should be selected carefully. A flexion deficit of the distal phalanx can be more disabling to the grip than extension deficit in the PIP, especially in the ulnar fingers. On the other hand reconstruction of the extensor apparatus at the PIP joint is difficult, and surgery must not jeopardize flexor function in an attempt to gain extension.

Treatment of a rheumatoid boutonnière deformity in stage 3 includes two distinct steps: correction of the deformities and repair of the extensor apparatus. Both the extension deficit of the PIP joint and the flexion deficit of the distal joint must be corrected. Correction of the flexion contracture at the PIP joint is usually achieved by splintage and exercises (Figure 38.21).

Extensor mechanism reconstruction is attempted, with the best chance of success when the interphalangeal joint contractions are passively corrected.

A liberation of the anterior structures may be considered. The fibrous flexor tendon sheath is opened at the level of pulley C1. Any tenosynovitis of the flexor tendons should be removed, and the freedom of the tendons should be tested.

Repair of the extensor apparatus includes shortening of the central extensor tendon and correction of the volar subluxation of the lateral extensor tendons (Figures 38.22 and 38.23) (see also Figures 3.25–3.27 in Chapter 3).

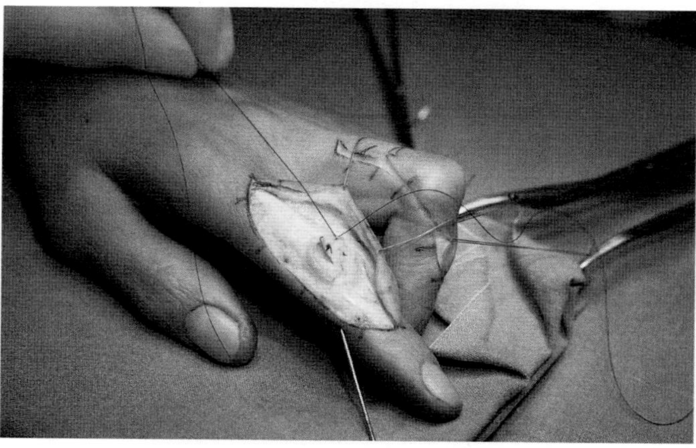

Figure 38.22

Shortening of the central extensor tendon and correction of the volar subluxation of the lateral extensor tendons on the index finger. The long finger is then operated.

- **Stage 4.** Radiography shows significant articular lesions at the PIP level. In cases of severe fixed flexion deformity of the PIP joint, arthrodesis of the PIP joint in a functional position is a reliable procedure. It can be combined with an oblique tenotomy of the two lateral extensor tendons to obtain flexion of the distal phalanx.

Arthroplasty of the PIP joint provides another alternative when the extensor system is salvageable.

Tenotomy of the lateral extensor tendons can also be done alone if the lack of the distal joint flexion is more disabling than the lack of PIP joint extension (see Figure 3.29 in Chapter 3, Late extensor mechanism repair).

At the distal interphalangeal joint level

- **Stage 1.** Mallet deformity with no limitation of passive motion and absence of deformity at the PIP joint. This is treated by synoviorthesis and splintage.
- **Stage 2.** Tenodesis effect: DIP joint flexion with PIP joint hyperextension. The best solution is a DIP joint arthrodesis in slight flexion.
- **Stages 3 and 4.** Fixed deformity. Persistent symptomatic deformity may benefit from fusion of the distal joint.

If pronounced, lateral deviation of the distal phalanx will also benefit from fusion, which gives a good cosmetic result.

Surgical indications in the thumb ray

Surgical joint synovectomies are rarely indicated as a single procedure because of their high recurrence rate. They are nearly always associated with other procedures for correction of a deformity. Depending on the site of the lesion, different types of thumb deformities have been described, the most common being the boutonnière and the swan neck. The restoration of a functional thumb requires that one of two proximal joints, the MP or the first carpometacarpal joint, be mobile and painless. In all cases, the aim of the surgical treatment is to limit fusion to one single joint. However, a double arthrodesis is possible on the two distal joints.

The most commonly used procedures on a rheumatoid thumb are:

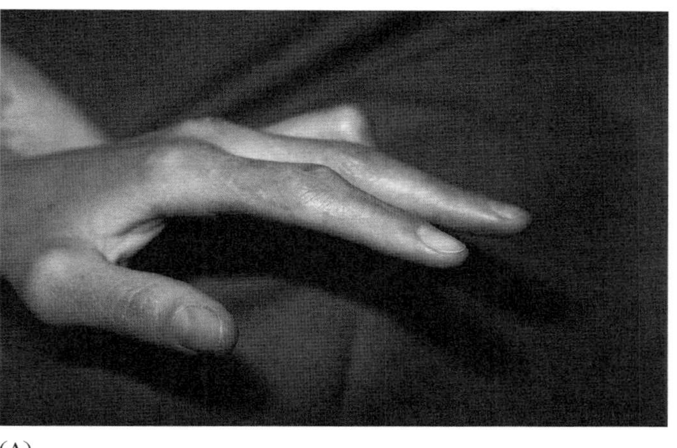
(A)

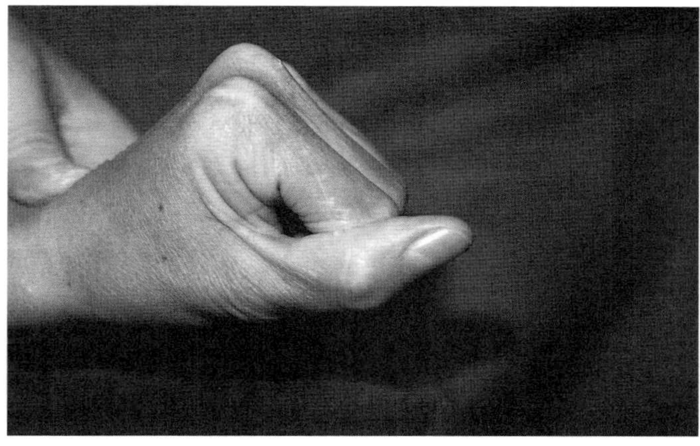
(B)

Figure 38.23
Results after extensor mechanism repair. (A and B) Full extension and flexion of the index and long fingers.

- IP level, arthrodesis.
- MP level, soft tissue procedures, capsulodesis, arthrodesis, MP flexible implant arthroplasty may be performed when arthrodesis is contraindicated.

At the carpometacarpal level, implant arthroplasty has limited indications because of the frequent fragmentation of the implant. We prefer to perform a resection arthroplasty (Tubiana 1998). The space between the metacarpal and the carpus is filled by a tendon, folded in an anchovy fashion. Advancement of the abductor pollicus longus insertion on the metacarpal will maintain its abduction (Figure 38.24).

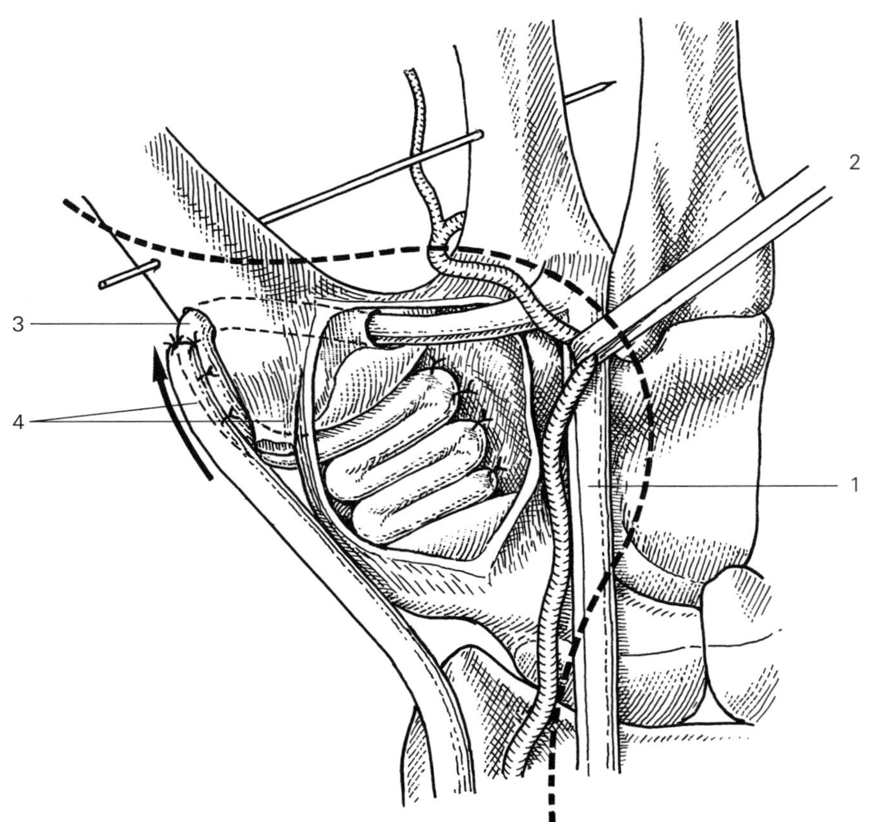

Figure 38.24
Trapeziometacarpal resection arthroplasty.

1. ECRL tendon. A long strip is taken from the radial side of the ECRL tendon
2. Radial artery
3. The ECRL strip, still inserted on the base of the second MP, is passed obliquely through the base of the first MP, from the ulnar side of the articular surface to the radial side of the bone (approx 1.5 cm distal from the articular surface). It is then used for the fibrous interposition and firmly sutured to the joint capsule
4. Advancement of the APL insertion and fixation to the ECRL tendon strip

Planning of the operating program

For each patient, several surgical programs are possible, but prudence demands that the number of procedures be kept to a minimum.

Progress in anesthesia, especially the increased use of regional anesthetic techniques, has considerably reduced its risks.

Order of intervention

When many sites need surgery it is recommended to begin with a tenosynovectomy of the flexor tendons at the wrist and digits. Thus, any nerve compression and associated pain are relieved, and at the same time the most important tendons of the hand are protected, and their range of motion is improved. This is an indispensable step before any procedure aimed at the recovery of the mobility of the finger joints is carried out. The second stage consists of extensor tendon tenosynovectomy associated with a dorsal wrist synovectomy and stabilization.

Reconstructive surgery on the joints should have a certain order. It is logical to start with the proximal joint, as wrist deformities have repercussions on the distal joints. In the same operating session, a procedure can be undertaken on the thumb.

We often combine a bony resection (the distal ulna) with an arthrodesis at another joint, in order to make use of the excised bone as a graft.

The third operation can be used for arthroplasty of the MP joints of the fingers, and any further procedures at the interphalangeal level. Again, it is necessary to follow a logical order. If there is a marked flexion contracture at the PIP joints, the correction of the PIP joint deformity must precede that of the MP joint arthroplasty, as the persistence of a PIP flexion deformity adversely affects the recuperation of MP joint flexion. However, a stiffness in extension of the PIP joint favors the recuperation of MP joint flexion, and the correction of a swan neck deformity must follow or be performed simultaneously with the MP joint arthroplasty.

The order should be flexible enough to be adapted to the needs of each patient. In general young people make heavy demands on their hands. The indications for implant arthroplasties should be carefully weighed; they should often be avoided. In the elderly patient, it is preferable to limit surgery to simple and effective procedures that do not need long periods of rehabilitation.

The operative program should obviously include the other hand. The first hand to be operated upon should be the most painful or that in which the lesions are the most threatening. The next operation will be on the other hand.

Rheumatoid involvement in the other areas such as the cervical spine, the proximal joints of the upper limb and the lower limbs should also be borne in mind and preferably treated before the hand.

Association with physiotherapy

The treatment of rheumatoid arthritis does not consist solely of the application of a basic effective treatment that is well tolerated by the patient in correcting deformities to improve function. It is also necessary to maintain these corrections, which is the main role of the physiotherapist. Thermoplastic orthesis adapted to the patient allows joints to rest and avoid deformity. Rehabilitation and its associated equipment are essential in the postoperative period. Occupational therapy has a very useful role in the re-education of the patient in the activities of daily living in such a way as to protect fragile joints.

References

Allieu Y (1996) Traitement chirurgical du poignet rhumatoïde. In: *La Main et le Poignet Rhumatoïdes*, Monographie du GEM (Expansion Scientifique Française: Paris) 63–79.

Black RM, Boswick JA Jr, Wiedel J (1977) Dislocation of the wrist in rheumatoid arthritis. The relationship to distal ulnar resection, *Clin Orthop* **124**: 84.

Chamay A, Della Santa D, Vilaseca A (1983) L'arthrodèse radio-lunaire, facteur de stabilité du poignet rhumatoïde, *Ann Chir Main* **2**: 5–17.

Della Santa D, Chamay A (1995) Radiological evolution of the rheumatoid wrist after radio lunate arthrodesis, *J Hand Surg* **20B**: 146–54.

Fourastier J, Langlais F, Colmar M (1992) Translation cubitale du carpe après chirurgie du poignet rhumatoïde, *Rev Chir Orthop Rep App Moteur* **78**: 176–85.

Fowler SB (1949) Extensor apparatus of the digits, *J Bone Joint Surg* **31B**: 477.

Fowler SB, as quoted by Littles JW in Principles of reconstructive surgery of the hand. In: Converse JM (ed) (1964) *Reconstructive Plastic Surgery* (WB Saunders: Philadelphia) 1630–1.

Gainor BJ, Schaberg J (1985) The rheumatoid wrist after resection of the distal ulna, *J Hand Surg* **10A**: 837–44.

Gschwend N, Kentsch A (1985) Late results of synovectomy of wrist, MCP and PIP joints. Multicenter Study, *Clin Rheum* **4**: 23–5.

Hodgson SP, Stanley JK, Muirhead A (1989) The Wrightington classification of rheumatoid wrist X-rays: a guide to surgical management, *J Hand Surg* **14B**: 451–5.

Mannerfelt L (1984) Surgical treatment of the rheumatoid wrist and aspects of the natural course when untreated, *Clin Rheum Dis* **10**: 549–70.

Nalebuff EA, Terrono A (1999) Surgical techniques. In: Tubiana R, ed, *The Hand*, vol V (WB Saunders: Philadelphia) 226–69.

Sauvé A, Kapandji M (1936) Une nouvelle technique de traitement chirurgical des luxations récidivantes de l'extrémité inférieure du cubitus, *J Chir* **47**: 589–94.

Simmen BR, Huber H (1992) The rheumatoid wrist: a new classification related to the type of the natural course and its consequences for surgical therapy. In: Simmen BE, ed, *The Wrist in Rheumatoid Arthritis* (Karger: Basel).

Souter WA (1979) Planning treatment of the rheumatoid hand, *The Hand* **II**: 3.

Stanley JK, Tobat AR (1993) Long term results of Swanson silastic arthroplasty in the rheumatoid wrist, *J Hand Surg* **18B**: 381–8.

Swanson AB (1972) Flexible implant arthroplasty for the arthritic finger joints: rationale, technique and results of treatment, *J Bone Joint Surg* **54A**: 435–55.

Swanson AB (1981) Implant arthroplasty in the hand and upper extremity and its future, *Surg Clin North Am* **61**: 369.

Taleisnik J (1992) The Sauvé–Kapandji procedure, *Clin Orthop Rel Res* **275**: 110–23.

Tubiana R (1990) Technique of dorsal synovectomy on the rheumatoid wrist, *Ann Chir Main* **9**: 138–45.

Tubiana R (1998) Arthroplastie de la base du premier métacarpien avec interposition d'une bandelette du premier radial (ECRL), *La Main* **3**: 267–8.

Van Gemert AM, Spauwen PH (1994) Radiological evaluation of the long-term effects of resection of the distal ulna in rheumatoid arthritis, *J Hand Surg* **19B**: 330–3.

Vincent KA, Szabo RM, Agge JM (1993) The Sauvé–Kapandji procedure for reconstruction of the rheumatoid distal radio ulnar joint, *J Hand Surg* **18A**: 978–83.

Wilson YG, Sykes PJ, Niranja NS (1993) Long-term follow-up of Swanson's arthroplasty of the metacarpophalangeal joints in rheumatoid arthritis, *J Hand Surg* **18B**: 81.

39 Tendinitis of the wrist and epicondylitis

D Le Viet and Z Dailiana

Tendinitis is an inflammatory process, usually of traumatic origin (repeated microtrauma), affecting the tendons and their insertions as well as the synovial sheaths. The tendons most commonly affected are the longer and thinner ones, as they are submitted to quick movements and angulations and thus the frequency of tendinitis at the level of the wrist and hand is relatively high.

Non-operative treatment must be focused on the prevention and especially the avoidance of aggravating activities such as repetitive professional activities or sports movements. Conservative measures, including non-steroidal anti-inflammatory drugs (NSAIDs), splints, and physical therapy must be always applied before operative treatment is suggested. Surgical techniques for the treatment of the various forms of tenosynovitis of the wrist will be presented in detail along with their results.

Physical findings

The symptoms are often specific and include pain accentuated by flexion and extension against resistance and during palpation of the tendon. Painful swelling associated with crepitus may also be observed, as well as pain and signs of local inflammation at the level of insertion of the tendon. The treatment is primarily conservative, with splints for immobilization of the wrist, NSAIDs, and physical therapy. Cessation of the provocative movement is a very important element of the treatment. The modification of sports equipment (racquets, gloves, etc.) is also a basic part of the preventive treatment.

The lesions will be described from the palmar to the dorsal side of the wrist. Flexor carpi radialis tendinitis, the de Quervain's tenosynovitis, extensor carpi ulnaris tendinitis and the flexor carpi ulnaris tendinitis will be presented in detail, whereas the less common lesions will be described briefly.

Flexor carpi radialis (FCR) tendinitis

Although FCR tendinitis was described by Fitton et al in 1968 it remains a relatively unknown condition with ill-defined pathophysiology. The 30° angulation at the course of the carpal component of the FCR tendon and the axial rotation of its fibers are related to this pathologic condition (Lantieri et al 1993). Any modification in the architecture of the tunnel surrounding the FCR and especially scapho-trapezial-trapezoid (STT) joint arthritis may provoke this tendinitis (Figure 39.1). Communication of the scapho-trapezial joint with the FCR tunnel is a common surgical finding in cases of FCR tendinitis.

The incidence of FCR tendinitis is probably underestimated owing to ignorance of this condition and its frequent association with other pathologic conditions of the wrist. The majority of authors agree that treatment of FCR tendinitis is basically conservative with NSAIDs, splinting, and eventually local corticosteroid injections. Treatment becomes complicated after rupture of the tendon due to prolonged FCR tendinitis and thus surgical treatment should be suggested in cases of failure of conservative treatment.

Operative technique

With the exception of cases requiring treatment of associated conditions of the wrist, the surgical technique is typical. Through an anterior forearm-palmar approach

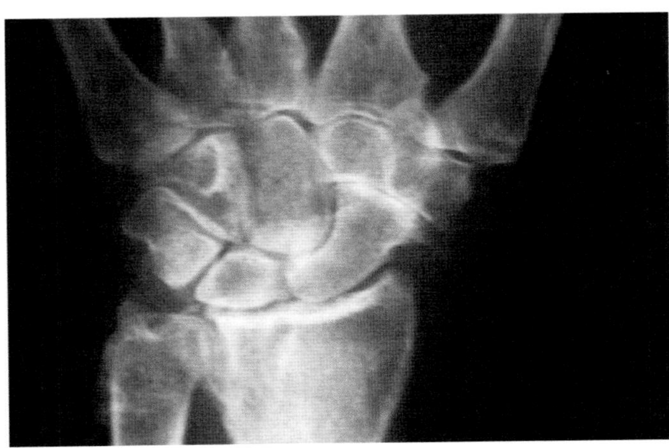

Figure 39.1
Radiograph depicting the STT joint arthritis that provokes FCR tendinitis.

the carpal tunnel is opened medially to the palmaris longus tendon and the palmar cutaneous branch of the median nerve is dissected and retracted. At the lateral part of the carpal tunnel, the fibro-osseous tunnel of the tendon is found with the aid of a fine and blunt instrument inserted from its proximal orifice. After dividing the tunnel over this instrument the tendon is dislocated and retracted. The synovial tissue is often hyperplastic and inflamed and it must be separated from the tendon and the fibro-osseous tunnel before resection. Histologic examination of the synovial tissue reveals non-specific inflammatory lesions only. The surgical findings are almost identical in every procedure. In general the tendon is thinner and less glossy than normal. The constant finding of one or more ulcerations, usually lateral, at the level of the scapho-trapezial space, is associated with abnormal tendon adhesions to the fibro-osseous tunnel. The ulcerations are related to the presence of trapezial or most frequently scaphoid spurs, which must be excised before the closure of the joint. The tendon is then reinserted in the fibro-osseous tunnel and the absence of dislocation during ulnar deviation must always be verified. When direct closure of the tunnel is impossible, a small rotation flap from the lateral borders of the tunnel can be used. Postoperatively the wrist is immobilized with a forearm-palmar splint.

Patients and methods

Twenty-seven patients, 25 female and 2 male, with 28 cases of FCR tenosynovitis were operated between 1984 and 1992, by the same surgeon (Kerboull and Le Viet 1995). Their mean age was 56.6 years (± 11.2 years; range 36–80 years) and the mean duration of tendinitis was 13 months (± 6 months; range 3 months to 4 years). All the patients underwent conservative treatment for a sufficient period; however, conservative treatment did not lead to remission of symptoms. Three patients had previously been operated for a misdiagnosed anterior synovial cyst of the wrist that subsequently recurred.

Wrist flexion against resistance was painful in 27 cases and an anterior swelling over the radial aspect of the wrist, mimicking a synovial cyst, was noted in the majority of cases (Figure 39.2). In 2 cases FCR tendinitis was an isolated condition of the wrist and in the other 26 cases it was associated with one or more of the following conditions: carpal tunnel syndrome in 11 cases, basal joint arthritis in 10 and STT joint arthritis in 10 cases. The basic radiographic evaluation included wrist X-rays in two planes.

Results

Complete relief from pain was noted in 18 cases. In five cases pain was related to activity and in three cases it

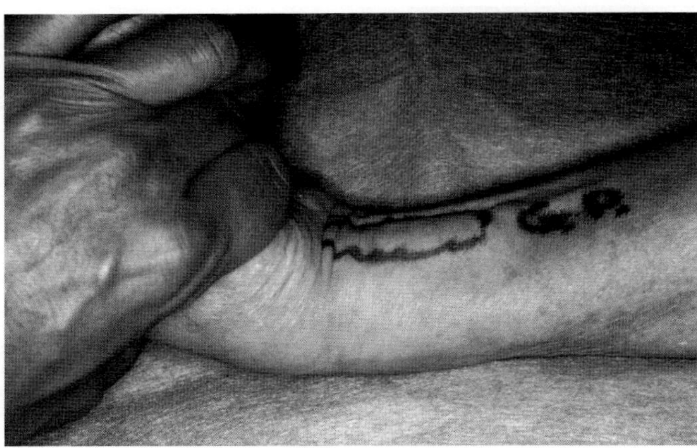

Figure 39.2

Typical aspect of FCR tendinitis with painful wrist flexion against resistance and polylobed synovial swelling around the distal FCR.

was provoked by the palpation of the scar. In the latter cases pain was probably related to irritation of the palmar cutaneous branch of the median nerve. Recurrence of pain was noted in two patients, within the first postoperative year. In total, results were excellent in 18 cases, good in 5 and fair in 3 cases, whereas the 2 cases that failed had to be reoperated.

Discussion

The diagnosis of FCR tendinitis is basically clinical. The condition must be suspected in the presence of anterior radial wrist pain, especially when it is provoked or aggravated during resisted wrist flexion. The presence of a synovial mass (Le Viet 1991), although not a constant finding, reinforces the diagnostic hypothesis. Several authors have described specific signs. Foucher (1989) (Gazaria and Foucher 1992) has underlined the presence of dysesthesia in the territory of the palmar cutaneous branch of the median nerve, which was found in 25% of his series of 24 cases. In the last 10 patients of our series that were evaluated after the aforementioned publication the latter sign was found three times, confirming Foucher's observations. Wood and Dobyns (1986) insisted on the presence of crepitus over the tendon without defining the frequency of this sign. This sign was only observed once in our series in a case with very significant synovitis. Sometimes the diagnosis is difficult, especially in the presence of associated conditions with more prominent symptoms. In these cases the lesions can be precisely depicted with the use of additional imaging evaluation such as computed tomography (CT) and magnetic resonance imaging (MRI) (Figure 39.3).

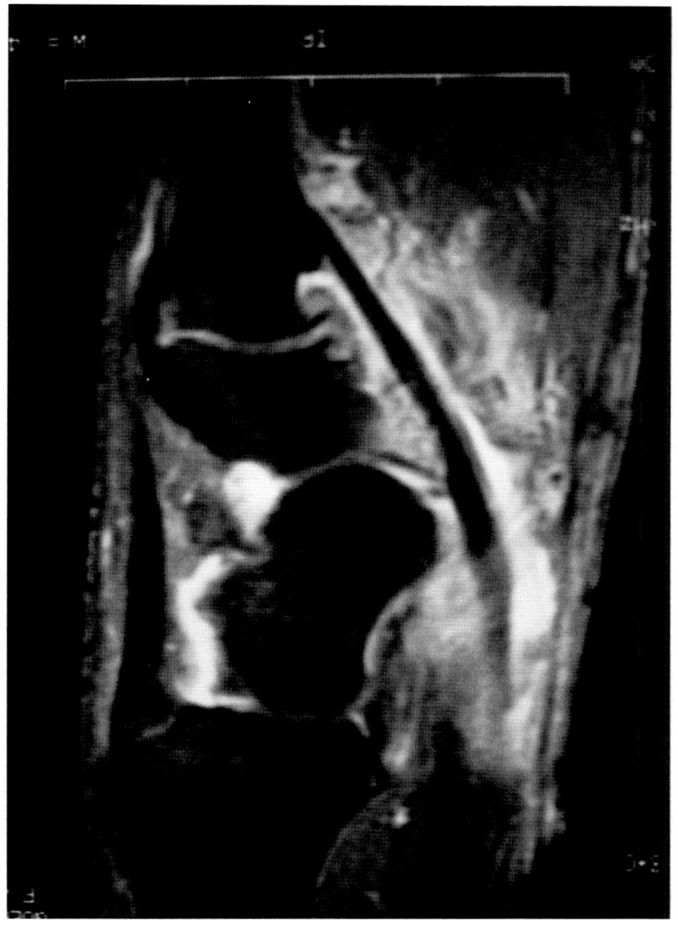

Figure 39.3
MRI depicting the distal synovitis in the carpal tunnel, around the FCR.

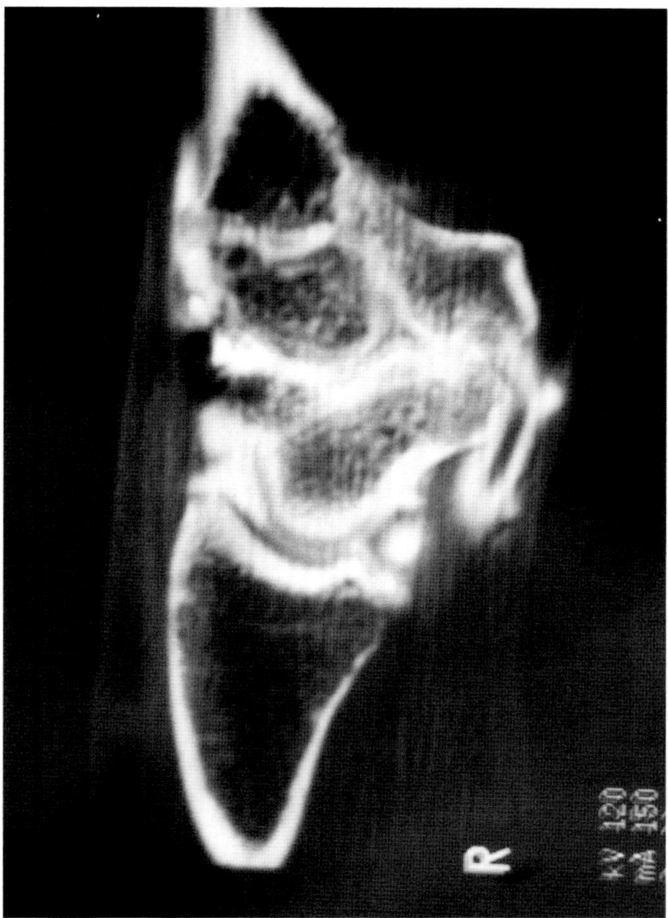

Figure 39.4
The communication between the STT joint and the FCR tunnel is depicted in this CT scan.

FCR tendinitis is most frequent in women and is not related to a specific professional activity or a sport. The mean age of the patients does not vary significantly in the different studies; patients are usually around the age of 50, although sometimes the condition was described in much younger patients. According to Fitton et al (1968) this condition affects female patients over 50 years of age; the average age of our patients was 56 years.

Repeated microtrauma is considered the major etiologic factor of this condition, whereas the hypothesis of an inflammatory synovial or tendinous process as a potential etiologic factor seems less likely. Degenerative arthritic lesions in contact with the tendon's tunnel could be the principal source of the tendon lesions, explaining the predominance of these lesions after the age of 50. Dissection of this region reveals that the fibro-osseous tunnel and the scapho-trapezial and trapezio-metacarpal joints have common elements: the ligaments and capsules that stabilize these joints are also involved in the structure of the floor of the fibro-osseous tunnel. As a result of this proximity the mechanism of the lesion is probably double: chemical and mechanical. Fitton et al (1968) hypothesized that degradation products from the destruction of the joint are released after the opening of the capsule in the tendon tunnel and Carstam et al (1968) confirmed this hypothesis with an arthrographic study of patients suffering from scapho-trapezial arthritis, which showed a communication between the joint and the tendon tunnel in 11 of 12 arthrograms (Figure 39.4).

Since FCR tendinitis is etiologically linked with lateral wrist arthritis it is more reasonable to use a dorsal approach for local steroid injections so as to treat the tendinitis and its probable cause simultaneously (under radiographic control). Injection of a contrast medium will confirm the communication.

Although the results of the present series confirm the efficacy of surgical treatment, it must be underlined that in the majority of cases, FCR tendinitis is relieved with non-operative measures and thus the surgical treatment should be reserved for failures of conservative treatment.

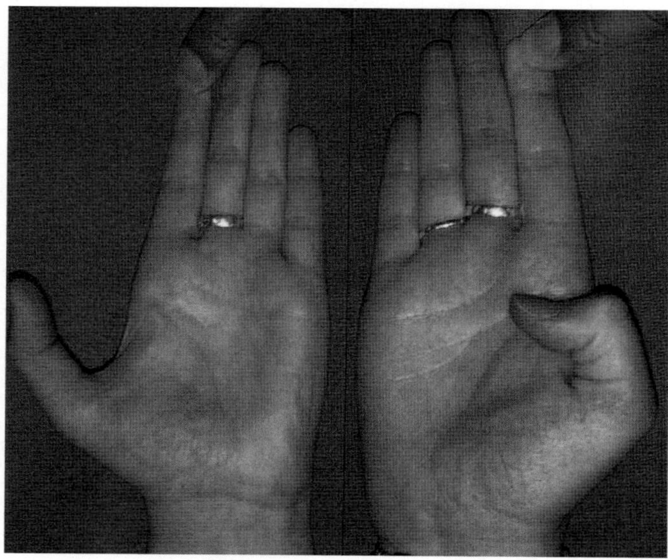

Figure 39.5

Clinical aspect of Lindburg's syndrome: inability of thumb flexion when the index is extended.

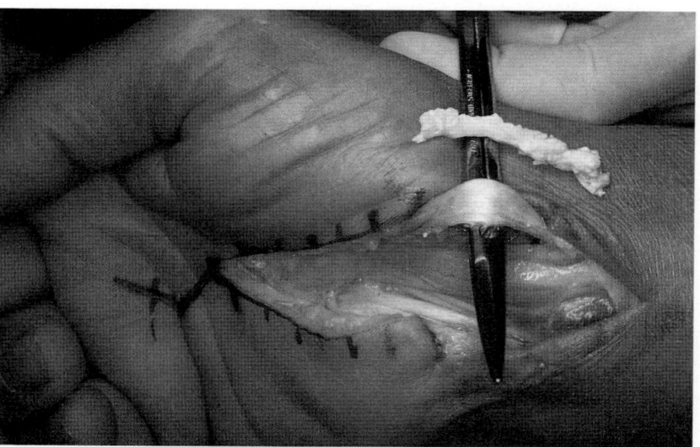

Figure 39.6

Tendinitis of the flexor profundus of the index finger: excision of a tendon strip that was ulcerated from the protruding lunate.

Flexor tenosynovitis

Tenosynovitis of the digital flexors must be explored in young patients. Although the carpal tunnel syndrome is most commonly idiopathic in female patients after menopause, in younger patients it is often due to an osseous or muscle anomaly. Surgical treatment of flexor tenosynovitis includes synovectomy after opening and exploration of the carpal tunnel for muscular anomalies (Le Viet 1995), supernumerary muscles, tendon interconnections (Figure 39.5), lumbrical muscles with proximal insertion or muscle bellies descending distally.

Flexor tendinitis often occurs after wrist injuries with osseous or ligamentous lesions. In these cases the following conditions must be excluded: hypertrophic callus formation, misdiagnosed lunate dislocation, Kienböck's disease, and carpal (especially DISI) instability. Lunate deviation towards the carpal tunnel may lead to an erosion of the base of the carpal tunnel and to a protrusion, injuring the dorsal aspect of the flexor tendons during flexion and extension, that justifies surgical treatment of the resulting painful tendinitis (Figure 39.6).

Tendinitis of the fourth and fifth digital flexors may be the result of an underlying non-union of the hook of the hamate (Carter 1977, Egawa 1983, Le Viet 1993, Stark 1977), necessitating its surgical removal (Figure 39.7). Non-union of the hook of the hamate is a rare condition, representing 2% of fractures of carpal bones (Allieu et al 1988). Due to the difficulty of imaging of the hamate, the fracture is often missed during the initial diagnostic evaluation, leading to a non-union (Nisenfield 1974). Non-unions of the hook of hamate and their subsequent nerve

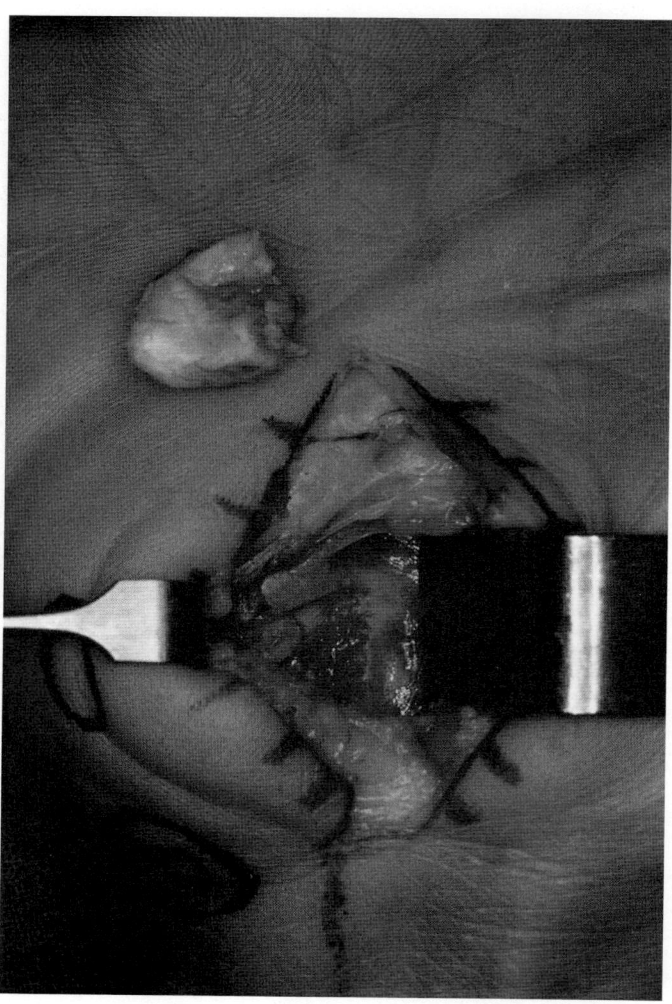

Figure 39.7

Removal of the hook of hamate in a patient with hamate non-union and signs of flexor tendinitis.

(Baird and Friedlenberg 1968, Manske 1978, Chaise and Sedel 1983) and tendinous (Crosby and Linscheid 1974, Tessier et al 1983) lesions often complicate sports injuries of the dominant (tennis) or the non-dominant (golf) upper extremity (Rodineau and Saillant 1987). For diagnostic evaluation of non-unions of the hook of hamate, CT is the examination of choice (Murray 1979).

Flexor carpi ulnaris (FCU) tendinitis

FCU tendinitis often mimics an infection, with erythema over the FCU and is probably a form of the hydroxyapatite deposition disease, described by Amor et al (1977). In the presence of FCU tendinitis the diagnostic investigation must include examination of the pisiform and of the surrounding area for local irritation, arthritis, and calcific deposits.

FCU tendinitis can be isolated but most frequently it is associated with pisiform lesions or pisotriquetral arthritis. The first cases of pisotriquetral arthritis were simultaneously described in 1951 by Jenkins and Lecocq. The pisiform has been described as the patella of the wrist joint by many authors, as it increases the lever arm of FCU according to Laude et al (1979). Its mobility depends on the FCU and, according to Ferpel et al (1992), the ligaments play only a small role in the stabilization of the pisiform.

Pisotriquetral arthritis can be attributed to pisiform instability, described by Helal in 1978 as 'racquet player's pisiform' or it can be post-traumatic. A history of injury has been reported in different percentages by several authors; Carroll and Coyle (1985) reported 43% of previous injury in a series of 67 cases.

The percentage of FCU tendinitis associated with pisiform lesions or arthritis ranged from 4% to 47% in the series reported by Carroll and Coyle (1985) and Palmieri (1982), respectively. Pain in the ulnar side of the wrist, increasing with local palpation and wrist movements in radial and ulnar deviation, is typical of this condition. Pain is accentuated by wrist flexion against resistance and by pronation-supination movements. Transverse sliding of the pisiform on the wrist leads to painful crepitus equivalent to the finding in the knee joint.

Flexor tendon ruptures have been reported by Lutz and Monsivais (1988) and Takami et al (1991); they are analogous to the tendon ruptures observed in cases of non-unions of the hook of hamate (Crosby and Linscheid 1974, Tessier et al 1983).

In several cases, the most important finding is a synovial cyst on the medial side of the wrist (Figure 39.8), between the flexor and the extensor carpi ulnaris, revealing pisotriquetral arthritis. Pain radiating to the fingers is another sign, reported in 50% of the cases in Caroll and Coyle's series (Carroll and Coyle 1985) and is associated with ulnar nerve irritation.

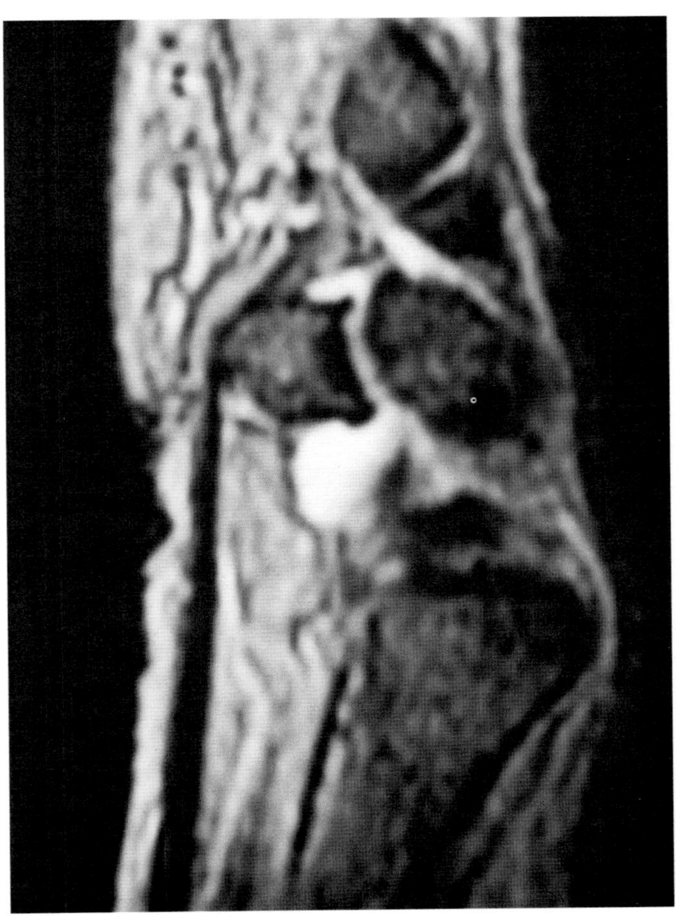

Figure 39.8
A synovial cyst on the medial side of the wrist, arising from the pisotriquetral joint, is visible on the MRI.

Although pisotriquetral arthritis can be minimally or not at all disturbing, conservative treatment with splints and injections is not really effective once this condition becomes painful. Failed non-operative treatment of 6 months duration must be followed by a surgical procedure to avoid secondary complications such as ulnar nerve lesions or ruptures of the profundus flexors of the ring and little fingers due to local irritation from the exostoses. On the other hand, conservative treatment is successful in the majority of cases of FCU tendinitis and surgical treatment is necessary in very few cases. However, FCU tendinitis and pisotriquetral arthritis are two entities that must be differentiated, as they require different treatment approaches.

Surgical treatment

For surgical treatment of FCU tendinitis an anteromedial approach is used through a longitudinal incision over the

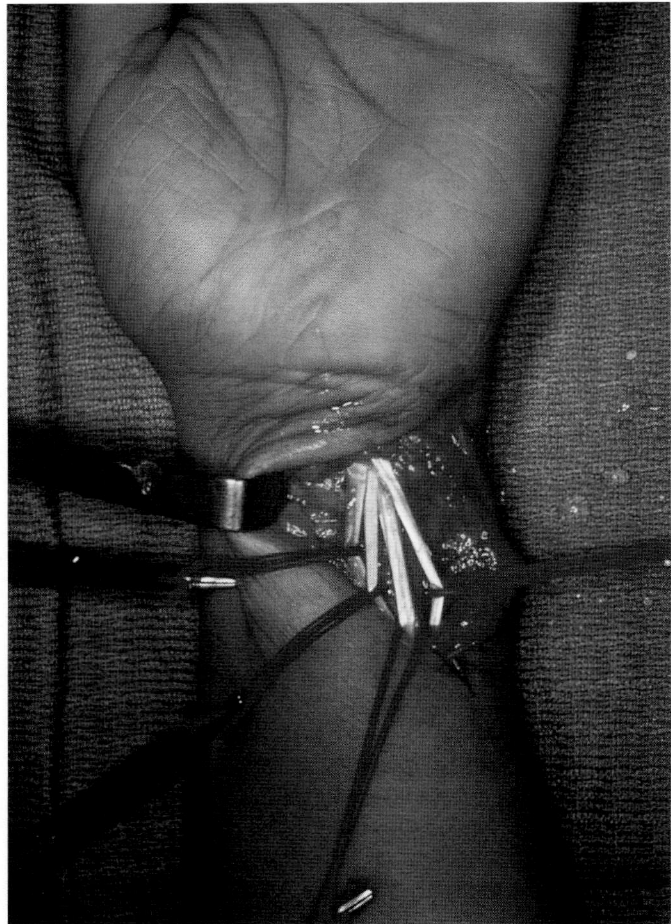

Figure 39.9
FCU tendinitis treated by longitudinal division of the tendon into four strips.

FCU tendon, whereas in cases with associated pisiform lesions a transverse incision over the wrist flexion crease, extended towards Guyon's canal, is indicated.

Complete synovectomy of the FCU is the first step of the procedure, revealing the tendon, which is often irregular, ulcerated, or hemorrhagic. If the synovium is not markedly hypertrophied the tendon's substance must be explored for necrotic zones, through multiple longitudinal incisions and division of the tendon into four or five strips (Figure 39.9). The necrotic zones can be excised then and with the healing process the caliber of the longitudinally divided tendon will increase and the tendon will be reinforced. After skin closure the wrist must be immobilized with a plaster splint for a period ranging from 2 to 4 weeks, according to the intraoperative findings.

Several authors described pisotriquetral arthrodesis for the treatment of pisotriquetral arthritis. Among them, Lutz and Monsivais (1988) and McEwen Smith (1954) have the most significant experience; the latter performed four arthrodeses and eventually removed the pisiform in a failed case with non-union.

However, the most commonly recommended treatment is subperiosteal dissection and excision of the pisiform (Bellapia 1992). The incision is usually longitudinal on the forearm, over the FCU. It becomes zig-zag on the flexion crease of the wrist and finally follows the axis of the fourth metacarpal on the palm. Several authors preserve the piso-hamate and piso-metacarpal ligaments in order to avoid a reduction of strength and motion. The authors of the present chapter open the Guyon's canal and dissect the bundle to avoid ulnar nerve lesions, before subperiosteal excision of the pisiform. With this technique division of the piso-hamate ligament is inevitable; however, no major consequences have been noted. At the end of the procedure the continuity of the FCU tendon to the piso-hamate and piso-metacarpal ligaments is preserved with interrupted sutures of the palmar periosteum of the pisiform, which was incised longitudinally. After a 3-week period of immobilization with a plaster splint, physical therapy is indicated.

Conclusion

Isolated tendinitis of FCU is very rarely treated surgically. Pisotriquetral arthritis, on the other hand, is a relatively unknown, usually post-traumatic entity. Although pisotriquetral arthritis is probably frequent, the painful or debilitating clinical manifestations are rare and often associated with FCU tendinitis.

Conservative treatment is rarely effective after the appearance of pain and functional limitation. For cases with persistent pain after appropriate non-operative treatment, the recommended surgical treatment is the subperiosteal excision of the pisiform. This procedure offers very satisfactory pain relief, although postoperatively the ulnar nerve is left unprotected during wrist hyperextension.

de Quervain's disease

This stenosing tenosynovitis of the first dorsal compartment of the wrist is the expression of the discrepancy of the volumes of extensor pollicis brevis (EPB) and abductor pollicis longus (APL) tendons and the dimensions of the fibro-osseous tunnel of the first dorsal compartment.

de Quervain, a Swiss surgeon and assistant of Kocher, described the homonymous entity in 1895.

Clinical findings

Patients always present with pain and soft tissue swelling at the radial styloid (Figure 39.10). Finkelstein's test

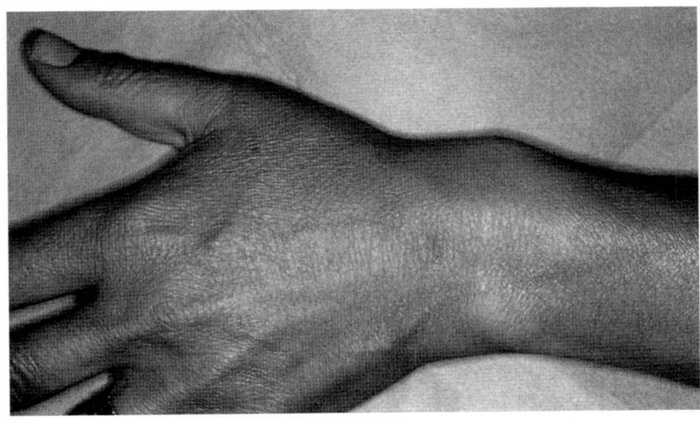

Figure 39.10
Lateral soft tissue swelling, typical of de Quervain's tenosynovitis.

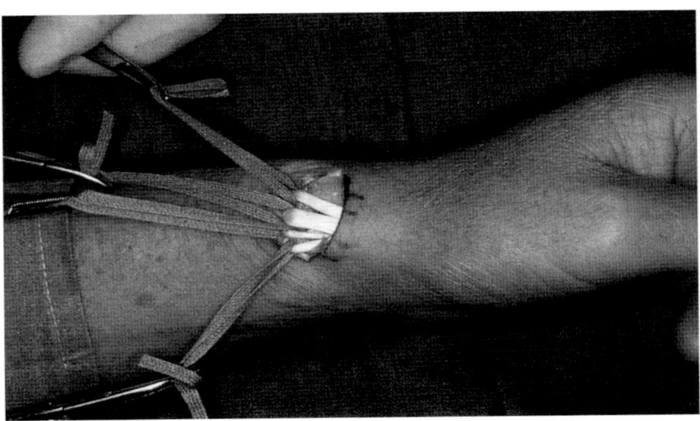

Figure 39.11
APL tendon with multiple (four) slips.

(Finkelstein 1930) is theoretically a pathognomonic test, which reproduces the pain through hyperextension of the dorsal thumb tendons. In this test the thumb is flexed into the palm and remains adducted while the wrist is deviated ulnarly, stretching the APL and EPB tendons.

Wartenberg's neuropathy (Wartenberg 1932) is sometimes associated with this condition; in this case the nerve must be dissected free during the surgical procedure to avoid a postoperative aggravation of the neuropathy. Wartenberg's neuropathy can be also exacerbated after compression of the nerve by a watch bracelet, as described by Matzdorff (1926).

Surgical technique

The recommended technique consists of a horizontal approach and preservation of the anterior flap of the sheath. After a transverse incision on the radial wrist crease, over the soft tissue swelling, the radial nerve and its branches are identified and protected to avoid a postoperative neuroma. Owing to the limited space available, the transverse incision requires detailed knowledge of the anatomy of the radial nerve.

The first dorsal compartment is identified then; it is usually inflated and sometimes filled with synovial tissue. The sheath is opened longitudinally, revealing the EPB tendon and the APL tendon(s). The first dorsal compartment is very often duplicated, partially or totally, necessitating exploration for a sagittal septum. The APL can have as many as five tendon slips (Figure 39.11) but most frequently it has two slips. The dorsal aspect of the first compartment is then excised. To avoid volar subluxation of the tendons during flexion, the anterior flap of the sheath is fixed to the skin during skin closure with an intradermal suture (Figure 39.12). This technique can be used only if the radial nerve is not close to the level of fixation. In cases with associated Wartenberg's neuropathy a longitudinal incision, offering a better aspect of the radial nerve, is recommended.

Discussion

Conservative treatment with local corticosteroid injections can be complicated by skin and subcutaneous atrophy and Wartenberg's neuropathy. Because of these complications Woods (1964) recommended that the surgical procedure should be performed without delay. Although the longitudinal incision provides ample space for surgical exploration it can be complicated by a hypertrophic and unsightly scar and by a painful and audible APL dislocation.

Several surgeons recommended different techniques to avoid dislocation of the tendons: Codega (1987) suggested reconstruction with the whole detached pulley, whereas Kapandji (1990) recommended an augmenting pulley plasty technique, similar to the one used for the flexor tendons.

Technical errors can lead to formation of neuromas, whereas radial nerve irritation can be observed when the posterior part of the pulley is not excised. Allegado and Meals (1979) reported a case of compression of the superficial branch of the radial nerve from the remaining posterior pulley during extension, as it was pushed by the underlying protruding tendons.

Conclusion

Transverse incision and fixation of a flap of the sheath guarantee that a good esthetic and functional result

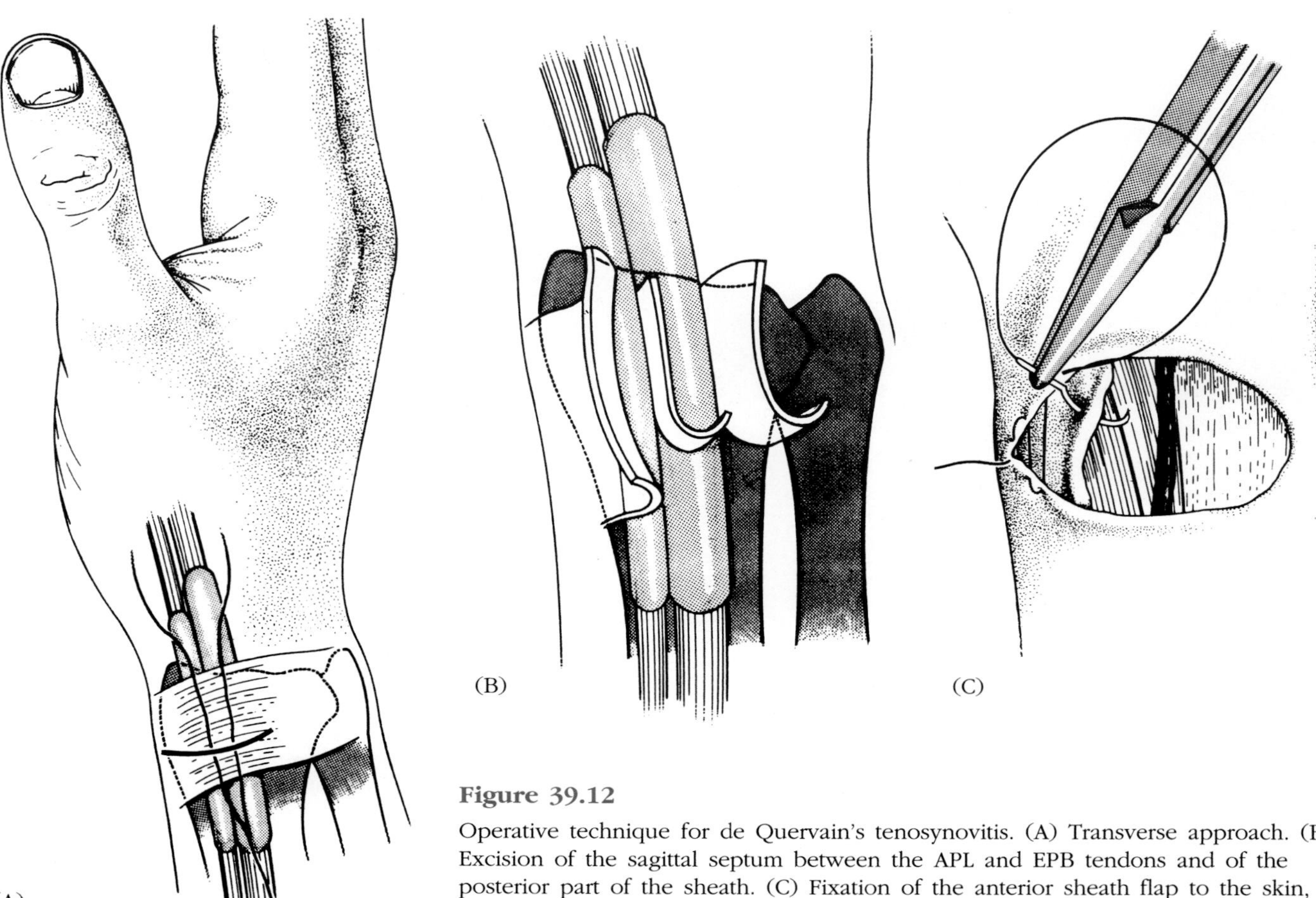

Figure 39.12

Operative technique for de Quervain's tenosynovitis. (A) Transverse approach. (B) Excision of the sagittal septum between the APL and EPB tendons and of the posterior part of the sheath. (C) Fixation of the anterior sheath flap to the skin, during skin closure with an intradermal suture.

(Figure 39.13) is obtained in a short time, whereas treatment of sequelae of de Quervain's disease is often disappointing. Complications such as the hypertrophic and unsightly scar, neuromas and anterior dislocation of the APL can be avoided by knowledge of the relevant anatomy, meticulous dissection, and preservation of the anterior part of the sheath.

Radial styloiditis

Radial styloiditis is a tendinitis at the level of insertion of the brachioradialis muscle. The absence of exacerbation of symptoms during mobilization of the thumb ray differentiates this entity from de Quervain's disease. The brachioradialis tendon has very limited mobility and thus this tendinitis is very rare. Usually the symptoms are due to osseous irritation at the level of insertion of the tendon and sometimes a detached osseous fragment is observed (Figure 39.14). The condition responds very well to conservative treatment with resting and steroid injections and surgical treatment is only indicated in exceptional cases.

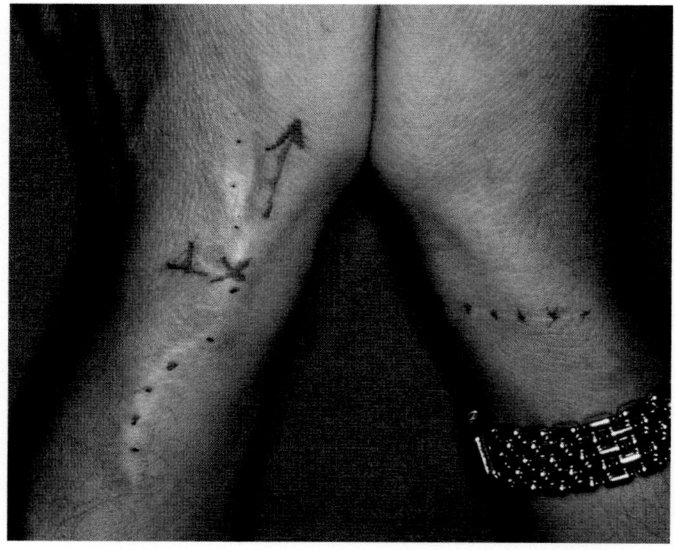

Figure 39.13

Result of two different techniques on the same patient: on the left, a hypertrophic and unsightly scar along with a Tinel sign (T) after a longitudinal incision and on the right the result after a transverse incision.

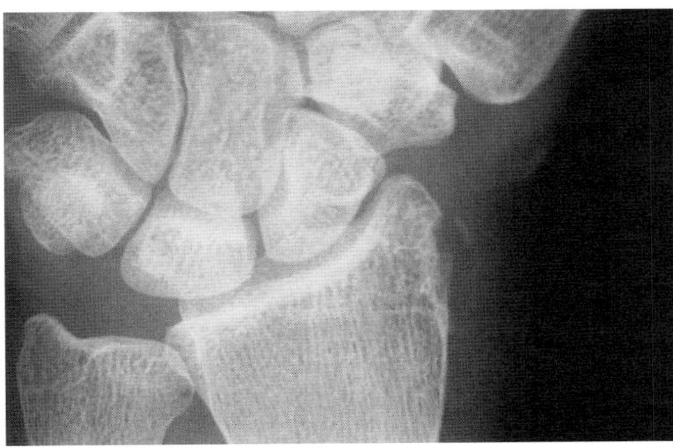

Figure 39.14
Radial styloiditis with detachment of a small osseous fragment from the lateral part of the radial styloid.

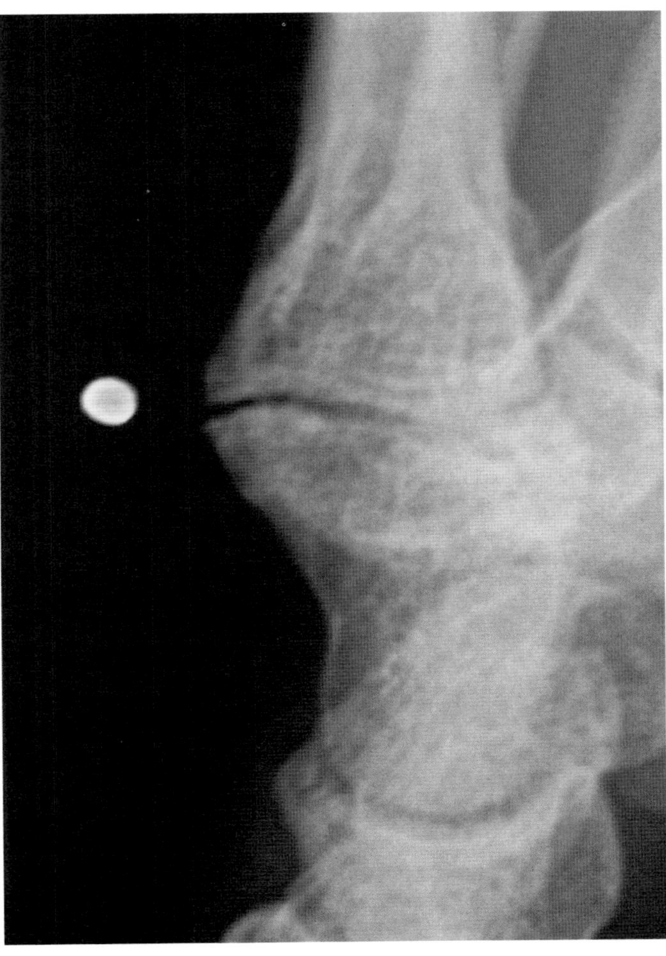

Figure 39.15
'Carpal boss': carpometacarpal exostosis between the base of the capitate and the third metacarpal.

Tenosynovitis of the radial extensors

Tenosynovitis of the radial wrist extensors – extensor carpi radialis longus (ECRL) and brevis (ECRB) – is characterized by pain in palpation and in wrist extension against resistance. The pain is localized at the level of the distal insertion of the radial wrist extensors at the base of the second and third metacarpal. A 'carpal boss' described by Fiolle (1931) is often associated with this condition and the imaging evaluation must include special wrist views of 3/4, to depict the carpometacarpal exostosis of the second or third ray (Figure 39.15) and the carpometacarpal arthritis that often accompanies it (Le Viet 1995). Another etiologic factor that must be evaluated in wrist radiographs is the additional bone 'os styloidium' intercalated between the trapezoid and the metacarpal. Commonly associated conditions are bursitis at the level of insertion of the radial extensors and tendinitis of the index extensors. The index extensors are irritated by osseous anomalies during radial-ulnar wrist deviation. In cases of bursitis at the level of insertion pain is aggravated by index or wrist extension against resistance. Cuono (Cuono and Watson 1979, Lenoble and Foucher 1992) described a cuneiform excision for surgical treatment of the carpal boss. The surgical techniques for the treatment of insertional tenosynovitis and of tendinitis of the radial extensors at the lateral forearm differ.

For the most frequent insertional tenosynovitis associated with a carpal boss, a transverse incision is performed on the top of the curve. The exostosis is then identified, the trapezoid-metacarpal space is explored and the os styloidium is excised if present. The cuneiform excision of the exostosis related to the trapezoid and the second metacarpal at the carpometacarpal level is performed with an osteotome (Figure 39.16). Special care is needed to avoid disinsertion of the ECRL or ECRB and to close the periosteum of this region at the end of the procedure.

Postoperative immobilization with the wrist in functional position for 4 weeks is necessary to avoid secondary ruptures of the ECRL or ECRB after potential damage of their insertions during the excision of the exostosis.

In cases of ECRL or ECRB tendinitis, the incision is dorsolateral at the lower aspect of the forearm. After identification and protection of the sensory branch of the radial nerve and retraction of the EPB and APL, the radial wrist extensors are identified. Complete synovectomy of the two tendons is then performed (Figure 39.17) and the tendons are split into several strips if tendinous lesions are observed intraoperatively. Postoperatively, the wrist is immobilized with a plaster splint for a minimum period of 2 weeks.

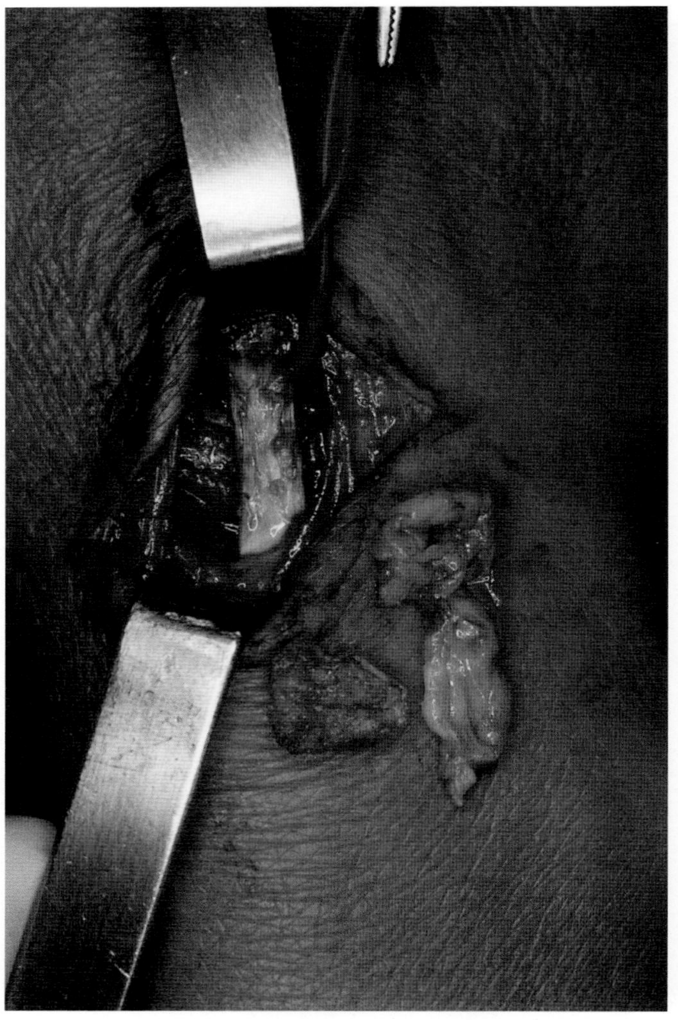

Figure 39.16

Excision of the carpal boss. The ECRL tendon is exposed and excision of the inflamed bursa along with the removal of the bone can be seen.

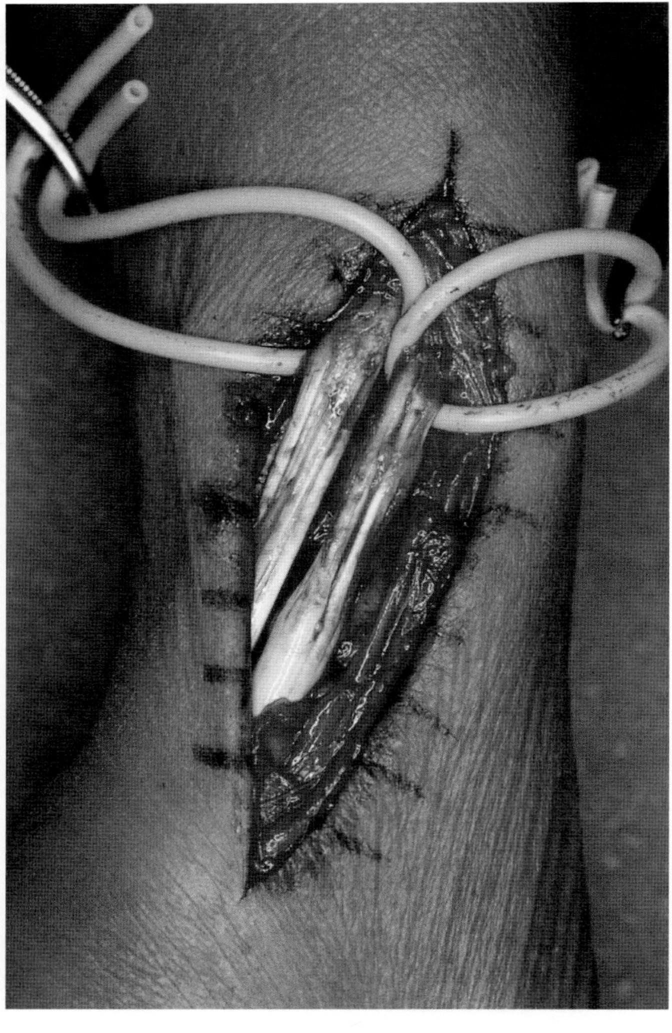

Figure 39.17

Synovectomy for the treatment of tendinitis of the radial wrist extensors (ECRL and ECRB).

Intersection syndrome

Wrist intersection syndrome is not a true tendinitis but an inflammatory condition of the bursa that is located between the radial wrist extensors, the APL and the lateral radius ('squeaker's wrist'). Pain is located at the lateral distal forearm, 6–8 cm from the radial styloid and is often exacerbated by pressure and accompanied by local swelling and crepitus (Figure 39.18).

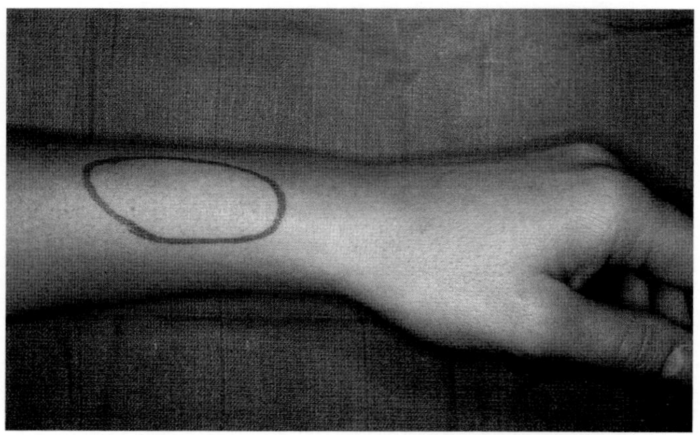

Figure 39.18

Intersection syndrome with painful crepitus at the forearm.

Surgical treatment

In cases of failure of conservative treatment the recommended surgical procedure is relatively simple. The

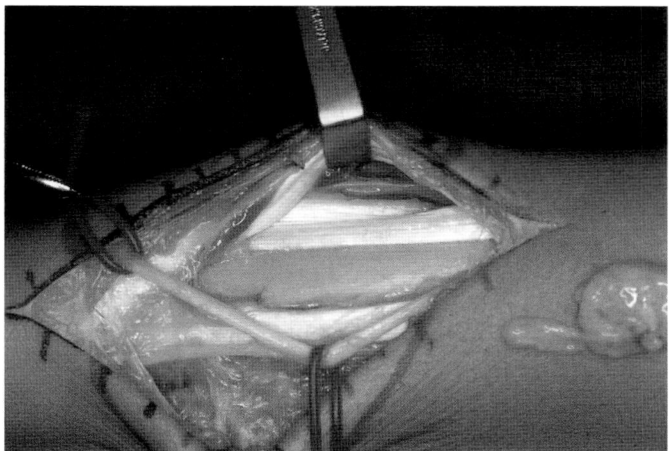

Figure 39.19
Excision of the inflammatory bursa (B) located between the radial wrist extensors (ECRL and B), the abductor pollicis longus, and the lateral radius.

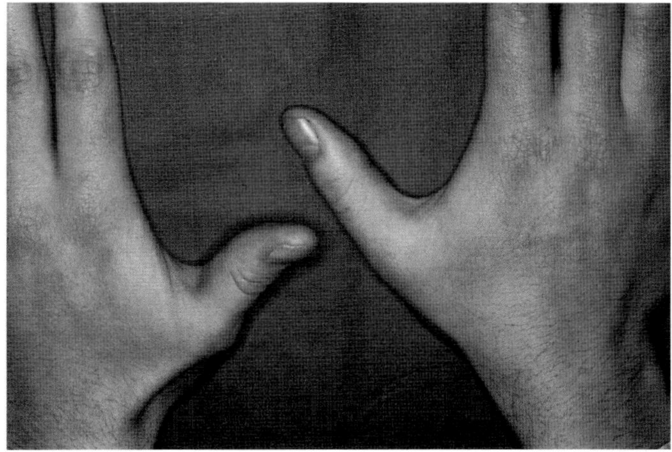

Figure 39.20
EPL rupture with loss of extension-retroposition of the thumb.

lateral incision is centered over the soft tissue swelling, revealing bursal inflammation after identification and protection of the sensory branch of the radial nerve. The bursa is adherent to the lateral radius and is located between the radial extensors of the wrist and the APL that crosses them obliquely. Communication of the profundus surface of the bursa with the radial extensors and the APL is a common operative finding (Figure 39.19). Degenerative tendon lesions were not observed in our cases, in contrast to the findings of other authors (Codega 1987). After closure of the skin the wrist is immobilized with a splint for 15 days. The surgical procedure is always effective for treatment of cases that are resistant to conservative measures.

Discussion

Several terms have been used to describe the intersection syndrome: crossroad syndrome, tendinitis of the radial wrist extensors, peritendinitis crepitans, and finally 'squeaker's wrist' or 'ai crépitant' (Tillaux used the latter term to describe the crepitus in the distal lateral forearm). Although it has been inaccurately considered a tendinitis of the radial wrist extensors for a long period, Wood and Linscheid (1973) insisted on the presence of an adventitial bursa between the radial wrist extensor tendons and the APL muscle, which had been first described in 1788 by Monro in a series of 33 bursae of the upper extremity.

The onset of intersection syndrome is usually acute in young patients, after an unusual effort or repetitive trauma. The soft tissue swelling is located at the dorsal aspect of the lower forearm and the palpation is painful. Subcutaneous crepitus accompanies the wrist movements in flexion-extension and in pronation-supination. Wrist movements are painful, especially extension of the wrist against resistance.

Conservative treatment with the use of wrist splints is usually very effective and NSAIDs or steroid injections are seldom needed. Very few cases are resistant to conservative measures and their treatment necessitates surgical exploration. Thus, the number of surgically treated cases reported in the literature is limited. In 1990, the authors of the present chapter published a series of three cases of intersection syndrome treated surgically (Le Viet et al 1990) and since then they have operated another two cases. The symptoms were related to sports injuries in three cases, including one golf and two tennis injuries. After an initial period of conservative treatment that failed to relieve the symptoms of these patients, complete functional restoration was noted after the surgical procedure and the symptoms disappeared.

The differential diagnosis includes de Quervain's tenosynovitis and insertional tenosynovitis of the radial wrist extensors. Although the Finkelstein test is considered pathognomonic for de Quervain's disease, it is often positive in cases of intersection syndrome; however, the pain is more proximal in the latter case.

Extensor pollicis longus (EPL) tendinitis

This entity is related to repetitive injuries and distal radius fractures. The condition must be diagnosed before the rupture of the EPL, which is characterized by the inability of the patient to extend the thumb above a flat surface on which the hand is placed for examination. In cases of EPL rupture, the tendon cannot be palpated in the snuffbox while extension of the thumb is attempted (Figure 39.20). Surgical treatment is indicated in cases with functional limitation.

Surgical treatment

The dorsal curved incision is centered over the EPL tendon. Before tendon rupture, the surgical treatment consists of synovectomy after opening of the third compartment in combination with excision of Lister's tubercle. The EPL is then re-routed, following a direct course on the dorsal aspect of the second compartment after opening of the septum between the second and third dorsal compartments (Figure 39.21). The extensor retinaculum is then closed over the EPL.

After tendon rupture, the most common surgical finding is a distal segment of the tendon located in the snuffbox and a proximal segment retracted in the forearm. In recent injuries, secondary repair can be attempted with the use of palmaris longus tendon graft. However, in most cases a transfer of the extensor indicis proprius (EIP), after division of the tendon at the metacarpophalangeal joint level, is indicated.

Finally, conservative measures for the treatment of EPL tendinitis diagnosed before rupture of the tendon should not include steroid injections, since these could induce rupture of the tendon.

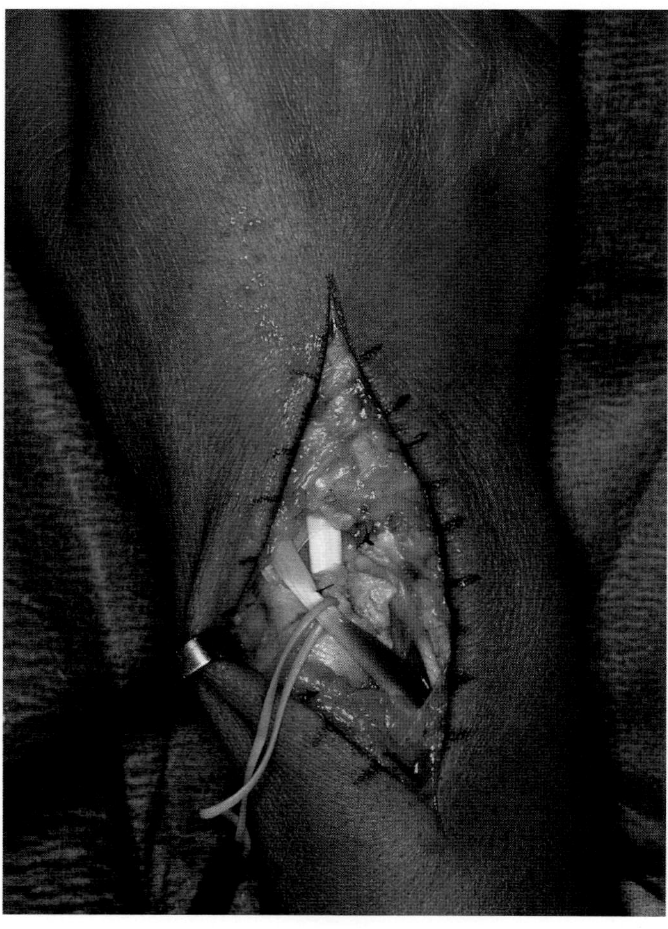

Figure 39.21

EPL re-routed over the ECRL and ECRB after excision of Lister's tubercle.

Tendinitis of the common digital extensors

Repetitive injury of the dorsal wrist is the most common cause of this tendinitis. The treatment is most often conservative and consists of splinting, although sometimes a synovectomy is necessary. Tenosynovitis of the digital extensors is uncommon and patients should be evaluated for associated diseases (rheumatoid arthritis, tuberculosis) in the absence of a specific etiology, such as trauma.

Finally, tenosynovitis of the extensor indicis proprius (Ritter and Inglis 1969) and extensor digiti quinti proprius (Drury 1955) also exist as isolated but rare entities (Figure 39.22).

Extensor carpi ulnaris (ECU) tendinitis

The stability of the ulnar head relies on the sixth dorsal compartment, which comprises the ECU tendon (Spinner and Kaplan 1970). On the dorsal-medial side of the ulnar head, the ECU is restrained in an approximately 1.5 cm long fibro-osseous tunnel. The ECU sheath is distinct

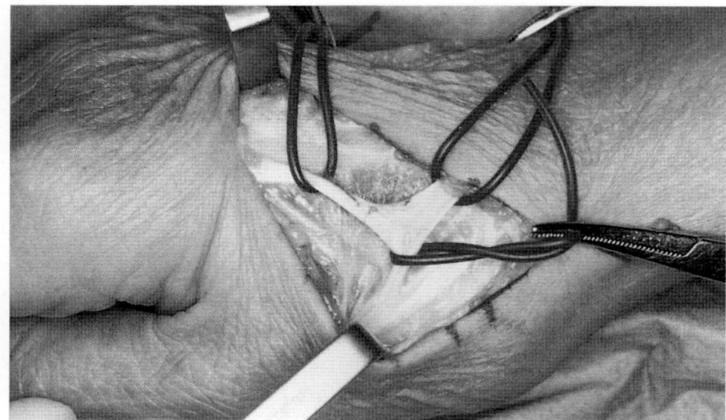

Figure 39.22

Extensor indicis proprius tendinitis due to abnormal connection of the extensor pollicis longus and the extensor indicis proprius.

from the overlying extensor retinaculum, which is a basic element of the remaining five dorsal compartments. The position of the ECU is variable owing to the mobility of the ulnar head during pronation and supination. In pronation a gap between the ECU and the adjacent extensor digiti quinti proprius is palpable, whereas in full supination the two compartments are in close contact and no gap can be palpated.

Materials and methods

Our series of 26 traumatic lesions of the ECU in the wrist consists of 18 dislocations and 8 cases of tendinitis (Montalvan and Le Viet 1997). There were 25 patients in our series, 8 male and 17 female; a female patient underwent a bilateral procedure. Nine of the 26 cases were related to sports injuries and especially to tennis injuries (7 cases) (Chard 1987, Kiefhaber 1992, Osterman 1988). ECU dislocations associated with rheumatoid polyarthritis were excluded from this study.

The mean age of the patients in our series was 31.7 years, ranging from 17.7 to 69.1 years and the follow-up period ranged from 18 to 87.8 months with a mean period of 45.8 months. The right side was affected in 19 cases and the left in 7 cases.

Dickson and Luckey first described the ECU tendinitis in 1948. In our series, ECU tendinitis was surgically treated either by release of the radial aspect of the fibro-osseous tunnel (in three cases), followed by suture of the remaining ulnar fibrous flap to the dorsal retinaculum to avoid subluxation of ECU, as proposed by Hajj and Wood (1986) or by division of the ECU into strips, in the cases where the fibro-osseous tunnel could be preserved.

In all 18 cases of ECU dislocation, the tendon was reattached to its fibro-osseous tunnel at the dorsal aspect of the ulnar head. In the first three cases the flap for reconstruction of the ECU tunnel was elevated from the dorsal retinaculum and remained attached to it, as described by Spinner and Kaplan (1970) and Burkhard et al (1982). In the next 15 cases a free flap from the dorsal retinaculum was fixed on the two sides of the ulnar osseous canal (Figure 39.23), followed by reconstruction of the overlying dorsal retinaculum. The latter technique, performed by Eckhardt and Palmer (1981) in four cases and by Loty et al (1986) in one case, reconstructs both planes of ECU.

Remarkable synovitis was noted in 18 cases in our series, whereas tendon lesions justifying a synovectomy and division of the tendon in four or five strips were found in five cases. Finally an ECU rupture was observed in one case.

Results

Results were very good in 14 cases and the patients returned to their previous activities, without limitation of mobility or grip strength. In eight cases results were good, with normal range of movement (ROM) but with a loss of grip strength greater than 30% in comparison with the contralateral wrist. Finally, results were fair in three cases and in the one case that failed, recurrence of ECU tendinitis necessitated a reoperation. Although two patients were lost during follow-up, their initial postoperative evaluation performed at 8.7 and 14 months respectively, was sufficient and they were not excluded from the study.

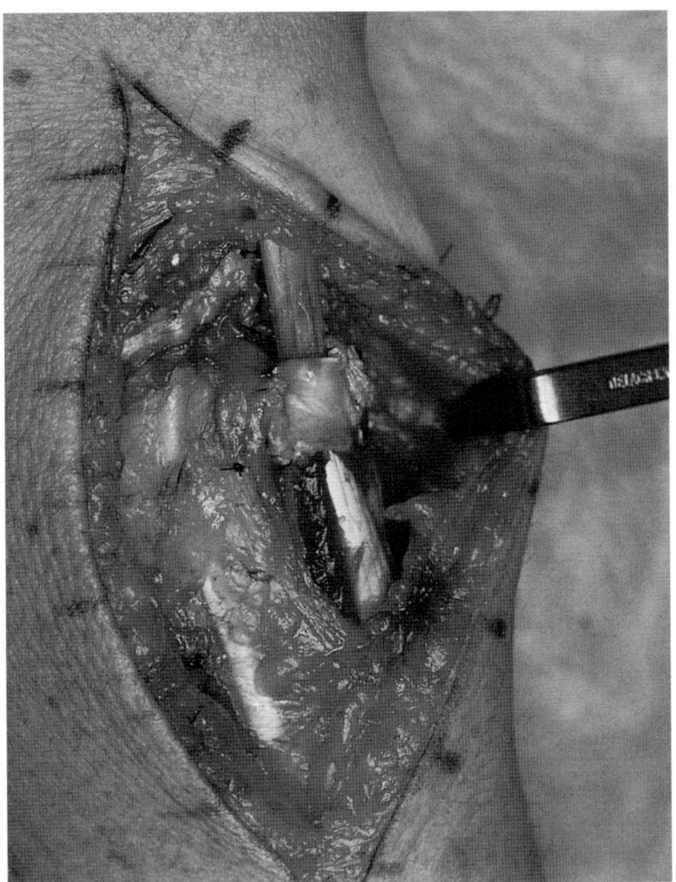

Figure 39.23
Free flap from the dorsal retinaculum fixed on the sides of the ulnar osseous trough to reconstruct the fibro-osseous tunnel of the ECU.

Discussion

Instability of the ECU after the rupture of the medial wall of the tunnel is a frequent lesion that has been described by many authors. Instability usually occurs after injuries in supination, palmar flexion, and ulnar deviation (Rayank Ghazi 1983).

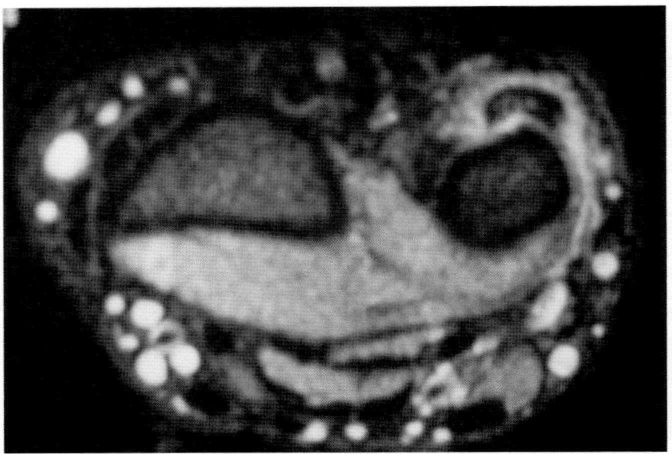

Figure 39.24

MRI depicting subluxation of the ECU on the medial side of the ulnar head, surrounded by synovitis.

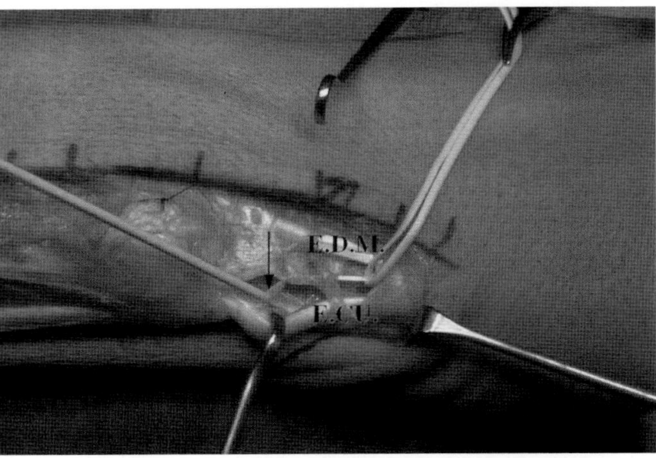

Figure 39.25

Intraoperative aspect of Barfred's syndrome (abnormal tendon band connecting the ECU and the extensor digiti quinti proprius).

According to the experience of the authors of the present chapter, in several cases and especially in cases related to sports, a period of tenosynovitis is often noted before rupture of the fibro-osseous tunnel (Montalvan and Le Viet 1997). This lesion has been reported in relation to several sports such as tennis, golf, weightlifting, and rodeo riders.

Hajj and Wood (1986), among other authors, have described a simple technique for the release of the radial wall of the fibro-osseous tunnel of the ECU, for the treatment of stenosis of the sixth dorsal compartment with tenosynovitis. They reported excellent results after surgical decompression of the sixth dorsal compartment in all three cases that they operated.

Nachinolcar and Khanolkar (1988) reported an important series of ECU tendinitis, comprising 72 cases; 63 of the 72 cases were treated surgically with a limited procedure. According to these authors, the excision of the fibro-osseous tunnel of the ECU always led to excellent results.

Due to the ECU tenosynovitis and the tendon enlargement, the fibro-osseous tunnel of the sixth dorsal compartment is dilated (Figure 39.24) and the ulnar wall is ruptured in response to repetitive injuring movements, leading to palmar subluxation of the ECU tendon. Thus, surgical treatment of ECU tendinitis before rupture of the ulnar wall of the tunnel is essential. At the pre-rupture stage, the simple release of the radial aspect of the fibro-osseous tunnel is a reasonable procedure and should be combined with tenodesis to avoid ulnar and palmar subluxation of the tendon. Surgical treatment of ECU tenosynovitis in the pre-subluxation stage also includes synovectomy and division of the tendon into several strips in cases with associated synovitis or tendon lesions. In the majority of cases the fibro-osseous tunnel of the ECU can be preserved while the latter procedures are performed.

After rupture of the ulnar wall of the tunnel and ulnar-palmar dislocation of the ECU, reconstruction of the fibro-osseous tunnel is necessary. Following surgical treatment of the tendinous lesions, a free flap raised from the extensor retinaculum is attached to the medial and lateral side of the ulnar head groove and the tunnel is reconstructed.

Finally, after prolonged tendinitis of the ECU, a tendon rupture may occur. Moran and Ruby (1992) reported good results of surgical treatment of two non-rheumatoid ECU ruptures, with the use of a tendon graft. In 1987 Chun and Palmer reported a painful wrist condition related to partial rupture of the ECU. Our series of patients includes a female professional tennis player (ranked 50th in the world) who suffered from ECU tendinitis for a long period and had been treated with multiple steroid injections before an acute pain during a backhand movement prohibited any further practice of the sport. After a period of absence from the tennis courts of 1.5 months, the surgical procedure revealed a rupture of the ECU which had not been depicted in any of the preoperative imaging examinations, including radiographs, CT, and MRI. The continuity of the tendon was restored with the use of a palmaris longus tendon graft, while the fibro-osseous tunnel was reconstructed with the use of a flap from the extensor retinaculum. After 6 months of absence from the tennis courts the patient returned to her professional activities, to the same competition level that she was at before her injury.

Finally, another cause of pain and synovitis is an abnormal tendon band extending between the ECU and the extensor digiti quinti proprius (Figure 39.25), as described by Barfred and Adamsen (1986). Due to the different length and course of the ECU (3 cm) and the extensor digiti quinti proprius (5 cm) this band may prohibit the simultaneous flexion of the wrist and little finger. Simple excision of the band along with synovectomy led to excellent results in the cases operated by the authors of this chapter.

Conclusion

The majority of cases of wrist tendinitis and tendinopathy can be treated conservatively with wrist splints and local and systemic administration of anti-inflammatory drugs. The splints must be adapted to each pathologic entity and must allow muscle relaxation provided by wrist flexion for the palmar pathologic conditions and by wrist extension for the dorsal conditions. Avoidance of aggravating repetitive movements is also a basic element of conservative treatment.

Surgical treatment should be limited to cases that have proved resistant to conservative treatment for a sufficient period, but before the development of irreversible tendon lesions that may lead to tendon ruptures with poor functional prognosis. The period of postoperative splint immobilization must be adapted to the intraoperative findings; however, this should not be shorter than 15 days.

Epicondylitis

Epicondylitis is a common pathologic condition of the elbow, involving the musculotendinous origins of the forearm flexors or extensors. Lateral epicondylitis or 'tennis elbow' is a tendinitis of the forearm extensors, whereas medial epicondylitis or 'golfer's elbow' involves the flexor-pronator origin.

Although both conditions occur in the fourth and fifth decades of life and are considered overuse syndromes, lateral epicondylitis occurs much more frequently than medial epicondylitis. The repetitive movements of the wrist and elbow result in micro tears in the musculotendinous substance and in degenerative changes, usually located within the extensor carpi radialis brevis for lateral epicondylitis and within the pronator teres and flexor carpi radialis for medial epicondylitis (Coonrad and Hooper 1973, Jobe and Ciccotti 1994, Froimson 1999).

Clinical findings

Lateral epicondylitis is characterized by pain at the lateral epicondyle, radiating to the forearm, with gradual onset, usually following repetitive movements in wrist extension. The symptoms are aggravated by resisted wrist extension, and palpation reveals an area of maximal tenderness just distal to the lateral epicondyle.

Patients suffering from medial epicondylitis present with pain and tenderness on the origin of the forearm flexors in the area of the medial epicondyle. Pain in this situation is aggravated by resisted wrist flexion with the elbow extended.

Evaluation of the entire upper extremity and the neck region is necessary to exclude other conditions such as cervical radiculopathy, nerve compression syndromes, and disorders of the elbow joint (Bennett 1994, Jobe and Ciccotti 1994).

Treatment

Epicondylitis usually responds to cessation of the provoking activities and to conservative measures including rest, NSAIDs, and forearm bands. Physical therapy modalities such as ultrasound, electric stimulation, and heat have also been used for the treatment of epicondylitis. Finally, local steroid-anesthetic injections can be used in resistant cases. Modification of equipment used in sports and of causative activities is imperative for the prevention of recurrences.

Surgical treatment is indicated for cases not responding to a well-conducted period of conservative treatment of 6–12 months duration. The procedures used can be classified as intra-articular or extra-articular (Coonrad and Hooper 1973, Wittenberg et al 1992, Bennett 1994, Jobe and Ciccotti 1994, Kurvers and Verhaar 1995, Froimson 1999). The latter include three types of operations: release of the extensor or flexor origin from the lateral or medial epicondyle, excision of the pathologic tendon and granulation tissue from the lateral or medial epicondyle with reconstruction of the extensor and flexor origin, respectively, and finally, distal lengthening of the extensor carpi radialis brevis tendon for lateral epicondylitis.

In conclusion, lateral and medial epicondylitis, 'tennis' and 'golfer's' elbow, respectively, are common pathologic conditions of the elbow, resulting from tears in the musculotendinous origins of the forearm extensors or flexors. Lateral epicondylitis is much more frequent than medial epicondylitis, but both conditions occur in the fourth and fifth decades of life. Lateral and medial epicondylitis usually respond to conservative treatment with rest, NSAIDs, forearm bands, physical therapy, or local steroid-anesthetic injections. Surgical treatment is only indicated in cases that are resistant to a well-conducted and prolonged period of conservative treatment. The most common extra-articular procedures are release of the extensor or flexor origin from the (lateral or medial) epicondyle and excision of the pathologic tendon and granulation tissue from the (lateral or medial) epicondyle with reconstruction of the extensor and flexor origin.

References

Alegado RB, Meals RA (1979) An unusual complication following surgical treatment of de Quervain's disease, *J Hand Surg* **3A**: 185–6.

Allieu Y, Benichou M, Touchais S (1988) Fracture des os du carpe. In: *Encycl Med Chir, App. Locomoteur* (Elsevier: Paris).

Amor B, Cherot A, Delbarre F (1977) Le rhumatisme à hydroxyapatite. La maladie des calcifications multiples, *Rev Rhum* **44**: 301–8.

Baird DB, Friedlenberg ZB (1968) Delayed ulnar nerve palsy following a fracture of the hamate, *J Bone Joint Surg* **50A**: 570–2.

Barfred T, Adamsen S (1986) Duplication of the extensor carpi ulnaris tendon, *J Hand Surg* **11A**: 423–5.

Bellapia PP, Burke FD (1992) Excision of the pisiform in piso pisiforme ostéoarthritis, *J Hand Surg* **17B**: 133–6.

Bennett JB (1994) Lateral and medial epicondylitis, *Hand Clin* **10**: 157–63.

Burkhart SS, Wood MB, Linscheid RL (1982) Posttraumatic recurrent subluxation of the extensor carpi ulnaris tendon, *J Hand Surg* **7A**: 1–3.

Carroll RE, Coyle MP (1985) Dysfunction of the piso pisiforme joint: treatment by excision of the pisiform, *J Hand Surg* **10A**: 703–7.

Carstam N, Eiken O, Andren L (1968) Osteoarthritis of the trapezio-scaphoid joint, *Acta Orthop Scand* **39**: 354–8.

Carter PR, Eaton RG, Littler JW (1977) Ununited fracture of the hamate, *J Bone Joint Surg* **59A**: 583–8.

Chaise F, Sedel L (1983) Les compressions isolées de la branche motrice du nerf cubital, *Ann Chir Main* **2**: 33–7.

Chard MD, Lachmann SM (1987) Racquet sports – patterns of injury presenting to a sports injury clinic, *Br J Sports Med* **21**: 150–3.

Chun S, Palmer AK (1987) Chronic ulnar wrist pain secondary to partial rupture of the extensor carpi ulnaris tendon, *J Hand Surg* **12A**: 1032–5.

Codega G (1987) Tecnica chirurgica nella malattia di De Quervain. In: *La Patologia del Polso* (Piccin Nuova Libraria: Padua).

Coonrad RW, Hooper WR (1973) Tennis elbow: its course, natural history, conservative and surgical management, *J Bone Joint Surg* **55A**: 1177–82.

Crosby EB, Linscheid RL (1974) Rupture of the flexor profundus tendon of the ring finger secondary to ancient fracture of the hook of the hamate: review of the literature and report of two cases, *J Bone Joint Surg* **56A**: 1076–8.

Cuono CB, Watson HK (1979) The carpal bos: surgical treatment and etiological considerations, *Plast Reconstr Surg* **63**: 88–93.

de Quervain F (1895) Uber eine Form von chronischen Tendovaginitis, *Korresp-Bl Schweiz Arz* **25**: 389–94.

Dickson DD, Luckey CA (1948) Tenosynovitis of the extensor carpi ulnaris tendon sheath, *J Bone Joint Surg* **30A**: 903–7.

Drury BJ (1955) Tendovaginitis of extensor digiti quinti proprius, *J Bone Joint Surg* **37A**: 407.

Eckhardt WA, Palmer AK (1981) Recurrent dislocation of extensor carpi ulnaris tendon, *J Hand Surg* **6A**: 629–31.

Egawa M, Asai T (1983) Fracture of the hook of the hamate: report of six cases and the suitability of computerized tomography, *J Hand Surg* **8**: 393–8.

Ferpel V, Rooze M, Louryan S, Lemort M (1992) Bi- and three-dimensional CT study of carpal bone motion occuring in lateral deviation, *Surg Radiol Anat* **14**: 341–8.

Finkelstein H (1930) Stenosing tendovaginitis at the radial styloid process, *J Bone Joint Surg* **12A**: 509–39.

Fiolle J (1931) Le carpe bossu, *Soc Nat Chir* **57**: 1687.

Fitton JM, Shea FW, Goldie W (1968) Lesion of the flexor carpi radialis tendon and its sheath causing pain at the wrist, *J Bone Joint Surg* **50B**: 359–63.

Foucher G (1989) Tendinites de la main et du poignet. In: *Pathologie Tendineuse de la Main* (Masson: Paris) 147–55.

Froimson AI (1999) Tennis elbow. In: Green DP, Hotchkiss RN, Pederson WC, eds, *Green's Operative Hand Surgery*, 4th edn (Churchill Livingstone: New York) 683–8.

Gazarian A, Foucher G (1992) La tendinite du grand palmaire. A propos de vingt-quatre cas, *Ann Chir Main* **11**: 14–17.

Hajj AA, Wood MB (1986) Stenosing tenosynovitis of the extensor carpi ulnaris, *J Hand Surg* **11A**: 519–20.

Helal B (1978) Racquet player's pisiform, *The Hand* **10**: 87–90.

Jenkins SA (1951) Osteoarthritis of the pisiform-triquetral joint. Report of three cases, *J Bone Joint Surg* **33B**: 532–4.

Jobe FW, Ciccotti MG (1994) Lateral and medial epicondylitis of the elbow, *J Am Acad Orthop Surg* **2**: 1–8.

Kapandji AI (1990) Plastie d'agrandissement de la coulisse radio-styloïdienne dans le traitement de la ténosynovite de De Quervain, *Ann Chir Main Memb Super* **9**: 42–6.

Kerboull L, Le Viet D (1995) La tendinite du grand palmaire. Physiopathogénie et résultats du traitement chirurgical. A propos de 28 cas, *Ann Chir Main* **14**: 135–41.

Kiefhaber TR, Stern PJ (1992) Upper extremity tendinitis and overuse syndromes in the athlete, *Clinics in Sports Medicine* **11**: 32–48.

Kurvers H, Verhaar J (1995) The results of operative treatment of medial epicondylitis, *J Bone Joint Surg* **77A**: 1374–9.

Lantieri L, Hennebert H, Le Viet D, Guerin-Surville H (1993) A study of the orientation of the fibers of the flexor carpi radialis tendon: anatomy and clinical applications, *Surg Radiol Anat* **15**: 85–9.

Laude M, Legars D, Boudin G (1979) Anatomie fontionnelle du pisiforme, *Bull Assoc Anat (Nancy)* **63**: 451–8.

Lecocq EA (1951) Traumatic arthritis of the pisiform-triangular joint. A case report, *Western Journal of Surgery, Obstetrics and Gynaecology* **59**: 357.

Lenoble E, Foucher G (1992) [The carpal boss], *Ann Chir Main* **11**: 46–50.

Le Viet D (1991) Les kystes dits synoviaux du poignet et de la main. In: *Cahiers d'Enseignement de la Société Française de Chirurgie de la Main* (Expansion Scientifique Française: Paris) 49–58.

Le Viet D (1995) Les tendinites et apophysites du poignet. In: *Cahiers d'Enseignement de la Société Française de Chirurgie de la Main* (Expansion Scientifique Française: Paris) 49–60.

Le Viet D, Montalvan B, Rodineau J (1990) Syndrome de l'intersection à l'avant-bras, *J Traumatol Sport* **7**: 185–8.

Le Viet D, Lantieri L, Bouvet R (1993) La pseudarthrose de l'apophyse unciforme de l'os crochu. Nonunion of the hamate. Review of the literature and report of 10 cases, *Rev Chir Orthop* **79**: 192–8.

Loty B, Meunier B, Mazas F (1986) Luxation traumatique isolée du tendon cubital postérieur, *Rev Chir Orthop* **72**: 219–22.

Lutz RA, Monsivais JJ (1988) Piso-pisiforme arthrosis as a cause of rupture of the profundus tendon of the little finger, *J Hand Surg* **13B**: 102–3.

McEwen Smith A (1954) Sprain of the pisiform-pisiforme joint. Report of 6 cases, *J Bone Joint Surg* **36B**: 618–21.

Mandelbaum BR, Bartolozzi AR, Davis CA. Teurlings L, Bragonier B (1989) Wrist pain syndrome in the gymnast. Pathogenetic, diagnostic, and therapeutic considerations, *Am J Sports Med* **17**: 305–17.

Manske PR (1978) Fracture of the hook of the hamate presenting a carpal tunnel syndrome, *The Hand* **10**: 181–3.

Matzdorff P (1926) Zwei seltene falle von peripherer sensibler lahmung, *Klin Wochenschr* **5**: 1187.

Monro A (1788) *Description of all the Bursae Mucosae of the Human Body* (Elliot TK: Edinburgh).

Montalvan B, Le Viet D (1997) Subluxation et luxation du cubital postérieur chez le joueur de tennis. In: Simon L, Revel M, Rodineau J, eds, *Main et Médecine Orthopédique* (Masson: Paris) 238–47.

Moran S, Ruby LK (1992) Nonrheumatoid closed rupture of extensor carpi ulnaris tendon, *J Hand Surg* **17A**: 281–3.

Murray WT, Meuller PR, Rosenthal DI, Jauernek RR (1979) Fracture of the hook of the hamate, *Am J Roentgenol* **133**: 899–903.

Nachinocar UG, Khanolkar KB (1988) Stenosing tenovaginitis of extensor carpi ulnaris: brief report, *J Bone Joint Surg* **70B**: 839.

Nisenfield FG, Neviaser RJ (1974) Fracture of the hook of the hamate: a diagnosis easily missed, *J Trauma* **14**: 612–16.

Osterman LA, Moskowe L, Low DW (1988) Soft-tissue injuries of the hand and wrist in racquet sports, *Clin Sports Med* **7**: 329–35.

Palmieri TJ (1982) The excision of painful pisiform bone fractures, *Orthop Rev* **11**: 99–103.

Rayank Ghazi M (1983) Recurrent dislocation of the extensor carpi ulnaris in athletes, *Am J Sports Med* **11**: 183–4.

Ritter MA, Inglis AE (1969) The extensor indicis proprius syndrome, *J Bone Joint Surg* **51A**: 645–8.

Rodineau J, Saillant G (1987) La fracture de l'apophyse unciforme de l'os crochu en traumatologie du sport, *Rev Chir Orthop* **73** (Suppl 2): 103–5.

Spinner M, Kaplan EB (1970) Extensor carpi ulnaris. Its relationship to the stability of the distal radio-ulnar joint, *Clin Orthop* **68**: 124–9.

Stark MH, Jobe FW, Boyes JH, Ashworth CR (1977) Fractures of the hook of the hamate in athletes, *J Bone Joint Surg* **59A**: 575–82.

Takami H, Takahashi S, Ando M, Kabata K (1991) Rupture of the flexor tendon secondary to osteoarthritis of the pisopisiforme joint: case report, *J Trauma* **31**: 1703–6.

Tessier J, Escarre PH, Asencio G, Gomis R, Allieu Y (1983) Rupture des tendons fléchisseurs de l'auriculaire sur fracture de l'apophyse unciforme de l'os crochu: à propos de 2 cas, *Ann Chir Main* **2**: 319–27.

Wartenberg Z (1932) Cheiralgia paresthesica (Isolierte neuritis des ramus superficialis nervi radialis), *Ger Neurol Psychiat* **141**: 145–55.

Wittenberg RH, Schaal S, Muhr G (1992) Surgical treatment of persistent elbow epicondylitis, *Clin Orthop* **278**: 73–80.

Wood MB, Dobyns JH (1986) Sports-related extra articular wrist syndromes, *Clin Orthop* **202**: 93–101.

Wood MB, Linscheid RL (1973) Abductor pollicis longus bursitis, *Clin Orthop* **93**: 293–6.

Woods THE (1964) De Quervain's disease: a plea for early operation, *Br J Surg* **57**: 358–9.

V Other conditions

40 Occupational disorders in the upper extremity

Frank D Burke

The association between work and upper limb complaints remains contentious, with widespread disagreement between clinicians as to causation in many instances. There are a variety of reasons creating this disparity of view.

National perceptions of injury at work have developed independently over the last 100 years. These developments have been moulded by the local occupational health concerns and the legal framework within a particular country. On occasions, this has produced radically different attitudes to causation by work across national boundaries. In the United Kingdom, the principle consequence of the use of vibrating tools at work is considered to be a vasospastic complaint to the hands (vibration white finger). Bone changes are considered to be rarely seen. Other countries in Europe have considered vibration disease to bone to be a common manifestation which merits compensation.

The subject is studied by a variety of specialists, including epidemiologists, surgeons, rheumatologists, occupational physicians, ergonomists, occupational therapists and physiotherapists. The assessment techniques are diverse between investigator groups, making comparison and collaboration between professions difficult.

From the strictly philosophical point of view, the epidemiologic approach has certain advantages. Whole populations (geographical or industrial) may be assessed at a specific point in time (a cross-sectional study) or a group may be assessed over a period of time (a cohorts' study). Groups can be compared with controls (a case control study). The data are then submitted to statistical analysis to reveal normal rates of presentation of upper limb disorders, and to identify an increased incidence for at risk occupations. Such studies may attempt complete analysis of the working or local population, but there are inherent weaknesses to this form of study. Cross-sectional studies may not identify temporary changes in practice or adequately assess length of exposure. Diagnostic criteria might not be rigorous (weak case definition). It is not uncommon for such studies to rely on patient questionnaires or nurse evaluation of physical signs for diagnosis (which has the effect of further limiting diagnostic accuracy). Several specific upper limb complaints may be amalgamated into a larger group for statistical purposes. The study then becomes less specific in its area of investigation, and the amalgamation of groups may have the effect of hiding a subgroup association with work. A job title may be used as a quick and easy assessment of upper limb function at work. However, the correlation between job title and the range of upper limb movements, and power requirement in individual cases may be extremely poor.

The clinician's assessment makes no attempt at the overview. It seeks to advance knowledge on work causation by precise diagnosis of the limited number of cases referred for an opinion. The assessor is commonly an experienced physician or surgeon. Diagnosis is further enhanced by the availability of provocative tests and clinical investigations. An epidemiological assessment of workers with pain at the base of the thumb might consider the entire group as suffering from de Quervain's tenovaginitis. A clinician's assessment of a similar group may wish to remove all patients with arthritis of the first carpometacarpal (CMC) joint and the scaphotrapezial joint, or patients with a scaphoid nonunion, and may require specific physical signs for validation of a diagnosis of de Quervain's syndrome. Laxity of the ligaments supporting the first carpometacarpal joint is a common cause of pain at the thumb base amongst young females. Stress testing the first CMC joint readily differentiates laxity from de Quervain's tenovaginitis.

Surgeons commonly have the additional benefit of direct visualization of the involved structures at operative exploration, with perhaps a local biopsy to evaluate the underlying pathological process. There is a resurgence of interest in the basic science of common upper limb disorders. However, there is still a paucity of histological data concerning upper limb disorders, and many clinicians see further studies in this area as crucial to the understanding of causation in possible work-related upper limb disorders.

The ergonomic assessment shares with clinical medicine rather more art than science. Neither profession has a sufficiently large core of knowledge at present. This can allow two competent, unbiased ergonomists or clinicians to hold diametrically opposed views on work causation in many cases. The validity of accepted tolerances for workplace activity in terms of frequency of use, joint range, force or workplace design are often no more than a best guess, which takes little account of the effect of age, stature and general fitness.

The legal perspective also moulds attitudes to work-related upper limb disorders. In the UK, judgement is based on the balance of probability. The medical experts are not asked to state with certainty whether a condition was caused by work, they are simply asked whether it is more or less likely. Alternative systems have a threshold for acceptance which extends below a 51% likelihood. Legal processes in some countries are adversarial in nature or, alternatively, systems may be adjudicated through the use of a tribunal.

The psychological perspective cannot be discounted when considering a possible association between work and an upper limb disorder. Brown (1982) reminds us that motivation of the patient is more important to hand function than the actual number of available digits. Injury at work is often perceived as an assault, particularly if employer/employee relationships in the work place are polarized. A sense of aggrievement may markedly effect outcome (Paterson and Burke 1995). The possibility of personal financial gain almost inevitably affects the claimant's attitude to the injury. Compensation for personal injury is a desirable social practice, but it would be naive to assume that it did not produce its own problems in some cases. The counter-productive effect of the 'greenback poultice' has been well described by Grunert et al (1992) in two cohorts of patients (half injured in the home and half at the workplace). Both groups were assessed for their views as to the effect of personal error or fatigue in the cause of their injury while still in the Accident and Emergency room. The same assessment was made again 6 months later. Occupationally injured patients initially reported 46% personal error, but a significant number revised their view at 6 months with only 6% reporting personal error at that stage. The results among the non-occupationally injured patients were quite different; 71% admitting to personal error at the outset with little alteration in their attitude in the months that followed (66% retained that view when assessed later).

Meyer (1993) in a personal communication had the experience of treating over 30 patients with upper limb injuries of consequence at work. All were subsequently surreptitiously videoed by insurance carriers to assess their informal use of the hand. Meyer concluded that in all but one case they exhibited more ability on the video than they were prepared to admit at clinical assessment. The remaining patient in the series had a plaster cast to the forearm when the video was made and no conclusion could, therefore, be drawn on this case! In these circumstances, patients may feign additional disability to their doctor, but elsewhere will make full use of the available function. However, a minority of patients in such circumstances apparently live out more extensive disability at all times. This is perhaps more likely to occur in the presence of established psychological disease. It may suit a patient to live out a role of increased disability that places them at the centre of a supportive family group. Legal processes unfold slowly in many countries and a claimant in such circumstances may live out a role of excessive disability for several years before compensation is gained. It is uncertain whether the claimant is then capable of putting the issue behind him and capitalizing on all available remaining function to the limb. Brown (1991) advises that litigation be resolved as swiftly as possible to minimize the risk of the compensation process creating additional disability.

Psychology plays an extremely important role in the assessment of response to upper limb injury. It is not uncommon for patients to manifest psychological problems through an upper limb complaint. Hand surgeons should always be vigilant to identify patients with factitious injury (self-induced lacerations or insertion of foreign bodies or noxious fluids). The problem may take the form of a bona fide hand injury which is subsequently tampered with by the patient (the wound that does not heal). Secretan's syndrome (peritendonous fibrosis) is considered to be caused by percussion to the dorsal aspect of the hand, consciously or subconsciously. A small number of patients present with progressive 'flexion contractures' to the fingers (Figure 40.1). The problem is usually restricted to the ring and little fingers. This has the effect of creating a problem for which the patient needs help (the 'contracture' to the ring and little fingers), yet leaves fine manipulative skills (thumb, index and middle fingers) available for use.

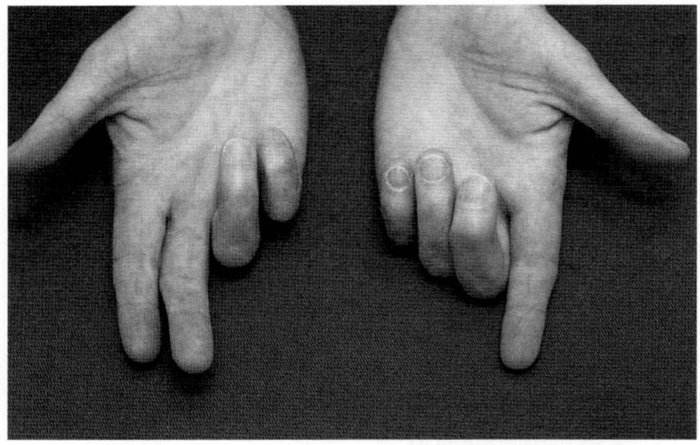

Figure 40.1
The psycho-flexed hand.

Criteria for assessing a work-related upper limb disorder

1. A specific and consistent upper limb diagnosis with symptoms and signs that do not flit about the upper limb. Generalized limb pain or fatigue should not be present.
2. The hand and upper limb movements required at work, and the force and frequency of the activity, should logically put the structure nominated by the specific diagnosis at risk.
3. A change in working practice around the time the symptoms developed. This may take the form of a new worker starting a repetitive job or an experienced worker returning to repetitive duties after a holiday or maternity leave. There may be a reduction in staffing of operatives servicing a conveyor belt with a steady output (in effect increasing personal activity). Alternatively, the work rate in terms of products processed per minute may have been increased.
4. The symptoms should ease on removing the operative from the activity in question, and increase on returning to such duties. Discomfort would commonly ease over a weekend and recur during Monday's shift.
5. A clustering of a specific diagnosis with several patients doing the same duties experiencing the same specific upper limb complaint. It is not uncommon for several workers from a company to present for assessment at the same time. However, they often have a variety of specific upper limb conditions or diffuse complaints that defy precise diagnosis. A clustering of cases is only supportive of work causation if a specific diagnosis is involved, and the activities at work would be likely to put those structures at risk.

Review of available documentation

If there has been a specific incident at work, inspection of the earliest records is essential. These documents are commonly drawn together before the thought of compensation has been considered. They, therefore, probably represent the least biased documents from all points of view. The earliest records might include an incident report from the factory, the assessment in the Accident and Emergency Department or from the family doctor. It is important to obtain all the previous medical family doctor records in these cases. The claimant may be seeking compensation for an upper limb condition which did not develop at the alleged time of onset, but was simply a recurrence or continuation of existing difficulties. It is not uncommon to find details of the mechanism of injury in the Accident and Emergency records which are at variance to the view subsequently put forward when a claim is being raised. Alternatively, the earliest family doctor records may reveal the cause of the injury to be other than work (for example, injury while working out in a gym).

Subsequent documents may reveal hospital referral with clinical examination by specialists in terms of symptoms and signs. Physiotherapy and occupational therapy reports are also very valuable in formulating a view as to diagnosis and causation. Operations may have been required, permitting visualization of damaged structures or biopsies revealing the pathological process involved.

Hobbies and sports may be an alternative cause of upper limb complaints. Claimants may be reluctant to discuss these areas. A simple request – do you perform any sports or hobbies? – will commonly produce a response in the negative. However, if the question is flighted along the lines of – does your current problem restrict you in carrying out your hobbies and sports? – a more comprehensive assessment of their non-work activities may become apparent!

Examination of the upper limb

Appearance

- Are there callosities to the palm, indicating adequate use?
- Is there swelling at the base of the thumb, suggestive of osteoarthritis of the first CMC joint (Figure 40.2)?

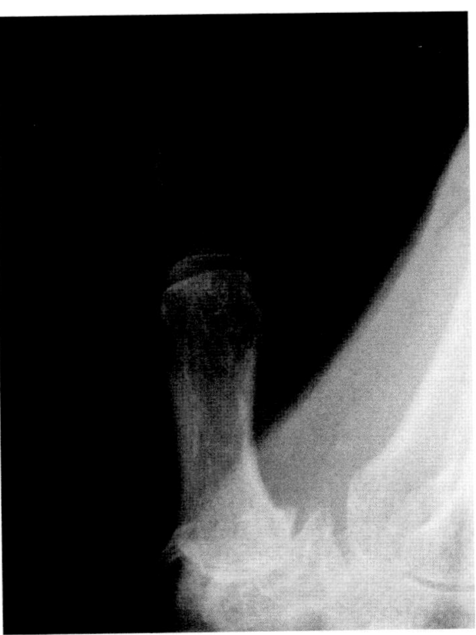

Figure 40.2

Osteoarthritis to the first carpometacarpal joint.

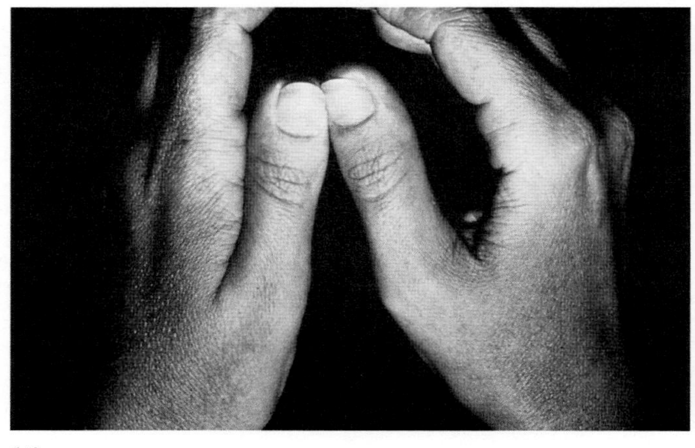
(A)

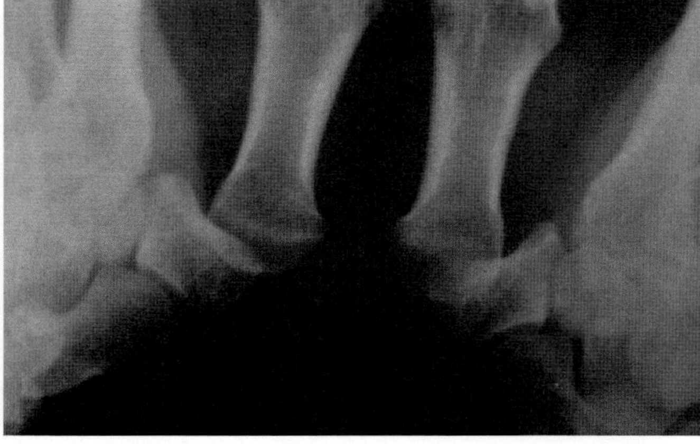
(B)

Figure 40.3
Ligamentous laxity of the first carpometacarpal joint: (A) The thumbs pressed together, creating a subluxing force to the first CMC joint; (B) subluxation demonstrated at the first CMC joint at the thumb bases.

- Are the pulps of the fingers atrophic, and the skin ridges absent, consistent with nerve injury?
- Is the skin thin, and apparently poorly used?
- If a splint is allegedly used continually, does it look dirty and used, and in summer months is the skin under the splint paler than the surrounding areas?
- Are movements of the digits slow and laborious, and is there a consistency of range?
- Are informal movements during the assessment indicative of a wider range than when specifically measured?

Palpation

- Is the extensor tendon under load when the patient is asked to exhibit maximal flexion of the fingers?
- Is there any crepitus over tendons or tenderness related to specific structures?
- Forearm circumference measurements – a standard number of centimetres proximal to the ulna styloid will give an objective assessment of forearm muscle bulk.
- Is sensibility reduced to light touch or monofilament devices?
- Does it lie within an accepted nerve area, or is it more in keeping with a glove and stocking distribution?
- Grip strength on the JAMAR dynamometer at the second setting is also worthwhile. Three measurements of maximal grip strength should cluster within 10% (Bechtol 1954). Hildreth et al (1989) recommend a rapid exchange grip test of six assessments (three right, three left alternating). Power pinch between thumb and index finger is performed in a similar manner.
- Ligamentous laxity to the first carpometacarpal joint is an important cause of discomfort at the base of the thumb, particularly in younger females. The joint should be stressed to assess laxity and discomfort (Figures 40.3A and B).

Investigations

X-rays may reveal osteoarthritis at the base of the first metacarpal or the scaphotrapezial joint, or scaphoid non-union in cases of radial border wrist pain. Keinbock's disease or impingement syndrome arising from an over-long ulna styloid may cause more central or ulna border wrist pain. A 30° supinated lateral documents the pisotriquetral joint and may reveal an osteoarthritic joint as a cause of ulna border wrist pain. Nerve conduction studies offer objective assessment of nerve function. Normal results do not exclude minor sensory complaints, but would disprove any significant loss of faculty through nerve injury.

A security video may be requested by insurance carriers who wish to obtain information on the informal use of the patient's hand. It can be particularly important where a young patient claims substantial disability in the absence of physical findings. The quantum in such cases is extremely high. A video in such circumstances can help all parties to come to an agreement as to the degree of continuing loss of function.

Upper limb disorders

Tennis elbow

The British Orthopaedic Association report to the Industrial Injuries Advisory Council in 1992 reviewed the available literature and did not feel there was evidence that tennis elbow was more frequent in manual workers, nor was it associated with any particular working activity. Dimberg's paper (1987) is widely quoted in legal cases concerning tennis elbow potentially caused by work. This reveals a majority of cases involving the dominant arm and a higher prevalence with advancing age. Heavy manual workers did not have a statistically significant increased incidence of the disorder. Diagnostic criteria require pain or tenderness to the lateral epicondyle or to the muscular tendinous area just distal to the bone. Pain in the appropriate area on resisted extension of the wrist is considered mandatory to sustain a diagnosis of tennis elbow. Dimberg considered that a minority of the patients he investigated (35%) probably had tennis elbow arising from their activities at work. He considered that 27% arose from hobbies and other leisure activities, and 8% from tennis. No cause was found for the remaining 30%. The condition is considered to be frequently constitutional in nature, arising from degenerative processes in the extensor origin as it inserts into the bone. Many doctors would allow a minority of tennis elbows to have arisen from an acute injury to the extensor origin close to the insertion to bone. The condition may also arise from forceful supination or dorsiflexion of the arm. Tennis elbow may be provoked by lifting heavy objects away from the body with the elbow in a fairly extended position. The forces acting through the extensor origin during such an activity are extremely high, which may lead to tissue failure – particularly in situations where degenerative changes to the extensor insertion into bone have already taken place.

Golfer's elbow is generally considered to be a similar process involving the flexor origin in the area of the medial epicondyle. Diagnostic criteria again require tenderness directly over the medial epicondyle or within 2 or 3 cm distally. Pain should be provoked in the appropriate area on resisted flexion of the wrist.

Radial tunnel syndrome has been put forward as a condition which may arise from activities at work. The condition is caused by radial or posterior interosseous nerve compression at or around the arcade of Frohse between the two heads of supinator. Regrettably, nerve conduction studies are not considered diagnostic in confirming the presence or the absence of radial tunnel syndrome. Diagnostic criteria include pain in the proximal radial forearm, tenderness over the radial tunnel (somewhat more distal and more medial than tennis elbow), pain during resisted forearm supination and pain during the resisted middle finger extension test. Lawrence et al (1995) considered that patients with occupations requiring repetitive manual tasks seemed to be particularly at risk for developing radial tunnel syndrome, and justified the statement with a literature review which suggested a high incidence among manual workers, and an absence of radial tunnel syndrome in people who are retired. The dominant hand was noted to be affected in 89% of patients. They postulate repeated prono-supination under load or forceful wrist extension to cause the condition (Stuley 1996). To date, the condition has been investigated in only relatively small patient groups, and there is no firm evidence that radial tunnel syndrome is occupationally induced.

Tenosynovitis of the wrist extensors

Thompson et al (1951) reported an extensive series of over 500 cases from the Vauxhall Motor Company. The tendons most commonly affected were the radial wrist extensors. He considered the condition to be peritendonitis crepitans which did not involve the extensor tendon sheath, but more proximally at the musculotendinous junction, 4 cm or more proximal to the radial styloid. Onset was provoked by a change in working practice, a return to work after absence, specific local injury or simply repetitive movements under load and at speed. A short period of splintage resolved almost all the patients' difficulties.

More recently, Grundberg and Reagan (1985) reported on a proximal intersection syndrome where the muscle bellies of the abductor pollicis longus and extensor pollicis brevis crossed the common wrist extensors. The swelling is 4 cm proximal to the radial styloid in a similar position to that described by Thompson et al. They consider the condition to be a stenosing tenosynovitis of the radial wrist extensors. They found that 60% of patients obtained permanent relief with non-operative intervention (splintage or steroid injections to the second dorsal compartment). Decompression of the second dorsal compartment revealed acute or chronic synovitis. There is an acceptance that peritendonitis crepitans or proximal intersection syndrome can be caused by activities at work, particularly if the aetiological factors that Thompson et al reported on are present. Diagnostic criteria for extensor tenosynovitis require local swelling, with or without tenderness, in the area of the appropriate extensor compartment. Crepitus is diagnostic.

Silverstein et al (1987) consider that the epidemiological evidence for hand/wrist tendonitis being work-related is reasonably convincing. However, many of the studies involved make no distinction between the extensor compartment involved and in particular do not discriminate between de Quervain's tenovaginitis and tenosynovitis involving alternative compartments.

De Quervain's tenovaginitis

De Quervain's syndrome has attracted renewed interest in recent years and many hand surgeons consider it should be regarded as an entirely separate entity to extensor tendon tenosynovitis. Biopsy of the first extensor sheath has failed to reveal any evidence of inflammation. The thickened tissue reveals increased vascularity and myxomatous tissue with chondroid metaplasia (Ippolito et al 1985). Jackson et al (1986) identified anatomical abnormalities in 27 out of 40 patients with de Quervain's tenovaginitis. The number of tendons differed from what was considered standard with complete or partial septation in 40% of cases. They found that septation of the first extensor compartment was more common in patients with de Quervain's disease than in the general population, and considered that this anatomical abnormality was involved in the aetiology of de Quervain's disease. Witt et al (1991) found steroid injections to be very helpful in relieving de Quervain's tenovaginitis. A minority of patients had recurrent problems; 33 unresolved cases were explored and no less than 73% had a separate compartment for extensor pollicis brevis. The prevalence of a separate compartment was in their view significantly higher than in the general population. The occupations of the patients in their series did not appear to indict any particular form of activity. The diagnostic criterion for de Quervain's tenovaginitis is localized swelling (Figure 40.4), with or without tenderness, to the first extensor compartment. Crepitus is again diagnostic.

Epidemiologists and occupational physicians rarely classify de Quervain's tenovaginitis separately, and there are few papers from those areas that specifically seek to offer a view as to whether the condition is caused by work. Pain at the base of the wrist on the radial border may be considered an adequate diagnostic criterion for de Quervain's syndrome. However, the very high prevalence of degenerative arthritis to the base of the thumb in post-menopausal women (Armstrong et al 1994) considerably undermines radial wrist pain alone as the criterion for diagnosis of de Quervain's syndrome. Armstrong and colleagues identified the prevalence of osteoarthritis at the base of the thumb at 28%, and observed that 55% of patients with combined carpometacarpal and scaphotrapezial arthritis complained of basal thumb pain.

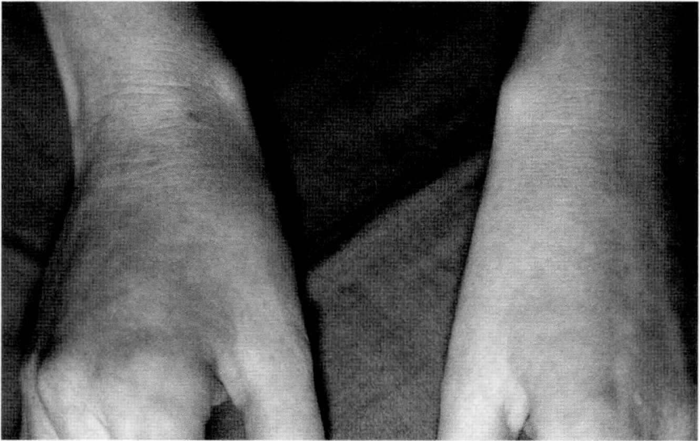

Figure 40.4
De Quervain's tenovaginitis of the first extensor sheath.

Flexor tenosynovitis

The condition is less easy to diagnose. Swelling is less obvious and crepitus is rare. Isolated tenosynovitis involving the flexor carpi ulnaris or the flexor carpi radialis is probably the most obvious in presentation because of their proximity to the skin. Tenosynovitis involving the digital flexors is infrequently seen.

Flexor tenosynovitis and carpal tunnel syndrome

In the UK, carpal tunnel syndrome is on occasions considered a work-related upper limb disorder. The association is made on the basis that the patient has flexor tenosynovitis arising from work creating carpal tunnel syndrome as a secondary event. The association is questioned by Kerr et al (1992) and Badalamente (1994). Kerr reviewed 625 patients with chronic idiopathic carpal tunnel syndrome and obtained synovial biopsies when decompression was performed. Only 23 (4%) showed chronic inflammation on synovial biopsy and one patient (0.2%) revealed evidence of acute inflammation. In a similar study Badalamente reviewed the synovium of 125 patients and found no evidence of tenosynovitis in any specimen. The concept of flexor tenosynovitis playing a role in the development of carpal tunnel syndrome remains questionable.

Carpal tunnel syndrome and work

There are several epidemiologic studies suggesting an association between carpal tunnel syndrome and work. Perhaps the most authoritative is by Silverstein et al (1987), which reviewed 652 active workers. Their jobs were assessed for hand force and repetitiveness. The authors concluded that carpal tunnel syndrome was strongly associated with high force, highly repetitive work and to a lesser extent highly repetitive work alone irrespective of other factors. However, the British Orthopaedic Association Working Party (Barton et al 1992) considered that there was little evidence to support the view that the majority of patients with carpal tunnel syndrome were suffering from a work-related upper limb disorder. They acknowledged that work might on rare occasions cause carpal tunnel syndrome, but felt that the vast majority of cases were not caused by work. They did, however, acknowledge that work might exacerbate the symptoms in someone with pre-existing carpal tunnel syndrome. Nathan and Keniston (1993) and Stallings et al (1997) investigated carpal tunnel syndrome against the patients' general physical condition. They concluded that being overweight, older and physically inactive were major risk factors. Burke et al (1997) investigated the incidence of carpal tunnel syndrome in a local population of 400,000. The incidence of carpal tunnel syndrome in working females was lower than the incidence in non-working females of working age (93 per 100,000 of population per year compared with 147 per 100,000 for the economically inactive group). The results do not exclude the possibility of carpal tunnel syndrome being caused by work, but do suggest that an association with work is unusual.

Carpal tunnel syndrome and vibration white finger

Vibration injury to the hand takes two main forms. There is a vasospastic variety, characterized by the development of episodic blanching of the digits (vibration white finger). Alternatively, a peripheral neuropathy may become apparent. Vibration white finger was accepted by the Department of Health and Social Security of the UK as a compensatable disease in 1985. Nineteen patients were assessed for compensation in Boyle et al's (1988) study. No less than 63% had carpal tunnel syndrome, confirmed by nerve conduction studies. The effect of carpal tunnel decompression in this group was of interest. Savage et al (1990) subsequently reported that eight of the group were treated by surgical decompression of the carpal tunnel. On review 6 months later, all symptoms of carpal tunnel syndrome had improved, and half the patients considered that the vibration white finger symptoms were also improved. On the limited evidence available, it seems reasonable to conclude that there is an association between carpal tunnel syndrome and vibration white finger. Decompression of the nerve is of neurological and sometimes vascular benefit. The progress of the white finger is halted by transfer to duties that avoid use of vibrating tools (Figure 40.5). Some patients improve slowly thereafter, others observe neither improvement nor deterioration.

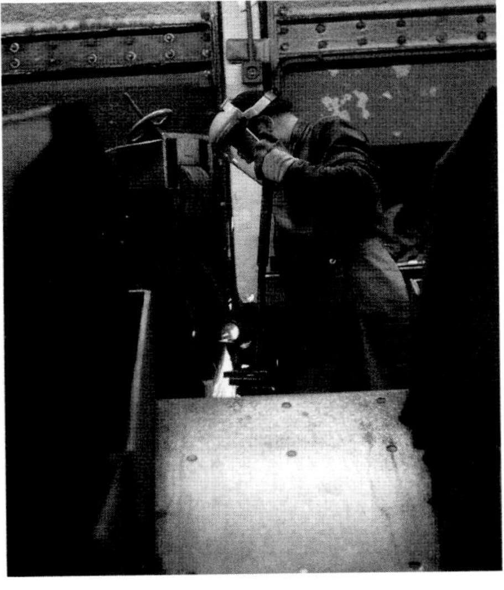

Figure 40.5

A fettler smoothing off castings in a foundry. The persistent vibration places him at risk for developing vibration white finger.

Ganglia arising from the wrist joint and flexor tendon sheath

The British Orthopaedic Association Working Party (Barton et al 1992) did not find any compelling evidence to suggest that ganglia were caused by work. They cited Barnes et al (1964) to justify their view. More recently Al Khawashki and Hooper (1997) also considered there was no relationship to repeated occupational trauma.

Trigger finger

The pathobiology of trigger finger has been investigated by Sampson et al (1991). Histological analysis of 65 patients with trigger digits revealed no evidence of a synovial cell layer at the level of the A1 pulley. Tenosynovitis did not appear to play a role in causation. The underlying pathological process was characterized by fibro-cartilaginous metaplasia. It is unclear whether this adaptive or degenerative process is associated with heavy use of the hand. The limited available literature on this condition does not offer a reasonable case for work association at present.

Osteoarthritis to the first carpometacarpal joint

To date, there is no convincing evidence that osteoarthritis to the first carpometacarpal joint is the consequence

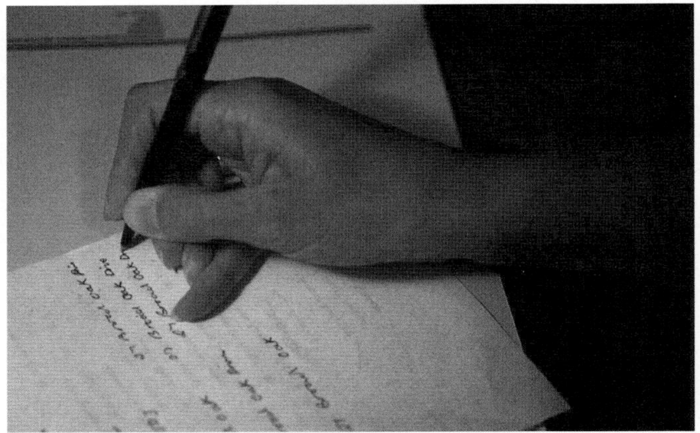

Figure 40.6
Writer's cramp. The fingers are drawn into excessive flexion shortly after starting to write.

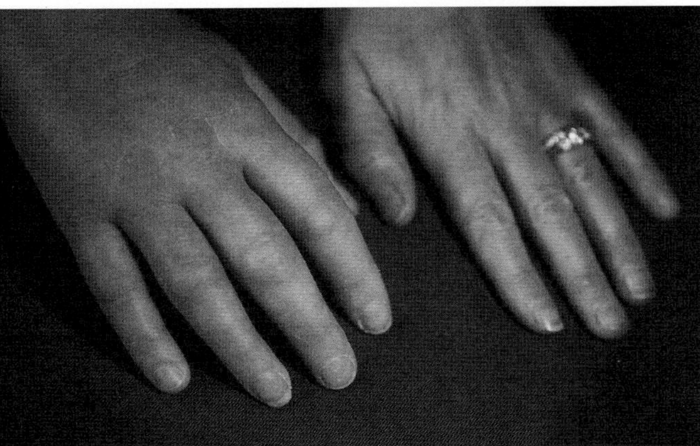

Figure 40.7
Complex regional pain syndrome (type I) involving the hand.

of repetitive use of the hand. Lawrence (1961) suggested that there might be an association, but analysis of working activity was poor. Pellegrini (1991) considers that the high prevalence of osteoarthritis at the base of the thumb in post-menopausal females probably relates to those patients experiencing undue ligamentous laxity at the CMC joint in their teens and twenties, rather than any specific activities at work thereafter.

Writer's cramp (or musician's cramp)

This is a relatively rare condition and is considered to be a focal dystonia. It is characterized by a contraction of the agonist and antagonist muscles in the forearm and hand. It is brought on by a specific activity (writing or playing a musical instrument). The hand only demonstrates lack of coordination during the specific activity, and the joints are commonly drawn into bizarre postures (Figure 40.6). The problem does not arise during normal activities, and is not of itself painful, although there may be an ache. Rhoad and Stern (1993) consider that botulinum toxin injections are a promising therapeutic advance. This rare condition should not be confused with complex regional pain syndromes (which are characterized by pain rather than an ache, muscle tenderness and fatigue, and are triggered by a wide variety of manual activities).

Complex regional pain syndrome

Patients with chronic arm pain, in the absence of physical signs, are sometimes considered to be suffering from reflex sympathetic dystrophy. Reflex sympathetic dystrophy has in recent times been reclassified as complex regional pain syndrome type I. CRPS type I is defined on the basis of four diagnostic criteria (Glynn 1995):

1. The presence of an initiating noxious event or a cause of immobilization.
2. Continuing pain or hyperalgesia with the pain disproportionate to any inciting event.
3. Evidence at some time of oedema, changes in skin blood flow or abnormal sudomotor activity in the region of the pain (Figure 40.7).
4. The diagnosis is excluded by the existence of conditions that would otherwise account for the degree of pain and discomfort.

Criteria 2, 3 and 4 must be present to confirm the diagnosis. Hyperalgesia, and at some time oedema or abnormal sudomotor activity, must be present to sustain the diagnosis. CRPS type 1 is usually obvious in the more severe cases, but difficulty with the classification of milder cases occurs frequently. The uncertainty with diagnosis bedevils assessment of treatment protocols and restricts research in this area.

References

Al Khawashki H, Hooper G (1997). Distribution of fibrous flexor sheath ganglion, *J Hand Surgy* **22B**: 226–7.

Armstrong AL, Hunter JB, Davis TRC (1994). The prevalence of degenerative arthritis of the base of the thumb in post-menopausal women, *J Hand Surg* **19B**: 340–1.

Badalamente MA (1994) Correspondence Newsletter. American Society for Surgery of the Hand, No. 148.

Barnes, WE, Larsen RD, Posch JL (1964). Review of ganglion of the

wrist and hand with analysis of surgical technique, *Plast Reconstr Surg* **34**: 570–8.
Barton NJ, Hooper G, Noble J, Steel WM (1992). Occupational causes of disorders in the upper limb, *Br Med J* **304**: 309–11.
Bechtol C (1954) The use of a dynamometer with adjustable hand spacings, *J Bone Joint Surg* **36A**: 820–4.
Boyle JC, Smith NJ, Burke FD (1988) Vibration white finger, *J Hand Surg* **13B**: 171–6.
Brown P (1982) Less than 10 – surgeons with amputated fingers, *J Hand Surg* **7**: 31–7.
Brown P (1991) The role of motivation in the recovery of the hand. In: Kasdan ML, ed., *Occupational Hand and Upper Extremity Injuries and Diseases* (Hanley and Belfus: Philadelphia) 1–11.
Burke FD, Dias J, Webster H (1997) Median nerve compression syndrome at the wrist. In: Hunter J, Sneider L, Mackin E, eds, *Tendon and Nerve Surgery in the Hand. A Third Decade* (Mosby: St Louis) 145–8.
Dimberg L (1987) The prevalence and causation of tennis elbow (lateral humeral epicondylitis) in a population of workers in an engineering industry, *Ergonomics* **30**: 573–80.
Glyn C (1995) Complex regional pain syndrome type I. Reflex sympathetic dystrophy and complex regional pain syndrome type 2 – causalgia, *Pain Reviews* **2**: 292–7.
Grundberg AB, Reagan DS (1985) Pathologic anatomy of the forearm: intersection syndrome, *J Hand Surg* **10A**: 299–302.
Grunert BK, Hargarten SW, Matloub HS et al (1992) Predictive value of psychological screening in acute hand injuries, *J Hand Surg* **17A**: 196–9.
Hildreth DH, Briedenback WC, Lister GD, Hodges AD (1989) Detection of submaximal effort by use of the rapid exchange grip, *J Hand Surg* **14A**: 742–5.
Ippolito E, Postacchini F, Scola E et al (1985) De Quervain's disease, *Int Orthop* **9**: 41–7.
Jackson WT, Viegas SF, Coon TM et al (1986). Anatomical variations in the first extensor compartment of the wrist, *J Bone Joint Surg* **68A**: 923–6.
Kerr CD, Sybert DR, Albarracin NS (1992) An analysis of the flexor synovium in idiopathic carpal tunnel ryndrome. Report of 625 cases, *J Hand Surg* **17A**: 1028–30.
Lawrence JS (1961) Rheumatism in cotton operatives, *Br J Ind Med* **18**: 270–6.
Lawrence T, Mobbs P, Fortems Y, Stanley JK (1995) Radial tunnel syndrome, *J Hand Surg* **20B**: 454–9.
Meyer FN (1993) Correspondence Newsletter. American Society for Surgery of the Hand, No. 131.
Nathan PA, Keniston RC (1993) Carpal tunnel syndrome and its relationship to general physical condition, *Hand Clin* **9**: 253–61.
Paterson MC, Burke, FD (1995) Psychosocial consequences of upper limb injury, *J Hand Surg* **20B**: 776–81.
Pellegrini VD (1991) Osteoarthritis of the trapezio-metacarpal joint. The pathophysiology of articular cartilage degeneration. 1. Anatomy and pathology of the ageing joint, *J Hand Surg* **16A**: 967–74.
Rhoad RC, Stern PJ (1993) Writer's cramp. A focal dystonia. Aetiology diagnosis and treatment, *J Hand Surg* **18A**: 542–4.
Sampson SP, Badalamente MA, Hurst LC, Seidman J (1991) Pathobiology of human A1 pulley in trigger finger, *J Hand Surg* **16A**: 714–21.
Savage R, Burke FD, Smith NJ, Hopper I (1990) Carpal tunnel syndrome in association with vibration white finger, *J Hand Surg* **15B**: 100–3.
Silverstein BA, Fine LJ, Armstrong TJ (1987) Occupational factors and carpal tunnel syndrome, *Am J Ind Med* **11**: 343–58.
Stallings SP, Kasdan ML, Saergel TM, Corwin HM (1997) A case control study of obesity as a risk factor for carpal tunnel syndrome in a population of 600 patients presenting for independent medical examination, *J Hand Surg* **22A**: 211–15.
Stanley JK (1996) Letter to Editor, *J Hand Surg* **21B**: 562.
Thompson AR, Plewes LW, Shaw EG (1951) Peritendonitis crepitans and simple tenosynovitis. A clinical study of 544 cases in industry, *Br J Ind Med* **8**: 150–8.
Witt J, Pess G, Gelberman R (1991) Treatment of De Quervain's tenosynovitis, *J Bone Joint Surg* **73A**: 219–22.

41 Soft tissue and bone tumors of the hand

C Leclercq

The actual incidence of hand tumours is rather difficult to assess, because their management is spread out among a number of specialists. Even nowadays, a lot of tumors of the hand are treated by many different specialists: cutaneous tumors are mostly dealt with by dermatologists or plastic surgeons, whereas bone tumors are usually referred to orthopedic surgeons. Also the definition of 'tumors' is rather vague, and a number of non-tumoral lesions, such as ganglia, inclusion cysts, even Dupuytren's disease, are often included in series of hand tumors.

The largest reported series are by Haber et al (1965: 2321 cases) which includes 507 Dupuytren's diseases and a number of post-traumatic neuromas, Posch (1956: 679 cases), Bogumill et al (1975), Johnson (1985: 543 cases), and Glicenstein et al (1988: 471 cases). A recent survey of all tumors operated in a large hand surgery centre (Institut de la Main) between 1995 and 2002, reported 1952 cases (Mateva and Leclercq 2003). The vast majority of hand tumors are located in the soft tissues (Table 41.1). About half of them are ganglia (1024), the next most frequent being mucous cysts (192), pigmented villonodular synovitis (173) and glomus tumors (79). The breakdown into each kind of tumor is reported in Table 41.2. This article will not deal with cutaneous tumors, which do not display specific features at the level of the hand as compared to other locations, but will be devoted to soft tissue and bone tumors, some of which are very specific to the hand.

Table 41.1 *Series of l'Institut de la Main: location of hand tumors in the different tissues*

Location	*Percentage*
Cutaneous tumors	5.53
Soft tissue tumors	87.8
Bone tumors	6.66

Table 41.2 *Series of l'Institut de la Main: the eight most frequent tumors*

Tumor	*Number*	*%*
Ganglion	1024	70
Mucous cyst	192	9.8
Pigmented villonodular synovitis	173	8.8
Glomus tumor	79	4
Chondroma	73	3.5
Schwannoma	44	2.2
Epidermal cyst	41	2.1
Fibroma	23	1.1

Soft tissue tumors

The word 'tumor' should be taken here in its broadest sense, because a large number of these lesions are not true tumors, but rather pseudo-tumors.

Soft tissue tumors represent on average 70% of all hand tumors. They consist mostly of ganglia, mucous cysts, pigmented villonodular synovitis, lipomas and glomus tumors. Nerve, vascular, and fibrous tumors are less frequent.

Symptoms of soft tissue tumors are not specific, made of a spontaneous swelling, occasionally noted after a local trauma. Sometimes the swelling is painful. Functional impairment is usually associated with pain, or localization near a joint.

Ganglia

Ganglia are the most common tumors in the hand. This is a benign neoplasm which develops adjacent to joints and tendon sheaths. It is formed of a wall which resembles synovial tissue, but is exempt of any pathological process, containing a viscous fluid. They are more common in women, and most prevalent in the second and third decades of life.

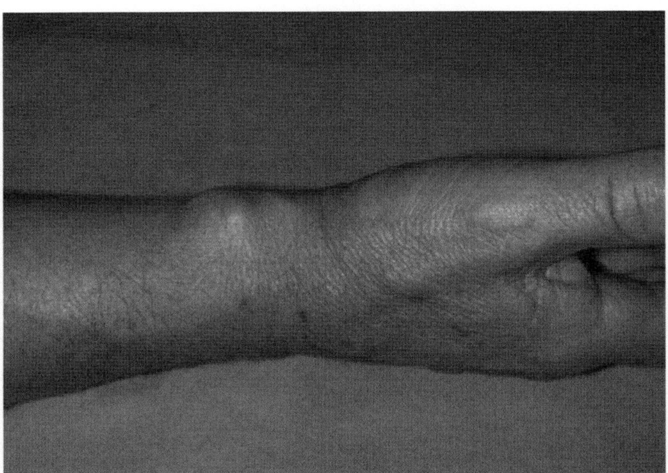

Figure 41.1
Ganglion on the palmar aspect of the wrist.

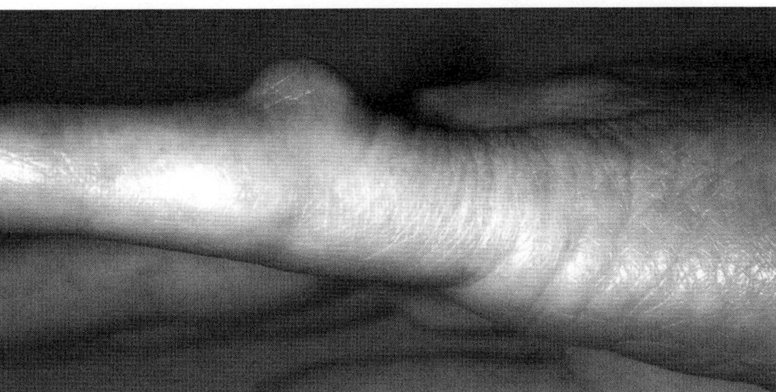

(A)

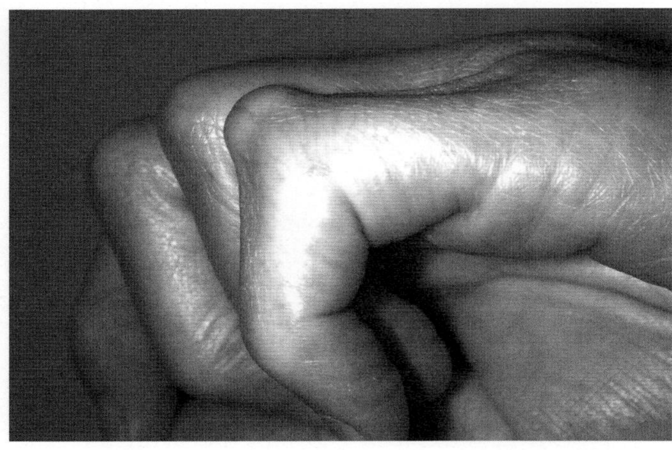

(B)

Figure 41.2
Ganglion located on the dorsal aspect of the PIP joint (A), interfering with full flexion (B).

The swelling often appears spontaneously, occasionally following an injury. Usually hard and tense, the swelling may become soft and may even disappear spontaneously.

Ganglia are most commonly located at the wrist, either dorsal or palmar, less commonly on the flexor tendon sheaths, extensor tendons, or near a finger joint. Ganglia on the dorsal aspect of the wrist are usually located in the scapholunate area, appearing between the third and the fourth dorsal compartments. Occasionally they are located in the anatomical snuffbox or other dorsal wrist compartments. They may be painful, especially during hyperextension of the wrist, but they are usually not troublesome, except for their cosmetic aspect. The possibility of an intracapsular dorsal ganglion should always be considered when confronted with isolated chronic wrist pain without apparent swelling. Ultrasound or magnetic resonance imaging (MRI) will usually visualize the ganglion.

Ganglions are less often located on the palmar aspect of the wrist (Figure 41.1). They are often located near the radial artery, and may produce a functional obstruction of the artery, best investigated by Allen's test. They may also be located in Guyon's canal which may result in an ulnar nerve compression.

Ganglia arising from the flexor tendon sheaths generally occur at the metacarpophalangeal (MP) level, most commonly in the middle finger. The swelling is usually small, firm, and independent of the flexor tendon motion. It is often tender on pressure, and may prevent powerful grasp. Digital ganglia are less common. They are mainly found on the dorsal aspect of the proximal interphalangeal joint, between the central tendon and the lateral band. They may interfere with full finger flexion (Figure 41.2).

Ganglia may also be located inside a bone, and the most frequent occurrence is in the lunate or in the scaphoid bones (Figure 41.3).

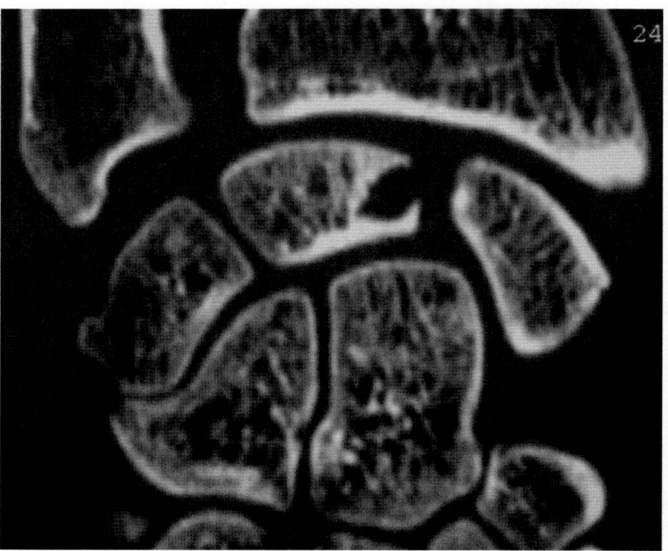

Figure 41.3
Intraosseous ganglion, located in the lunate (CT scan).

The diagnosis of a ganglion is usually straightforward, and no complementary investigations are required. When necessary, ultrasound imaging will confirm the liquid nature of the swelling, and MRI will establish its articular or tendinous origin.

Pathologic anatomy

The clinical swelling represents only the outer part of the lesion, which is prolonged deeply by a pedicle of variable length to the real origin of the ganglion. The existence of a communication between the ganglion and the joint cavity has been widely debated. Razemon (1983) reported no evidence of a communication on 300 ganglia, but found multiple neighboring microganglia. His hypothesis is that rather than dosing from a hernia, ganglia come from a degeneration or mucous secretion of the para-articular connective tissue. The thick wall contains many small cysts, one of which develops by the coalescence of several small cysts. Microscopically, the wall of the cyst consists of connective tissue with no synovial lining, which persuaded several authors to reject the term 'synovial cyst'. Study of the pericystic articular capsule frequently reveals adjacent microcysts caused by a myxoid infiltration, and devoid of a true wall.

Treatment

Many different treatments have been advocated, they carry the same risk of recurrence, which is the only true complication of this condition.

Abstaining can be justified as long as the ganglion is not bothersome to the patient. In a number of cases, a spontaneous and permanent regression can occur.

Compression bursting can be performed on a tense ganglion of the dorsal wrist. The compression is performed with a flat, hard object (coin, thumb, hammer, family Bible! . . .), and results in a in a large tear in the cyst wall, with the synovial fluid spreading into the surrounding tissues. The rate of recurrence is high, but some authors remain faithful to the technique, confident that a permanent cure may be obtained after several burstings.

Aspiration alone, or combined with the injection of a variety of substances, often produces a high recurrence rate. This rate can be reduced by immobilizing the wrist in a splint for 3 weeks after the injection (Richman and Gelberman 1987).

Surgical excision of the ganglion appears to be the most effective treatment. Excision should include all of the ganglion and its pedicle down to the affected capsule. Following Razemon (1983), we resect an additional collar of pericystic capsule 2–4 cm² large, then immobilize the wrist for 2 weeks in a splint to avoid capsular retraction. Series from the literature report recurrence rates between 3 and 20% after surgical excision.

Removal of a palmar wrist ganglion must be performed with care so as to avoid an injury to the radial artery, which may be deviated by or even enclosed in the cyst. First the artery should be identified proximally then the dissection should be performed under magnifying loops.

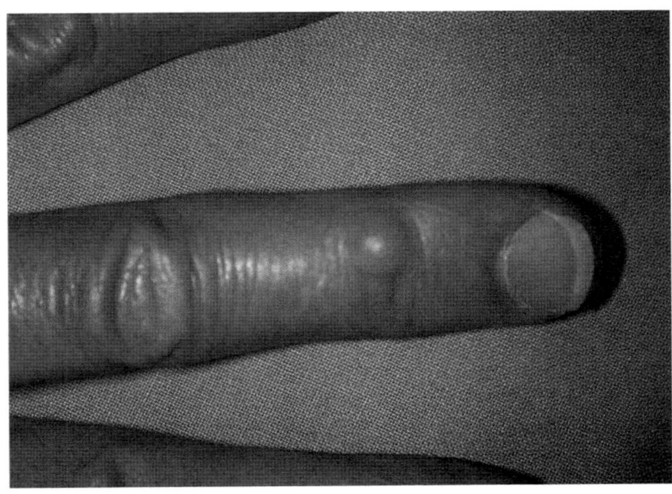

Figure 41.4
Mucous cyst.

Mucous cysts

Initially described by Hyde in 1883, mucous cysts were considered to be a form of ganglion, however, they have some specific features. They are almost exclusively located on the dorsal aspect of the distal interphalangeal joint (DIP) joint usually dorso-laterally, and present as a small, rounded, usually painless swelling (Figure 41.4). If they lie on the nail matrix, a nail deformity is often associated. The cyst is adherent to the overlying skin, which may become thinned, and may even ulcerate, releasing a thick fluid. They affect mostly the 50- and 60-year age groups. There is a high prevalence of associated osteoarthritis of the DIP joint.

The histology is similar to that of a ganglion, with a connective tissue pseudo-capsule containing a mucous material.

As regards their pathogenesis, no consensus has been reached. Several studies have demonstrated a constant communication between the cyst and the underlying DIP joint (Kleinert et al 1972, Newmeyer et al 1974).

The treatment of choice is surgical excision. Abstaining carries a risk of fistulization and secondary infectious arthritis. Aspiration combined with injection of various substances carries a high risk of recurrences.

Excision should include the skin when it is thinned, the cyst, and its pedicle, which may run underneath the extensor tendon. Kleinert et al (1972) recommend a routine synovectomy, and excision of osteophytes. Direct

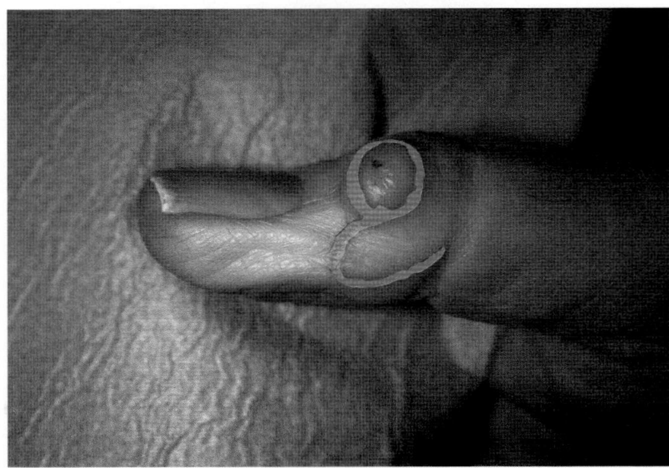

Figure 41.5
Planning of a rotation flap to cover the skin defect after excision of a mucous cyst.

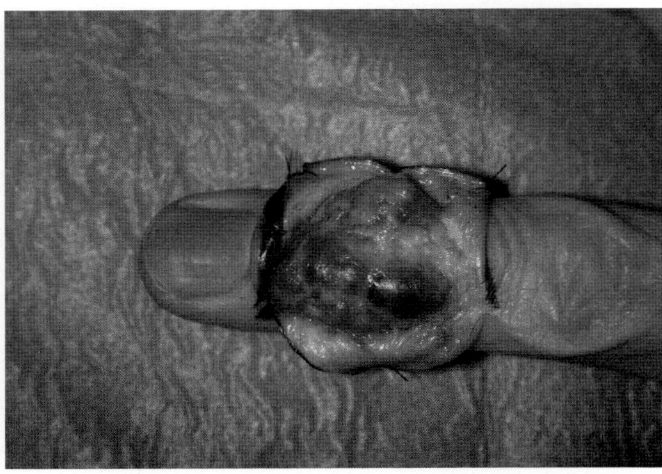

Figure 41.6
Pigmented nodular synovitis of the DIP joint: intraoperative view.

skin suture may be impossible after skin resection, requiring a local rotation flap from the lateral aspect of the finger, or the use of a full-thickness skin graft (Figure 41.5).

Pigmented villonodular synovitis

The third most common tumor after ganglia and mucous cysts, giant cell tumors of the tendon sheaths remain the subject of an unresolved terminological and etiologic debate. They have successively been called:

- tendon sheath cancer
- tendon sheath myeloma
- giant cell tumor
- xanthoma
- myeloxanthoma
- villous arthritis
- myeloplastic tumor
- benign synovioma.

The most currently accepted denomination is 'pigmented (villo-)nodular synovitis'.

Most common in women between 40 and 60 years of age, this benign tumor occurs often on the palmar aspects of the fingers, usually in the vicinity of the DIP joint. It may, however, occur in other age groups and anatomic sites in the hand. The swelling may appear rather abruptly. It is usually painless. The overlying skin is normal, but more or less adherent to the underlying tumor. This, together with a firm and irregular consistency suggests the diagnosis. Radiographs may show a bony erosion caused by compression of the swelling on the bone cortex, and a small area of radiolucency at the bony insertion of the synovial membrane. If left untreated, the lesion spreads progressively around the joint, growing to the dorsal aspect of the phalanx; and making complete excision more challenging.

Complete excision is curative, most of the so-called 'recurrences' being due to an initially incomplete excision. If the tumor has spread around the joint, several skin incisions may be necessary. The macroscopic aspect of the pigmented nodular synovitis is very characteristic, pseudo-encapsulated, yellow-brownish, consisting of irregular lobulated nodules (Figure 41.6). The pseudo-capsule is often adherent to the skin, and the tumor often infiltrates beneath the tendons down to the joint capsule, to which it may adhere, but it rarely enters the joint itself.

Some invasive forms may penetrate the bone, especially near the capsular insertions around the joint. Standard X-rays then reveal periarticular geodes similar to those observed in villonodular synovitis of the knee. No malignant transformation has been described.

Macroscopic examination shows the tumor to be made of numerous cellular elements loosely arranged in the connective tissue:

- macrophages, containing hemosiderin inclusion, responsible for the yellow-brownish color of the lesion;
- multinucleate giant cells, which resemble osteoclasts;
- xanthomatous cells containing lipid inclusions.

Lipoma

The hand is not a common site of of lipomas (1%). Most lipomas of the hand have no distinctive features from

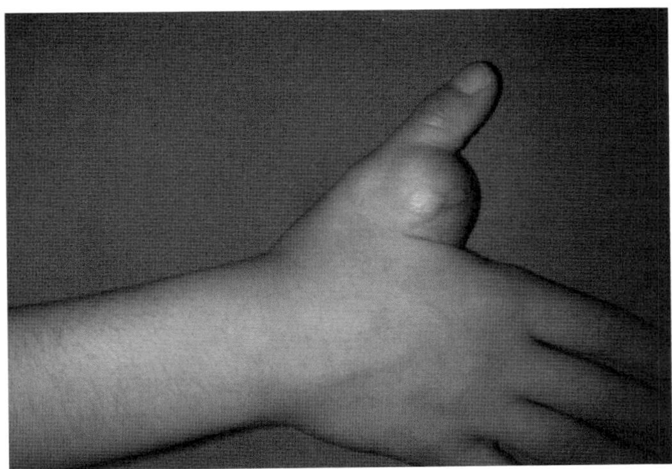

Figure 41.7
Lipoma of the first web in a 7-year-old child.

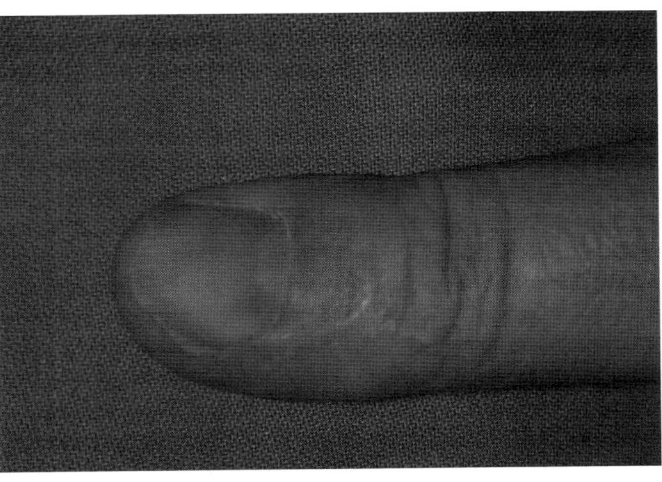

Figure 41.8
Glomus tumor: red coloration at the base of the nail, and distal nail groove.

those found elsewhere. They may be superficial, underlying the skin (Fig 41.7), or deep (subfascial, intramuscular, or periosteal). They are more commonly located on the palmar aspect of the hand. Clinical signs are non-specific, depending on the site and size of the swelling.

There are two specific locations of lipomas in the hand:

- The interosseous lipoma, developing both palmarly and dorsally, which may require two surgical approaches.
- The lipoma of tendon sheaths, which spreads inside flexor tendon sheaths, sometimes branching into several digits.

Some lipomas may reach very large sizes.

Standard X-rays may show a slightly visible homogeneous mass; ultrasound imaging is usually able to determine the lipomatous nature of the swelling. MRI may be needed in very large lesions, and when an interosseous lipoma or a lipoma of tendon sheaths is suspected.

Surgical excision is easy for superficial lesions, which can be enucleated through a small skin incision. Extensive lipomas such as those described above may prove much more challenging, the interosseous type requiring dissection and protection of the neurovascular bundles, and the tendon sheath type requiring extensive dissection of the sheath and pulleys. Recurrence is rare and usually the result of an incomplete excision, or else a misleading liposarcoma.

Liposarcomas are rare in the hand (0.5–1% of all liposarcomas). Even if the clinical signs are suggestive of a lipoma, the plume-like aspect, with areas of necrosis and hemorrhage indicates malignancy. The histologic grading is an important prognosticator, with a survival rate of 75% for differentiated types, falling to 30% in the anaplastic type.

Glomus tumor

Glomus tumors, or glomangiomas, account for 1–4% of all hand tumors. Probably initially described by Wood in 1812, they consist of hypertrophy of the neuromyoarterial glomus, and may occur anywhere the glomi are normally present, that is essentially the cutaneous sublayers, mostly in the digital extremity (pulp and nailbed areas).

Three symptoms are pathognomonic of the lesion (Carroll and Berman 1972):

- spontaneous localized pain, with proximal radiation, and hyperalgic paroxysms;
- severe tenderness, even on light touch, which may render clinical examination difficult;
- intolerance to changes in temperature, and especially to cold.

Observation may reveal the tumor as a localized, deep red coloration in the nailbed or the pulp skin. Nailbed localizations may cause a nail groove (Figure 41.8).

The diagnosis is very often overlooked for many years (average 7 years in the literature), and in the meantime, patients often undergo aggressive adverse treatments because the pain is so strong (e.g. psychiatry, amputation), and no treatment can improve it except surgical excision.

Clinical findings are usually suggestive enough to ascertain a positive diagnosis of glomus tumor. Standard X-rays may reveal a small cortical notch when the tumor is lying on it. Before the advent of MRI, the only way to actually visualize it was arteriography. Both methods show a small rounded mass, highly vascular, made up of a bunch of fine entangled vessels (Figure 41.9). This type of imaging is necessary only in doubtful cases, or when a double or multiple localization is suspected.

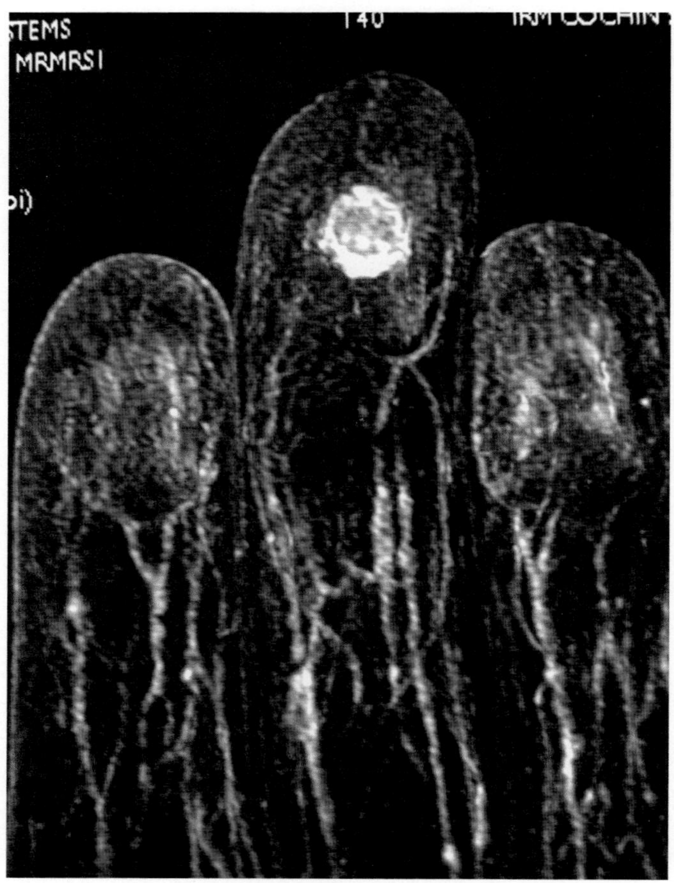

Figure 41.9
Glomus tumor: MRI scan.

Surgery is immediately curative, provided that it achieves complete removal of the tumor. Nailbed lesions can be removed through a trans-ungual approach, which is easier, but is likely to lead to nail growth disturbance, or preferably through a latero-dorsal approach, raising the nail and the nailbed from the periosteum. The glomus tumor appears as a small rounded, soft and beige mass, easily cleavable from the surrounding structures, but fragile, which carries a risk of leaving a tumor remnant behind. The surrounding tissues should always be explored for a second tumor. Some cases of double lesions, one in the pulp and one in the nailbed, have been described.

Postoperatively, the immediate disappearance of the pain is characteristic. If identical pain recurs very shortly, this is suggestive of an incomplete removal, or a second tumor. In such a case, MRI studies are necessary.

Vascular tumors

This heterogeneous group, which includes arterial, venous, capillary, and lymphatic lesions, has been subdivided by Merland (1982) into angiodysplasias and congenital or acquired vascular anomalies, and the very rare true vascular tumors.

Angiodysplasias

Because of their contrasting behavior, it is possible to distinguish immature angiomas, which regress spontaneously, and mature angiomas that have no tendency to regress.

Immature angiomas appear during the first months of life. They may be tuberous, purely dermic, or subcutaneous with normal overlying skin. Their natural history includes three phases: an increase that is maximal around the sixth month of life, a static phase until the twentieth month, and a slow regression phase, which may last until the sixth or seventh year and ends up with complete regression in about 90% of children

Mature angiomas are classified according to the type of vascular tissue affected. They may be capillary, capillovenous, venous, arterial, or lymphatic.

Capillary angiomas include telangiectasias (a central vivid red point with fine, spreading branches), angiokeratomas (small, dark-red structures covered by hyperkeratosis), and flat angiomas (the classic 'port wine' stain), found mostly on the face and limbs. These are very difficult to treat because surgical excision leaves significant esthetic sequelae and argon laser treatment may cause pigmentation and keloid scarring.

Capillovenous angiomas produce a bluish subcutaneous swelling, covered by a normal skin, which may progressively increase in size (Figure 41.10). On physical examination, there is neither a palpable thrill nor a murmur. Their size is variable, from a few mm^3 to a large lesion involving several fingers.

Arteriography, necessary for the larger lesions, has been supplanted by angio-MRI; it is an important diagnostic and therapeutic tool. The lesion looks like a bunch of grapes (Figure 41.11). The treatment of large lesions is difficult. Embolization carries a risk of digital necrosis, and surgical excision – made difficult by the lack of a plane of dissection and the number of affected pedicles – is only recommended in the localized forms.

Venous angiomas include *cavernous angioma*, which is a simple ectasia arising from a vein and can be easily removed or ligated, and *dilatation of large veins*, which is much more difficult to treat.

Arterial angiomas may be in the form of arterial aneurysm or arteriovenous angioma.

- Arterial aneurysms can be 'false' when they arise from a hematoma resulting from an arterial laceration. The lesion is saccular and histologically has neither elastic nor muscular fibers. 'True' aneurysms, more commonly found in the hand, are due to a dilation of the arterial lumen. The lesion is fusiform, and its wall contains elastic and muscular fibers. In both cases, physical examination finds the lesion to

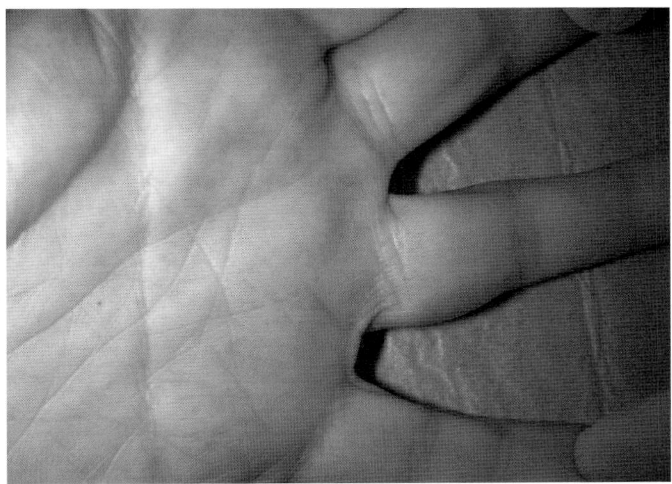

Figure 41.10
Clinical aspect of a capillovenous angioma.

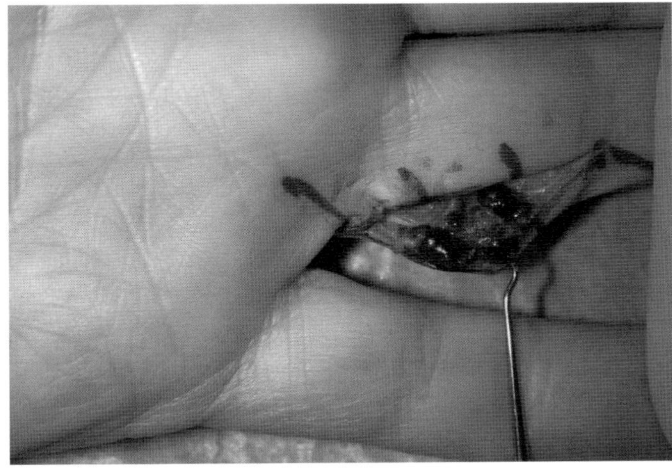

Figure 41.11
Intraoperative view of the capillovenous angioma shown in Figure 41.10.

be pulsatile with a systolic thrill. The distal vascular status is assessed by palpating the pulse, and Allen's test; occasionally a Doppler study or an arteriogram is required. Surgical treatment consists of excision of the lesion. If there is a satisfactory collateral blood supply, microsurgical reconstruction may not be required.

- Arteriovenous malformations are abnormal communications, or shunts, between an artery and a vein which may be of traumatic or congenital origin. They may remain latent until a second injury. A venous dilation in the hand is suggestive. There is a characteristic thrill, a bruit, and an increase in local temperature. Arteriogram or angio-MRI reveals the site of the communicating vessels and the marked, excessively rapid venous return.

Surgery must be decided on cautiously in the congenital forms of arteriovenous malformations because of the large number of shunting vessels and the possibility of other latent shunts.

Lymphangiomas are relatively rare. They may be superficial and circumscribed or deep. Surgery involves a risk of postoperative lymph fistula.

True vascular tumors

These tumors are extremely rare. They include hemangioendothelioma, hemangiopericytoma, angioleiomyoma, and malignant tumors (angiosarcoma and lymphangiosarcoma).

The first two of these usually behave aggressively, and histologic differentiation with a malignant tumor is often difficult. They require careful and frequent follow-up after surgical excision.

Fibroma and fibromatosis

Fibromatous tumors may classified into:

- fibromas, solitary, small and superficial lesions characterized by a fibroblastic and histiocytic proliferation;
- fibromatosis, a heterogeneous group in which the tumors are larger, deeper, and usually multiple.

Fibroma

The term 'histiocytary fibroma' is now commonly used for both cutaneous fibromas, histiocytomas and histiocytofibromas, which differ only in histologic features. These lesions are probably more common in the hand than usually reported (Stack 1960, 1%; Haber et al 1965, 0.5%) because of their insignificance. They are small, benign, painless lesions, several millimeters in diameter, encased in the skin. Surgery is not routinely indicated, except for pain, cosmesis, or functional impairment.

Fibromatosis

Fibromatoses are classified into juvenile, adult, and pseudosarcomatous types.

Juvenile fibromatosis

There are classically two different types of juvenile fibromatoses:

1. Reye's benign juvenile digital fibromatosis (Reye 1956), which appears in the second or third year of life. These are multiple intradermic nodules measur-

ing 1–2 cm in diameter, located mainly in the fingers but occasionally in the toes, and growing slowly. Their natural course is always benign. Radiographs may occasionally show associated skeletal anomalies, especially brachymetacarpy (Bloem et al 1974, Lakhanpal et al 1978). Histologically, there is a typical fibroconnective tissue proliferation with characteristic intracytoplasmic inclusion bodies. There is controversy regarding treatment because of the very high rate of recurrence after excision. Biopsy can be useful to confirm the diagnosis. Operative excision is necessary in those cases with functional disturbance, or to preserve a nail.

2. Keasbey's palmoplantar aponeurotic fibromatosis (Keasbey and Panselau 1961) differs in that it appears later in life (infants and adolescence), it involves mainly the palms of the hands and the soles of the feet, and it affects deeper structures (Allen and Enzinger 1970). The recurrence rate is also quite high. Histologic confirmation is occasionally difficult because the cellular abundance and hyperchromatic cells may suggest a malignant lesion.

As for Reye's fibromatosis, treatment must allow for the benign nature of the lesion, and the high risk of recurrence should not lead to mutilating surgery.

Adult fibromatosis
Aside from Dupuytren's disease, adult fibromatoses consist of three lesions:

1. Acquired fibrokeratomas are small, painless, isolated nodules that are surrounded by a pathognomic hyperkeratotic ring (Bart et al 1968). They involve the fingers and may occasionally elevate a fingernail.
2. Koenen's tumors are almost exclusively reported in Bourneville's tuberous sclerosis (a hereditary condition including visceral tumors and malformations, neuropsychiatric problems, ocular lesions, and mucocutaneous signs) (Koenen 1932). These are small lesions, grey or pink, rounded or like wheat grains, usually multiple and almost always located in the nailfold. However, a few cases of isolated Koenen's tumors have been described (Martin 1981).
3. Finger knuckle pads are oval swellings on the dorsal aspect of the proximal interphalangeal (PIP) joints (Garrod 1893). They are often, but not exclusively, associated with Dupuytren's disease, of which they are one of the ectopic lesions. Surgery is indicated when they are troublesome. Because of the infiltrating nature of the lesion and the high rate of recurrence, it is advisable to excise the affected skin, and perform either a local flap or a full-thickness skin graft.

Pseudosarcomatous fibromatosis
Pseudosarcomatous fibromatoses are benign tumors that invade local structures without the potential for metastatic spread. They are represented by two types of lesions.

1. Nodular fasciitis develops from fascias and is seen more often in the forearm than in the hand or wrist. There is a rapid appearance of an isolated, uninodular, or multinodular, firm and sensitive, even tender lesion, which is more or less fixed to the surrounding tissues. These worrying symptoms usually lead to an early surgical removal, revealing a gray or whitish irregular lesion, ill-defined, possibly infiltrating the surrounding tissues. Histologic diagnosis is difficult, and there is a high rate of confusion with a malignant lesion, which can result in unnecessary, mutilating surgery (Price et al 1961).

   Surgical excision is usually curative. Some multinodular forms may even regress spontaneously.
2. Desmoid tumors occur mostly in the abdominal cavity. In the limbs (28% of the extra-abdominal sites) (Das Gupta et al 1969), it involves manly the girdles, and distal lesions are exceptional. Occurring preferentially in young females it manifests as a solitary, deep, firm, painless swelling. Soft tissue radiographs may demonstrate a single homogeneous opacity.

The diagnosis is made histologically: macroscopically, the lesion is dense, whitish, non-encapsulate and difficult to separate from the surrounding tissues: microscopically, the presence of few but normal mitoses allows it to be differentiated from a fibrosarcoma.

Frequent adhesions to surrounding tissues make complete excision difficult, and the surgeon may have to decide between an incomplete excision which carries a risk of recurrence, and a rigorous but mutilating excision for this benign tumor.

Soft tissue chondroma

As opposed to the bony chondromas, soft tissue chondromas are rare. They are usually found near a joint or tendon sheath, as a multilobular tender swelling, independent from surrounding structures. In the hand, they are more commonly found in the fingers, exceptionally in the thumb (Dahlin and Salvodor 1974a).

Radiography may show scattered calcifications within the tumor.

The macroscopic appearance at surgery is very suggestive, with a multilobular and well delineated cartilaginous tissue.

Histologic findings may simulate those of a malignant tumor. However, this benign tumor never undergoes secondary malignancy.

Recurrence after surgical excision is not infrequent (estimated at 20%). It has been observed to take place in the less differentiated histologic forms. Lichtenstein and Goldman (1964) advised thorough histologic examination and a more extensive excision in the less differentiated forms.

Muscle tumors

Leiomyoma

Leiomyoma is a benign lesion arising from smooth muscle fibers. Neviaser and Newman (1977) reported 84 upper limb lesions, of which 2 were located in the wrist and 12 in the hand.

It occurs at all ages, and equally in both sexes. Clinically, there is a single or multiple nodules, several millimeters in size, characterized by two elements: (1) pain, often spontaneous and paroxysmal, always relieved by pressure and (2) painful hardening in the cold and after palpation.

When multiple, the lesion is more superficial, embedded in the dermis, very painful and often pruriginous. These forms have been said to originate from the hair erector muscles and sweat glands. The solitary lesions are deeper, may be painless, and are said to originate from the vascular walls.

Excision is curative.

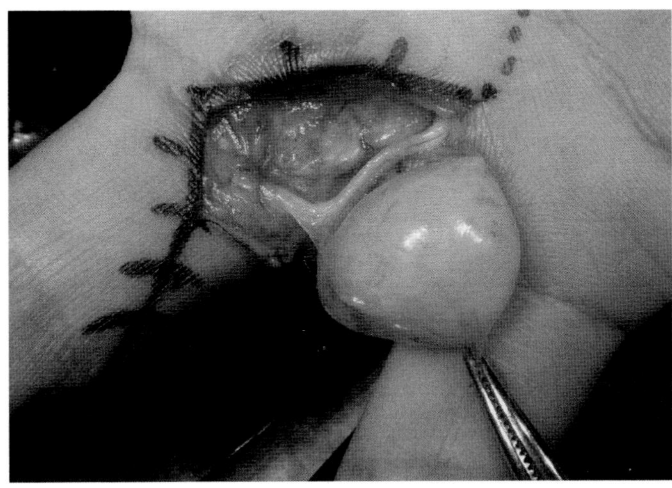

Figure 41.12

Intraoperative view of a schwannoma: the collateral nerve runs on the surface of the schwannoma.

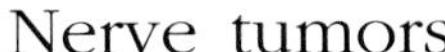

Nerve tumors

Nerve tumors represent 2.5% of all soft tissue tumors in the hand (thus making up 1.8% of all hand tumors).

There is a certain confusion in their terminology arising from histologic difficulties. Normally, three distinct types of tumors are recognized, all originating from the Schwann cell and occasionally from the endoneural and perineural fibroblasts:

- schwannomas
- neurofibromas
- malignant nerve tumors,

to which were added two more recent entities, fibrolipomas and pacinomas.

Schwannomas

It has long been difficult to differentiate schwannomas and neurofibromas until Stout (1949) demonstrated the difference between the two tumors, but some etiopathogenic problems remain.

The schwannoma, still sometimes called neurilemmoma, is the most frequent tumor of the nerves. The typical picture is a solitary swelling, regular and firm, which may be mobile transversally but not longitudinally. Often located on the anterior aspect of the forearm or the fingers, the schwannoma is most often asymptomatic, and signs of nerve irritation are rare; indeed, Tinel's sign is usually missing.

At surgery, the macroscopic appearance is quite characteristic. The tumor is within the nerve trunk, but it is well encapsulated and does not invade the surrounding fascicles, which are spread out on the surface of the schwannoma (Figure 41.12). Complete excision under loop magnification is usually easy without any damage to the adjacent fascicles.

Histologically, there are two types of schwannomas. Type Antoni A has a characteristic palisade arrangement, forming Verocay bodies; type Antoni B has no characteristic arrangement. Some authors believe that these two types are just different stages of development found within the same tumor.

The normal course of schwannoma is slow and benign, and possible signs of compression are more commonly due to the location of the tumor than to its size.

Several cases of multiple schwannomas on the same nerve trunk have been described (Phalen 1976).

Neurofibromas

Rarely solitary and found most often as part of von Recklinghausen's disease, neurofibromas may be found in two forms, cutaneous and nervous.

- The cutaneous neurofibroma (molluscum fibrosum) is not a real nerve tumor, but is found at the end of a cutaneous nerve branch. Usually located on the dorsal aspects of the hand and fingers, it is a small and soft swelling, covered by pigmented skin. It is most commonly multiple.
- The neurofibroma proper is a solitary lesion, but it may also form several swellings on the same nerve, like beads on a chain. As opposed to schwannomas, it may become very large, producing distal signs of neurological impairment. On palpation, the neurofibroma is firm but heterogeneous.

Diagnosis is easy when the patient is known to have von Recklinghausen's disease. Otherwise, the macroscopic appearance may be suggestive, with the tumor centrally located inside the nerve, whitish, edematous, heterogeneous, and occasionally brain-like. Two specific elements are characteristic:

1. Some fascicles are included inside the tumor (as compared with schwannoma, where the fascicles are displaced or stretched but never invaded).
2. When opening the tumor, there are no cystic or necrotic areas as may be found in a schwannoma.

Microscopically, there is no characteristic cellular organization, unlike the schwannoma. Many misleading features exist and, in the absence of von Recklinghausen's disease, the histological diagnosis is sometimes difficult to ascertain.

Treatment of neurofibroma is difficult: ideally the tumor should be excised completely, without any nerve damage. However, the tumor is not well encapsulated, and nerve fibers may enter it. The indications for nerve excision must be carefully evaluated. If the tumor is obviously benign, in a case of known von Recklinghausen's disease, it should not be excised unless it is significantly troublesome. If the tumor is first discovered to be a neurofibroma at surgery, dissection should be performed using a microscope, reducing nerve damage to a minimum (Strickland and Steinchen 1977). On some occasions one has to perform an incomplete resection when faced with a undissectable tumor in a large nerve trunk.

Clinical suggestion of malignant transformation is, on the contrary, an absolute indication for excision surgery. This may be suspected when there is a rapid increase in size, the onset of pain, or early recurrence after surgery; malignant changes have occurred in 13–22% in the literature.

Fibrolipoma of the median nerve

Reported simultaneously by several authors (Brunelli 1964, Mikhail 1964, Pulvertaft 1964, Yeoman 1964), fibrolipoma of the median nerve is not a true tumor but more accurately a benign fibro-adipose infiltration of the nerve. Initially reported in the median nerve (about 30 cases reported in the world literature), it has now also been reported in the ulnar nerve. It usually manifests as a soft swelling in the palm, which has been present since childhood. Often asymptomatic, it may be bilobular on each side of the carpal tunnel. There may be paresthesia in the median nerve distribution (which in a child should suggest the diagnosis).

Macroscopic examination reveals a yellowish-white, fusiform tumor encasing the median nerve, usually ending at the nerve division into its terminal branches. Histology is characteristic, showing a proliferation of adipose cells and fibrous tissue, spreading apart the nerve fascicles to which it is intimately adherent. All parts of the nerve (epineurium, perineurium, and endoneurium) may be affected by the infiltration.

Surgical treatment is often limited to opening the carpal tunnel and excising a small fragment of the tumor for diagnostic purposes (Patel et al 1979). This procedure usually alleviates the symptoms. Complete excision and nerve grafting seems too invasive a procedure for this benign lesion. Some interesting results have been reported after microsurgical decortication (Terzis et al 1978).

Pacinian tumor

Hyperplasia of the pacinian corpuscles has been reported on several occasions in the medical literature (Zweig and Burn 1968, Hart et al 1971). This lesion usually involves the pulp. It presents as a discrete swelling associated with severe and resistant pain.

Surgical exploration reveals a group or bunch of pearly white nodules arising from the collateral nerve, joined to it by a fine pedicle. Histology confirms hypertrophy and hyperplasia of the pacinian corpuscles.

Recurrence is very frequent after excision (Chavoin et al 1980).

Bone tumors

Bone tumors account for 1–5.4% of all tumors of the hand in the literature. Of the 1952 hand tumors operated at l'Institut de la Main, 122 occurred in bone (Mateva and Leclercq 2003).

Current classifications are based on that of Lichtenstein and Goldman (1964), which refers to both the cellular components of the tumor and the tissue in which it occurs. In terms of cellular components, the majority of bone tumors arising in the hand are cartilaginous, including chondroma (the most frequent), osteochondroma, chondroblastoma, chondrosarcoma, and chondromixoid fibroma (which includes both cartilaginous and fibrous cells). Tumors deriving from bone cells include osteoid osteoma, osteoblastoma, and osteosarcoma. Fibrous tumors include fibrous dysplasia and fibrosarcoma.

Chondroma

Chondroma is the most frequent cartilaginous tumor. It affects predominantly the hand (Dahlin and Salvador 1974a; Mirra 1980). Campanacci's series (1990) of chondromas includes 334 cases, of which 233 occurred in the hand. It is also the most frequent bone tumor in the hand (Campbell 1995: 42/80). The series of l'Institut de la Main comprises 70 chondromas, out of 120 bone tumors (Mateva and Leclercq 2003). The largest

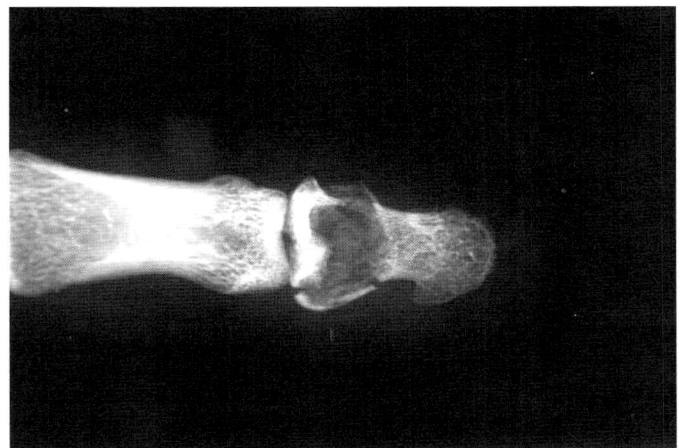

Figure 41.13
Pathologic fracture of a chondroma of the distal phalanx.

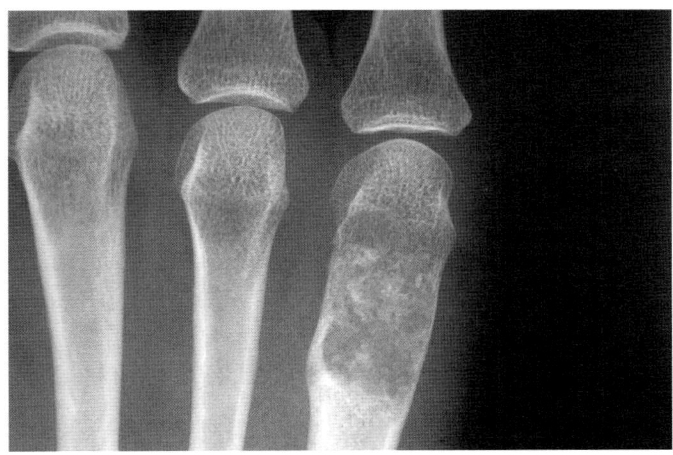

Figure 41.14
Chondroma of the fifth metacarpal, punctuated with calcifications.

published series of chondromas of the hand are by Takigawa (1971: 110 cases), Tomeno and Forest (1974: 29 cases), Noble and Lamb (1974: 40 cases), and Alawneh et al (1977: 33 cases).

Chondromas occur predominantly in adult life (average 40 years), except for multiple chondromas, which are usually detected in childhood. Some series report a higher feminine prevalence. This was very significant in our series (56 female/70). They affect predominantly the ulnar fingers, but do occur on all fingers. The bones involved are mainly the proximal and middle phalanges (respectively 45 and 22%), then the metacarpals (23%) and the distal phalanx (8%) (Glicenstein et al 1988). The wrist is very rarely involved (1%).

The tumor may be revealed by a pathologic fracture (50–75% in the different series) (Figure 41.13), or a swelling (30–57%). When present, the swelling is of a hard, bony consistency, with regular contours. Associated pain is not always present, and rarely the main symptom. In 4–20% of cases, the chondroma is asymptomatic, and is revealed by an X-ray performed for another reason.

The typical radiographic aspect of a chondroma is central, round, and purely osteolytic, usually developed near the metaphysis. In early cases the bone contour is normal, but as it grows, the chondroma may thin the bone cortex, and even expand the bone contour, which looks ultimately 'blown-out'. However, the cortex is never invaded or ruptured, except in the event of a pathologic fracture, and a thin sclerotic rim usually surrounds the chondroma. Small punctiform calcifications may appear inside the lesion as it matures (Figure 41.14). Takigawa (1971) has classified five different locations of the chondroma within the bone: central (58%), eccentric (19%), combined (several lesions in the same bone, 21%), polycentric (11%), and giant (3%). Another type was described by Lichtenstein and Hall in 1952, the juxta-cortical chondroma, which develops between the bone and the periosteum. X-rays show a cortical erosion, and the chondroma itself is visible as small punctuate calcifications in the adjacent soft tissues, sometimes surrounded by a thin sclerous rim.

The macroscopic findings are typical, with a thinned but intact cortex easily opened with a surgical blade, and in the often lobulated cavity, a soft whitish cartilaginous tissue, with foci of calcifications. The histological appearance is that of regular cartilaginous lobules, separated by poorly vascularized fibrous septa. The chondrocytes are normal in number and appearance, with small nuclei of poor chromatic density and few mitoses, scattered in a hyaline or mixoid stroma. Occasionally, there are binucleate cells and hypercellularity.

Recent genetic investigations (Tallini et al 2002) have shown frequent chromosomal abnormalities in cartilaginous tumors, with different anomalous patterns for each type of tumor.

The spontaneous course of chondroma is slow, and may evolve towards stabilization, and even involution of the lesion. There have been some reports of malignant change into a chondrosarcoma (Culver 1975, Justis 1983, Wu 1983, Bonneviale 1988). Classically, the chondroma becomes painful with a rapid increase in size. Radiographs show an enlargement of the lytic area, with cortical rupture and spreading into the soft tissues. However, none of these signs are significant, as demonstrated by comparative studies of large series of chondromas and chondrosarcomas (Bauer et al 1995, Geirnaerdt et al 1997, Cawte et al 1998). Moreover, the histology is not always decisive, as chondromas may display hypercellularity and binucleate cells, and chondrosarcomas may have few mitoses. So it may be that true primitive chondrosarcomas are sometimes initially mistaken for chondromas.

Curettage is the treatment of choice for solitary chondromas. Most authors pack the residual cavity with cancellous bone (Takigawa 1971), bank bone (Jewusiak et al 1971), or artificial bone. Some advise against surgery (Noble and Lamb 1974), and advocate regular clinical and radiological control. They have shown that clinical results are best without treatment. Recurrence after surgical treatment has been reported. This is generally due to incomplete removal of the cartilaginous tissue, and is evidenced by the reappearance of a lytic area on standard X-rays. Reoperation is required in those cases, with careful histologic examination of the whole specimen, as it must arouse the suspicion of an initial failure to recognize a chondrosarcoma.

Multiple chondromas

Multiple chondromas can occur as several chondromas on the same bone ('combined' chondromas), on the same hand ('multiple' chondromas) (Figure 41.15), or involve an entire half of the body ('multiple hereditary enchondromatosis of Ollier'). The hand is frequently involved in this last form, with impairing deformities, limitations of joint motion, and multiple fractures. The risk of malignant change is much higher than in solitary chondromas (up to 50%), and should be suspected when a lesion becomes painful, and/or increases rapidly in size. Radiographic changes include cortex rupture, invasion of the soft tissues, and a periosteal reaction with bone spicules. A biopsy must be performed at the edge of the changing tumor.

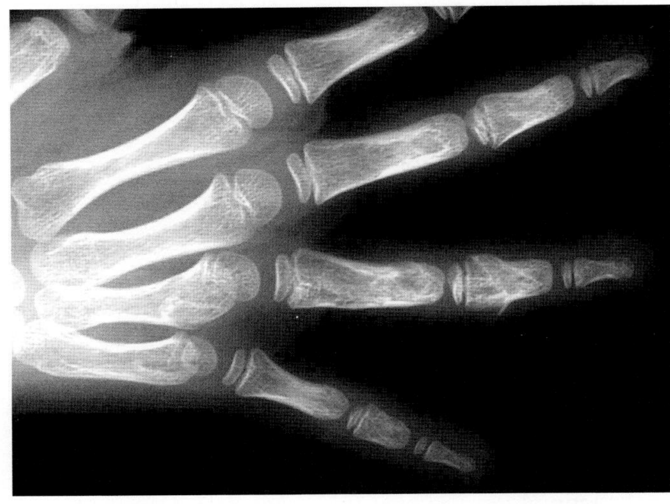

Figure 41.15
Multiple chondromas on the fourth and fifth rays.

Osteochondroma

Also termed solitary osteogenic exostosis or 'ecchondroma', the osteochondroma is a benign tumor arising from the growth plate, and its name is derived from its dual content, both bony and cartilaginous. It is the most frequent tumor in the skeleton (Dahlin 1973), affecting mainly the lower metaphysis of the femur and upper metaphysis of the humerus, and the second most frequent in the hand.

Osteochondroma develops in bones during growth, and affects mostly young people (10–30 years) of both sexes. It occurs frequently as a painless swelling, usually located distally in the metacarpals, or proximally in the phalanges. A specific location is the subungual exostosis, more common in the toes than in the fingers, which elevates and deforms the nail plate. Carpal osteochondromas are very rare (Medland and Sprague 1979, Bellemere et al 1994). In 10% of cases the osteochondroma is asymptomatic, discovered on X-rays performed for another reason.

Only the bony component of the lesion is visible radiologically, therefore the radiological image is smaller than the actual swelling. It presents as a bony excrescence, which may be either pedunculated, and easily visualized, or sessile, and may require multiple views in order to visualize its basis. The trabecula of cancellous bone is continuous from the normal bone into the tumor, signing the diagnosis (Figure 41.16). The density of bone within the tumor is usually normal, with sometimes denser streaks of calcification. The contour of the cartilaginous cap may be visible, when mature, as a dotted line.

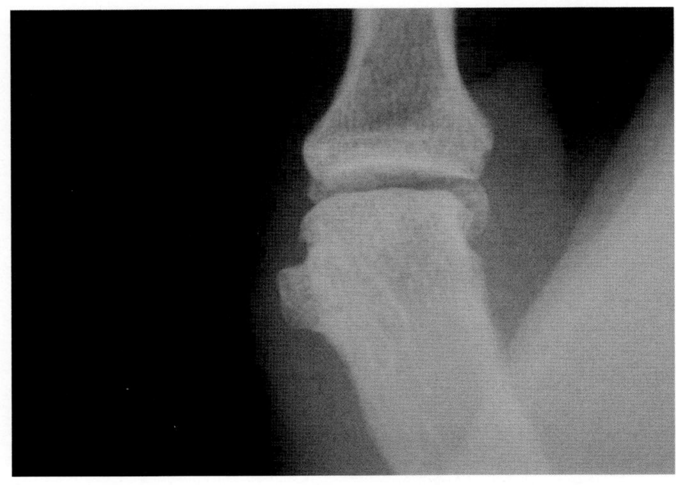

Figure 41.16
Metacarpal osteochondroma.

The macroscopic aspect of osteochondroma at surgery is that of a whitish tumor with a regular rounded contour covered with a sometimes adherent periosteum. This is the cartilaginous cap, which covers the bony component, and may conceal the base of the tumor. If the specimen is opened there is a clear distinction between the peripheral cartilaginous area, and the bony base, made of irregular cancellous bone, surrounded by a thin cortex in continuity with the normal bone cortex.

The histological diagnosis is made on examination of the cartilaginous cap. It is composed of cartilage cells of variable density, some of which may be binucleate, but with regular nuclei. The deep portion of the cartilage is the site of intense vascular activity, with calcification and enchondral ossification leading to the formation of mature cancellous bone which includes areas of persistent calcification.

Osteochondromas undergo changes at the end of skeletal growth: the cartilaginous cap thins, becomes less cellular, and may even disappear. Ossifications may appear inside the tumor (Chrisman and Goldenberg 1968)

As regards diagnosis, the radiological aspect may be suggestive of other bone tumors, such as a periosteal chondroma or even chondrosarcoma, but visualization of the base of implantation, the regular cortical dehiscence, and continuity of the cancellous bone is strongly suggestive of an osteochondroma.

It is generally agreed that osteochondromas should be removed only if they are functionally impairing. Impairment is more frequent in the hand than in other locations (proximal humerus). Whenever possible, it is preferable to wait until skeletal maturation for excision, so as to avoid recurrence.

Removal of the osteochondroma must include the periosteum, and the whole tumor with its base, without any attempt at dissecting these elements from each other.

Malignant degeneration has been reported (Dahlin 1973, Ogose et al 1997) in the form of chondrosarcoma. One should be suspicious of an osteochondroma which becomes symptomatic in an adult, or grows rapidly. X-rays are suggestive if they show peritumoral calcifications or lacunae in the base of implantation (indicative of cartilaginous foci penetrating the normal bone). Histology typically shows irregular nuclei with binucleation, cytolysis and numerous mitoses, but it may be difficult to distinguish between a benign osteochondroma and a well-differentiated chondrosarcoma.

Subungual exostosis

Localization of an osteochondroma at the tip of the distal phalanx is frequent, and has sometimes been regarded as a separate entity (Landon et al 1979). It is much more frequent in the foot than in the hand (Hoehn and Coletta 1992). In a review of the literature, Carroll et al (1992) found only 34 positively identified cases in the hand.

It occurs at all ages, but finger exostoses have been reported to occur later in life than toe localizations (Dahlin 1973). It usually presents as a solitary swelling that is painful, and elevates the tip of the nail or one of its lateral margins. It may produce nail dystrophy, or even ulceration of the nail (Ganzhorn et al 1981), often associated with a chronic infection. It may also be pigmented, suggesting a melanonychia. This multiform presentation may suggest many different diagnoses, such as botriomycoma, onychomycosis, epithelioma, wart, glomus tumor, or even a melanoma, until X-rays are performed.

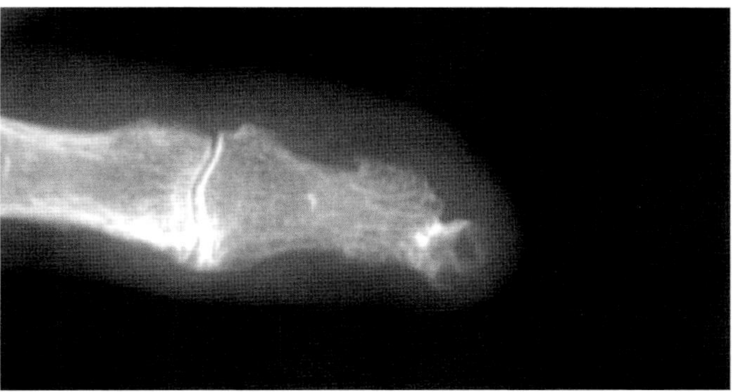

(A)

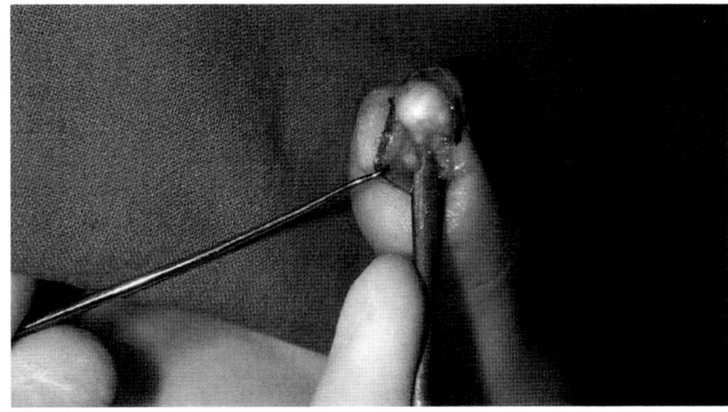

(B)

Figure 41.17
(A) Subungual exostosis: radiographic aspect.
(B) Intraoperative view.

Radiographic imaging evidences an excrescence of the tuft of the distal phalanx, made of trabecular bone in continuity with the trabeculae of the phalangeal tuft. This excrescence is bounded by a cortex continuous with that of the tuft, except at its distal end, where there is no definite boundary between the cancellous bone and the soft tissues (Figure 41.17A). The gross and histological appearance of subungual exostosis is identical with those of osteochondroma; yet a definite history of injury has been reported in a number of cases (Dahlin 1973).

Treatment of a subungual exostosis does not differ from other osteochondromata, except for the surgical approach. If the lesion is lateral, a skin incision adjacent to the lateral fold can be performed, raising the nail and nailbed together. If the lesion is central, one may have to remove the nail, then carefully elevate the nailbed from the periosteum, in continuity with the matrix. If the lesion is distal, it may be approached through a distal pulp incision (Figure 41.17B). When there is extensive ulceration of the nailbed, it may have to be replaced (nailbed graft from a toe).

To the best of our knowledge, no case of sarcomatous degeneration of subungual exostosis has been reported so far.

Multiple exostoses

Osteochondromatosis is a rare disorder of a hereditary nature, with autosomal dominant transmission. Osteochondromata appear in early childhood, usually located at the distal end of enchondral bones. They are generally bilateral and roughly symmetrical, and may induce various growth deformities.

In the upper limb, the most frequent is the distal ulnar localization (Shapiro et al 1979), producing a severe wrist deformity with radial club hand, limitation of pro-supination, and dislocation of the radial head (Bessel-Hagen disease). In the hand, they induce metaphyseal protuberances, but rarely induce joint limitation.

Multiple exostoses usually cease to grow at the end of skeletal maturation.

In view of the frequency of malignant changes, it is advocated that any exostosis which becomes painful, increases in size, or undergoes radiological modifications should be removed when skeletal maturation is complete. Other than this specific circumstance, only disturbing lesions should be removed.

Chondroblastoma

Chondroblastoma is a rare bone tumor, probably of cartilaginous origin. Although classically benign, several cases of lung dissemination have been reported. It is exceptionally located in the hand (Bloem and Mulder 1985). In his major series of 465 chondroblastomas, Mirra (1980) reported eight cases in the hand. Cases have been reported mainly in metacarpals (Bliss and Mann 1985), and rarely in carpal bones (Tountas and Cobb 1992) or phalanges (Peh et al 2000).

The clinical presentation of a chondroblastoma in the hand is very similar to that of a chondroma. Occasionally pain is present, often due to a fractured lesion (Neviaser and Wilson 1972). The radiographic aspect, again, may mimic a chondroma, with a clear, multilobulated image initially limited to the metaphysis, but sometimes affecting the entire bone, with possible expansion and thinning of the cortex. The lesion is usually surrounded by a thin sclerotic rim, and can be punctuated by small calcifications.

In a number of cases, the diagnosis is not considered until surgical approach, which reveals a soft reddish, semi-fluid tissue, with grayish and hemorrhagic zones, very distinct from the whitish cartilaginous tissue of a chondroma, which histologic examination will show to be a chondroblastoma, based on the two cellular populations (chondroblasts and giant cells) surrounded by calcified foci, and the islands of hyaline cartilage away from the cellular areas. Recommended treatment is curettage and packing with cancellous bone. In those cases where the lesion involves the whole bone, it has been advocated that bone excision and reconstruction with a cortico-cancellous graft, or a toe phalanx be performed. Recurrence after curettage has been reported to be 5%.

There have been several reports of malignant degeneration of chondroblastoma, with invasion of the soft tissues, and lung metastases, but in a number of cases, this followed radiation therapy (Mirra 1980), and it is not clear which is responsible for the malignancy. To our knowledge, no such malignant change has been reported in the hand.

Chondrosarcoma

Chondrosarcoma was first reported in the hand by Lichtenstein and Jaffe (1943), who described a lesion of the proximal phalanx of the index finger.

The main and most characteristic feature is a slowly but steadily increasing swelling, usually painless, developing in an adult over the age of 50 years, and which can reach a considerable size. In the hand, it is often located on either side of the MP joint (distal metacarpal, or proximal part of the proximal phalanx), and preferably on the fifth ray.

Radiographic features include a large lytic area in the bone, irregular, with disseminated calcifications. Bone contours are irregular, with a possible cortex rupture and spreading of the lesion into the soft tissues (Figure 41.18).

Macroscopically, chondrosarcoma presents as a bluish-white lobulated cartilaginous substance, with softer gelatinous areas. The differential histologic diagnosis may be very difficult, as the typical aspect of hypercellularity with binucleated cells and swollen nuclei containing visible mitosis may also be found in chondromas, and as cortex rupture may be missing. In most cases the histologic grading of chondrosarcomas of the hand is a grade 1. In some cases with clinical and radiographic features resembling chondrosarcomas, but with histologic features typical of chondromas, the term 'aggressive chondroma' has been coined.

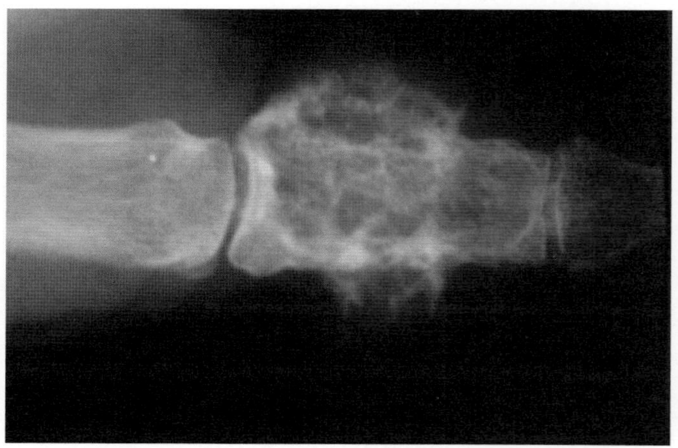

Figure 41.18

Radiographic appearance of a chondrosarcoma of the thumb.

Spontaneous evolution of these lesions in the hand is unusual as compared with other chondrosarcomas, as they grow very slowly over the years, with very little metastasis (Bovee et al 1999), and have a fairly low rate of recurrence after curettage (9–33%). This has led Mankin (1999) to view them as a separate entity which he has termed 'primitive non-metastasing chondrosarcomas of the fingers'.

It is not clear from the literature whether chondrosarcomas may be derived from chondromas or not. Three articles in the literature have compared features of both tumors (Bauer et al 1995, Geirnaerdt et al 1997, Cawte et al 1998) and have concluded that it was impossible to differentiate them both clinically and radiographically, and that histologic differentiation was not reliable in a number of cases. Moreover, a review of the large series of chondrosarcomas of the hands (and feet) reveals that malignant degeneration of a benign lesion, which occurred in 0–22% of cases, was never secondary to a solitary chondroma, but rather to either a chondromatosis, an osteochondroma, or an osteochondromatosis (Dahlin and Salvador 1974b, Palmieri 1984, Ogose et al 1997, Cawte et al 1998).

Most authors agree that amputation is justified for chondrosarcomata of the tubular bones of the hand. However, in view of the low aggressive course of this lesion, bone excision may be justified when there is no cortical rupture and invasion of the adjacent soft tissues. Whenever the preoperative diagnosis is uncertain, it is preferable to perform an excision biopsy rather than a single biopsy, as chondrosarcoma may contain juxtapositions of chondromatous and chondrosarcomatous areas. In such a case, the skin incision must be planned according to a possible secondary amputation through the same approach.

Osteoid osteoma

Osteoid osteoma is a benign tumor of bony origin. Initially reported by Heine in 1927, it was fully described by Jaffe in 1935. It is a relatively common lesion – 10% of benign bone tumors according to Dahlin (1973) – but does not often involve the hand (6–10%). In the series of l'Institut de la Main, it accounted for 9 of the 122 bone tumors.

Carroll published the first series of osteoid osteoma in the hand (six cases) in 1953. Thereafter, limited series have been reported (Braun et al 1979: 10 cases, Ambrosia et al 1987: 19 cases, Bednar et al 1993: 24 cases, Marcuzzi et al 2002: 18 cases), with the exception of the multicenter study by Allieu and Lussiez (1988), reporting 46 cases.

Osteoid osteoma is a lesion of the young, occurring mainly between 10 and 30 years, but cases have been described in the elderly (Tubiana et al 1978). It affects males twice as often as females. Although there is a predilection for the long bones, it may be found virtually anywhere in the skeleton. In the hand it preferentially involves the phalanges (mainly proximal and distal, 50%), then the metacarpals and the carpus (25% each). The scaphoid is the most frequently affected carpal bone. Localization at the distal radial epiphysis is very uncommon (Blair and Kube 1977). Pain is the cardinal symptom, typically continuous, very intense, localized, predominantly nocturnal, relieved by aspirin and non-steroidal anti-inflammatory agents. The pain may be absent in tubular bones (Lawrie et al 1970, de Smet et al 1998, Basu et al 1999), or it may be rather diffuse. Swelling is a constant finding in phalanges, but may be absent in the metacarpals or the carpus. It consists of a hypertrophy of the soft parts, deforming the finger to a 'teat' in the proximal phalanx, and a 'barrel' in the middle phalanx. In the distal phalanx, the combination of global swelling and clubbing produces a misleading deformity (Giannikas et al 1977, Bowen et al 1987). For some time the swelling may remain the only feature, preceding the onset of pain by several months or even years, making the diagnostic search very difficult. Herndon et al (1974) reported a case of carpal tunnel syndrome revealing an osteoid osteoma of the hamate.

Radiographic imaging confirms the diagnosis of osteoid osteoma, when the typical 'nidus' is present; this is a central, rounded, radiolucent zone, a few millimeters in diameter, surrounded by a dense area of sclerosis. Within the nidus there may be a central calcified image, the nucleus, producing the typical 'rosette' appearance, but the radiographic image varies with the site of the osteoid osteoma within the bone:

- Cortical osteoid osteomas display a localized thickening of the bone cortex, sometimes so thick that it conceals the nidus requiring oblique views. Some

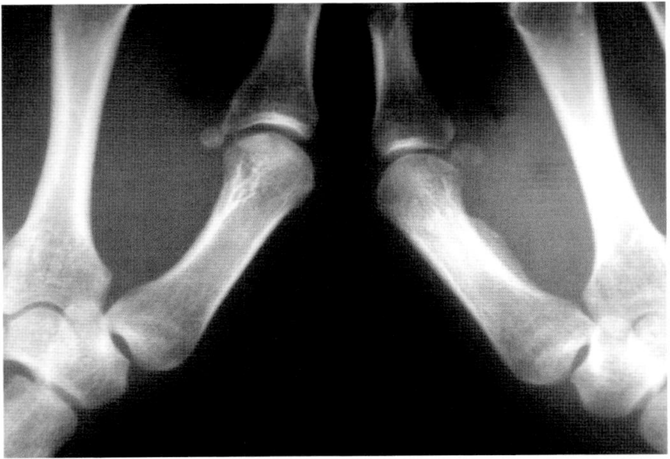

Figure 41.19

Comparative aspect of a cortical osteoid osteoma (right) of the first metacarpal, and the normal contralateral thumb (left).

images are very deceptive (De Smet and Fabry 1995): e.g. global hypertrophy of the bony segment (Braun et al 1979), bony condensation away from the nidus (Figure 41.19).

- In cancellous osteoid osteoma, such as in the carpus, the nidus may be absent, and the sclerosis may be limited to a narrow opaque band.
- In subperiosteal osteoid osteoma, there is little if any peripheral sclerosis, and the nidus raises the periosteum (Crosby and Murphy 1988).

Double nidus has been reported in a proximal phalanx (Allieu et al 1989), and in a scaphoid (Muren et al 1991).

In doubtful cases, three-phase bone scan displays a highly positive image, which, although non-specific, confirms the bony origin of the lesion. It is helpful in localizing the site of the osteoid osteoma in the carpus and the proximal metacarpus (Bohne et al 1975). It has been reported to be negative in some cases (Leroy and Couturaud 1980).

Before computed tomography (CT) was available, angiography was helpful in the diagnosis of osteoid osteoma (O'Hara et al 1975, Van Rompaey et al 1986), showing hypervascularity of the surrounding soft parts, and early opacification of the nidus. Nowadays CT scan is the most accurate diagnostic tool, as it clearly shows the nidus itself, and the peripheral sclerotic reaction (Figure 41.20).

Several other diagnoses may be considered as long as the nidus has not been evidenced: e.g. glomus tumor, osteomyelitis, arthritis.

The macroscopic appearance of osteoid osteoma is that of a small rounded, reddish-brown, or else grayish focus, rarely exceeding 5 mm in the hand, surrounded by a sclerotic area which may be so dense as to hinder identification of the nidus. Thus there is a need in some cases for intraoperative localization of the nidus, with radionuclide imaging (Gartsman and Ranawat 1984, Todd et al 1989). The microscopic diagnosis is usually straightforward. Some aspects may be confused with an osteoblastoma, but the clinical and radiologic picture is very different (Gitelis and Schajowicz 1989).

Treatment of osteoid osteoma is simple and well established: it consists of an 'en-bloc' resection of the nidus. This is usually rather easy to perform at the phalangeal level, where the nidus can usually be precisely localized, but this may prove much more difficult at the wrist level, and may require intraoperative imaging (see above). Intraoperative radiographs of the excised specimen will confirm that it includes the whole nidus.

In juxta-articular osteoid osteoma, removal of the nidus may alter the articular surface, with potential joint stiffness.

The immediate postoperative course is marked by a spectacular reduction of pain, usually so dramatic that the persistence of any painful phenomenon after cessation of the normal postoperative pain should suggest incomplete excision of the osteoid osteoma. In phalangeal localizations, swelling of the soft tissues may be slow to subside, and in the distal phalanx, clubbing of the nail may remain despite complete removal of the lesion.

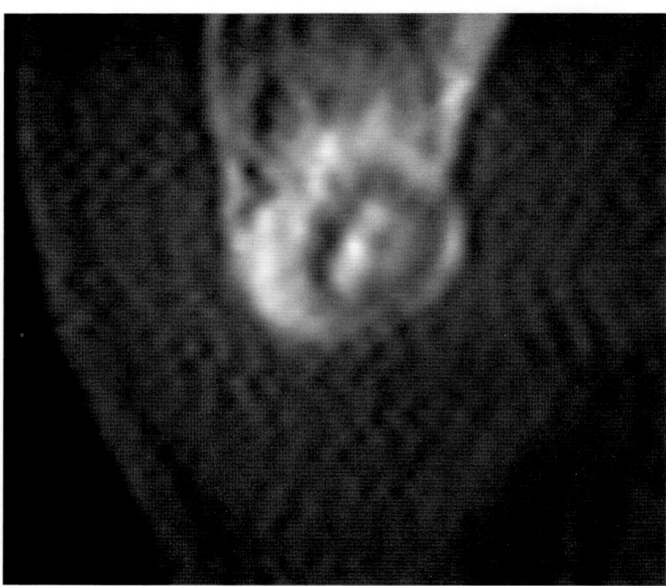

Figure 41.20
CT scan clearly shows the nidus of the osteoid osteoma.

Giant cell tumor

Giant cell tumors (GCT) were defined by Jaffe et al (1940), and many large series have been published since (Goldenberg et al 1970: 222 cases, Dahlin et al 1970: 195 cases). It affects predominantly the epiphysis of long bones.

It is quite rare in the hand. Averill (1980) collected 20 large series, amounting to 1288 giant cell tumors, of which 31 (2%) were located in the hand. They added a personal series of 28 cases in the hand. Wold (1984) reported 43 GCT of the small bones of the hands and feet, Athanasian (1997) reported the Mayo Clinic experience over a 50-year period, with 13 cases, and Biscaglia (2000) reported the Rizolli Institute experience over the same period, comprising 8 cases. Localization to the distal radius is more frequent.

Giant cell tumors affect young adults, with a slight female predominance. They have been reported in children, although rarely (Krajca-Radcliffe 1994). The tumor occurs mainly in the epiphysis of long bones: phalanges 50%, metacarpals 45%. Carpal lesions are very rare (Fitzpatrick and Bullough 1977, Athanasian 1997). The tumor is usually revealed by a localized, dull, persistent pain. Swelling occurs later along the course of the tumor.

Hand localizations occur in younger patients, with a female predominance, and display a more aggressive course, with a mean duration of symptoms before presentation shorter than at other sites (Athanasian 1997, Biscaglia 2000). They have also been reported as more frequently multicentric (18%), and some authors advocate a bone scan when these tumors occur in the hand (Averill 1980, Wold 1984). They tend to recur more than GCT at other sites, and to have a higher metastatic potential to the lungs.

On standard radiographs, there is a lytic radiolucent image with sharp boundaries, and without any peripheral sclerosis. It is usually epiphyseal, expanding both towards the metaphysis and the subchondral bone. The cortex is thinned, and may be perforated, or fractured. Intra-tumoral calcifications are rare. In the hand, radiographically advanced disease is common (Athanasian 1997), and it is common to find a tumor which has invaded the whole epiphysis.

Macroscopically, the thin periosteum covers a brown or dark-red friable tissue of vascular appearance, with yellowish-gray zones of necrosis.

Histologically there is a meshwork of round, oval or fusiform cells, and giant cells arranged in a more or less loose intercellular stroma. Three histologic grades have been established by Jaffe (1940), according to the amount of giant cells, the cellularity, and the number of mitoses. However, its prognostic value is questioned, as malignant changes and metastases have been reported to occur in all three grades (Lopez-Barea 1992).

GCT is a bone tumor, non-neoplastic in origin. It is known as a benign tumor, but malignancy may occur, especially after a recurrence. Metastases to the lungs have been reported, but they may be benign.

The diagnosis of GCT may be mistaken for that of other osteolytic lesions containing giant cells: giant cell reparative granulomas, and aneurysmal bone cysts (Wold 1984, Johnston 1987). The clinical and radiologic features of the three lesions overlap so much that the definitive diagnosis can be established only by histologic examination (Picci 1986, Biscaglia 2000).

A review of the literature indicated that two-thirds of the giant cell tumors of small bones, 39% of the giant cell reparative granulomas, and 33% of the aneurysmal bone cysts recurred (Dahlin 1987). This difference in recurrence makes it even more important to distinguish these three lesions.

Treatment by curettage leads to a high rate of recurrence (79–86%) (Averill 1980, Athanasian 1997). It is preferable to perform a wide excision or ray resection.

Aneurysmal bone cyst

Aneurysmal bone cyst (ABC) is a rare bone dystrophy, with a predilection for long bones, and the spine. Involvement of the hand is rare. Fuhs and Herndon (1979) found 17 lesions of the hand in 516 cases reported in the literature (3%); Frassica (1988) identified only 2 cases out 208 ABC filed at their institution. Most reports on hand ABCs describe isolated cases.

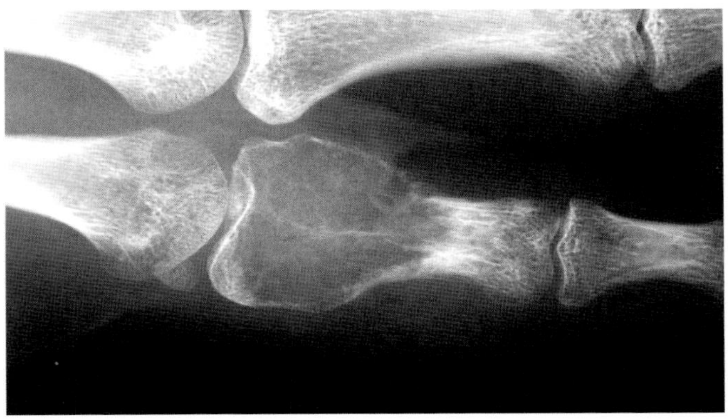

Figure 41.21
Aneurysmal bone cyst of the proximal phalanx (courtesy of Prof Alain Gilbert).

The clinical and radiologic features are very similar to those of giant cell tumors (see above), although they initially affect the metaphysis rather than the epiphysis, and in mature ABCs, there may be a trabecular appearance, with intracystic calcifications (Figure 41.21). Alnot et al (1983) reported a juxta-cortical metacarpal lesion.

Macroscopic appearance is that of a 'sponge filled with blood'; it is lined with a distinct membrane, unlike GCT. Microscopically, the cavities are separated by septa of fibrous tissue containing macrophages, multinucleate giant cells and osteoid cells. The septa are covered with endothelial cells, but without muscle or elastic cells.

Several authors have reported the presence of another benign tumor in the vicinity of the cyst (Koskinen and Visuri 1976).

Curettage has been advocated as the treatment of choice, but it carries the risk of profuse peroperative bleeding, which is difficult to control until the whole of the cyst has been removed. It also carries a higher risk of recurrence than resection. Sometimes the bone is so blown out that en-bloc resection and bone grafting is the most appropriate treatment (Barbieri 1984).

References

Alawneh I, Giovanini A, Willmen HR, Peters H, Kuhnelt F, Scubert HJ (1977) Enchondroma of the hand, *Int Surg* **62**: 218–19.

Allen PW, Enzinger FM (1970) Juvenile aponeurotic fibroma, *Cancer* **26**: 857–67.

Allieu Y, Lussiez B, Benichou M, Cenac P (1989) A double nidus osteoid osteoma in a finger, *J Hand Surg [Am]* **14**: 538–41.

Allieu Y, et al (1989) A double nidus osteoid osteoma in a finger, *J Hand Surg [Am]* **14**: 538–41.

Alnot JY, Badelon O, Grossin M, Bocquet J (1983) Kyste anévrysmal "juxta-cortical" du troisième métacarpien, *Ann Chir* **2**: 358.

Ambrosia JM, Wold LE, Amadio PC (1987) Osteoid osteoma of the hand and wrist, *J Hand Surg [Am]* **12**: 794–800.

Athanasian EA, Wold LE, Amadio PC (1997) Giant cell tumors of the bones of the hand, *J Hand Surg [Am]* **22**: 91–8.

Averill RM, Smith RJ, Campbell CJ (1980) Giant-cell tumors of the bones of the hand, *J Hand Surg [Am]* **5**: 39–50.

Barbieri CH (1984) Aneurysmal bone cyst of the hand. An unusual situation, *J Hand Surg* **9B**: 89.

Bart RS, Andrade R, Kopf AW, Leider M (1968) Acquired digital fibrokeratoma, *Arch Dermatol* **97**: 120–9.

Basu S, Basu P, Dowell JK (1999) Painless osteoid osteoma in a metacarpal, *J Hand Surg [Br]* **24**: 133–4.

Bauer HC, Brosjo O, Kreicbergs A, Lindholm J (1995) Low risk of recurrence of enchondroma and low-grade chondrosarcoma in extremities. 80 patients followed for 2–25 years. *Acta Orthop Scand* **66**: 283–8.

Bednar MS, McCormack RR Jr, Glasser D, Weiland AJ (1993) Osteoid osteoma of the upper extremity, *J Hand Surg [Am]* **18**: 1019–25.

Bellemere P, Chaise F, Friol JP, Gaisne E (1994) [Solitary carpal osteochondroma. Apropos of a case] [Article in French], *Ann Chir Main Memb Super* **13**: 179–83.

Biscaglia R, Bacchini P, Bertoni F (2000) Giant cell tumor of the bones of the hand and foot, *Cancer* **88**: 2022–32.

Blair WF, Kube WJ (1977) Osteoid osteoma in a distal radial epiphysis. Case report, *Clin Orthop* **126**: 160–1.

Bliss D, Mann R (1985) Chondroblastoma of a metacarpal. Report of a case and review of the literature, *Clin Orthop* **194**: 211–13.

Bloem J, Mulder J (1985) Chondroblastoma: a clinical and radiological study of 104 cases, *Skeletal Radiol* **14**: 1–9.

Bloem JJ, Vuzevski VD, Huffstad AJC (1974) Recurring digital fibroma of infancy, *J Bone Joint Surg [Br]* **56**: 746–51.

Bogumill GP, Sullivan DJ, Baker GI (1975) Tumors of the hand, *Clin Orthop* **108**: 214–22.

Bohne WH, Levine DB, Lyden JP (1975) 18-F scintimetric diagnosis of osteoid osteoma of the carpal scaphoid bone, *Clin Orthop* **107**: 156–8.

Bonnevialle P, Mansat M, Durroux R, Devallet P, Rongieres M (1988) Chondromas of the hand. A report of thirty-five cases [Article in English, French], *Ann Chir Main* **7**: 32–44.

Bovee JV, Van Der Heul RO, Taminiau AH, Hogendoorn PC (1999) Chondrosarcoma of the phalanx: a locally aggressive lesion with minimal metastatic potential: a report of 35 cases and a review of the literature, *Cancer* **86**: 1724–32.

Bowen CV, Dzus AK, Hardy DA (1987) Osteoid osteomata of the distal phalanx, *J Hand Surg [Br]* **12**: 387–90.

Braun S, Chevrot A, Tomeno B et al (1979) [Phalangeal osteoid osteoma (13 cases)], *Rev Rhum Mal Osteoartic* **46**: 225–33 (in French).

Brunelli G (1964) Lipoma interfibrillare del nervo mediano con sindrome da compressione nel canale del carpo, *Minerva Ortop* **15**: 211–17.

Campanacci M (1990) Solitary chondroma. In: *Bone and Soft Tissue Tumors* (Springer Verlag: Wien and New York) 213–24.

Campbell DA, Millner PA, Dreghom CR (1995) Primary bone tumours of the hand and wrist, *J Hand Surg [Br]* **20**: 5–7.

Caroll RE (1953) Osteoid osteoma in the hand, *J Bone Joint Surg [Am]* **35**: 888–93.

Caroll RE, Berman AT (1972) Glomus tumors of the hand, *J Bone Joint Surg [Am]* **54**: 691–703.

Carroll R, Chance J, Inan Y (1992) Subungual exostosis in the hand, *J Hand Surg* **17B**: 569–74.

Cawte TG, Steiner GC, Beltran J, Dorfman HG (1998) Chondrosarcoma of the short tubular bones of the hands and feet, *Skeletal Radiol* **27**: 625–32.

Chavoin JP, Durrous R, Mansat M et al (1980) Prolifération tumorale douloureuse des corpuscules de Pacini au niveau de la main, *Ann Chir* **34**: 738.

Chrisman OD, Goldenberg RR (1968) Untreated solitary osteochondroma, *J Bone Joint Surg [Am]* **50**: 508.

Crosby LA, Murphy RP (1988) Subperiosteal osteoid osteoma of the distal phalanx of the thumb, *J Hand Surg [Am]* **13**: 923–5.

Culver JE Jr, Sweet DE, McCue FC (1975) Chondrosarcoma of the hand arising from a pre-existent benign solitary enchondroma, *Clin Orthop* **113**: 128–31.

Dahlin DC (1987) Giant-cell-bearing lesions of bone of the hands, *Hand Clin* **3**: 291–7.

Dahlin DC (1973) *Bone Tumors*, 2nd edn (Charles C Thomas: Springfield, IL).

Dahlin DC, Salvador AH (1974a) Cartilaginous tumors of the soft tissues of the hands and feet, *Mayo Clin Proc* **48**: 721–6.

Dahlin D, Salvador A (1974b) Chondrosarcomas of bones of the hands and feet – a study of 30 cases, *Cancer* **34**: 755–60.

Dahlin DC, Cupps RE, Johnson EW (1970) Giant cell tumor: a study of 195 cases, *Cancer* **25**: 1051.

Das Gupta RK, Brasfield RD, O'Hara J (1969) Extra-abdominal desmoids: a clinicopathological study, *Ann Surg* **170**: 109–21.

De Smet L, Fabry G (1995) Osteoid osteoma of the hand and carpus: peculiar presentations and imaging, *Acta Orthop Belg* **61**: 113–16.

De Smet L, Spaepen D, Zachee B, Fabry G (1998) Painless osteoid osteoma of the finger in a child. Case report, *Chir Main* **17**: 143–6.

Fitzpatrick DJ, Bullough PG (1977) Giant cell tumor of the lunate bone: a case report, *J Hand Surg* **2**: 269.

Frassica FJ, Amadio PC, Wold LE, Beabout JW (1988) Aneurysmal bone cyst: clinicopathologic features and treatment of ten cases involving the hand, *Hand Surg [Am]* **13**: 676–83.

Fuhs S, Herndon J (1979) Aneurymal bone cyst involving the hand: two cases, *J Hand Surg* **4**: 152.

Ganzhorn RW, Bahri G, Horowitz M (1981) Osteochondroma of the distal phalanx, *J Hand Surg* **6**: 625.

Garrod AE (1893) On an unusual form of nodule upon the joints of finger, *St Barth Hosp Rep* **29**: 157–61.

Gartsman GM, Ranawat CS (1984) Treatment of osteoid osteoma of the proximal phalanx by use of cryosurgery, *J Hand Surg [Am]* **9**: 275–7.

Geirnaerdt MJ, Hermans J, Bloem JL et al (1997) Usefulness of radiography in differentiating enchondroma from central grade 1 chondrosarcoma, *AJR Am J Roentgenol* **169**: 1097–104.

Giannikas A, Papachristou G, Tiniakas G, Chrysafidis G, Hartofilakidis-Garofalidis G (1977) Osteoid osteoma of the terminal phalanges, *Hand* **9**: 295–300.

Gitelis S, Schajowicz F (1989) Osteoid osteoma and osteoblastoma, *Orthop Clin North Am* **20**: 313–25.

Glicenstein J, Ohana J, Leclercq C (1988) *Tumors of the Hand* (Springer-Verlag: Berlin).

Goldenberg R, Campbell CJ, Bonfiglio M (1970) Giant cell tumor of bone. An analysis of 218 cases, *J Bone Joint Surg [Am]* **52**: 619–64.

Haber MH, Alter AH, Wheelock MC (1965) Tumors of the hand, *Surg Gynecol Obstet* **121**: 1073–80.

Hart WR, Thompson NW, Hildreth DH, Abell MR (1971) Hyperplastic pacinian corpuscles: a cause of digital pain, *Surgery* **70**: 730.

Heine J (1927) Einheilender Knochensequester an der Grundphalanx des Ringfingers, *Arch Klein Chir* **146**: 737.

Herndon JH, Eaton RG, Littler JW (1974) Carpal-tunnel syndrome. An unusual presentation of osteoid-osteoma of the capitate, *J Bone Joint Surg Am* **56**: 1715–18.

Hoehn J, Coletta C (1992) Subungual exostosis of the fingers, *J Hand Surg* **17A**: 468–71.

Jaffe HL (1935) Osteoid osteoma: a benign ostoblastic tumor composed of osteoid and atypical bone, *Arch Surg* 31: 709–28.

Jaffe HL, Lichtenstein L, Portis R (1940) Giant cell tumor of bone. Its pathological appearance, grading supposed variance, *Arch Pathol* **30**: 993.

Jewusiak EM, Spence KF, Sell KW (1971) Solitary benign enchondroma of the long bones of the hand, *J Bone Joint Surg [Am]* **53**: 1587–90.

Johnson J, Kilgore E, Newmeyer W (1985) Tumorous lesions of the hand, *J Hand Surg [Am]* **10**: 284–6.

Johnston AD (1987) Aneurysmal bone cyst of the hand, *Hand Clin* **3**: 299–310.

Justis EJ Jr, Dart RC (1983) Chondrosarcoma of the hand with metastasis: a review of the literature and case report, *J Hand Surg [Am]* **8**: 320–4.

Keasbey LE, Panselau HA (1961) The aponeurotic fibroma, *Clin Orthop* **19**: 115–31.

Kleinert H, Kutz J, Fishman J, McGraw L (1972) Etiology and treatment of the so-called mucous cyst of the finger, *J Bone Joint Surg [Am]* **54**: 1455–8.

Koenen J (1932) Eine familare hereditare Form von tuberoser Sklerose, *Acta Psychiatr Scand* **1**: 813–21.

Koskinen EV, Visuri TI, Holmstrom T, Roukkula MA (1976) Aneurysmal bone cyst. Evaluation of resection and of curettage in 20 cases, *Clin Orthop* **118**: 136–46.

Krajca-Radcliffe JB, Thomas JR, Nicholas RW (1994) Giant-cell tumor of bone: a rare entity in the hands of children, *J Pediatr Orthop* **14**: 776–80.

Lakhanpal VP, Yalau SS, Sastry RK, Krishnamurthy CS (1978) Recurring digital fibromas of infancy: a case report, *Acta Orthop Scand* **49**: 147–50.

Landon GC, Johnson KA, Dahlin DC (1979) Subungual exostoses, *J Bone Joint Surg [Am]* **61**: 256–9.

Lawrie TR, Aterman K, Sinclair AM (1970) Painless osteoid osteoma. A report of two cases, *J Bone Joint Surg [Am]* **52**: 1357–63.

Leroy V, Couturaud M, Lathelize H et al (1980) [La scintigraphic osseuse est-elle si fiable dans la recherche de l'ostéome ostéoïde?], *Rev Rhum Mal Osteoartic* **47**: 53–6 (in French).

Lichenstein L, Goldman E (1964) Cartilage tumors in soft tissues, particularly in the hand and foot, *Cancer* **17**: 1203–8.

Lichtenstein L, Hall JE (1952) Periostal chondroma, *J Bone Joint Surg [Am]* **34**: 691–7.

Lichtenstein L, Jaffe HL (1943) Chondrosarcoma of bone, *Am J Pathol* **19**: 553–90.

Lopez-Barea F, Rodriguez-Peralto JL, Garcia-Giron J, Guemes-Gordo F (1992) Benign metastasizing giant-cell tumor of the hand. Report of a case and review of the literature, *Clin Orthop* **274**: 270–4.

Mankin H (1999) Chondrosarcomas of digits: are they really malignant?, *Cancer* **86**: 1635–7.

Marcuzzi A, Acciaro AL, Landi A (2002) Osteoid osteoma of the hand and wrist, *J Hand Surg [Br]* **27**: 440–3.

Martin B (1981) Les tumeurs de Koenen, Thesis, Faculté de Médecine Broussais, Hôtel Dieu.

Mateva E, Leclercq C (2003) Tumors of the hand: a consecutive series of 1952 cases. Personal communication: Symposium of l'Institut de la Main: 'Tumors of the hand and upper extremity', March 2003, Paris.

Medlar R, Sprague H (1979) Osteochondroma of the carpal scaphoid, *J Hand Surg* **4**: 150.

Merland JJ, Natali J, Drouet L et al (1982) *Les Angiomes et Malformations Vasculaires*, Paris: Editions Medicorama.

Mikhail IK (1964) Median nerve lipoma in the hand, *J Bone Joint Surg [Br]* **46**: 726–30.

Mirra JM, ed (1980) *Bone tumors. Diagnosis and treatment. Chondroblastoma* (Lippincott: Philadelphia) 219–33.

Muren C, Hoglund M, Engkvist O, Juhlin L (1991) Osteoid osteomas of the hand. Report of three cases and review of the literature, *Acta Radiol* **32**: 62–6.

Nevasier RJ, Newman W (1977) Dermal angiomyoma of the upper extremity, *J Hand Surg* **2**: 271–4.

Nevasier RJ, Wilson J (1972) Benign chondroblastoma in the finger, *J Bone Joint Surg [Am]* **54**: 389–92.

Newmeyer WL, Kilgore ES, Graham WP (1974) Mucous cysts: the dorsal distal interphalangeal joint ganglion, *Plast Reconstr Surg* **53**: 313–15.

Noble J, Lamb DW (1974) Enchondromata of bones of the hand. A review of 40 cases, *Hand* **6**: 275–84.

Ogose A, et al (1997) Chondrosarcoma of small bones of the hands and feet, *Cancer* **80**: 50–9.

O'Hara JP, 3rd, et al (1975) Angiography in the diagnosis of osteoid-osteoma of the hand, *J Bone Joint Surg [Am]* **57**: 163–6.

Palmieri T (1984) Chondrosarcoma of the hand, *J Hand Surg* **9A**: 332–8.

Patel ME, Silver JW, Lipton DE, Pearlman HS (1979) Lipofibroma of the median nerve in the palm and digits of the hand, *J Bone Joint Surg [Am]* **61**: 393–7.

Peh W, Shek T, Ip W (2000) Metadiaphyseal chondroblastoma of the thumb, *Skeletal Radiol* **29**: 176–80.

Phalen GS (1976) Neurilemmomas of the forearm and hand, *Clin Orthop* **114**: 219–22.

Picci P, Baldini N, Sudanese A, Boriani S, Campanacci M (1986) Giant cell reparative granuloma and other giant cell lesions of the bones of the hands and feet, *Skeletal Radiol* **15**: 415–21.

Posch JL (1956) Tumors of the hand, *J Bone Joint Surg [Am]* **38**: 517–39.

Price EB, Silliphant WM, Shuman R (1961) Nodular fasciitis: a clinicopathologic analysis of 65 cases, *Am J Clin Pathol* **35**: 122–36.

Pulvertaft RG (1964) Unusual tumors of the median nerve: report of two cases, *J Bone Joint Surg [Br]* **46**: 731–3.

Razemon JP (1983) Traitement chirurgical des kystes dits synoviaux du poignet avec exérèse capsulaire. A propos de 300 observations, *Ann Chir Main* **2**: 230–43.

Reye RDK (1956) A consideration of certain subnormal "fibromatous tumors" of infancy, *J Pathol* **72**: 149–54.

Richman JA, Gelberman RH, Engber WD, Salamon PB, Bean DJ (1987) Ganglions of the wrist and digits: results of treatment by aspiration and cyst wall puncture, *Hand Surg [Am]* **12**: 1041–3.

Shapiro F, Simon S, Glimcher M (1979) Hereditary multiple exostoses, *J Bone Joint Surg [Am]* **61**: 815.

Stout AP (1949) Tumors of peripheral nerves. In: *Atlas of Tumor Pathology*, sect 2, fasc 6 (Armed Forces Institute of Pathology: Washington).

Strickland JW, Steinchen JB (1977) Nerve tumors of the hand and forearm, *J Hand Surg* **2**: 285–91.

Takigawa K (1971) Chondroma of the bones of the hand. A review of 110 cases, *J Bone Joint Surg [Am]* **53**: 1591–600.

Tallini G, Dorfman H, Brys P et al (2002) Correlation between clinicopathological features and karyotype in 100 cartilaginous and chordoid tumours. A report from the Chromosomes and Morphology (CHAMP) Collaborative Study Group, *J Pathol* **196**: 194–203.

Terzis JK, Daniel RK, William HB, Spencer PS (1978) Benign fatty tumors of the peripheral nerves, *Ann Plast Surg* **1**: 193–216.

Todd BD, Godfrey LW, Bodley RN (1989) Intraoperative radioactive localization of an osteoid osteoma: a useful variation in technique, *Br J Radiol* **62**: 187–9.

Tomeno B, Forest M (1974) Chondromes des members. In: Meary R, ed, *Tumeurs Bénignes Osseuses et Dystrophies Pseudo-tumorales*, Monographies des Annales de Chirurgie (Expansion Scientifique: Paris) 21–6.

Tountas C, Cobb S (1992) Chondroblastoma of the lunate: a case report, *J Hand Surg* **17A**: 466–7.

Tubiana R, Menkes CJ, de Seze S (1978) Localisation carpienne de l'ostéome ostéoïde, *Rev Rhum Mal Osteoartic* **45**: 133–5.

Van Rompaey W, Vereycken H, De Schepper A (1986) Diagnosis of osteoid osteoma by digital subtraction angiography, *ROFO Fortschr Geb Rontgenstr Nuklearmed* **145**: 578–81.

Wood W (1812) On painful subcutaneous tubercle, *Edinburgh Med J* **8**: 283.

Wold LE, Swee RG (1984) Giant cell tumor of the small bones of the hands and feet, *Semin Diagn Pathol* **1**: 173–84.

Wu KK, Frost HM, Guise EE (1983) A chondrosarcoma of the hand arising from an asymptomatic benign solitary enchondroma of 40 years' duration, *J Hand Surg [Am]* **8**: 317–19.

Yeoman PM (1964) Fatty infiltrations of the median nerve, *J Bone Joint Surg [Br]* **46**: 737–9.

Zweig J, Burn H (1968) Compression of digital nerves by Pacinian corpuscles, *J Bone Joint Surg [Am]* **50**: 999–1001.

Index

Page numbers in *italics* indicate figures or tables.